CURRENT

Diagnosis & Treatment in

Gastroenterology

a **LANGE** medical book

CURRENT

Diagnosis & Treatment in
Gastroenterology

Edited by

James H. Grendell, MD
Professor of Medicine
Chief, Division of Digestive Diseases
Department of Medicine
Cornell University Medical College
Attending Physician
New York Hospital

Kenneth R. McQuaid, MD
Associate Professor of Clinical Medicine
University of California, San Francisco
Director, GI Endoscopy
San Francisco Veterans Affairs Medical Center

Scott L. Friedman, MD
Associate Professor of Medicine
University of California, San Francisco
Attending Gastroenterologist
San Francisco General Hospital

APPLETON & LANGE
Stamford, Connecticut

Copyright © 1996 by Appleton & Lange
A Simon & Schuster Company

96 97 98 99 / 10 9 8 7 6 5 4 3 2 1

Prentice Hall International (UK) LImited, *London*
Prentice Hall of Australia Pty. Limited, *Sydney*
Prentice Hall Canada, Inc., *Toronto*
Prentice hall Hispanomericana, S.A., *Mexico*
Prentice Hall of India Private Limited, *New Delhi*
Prentice Hall of Japan, Inc., *Tokyo*
Simon & Schuster Asia Pte. Ltd., *Singapore*
Editora Prentice Hall do Brasil Ltda., *Rio de Janeiro*
Prentice Hall, *Englewood Cliffs, New Jersey*

ISBN: 0–8385–1448–0

ISBN 0-8385-1448-0

90000

9 780838 514481

Acquisitions Editor: Shelley Reinhardt
Production Editor: Todd Miller
Senior Art Coordinator: Maggie Belis Darrow

PRINTED IN THE UNITED STATES OF AMERICA

Table of Contents

Authors

Thomas L. Abell, MD
Associate Professor of Medicine, University of Tennessee College of Medicine, Memphis
Gastrointestinal Problems in Pregnancy

Paul C. Adams, MD
Associate Professor of Medicine, University of Western Ontario School of Medicine, and University Hospital, London, Ontario, Canada
Metal Overload Diseases

Siamak A. Adibi, MD, PhD
Professor of Medicine, and Director, Clinical Research Unit, University of Pittsburgh School of Medicine, Pittsburgh
Nutritional Disorders and Their Treatment in Diseases of Gastrointestinal Tract

Nathan M. Bass, MD, PhD
Associate Professor, Department of Medicine, University of California, San Francisco; Attending Physician, University of California, San Francisco Hospitals & Clinics
Drug Induced Liver Disease

Paul M. Basuk, MD
Assistant Professor of Medicine, The Mount Sinai Hospital, New York, New York
Tumors of the Ampulla and Bile Ducts

Bhupinder N. Bhandari, MD, MRCP
Senior Fellow in Gastroenterology and Hepatology, University of California, San Francisco
Viral Hepatitis

D. Montgomery Bissell, MD
Professor of Medicine, University of California, San Francisco; Attending Physician, San Francisco General Hospital and University of California Hospitals, San Francisco.
Hepatic Porphyrias

Kurt O. Bodily, MD
Associate, Division of Gastroenterology, Duke University Medical Center, Durham
Approach to the Patient with Suspected Liver Disease

Lawrence J. Brandt, MD, FACP, FACG
Professor of Medicine, Albert Einstein College of Medicine; Director, Division of Gastroenterology, Department of Medicine, Moses Division, Montefiore Medical Center, and North Bronx Hospitals, Bronx, New York
Mesenteric Vascular Disease

Scott R. Brazer, MD, MHS
Assistant Professor of Medicine, Duke University Medical Center, Durham
Esophageal Motility Disorders & Noncardiac Chest Pain

Robert S. Bresalier, MD
Director of Gastrointestinal Oncology, Henry Ford Health Sciences Center, Detroit; Associate Professor of Medicine, University of Michigan School of Medicine, Ann Arbor
Malignant & Premalignant Lesions of the Colon

Michael Camilleri, MD
Professor of Medicine, Mayo Graduate School of Medicine, Rochester, Minnesota; Consultant in Gastroenterology and Physiology and Biostatitistics, Mayo Clinic, Rochester, Minnesota
Motility Disorders of the Stomach & Small Intestine

John P. Cello, MD
Professor of Medicine and Surgery, University of California, San Francisco; Chief, Gastroenterology, San Francisco General Hospital, San Francisco, California
Tumors of the Pancreas

Albert J. Czaja, MD
Professor of Medicine, Mayo School of Medicine, Rochester, Minnesota; Consultant in Gastroenterology, Mayo Clinic, Rochester, Minnesota
Chronic Nonviral Liver Disease

Christine B. Dalton, PA-C
Division of Gastroenterology, Duke University Medical Center, Durham
Esophageal Motility Disorder & Noncardiac Chest Pain

Anna Mae Diehl, MD
Associate Professor, Department of Medicine, Johns Hopkins University School of Medicine, Baltimore
Complications of Chronic Liver Disease

David J. Ellis, MD
Senior Fellow in Gastroenterology, Montefiore Medical Center, Bronx, New York
Mesenteric Vascular Disease

J. Gregory Fitz, MD
Associate Professor of Medicine, Duke University Medical Center, Durham
Approach to the Patient with Suspected Liver Disease

Jaquelyn F. Fleckenstein, MD
Assistant Professor of Medicine, Division of Gastroenterology and Hepatology, Department of Medicine, Johns Hopkins University School of Medicine, Baltimore
Complications of Chronic Liver Disease

Chris E. Forsmark, MD
Assistant Professor of Medicine, Division of Gastroenterology, Hepatology, and Nutrition, University of Florida College of Medicine, Gainesville
Chronic Pancreatitis and Pancreatic Insufficiency

Scott L. Friedman, MD
Associate Professor of Medicine, University of California, San Francisco; Attending Gastroenterologist, San Francisco General Hospital, San Francisco
Liver & Biliary Disease in HIV Infection

Ira S. Goldman, MD
Associate Professor of Clinical Medicine, Cornell University Medical College, and Associate Attending Physician, North Shore University Hospital-Cornell University Medical College, Manhasset, New York
Infections of the Liver

James H. Grendell, MD
Professor of Medicine, Chief, Division of Digestive Diseases, Cornell University Medical College; Attending Physician, New York Hospital
Miscellaneous Disorders of the Stomach & Small Intestine; Acute Pancreatitis

Samuel B. Ho, MD
Assistant Professor of Medicine, University of Minnesota School of Medicine, Minneapolis; Staff Physician, Gastroenterology Section, Veterans Affairs Medical Center, Minneapolis
Tumors of the Stomach & Small Intestine

Ira M. Jacobson, MD
Associate Clinical Professor of Medicine, Cornell University Medical College; Associate Attending Physician, New York Hospital, New York
Gallstones

Dennis M. Jensen, MD
Professor of Medicine, University of California, Los Angeles School of Medicine, Los Angeles
Acute Upper Gastrointestinal Bleeding

Rome Jutabha, MD
Assistant Professor of Medicine, University of California, Los Angeles School of Medicine, Los Angeles
Acute Upper Gastrointestinal Bleeding

David J. Kearney, MD
Fellow in Gastroenterology, University of California, San Francisco
Approach to the Patient with Gastrointestinal Disease

Emmet B. Keeffe, MD
Professor of Medicine, Stanford University School of Medicine; Director, Liver Transplant Program, and Chief of Clinical Gastroenterology, Stanford University Medical Center, Stanford.
Fulminant Liver Disease

Johannes Koch, MD
Assistant Clinical Professor of Medicine and Radiology, University of California, San Francisco
Esophageal Tumors

Richard A. Kozarek, MD
Chief of Gastroenterology, Virginia Mason Clinic, Seattle, Washington; Clinical Professor of Medicine, University of Washington School of Medicine, Seattle
Endoscopic Management of Biliary and Pancreatic Diseases

Douglas R. LaBrecque, MD
Professor of Medicine, University of Iowa College of Medicine, Iowa City; Director, Liver Service, Iowa Hospitals & Clinics; Chief, Gastroenterology and Hepatology, Veterans Affairs Medical Center, Iowa City
Mass Lesions & Neoplasia of the Liver

John R. Lake, MD
Associate Professor of Medicine, Department of Medicine, and Liver Transplantation Program, University of California, San Francisco
Liver Transplantation

Bret A. Lashner, MD, MPH
Director, Center for Inflammatory Bowel Disease, Cleveland Clinic Foundation, Cleveland
Miscellaneous Diseases of the Colon

Joel E. Lavine, MD, PhD
Assistant Professor of Pediatrics, Harvard Medical School; Attending Physician in Gastroenterology, Children's Hospital, Boston
Pediatric Liver Diseases

Keith D. Lindor, MD
Associate Professor, Mayo Medical School, Rochester, Minnesota
Primary Disease of the Bile Ducts

Kip D. Lyche, MD
Assistant Clinical Professor of Medicine, and Medical Director, Gastrointestinal Endoscopy, University of California, San Diego School of Medicine, La Jolla
Miscellaneous Diseases of the Peritoneum & Mesentery

Jacquelyn J. Maher, MD
Assistant Professor of Medicine, University of California, San Francisco; Attending Physician in Medicine and Gastroenterology, San Francisco General Hospital, San Francisco
Alcoholic Liver Disease

Victoria R. Masakowski, MD, PhD
Instructor in Medicine, Harvard Medical School, and Children's Hospital, Boston
Pediatric Liver Disease

Denis M. McCarthy, MD, MSc, FACP
Professor of Medicine, and Chief, Division of Gastroenterology and Hepatology, University of New Mexico School of Medicine, Albuquerque; Chief of Gastroenterology, USAF-VA Medical Center, Albuquerque
Peptic Ulcer Disease

George B. McDonald, MD
Professor of Medicine, University of Washington School of Medicine, Seattle; Member, Clinical Research Division, Fred Hutchinson Cancer Research Center, Seattle
Hepatic Complications of Bone Marrow Transplantation

Kenneth R. McQuaid, MD
Associate Professor of Clinical Medicine, University of California, San Francisco; Director, GI Endoscopy, San Francisco Veterans Affairs Medical Center
Approach to the Patient with Gastrointestinal Disease; Dyspepsia & Nonulcer Dyspepsia

Sean J. Mulvihill, MD
Associate Professor, Department of Surgery, and Chief of General Surgery, University of California Medical Center, San Francisco
Minimally Invasive Surgery for Gastrointestinal Diseases

Said I. Nabhan, MD
Fellow in Gastroenterology and Hepatology, University of Tennessee College of Medicine, Memphis
Gastrointestinal Complications of Pregnancy

Brent A. Neuschwander-Tetri, MD
Assistant Professor, Department of Internal Medicine, St. Louis University School of Medicine, St. Louis
The Liver in Systemic Disease

Michael D. O'Brien, MD
Fellow in Gastroenterology, Mayo Medical School, Rochester, Minnesota
Motility Disorders of the Stomach & Small Intestine

Roderick C. Rapier, MD
Instructor, Department of Internal Medicine, and Fellow in Gastroenterology, University of California, San Diego School of Medicine, La Jolla
Gastrointestinal Problems of the Elderly

Jonathan Lee Riegler, MD
Assistant Medical Director, Liver Transplant Service, Wilford Hall Medical Center, Lackland AFB, Texas
Liver Transplantation

Don C. Rockey, MD
Assistant Professor of Medicine, University of California, San Francisco
Chronic Gastrointestinal Bleeding

Thomas J. Savides, MD
Assistant Clinical Professor of Medicine, University of California, San Diego School of Medicine, La Jolla
Acute Lower Gastrointestinal Bleeding

Lawrence R. Schiller, MD
Director, Gastrointestinal Physiology Laboratory, Baylor University Medical Center, Dallas
Malabsorption Disorders

Stuart Jon Spechler, MD
Director of Center for Swallowing Disorders, Division of Gastroenterology, Beth Israel Hospital, Boston; Associate Professor of Medicine, Harvard School of Medicine, Boston
Gastroesophageal Reflux Disease & Its Complications

Bruce E. Stabile, MD
Professor of Surgery, University of California, Los Angeles School of Medicine, Los Angeles; Chairman, Department of Surgery, Harbor-UCLA Medical Center, Torrance
Diverticular Disease of the Colon

Nicholas J. Talley, MD, PhD
Professor of Medicine, University of Sydney; Napean Hospital, Penrith, Australia
Functional Gastrointestinal Disorders

Rebecca W. Van Dyke, MD
Associate Professor of Medicine, University of Michigan School of Medicine, Ann Arbor
Liver Disease in Pregnancy

Anne H. Wang, MD
Assistant Clinical Professor of Medicine, University of California, San Francisco
Acute Diarrheal Disease

Mark Lane Welton, MD
Assistant Professor of Surgery, University of California, San Francisco
Anorectal Diseases

C. Mel Wilcox, MD
Associate Professor, Gastroenterology & Hepatology Division, University of Alabama, Birmingham
AIDS & the Gastrointestinal Tract

Robert F. Willenbucher, MD
Assistant Professor of Medicine, University of California, San Francisco; Director, Center for Inflammatory Bowel Disease, UCSF-Mount Zion Medical Center, San Francisco
Inflammatory Bowel Disease

Teresa L. Wright, MD
Chief, Gastroenterology Section, San Francisco Veterans Affairs Medical Center; Associate Professor of Medicine, University of California, San Francisco
Viral Hepatitis

Wallace C. Wu, MD, MBBS
Professor of Medicine (Gastroenterology), Bowman Gray School of Medicine, Winston-Salem
Miscellaneous Disorders of the Esophagus

Judy Yee, MD
Assistant Professor in Residence, Department of Radiology, University of California, San Francisco; Chief, CT/GI Radiology, San Francisco Veterans Affairs Medical Center
Imaging Studies in Gastrointestinal & Liver Diseases

Laurence Yee, MD
Research Fellow, Department of Surgery, University of California, San Francisco
Minimally Invasive Surgery for Gastrointestinal Diseases

Rowen K. Zetterman, MD
Professor, Department of Internal Medicine, University of Nebraska Medical Center, Omaha
Cystic Diseases of the Bile Duct & Liver

Preface

Current Diagnosis and Treatment in Gastroenterology is the first edition of a single-source reference for practitioners in both hospital and ambulatory settings, responding to a need for an up-to-date and accessible text covering all aspects of gastrointestinal and liver diseases with emphasis on practical features of diagnosis and patient management.

OUTSTANDING FEATURES

• Incorporation of up-to-date, cost-effective diagnostic approaches and therapeutic strategies.
• Comprehensive coverage of all major clinical aspects of gastrointestinal, hepatic, biliary and pancreatic diseases.
• Authors are all experts who are currently directly involved in patient care and clinical teaching.
• Concise, readable format affording efficient use in various practice settings.
• Inexpensively priced.

INTENDED AUDIENCE

Medical students and house officers will find the concise, clinically oriented descriptions of diseases and their management useful on a daily basis for both the care of patients and preparation for rounds and clinical conferences.

Surgeons, family physicians, and internists who are not gastroenterologists will find this book helpful as an easy-to-use, ready reference and review.

Nurses, nurse practitioners, physician's assistants, and other health care providers will appreciate the concise approach to clinical problems combined with clear descriptions of the principles underlying the diagnosis and treatment of digestive diseases.

ORGANIZATION

The first chapter of CDTG presents information on the general approach to the patient with symptoms and signs of gastrointestinal disease. Chapters 2–12 are symptom-oriented or relate to disease processes involving more than one organ such as gastrointestinal bleeding, acute diarrhea, functional disorders, and AIDS as well as gastrointestinal problems related to pregnancy and aging. Chapter 13 covers the evaluation and treatment of nutritional disorders. The rapidly evolving use of minimally invasive surgery for gastrointestinal diseases is summarized in Chapter 14. Chapter 15 describes the use of imaging studies for both gastrointestinal and liver diseases, and Chapter 16 the endoscopic management of biliary and pancreatic disease. Chapters 17–33 are organized by organ, providing information on diseases of the esophagus (Chapters 17–20), stomach and small intestine (Chapters 21–26), colon and rectum (Chapters 27–30), and pancreas (Chapters 31–33).

The final twenty-one chapters (34–54) consider diseases of the liver and bile ducts, beginning with a chapter on the approach to the patient with suspected liver disease. The subsequent chapters provide information on diseases of the liver and bile ducts both on the basis of etiology (e.g., viral hepatitis, alcoholic liver disease) and on their impact on specific groups of patients (liver disease in children, during pregnancy, and following bone marrow transplantation). Individual chapters are also directed at liver failure, the liver in systemic disease, and liver transplantation.

ACKNOWLEDGMENTS

We would like to thank our chapter authors for their participation and the editorial staff of Appleton & Lange for their expert assistance in bringing this first edition from concept to reality.

James H. Grendell, MD
Kenneth R. McQuaid, MD
Scott L. Friedman, MD

New York and San Francisco
October 1995

Section I
General Approach to Gastrointestinal Diseases

Approach to the Patient
with Gastrointestinal Disorders*

1

David J. Kearney, MD, & Kenneth R. McQuaid, MD

The primary functions of the gastrointestinal tract are the efficient processing of ingested nutrients and fluids and the elimination of undigested waste. The disruption of this process leads to a number of complaints. The cardinal symptoms that suggest gastrointestinal pathology are heartburn, dyspepsia, problems of swallowing (odynophagia and dysphagia), chest pain, hiccups, nausea and vomiting, gas, diarrhea, constipation, abdominal pain, weight loss, and occult or overt gastrointestinal bleeding. These symptoms may be attributable to problems intrinsic to the gastrointestinal tract or may be a manifestation of a systemic disorder. The complaints may represent minor problems that are easily corrected by a change in diet or lifestyle, or may be indicative of serious pathology. In this chapter, the approach to each of these symptoms will be addressed. For a discussion of the specific disease processes giving rise to these symptoms, the reader will be referred to the pertinent chapters.

SYMPTOMS OF ESOPHAGEAL DISEASE

The clinical history is extremely important in the diagnosis of esophageal disease. Complaints of heartburn, dysphagia and odynophagia are highly specific and virtually always indicate an esophageal cause of symptoms. Less specific complaints that may be sometimes attributable to esophageal dysfunction include chest pain, belching, and hiccups. The approach to dysphagia and hiccups is discussed in subsequent sections.

Heartburn
Heartburn (pyrosis) is the classic symptom of gastroesophageal reflux disease (GERD). It usually is

described as a feeling of substernal burning, that radiates upwards from the epigastrium toward the neck. Patients may use a number of other synonyms, including "indigestion" and "acid regurgitation." Because heartburn is caused by the regurgitation of gastric acidic contents into the esophagus, it is generally improved, albeit transiently, by antacids. Heartburn most commonly occurs within 1 hour of meals or within 2 hours of reclining, especially if the patient has eaten a late meal or snack. Heartburn may be precipitated by certain foods that either decrease the lower esophageal sphincter pressure or cause direct mucosal irritation of the esophagus. It may also be precipitated by maneuvers that increase intra-abdominal pressure (eg, lifting, bending, and exercise). Cigarettes and alcoholic beverages potentiate heartburn by lowering the lower esophageal sphincter pressure. The clinical diagnosis of GERD based on the patient's overall symptoms has a relatively high sensitivity of approximately 80% but a specificity of only 60%. In contrast, when heartburn clearly dominates the patient's complaints, the specificity increases to 90% with a positive predictive value for GERD of 80%. In other words, those patients with a primary complaint of heartburn likely have GERD. However, in patients who complain of a number symptoms including heartburn and other associated dyspeptic symptoms, the diagnosis of GERD is less certain.

Regurgitation
Regurgitation describes the sudden, spontaneous reflux of small volumes of bitter tasting acidic material into the mouth. It most commonly occurs after meals, especially when bending over or at night. It is present in approximately two-thirds of patients with GERD but also occurs intermittently in up to one-half of healthy adults. It is distinguished from vomiting by the absence of nausea or retching.

Regurgitation must be differentiated from **rumination,** which is the involuntary regurgitation of recently ingested food, often solid, into the mouth with subsequent remastication and reswallowing. Rumina-

*Selected sections of this chapter have been reprinted from McQuaid KM: Alimentary Tract. In: *Current Medical Diagnosis & Treatment 1996.* Tierney LM Jr, McPhee SJ, Papadakis MA (editors). Appleton & Lange, 1996.

tion usually occurs within 15–30 minutes after meals. It may occur in healthy people after hastily eating large meals and in patients with bulimia. It is also seen in patients with severe psychiatric problems or the severely retarded.

Odynophagia

Odynophagia is substernal pain on swallowing that may limit oral intake. It may be sharp or dull but usually reflects severe erosive disease. It is most commonly associated with infectious esophagitis resulting from *Candida*, herpes, and cytomegalovirus, especially in immunocompromised patients (eg, AIDS). Odynophagia may also be caused by corrosive injury owing to caustic ingestions and by pill-induced ulcers (Table 1–1). Rarely, it may be caused by severe erosive esophagitis resulting from GERD or esophageal carcinoma.

Chest Pain

Recurrent chest pain resembling angina pectoris can originate from problems in the esophagus. Cardiac diseases (eg, coronary ischemia, coronary spasm, mitral valve prolapse, and microvascular angina) must be excluded definitively in patients with typical or atypical angina. Approximately one-third of patients with chest pain who undergo cardiac catheterization have normal epicardial arteries and, therefore, are presumed to have a noncardiac source of pain. Causes of noncardiac chest pain include chest wall or thoracic spine pain, psychiatric problems (eg, depression and panic disorder), and esophageal dysfunction. Esophageal causes of chest pain include acid reflux (in up to 50% of patients), esophageal

Table 1–1. Causes of odynophagia.

Pill esophagitis
  Antibiotics
    Doxycycline
    Tetracycline
    Clindamycin
  Antivirals
    Zidovudine
    Zalcitabine
  Nonsteroidal anti-inflammatory drugs
  Others
    Potassium chloride pills
    Quinidine
    Ferrous sulfate
    Ascorbic acid
    Phenytoin
    Theophylline
Infectious esophagitis
  Candida albicans
  Herpes simplex
  Cytomegalovirus
Corrosive esophagitis
Severe reflux esophagitis
Nonspecific ulcerations
  Primarily in AIDS

motility disorders, abnormal visceral nocioception, and esophageal distention (see Chapter 18).

The clinical history is unreliable in distinguishing cardiac from esophageal causes of chest pain. Esophageal chest pain may present as typical angina with symptoms of substernal squeezing or a burning pain that may radiate to the neck, jaw, or arm. It may be precipitated by exercise or emotional tension and may be relieved by nitroglycerin. More commonly, however, esophageal chest pain presents with features that do not characterize cardiac ischemia, including pain that occurs during sleep, lasts for hours to days, or pain precipitated by hot or cold liquids or meals. The majority of patients with esophageal chest pain report other symptoms compatible with esophageal disease, such as heartburn, regurgitation, or dysphagia. These symptoms, however, are present in up to one-half of patients with cardiac chest pain.

Clinical Evaluation

A. Signs: The physical examination is almost always normal in patients with the above esophageal symptoms. Signs of weight loss, and overt or occult gastrointestinal bleeding warrant further diagnostic tests to exclude complicated gastroesophageal reflux disease, a gastric or esophageal malignancy, or other gastrointestinal pathology.

B. Diagnostic Studies:

1. Upper endoscopy–Endoscopy is the study of choice for evaluating persistent heartburn, odynophagia, and structural abnormalities detected on barium esophagography. In addition to providing a direct image, it allows the clinician to biopsy mucosal abnormalities (such as Barrett's esophagus) and dilate esophageal strictures or rings.

2. Video esophagography–Oropharyngeal dysphagia is best evaluated with a rapid sequence, videoesophogram. It is the initial diagnostic study of choice in most patients with oropharyngeal dysphagia (see section under, "Dysphagia").

3. Barium esophagography–Patients with esophageal dysphagia usually are evaluated first with a radiographic barium study to differentiate between mechanical lesions and esophageal motility disorders. Although this study provides limited information about esophageal motility, it can provide strong clues to the diagnosis of certain motility disorders (eg, achalasia, diffuse esophageal spasm, and scleroderma esophagus). In patients in whom there is a high suspicion of a mechanical lesion, many clinicians will proceed to an endoscopic evaluation without a barium study (see following section, "Dysphagia").

4. Esophageal manometry–Esophageal motility of the body and lower esophageal sphincter is best studied using manometric techniques. A small pressure-sensing catheter assembly is passed nasally into the esophagus, allowing manometric assessment of the lower and upper esophageal sphincters and esophageal body. In practical use, it provides information about limited aspects of esophageal physiology, specifically the function of the lower esophageal sphincter and integrity of esophageal peristalsis. It is most useful to document impaired lower esophageal sphincter relaxation, weak or absent esophageal peristalsis, and disordered peristalsis. Thus, manometry appears to be useful in specific clinical situations, and guidelines for its use have been recently established. It is indicated to establish the diagnosis in suspected cases of achalasia or diffuse esophageal spasm after more common causes of esophageal symptoms have been excluded by upper endoscopy or barium esophagography. This technique may be indicated rarely to document esophageal motor abnormalities in patients with suspected systemic diseases (eg, scleroderma) when this determination would help establish a definitive diagnosis. In patients undergoing fundoplication for gastroesophageal reflux, it should be performed preoperatively to document adequate peristaltic function. Finally, it is often employed to determine the location of the lower esophageal sphincter before placing an esophageal probe for continuous pH monitoring (usually located 5 cm above the lower esophageal sphincter).

Manometry is not useful in the diagnosis of gastroesophageal reflux disease. Although it previously was employed in the evaluation of noncardiac chest pain, it is recognized now to be of limited usefulness in this setting because of the low likelihood of determining any clinically significant motility disorders.

5. Ambulatory esophageal pH monitoring– Esophageal pH may be monitored continuously by means of a small pH probe, which is passed transnasally and attached to a small, portable pH recording device. The probe and recorder are worn by the patient for up to 24 hours. The recording can be analyzed to determine a number of parameters. The most clinically useful information has been the amount of gastroesophageal acid reflux (measured percent time below pH 4) in the upright and supine positions and for the total reporting period. Because a certain amount of acid reflux occurs in everyone, the definition of normal and abnormal values is somewhat arbitrary. Normal values are derived from studies of asymptomatic volunteers and vary between studies. In general, normal values of acid reflux (percent time below pH 4) are less than 8.1% in the upright position, less than 3.0% in the supine position, and less than 5.5% for the total 24-hour period. The ambulatory pH study also is useful to determine whether a patient's symptoms correlate with documented episodes of acid reflux. A symptom index of greater than 50% (number of symptoms with pH<4÷ total number of symptoms) × 100% is deemed significant.

Although ambulatory pH monitoring is the best means of diagnosing abnormal amounts of acid gas-

troesophageal reflux, it is seldom needed in the evaluation of patients with uncomplicated GERD who respond to typical therapy. For patients with typical symptoms who do not respond to standard therapies and who do not have evidence of reflux esophagitis on endoscopy, ambulatory monitoring may be useful in confirming or excluding GERD. Its principal value is in diagnosing GERD in patients with atypical symptoms that may be attributable to underlying GERD (eg, including noncardiac chest pain, hoarseness, chronic cough, asthma, and aspiration pneumonia). Finally, ambulatory monitoring is useful in patients with GERD before performing antireflux surgery to document the severity of reflux, especially if symptoms are ambiguous or atypical.

DYSPHAGIA

General Considerations

Dysphagia refers to a sensation of impaired passage of food from the mouth to the stomach. Patients commonly complain that the food "sticks" or "gets stuck" as it goes down the esophagus. Dysphagia must be distinguished from **odynophagia** (painful swallowing) and **globus** (a sensation of a lump in the throat), which involve different differential diagnoses. A carefully taken history will allow a correct diagnosis in approximately 80% of patients presenting with dysphagia.

Dysphagia may result from an abnormality at each stage of the swallowing process. The normal act of swallowing may be divided into oropharyngeal, and esophageal stages. The oropharyngeal phase involves the process of chewing and mixing solid food with saliva so that individual food particles are sufficiently reduced in size and lubricated to allow easy passage through the pharynx and esophagus. With the voluntary initiation of swallowing, the food bolus is propelled posteriorly by the tongue into the pharynx. A rapid series of carefully orchestrated involuntary events follow in which the soft palate and larynx close (to prevent nasal regurgitation and aspiration), the upper esophageal sphincter opens, and a wave of pharyngeal peristalsis propels the food bolus into the upper esophagus. This involuntary process of food bolus transfer is controlled by the swallowing center located in the medulla oblongata. Respiration is inhibited centrally during the act of swallowing. Afferent input to the swallowing center is provided by cranial nerves V, X, and XI, and efferent motor function is provided by cranial nerves V, VII, IX, X, and XII. Once the food bolus has reached the upper esophagus, the esophageal phase of swallowing takes place. A primary peristaltic wave propels the food bolus down the esophagus. The lower esophageal sphincter relaxes in anticipation of the peristaltic wave, allowing passage of the food bolus into the stomach.

Dysphagia is usually classified as oropharyngeal

or esophageal in origin. Oropharyngeal dysphagia (also termed transfer dysphagia) is produced by an abnormality in the preparation or transfer of food from the mouth to the upper esophagus, whereas esophageal dysphagia is caused by a mechanical or motor abnormality of the esophagus which impairs movement of the food bolus through the esophagus into the stomach.

Clinical Findings

A. Symptoms and Signs: Oropharyngeal and esophageal dysphagia may be distinguished by a careful history and physical examination (Figure 1–1).

1. Oropharyngeal dysphagia–Patients with oropharyngeal dysphagia experience difficulty transferring a food bolus from the mouth to the esophagus. This may occur as a result of poor motor control of the tongue, jaw, or other oral structures or may be due to an abnormality of the swallowing reflex. Symptoms suggesting an oropharyngeal cause of dysphagia include nasal regurgitation, coughing dur-

ing swallowing, or difficulty initiating a swallow. A speech disorder, cranial nerve deficits, abnormalities of motor function of the limbs or a history of a recent cerebrovascular accident are frequently present. Oropharyngeal dysphagia is most commonly caused by neurologic or muscular disorders that are readily apparent at the time of physical examination. A small proportion of patients have symptoms produced by a structural abnormality of the pharyngeal region. A complaint of transfer dysphagia with regurgitation of undigested food contents, halitosis, or nocturnal coughing suggests a Zenker's diverticulum. Table 1–2 lists the neurologic, motor, local/structural and motility disorders which may cause oropharyngeal dysphagia.

Inspection of the oral cavity should be performed in patients complaining of oropharyngeal dysphagia paying particular attention to mucosal ulcerations, mass lesions, and dentition. Neurologic testing of the cranial nerves involved in swallowing (sensory: V, IX, X and motor: V, VII, X, XI and XII) is important to rule out a neurologic deficit contributing to dys-

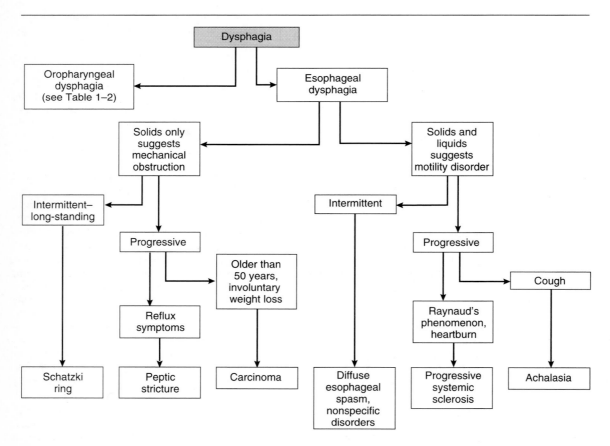

Figure 1–1. Algorithm illustrating the differential diagnosis for dysphagia. (Modified, with permission, from Castell DO: Esophagus: Overview and symptom assessment. In: *The Esophagus.* Castell DO (editor). Little, Brown, & Company, 1992.)

Table 1–2. Causes of dysphagia.

Oropharyngeal Dysphagia

Neurologic disorders
  Cerebrovascular accident (especially brainstem)
  Parkinson's disease
  Multiple sclerosis
  Brainstem tumors
  Bulbar poliomyelitis
  Peripheral neuropathies
  Huntington's disease
Diseases of myoneural junction
  Myasthenia gravis
  Eaton-Lambert syndrome
  Botulism
Muscular disorders
  Muscular dystrophies
  Dermatomyositis/Polymyositis
  Sarcoidosis
  Metabolic myopathies (hypo- or hyperthyroidism)
  Amyloidosis
  Steroid-induced myopathy
Structural abnormalities
  Oropharyngeal neoplasms
  Extrinsic compression (cervical osteophytes, thyromegaly)
  Esophageal web
  Zenker's diverticulum
Upper esophageal sphincter (UES) dysfunction
  Cricopharyngeal achalasia
  Hypertensive UES

Esophageal Dysphagia

Intrinsic mechanical abnormalities
  Peptic (reflux-induced) stricture
  Esophageal carcinoma
  Esophageal webs/rings
  Schatzki ring
  Esophageal diverticula
Extrinsic esophageal compression
  Mediastinal tumors
  Vascular compression
  Cervical osteophytes
Esophageal motility disorders
  Achalasia
  Diffuse esophageal spasm
  Hypertensive lower esophageal sphincter
  Nonspecific motility disorders
  Chagas' disease
  Scleroderma/Progressive systemic sclerosis
  Severe gastroesophageal reflux disease

---

phagia. Examination of the neck is performed to exclude mass lesions or thyromegaly. Inspection of the limbs may show characteristic skin changes suggesting scleroderma or weakness suggesting a neuromuscular disorder. Patients with oropharyngeal dysphagia and hoarseness should be referred for otolaryngology consultation and direct laryngoscopy.

2. Esophageal dysphagia–Patients with esophageal dysphagia are able to transfer food from the mouth into the upper esophagus, but experience a sensation of food "hanging up" or "sticking" after it is swallowed. Esophageal dysphagia may be caused by two general categories of disease processes: (1) A structural or mechanical process impairing movement of a food bolus through the esophageal lumen (including structural abnormalities originating in the esophagus or extrinsically impinging upon the esoph-

agus). (2) Motility disorders of the esophagus. Table 1–2 lists diseases that may cause esophageal dysphagia. These etiologies may be differentiated by several historical points.

a. Solid versus liquid dysphagia–Dysphagia to solids alone suggests a mechanical or structural abnormality, whereas dysphagia to both solids and liquids suggests a neuromuscular disturbance.

b. Intermittent versus progressive symptoms–A long history of intermittent dysphagia to solids (particularly steak or bread) suggests a fixed esophageal ring or web, which has not changed in size. In contrast, progressively worsening of solid food dysphagia suggests a peptic stricture, neoplasm, or achalasia.

c. Associated symptoms–An associated history of heartburn or acid regurgitation suggest scleroderma or a peptic stricture as the underlying abnormality. Suspicion of an esophageal neoplasm should be heightened among older patients presenting with weight loss and a history of alcohol or tobacco use. Regurgitation of undigested food in association with coughing while in the recumbent position or recurrent pneumonia suggest achalasia. Associated symptoms of chest pain with intermittent dysphagia may indicate diffuse esophageal spasm or achalasia. Patients with AIDS may have dysphagia from opportunistic infections or mass lesions (eg, Kaposi's sarcoma and lymphoma) (see Chapter 2).

The physical examination usually is unremarkable in patients with esophageal dysphagia. Profound weight loss may be seen in patients with advanced esophageal malignancy or achalasia, but is uncommon in other benign conditions. The presence of a positive fecal occult blood test may be found in malignancy or reflux esophagitis.

B. Diagnostic Studies: Patients with dysphagia require a diagnostic evaluation to determine the cause. The available diagnostic tests include upper gastrointestinal endoscopy, barium esophagography (with or without videofluoroscopic assessment of swallowing) and esophageal manometry. Patients with oropharyngeal dysphagia should undergo a videofluoroscopic examination of deglutition. During this examination, barium of various consistencies is ingested by the patient and the swallowing sequence is recorded fluoroscopically. Anatomic and structural defects, as well as discoordination of muscular movements may be identified. This examination may also aid in nutritional management by determining the food consistency most easily swallowed by the patient as well as head and body positions that facilitate swallowing.

Patients with esophageal dysphagia may undergo either endoscopy or a barium swallow as the initial diagnostic evaluation. Under most circumstances, a barium swallow is favored as the initial study because it provides information about both structural lesions (strictures, tumors, rings or webs, cervical osteophytes) and esophageal motility. Endoscopy may overlook subtle mucosal rings or webs and is a poor means of assessing esophageal motility. However, for patients with persistent heartburn (suggesting a peptic stricture) or with significant weight loss (suggesting malignancy) endoscopy may be the study of first choice because it permits mucosal biopsy and dilation, as deemed necessary. Patients with suspected peptic strictures identified on barium swallow must undergo endoscopy in order to rule out esophageal carcinoma. Patients with lesions found on barium swallow which suggest carcinoma also must undergo endoscopy with biopsy for confirmation. Esophageal rings or webs identified on barium studies may benefit from endoscopic dilation and disruption, and thus should be referred for endoscopy as well. Findings suggesting achalasia on barium swallow (a dilated aperistaltic esophageal body and narrowed distal esophagus) warrant referral for esophageal manometry and endoscopy to exclude secondary causes of achalasia. Simultaneous nonperistaltic contractions seen on barium swallow suggest diffuse esophageal spasm, and manometry may be considered. The reader is referred to Chapters 17, 18, 19 for a full discussion of the management of esophageal strictures, malignant neoplasms, and motility disorders.

DYSPEPSIA

Dyspepsia is a vague, imprecise term that refers to a group of upper abdominal or epigastric symptoms such as pain, nausea, bloating, burping, early satiety, heartburn, regurgitation or, simply, "indigestion." Dyspeptic symptoms are prevalent in one-fourth of the adult population. The majority of people, however, never seek medical attention for their symptoms. In medical practice, it is among the most common complaints evaluated by both general practitioners and gastroenterologists. A full discussion of dyspepsia and nonulcer dyspepsia is provided in Chapter 22.

Etiology

Dyspepsia may arise from a host of conditions, the most common are:

1. Luminal gastrointestinal tract (eg, gastroesophageal reflux disease, peptic ulcer disease, gastric neoplasms, gastroparesis, lactose intolerance). (Note: *Helicobacter pylori*-associated gastritis has not been proven to be a cause of chronic dyspepsia.)
2. Medications including alcohol, caffeine, iron, niacin, nonsteroidal anti-inflammatory drugs (NSAIDs), antibiotics, theophylline, and digitalis.
3. Pancreatic disease (eg, pancreatic carcinoma, chronic pancreatitis).

4. Biliary tract disease (eg, cholelithiasis, choledocholithiasis, sphincter of Oddi dysfunction).
5. Systemic conditions including pregnancy, diabetes mellitus, intra-abdominal malignancy, coronary ischemia, thyroid disease.
6. Nonulcer dyspepsia is present in up to one-half of dyspeptic patients. A cause of the symptoms cannot be determined from endoscopy or abdominal sonography. Symptoms in these patients may arise from a complex interaction of psychological factors, abnormal visceral pain perception, and disordered gastric motility.

Clinical Findings

A. Symptoms and Signs: The clinical history is of limited usefulness in distinguishing among the causes of dyspepsia. A complete drug and dietary history (including lactose) should be taken. Patients should be asked about the character and location of pain, its pattern of radiation, whether it is constant or intermittent, and factors that alleviate it. Predominant substernal burning (heartburn) and regurgitation is highly specific for gastroesophageal reflux disease (see preceding section, "Heartburn"). The epigastrium is the most common site of pain in dyspepsia of all other causes, including biliary tract disease. Peptic ulcer disease is more likely with episodic bouts of rhythmic, gnawing epigastric pain that occurs between meals or at night. The pain is relieved by antacids or food; however at least one-half of ulcer patients do not give this classical history. Irregular, intermittent right upper quadrant or epigastric pain that is precipitated by meals and has a crescendo–decrescendo pattern is suggestive of biliary disease. Constant, vague epigastric pain associated with weight loss is suspicious for pancreatic disease. Finally, nonulcer dyspepsia is more likely in younger patients with chronic, vague epigastric pain associated with a variety of other complaints such as bloating and distention. Although these clinical features of dyspepsia may provide clues to the cause, they are nonspecific and cannot be relied upon to make anything other than a speculative diagnosis.

A complete physical examination is mandatory in dyspeptic patients including stool occult blood testing. The majority of patients have an entirely normal examination. Signs of organic disease such as weight loss, organomegaly, abdominal mass, or positive fecal occult blood mandate further investigation. Initial laboratory work should include a complete blood cell count (CBC) and a screening biochemical and liver chemistry panel.

B. Diagnostic Studies: Because the history and physical examination are nonspecific, a diagnosis of dyspepsia in most cases requires special examinations. Upper endoscopy is highly accurate at diagnosing peptic ulcer disease, erosive gastroesophageal reflux disease, and gastric neoplasms. However, at least one-half of patients with dyspepsia have normal or nonspecific findings on endoscopy. Although barium upper gastrointestinal series is less expensive, it is less accurate and a suboptimal means of evaluating patients with dyspepsia. Abdominal ultrasonography should be obtained only when biliary or pancreatic disease is suspected. Computed tomography (CT) or magnetic resonance imaging (MRI) should only be obtained when there is a strong suspicion of intra-abdominal diseases or to pursue abnormal findings on ultrasonography.

The decision as to when and how to investigate the dyspeptic patient depends on a number of factors. Patients who are older than 45 years with new onset dyspepsia, have physical or laboratory abnormalities, or are from regions endemic for gastric cancer, should undergo a diagnostic endoscopy. In patients younger than 45 years of age with normal physical and laboratory examinations (in whom the risk of malignancy is low) the optimal approach is controversial. Until recently, an empiric trial of therapy with H_2-receptor antagonists was recommended. In patients who failed to improve or had persistent symptoms, further diagnostic evaluation with endoscopy was recommended. With the recognition of the pivotal role of *H pylori* in peptic ulcer disease, the merits of these guidelines are called into question. Some clinicians now recommend early endoscopy in patients with acute dyspepsia to diagnose peptic ulcer disease and *H pylori* infection so that definitive antibacterial therapy can be given and the ulcer diathesis eliminated.

Other clinicians recommend screening patients with dyspepsia for *H pylori* infection with noninvasive tests, eg, serology or urease breath tests. Patients with evidence of *H pylori* infection could be treated empirically with antibacterial therapy. Patients who are negative for *H pylori* infection or who fail to respond to anti-*H pylori* treatment likely have nonulcer dyspepsia. Further diagnostic tests are unlikely to reveal significant abnormalities. A full discussion of these issues is discussed in Chapter 22.

HICCUPS

Hiccups is a complex reflex pattern characterized by a sudden contraction of the inspiratory muscles which is terminated with an abrupt closure of the glottis, resulting in the characteristic "hiccup" sound. A brain stem "hiccup center" receives afferent activity from the CNS, vagus, or phrenic nerves and coordinates efferent activity via multiple nerves to the respiratory center and to the diaphragm (phrenic nerve), glottis (vagus nerve), scalenes (cervical plexus) and intercostals (thoracic nerves). Though usually a benign and self-limited annoyance, they may be persistent and occasionally reflect serious underlying illness. Chronic hiccups appear to be without major consequences. Reports that hiccups lead to

exhaustion, weight loss or death are unsubstantiated. In patients on mechanical ventilation, hiccups can trigger a full respiratory cycle and result in respiratory alkalosis.

Causes of benign, self-limited hiccups include gastric distention (eg, carbonated beverages, air swallowing, overeating), sudden temperature changes (eg, hot or cold liquids, cold shower), alcohol ingestion, and psychogenic causes (eg, excitement, stress, laughing). Over one hundred causes of recurrent or persistent hiccups have been identified. These may be grouped into the following categories:

- CNS–neoplasms, infections, cerebrovascular accident, trauma
- Metabolic–uremia, hypocarbia (hyperventilation), electrolyte imbalance
- Irritation of vagus or phrenic nerve–
  Head and neck: foreign body in ear, goiter, neoplasms
  Thorax: pneumonia, empyema, neoplasms, myocardial infarction, pericarditis, aneurysm, esophageal obstruction, reflux esophagitis
  Abdomen: subphrenic abscess, hepatomegaly, hepatitis, cholecystitis, gastric distention, gastric neoplasm, pancreatitis, or pancreatic malignancy
- Surgical–general anesthesia, postoperative
- Psychogenic and idiopathic.

Clinical Findings

Patients with self-limited hiccups require no evaluation. Evaluation of the patient with persistent hiccups should include a history and physical examination (including neurologic examination), CBC, electrolytes, liver chemistry tests, and a chest radiograph. When the cause remains unclear, further testing may include CT of the chest and abdomen, echocardiography, bronchoscopy, and upper endoscopy.

Treatment

A number of simple remedies work by interrupting the reflex arc and may be helpful in patients with acute, benign hiccups:

1. Irritation of the nasopharynx—tongue traction, lifting uvula with spoon, catheter stimulation of the nasopharynx, and eating 1 tsp of dry granulated sugar or a lemon wedge in Angostura bitters.
2. Interruption of respiratory cycle—breath holding, valsalva, sneezing, gasping (frightful stimulus), rebreathing into a bag.
3. Irritation of vagus—supraorbital pressure, carotid massage.
4. Irritation of diaphragm—holding knees to chest, continuous positive airway pressure (CPAP) during mechanical ventilation;
5. Relief of gastric distention—belching, nasogastric tube.

In patients with persistent hiccups, therapy should be directed at relieving the predisposing cause.

A number of drugs have been touted as being useful in the treatment of hiccups, but none has ever been tested in a controlled fashion. Chlorpromazine 25–50 mg orally or intramuscularly is most commonly used. Other agents that have been reported to be effective in some cases include: anticonvulsants (phenytoin, carbamazepine), metoclopramide, baclofen, nifedipine, and, occasionally, anesthesia. Unilateral phrenic nerve crushing may weaken the intensity but may not ablate hiccups, which have bilateral diaphragmatic involvement.

GASTROINTESTINAL GAS

Belching

Belching or **burping** is the voluntary or involuntary eructation of gas from the stomach or esophagus. The belch reflex consists of relaxation of the lower esophageal sphincter and gaseous reflux into the esophagus, followed by relaxation of the upper esophageal sphincter with gas expulsion. Belching occurs most frequently after meals, when gastric distention results in transient lower esophageal sphincter relaxation. It is more commonly seen in patients with GERD. Belching is restricted in the supine position because of the formation of a fluid "trap" at the gastroesophageal junction. It is also restricted after surgical fundoplication.

Virtually all gas in the stomach comes from swallowed air. Each swallow draws 3–5 ml of air into the upper gastrointestinal tract, 80% of which is nitrogen. Swallowing of excessive amounts of air may result in distention, belching, flatulence, and abdominal pain. Increased air swallowing may occur with gum chewing, smoking, rapid eating, and the ingestion of carbonated beverages. In addition, some patients may consciously or unconsciously engage in forceful air swallowing (aerophagia). Conscious aerophagia occurs primarily in institutionalized or psychotic patients. (It is also a common parlor trick, usually performed by adolescent boys to generate loud, obnoxious eructations.) It may also occur subconsciously in anxious adults who relax the UES and draw air into the esophagus with negative intrathoracic pressure.

Belching is a normal physiologic reflex and does not denote gastrointestinal pathology per se. Chronic excessive belching is almost always caused by aerophagia. Evaluation of belching should be restricted to patients with other complaints (eg, dysphagia, distention, early satiety or vomiting) that suggest more serious problems. Aerophagia and belching may be reduced by simple behavioral changes. These include chewing and eating food slowly, not drinking through a straw, and not chewing gum. In severe cases formal behavioral modification may be tried.

Flatus

The rate and volume of excretion of intestinal gas per rectum is highly variable. Normal volumes range from 500–1500 ml/day and the normal number of passages of gas per rectum ranges from 6–20 times/d. Intestinal flatus is derived from two sources: swallowed air and bacterial fermentation of undigested carbohydrates. Oxygen from swallowed air is readily absorbed, but no appreciable nitrogen absorption occurs because the partial pressure of nitrogen in the gut and blood are similar. Swallowed air (nitrogen) that is not belched passes through the gut and leaves as flatus. Swallowed air may contribute up to 400 mL of flatus/d. Bacterial fermentation of undigested carbohydrates leads to the additional production of gas, particularly the odorless gases hydrogen and methane. Except for situations in which there is bacterial overgrowth in the small intestine, the majority of fermentation takes place in the colon. Under normal circumstances, a small amount of fermentable substrates reach the colon. These include lactose, fructose, bean starch, and complex carbohydrates derived from wheat, oats, corn, and potatoes. Gas production may be increased dramatically with diseases of malabsorption (eg, celiac sprue), or after ingestion of poorly absorbed carbohydrates (eg, lactose, lactulose, sorbitol). Gases derived from plant carbohydrates have little odor. In contrast, the digestion of meats and eggs may give rise to small quantities of odorous gases.

To determine normal from abnormal amounts of flatus can be difficult. In most cases no formal evaluation is needed. A work up for malabsorption should be undertaken in patients who have diarrhea or signs or weight loss or anemia. An initial trial of a lactose-free diet should be given. Common gas producing foods should be reviewed and the patient given an elimination trial. These include brown beans, cauliflower, brussel sprouts, broccoli, cabbage, onions, beer, red wine, and coffee. For patients with persistent complaints, fructose and complex carbohydrates may be eliminated, but such restrictive diets are unacceptable to most patients. The usefulness of activated charcoal or simethicone is dubious. The nonprescription agent "Beano" (alpha-galactosidase) reduces gas production after the ingestion of baked beans.

The complaints of chronic abdominal distention or bloating are common but do not correlate with increased intra-abdominal gas or gas production. The majority of these patients have an underlying functional gastrointestinal disorder, eg, irritable bowel syndrome or nonulcer dyspepsia.

NAUSEA & VOMITING

Nausea and vomiting are extremely common symptoms that may reflect benign, self-limited illness or life-threatening disease. **Nausea** is a vague, intensely disagreeable sensation of sickness or "queasiness" that may be followed by vomiting. **Vomiting** is the forceful expulsion of gastric contents through a relaxed upper esophageal sphincter and open mouth, which is brought on by coordinated gastric, abdominal, and thoracic contractions. It is often preceded by nausea and by **retching,** spasmodic respiratory and abdominal movements (dry heaves). Vomiting should be distinguished from regurgitation and rumination (see preceding section under, "Symptoms of Esophageal Disease").

The act of vomiting is controlled by a center in the medulla that coordinates the respiratory, salivary, and vasomotor centers and the vagus nervous innervation of the gastrointestinal tract. The vomiting center may be stimulated by four different sources of afferent input:

1. Afferent vagal fibers (rich in serotonin 5-HT_3 receptors) and splanchnic fibers from the gastrointestinal viscera; these may be stimulated by biliary or gastrointestinal distention, mucosal or peritoneal irritation or infections.
2. The vestibular system; this may be stimulated by motion or infections. These fibers have high concentrations of histamine H_1 and muscarinic cholinergic receptors.
3. Higher CNS centers; CNS disorders or certain sights, smells, or emotional experiences may result in vomiting. For example, patients receiving chemotherapy may develop vomiting in anticipation of the treatment.
4. The "chemoreceptor trigger zone" (CTZ) located outside the blood-brain barrier in the area postrema of the medulla; this area has chemoreceptors that may be stimulated by drugs and chemotherapeutic agents, toxins, hypoxia, uremia, acidosis, and radiation therapy. This region is rich in serotonin $5HT_3$ and dopamine D2 receptors. A list of the causes of vomiting are many, a simplified list is provided in Table 1–3.

Complications of vomiting include dehydration, hypokalemia, metabolic alkalosis, pulmonary aspiration, rupture of the esophagus (Boerhaave's syndrome) and bleeding secondary to a mucosal tear at the gastroesophageal junction (Mallory-Weiss syndrome).

Clinical Findings
  A. Symptoms and Signs: The history and physical examination are important in distinguishing among the causes of vomiting. Acute symptoms without abdominal pain are typically caused by food poisoning, infectious gastroenteritis, or drugs. Inquiry should be made into recent changes in medications, food ingestions, other viral symptoms of malaise or diarrhea, or similar illness in family mem-

bers. The acute onset of severe pain and vomiting suggests peritoneal irritation, acute intestinal obstruction, or pancreaticobiliary disease. Examination may reveal fever, focal tenderness, guarding or rebound tenderness. Chronic vomiting suggests pregnancy, gastric outlet obstruction, gastroparesis, intestinal dysmotility, psychogenic disorders, CNS diseases or systemic disorders.

The timing of vomiting in relation to meals and the nature of the emesis may provide clues to the cause. Vomiting immediately after meals suggests bulimia or psychogenic causes but may also occur in pyloric stenosis from peptic ulcer disease. Vomiting undigested food 1 to several hours after meals suggests gastroparesis (eg, diabetes or postvagotomy) or a gastric outlet obstruction resulting from peptic ulcer disease or malignant neoplasm. Physical examination in these patients may reveal a succussion splash. Vomiting that occurs in the early morning may be seen in pregnancy, alcoholism, uremia, and with increased intracranial pressure. Patients with either acute or chronic symptoms should be asked about neurologic symptoms, such as headaches, stiff neck, vertigo, and focal paresthesias or weakness. Vomitus that contains truly undigested food is seen in patients with achalasia. Otherwise, the presence of food contents suggests gastric outlet obstruction, proximal small intestine obstruction, or gastroparesis.

Evidence of dehydration should be sought, including orthostatic vital signs, skin turgor, and appearance of mucous membranes. Evidence of weight loss or a palpable abdominal mass raise the suspicion of malignant neoplasm. Abdominal distention raises suspicion of small intestinal obstruction. A succussion splash may be present with gastric outlet obstruction or gastroparesis. Hernial orifices should be examined with careful attention to surgical scars. A careful neurologic and fundoscopic examination are required.

  B. Laboratory Findings: Prolonged vomiting may result in metabolic imbalances. The most common imbalances are metabolic alkalosis, hypokalemia, and either hyponatremia or hypernatremia. Prerenal azotemia may be present.

  C. Special Examinations: In acute vomiting, a flat and upright abdominal radiograph are obtained in patients with severe pain or suspicion of mechanical obstruction to look for free intraperitoneal air or dilated loops of small bowel. In patients with suspected mechanical small intestinal or gastric obstruction, a nasogastric tube should be placed for relief of symptoms. Aspiration of more than 200 mL of residual material in a fasting patient suggests obstruction or gastroparesis. This may be confirmed by a saline load test showing more than 400 mL residual on gastric aspiration performed 30 minutes after nasogastric instillation of 750 mL of normal saline. The cause of the gastric outlet obstruction is best demonstrated by upper endoscopy. Gastroparesis is confirmed by nu-

Table 1–3. Causes of nausea and vomiting.

Acute Nausea and Vomiting	
1. Infectious 　Viral gastroenteritis 　　Norwalk agent 　　Rotavirus 　Toxin-mediated (food poisoning) 　　*Staphylococcus aureus* 　　*Bacillus cereus* 　　*Clostridia perfringens* 　Acute systemic infections 　Infections in immunocompromised hosts 2. Gastrointestinal Mechanical Obstruction 　Acute gastric outlet obstruction 　　Pyloric channel ulcer 　Extrinsic small bowel obstruction 　　Incarcerated hernia 　　　Inguinal, femoral, obturator, umbilical, incisional 　　Volvulus 　　Adhesions 　　Malrotation 　　Internal hernias 　Intrinsic small bowel obstruction 　　Crohn's disease 　　Small intestinal tumors 　　Radiation stricture 　　Foreign body (gallstone ileus) 　　Intussusception 　　Meckel's diverticulum 　Ileus 　　Postoperative 　　Medical illness	3. Visceral Pain 　Appendicitis 　Acute pancreatitis 　Acute cholecystitis 　Mesenteric ischemia 　Peritonitis of any cause 4. Central Nervous System 　Motion sickness 　Labyrinthitis (Meniere's) 　Migraine headaches 　Increased intracranial pressure 　CNS trauma 　CNS tumors or pseudotumors 　Meningitis, encephalitis 5. Systemic Conditions 　Pregnancy 　Myocardial infarction 　Renal failure 　Diabetic ketoacidosis 　Radiation therapy 　Reye's syndrome (children) 6. Medications/Topical Irritation 　Chemotherapeutic agents 　Nonsteroidal anti-inflammatory drugs 　Antibiotics 　Digoxin 　Theophylline 　Narcotics 　Niacin 　Heavy ethanol ingestion

Chronic Nausea and Vomiting	
1. Gastrointestinal Mechanical Obstruction 　Chronic gastric outlet obstruction 　　Chronic peptic ulcer disease 　　Gastric tumor 　　Crohn's disease with duodenal stricture 　　Pancreatic cancer with duodenal obstruction 　Small intestine obstruction 　　Peritoneal carcinomatosis 2. Motility Disorders 　Gastroparesis 　　Diabetes mellitus 　　Collagen vascular disorders (scleroderma) 　　Postvagotomy 　　Medication-induced 　　Idiopathic	Small intestine motility disorders 　　Chronic intestinal pseudo-obstruction 　　Familial visceral myoneuropathy 　　Paraneoplastic syndromes 　　Amyloidosis 3. Psychogenic 　Bulimia 　Psychogenic 4. Others 　Increased intracranial pressure 　Metabolic: hyperthyroidism, renal failure, Addison's 　Medications

clear scintigraphic studies which show delayed gastric emptying and either upper endoscopy or barium upper gastrointestinal series showing no evidence of mechanical gastric outlet obstruction. Abnormal liver function tests or amylase suggests pancreaticobiliary disease, which may be investigated with an abdominal sonogram or CT. CNS symptoms warrant CT or MRI imaging of the brain.

Treatment

A. General Measures: The treatment of vomiting should be directed primarily at finding and correcting the underlying cause. Most causes of acute vomiting are mild, self-limited and require no specific treatment. Patients should ingest clear liquids (broths, tea, soups, carbonated beverages) and small quantities of dry foods (soda crackers). For more severe acute vomiting, hospitalization is required. Because of the inability to eat and loss of gastric fluids, patients may become dehydrated and develop hypokalemia and metabolic alkalosis. Intravenous 0.45% saline with 20 meq/L potassium is given in most cases to maintain hydration. A nasogastric suction tube for gastric decompression improves patient comfort and permits monitoring of fluid loss.

B. Antiemetic Medications: Medications may be given either to prevent or to control vomiting. Given the complexity of the various pathways that control and stimulate vomiting, it is not surprising that no single medication is effective in all patients.

Combinations of drugs from different classes may provide better control of symptoms with less toxicity in some patients. The medications listed in Table 1–4 should be avoided in pregnancy.

1. Serotonin 5-HT$_3$ receptor antagonists– These are the newest family of antiemetic drugs; ondansetron and granisetron are currently available. When initiated prior to treatment, it is highly effective in the prevention of chemotherapy-induced emesis. Its efficacy in other situations is less well studied.

2. Dopamine antagonists–The phenothiazines, butyrophenones and substituted benzamides have antiemetic properties which is due, at least in part, to dopaminergic blockade as well as sedative effects. High doses of these agents are associated with antidopaminergic side effects, including extrapyramidal reactions and depression. These agents are commonly used antiemetics for a variety of situations.

3. Antihistamines–These have weak antiemetic properties, but are useful in the prevention of vomiting due to motion sickness.

4. Sedatives–Benzodiazepines may be helpful in patients with psychogenetic and anticipatory vomiting.

5. Corticosteroids–These may be used in combination with other agents in the treatment of chemotherapy-induced vomiting.

6. Dronabinol (tetrahydrocannabinol)–One of the major substances in marijuana, this agent has been found empirically to have antiemetic properties. The mechanism is unknown. It is used for the control of nausea and vomiting related to chemotherapy. The dose is 5–15 mg/m^2, given 1–3 hours prechemotherapy and every 3–4 hours as needed after chemotherapy is given.

DIARRHEA

Diarrhea is a common symptom that can range in severity from an acute, self-limited annoyance to a severe, life-threatening illness. Patients may use the term **diarrhea** to refer to an increased frequency of bowel movement, increased stool liquidity, a sense of fecal urgency, or incontinence. To properly evaluate the complaint, the physician must determine the patient's normal bowel pattern and the nature of the current symptoms.

In the normal state, approximately 10 L of fluid enter the duodenum daily, of which all but 1.0 L are absorbed by the small intestine. The colon resorbs most of the remaining fluid, with only 100 mL lost in the stool. From a medical standpoint, diarrhea is defined as a stool weight of more than 250 g/24 h. In clinical practice, quantification of stool weight is necessary only in some patients with chronic diarrhea. In most cases the practical definition of diarrhea is an increased stool frequency (> 2–3 times/d) or liquidity.

The causes of diarrhea are myriad. In clinical practice it is helpful to distinguish acute from chronic diarrhea, as the evaluation and treatment is entirely dif-

Table 1–4. Antiemetic dosing regimens.

	Dosage	Route
Serotonin 5-HT$_3$ antagonist[1]		
Ondansetron	32 mg over 15 min beginning 15 minutes before chemotherapy; 4 mg over 2–5 min for postoperative vomiting	IV
	8 mg tid	PO
Granisetron	10 mcg/kg over 5 minutes, 30 min before chemotherapy	IV
Dopamine antagonists		
Prochlorperazine	5–10 mg every 4–6 hours	PO, IM
	25 mg suppository every 6 hours	PR
Promethazine	25 mg every 4–6 hours	PO, IM, PR
Droperidol	1–2.5 mg	IV
Metoclopramide	10–20 mg every 6 hours	PO
	0.5–2 mg/kg every 6–8 hours	IV
Antihistamines/Anticholinergics		
Diphenhydramine	25–50 mg every 4–6 hours	PO, IM, IV
Scopalamine patch	1.5 mg every 3 days	Patch
Dimenhydrinate	50 mg every 4 hours	PO
Meclizine	25–50 mg q24 hours	PO
Sedatives/CNS altering agents		
Diazepam[2]	2–5 mg every 4–6 hours	PO, IV
Lorazepam[2]	1–2 mg every 4–6 hours	PO, IV
Dronabinol[3]	5 mg/m2 1 hour before chemotherapy and every 2–4 hours prn	PO

[1]Approved for prevention of chemotherapy-induced nausea and vomiting and for treatment of postoperative nausea and vomiting. Use in other situations requires further study.
[2]Useful when given before chemotherapy in patients with anticipatory vomiting.
[3]Used primarily in the treatment of nausea and vomiting associated with chemotherapy; usefulness in other situations requires further study.

ferent. A complete list of causes is given in the Table 1–5.

1. ACUTE DIARRHEA

Etiology & Clinical Findings

Diarrhea that is acute in onset and present for less than 3 weeks is most commonly caused by infectious agents, bacterial toxins (either ingested preformed in food or produced in gut), or drugs. Epidemiologic information may provide clues to the causative agent. Similar recent illness in family members suggests an infectious origin. Recent ingestion of improperly stored or prepared food implicates food poisoning, especially if other people were similarly affected. Exposure to unpurified water (camping, swimming) may result in infection with *Giardia* or *Cryptosporidium*. Recent foreign travel suggests "traveler's diarrhea." Antibiotic usage within the preceding several weeks increases the likelihood of *C difficile* colitis. Finally, risk factors for HIV infection or sexually transmitted diseases should be determined. Patients practicing unprotected anal intercourse are at risk for a variety of infections, including gonorrhea, syphilis, lymphogranuloma venereum, and herpes simplex. A variety of medications may cause diarrhea through various mechanisms and should not be overlooked. A full discussion of AIDS-associated diarrhea and acute diarrhea is provided in Chapters 2 and 8, respectively.

The nature of the diarrhea helps distinguish among different infectious causes (Table 1–5).

A. Noninflammatory Diarrhea: Watery, non-bloody diarrhea associated with periumbilical cramps, bloating, nausea or vomiting suggests a small bowel enteritis caused by either a toxin-producing bacterium (enterotoxigenic *E coli* [ETEC], *S aureaus*, *B cereus*, *C perfringens*) or other agents (viruses, *Giardia*) that disrupt the normal absorption and secretory process in the small intestine. Prominent vomiting suggests viral enteritis or *S aureus* food poisoning. Though typically mild, the diarrhea (which originates in the small intestine) may be voluminous (ranging from 10 to 200 mL/kg/24h) and result in dehydration with hypokalemia and metabolic acidosis due to loss of HCO_3^- in the stool (eg, cholera). Because tissue invasion dose not occur, fecal leukocytes are not present.

B. Inflammatory Diarrhea: The presence of fever and bloody diarrhea (dysentery) indicates colonic tissue damage caused by invasion (shigellosis, salmonellosis, *Campylobacter*, *Yersinia*, amebiasis) or a toxin (*C difficile*, *E coli* 0157:H7). Because these different organisms involve predominantly the colon, the diarrhea is small in volume (<1L/d) and associated with left lower quadrant cramps, urgency and tenesmus. Fecal leukocytes are present in infections with invasive organisms. *E coli* 0157:H7 is a toxigenic, noninvasive organism that may be acquired from contaminated meat and has resulted in several outbreaks of an acute, often severe,

Table 1–5. Causes of acute diarrhea.

Noninflammatory Diarrhea[1]	Inflammatory Diarrhea[2]
Viral	**Viral**
Norwalk virus	Cytomegalovirus[3]
Rotavirus	**Bacterial**
Protozoa	**1. Cytotoxin production**
Giardia lamblia	*E coli* O157:H7 (Enterohemorrhagic)
Crytosporidium	*Vibrio parahaemolyticus*
Bacterial	*Clostridium difficile*
1. Preformed enterotoxin	**2. Mucosal invasion**
Staphylococcus aureus	*Shigella*
Bacillus cereus	*Salmonella sp.*
Clostridium perfringens	Enteroinvasive *E coli*
2. Intra-intestinal enterotoxin production	*Aeromonal*
E coli (enterotoxigenic)	*Yersinia enterocolitica*
Vibrio cholerae	*Plesimonal*
New medications	**3. Bacterial proctitis**
Fecal impaction	*Chlamydia*
	N gonorrhoeae
	Protozoal
	Entamoeba histolytica
	Intestinal ischemia
	Inflammatory bowel disease
	Radiation colitis

[1]Noninflammatory: Fever absent. Stool without evidence of blood or fecal leukocytes.
[2]Inflammatory diarrhea: Often with systemic features, including fever. Fecal leukocytes with or without gross blood usually present. (**Note:** Fecal leukocytes are variable in *Salmonella, Yersinia, V parahaemolytica, C difficile,* and *Aeromonas*.)
[3]Most commonly in immunocompromised patients, especially AIDS. Full causes of AIDS-associated diarrhea are discussed in Chapter 2.

hemorrhagic colitis. Most of these outbreaks have been traced to contaminated ground beef (eg, hamburger, salami), which has been improperly prepared. It now is believed to be the most common cause of infectious bloody diarrhea in adults and the most common cause of hemolytic uremic syndrome in children. In immunocompromised and HIV-infected patients, CMV may result in intestinal ulceration with watery or bloody diarrhea. Infectious dysentery must be distinguished from acute ulcerative colitis, which may also present acutely with fever, abdominal pain and bloody diarrhea.

C. Enteric Fever: A severe systemic illness manifested initially by prolonged high fevers, prostration, confusion, respiratory symptoms followed by abdominal tenderness, diarrhea and a rash is due to infection with *S typhi* or *parathyphi,* which causes bacteremia and multiorgan dysfunction.

Evaluation

In over 90% of patients with acute diarrhea, the illness is mild and self-limited and responds within 5 days to simple rehydration therapy or symptomatic antidiarrheal agents. In such cases, a laboratory investigation to determine the causative agent is unnecessary because it is costly, often unrevealing, and does not affect therapy or outcome. Indeed, the isolation rate of bacterial pathogens from stool cultures in patients with acute diarrhea is less than 3%. Thus, the goal of initial evaluation is to distinguish these patients from those with more serious illness. In many outpatient clinics, a microscopic examination of the stool for fecal leukocytes is obtained in order to distinguish noninflammatory from inflammatory diarrhea. This test is easily performed and inexpensive. The presence of leukocytes suggests an inflammatory diarrhea and warrants a stool bacterial culture.

Patients with signs of inflammatory diarrhea manifested by any of the following require prompt medical attention: high fever (>38.5 °C [101.3 °F]), bloody diarrhea, abdominal pain, or diarrhea not improving after 4–5 days. Similarly, patients with symptoms of dehydration must be evaluated (excessive thirst, dry mouth, decreased urination, weakness, lethargy). Physical examination should note the patient's general appearance, mental status, volume status, and the presence of abdominal tenderness or peritonitis. Peritoneal findings may be present in *C difficile* and enterohemorrhagic *E coli.* Hospitalization is required in patients with severe dehydration, toxicity, or abdominal pain. Stool specimens should be collected from patients in order to examine for fecal leukocytes and bacterial cultures (Table 1–5). The rate of positive bacterial cultures in patients with dysentery symptoms is 60–75%. A wet mount examination of the stool for amebiasis also should be performed in patients with dysentery who have recently travelled to endemic areas or those who are homosexual. In patients with a history of an-

tibiotic exposure, a stool sample should be sent for *C difficile* toxin testing. If *E coli* 0157:H7 is suspected, the laboratory must be alerted to do specific serotyping. In patients with diarrhea that persists for longer than 10 days, three stool examinations for ova and parasites also should be performed. Rectal swabs may be sent to a laboratory for *Chlamydia,* gonorrhea, and herpes simplex virus testing in sexually active patients with severe proctitis symptoms.

Sigmoidoscopy is warranted acutely in patients with symptoms of severe proctitis (tenesmus, discharge, rectal pain) and in patients with suspected *C difficile* colitis who appear ill. It may also be helpful in distinguishing infectious diarrhea from ulcerative colitis or ischemic colitis, especially in patients with bloody diarrhea.

Treatment

A. Diet: The overwhelming majority of adults have mild diarrhea that will not lead to dehydration provided the patient takes adequate oral fluids containing carbohydrates and electrolytes. Patients will find it more comfortable to rest the bowel by avoiding high fiber foods, fats, milk products, caffeine, and alcohol. Frequent feedings of fruit drinks, tea, de-fizzed carbonated beverages and soft, easily digested foods (eg, soups, crackers) are encouraged.

B. Rehydration: In more severe diarrhea, dehydration can occur quickly, especially in children. Oral rehydration therapy containing glucose, Na^+, K^+, Cl^-, and bicarbonate or citrate is preferred in most cases to intravenous fluids because it is inexpensive, safe, and highly effective in almost all awake patients. An easy mixture is 1/2 tsp salt (3.5 g), 1 tsp baking soda (2.5 g $NaHCO_3$) 8 tsp sugar (40 g) and 8 oz of orange juice (1.5 g KCl) may be diluted to 1 L with water. Alternatively, oral electrolyte solutions are readily available. Fluids should be given at rates of 50–200 mL/kg/24h, depending on the hydration status. Intravenous fluids (lactated Ringer's solution) is preferred acutely in patients with severe dehydration.

C. Symptomatic Agents: Antidiarrheal agents may be used safely in patients with mild to moderate diarrheal illnesses to improve patient comfort. Opiate agents help decrease the stool number and liquidity and control fecal urgency. However, they should not be used in patients with bloody diarrhea, high fever, or systemic toxicity for fear of worsening the disease. Similarly, they should be discontinued in patients whose diarrhea is worsening despite therapy. With these provisos, these agents provide excellent symptomatic relief. Loperamide is the preferred agent; 4 mg is given initially, followed by 2 mg after each loose stool (maximum: 16 mg/24 h).

Bismuth subsalicylate (PeptoBismol), 2 tablets or 30 mL four times daily reduces symptoms in patients with traveler's diarrhea because of its anti-inflammatory and antibacterial properties; its role in other settings is poorly studied. Scores of other agents touted for their antidiarrheal action have undergone little or no controlled testing but appear to have minimal or no symptomatic benefit (lactobacilli, kaolin, pectin). Anticholinergic agents are contraindicated in acute diarrhea (eg, atropine).

D. Antibiotic Therapy:

1. Empiric treatment–As the overwhelming majority of patients have mild, self-limited disease due to viruses or noninvasive bacteria, empiric antibiotic treatment of all patients with acute diarrhea is not warranted. Even patients with inflammatory diarrhea caused by invasive pathogens most often have mild disease that will resolve within several days without specific treatment. Conversely, in patients who appear to have signs of an invasive pathogen with moderate to severe symptoms of fever, tenesmus, bloody stools, and positive fecal leukocytes, empiric treatment is recommended while the stool bacterial culture is incubating. The drugs of choice are the flouroquinolones (ciprofloxacin 500 mg twice daily) for 5–7 days. These agents have good antibiotic coverage against most invasive bacterial pathogens, including *Shigella, Salmonella, Campylobacter, Yersinia,* and *Aeromonas.* Alternative agents are trimethoprim/sulfamethoxazole 160/800 mg twice daily or erythromycin 250–500 mg four times daily.

2. Specific antimicrobial treatment–Antibiotics are not generally recommended in patients with nontyphoid *Salmonella, Campylobacter,* or *Yersinia* except in severe or prolonged disease because they have not been shown to hasten recovery or reduce the period of fecal bacterial excretion. The infectious diarrheas for which treatment is clearly recommended are *Shigella,* cholera, extraintestinal salmonellosis, "traveler's" diarrhea, *C difficile, Giardia, Entamoeba histolytica,* and the sexually transmitted infections (gonorrhea, syphilis, *Chlamydia,* and herpes simplex infection). Specific treatment of these organisms is discussed in Chapter 8.

2. CHRONIC DIARRHEA

Etiology

The causes of chronic diarrhea may be grouped into six major pathophysiologic categories (Table 1–6):

A. Osmotic: As stool leaves the colon, the fecal osmolality is equal to the serum osmolality, ie, approximately 290 mosm/kg. Under normal circumstances, the major osmoles are Na^+, K^+, Cl^-, and bicarbonate. The stool osmolality may be estimated by multiplying the stool $(Na^+ + K^+) \times 2$ (multiplied by two to account for the anions). The osmotic gap is the difference between the *measured* osmolality of the stool (or serum) and the *estimated* stool osmolality and is normally less than 50 mosm/kg. An increased osmotic gap implies the diarrhea is caused by

Table 1–6. Causes of chronic diarrhea.

Osmotic Diarrhea

Lactose intolerance
Medications: sorbitol, lactulose, antacids
Factitious: magnesium laxatives or sodium sulfate laxatives
Clues: Stool volume decreases with fasting; increased osmotic gap greater than 50 mosm/L.

Malabsorptive Conditions

Intestinal mucosal diseases: celiac sprue, Whipple's disease, eosinophilic gastroenteritis, Crohn's disease, small bowel resection
Lymphatic obstruction
Pancreatic disease: chronic pancreatitis, pancreatic carcinoma
Small bowel bacterial overgrowth: motility disorders (vagotomy, scleroderma, diabetes), colonic-enteric fistulas, small intestinal diverticula
Clues: Weight loss, fecal fat greater than 7–10 g/24 h stool collection, anemia, hypoalbuminemia.

Secretory Diarrhea

Hormonal secretion: VIPoma, carcinoid, medullary carcinoma of thyroid, Zollinger-Ellison syndrome (gastrinoma)
Bile salt malabsorption: ileal resection, Crohn's disease
Medications
Factitious: phenolphthalein, cascara, senna
Villous adenoma
Clues: Large volume (>1L/d); little change with fasting (except with bile salt diarrhea); normal stool osmotic gap.

Inflammatory Conditions

Ulcerative colitis
Crohn's disease
Microscopic colitis
Radiation enteritis
Malignancy: lymphoma, adenocarcinoma
Clues: Fever, hematochezia or abdominal pain (absent in microscopic colitis).

Motility Disorders

Postsurgical: vagotomy, partial gastrectomy
Systemic disorders: scleroderma, diabetes mellitus, hyperthyroidism
Irritable bowel syndrome

ingestion or malabsorption of an osmotically active substance. The most common causes of osmotic diarrhea are: disaccharidase deficiency (lactase deficiency), laxative abuse, and malabsorption syndromes (see following section). Osmotic diarrheas resolve during fasting. Osmotic diarrheas caused by malabsorbed carbohydrates are characterized by abdominal distention, bloating and flatulence resulting from increased colonic gas production.

Disaccharidase deficiencies are extremely common and should always be considered in patients with chronic diarrhea. Lactase deficiency occurs in three-fourths of non-white adults and up to 25% of white adults. It may also be acquired after viral gastroenteritis, a medical illness, or gastrointestinal surgery. Sorbitol is a commonly used as a sweetener in gums, candies, and some medications that may cause diarrhea in some patients. The diagnosis of sorbitol or lactose malabsorption may be established by an elimination trial for 2–3 weeks. The diagnosis may be confirmed by measuring a rise in breath hydrogen of more than 20 ppm after lactose or sorbitol ingestion, but this is seldom necessary.

Ingestion of magnesium or phosphate containing compounds (laxatives, antacids) should be considered in enigmatic diarrhea. Surreptitious use should be considered especially in young women with possible eating disorders and patients with psychiatric problems, a long history of vague or mysterious medical ailments, or employment in the medical field.

B. Malabsorptive Conditions: The major causes of malabsorption are small mucosal intestinal diseases, intestinal resections, lymphatic obstruction, small intestinal bacterial overgrowth and pancreatic insufficiency. The hallmarks of malabsorption are weight loss, osmotic diarrhea and nutrient deficiencies. Significant diarrhea in the absence of weight loss is unlikely to be malabsorption. The physical and laboratory abnormalities related to deficiencies of vitamins or minerals are discussed elsewhere. Briefly, they include anemia (micro- or macrocytic), hypoalbuminemia, low serum cholesterol, hypocalcemia, and an elevated prothrombin time.

In patients with suspected malabsorption, a quantification of the stool fecal fat should be performed. In patients with more than 10 g/24 h of fecal fat, further workup for malabsorption is indicated (see Chapter 24).

C. Secretory Conditions: Increased intestinal secretion or decreased absorption results in a watery diarrhea that may be large in volume (1–10 L/d) but has a normal osmotic gap. There is little change in stool output during the fasting state. In serious conditions, significant dehydration and electrolyte imbalance may develop. Major causes include endocrine tumors (stimulating intestinal or pancreatic secretion), bile salt malabsorption (stimulating colonic secretion), and laxative abuse.

D. Inflammatory Conditions: Diarrhea is present in the majority of patients with inflammatory bowel disease (eg, ulcerative colitis, Crohn's, microscopic colitis). A variety of other symptoms may be present including abdominal pain, fever, weight loss, and hematochezia (see Chapter 7).

E. Motility Disorders: Abnormal intestinal motility secondary to systemic disorders or surgery may result in diarrhea due to rapid transit or to stasis of intestinal contents with bacterial overgrowth resulting in malabsorption.

Perhaps the most common cause of chronic diarrhea is irritable bowel syndrome. In this idiopathic, chronic condition, patients have a variety of complaints including abdominal pain (often relieved by defecation), bloating, and disturbed defecation with fluctuating stool consistency and frequency (see Chapter 7). Although many of these patients complain of diarrhea, the majority, in fact, have a normal stool weight (see Chapter 6).

F. Chronic Infections: Chronic parasitic infections may cause diarrhea through a number of mechanisms. Although the list of parasitic organisms is lengthy, agents most commonly associated with diarrhea include the protozoans, *Giardia* and *E histolytica,* and the intestinal nematodes.

Immunocompromised patients, especially those with AIDS, are susceptible to a number of infectious agents that can cause acute or chronic diarrhea (see Chapter 2). Chronic diarrhea in AIDS patients is commonly caused by *Microsporidia, Cryptosporidia,* cytomegalovirus, *Isosopora belli,* and *Mycobacterium avium-intracellulare* (MAC).

Evaluation

The list of diagnostic tests available for the evaluation of chronic diarrhea is exhaustive. In most cases however a careful history and physical examination suggest the underlying pathophysiologic category which guides the subsequent diagnostic work up (Figure 1–2). The following tests are commonly employed in the evaluation of chronic diarrhea.

A. Stool Analysis:

1. Twenty-four-hour stool collection for weight and quantitative fecal fat–A stool weight of more than 300 g/24 h confirms the presence of diarrhea, justifying further workup. A weight greater than 1000–1500 g suggests a secretory process. A fecal fat exceeding 10 g/24 h indicates a malabsorptive process.

2. Stool osmolality–An osmotic gap confirms osmotic diarrhea. A stool osmolality less than the serum osmolality implies that water or urine has been added to the specimen (factitious diarrhea).

3. Stool laxative screen–In suspected laxative abuse, stool magnesium, phosphate, and sulfate levels may be ordered. Phenolphthalein is indicated by the presence of a bright red color after alkalinization of the stool. Bisacodyl can be detected in the urine.

4. Fecal leukocytes–The presence of leukocytes in a stool sample implies an underlying inflammatory diarrhea.

5. Stool for ova and parasites–In normal hosts, *Giardia* and *E histolytica* are considered.

B. Laboratory Tests:

1. Routine tests–CBC, serum electrolytes, liver chemistry tests, calcium, phosphorus, albumin, TSH, total T_4, β-carotene and protime should be obtained. Anemia occurs in malabsorption (B_{12}, folate, iron) and inflammatory conditions. Hypoalbuminemia is present in malabsorption, protein losing enteropathies, and inflammatory diseases. Hyponatremia and non-anion gap metabolic acidosis may occur in profound secretory diarrheas. Malabsorption of fat soluble vitamins may result in an abnormal protime, low calcium, low carotene or abnormal alkaline phosphatase.

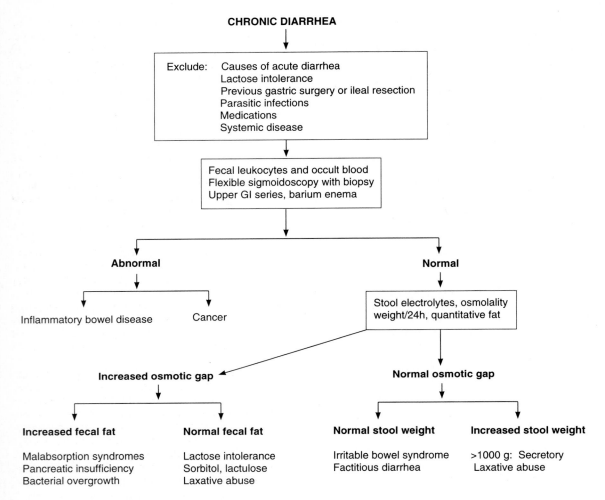

Figure 1–2. Decision diagram for diagnosing causes of chronic diarrhea. (Reproduced, with permission, from McQuaid KR: Alimentary Tract. In: *Current Medical Diagnosis & Treatment 1996.* Tierney LM Jr, McPhee SJ, Papadakis MA (editors). Appleton & Lange, 1996.)

2. Specific laboratory tests—In patients with suspected secretory diarrhea, serum VIP (VIPoma), gastrin (Zollinger-Ellison), calcitonin (medullary thyroid carcinoma), cortisol (Addison's), and urinary 5-HIAA (carcinoid) levels should be obtained.

C. Proctosigmoidoscopy with Mucosal Biopsy: Examination may be helpful in detecting inflammatory bowel disease (including microscopic colitis) and melanosis coli, which indicates chronic use of anthraquinone laxatives.

D. Imaging Studies: After the above studies have been performed, the cause of the diarrhea will generally be clear and further imaging studies can be ordered as indicated. Calcification on a plain abdominal radiograph confirms chronic pancreatitis. An upper gastrointestinal series or enteroclysis study is helpful in evaluating Crohn's disease, lymphoma, or carcinoid. Colonoscopy is helpful in evaluating for colonic inflammation resulting from inflammatory bowel disease. Upper endoscopy with small bowel biopsy is useful in suspected malabsorption due to mucosal diseases. Upper endoscopy with a duodenal aspirate and small bowel biopsy is also useful in patients with AIDS and to document *Cryptosporidum, Microsporidia,* and MAC infection. Abdominal CT is helpful to detect chronic pancreatitis or pancreatic endocrine tumors.

Treatment

Treatment of chronic diarrhea is directed at the underlying condition. A number of antidiarrheal agents may be used in certain situations in patients with chronic diarrheal conditions and are listed below:

A. Narcotic Analogues: These may be used safely in most patients with chronic, stable symptoms.

1. **Loperamide**–4 mg initially; then 2 mg after each loose stool (maximum dose: 16mg/d).
2. **Diphenoxylate with atropine**–One tablet three to four times daily.
   B. Narcotics: Because of their addictive potential these are generally avoided except in cases of chronic, intractable diarrhea.
1. **Codeine**–15–60 mg every 4 hours, as needed.
2. **Paregoric**–4–8 ml after liquid bowel movement.
   C. Other Agents:
1. **Clonidine**–α_2 adrenergic agonists inhibits intestinal electrolyte secretion. A clonidine patch that administers 1 mg/d for 7 days may be useful in some patients with secretory diarrheas, *Cryptosporidia,* and diabetes.
2. **Octreotide**–This somatostatin analogue stimulates intestinal fluid and electrolyte absorption and inhibits secretion. Furthermore, it inhibits the release of gastrointestinal peptides. It is very useful in treating secretory diarrheas due to VIPoma and carcinoid and in some cases of diarrhea associated with AIDS. Effective doses range from 50 to 250 µg subcutaneously three times daily.
3. **Cholestyramine**–This bile salt binding resin may be useful in patients with bile salt induced diarrhea secondary to intestinal resection or ileal disease. A dose of 4 g one to three times daily is recommended.

CONSTIPATION

Constipation is best described as a perception of abnormal defecation that may include decreased frequency of bowel movements, a sensation of incomplete evacuation, painful defecation, straining, or the presence of hard stools. The frequency of "normal" bowel movements is broad, ranging from 3 to 12 per week. Thus, in many patients the complaint of constipation may reflect a mistaken perception of what constitutes a normal bowel habit. From a medical perspective, constipation is present when a patient has fewer than three bowel movements per week or has excessive straining at defecation. Constipation is more common among women than men, and surveys of the American population have indicated a prevalence of constipation ranging from 3 to 20%, depending on the criteria used. A marked increase in the subjective complaint of constipation occurs with advanced age. Constipation is among the most common complaints encountered by primary care physicians and gastroenterologists, and the economic resources directed toward the evaluation and treatment of constipation are considerable. A knowledge of the causes and treatment of constipation allows determination of the appropriate type and extent of workup required for this common complaint.

The primary functions of the colon are the storage and conversion of liquid chyme to solid fecal bulk and the timely elimination of fecal contents. Approximately 1 L of liquid chyme passes daily through the ileocecal valve into the colon. Through a process of active colonic resorption of fluid and electrolytes and the activity of gut bacteria, this is converted to approximately 200 g of solid fecal waste. The colon may be divided into three functional regions: the proximal colon, the distal colon, and the rectum. In the proximal colon, which extends from the cecum to the hepatic flexure, fecal chyme is churned and mixed by rhythmic segmental and retrograde contractions that retard fecal passage and permit fluid resorption. Thus, this segment serves an important reservoir function. Intermittently, orthograde contractions occur that propel solid contents forward into the more distal colon. In the segment from the transverse colon to the rectosigmoid junction, orthograde rhythmic contractions occur that gradually move the more solid contents towards the rectum, allowing further fluid resorption. Two to three times daily there is a large propulsive movement that propels a larger amount of fecal contents distally. The rectum appears to fill slowly with solid contents from the sigmoid and serves as a storage area until elimination is convenient.

The process of defecation involves a complex array of autonomic and voluntary mechanisms. To permit defecation, the natural barriers to involuntary elimination must be overcome. Under normal circumstances, continence is assisted by the pelvic floor muscles (puborectalis and pubococcygeus), striated muscles that are innervated by the pudendal nerve and are under voluntary control. These muscles form a sling around the rectum to form an acute anorectal angle. In addition, the internal anal sphincter, which is under involuntary control, is tonically contracted. When the rectum becomes distended, the internal anal sphincter relaxes, due to spinal and intramural inhibitory reflexes. If elimination is not desired, voluntary contraction of the pelvic floor muscles and external sphincter prevents defecation until the internal anal sphincter tone returns. When defecation is desired, voluntary relaxation of the pelvic floor permits perineal descent and straightening of the anorectal angle. This is facilitated by assuming a squatting or sitting position. A valsalva maneuver to increase intra-abdominal pressure in conjunction with a mass rectal contraction permits evacuation.

Etiology

Given the complexity of colonic function and the defecatory process, constipation can occur for a variety of reasons. Constipation may occur as a result of abnormal motor function of the large intestine, which may be due to systemic disease, medications, or primary motor disorders of the bowel. Alternatively, abnormalities of the muscular structures of the anorectum (pelvic floor dysfunction) may lead to abnormal defecation and complaints of constipation.

A. Poor Dietary and Toilet Habits: The overwhelming majority of constipated patients have mild symptoms that cannot be attributed to any structural abnormalities, intestinal motility disturbances or systemic disease. Careful dietary review reveals that most of these patients do not consume adequate dietary fiber or fluids. Many patients ignore nature's "call to stool." In addition, immobility produced by chronic illness may lead to fecal retention and loss of rectal sensory cues to defecate, resulting in fecal impaction. The elderly in particular are predisposed to constipation because of a combination of poor eating habits, the use of medications that are constipating, decreased colonic motility, and physical limitations that may restrict ease of access to a bathroom or the ability to sit for defecation.

B. Systemic Diseases that may Cause Constipation: A variety of neurologic, endocrinologic, metabolic, and collagen vascular disorders may cause constipation (Table 1–7).

C. Medications: A number of medications may produce constipation (Table 1–7).

D. Structural Abnormalities: Colonic lesions that obstruct fecal passage must be excluded in patients with constipation. Particular concern is raised in younger patients with lifelong constipation for Hirschsprung's disease and in patients over 45 with new-onset constipation for malignancy.

E. Idiopathic Constipation: The vast majority of patients with refractory constipation do not have an identifiable systemic disease or medication to which constipation may be attributed, and thus fall into this category. These patients may be further classified according to findings on colonic transit studies and studies of rectosphincteric function (see following section, "Diagnostic Studies").

1. Colonic inertia–Some patients have an idiopathic delay in large bowel transit. Severe colonic inertia is more common in women, some of whom have a history of abuse or psychosocial problems. Colonic inertia may be part of a more generalized gastrointestinal dysmotility syndrome. It can also be caused by years of cathartic abuse.

2. Pelvic floor dysfunction (also termed outlet obstruction)–An abnormality in the relaxation of the puborectalis or sphincteric mechanism resulting in impaired evacuation of the rectum may occur with or without an abnormality of colonic transit. This most commonly affects women. Defecatory difficulties can be a result of a variety of anatomic problems that impede or obstruct flow, some of which may benefit from surgery. In other patients there is a failure to relax the pelvic floor during straining (anismus).

3. Constipation with normal colonic transit–This is most often due to irritable bowel syndrome.

Clinical Findings

A. Symptoms and Signs: The first step in the

Table 1–7. Causes of constipation in adults.

Lifestyle
  Low fiber
  Inadequate fluids
  Poor toilet habits
  Inability to sit on toilet
  Inadequate exercise
Medications
  Anticholinergics
    Antidepressants
    Neuroleptic agents
    Antihistamines
    Antiparkinsonian drugs
  Antihypertensives
    Calcium channel blockers
    Clonidine
  Cation-containing agents
    Iron supplements
    Calcium supplements
    Aluminum-containing antacids, sucralfate
  Opiates
    Morphine
    Codeine
    Diphenoxylate
Structural abnormalities
  Perianal disease: fissure, thrombosed hemorrhoid
  Obstructing colonic carcinoma
  Colonic stricture: diverticular, radiation, ischemia
  Idiopathic megarectum
Systemic disease
  Metabolic and endocrine
    Hypothyroidism
    Hypercalcemia
    Chronic renal failure
    Diabetes mellitus
  Neurologic disorders
    Spinal cord lesions
    Multiple sclerosis
    Parkinson's disease
    Hirschsprung's disease
    Autonomic neuropathy
    Prior pelvic surgery with disruption of parasympathetics
  Others
    Amyloidosis
    Dermatomyositis
    Progressive systemic sclerosis
    Depression
    Dementia
Causes of refractory constipation
  Slow colonic transit
    Idiopathic
    Chronic intestinal pseudo-obstruction
  Anorectal outlet disorders
    Rectocoele
    Rectal intussusception
    Rectal prolapse
    Perineal descent
    Anismus

evaluation of a patient complaining of constipation is to better define the nature of the symptoms. Patients complaining of constipation may have widely varying attitudes regarding what constitutes normal bowel habits. The frequency of defecation, as well as a history of painful evacuation, incomplete evacuation, small hard stools, or rectal bleeding should be sought. Excessive straining, the need to digitally extract stool, persistent rectal fullness, and pelvic floor descent suggest pelvic floor dysfunction. The chronicity of the symptoms is perhaps the most important historical question. A recent change in bowel habits makes an identifiable cause more likely and requires investigation, whereas longstanding complaints suggest a functional origin. The patient should be questioned regarding toilet habits, including the time of day and duration of use. A history of dietary habits with emphasis on fiber intake should be obtained. The patient should also be questioned about symptoms that may suggest irritable bowel syndrome. Irritable bowel syndrome may result in constipation along with complaints of lower abdominal pain, distention, passage of mucus per rectum, a sensation of incomplete evacuation, and increased frequency and fluidity of stools with the onset of abdominal discomfort. Questions directed at detection of depression are appropriate in the evaluation of constipation. A thorough review of prescription and nonprescription medications should be performed, with special attention to use of laxative preparations.

In the majority of patients with constipation the physical examination is normal. Signs of systemic diseases, such as diabetes mellitus or hypothyroidism, should be sought. Distended bowel loops or a palpable abdominal mass suggest malignancy. The rectal examination may detect the presence of occult blood, rectal masses, anal fissures, fecal impaction, abnormal sphincter tone or rectal prolapse. The sensation of the perineal area and the "anal wink" (a reflex contraction of the sphincter upon pinprick stimulation of the perianal area) reflex should be tested.

B. Diagnostic Studies:

1. Routine studies–Initial laboratory studies include a screening blood count, chemistry panel, tests of thyroid function, and serum calcium. The selection of patients for further investigation depends on the patient's age, chronicity of symptoms, and the presence of occult or gross bleeding. Patients with a recent change in bowel habits, weight loss, or evidence of rectal bleeding require examination with flexible sigmoidoscopy and barium enema (or colonoscopy) to exclude mass lesions or stricture. Patients lacking these features who are 45 years of age or older should undergo a flexible sigmoidoscopy followed by an empiric trial of fiber supplementation and general measures (see following section) if the flexible sigmoidoscopy is unrevealing. Patients younger than 45 years of age should initially be managed by a trial of fiber supplementation.

2. Specific studies–Studies of colonic motility and rectosphincteric function should be reserved for patients with severe symptoms who fail conservative measures of treatment, and who have had structural abnormalities ruled out with a colonoscopic or barium enema examination. This group of patients with intractable constipation constitutes a small proportion (estimated at < 1%) of the total population of patients with constipation.

a. Colonic transit study–The initial test of colonic motility performed should be a **radiopaque marker intestinal transit study.** This is a simple technique that allows assessment of overall colonic motor function. Patients should be on a high fiber diet but should not use laxatives or enemas during the study. The simplest technique involves the ingestion of 24 radiopaque markers at time zero followed by a single abdominal radiograph 5 days later. In a normal study, 80% of the markers are evacuated by the fifth day. A modification of this protocol allows assessment of segmental colonic function by having patients ingest 24 markers on 3 consecutive days followed by radiographs on fourth and seventh days. The total number of markers remaining on these radiographs are totalled, yielding an approximation of total colonic transit time. In addition, the markers in the right colon, left colon, and rectosigmoid can be tallied to give segmental transit times. Normal colonic transit time is approximately 35 hours; more than 72 hours is significantly abnormal. Patients with abnormal transit studies have what has been termed **colonic inertia.**

The usefulness of a radiopaque marker transit study lies in its ability to identify patients who complain of constipation but have normal colonic motility. Some of these patients may have irritable bowel syndrome, and there appears to be a higher frequency of abnormalities on psychological testing in these patients as well. Patients with normal clearance of radiopaque markers do not require further colonic evaluation.

Scintigraphic techniques have also been developed in order to assess colonic function, and appear to correlate well with radiopaque marker transit studies. While scintigraphic techniques are advantageous because of the ability to assess gastric and small bowel motor function in addition to colonic function, the use of this technique is likely to be limited by the higher cost and the need for nuclear medicine isotopes and equipment.

b. Studies of pelvic floor function–Patients with symptoms suggesting an abnormality of the process of defecation (eg, digital extraction of stool, excessive straining) should undergo specialized studies to rule out pelvic floor dysfunction. The simplest test of pelvic floor dysfunction is to ask the patient to attempt to expel the examiner's finger during digital rectal examination. The puborectalis muscle should normally move posteriorly during this maneuver. Other specialized studies available to rule out pelvic floor dysfunction include the balloon expulsion test, anorectal manometry, and defecography. The balloon expulsion test involves inserting a urinary catheter into the patient's rectum and inflating it to approximately 50 ml. Inability of the patient to expel the balloon is predictive of pelvic floor dysfunction. Defecography involves instillation of barium of stool consistency into the patient's rectum and fluoroscopically assessing rectal evacuation as the patient sits on a commode. This may allow the diagnosis of anatomic abnormalities such as a abnormal perineal descent, rectocele, and intussusception, which in some cases benefit from surgery. In addition, abnormal contraction of the pelvic muscles during attempts at defecation can be identified, a condition known as **anismus** or **pelvic floor dyssynergia.** This latter condition may benefit from biofeedback therapy. Anorectal manometry may rarely lead to the diagnosis of adult onset Hirschprung's disease (as evidenced by failure of rectal balloon distention to cause relaxation of the internal anal sphincter) and may also show evidence of abnormally high anal sphincter pressure suggesting anismus or evidence of decreased rectal sensation. An algorithm suggesting the appropriate use of these studies is shown in Figure 1–3.

Treatment of Chronic Constipation

A. General Measures: Attempts should be made to minimize use of any medications known to cause constipation, and to correct any metabolic abnormalities (eg, hypothyroidism). Regular exercise and an increase in fluid intake (at least 1500 ml/day) may also be beneficial. Patients should be encouraged to attempt defecation each day for 10–15 minutes approximately 30 minutes following breakfast.

B. Dietary Modification: An increase in dietary fiber to between 20 and 30 g daily is the mainstay of therapy. Fiber serves to increase stool bulk and water content. This may be partially accomplished through an increase in the intake of fruits, vegetables, or high-fiber breakfast cereals, but a bulk-forming laxative is usually required. Although fiber benefits the majority of patients, it does not benefit those with severe colonic inertia or outlet disorders.

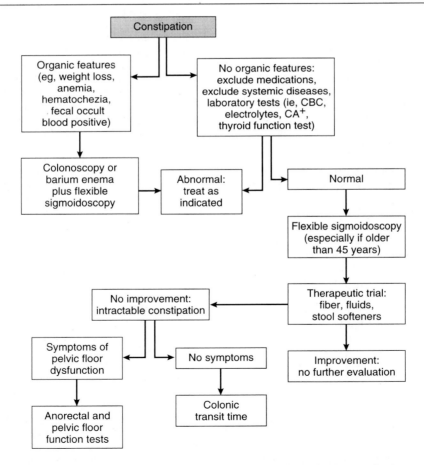

Figure 1–3. Algorithm suggesting appropriate diagnostic studies for constipation.

1. Bran powder–Between one and 2 tbsp of bran powder twice daily mixed with fluids or sprinkled over foods is an inexpensive means of providing 10–20 g/d of fiber.

2. Fiber supplements–A variety of pharmaceutical supplements are available; they are, however, more expensive than bran powder. Preparations include psyllium 3.4 g and methylcellulose 2g, one to three times daily (both are natural fibers derived from vegetable matter). Polycarbophil, 1 g one to four times daily, is a synthetic fiber that may be less gas producing than natural fibers.

C. Pharmacologic Therapy: With the exception of the bulk (fiber) forming laxatives, attempts should be made to minimize the regular use of laxative preparations. In patients with continued symptoms despite general measures and a bulk forming laxative, addition of a small daily dose of a hyperosmotic laxative may be effective with minimal risk of long-term use.

1. Osmotic laxatives–These agents may be used to soften stools. They are commonly employed in elderly nonambulatory patients or institutionalized patients to prevent constipation and fecal impaction. They may be used safely long-term and do not induced dependency. These agents are typically titrated to a dose that results in soft to semi-liquid stools.

a. Nonabsorbable sugars–Lactulose or sorbitol, 15–60 ml daily. Sorbitol is as effective as lactulose and is considerably less expensive. The malaborbed sugars may result in significant bloating, cramps, and flatulence.

b. Saline laxatives–Magnesium hydroxide (milk of magnesia), 15–30 ml daily. Hypermagnesemia may result in patients with impaired renal function.

2. Emollient laxatives–Docusate sodium (50–200 mg/d) or mineral oil (1–2 tbsp/d) may be given orally to promote stool softening. Mineral oil should be avoided in patients with decreased neurologic function owing to the risk of aspiration with pneumonitis.

3. Cisapride–This serotonin 5-HT$_4$ agonist is a promotility agent that has been shown to increase colonic motility in humans. Early results of double-blind placebo controlled trials have shown an increase in frequency of bowel movements in treated patients compared with controls. Further studies are needed to better define the efficacy of this new agent in patients with refractory constipation.

Treatment of Refractory Constipation

A. Biofeedback: In patients with pelvic floor dyssynergia (anismus) biofeedback appears to be effective in up to two thirds of patients, particularly children. A visual feedback signal (most commonly the external anal sphincter electromyography [EMG] reading) is provided for the patient so that the relaxation of the pelvic floor structures may be achieved during attempts at defecation.

B. Surgery: Selected patients with colonic inertia and severe symptoms who fail a trial of medical therapy have been shown to benefit from a subtotal colectomy with ileorectal anastomosis. Motility studies of the upper gastrointestinal tract must first be performed to rule out a generalized motility disturbance. Some anatomic problems (eg, rectal prolapse, vaginal rectocele) may benefit from surgical correction.

C. Psychiatric Referral: Patients with depression or a history of sexual abuse may benefit from psychiatric therapy.

Treatment of Acute Constipation

Normal people and patients with chronic constipation can become acutely constipated in response to acute medical or surgical illness, dietary changes, medications, or travel. If several days pass since the last movement, the therapies previously described for chronic constipation will not be sufficient to induce a prompt evacuation and relief of discomfort. In such cases, cathartic or osmotic laxatives or enemas may be given. (**Caution:** These agents should not be given to patients with a possible large bowel obstruction or fecal impaction).

A. Cathartic Laxatives: These agents stimulate fluid secretion and colonic contraction resulting in a bowel movement within 6–12 hours after oral ingestion or 15–60 minutes of rectal administration. They may causes severe cramps and diarrhea. Agents used in the medical setting include: cascara 4–8 mL orally, bisacodyl 5–15 mg orally or 10 mg suppository, and castor oil 15–45 mL orally. Senna and phenolthalein are common over the counter laxatives that are not generally prescribed. **Note:** Chronic use of any of these agents is discouraged and may result in loss of normal colonic neuromuscular function.

B. Osmotic Laxatives: Osmotic laxatives produce a prompt evacuation in 0.5–3 hours, generally with less discomfort than cathartic laxatives. They are used in the medical setting as a bowel purgative before surgery or colonic examinations. Preparations include: magnesium citrate 18 g/10 oz; magnesium sulphate 10–30 g "Epsom salts"); sodium phosphate 15–30 g (2–45 mL), and balanced polyethylence glycol lavage solution 1–4 L over one to four hours (GoLytely; Colyte).

C. Enemas: Enemas provide a simple and almost immediate means of relieving acute constipation. In some cases of severe constipation, it is best to treat with an enema first to promote comfortable fecal movement, before giving laxatives. Enemas vary in size and content: saline enemas 120–240 mL (non-irritating); tap water enemas 500–1000 mL (irritating). Oil retention enema 120 mL (useful for hard or impacted stool).

Treatment of Fecal Impaction

Severe impaction of stool in the rectal vault may result in obstruction of further fecal flow leading to a partial or complete large bowel obstruction. Predisposing factors include: severe psychiatric disease, prolonged bed rest and debility, neurogenic diseases of the colon, and spinal cord disorders. Clinical presentation includes decreased appetite, nausea, vomiting and abdominal pain and distention. There may be paradoxical "diarrhea" as liquid stool leaks around the impacted feces. Firm feces is palpable on digital examination in the rectal vault. Initial treatment is directed at relieving the impaction with enemas or digital disruption of the impacted fecal material. Care should be taken not to injure the anal sphincter. Rarely, spinal or general anesthesia is requires with manual disimpaction. Long-term care is directed at maintaining soft stools and regular bowel movements (see preceding section, "Treatment of Chronic Constipation").

WEIGHT LOSS

General Considerations

Involuntary loss of weight is a common complaint in general practice. A knowledge of the most common disease processes leading to decreased body weight is necessary in order to initiate an appropriate workup. The most important initial task is to document the presence of loss of weight. Approximately 50% of patients complaining of weight loss will not have had significant loss of weight when previous clinic records are available for documentation. The amount of weight loss considered significant is usually defined as loss of 5% of total body weight within the last 6 months. When previously documented weights are not available for comparison, a change in clothing size, independent corroboration of weight loss by a family member, or clear recall of specific weights by the patient may serve as reliable indicators of significant weight loss. Once a history of weight loss is ascertained, it is important to determine if the weight loss is truly involuntary, or is due to dieting or increased exercise.

Weight loss of at least 5% of total body weight represents a significant caloric deficit. Rapid changes in weight may suggest changes in hydration with loss of water accounting for the decrease in weight. When water loss is excluded, approximately 3500 kcals must be expended in order to lose 1 lb of body weight. Thus, a 160-pound man must have a caloric deficit of approximately 28,000 kcals in order to achieve an 8 lb (5%) decrease in body weight. Such a caloric deficit may be accomplished by decreased intake of food, increased metabolic rate, malabsorption of nutrients, or a combination of these factors. Patients without a clinically apparent condition which may account for weight loss require further investigation.

Etiology

The causes of weight loss are numerous. Tables 1–8 lists diseases or conditions affecting the intake of calories and the basal metabolic rate. Malabsorption produced by pancreatic exocrine insufficiency or small bowel mucosal disease may also produce weight loss. Previous studies reporting findings in patients undergoing investigation for weight loss have shown that the most common causes of unexplained weight loss are malignant neoplasms, gastrointestinal disease, and psychiatric disorders. In these studies, at least 25% of patients died within 1 year of initial evaluation. These studies also indicate that approximately one-fourth of patients with weight loss will not have a definable cause for their symptoms following investigation. These patients appear to have a better prognosis on long-term follow-up as compared with patients with an identifiable cause. The most common malignant neoplasms identified in patients with weight loss are gastrointestinal, lung, genitourinary, hematologic, breast, and oral cancers. The gastrointestinal diseases diagnosed included malabsorption, peptic ulcer disease, inflammatory

Table 1–8. Causes of weight loss.

Decreased Caloric Intake
  Anorexia
    Malignant neoplasm
    Medications
    Psychiatric disorders
    Chronic renal disease
    AIDS
    Chronic alcoholism
    Eating disorders
  Swallowing disorders
    Oropharyngeal dysphagia
    Esophageal strictures
  Abnormal taste
    Medications
    Malignant neoplasms
    Psychiatric disorders
    Zinc deficiency
  Postprandial pain
    Chronic pancreatitis
    Chronic mesenteric ischemia
    Partial gastric outlet obstruction
    Partial intestinal obstruction
    Gastric bezoar
Increased Metabolic Rate
    Chronic obstructive pulmonary disease
    Congestive heart failure
    Hyperthyroidism
    Chronic infections (TB, fungal, endocarditis)
    Advanced malignant neoplasms
    Diabetes mellitus
    AIDS
Decreased Caloric Absorption
    Intestinal malabsorption (Sprue, etc)
    Chronic pancreatitis
    Intestinal fistula
    Short bowel syndrome
    Bacterial overgrowth

bowel disease, diabetic enteropathy, motility disorders, cholelithiasis, and Zenker's diverticulum. More recent case series suggest that between 40 and 60% of patients may have psychiatric diagnoses as the origin of weight loss, most commonly depression.

Clinical Findings

A. Symptoms and Signs: A careful history and physical examination along with a limited number of screening studies will lead to a diagnosis in the vast majority of cases. Most patients presenting with unexplained weight loss have symptoms or signs that will direct the work-up. The history should include a careful review of systems. Pulmonary symptoms such as cough, shortness of breath or hemoptysis should be sought. Complaints such as fever, anorexia and weakness are nonspecific but should not be overlooked. Dyspnea on exertion, orthopnea and chest pain may indicate significant underlying cardiovascular disease. Hematuria warrants an evaluation for urologic tumor. Polydipsia, polyuria, or polyphagia may lead to the diagnosis of poorly controlled diabetes. Gastrointestinal complaints such as dysphagia, odynophagia, nausea, vomiting, hematemesis, abdominal pain, hematochezia, change in stool caliber and constipation should be sought. Diarrhea, especially with greasy, foul-smelling, or difficult to flush stools is suggestive of malabsorption of pancreatic insufficiency.

Behavioral disorders may account for weight loss and a history directed at diagnosis of these disorders is important. Depression is the most common psychological disorder associated with weight loss. Questions regarding sleep disturbances, anhedonia or anorexia may unveil this diagnosis. Schizophrenia or other psychotic disorders may be associated with delusional thinking about food and eating. Eating disorders such as anorexia nervosa and bulimia are quite common; however, patients often deny these behaviors.

Careful documentation of medications used by the patient should be performed in order to rule out medication-induced dysgeusia, anorexia, or dyspepsia. A strong family history of cancer may also serve to direct the workup. Smoking, alcohol, drug use, and risk factors for HIV infection should be recorded.

The physical examination should include a careful examination of the oral cavity to detect ulcerations, mass lesions, or poor dentition that may impair adequate oral intake. A search for lymphadenopathy should be performed as part of the evaluation for underlying disease. Evidence of obstructive lung disease, congestive heart failure as well as abdominal, breast, or pelvic masses may also be present. Digital rectal examination with stool guaiac testing may also direct further evaluation.

B. Diagnostic Studies: Further studies should be directed according to abnormalities detected on history and physical examination. For example, patients with symptoms of dysphagia, abdominal pain, or guaiac positive stool should undergo appropriate endoscopic or radiographic evaluation aimed at detection of underlying gastrointestinal pathology. In patients in whom the history and physical examination are unrevealing, further diagnostic evaluation usually includes a limited number of radiographic and laboratory studies. Initial studies should include an SMA-20, CBC, urinalysis, and chest x-ray. Fecal occult blood testing, thyroid function tests, and HIV testing should also be performed. If these studies are not helpful, an upper gastrointestinal series may be helpful. More than 80% of patients with an identifiable cause of weight loss have an abnormality on these screening laboratory or radiographic studies that suggests a diagnosis. CT of the abdomen or chest to detect occult malignant neoplasms, without symptoms or laboratory abnormalities suggestive of underlying disease, has a very low yield.

Prognosis

Patients who maintain their performance status despite weight loss and those without a significant smoking history are less likely to have a cause of weight loss identified on investigation. These patients generally have a good prognosis and are best managed by a period of observation. In contrast, patients who are heavy smokers, have a change in performance status, nausea or vomiting, a new or changed cough, or an abnormal physical examination are more likely to have significant underlying disease.

ABDOMINAL PAIN

A wide variety of disease states may cause abdominal pain. The origin of this symptom may be determined by a combination of historical factors, physical findings, laboratory values and radiographic findings. A thorough, systematic evaluation is necessary in order to avoid overlooking potentially life-threatening conditions. The most important point is to determine the nature of the symptoms—acute or chronic. Patients with the acute onset of abdominal pain require an efficient and expeditious evaluation. Before limiting the differential diagnosis to disease processes involving the abdomen, it is important to consider pulmonary processes and myocardial infarction as the underlying cause of the symptoms. An accurate history and physical examination are the most helpful tools available to help achieve a correct diagnosis.

1. ACUTE ABDOMINAL PAIN

Clinical Findings

A. Symptoms and Signs: The history should include information about the location, time-course, intensity, and character of the pain. Aggravating or alleviating factors should also be noted.

1. Location–Patients often have difficulty precisely describing the location of their abdominal pain. This is the result of several neuroanatomic factors. Sensation of the **abdominal viscera** is mediated by a network of afferent C fibers that are stimulated primarily by stretching, inflammation, or ischemia. The abdominal viscera lack the dense network of somatic afferent fibers found in the skin, which limits precise localization of stimuli. A single splanchnic afferent nerve may provide sensory input from several organs and enter the spinal cord at more than one level, further contributing to imprecise localization. Embryologically, most abdominal organs are derived from midline structures, and retain bilateral innervation. As a result of this bilateral innervation, most abdominal pain is poorly lateralized and is instead reported in the midline. The exception occurs when organs assume a more lateral position, such as the kidneys, ureters, ovaries, and gallbladder. For these organs, pain produced by disease states usually is experienced on the corresponding side of the involved organ.

The superior to inferior location of pain in the abdomen is an imprecise indicator of the organ involved, but may suggest a foregut, midgut or hindgut origin. Pain derived from foregut structures (eg, distal esophagus, stomach, proximal duodenum, liver, biliary system, and pancreas) most often presents with midline pain in the epigastrium. Pancreatic pain most often presents with pain in the midepigastrium or left side of the epigastrium with referred pain to the back.

Pain derived from the midgut structures (eg, small intestine, appendix, ascending colon, and proximal two-thirds of transverse colon) most often presents in a periumbilical location, although pain derived from the ileum (such as in Crohn's ileitis) may be localized to the right lower quadrant. Pain derived from hindgut organs (eg, distal transverse colon, descending colon, rectum, and sigmoid) most often present in the midline lower abdomen between the umbilicus and symphysis pubis.

Pain originating from the **parietal peritoneum** is usually much better localized. Somatic afferent nerve fibers allow more precise localization of stimuli. The parietal peritoneum does not have the characteristic bilateral innervation found in the abdominal viscera, and the density of nerve fibers in the parietal peritoneum is significantly greater than in the abdominal viscera. These factors allow better identification of the pain's origin when the parietal peritoneum is irritated by bile, urine, pus or luminal contents.

Referred pain is a term that describes pain localized to a site distant from the abdominal organ from which the pain originates. This occurs because of the common site of entry into the spinal cord of cutaneous sensory neurons and abdominal visceral afferents. Cutaneous and visceral afferents terminate on the same secondary neuron within the dorsal horn of the spinal cord, resulting in misinterpretation by the brain of the correct origin of the stimulus. For example, the biliary system is innervated by neurons terminating in segments T5–T9 of the spinal cord. Neurons derived from cutaneous dermatomes of the scapular area, back and shoulder also enter the spinal cord at T5–T9. Biliary disease may thus stimulate the same secondary neurons commonly stimulated by cutaneous afferents of the shoulder and scapular region, resulting in complaints of shoulder and back pain. Complaints of shoulder pain may also be noted when processes that irritate the diaphragm (including subdiaphragmatic blood, pus or masses, and pulmonary processes such as pneumonia) cause referred pain from the phrenic nerve (C3–C5). Associated findings in referred pain include skin hyperalgesia and increased tone of the abdominal wall muscles.

Visceral pain which is initially ill-defined and midline in location may shift as the adjacent parietal peritoneum becomes inflamed or irritated. This is classically the case in acute appendicitis, which often presents initially with periumbilical pain that migrates to the right lower quadrant as the parietal peritoneum becomes irritated. Similar migration of pain may occur in acute cholecystitis, which initially presents with pain in the epigastrium but shifts to the right upper quadrant as the disease progresses. Perforated peptic ulcer may present as epigastric pain that moves to the right lower quadrant as spilled luminal contents cause inflammation in the area of the right paracolic gutter.

2. Time-course–The onset of abdominal pain may be sudden (over seconds to minutes), rapidly progressive (over 1–2 hours), or gradual (over several hours) (Table 1–9). Sudden onset of abdominal pain suggests a catastrophic event such as a ruptured abdominal aneurysm, ruptured ectopic pregnancy, or perforated peptic ulcer. Pain that rapidly progresses over a few hours is seen typically in pancreatitis, cholecystitis, diverticulitis, bowel obstruction, renal or biliary colic, and mesenteric ischemia. Pain that progresses more slowly is more typical of peptic ulcer disease, distal small bowel obstruction, appendicitis, pyelonephritis, pelvic inflammatory disease, and malignant neoplasm, although it may be seen with many of the diagnoses in the more rapidly progressive categories as well. Pain occurring following the onset of vomiting often indicates a medical illness, whereas pain that precedes vomiting often indicates a surgical illness. Persistence of pain for over 6 hours after acute onset has a high likelihood of a surgical cause and requires admission for observation.

3. Intensity and description of pain–Certain characteristics of the type and severity of the pain may point toward a specific diagnosis. The pain of peptic ulcer disease is usually described as a dull, gnawing sensation of mild to moderate severity. Ex-

Table 1–9. Causes of acute abdominal pain.

Sudden onset (within seconds to minutes)
Perforated peptic ulcer
Ruptured aortic aneurysm
Ruptured abscess or hematoma
Esophageal rupture (Boerhaave's syndrome)
Ruptured ectopic pregnancy
Mesenteric infarction
Myocardial infarction

Rapidly progressive (within 1–2 hours)
Biliary colic
Cholecystitis
Renal colic
Proximal small bowel obstruction
Acute pancreatis
Diverticulitis
Appendicitis
Mesenteric ischemia

Gradual onset (over number of hours)
Appendicitis
Cholecystitis
Acute pancreatitis
Diverticulitis
Salpingitis
Peptic ulcer disease
Ectopic pregnancy (before rupture)
Pyelonephritis
Intra-abdominal abscess
Distal small bowel obstruction
Incarcerated hernia
Neoplasms with perforation
Inflammatory bowel disease

tremely intense pain of sudden onset suggests mesenteric ischemia or perforated peptic ulcer. "Colic" refers to episodic pain with intervening pain-free intervals. While renal colic often presents in this fashion, biliary pain typically presents with constant, steady pain without intervening pain-free intervals (the term biliary "colic" being somewhat of a misnomer). Pain that has a severe intensity and a "tearing" quality is commonly described in dissecting aneurysms.

4. Aggravating or alleviating factors—Actions that precipitate or improve the pain may help in determining the cause. Pain relieved by antacids suggests peptic ulcer disease or esophagitis. Pain worsened by movement suggests peritonitis, whereas constant movement by the patient in an attempt to find a comfortable position is commonly seen in bowel obstruction and renal colic. Patients with a retroperitoneal process (such as pancreatitis) commonly find partial relief by leaning forward, and aggravation by lying supine. Pain relieved by defecation may suggest a colonic source.

5. Physical examination—Examination of the abdomen is best performed before administration of narcotics or other medications that may affect the physical findings. The initial step is to observe the position and posture of the patient for clues that may suggest an underlying cause (as previously described). Vital signs may show tachycardia and hy-

potension indicative of intra-abdominal hemorrhage or septic shock. The fever of appendicitis, diverticulitis and cholecystitis is typically low-grade, whereas high fevers are seen in cases of cholangitis, urinary tract infections, pelvic inflammatory disease, or perforation of a viscus with frank peritonitis.

Inspection of the abdomen may reveal a distended abdomen suggesting bowel obstruction or the presence of ascites, whereas a scaphoid, tense abdomen is seen in cases of peritonitis. Auscultation of the abdomen should be performed before palpation or percussion so as not to interfere with the interpretation of bowel sounds. Absence of bowel sounds is a sign of diffuse peritonitis. Intermittent hyperactive bowel sounds occurring concurrently with worsening of pain suggests a bowel obstruction. High-pitched hyperactive bowel sounds may also be seen in gastroenteritis.

Percussion of the abdomen allows assessment of the presence of peritonitis. Pain produced by light tapping indicates inflammation of the parietal peritoneum. This pain may also be elicited by asking the patient to cough or by gently agitating the gurney upon which the patient is lying. A distended abdomen with tympany upon percussion suggests a bowel obstruction.

Palpation of the abdomen is performed in order to assess the presence of rigidity or guarding, as well as to localize the site of maximal tenderness. Tightening (rigidity) of the abdominal wall musculature occurs as a reflexive response to peritoneal inflammation. This may be assessed by gently compressing the abdominal wall musculature with both hands and assessing the relative softness or rigidity. Voluntary guarding refers to tightness or rigidity of the abdomen that relaxes when the patient is asked to take a deep breath, whereas involuntary guarding refers to rigidity of the abdominal wall musculature that does not relax in response to deep inspiration. Involuntary guarding is indicative of peritoneal inflammation. Palpation of the abdomen should start at the site most distant from where the patient localizes the pain, and gradually shifted toward the site of pain. The presence of a focal site of pain produced by palpation is a useful finding that helps to narrow the list of potentially involved organs. Tenderness over McBurney's point should be considered very strong evidence of appendicitis. Cholecystitis and salpingitis are often well-localized as well, and salpingitis may be confused with appendicitis. Patients with an unimpressive abdominal examination and complaints of severe, worsening pain should be suspected of having mesenteric infarction.

Murphy's sign refers to pain produced by deep inspiration during palpation of the right subcostal area and suggests acute cholecystitis. Pain produced by lightly punching the costovertebral angle ("punch tenderness") is often present in pyelonephritis. **Carnett's test** refers to the response of pain when the patient tenses the abdominal wall muscles by raising their head off the examination table. Worsening of pain during this maneuver suggests an abdominal wall source whereas improvement in the pain suggests a visceral origin. The **iliopsoas sign** refers to pain produced by passive extension of the leg and suggests a psoas abscess. The **obturator sign** refers to pain produced by rotation of the thigh in a flexed position. A rectal examination may reveal focal tenderness from an intra-abdominal abscess or appendicitis. A pelvic examination is mandatory in female patients to look for evidence of salpingitis or adnexal masses. The inguinal and femoral canals, umbilicus, and surgical scars should be evaluated for the presence of incarcerating hernias.

B. Laboratory Tests: Although the majority of diagnoses can be made from a careful history and physical examination, laboratory studies help to confirm the diagnosis in many cases. Initial studies should include a CBC with differential count, electrolytes, renal function tests, liver function tests, amylase, and urinalysis. Pregnancy testing should be performed in women of child-bearing age. Typing and cross-matching of blood should also be performed in any patient potentially requiring surgery. An arterial blood gas specimen should be obtained in patients with peritonitis, pancreatitis, ischemic bowel or hypotension to look for evidence of metabolic acidosis or hypoxemia.

A mildly elevated WBC count is a nonspecific finding found in many inflammatory conditions. Likewise, a mild elevation of the serum amylase may be found in many conditions presenting with acute abdominal pain and is a nonspecific finding.

C. Diagnostic Studies: Initial x-ray studies in patients presenting with acute abdominal pain should include an upright chest x-ray and supine and erect films of the abdomen in cases of suspected bowel obstruction, perforated viscus, mesenteric ischemia and renal colic. The chest x-ray may disclose subdiaphragmatic free air, evidence of a pulmonary infiltrate, spontaneous pneumothorax or sympathetic pleural effusion (owing to subdiaphragmatic infection or irritation).

Further x-ray studies may include angiography for patients suspected of having mesenteric ischemia, or contrast upper gastrointestinal studies for patients with possible perforated peptic ulcer (using a water soluble contrast agent in order to avoid barium peritonitis). Lower gastrointestinal contrast studies are useful in evaluating cases of suspected colonic obstruction, and may be used diagnostically as well as therapeutically in patients with suspected colonic volvulus.

Ultrasonography is useful in showing evidence of cholecystitis, biliary dilation, appendicitis, abdominal masses, hydronephrosis, pelvic inflammatory disease, and other conditions that may cause abdominal pain. CT provides better definition of the pancreas,

and also has the advantage of showing radiographic evidence of diverticulitis as well.

2. CHRONIC ABDOMINAL PAIN

Chronic abdominal pain is a very common complaint, and the origin of the discomfort is often difficult to determine. A wide variety of disease processes may cause intermittent or persistent abdominal symptoms. A useful method of categorizing abdominal pain is to distinguish between a history of discrete intermittent episodes of pain and nearly continuous discomfort. Separation of symptoms into these categories may help to narrow the differential diagnosis in many cases.

Chronic Intermittent Abdominal Pain

Pain that occurs in an intermittent pattern (lasting from minutes to hours) with intervening asymptomatic periods may be caused by several categories of disease. Often, the disorders causing intermittent discomfort are correctable conditions. Clues suggesting the underlying cause may be found by evaluating the history, physical examination, and laboratory or radiographic studies.

A. Clinical Findings:

1. Symptoms and signs—Biliary tract disease (including cholelithiasis, choledocholithiasis, and sphincter of Oddi dysfunction) leads to intermittent discomfort usually localized to the right upper quadrant or epigastrium. The pain of chronic pancreatitis may be episodic and be considered especially in patients with chronic alcohol ingestion. Pain that occurs at approximately monthly intervals should raise the suspicion of endometriosis or mittelschmerz. Postprandial abdominal discomfort suggests chronic intestinal ischemia or intermittent intestinal obstruction (eg, resulting from internal or abdominal wall hernias, adhesions, or Crohn's disease). Abdominal pain relieved by bowel movements or associated with increased frequency or looseness of stools suggests irritable bowel syndrome. A radiculopathy in diabetic patients may cause abdominal pain. Similarly, spinal compression fractures may lead to nerve compression syndromes causing pain. Medications recently started should also be noted. Recent use of barbiturates may precipitate acute intermittent porphyria. Diuretics, tetracycline, sulfonamides, 6-mercaptopurine and estrogen use may cause pancreatitis. Heavy metal poisoning may also cause abdominal pain.

The physical examination may reveal jaundice raising the possibility of biliary tract disease. A distended, tympanitic abdomen suggests a bowel obstruction. The presence of hernias should also be assessed. Right lower quadrant fullness or perianal disease may indicate Crohn's disease.

2. Laboratory and imaging studies—Routine

laboratory tests may provide evidence that supports the presence of an underlying disease process suspected in the history and physical examination. Anemia may be present in cases of inflammatory bowel disease or heavy metal poisoning. The liver function tests may be elevated in cases of symptomatic cholelithiasis or choledocholithiasis, although completely normal liver function tests may be seen as well. An elevated alkaline phosphatase and bilirubin suggest choledocholithiasis or sphincter of Oddi dysfunction. An elevated sedimentation rate (ESR) may indicate active inflammatory bowel disease or the presence of collagen vascular disease. A urine test for porphobilinogen should be sent in cases of suspected acute intermittent porphyria.

Plain films of the abdomen may show evidence of bowel obstruction from an internal hernia or intussusception. Pancreatic calcification establishes a diagnosis of chronic pancreatitis. Abdominal ultrasonography may reveal gallstones or a dilated biliary tree. CT of the abdomen provides an optimal image of the pancreas or intra-abdominal mass lesions. Colonoscopy is useful for ruling out cases of suspected colitis. Endoscopic retrograde cholangiopancreatography is indicated in cases of sphincter of Oddi dysfunction, choledocholithiasis, and in some cases of suspected chronic pancreatitis. The appropriate use of these modalities for each of these disorders is provided in the chapters discussing each of these disease processes.

Persistent Abdominal Pain

Chronic persistent abdominal pain (present much or all of the time) may be related to an underlying chronic disease or may be functional in origin. This complaint is an extremely common symptom among patients presenting to primary care physicians and gastroenterologists. A careful history is essential to guide the evaluation.

A. Clinical Findings:

1. Symptoms and signs–The history should define the location, character and aggravating or alleviating factors related to the symptoms. Pain or discomfort present in the upper abdomen (between the xiphoid process and umbilicus) may be classified as dyspepsia. Studies have shown that the clinical history is unable to reliably distinguish between peptic ulcer disease, gastroesophageal reflux disease, malignancy, or nonulcer dyspepsia as causes of dyspepsia (see preceding section, "Dyspepsia"). Pain in the abdomen that is relieved by bowel movements or that is associated with increased frequency or looseness of stools, a sense of incomplete evacuation, the presence of mucus in the stool or visible abdominal distention is a reliable indicator of irritable bowel syndrome. Signs and symptoms of psychiatric disorders that may be associated with functional bowel complaints should also be sought (see Chapter 6). Weight loss and anorexia should raise the possibility of underlying malignancy (see preceding section, "Weight Loss"). Chronic abdominal pain associated with steatorrhea, weight loss or a history of alcoholism may indicate chronic pancreatitis.

The physical examination is often unrevealing, but may show abnormalities that can direct the evaluation. Jaundice may suggest a pancreatic or biliary neoplasm. Palpation of abdominal mass lesions may lead to the diagnosis of a visceral neoplasm. The presence of ascites at the time of examination may be due to underlying liver disease, malignancy, or peritoneal disorders (see Chapter 10). A rectal examination may demonstrate occult blood, raising the question of peptic ulcer disease, inflammatory bowel disease, or an underlying neoplasm.

2. Laboratory and imaging studies–The appropriate use of laboratory and investigative studies in the evaluation of each disease category previously described is discussed in the respective chapters. The reader is directed to these chapters for a full discussion of the evaluation and management of each disorder.

REFERENCES

SYMPTOMS OF ESOPHAGEAL DISEASE

Browning TH: Diagnosis of chest pain of esophageal origin. A guideline of the Patient Care Committee of the American Gastroenterological Association. Dig Dis Sci 1990;35:289.

Castell DO (editor): Overview and symptom assessment. In: *The Esophagus.* Little, Brown, and Company, 1992.

Kahrilas P, Clouse R, Hogan W: Policy and Position Statement: American Gastroenterological Association technical review on the clinical use of esophageal manometry. Gastroenterology 1994;107:1865.

Klauser AG, Schindbleck NE, Muller-Lissner SA: Symptoms in gastro-oesophageal reflux disease. Lancet 1990;335:205.

Richter JE: *Ambulatory esophageal pH monitoring.* Igaku Shoin Medical Publishers, 1991.

DYSPEPSIA

Bytzer P, Hansen JM, Schaffalitzky de Muckadell OB: Empirical H_2-blocker therapy or prompt endoscopy in management of dyspepsia. Lancet 1994;3443: 811.

Jones RJ: When is endoscopy appropriate in dyspepsia? Am J Gastroenterol 1993;88:981.

Richter JE: Dyspepsia: Organic causes and differential characteristics from functional dyspepsia. Scand J Gastroenterol 1991;26;(Suppl 182):11.

Talley NJ: A critique of therapeutic trials in *Helicobac-*

ter pylori- positive functional dyspepsia. Gastroenterology 1994;106:1174.

Talley NJ: Non-ulcer dyspepsia: myths and realities. Aliment Pharmacol Ther 1991;5(Suppl 1):145.

Talley NJ et al: Lack of discriminant value of dyspepsia subgroups in patients referred for upper endoscopy. Gastroenterology 1993;105:1378.

HICCUPS

Lewis JH: Hiccups: Causes and cures. J Clin Gastroenterol 1985;7:539.

Strocchi A, Levitt MD: Alleviating intestinal gas. Contemp Int Med 1991;Jan:28.

GASTROINTESTINAL GAS

Strocchi A, Levitt MD: Intestinal gas. In: *Gastrointestinal Disease,* 5/e. Sleisenger MH, Fordtran JS (editors). Saunders, 1993.

NAUSEA AND VOMITING

Allan GS: Antiemetics. Gastroenterology Clin NA 1992;21:597.

Grunberg SM, Hesketh PH: Control of chemotherapy-induced emesis. N Engl J Med 1993;329:1790.

Hanson JS, McCallum RW: The diagnosis and management of nausea and vomiting. Am J Gastroenterol 1985;80:210.

Malagelada JR, Camilleri M: Unexplained vomiting: A diagnostic challenge. Ann Intern Med 1984;101:211.

DIARRHEA

Fedorak R, Rubinoff M: Basic investigation of a patient with diarrhea. In: *Diarrheal Diseases.* Michael Field (editor). Elsevier, 1991.

Guerrant RL, Bobak DA: Bacterial and protozoal gastroenteritis. N Engl J Med 1991;325:327.

Park SI, Giannella RA: Approach to the adult patient with acute diarrhea. Gastro Clin NA 1993;22:483.

CONSTIPATION

Camilleri M et al: Clinical management of intractable constipation. Ann Intern Med 1994;121:520.

Gattuso JM, Kamm MA: Review article: The management of constipation in adults. Aliment Pharmacol Ther 1993;7:487.

Talley NJ et al: Functional constipation and outlet delay: A population based study. Gastroenterology 1993;105:781.

WEIGHT LOSS

Martin KI, Sox HC Jr, Krupp Jr: Involuntary weight loss: Diagnostic and prognostic significance. Ann Intern Med 1981;95:568.

Rabinowitz M et al: Unintentional weight loss. A retrospective analysis of 154 cases. Arch Intern Med 1986;146:186.

ABDOMINAL PAIN

Bender JS: Approach to the acute abdomen. Med Clin NA 1989;73:1413.

Silen W: *Cope's early diagnosis of the acute abdomen,* 18/e. Oxford University Press, 1991.

Ridge JA, Way LH: Abdominal pain. In: *Gastrointestinal Disease,* 5/e. Sleisenger MH, Fordtran JS (editors). Saunders, 1993.

AIDS & the Gastrointestinal Tract

2

C. Mel Wilcox, MD

The gastrointestinal tract is one of the most common organ systems in which complications occur during the course of human immunodeficiency virus (HIV) infection. This prevalence can be explained largely by the direct link of the gut to the external environment and the importance of the mucosal immune system in preventing infection. In general, most opportunistic disorders are not seen until the CD4 lymphocyte count falls below 200/μL. Thus, in the evaluation of patients with HIV infection, the CD4 lymphocyte count is very helpful in either narrowing or expanding the differential diagnosis.

In the evaluation of the symptomatic patient, both opportunistic and nonopportunistic diseases always deserve consideration. As with all opportunistic infections in AIDS, relapse is frequent in diseases of the gastrointestinal tract, since antimicrobial therapy does not truly eradicate opportunistic organisms in the immunosuppressed. In many patients, therefore, life-long therapy may be necessary. Many of these disorders result in significant morbidity, but rarely mortality. Therefore, therapy is directed towards improving the quality of life. The long-term prognosis for most disorders is dictated primarily by the degree of underlying immunodeficiency.

DISEASES OF THE OROPHARYNX

Clinical Findings

Oropharyngeal disease is a frequently recognized complication in HIV-infected patients. The most common disorder involving the oropharynx is candidiasis (thrush) and frequently is the first manifestation of HIV infection. Candidiasis appears as multiple white to yellow plaques that may be focal or may completely coat the pharynx. Occasionally, candidiasis may be manifested by erythema in the absence of recognizable plaques.

Herpes simplex virus (HSV) stomatitis may present at any point during the course of HIV disease although it tends to be more severe with progression of immunodeficiency. Diffuse shallow oropharyngeal ulceration also involving the lips and nares is usually recognizable as HSV disease. Well-circumscribed focal ulcerations, which may be large and are typically painful, are usually of the aphthous type.

Other viruses occur less commonly. Epstein-Barr virus infection may produce oral hairy leukoplakia, which is manifested by whitish plaques on the lateral aspects of the tongue and is usually of no consequence. Cytomegalovirus (CMV) is a rare cause of oropharyngeal ulceration.

When oropharyngeal ulcers are very large, a fungal infection (histoplasmosis), or neoplasm (lymphoma) should be considered. Kaposi's sarcoma (KS) presents as a brownish-to-purple plaque or nodule on the hard or soft palate. Lymphoma appears as a mass-like lesion.

These entities can usually be distinguished by a thorough examination of the oropharynx. For oropharyngeal ulcers, biopsy may be required to exclude unusual infections or a neoplasm. The presence of these oropharyngeal lesions, especially when associated with esophageal symptoms (eg, odynophagia, dysphagia), should suggest coexisting esophageal disease. At many centers, oropharyngeal findings are used to guide empiric therapy for the patient with esophageal symptoms.

Treatment

Therapy will depend on the underlying etiology. Oropharyngeal candidiasis may be treated with short courses of antifungal agents, either local (clotrimazole troches) or oral systemic medications (ketoconazole, fluconazole, itraconazole). Corticosteroids are very efficacious for aphthous ulcers, however, long-term treatment is usually necessary due to recurrence.

DISEASES OF THE ESOPHAGUS

Esophageal disease is an important complication of acquired immunodeficiency syndrome (AIDS). At least one-third of HIV-infected patients experience esophageal symptoms at some point during the course of the disease. Opportunistic infections are by far the most common cause of esophageal disease (Table 2–1). In fact, opportunistic esophageal disease may be the initial manifestations of HIV infection. In addition, prophylactic medications used to prevent opportunistic infections have shifted the incidence of other diseases, including esophageal disorders. Both opportunistic and nonopportunistic causes, therefore, should always be considered when evaluating these patients.

CANDIDA

Essentials of Diagnosis

- Most common cause of esophageal disease.
- Most common symptoms: dysphagia or odynophagia, or both; however, infection may be asymptomatic.
- Diagnosis established by barium esophagography, endoscopy, or presumptively by a symptomatic response to empiric antifungal therapy.

General Considerations

Candida esophagitis is one of the most frequent opportunistic infections in patients with AIDS. Of HIV-infected patients with esophageal symptoms, Candida is the most common identifiable pathogen on endoscopy, occurring in up to 50% of patients. Oropharyngeal and esophageal candidiasis may be precipitated by the use of antibiotics or corticosteroids. In addition, Candida frequently coexists with other disease processes. Fungal cultures will usually yield *Candida albicans* and occasionally other Candida species or *Torulopsis glabrata*. Despite the vast numbers of yeasts involved in this infection, systemic dissemination does not occur, probably because the infection is limited to the superficial squamous epithelium.

Clinical Findings

A. Symptoms and Signs: The clinical presentation is broad, ranging from asymptomatic infection to severe symptoms with dehydration. Most commonly, **dysphagia** (difficulty in swallowing, de-

Table 2–1. Causes of esophageal disease in AIDS.

Common	Infrequent	Rare
Candida albicans	Herpes simplex	Bacteria
Cytomegalovirus	virus	Mycobacteria
Idiopathic ulcer	Gastroesophageal	Non-Candidal fungi
	reflux	Protozoa
	Kaposi's sarcoma	Lymphoma
	Pill-induced	
	esophagitis	

scribed as the sensation of food sticking or slow transit of a food bolus) is the primary complaint (Table 2–2). Less frequently, **odynophagia** (painful swallowing in the substernal area), heartburn, or spontaneous substernal chest pain may be reported. The presence of fever, nausea, vomiting and epigastric pain suggest some other cause.

The most important physical finding is the identification of oropharyngeal candidiasis. The prevalence of thrush is variable, ranging from 50–100% of symptomatic patients. The presence of thrush does not prove that Candida causes or contributes to the esophageal symptoms. Likewise, the absence of thrush does not exclude esophageal candidiasis.

B. Laboratory Findings: Candida esophagitis does not usually occur until the CD4 lymphocyte count falls to 300/μL or less. Additional laboratory abnormalities reflect the presence of other underlying processes.

C. Imaging: Barium esophagography is relatively insensitive for the detection of mild Candida esophagitis; however, most patients have severe disease at the time of diagnosis. The most common radiographic finding is diffuse mucosal irregularity resulting in a "shaggy" appearance mimicking diffuse ulceration (Figure 2–1). Focal disease or apparent mass lesions are unusual. A solitary ulceration in the absence of diffuse mucosal disease suggests a cause other than Candida.

D. Esophageal Brushings or Balloon Cytology: A cytology brush passed through a nasogastric tube, and a balloon cytology instrument used in a similar fashion, are reliable for the diagnosis and may abrogate the need for endoscopic or radiographic evaluation. Although sensitive and inexpensive, these diagnostic methods are rarely used, given the clinical practice of empiric oral systemic antifungal therapy for new-onset esophageal symptoms, and the fact that they will not reliably detect other causes, particularly in the patient with severe symptoms.

E. Endoscopy: Endoscopic evaluation is the most sensitive diagnostic method. The endoscopic appearance is pathognomonic consisting of multiple yellow plaques, which may be isolated or confluent involving the entire esophagus. Esophageal brushings of these plaques will confirm yeast forms typical of Candida. Endoscopic mucosal biopsies will also substantiate the diagnosis as well as exclude coexisting causes.

Differential Diagnosis

In the patient with dysphagia and odynophagia, exclusion of other opportunistic infections is important. The patient with mild dysphagia and odynophagia associated with thrush is likely to have Candida esophagitis. In contrast, the patient with severe odynophagia without dysphagia resulting in an inability to eat is less likely to have Candida esophagitis, regardless of the presence or absence of thrush. In

Table 2–2. Selected clinical features of common HIV-related esophageal disorders.

Feature	Etiology			
	Candida	**CMV**	**HSV**	**Idiopathic**
Oropharyngeal lesions				
Thrush	+++	+	+	+
Ulcer	– – –	+	++	+
Odynophagia	++	+++	+++	+++
Dysphagia	+++	+	+	+
Spontaneous chest pain	+	++	++	++
Fever	– – –	+	– – –	– – –
CD4 count (μL^3)	< 300	< 100	< 100	< 100
Radiography	Plaques	Ulcer	Ulcer	Ulcer
Endoscopy	Plaques	Ulcer	Ulcer	Ulcer
Diagnostic method	Empiric Rx Endoscopy	Endoscopy	Endoscopy	Endoscopy
Treatment	Fluconazole Ketoconazole Itraconazole	Ganciclovir Foscarnet	Acyclovir	Prednisone

Legends +++ = very common; ++ = Frequent; + = can occur; – – – = not seen.

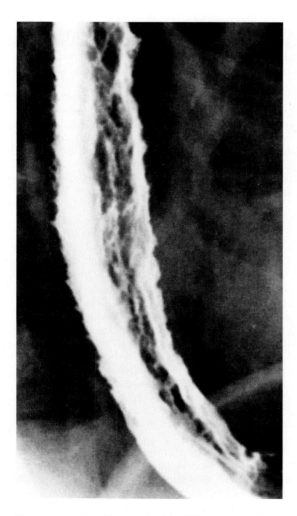

Figure 2–1. Candida esophagitis. Diffuse mucosal irregularity.

this setting, the most important causes to exclude are CMV esophagitis, idiopathic esophageal ulcer, and HSV esophagitis. Complicating the approach to diagnosis is the fact that Candida may coexist with other esophageal disorders.

Complications

In contrast to other opportunistic infections in the immunocompromised host, Candida esophagitis is not truly invasive and thus does not result in disseminated infection. Since histopathologic ulcer is distinctly uncommon, perforation does not occur. Bleeding is rare and only seen in patients with an underlying coagulopathy or coexisting ulceration from some other cause.

Treatment

A number of oral systemic antifungal agents have established efficacy (Table 2–2). Currently, fluconazole is the most commonly used agent, and results in a clinical cure in over 90% of patients. This drug is an ideal agent given the high rate of renal excretion, long half-life of over 30 hours, and minimal toxicity. Ketoconazole appears somewhat less effective than fluconazole but is only one-third the cost; hepatotoxicity secondary to ketoconazole has been recognized. Itraconazole also appears efficacious in limited studies. Anti-acid therapy will significantly decrease the absorption of ketoconazole and itraconazole and should not be given concomitantly. Patients with refractory oropharyngeal or esophageal candidiasis due to drug resistance may require systemic therapy with amphotericin B.

Prognosis

Candida esophagitis is not a fatal disease but a marker of significant immunodeficiency. The long-term prognosis, therefore, is related to other underlying diseases and the absolute level of immunodeficiency. Relapse is very frequent, usually occurring within 2–4 months after clinical cure. Although indefinite suppressive therapy is commonly prescribed, fluconazole once weekly or intermittent treatment for recurrent symptoms may lessen the likelihood of resistance, minimize side effects, and be more cost effective.

Bonacini M, Young T, Laine L: The causes of esophageal symptoms in human immunodeficiency virus infection. Arch Intern Med 1991;151:1567.

Connolly GM et al: Oesophageal symptoms, their causes, treatment, and prognosis in patients with the acquired immunodeficiencysyndrome. Gut 1989;30:1033.

Levine MS et al: Opportunistic esophagitis in AIDS: Radiographic diagnosis. Radiology 1987;165:815.

Lopez-Dupla M et al: Clinical, endoscopic, immunologic, and therapeutic aspects of oropharyngeal and esophageal candidiasis in HIV-infected patients: A survey of 114 cases. Am J Gastroenterol 1992;87:1771.

Parente F et al: Prevention of symptomatic recurrences of esophageal candidiasis in AIDS patients after the first episode: A prospective open study. Am J Gastroenterol 1994;89:416.

CYTOMEGALOVIRUS

Essentials of Diagnosis

- The most common viral cause of esophageal disease.
- Odynophagia almost uniformly present.
- Associated with concurrent extra-intestinal disease.
- Histopathologic identification of viral cytopathic effect the most specific means of diagnosis.

General Considerations

Prior exposure to CMV is almost uniform in HIV-infected patients. End-organ disease results from reactivation of latent infection. The reasons for reactivation in one organ as compared to other sites is unknown. Viremia can frequently be found, although its role in dissemination of disease is undefined. Concurrent disease of other gastrointestinal sites or the retina may be seen at the time of diagnosis, suggesting widespread reactivation or dissemination in some patients.

Clinical Findings

A. Symptoms and Signs: Odynophagia is the most consistent symptom. In contrast to Candida esophagitis, dysphagia is distinctly uncommon. The patient may disclose the presence of spontaneous (nonswallowing) substernal chest pain after close questioning. Heartburn is rare. Nausea, vomiting, and low-grade fever may be reported. Gastrointestinal bleeding can be the initial manifestation in the absence of significant esophageal symptoms. Concurrent intestinal and colonic disease may be suggested by the presence of diarrhea or abdominal pain. Altered vision may be an important clue to the presence of retinitis.

Physical findings are nonspecific. Concurrent oropharyngeal ulcerations are rare, however, thrush may be present.

B. Laboratory Findings: CMV gastrointestinal disease occurs in the setting of profound immunodeficiency; the CD4 lymphocyte count is almost always less than 100/μL and frequently less than 50/μL. Serologic studies for CMV antibody are not helpful, given the uniform positivity in these patients.

C. Imaging: Barium esophagography usually demonstrates one or more well-circumscribed ulcerations or a diffuse erosive pattern. Although characteristically large, ulcers may be variable in size and appearance, mimicking other disorders. Solitary or multiple large ulcers are not pathognomonic for CMV, but may be seen with the HIV-associated idiopathic esophageal ulcer (IEU) or pill-induced esophagitis. In contrast to Candida esophagitis, which has a more characteristic radiographic appearance, empiric antiviral therapy based on the radiographic findings alone is not appropriate, given the multiplicity of similar lesions. Computerized tomography (CT), obtained for other reasons, may also reveal marked thickening of the esophagus.

D. Endoscopy: Endoscopy is the diagnostic method of choice. Given the broad differential diagnosis of esophageal ulceration in these patients, endoscopy provides the opportunity for mucosal biopsy to establish a definitive diagnosis. As with esophagography, one or more well-circumscribed ulcers is the typical endoscopic finding. Multiple biopsies are required to reliably identify CMV cytopathic effect, as the inclusions may be few in number and atypical in appearance. Viral culture of biopsy specimens may be positive, but is less sensitive and specific than histopathologic examination.

Differential Diagnosis

CMV esophagitis must be distinguished from other causes of esophageal ulceration by endoscopic mucosal biopsy. An IEU is the most important lesion to exclude, given the similar clinical presentation, radiographic findings, and endoscopic features. Differentiation of these two disorders is important because they are managed differently. CMV is often missed when biopsy samples are inadequate or when viral cytopathic effect, which may be infrequent or atypical, has not been identified. In this situation, in situ hybridization or antibody staining can help to confirm the diagnosis. Pill-induced esophagitis, HSV esophagitis, and gastroesophageal reflux disease (GERD) can usually be excluded based on history, endoscopic findings, and histopathologic results.

Complications

These lesions result in significant morbidity related to pain. Dehydration requiring hospitalization may result from severe odynophagia. Gastrointestinal bleeding is well recognized in the absence of a coagulopathy. Perforation has not been reported. Strictures may occur following antiviral therapy.

Treatment

Currently, only parenteral agents are available. Ganciclovir and foscarnet yield a response rate of approximately 75% or greater. There have been no comparisons of these agents in gastrointestinal disease. Thus, choice of therapy should be based on the experience of the clinician with a particular agent and drug toxicity. Ganciclovir is most frequently associated with bone marrow suppression and resultant leukopenia. In contrast, foscarnet may result in reduced renal function; hydration with drug administration reduces the frequency of renal insufficiency. Reductions in serum calcium and magnesium are also frequent with foscarnet and may be symptomatic, requiring supplementation. Therapy should be given for approximately 2–3 weeks, depending on the clinical response. Life-long therapy may not be required in all patients, as a long-term remission may occur after ulcers have healed completely.

If the patient becomes asymptomatic and shows no signs of retinal disease, close clinical monitoring without maintenance therapy is appropriate. If symptoms reappear, endoscopy should be performed to document recurrence. Long-term therapy after relapse should be individualized. Ophthalmologic examination at the time of diagnosis or recurrence is mandatory to exclude retinal disease, as the presence of CMV retinitis mandates life-long treatment. Ganciclovir is administered at a dose of 5 mg/kg twice daily. Foscarnet can be given at 90 mg/kg twice daily. Elevation of serum creatinine during foscarnet therapy calls for a dose reduction. Myelosuppression with ganciclovir may be treated by giving bone marrow stimulators (G-CSF) or switching to foscarnet. Similarly, if significant renal insufficiency occurs during foscarnet therapy, a change to ganciclovir may be appropriate.

Prognosis

Despite successful therapy, the median survival for patients with CMV esophagitis is less than 1 year. Although rarely the cause of death, esophageal disease is a marker of severe immunodeficiency, with death resulting from other AIDS-related illnesses.

Goodgame R: Gastrointestinal cytomegalovirus disease. Ann Intern Med 1993;119:924.

Wilcox CM et al: Cytomegalovirus esophagitis in patients with AIDS. A clinical, endoscopic, and pathologic correlation. Ann Intern Med 1990;113:589.

HERPES SIMPLEX VIRUS ESOPHAGITIS

Essentials of Diagnosis

- Diagnosis confirmed by histopathologic or cytologic identification of viral cytopathic effect or by positive viral culture.

- Frequently associated with oropharyngeal ulceration.
- Relatively uncommon.

General Considerations

In contrast to its occurrence in the immunocompromised host after transplantation or chemotherapy, HSV esophagitis is relatively uncommon in HIV infection. This infrequency may only partially be explained by the use of chronic acyclovir therapy in these patients.

Clinical Findings

A. Symptoms and Signs: As with other causes of ulcerative esophagitis, odynophagia and substernal chest pain are the most frequent complaints. Dysphagia, heartburn, nausea, vomiting, and fever are uncommon. HSV stomatitis has a characteristic appearance and its presence may provide an important clue to the diagnosis. However, as with other ulcerative esophageal disorders, thrush may be concurrently seen.

B. Laboratory Findings: The CD4 lymphocyte count is usually low (less than 200 /μL).

C. Imaging: Barium esophagography most commonly demonstrates diffuse mucosal ulceration (Figure 2–2) or multiple well-circumscribed shallow ulcers with normal-appearing intervening mucosa. Large solitary ulcers are rare and more characteristic of CMV esophagitis or IEU.

D. Endoscopy: The most common endoscopic findings are a diffuse erosive esophagitis or multiple shallow ulcerations. Vesicles, which are the earliest manifestation, are rarely found, nor are large deep ulcers. At endoscopy, cytologic brushings and mucosal biopsies may be used to identify characteristic viral cytopathic effect. In the presence of diffuse erosive disease, diagnosis becomes more difficult as HSV cytopathic effect is only reliably identified in squamous cells. In this situation, immunohistochemical stains to identify viral antigens may assist in the histopathologic diagnosis. Viral culture may also be performed, although as with CMV esophagitis, sensitivity and specificity may be greater with cytology and histologic examination of biopsy specimens.

Differential Diagnosis

The most important causes to exclude are CMV esophagitis, IEU, and pill-induced esophagitis. As with other causes of ulcerative esophagitis, there are no truly pathognomonic radiographic or endoscopic features of HSV esophagitis; therefore, definitive diagnosis rests on the cytologic or histopathologic identification of viral cytopathic effect.

Treatment

Acyclovir is effective therapy, although resistance has been documented. Intravenous administration may be required when odynophagia is severe. The

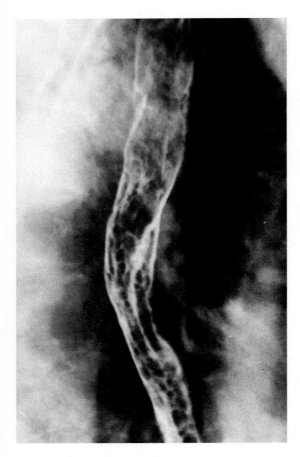

Figure 2–2. Herpes simplex virus esophagitis. Diffuse superficial ulceration in the middle and distal esophagus.

need for long-term therapy after diagnosis is not well established although such treatment is common. The recommended dose is 5 mg/kg every 8 hours. Foscarnet may be used for treatment failures.

Bagdades EK et al: Relationship between herpes simplex virus ulceration and CD4+ cell counts in patients with HIV infection. AIDS 1992;6:1317.
Levine MS et al: Herpes esophagitis: Sensitivity of double-contrast esophagography. AJR 1988;151:57.

IDIOPATHIC ESOPHAGEAL ULCERATION

Essentials of Diagnosis

- A common cause of esophageal ulceration.
- Diagnosis of exclusion.

General Considerations

Idiopathic esophageal ulceration is a frequent cause of esophageal ulceration. Although HIV has been identified by immunohistochemical techniques

in ulcer tissue from these patients, a similar prevalence of HIV has also been observed in other causes of esophageal disease, such as CMV. HIV has not been found in squamous epithelial cells, but rather, in rare inflammatory cells in the ulcer base. Thus, it is unclear what role HIV mucosal infection plays, if any, in the genesis of these lesions. It has also been postulated that these lesions may be an autoimmune phenomenon, which is frequently seen in these patients, or the result of some as yet unidentified pathogen. A careful drug history must be obtained to exclude pill-induced disease.

Clinical Findings

A. Symptoms and Signs: The clinical presentation is similar to other causes of ulcerative esophagitis: commonly, odynophagia (which is usually severe), substernal chest pain, and occasionally dehydration and weight loss. Concurrent oropharyngeal ulcerations are infrequent.

B. Laboratory Findings: Idiopathic esophageal ulceration is seen in the setting of profound immunodeficiency with the CD4 lymphocyte count usually less than $100/\mu L$. Self-limited esophageal ulcers have also been reported in patients with the HIV-associated seroconversion syndrome.

C. Imaging: Typical findings on barium esophagography include one or multiple well-circumscribed ulcerations that may be shallow or deep (Figure 2–3).

D. Endoscopy: The endoscopic appearance is one of single or multiple ulcerations of variable depth. As with CMV esophagitis, the intervening mucosa is normal. These findings are remarkably similar to CMV esophagitis. At the time of endoscopy, multiple biopsies of the ulcer base are necessary to exclude viral cytopathic effect.

Differential Diagnosis

The clinical, radiographic, and endoscopic findings are impossible to distinguish from CMV esophagitis. Multiple midesophageal ulcerations suggest a pill-induced esophagitis. Single or multiple distal ulcerations may mimic GERD; however, patients with GERD usually can be distinguished by a history of long-standing heartburn or regurgitation.

Complications

Sinus tract formation or fistulization to surrounding structures has been described, although frank perforation has not been reported. Bleeding may be seen.

Treatment

Corticosteroid therapy results in a dramatic response, with marked clinical improvement usually seen within the first few days of treatment. Prednisone administered at 40 mg/d orally, tapering 10 mg/wk for a 1-month course of treatment results in a

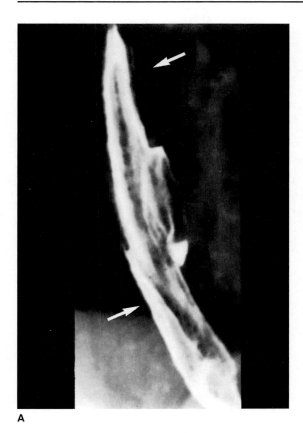

A

B

Figure 2–3. Idiopathic esophageal ulcer. **A:** Large deep ulcer in the mid esophagus **(arrow).** The smaller ulcer seen proximally represents barium collecting in a healed ulcer **(arrow).** Barium is also seen in a large healed distal ulcer **(arrow). B:** Endoscopic photograph of the large esophageal ulcer. The mucosa surrounding the ulcer is normal. The endoscopic appearance is also compatible with CMV esophagitis.

clinical and endoscopic cure rate of greater than 90%. Oral systemic antifungal therapy should be coadministered with prednisone to decrease the likelihood of symptomatic oropharyngeal or esophageal candidiasis, which may confuse assessment of the clinical response.

Prognosis

The long-term prognosis is related to the degree of immunodeficiency and the presence of other AIDS-defining illnesses. As with other opportunistic esophageal infections, IEU does not usually result in death. Relapse of IEU may be seen, usually occurring within the first several months after completion of therapy. Life-long low-dose corticosteroid therapy may be necessary for patients with frequent relapses to maintain a remission.

Smith PD et al: Esophageal disease in AIDS is associated with pathologic processes rather than mucosal human immunodeficiency virus type I. J Infect Dis 1993;167:547.

Wilcox CM, Schwartz DA: A pilot study of oral corticosteroid therapy for idiopathic esophageal ulcerations associated with human immunodeficiency virus infection. Am J Med 1992;93:131.

Wilcox CM, Schwartz DA: Endoscopic characterization of idiopathic esophageal ulceration associated with human immunodeficiency virus infection. J Clin Gastroenterol 1993;16:251.

MISCELLANEOUS DISORDERS

A variety of other opportunistic infections have been reported to involve the esophagus, including protozoa (cryptosporidia, *Pneumocystis carinii,*) bacteria (nocardia, actinomyces), mycobacteria, (*Mycobacterium avium* complex [MAC], *Mycobacterium tuberculosis* [TB]), as well as other fungi (*Histoplasma capsulatum*). These may be identified by appropriate histopathologic staining and culture of endoscopic biopsies. KS and non-Hodgkin's lymphoma (NHL) may also involve the esophagus. Nonopportunistic processes, which always demand consideration in the appropriate setting, include GERD and pill-induced esophagitis. Reflux disease typically presents with symptomatic heartburn and distal esophageal disease radiographically and endoscopically. Pill-induced esophagitis has been documented from a number of drugs; in these patients, zidovudine (ZDV) and zalcitabine (ddC) have been reported.

APPROACH TO INITIAL MANAGEMENT

For patients without a prior AIDS-defining illness, the CD4 lymphocyte count provides considerable guidance in considering the plausibility of an opportunistic esophageal disorder. Given the prevalence of

Candida esophagitis, the initial management of symptomatic patients usually consists of empiric oral systemic antifungal therapy, with fluconazole 100 mg daily after a 200-mg loading dose. This strategy may be employed in the presence or absence of thrush. In patients with severe esophageal symptoms associated with dehydration and weight loss, management should be individualized. For the patient without thrush, endoscopy may be appropriate to rapidly exclude ulcerative esophagitis.

Antifungal therapy with oral fluconazole usually results in rapid symptomatic improvement in the patient with Candida esophagitis and can be used as a diagnostic "test." In the absence of a prompt symptomatic improvement within 7–10 days of initiating treatment, endoscopy should be performed; barium esophagography or further empiric trials are not appropriate, given the high likelihood of ulcerative esophagitis requiring endoscopy with biopsy to exclude viral disease or IEU. Esophageal malignancy resulting from KS or NHL is uncommon, but may present with bleeding, or with dysphagia or odynophagia if the tumor is large and bulky. This suggested approach to management is summarized in Figure 2–4.

Connolly GM et al: Investigation of upper gastrointestinal symptoms in patients with AIDS. AIDS 1989;3:453.

Wilcox CM: Esophageal disease in the acquired immunodeficiency syndrome: Etiology, diagnosis, and management. Am J Med 1992;92:412.

DISEASES OF THE STOMACH

In contrast to esophageal disease, symptomatic gastric disorders are uncommon in these patients.

Diseases that affect the immunocompetent host, such as peptic ulcer, deserve consideration in the appropriate clinical setting, especially when the CD4 lymphocyte count is normal.

INFECTIONS & NEOPLASMS

Although a number of opportunistic pathogens have been documented to infect the stomach—including cryptosporidia, toxoplasma, fungi, leishmania, and *Pneumocystis carinii*; the most common opportunistic pathogen is CMV. These infections may be asymptomatic and found incidentally, or result in nausea, vomiting, epigastric pain, or gastrointestinal bleeding. As in the normal host, asymptomatic *Helicobacter pylori* gastritis is common.

Hypochlorhydria occurs in 40–67% of AIDS patients. Achlorhydria appears to be more common in those in the later stages of immunodeficiency. The pathophysiologic mechanisms underlying this reduced acid output are unknown but may include antiparietal cell antibodies or the gastric secretory failure described in other patients with severe systemic illnesses. Hypochlorhydria has important implications in relation to drug absorption and may predispose to gastrointestinal infections.

KS commonly involves the gastrointestinal tract, including the stomach; cutaneous disease is usually present. Although usually asymptomatic, KS may result in abdominal pain, obstruction, or bleeding when the lesions enlarge. NHL is usually symptomatic, presenting with obstruction or bleeding. Gastric adenocarcinoma is very rare.

Clinical Findings

A. Symptoms and Signs: Gastric infections usually cause nausea, vomiting, and epigastric pain. CMV may be associated with severe epigastric pain.

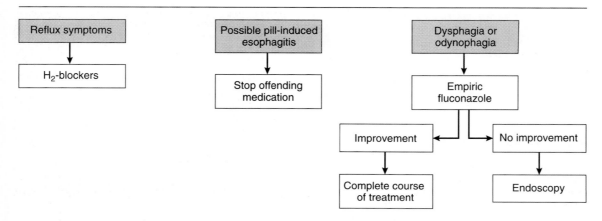

Figure 2–4. Suggested approach to the initial management of esophageal symptoms.

Bleeding results from ulcerative lesions (acid-peptic, nonsteroidal anti-inflammatory drug-induced, CMV) or neoplasms.

B. Laboratory Findings: Opportunistic infections should be suspected when the CD4 lymphocyte count is less than 200/μL.

C. Imaging: Upper gastrointestinal radiographic series may demonstrate thickened folds, indicative of gastritis. Gastric ulcers may have an acid-peptic etiology or be caused by CMV, neoplasms, or nonsteroidal anti-inflammatory drugs (NSAIDs). Large-mass lesions resembling neoplasms have been described from CMV. KS usually appears as a large ulcerated mass or multiple well-circumscribed lesions. NHL results in a mass lesion. CT may identify wall thickening with CMV (Figure 2–5) or neoplasms (Figure 2–6).

D. Endoscopy: In the patient with radiographic abnormalities and a low CD4 lymphocyte count, endoscopy with mucosal biopsy will often be required for diagnosis. The endoscopic appearance of KS is pathognomonic, and thus biopsy may not be required. Ulcerations should be biopsied to exclude an opportunistic infection or neoplasm.

Belitsos PC et al: Association of gastric hypoacidity with opportunistic enteric infections in patients with AIDS. J Infect Dis 1992;166:277.

Lake-Bakaar G et al: Gastric secretory failure in patients withthe acquired immunodeficiency syndrome (AIDS). Ann Intern Med 1988;109:502.

DISEASES OF THE PANCREAS

Essentials of Diagnosis

- Epigastric pain, nausea, and vomiting are the most common manifestations.
- Exclude treatable causes.

General Considerations

Elevation of the serum amylase concentration most commonly results from either increased levels of salivary amylase, macroamylasemia, or true pancreatic disease. Despite the fact that a variety of opportunistic infections and neoplasms have been documented to involve the pancreas, pancreatic disorders are an infrequent clinical problem. As with the normal host, an inflammatory process is the most common expression of pancreatic disease. Pancreatitis may be caused by opportunistic infections (cryptospordia, CMV, MAC, TB), drugs (pentamidine, didanosine [ddI]), alcohol, choledocholithiasis, or, less frequently, neoplasms. The underlying cause may be suggested by the clinical setting.

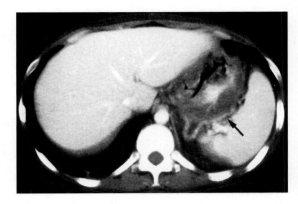

Figure 2–5. CMV gastritis. Dramatic thickening of the gastric wall with "dirty fat" involving the gastrosplenic ligament *(arrow).*

Clinical Findings

A. Symptoms and Signs: Nausea, vomiting, and epigastric pain are highly suggestive of pancreatitis. The pain will frequently radiate to the back. The pattern of pain is constant and usually severe in intensity. Low grade fever may be present.

B. Laboratory Findings: Pancreatic disease should be suspected when the amylase concentration exceeds two times the upper limits of normal. An elevation of serum lipase may help confirm a pancreatic origin of the amylase.

C. Imaging: Abdominal CT confirms the diagnosis of pancreatitis and identifies mass lesions or fluid collections. Pancreatic calcifications, retroperitoneal adenopathy, or other hepatic or splenic lesions may also be found by CT, further suggesting the underlying cause. CT-directed aspiration and biopsy of mass lesions or fluid collections with appropriate culture, staining, and pathologic evaluation may be nec-

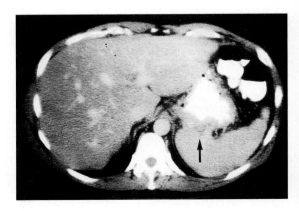

Figure 2–6. Gastric Kaposi's sarcoma. Nodularity and thickening primarily of the posterior gastric wall *(arrow).*

essary to exclude an infection or neoplasm. Ultrasound best excludes gallstones.

D. Endoscopy: Endoscopic retrograde cholangiopancreatography (ERCP) plays a valuable diagnostic and therapeutic role in the setting of suspected choledocholithiasis or in the jaundiced patient, as stones may be removed by endoscopic sphincterotomy and obstruction can be relieved by endoscopic stent placement, respectively.

Differential Diagnosis

The most likely cause depends on the clinical setting (eg, alcohol abuse or recent use of pentamidine). When the CD4 count is low, mass lesions or abscess may be related to opportunistic processes.

Complications

Complications of pancreatic disease in HIV infection are similar to those in the immunocompetent host. Chronic pancreatitis resulting from an opportunistic infection or neoplasm has not been described, probably as a result of short life expectancy.

Treatment

The treatment of pancreatitis depends on the cause. Reversible causes, such as alcohol and medications, should be excluded.

Prognosis

If a readily treatable process is found, the prognosis depends on the stage of immunodeficiency and the severity of the pancreatitis.

Bonacini M: Pancreatic involvement in human immunodeficiency virus infection. J Clin Gastroenterol 1991;13:58.

Murthy UK et al: Hyperamylasemia in patients with the acquired immunodeficiency syndrome. Am J Gastroenterol 1992;87:332.

DISEASES OF THE SMALL INTESTINE

Essentials of Diagnosis

- Most commonly manifested by diarrhea.
- Diarrhea usually of a large volume and can be associated with electrolyte disturbances and malabsorption.

General Considerations

The small bowel is a frequent target of both opportunistic and nonopportunistic infections. Although small intestinal infection may be asymptomatic, symptoms eventually develop as immunodeficiency progresses and the infection worsens. Diarrhea and malabsorption are usually the direct result of intestinal infection. However, functional and morphologic abnormalities, such as reductions in enzyme activity (eg, lactase) and enterocyte hypoproliferation and dysmaturation, respectively, have been documented in patients with AIDS in the absence of any identifiable infection. This has been termed **AIDS enteropathy.** These functional and morphologic abnormalities do not appear to result from direct HIV infection of the enterocyte, as HIV has only been found in inflammatory cells in the lamina propria. On routine light microscopic examination of small bowel biopsies, increased inflammatory cells in the lamina propria and mild atrophy may be seen. Electron microscopic examination can be used to identify microsporidia, although routine light microscopic examination of appropriately stained specimens will usually be diagnostic. Additional small intestinal disorders potentially contributing to this enteropathy include bacterial overgrowth, neuropathic changes of the enteric nervous system, and alteration in release of enteric peptides.

Clinical Findings

A. Symptoms and Signs: Opportunistic infections of the small bowel typically cause intestinal secretion and diarrhea, with stool volumes greater than 1 L/d. For example, cryptosporidial diarrhea can be massive, with loss of over 10 L of stool per day, resulting in severe electrolyte disturbances, dehydration, and malabsorption. MAC is associated with a less severe diarrhea; however, malabsorption may be striking, given the disordered mucosal architecture caused by diffuse infiltration of macrophage-engulfed organisms in the lamina propria (termed the pseudo-Whipple's syndrome). Weight loss and fever are common with disseminated MAC infection in the absence of identifiable intestinal disease. Intestinal microsporidiosis is associated with mild to moderate diarrhea and malabsorption. In asymptomatic patients, this pathogen may be an incidental finding on small bowel biopsy. Tuberculosis may result in mass lesions of the distal small bowel, causing obstructive symptoms or frank perforation. Infections afflicting the immunocompetent host, such as giardiasis, will present similarly in the immunocompromised.

Both well-recognized viruses (rotavirus, norwalk virus) and novel ones (picobirna, astra) have been documented and may be the cause of diarrhea when no diagnosis can be established by routine evaluation. CMV is infrequently isolated to the small bowel but may present with abdominal pain (perforation has been reported) or diarrhea.

KS is usually asymptomatic; bleeding or obstruction may occur when the lesions becomes large. NHL may present with bleeding or signs of obstruction, since these neoplasms are usually large when clinically evident.

B. Laboratory Findings: Evidence of malabsorption and malnutrition, such as hypoalbuminemia and hypocholesterolemia, may be present although these are nonspecific findings. Electrolyte disturbances such as hypokalemia and acidosis may reflect a secretory diarrhea. Blood cultures are important in providing indirect evidence for MAC or TB infection, and should be performed in the setting of persistent fever, weight loss, and diarrhea when the CD4 count is low (less than 100/µL).

C. Stool Analysis: Steatorrhea (positive qualitative fecal fat) may be found although it is nonspecific. Fecal leukocytes do not result from small bowel mucosal infection. At least three sets of fresh stool should be examined to more reliably exclude an infectious cause. Specific stains for cryptosporidia, isospora, and MAC should be performed. Routine ova and parasite examination will identify giardia, although multiple stool evaluations may be required to increase the diagnostic yield. Further development of immunofluorescent stains will help improve the diagnostic yield for cryptosporidia and microsporidia.

D. Imaging: Barium radiographic findings, such as bowel wall thickening, are often nonspecific; flocculation of barium results from failure of barium to adequately coat the mucosa as a result of excessive luminal fluid. Small bowel barium examination should not be routinely performed in the work-up of diarrhea as barium interferes with microscopic examination of the stool.

Abdominal CT may confirm the findings on the barium studies, such as small bowel thickening (Figure 2–7) or mass lesions (Figure 2–8); intra-abdominal and retroperitoneal adenopathy suggest mycobacterial diseases, NHL, or less frequently KS. Mass lesions may result from KS or NHL and are rarely infectious in etiology (TB, MAC).

E. Endoscopy: Because most small intestinal pathogens causing diarrhea can be found by evalua-

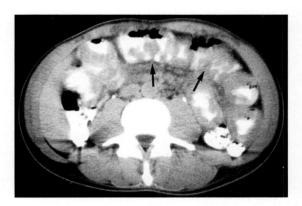

Figure 2–8. Non-Hodgkin's lymphoma involving the small intestine and colon. Loops of both small bowel **(arrow)** and colon are thickened. Multiple mass lesions are seen projecting into the colonic lumen **(arrow)**. Adenopathy is also present.

tion of multiple stool specimens, endoscopy with small bowel biopsy is infrequently required. Endoscopic evaluation is currently limited by the length of the endoscopes to the proximal small bowel (proximal jejunum). If multiple stool tests do not reveal a pathogen and small bowel infection is suspected clinically, endoscopically-directed small bowel biopsy may be helpful to diagnose cryptosporidia, microsporidia, or MAC. Characteristic endoscopic abnormalities can be seen with MAC (yellow plaques, bowel wall thickening) and neoplasms, eg, KS and NHL.

Differential Diagnosis

Although a variety of both small bowel and colonic pathogens may result in diarrhea (Table 2–3), the clinician can distinguish the location of infection (small bowel versus colon) and thus site of diarrhea by history, physical examination, and routine laboratory tests (Table 2–4). *Giardia lamblia,* occurring in both the immunocompetent and immunodeficient individual, typically results in upper gastrointestinal symptoms such as nausea, bloating, flatulence, and periumbilical cramps. Cryptosporidia and microsporidia may be difficult to differentiate clinically, although cryptosporidia usually results in more

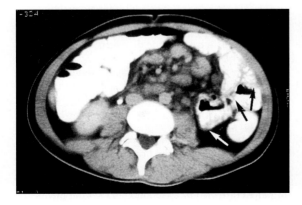

Figure 2–7. *Mycobacterium avium* complex enteritis. Thickening of the small bowel **(arrow)** associated with diffuse mesenteric and retroperitoneal adenopathy.

Table 2–3. Causes of diarrhea in AIDS.

Common	Infrequent	Rare
Cryptosporidiosis Cytomegalovirus Bacteria *Campylobacter* *C difficile* Giardiasis	Microsporidiosis *Mycobacterium avium* complex	Tuberculosis Histoplasmosis Amebiasis

Table 2–4. Clinical features assisting in the differentiation of a small bowel from colonic diarrhea.

Feature	Small Intestine	Colon
Stool frequency	Frequent	Frequent
Stool volume	Large	Small
Stool character	Watery	May be bloody
Electrolyte abnormalities	+++	− − −
Dehydration	++	− − −
Weight loss	+	+
Abdominal pain	+	++
Borborygmi	+	− − −
Upper gastrointestinal tract symptoms	+	− − −
Fecal leukocytes	Absent	Present with colitis

+++ = very common; ++ = frequent; + = can occur; − − − − = not seen.

significant diarrhea, and more commonly causes upper gastrointestinal symptoms (nausea). Significant epigastric and abdominal pain suggests CMV enteritis.

Regardless of the specific infectious causes, diarrhea tends to worsen with progression of immunodeficiency as the burden of pathogens increases. For example, cryptosporidia may cause only mild diarrhea or be asymptomatic when the CD4 count is greater than 200/μL; however, diarrhea can be massive and life-threatening when the CD4 count is less than 50/μL.

Complications

Small bowel infections, particularly cryptosporidia, may be complicated by severe dehydration and life-threatening electrolyte disturbances. Weight loss is almost uniform with opportunistic small bowel infections. Bleeding can result from large neoplasms and infections causing mucosal ulceration (CMV, TB, and rarely MAC).

Treatment

Antimicrobial therapy should be directed toward the identified pathogen. Either chemotherapy, radiation therapy, or both may be required for symptomatic neoplasms. Paromomycin has shown effectiveness in some patients with cryptosporidia. Metronidazole has not been uniformly effective for microsporidiosis, although albendazole holds promise. Multi-drug regimens may be efficacious in MAC. Overall, however, uniformly effective therapy for these pathogens is not available. Treatment of opportunistic infections does not truly eradicate the infection; therefore, life-long therapy will be required for responders.

Prognosis

Long-term survival is primarily dependent on the degree of immunodeficiency. The lack of a response to treatment may result in progressive malabsorption and weight loss contributing to death. Severe diarrhea associated with cryptosporidiosis has a very poor prognosis.

Bartlett JG, Belitsos PC, Sears CL: AIDS enteropathy. Clin Infect Dis 1992;15:726.
Connolly GM, Forbes A, Gazzard BG: Investigation of seemingly pathogen-negative diarrhoea in patients infected with HIV-1. Gut 1990;31:886.
Kotler DP et al: Small intestinal injury and parasitic diseases in AIDS. Ann Intern Med 1990;113:444.
Molina JM et al: Intestinal microsporidiosis in human immunodeficiency virus-infected patients with chronic unexplained diarrhea: Prevalence and clinical and biologic features. J Infect Dis 1993;167:217.
Petersen C: Cryptosporidiosis in patients infected with the human immunodeficiency virus. Clin Infect Dis 1992;15:903.
Rabeneck L: Diagnostic workup strategies for patients with HIV-related chronic diarrhea. J Clin Gastroenterol 1993;16:245.
Ullrich R et al: Small intestinal structure and function in patients infected with human immunodeficiency virus (HIV): Evidence for HIV-induced enteropathy. Ann Intern Med 1989;111:15.

DISEASES OF THE COLON

Infections are the most common cause of colonic disease, including both nonopportunistic (bacteria, protozoa) and opportunistic (viruses, mycobacteria, protozoa) causes. Abdominal pain, fever, bleeding, or perforation with peritonitis and an acute abdomen may be the initial manifestations of colonic disease.

BACTERIAL COLITIS

Essentials of Diagnosis

- A frequent cause of acute diarrhea.
- Watery or bloody diarrhea.
- May be associated with relapse, requiring long-term antibiotics in those with severe immunodeficiency.

General Considerations

The spectrum of bacterial pathogens causing colitis is similar to that in the normal host. The most frequently identified pathogen is *Campylobacter,* followed by *Salmonella* and *Shigella. Clostridium difficile* colitis is not infrequent and should always be considered in the appropriate setting. An increased risk for bacterial colitis may be seen in homosexual men engaging in oral-anal contact.

Clinical Findings

A. Symptoms and Signs: Bacterial colitis is associated with an acute diarrheal illness (less than 1 month in duration). The diarrhea is usually watery but may be bloody when colitis is severe. Lower abdominal pain and fever are frequent and may be prominent, suggesting peritonitis. Nausea and vomiting are uncommon.

Physical findings include fever and lower abdominal pain. Symptoms of proctitis (urgency, sense of incomplete evacuation, tenesmus, frequent low-volume stools) may be described. Digital rectal examination may demonstrate frank blood on the examining finger or a guaiac-positive stool.

B. Laboratory Findings: Bacterial colitis can occur at any stage of immunodeficiency. Electrolyte disturbances are infrequent, given that colitis does not typically cause a true secretory diarrhea, and may be positive, especially with *Salmonella*. Blood cultures should be performed in the patient with fever.

C. Stool Analysis: Submitting fresh stool for bacterial culture is essential. Stool staining with Gram's stain or methylene blue to evaluate for fecal leukocytes is mandatory. Their presence documents colitis. They are almost uniformly found in the setting of bacterial colitis including *C difficile*. *Clostridium difficile* toxin should be excluded on fresh stool in the patient recently receiving antibiotics or the patient developing diarrhea while hospitalized, especially when associated with fecal leukocytes. Occasionally, bacteremia may be found when stool cultures are negative.

D. Imaging: Routine abdominal radiographs are usually nonspecific, although in severe cases, thumbprinting or colonic dilation may be found. Barium enema examination plays no role in the evaluation of acute diarrhea, especially when bacterial colitis is suspected. As with small bowel disease, if barium enema is required for other reasons, all stool studies should be collected before the examination. In those with severe bacterial colitis, abdominal CT will often demonstrate colonic wall thickening.

E. Endoscopy: Flexible sigmoidoscopic examination of the distal colorectum may be diagnostic for *C difficile* colitis when multiple or confluent yellow plaques are seen. The endoscopic appearance of bacterial colitis is nondiagnostic, resembling CMV colitis or idiopathic inflammatory bowel disease (ulcerative colitis, Crohn's disease). Sigmoidoscopic examination should be performed in the patient with suspected colitis when multiple (at least three) stool cultures and *C difficile* toxin titer are negative. In the hospitalized patient with diarrhea and fecal leukocytes, early sigmoidoscopy may expedite diagnosis and treatment.

Differential Diagnosis

In the patient with acute diarrhea, differentiation between small bowel (ie, giardiasis) and colonic causes may be difficult. Pathogens involving the small bowel typically cause upper gastrointestinal symptoms, such as nausea, vomiting, bloating and distention, borborygmi, and periumbilical abdominal cramps. Colonic disorders result in lower abdominal or left-lower quadrant pain and tenderness. Urgency, sensation of incomplete evacuation, tenesmus, and frequent low-volume stools are highly suggestive of proctitis or distal colitis. In general, cryptosporidia, microsporidia and MAC cause small bowel disease and do not present acutely. Similarly, colonic processes such as CMV colitis or idiopathic inflammatory bowel disease are associated with chronic symptoms, however they may present acutely. These disorders can usually be differentiated by careful history, physical examination, and evaluation of multiple stool specimens, supplemented by sigmoidoscopic or colonoscopic evaluation where appropriate.

Treatment

The choice of definitive antimicrobial therapy depends on the culture and sensitivity results. Ciprofloxacin is the empiric therapy of choice for suspected bacterial colitis given the increasing bacterial resistance to trimethoprim-sulfamethoxazole. In contrast to the immunocompetent host with acute bacterial colitis, antibiotic therapy should be initiated in immunodeficient patients with documented bacterial colitis. *Clostridium difficile* colitis can be treated with metronidazole, with oral vancomycin reserved for patients with severe life-threatening disease.

Prognosis

Antibiotic therapy is effective. Long-term suppressive therapy may be required to prevent relapse if severe immunodeficiency is present, particularly for patients with *Salmonella*. *Clostridium difficile* colitis does not appear to be associated with more severe disease, refractoriness to antibiotics, or a higher rate of relapse than in immunocompetent patients.

Cappell MS, Philogene C: *Clostridium difficile* infection is a treatable cause of diarrhea in patients with advanced human immunodeficiency virus infection. Am J Gastroenterol 1993;88:891.

Laughon BE et al: Prevalence of enteric pathogens in homosexual men with and without acquired immunodeficiency syndrome. Gastroenterology 1988;94:984.

Rene E et al: Intestinal infections in patients with acquired immunodeficiency syndrome. A prospective study in 132 patients. Dig Dis Sci 1989;34:773.

Smith DP et al: Gastrointestinal infections in AIDS. Ann Intern Med 1992;116:63.

CYTOMEGALOVIRUS COLITIS

Essentials of Diagnosis

- The most common opportunistic cause of colonic disease.

- Usually presents as chronic diarrhea.
- Associated with extra-intestinal disease.
- Diagnosis most specific by histopathologic identification of viral cytopathic effect in mucosal biopsy specimens.

General Considerations

As with the identification of CMV in other gastrointestinal sites, extra-intestinal disease (ophthalmic disease) should be excluded at the time of diagnosis, given the implications for long-term management.

Clinical Findings

A. Symptoms and Signs: CMV colitis usually presents as a chronic (greater than 1 month) watery diarrhea in the setting of severe immunodeficiency. Fever, weight loss, and lower abdominal pain are common symptoms and signs. When the distal colorectum is involved, symptoms of proctitis may be reported. Gastrointestinal bleeding without diarrhea may be the initial manifestation of colitis. Other symptoms may be related to concurrent extra-intestinal CMV disease, such as altered vision in CMV retinitis. Concurrent symptomatic upper gastrointestinal disease is rare.

Physical findings are nonspecific. Digital rectal examination is usually unremarkable, although tenderness may be elicited with associated anorectal disease.

B. Laboratory Findings: CMV colitis almost always occurs when the CD4 lymphocyte count is severely reduced (< 100/μL). Serologic studies for CMV antibody are not helpful because they are uniformly positive in these patients.

C. Stool Analysis: The diagnosis should be suspected when multiple stool tests are negative in the setting of chronic diarrhea, weight loss, and severe immunodeficiency. Fecal leukocytes may be present with severe distal colitis.

D. Imaging: Routine abdominal radiographs are nonspecific. Barium enema examination should not be done for the routine evaluation of chronic diarrhea or if the diagnosis is suspected. Reported findings on barium enema however, include a pancolitis, segmental colitis, or focal ulcerations that may be segmental or diffuse. Abdominal CT usually demonstrates focal or diffuse colonic wall thickening depending on the extent of involvement (Figure 2–9). As with bacterial colitis, these CT findings are highly suggestive of colitis, but not specific for any particular cause.

E. Endoscopy: Endoscopic examination is necessary to establish the diagnosis. Viral cytopathic effect of CMV should be identified by histopathologic evaluation of biopsy specimens. Viral culture positivity of biopsy specimens is less sensitive and specific. In many patients, the region of disease will be continuous, beginning in the distal colorectum and

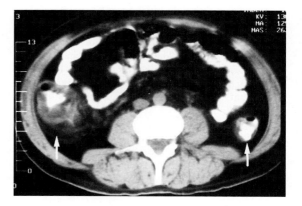

Figure 2–9. CMV colitis. The right colon and descending colon **(arrows)** are diffusely thickened. Similar findings may be seen with bacterial colitis.

extending proximally; thus, examination by sigmoidoscopy has a high yield. However, disease may be isolated to the right colon, thereby requiring full colonoscopy for diagnosis. Endoscopically, the most common appearance is a diffuse colitis mimicking bacterial colitis or idiopathic ulcerative colitis, or multiple ulcerations with normal-appearing intervening mucosa resembling Crohn's disease. Biopsies obtained throughout the colon may occasionally identify CMV in the absence of gross endoscopic abnormalities.

Differential Diagnosis

In the patient presenting with bloody diarrhea, lower abdominal pain, and fever, acute bacterial colitis should be excluded. Although CMV colitis may present with bloody diarrhea, it is more typically associated with a chronic watery diarrhea associated with weight loss and abdominal pain. *Clostridium difficile* colitis must be considered in those patients recently receiving antibiotics, or when the diarrhea develops during hospitalization. Patients presenting with acute diarrhea should have amebiasis excluded if they have travelled to an endemic area.

In the absence of colonic symptoms, differentiation from a small bowel diarrhea may be difficult; these patients should have multiple stool specimens evaluated to exclude bacterial and parasitic diseases before undergoing endoscopy. Iatrogenic causes should always be excluded: eg, antibiotics (without associated *C difficile* colitis), medications that contain magnesium or phosphate, which may precipitate diarrhea, and enteral feedings. A suggested approach for the evaluation of chronic diarrhea is provided in Figure 2–10.

Complications

Colonic perforation requires urgent surgical intervention. CMV colitis may also cause severe gastroin-

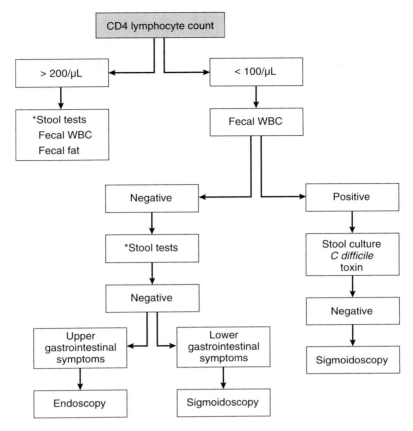

Figure 2–10. Suggested approach in the evaluation of chronic diarrhea. *At least 3 sets of fresh stool for ova and parasites, bacterial culture, and *C difficile* toxin.

testinal hemorrhage. Dehydration and electrolyte disturbances are rare unless a concurrent small bowel disease is present.

Treatment

Intravenous treatment with either ganciclovir or foscarnet is effective in approximately 75% of patients (see preceding section, "Diseases of the Esophagus"). Drug selection should be based on toxicity as well as the clinician's level of comfort in administering the agent. As with esophageal disease, there are no randomized studies comparing the efficacy of these two agents. In general, a longer course of treatment may be required for CMV colitis than for esophageal disease (usually 3–4 weeks), depending on the severity and extent of disease. As with esophageal disease, the need for life-long maintenance therapy is controversial. After a complete response, the patient should be followed clinically without maintenance anti-viral therapy. If relapse occurs, reinduction therapy followed by maintenance therapy should be initiated. Documentation of retinal disease at diagnosis or during follow-up requires life-long maintenance therapy.

Prognosis

Despite a clinical response, CMV colitis is a marker of poor long-term survival, the mean survival being approximately 8 months.

Dieterich DT, Rahmin M: Cytomegalovirus colitis in AIDS: Presentation in 44 patients and a review of the literature. J Acquir Immune Defic Syndr 1991;4(Suppl): S29.

Dieterich DT et al: Ganciclovir treatment of cytomegalovirus colitis in AIDS: A randomized double-blind, placebo-controlled multicenter study. J Infect Dis 1993;167:278.

MISCELLANEOUS COLONIC DISORDERS

Infections

A variety of other opportunistic pathogens have been reported to infect the colon in these patients, including *Pneumocystis carinii* and *Histoplasma capsulatum*. *Mycobacterium avium* complex may involve the colon, although usually in association with small bowel disease. Similarly, cryptosporidia may be identified on colonic biopsy but usually in association with small bowel infection. HSV infects squamous mucosa and therefore does not cause colitis; however, the distal colorectum may be involved in the setting of perianal disease.

Neoplasms

KS is the most common colonic neoplasm in HIV-infected patients. Colonic KS is usually associated with cutaneous disease as well as disease in the proximal gastrointestinal tract. Colonic KS, as with other gastrointestinal involvement, is most often clinically silent; however, bleeding, obstruction, or even perforation have been documented. NHL can involve the colon. These lesions are typically large, resulting in abdominal pain or obstruction; fever is often present (Figure 2–11). Barium enema examination or abdominal CT in the appropriate clinical setting may suggest the diagnosis. Colonic adenocarcinoma has also been reported in these patients. Colonoscopic biopsy will be required to make a definitive diagnosis of these neoplasms.

Idiopathic Inflammatory Bowel Disease

Given the prominent immunologic component of inflammatory bowel disease, the initial diagnosis of ulcerative colitis or Crohn's disease might be unexpected in these immunosuppressed patients. Interestingly, some HIV-infected patients with long-standing inflammatory bowel disease will have disease remission as the immunodeficiency progresses. Ulcerative colitis and Crohn's disease, therefore, are a diagnosis of exclusion in any HIV-infected patient with colitis. CMV colitis, bacterial colitis, and amebiasis should

also always be excluded, especially if corticosteroid therapy is to be given.

DISEASES OF THE ANORECTUM

Essentials of Diagnosis

- Pain that worsens with defecation is a common complaint.
- Bleeding is seen with hemorrhoids, fissures, or, rarely, tumors.

Clinical Findings

A. Symptoms and Signs: Anorectal disorders may cause significant morbidity, primarily as a result of pain. As with the general population, hemorrhoidal disease is the most common anorectal disorder and presents with anorectal pain or bleeding. Anal fissures cause anorectal pain, particularly with defecation, and may be associated with bleeding and rectal discharge. Fistulas, without any apparent underlying cause, may present with bleeding, pain, or discharge. Venereal diseases (syphilis, gonorrhea, chlamydia) should be suspected in the patient with symptoms of proctitis who engages in unprotected receptive anal intercourse.

CMV may cause solitary anorectal ulceration with severe pain or bleeding. HSV is associated with perianal disease; rarely, a distal proctitis may be seen.

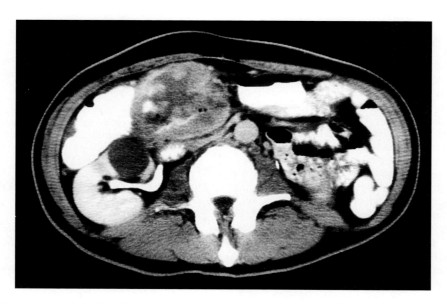

Figure 2–11. Colonic non-Hodgkin's lymphoma. Large mass lesion involving the proximal transverse colon.

Unexplained anorectal ulcerations have also been described in HIV-positive patients.

Neoplasms such as KS, NHL, cloacogenic carcinoma, and squamous cell carcinoma have been increasingly recognized. When these tumors ulcerate, pain and bleeding may occur; when they enlarge, obstruction results.

Physical examination plays an invaluable role in determining the underlying cause. Inspection of the perianal region may reveal ulcerations (neoplasms, infections such as HSV, CMV), mass lesions (KS, NHL, cloacogenic or squamous cell carcinoma) hemorrhoidal disease, or fissures. If digital rectal examination elicits exquisite tenderness, ulcerative disease of the anal canal is almost certainly present.

B. Endoscopy: These patients may need to be sedated to obtain an adequate evaluation; surgical proctoscopic examination may be necessary to obtain adequate biopsy samples. Sigmoidoscopic examination of the more proximal rectum may identify concurrent colitis or ulcers.

Treatment

Treatment depends on the underlying disorder. Local therapies and stool softeners are helpful for hemorrhoidal disease and fissures. When hemorrhoidal disease is precipitated by chronic diarrhea, antimotility agents to reduce stool frequency should be initiated. Medical therapy will be required for opportunistic infections. NHL responds to radiation therapy. Carcinomas respond poorly to therapy, although surgical excision has been used. Poor wound healing in the patient with severe immunodeficiency will limit the surgical options.

Melbye M et al: High incidence of anal cancer among AIDS patients. Lancet 1994;343:636.

Wilcox CM, Schwartz DA: Idiopathic anorectal ulceration in patients with human immunodeficiency virus infection. AmJ Gastroenterol 1994;89:599.

3   Acute Upper Gastrointestinal Bleeding

Rome Jutabha, MD, & Dennis M. Jensen, MD

This chapter discusses the diagnostic approach, acute and long-term management, and treatment options for acute upper gastrointestinal bleeding. **Acute upper gastrointestinal bleeding** refers to blood loss within the intraluminal gastrointestinal tract from any location between the upper esophagus to the duodenum at the ligament of Treitz. Specific causes of upper gastrointestinal bleeding will be reviewed and treatment modalities will be discussed (Tables 3–1 and 3–2).

The onset and severity of blood loss can range from intermittent and low-grade occult bleeding presenting as occult-blood-positive stools and iron deficiency anemia to very abrupt and massive blood loss presenting as hematemesis and hypovolemic shock. This discussion focuses on the medical and endoscopic management of severe, acute upper gastrointestinal bleeding that necessitates admission to an intensive care unit (ICU) and performance of emergency upper panendoscopy.

Acute upper gastrointestinal bleeding is responsible for significant morbidity and mortality. In addition, the costs to society in terms of hospital admission charges, lost work due to illness, and expense of maintenance therapy for prevention of rebleeding are staggering. Although there have been many advances in the past 50 years in critical care management, development of potent antisecretory medications, and new diagnostic and therapeutic technologies for acute upper gastrointestinal bleeding, the overall mortality rates have not changed significantly since 1945. More effective and safer endoscopic hemostasis modalities, such as thermal contact probes for control of nonvariceal hemorrhage and variceal band ligation for esophagogastric varices, have recently been developed and refined. Some of the randomized trials suggest improved morbidity and mortality rates for these new techniques as compared to traditional medical and surgical therapies.

By convention, upper gastrointestinal bleeding has been categorized as either variceal or nonvariceal in origin. **Gastroesophageal varices** are enlarged venous collateral channels that dilate as a consequence of portal hypertension. Varices gradually enlarge and eventually rupture, resulting in massive upper gastrointestinal hemorrhage. In contrast, **nonvariceal bleeding** results from disruption of esophageal or gastroduodenal mucosa with ulceration or erosion into an underlying vessel. Some examples of nonvariceal lesions responsible for upper gastrointestinal bleeding include Mallory-Weiss tears, gastroduodenal ulcers or tumors, and Dieulafoy's lesions.

Before the development of diagnostic endoscopy and therapeutic endoscopic hemostasis, the distinction between variceal and nonvariceal bleeding was of great importance because they were diagnosed and managed differently. Furthermore, before liver transplantation was an option, the long-term prognosis for variceal bleeders was dismal because of end-stage liver disease. Now, the basic principles of resuscitation and the acute management of active upper gastrointestinal bleeding are the same for all patients, regardless of the origin of bleeding. The approach to acute upper gastrointestinal bleeding will be discussed in detail in the next section of this chapter.

ACUTE MANAGEMENT OF SEVERE UPPER GASTROINTESTINAL BLEEDING

Patients experiencing severe upper gastrointestinal bleeding may present with dizziness, light-headedness, weakness, or pallor. They may also have palpitations, tachycardia, and hypotension. Patients may have anemia that is normochromic and normocytic. Blood loss is overt, demonstrated by vomiting or passing of blood in the stool.

The basic elements of the management of acute upper gastrointestinal bleeding include: (1) prompt patient resuscitation and stabilization, (2) assessment of the onset and severity of bleeding, (3) regional localization of the bleeding site, (4) determination of the most likely cause of upper gastrointestinal bleeding, (5) preparation for emergent upper panendoscopy, (6) control of active bleeding or treatment of lesions at high risk of rebleeding with therapeutic endoscopy, (7) minimization of treatment-related

Table 3–1. Causes of acute upper gastrointestinal bleeding.

Ulcerative, erosive, or inflammatory diseases
　　Peptic ulcer disease
　　　　Gastric or duodenal ulcer disease
　　　　Zollinger-Ellison syndrome
　　　　Gastroesophageal reflux disease
　　Stress ulcer
　　Infectious causes
　　　　Helicobacter pylori
　　　　Cytomegalovirus
　　　　Herpes simplex virus
　　Drug-induced erosions, ulcers, or bleeding
　　　　Aspirin
　　　　Nonsteroidal anti-inflammatory drugs (NSAIDs)
　　　　Pill-induced ulcer (tetracycline, quinidine, potassium
　　　　　　chloride tablets)
　　　　Anticoagulation therapy
Trauma
　　Mallory-Weiss tear
　　Foreign body ingestion
Vascular lesions
　　Varices
　　Angiomas and Osler-Weber-Rendu syndrome
　　Dieulafoy's lesion
　　Watermelon stomach (gastric antral vascular ectasia)
　　Portal hypertensive gastropathy
　　Aortoenteric fistula
　　Radiation-induced telangiectasia
Tumors
　　Benign
　　　　Leiomyoma
　　　　Lipoma
　　　　Polyp (hyperplastic, adenomatous, hamartomatous)
　　　　Blue rubber bleb nevus syndrome
　　Malignant
　　　　Adenocarcinoma
　　　　Leiomyosarcoma
　　　　Lymphoma
　　　　Kaposi's sarcoma
　　　　Carcinoid
　　　　Melanoma
　　　　Metastatic tumor
　　Miscellaneous
　　　　Hemobilia
　　　　Hemosuccus pancreaticus

Table 3–2. Therapeutic options for acute upper gastrointestinal hemorrhage.

Medical therapy
　　Peptic ulcer disease
　　　　Antisecretory therapy (H_2 receptor antagonist, proton
　　　　　　pump inhibitors)
　　　　Antacids
　　　　Sucralfate
　　　　Misoprostol
　　Gastroesophageal varices
　　　　Intravenous vasopressin with or without nitroglycerin
　　　　Intravenous octreotide
　　　　Balloon tamponade
Endoscopic therapy
　　Peptic ulcer disease
　　　　Thermal coagulation
　　　　　　Multipolar electrocoagulation (bicap or gold probe)
　　　　　　Heater probe
　　　　　　Laser therapy
　　　　Injection therapy
　　　　　　Epinephrine
　　　　　　Alcohol
　　　　Combination therapy: thermal coagulation and injection
　　Gastroesophageal varices
　　　　Injection sclerotherapy
　　　　Variceal band ligation
　　　　Cyanoacrylate injection
　　　　Combination therapy: sclerotherapy and band ligation
　　Tumors
　　　　Thermal probe (tumor, endoscopic bipolar, or heater
　　　　　　probe)
　　　　Laser ablation
　　　　Thermal balloon catheter
Surgical therapy
　　Nonvariceal (ulcer, tumor, or Mallory-Weiss tear)
　　Variceal
　　　　Portosystemic shunting
　　　　Esophageal transection and devascularization
　　　　Liver transplantation
Radiologic therapy
　　Peptic ulcer disease
　　　　Arterial embolization
　　　　Intra-arterial vasopressin infusion
　　Gastroesophageal varices
　　　　Embolization
　　　　Transjugular intrahepatic portosystemic shunting

complications, and (8) treatment of rebleeding episodes (Table 3–3).

PATIENT RESUSCITATION & STABILIZATION

The fundamental principles of emergency medicine apply to the patient presenting with acute upper gastrointestinal bleeding, namely, prompt assessment and establishment of the ABCs (airway, breathing, circulation). Elective endotracheal or nasotracheal intubation with or without mechanical ventilation is recommended before emergency endoscopy for patients with shock secondary to massive bleeding, ongoing hematemesis, severe agitation or altered mental status, or impaired respiratory status. This will facilitate both the diagnostic and therapeutic endoscopies and minimize the risk of aspiration. The en-

dotracheal tube can be removed after the effects of the premedication have worn off. In patients with hepatic encephalopathy, long-acting benzodiazepines should be avoided because they may exacerbate an already deteriorating mental status.

The importance of adequate resuscitation before diagnostic and therapeutic endoscopy cannot be overemphasized. Two large-caliber (18 gauge or larger) peripheral catheters should be inserted for intravenous access and volume replacement. High-risk patients (elderly or those with known cirrhosis or coronary artery disease) should receive packed red blood cell transfusion to maintain the hematocrit above 30%. Young and otherwise healthy patients should be transfused to maintain their hematocrit above 20%. Patients with a coagulopathy (prolonged prothrombin time) or low platelet count should be transfused with fresh frozen plasma and platelets, respectively.

Table 3–3. Management approach for acute upper gastrointestinal hemorrhage.

Acute management
  Patient stabilization (ABCs)[1]
    Respiratory stabilization (consider endotracheal intubation if altered respiratory status or ongoing hematemesis)
    Intravenous access
    Intravascular volume replacement
    Transfusions
      Packed red blood cells
      Fresh frozen plasma
      Platelets
  Focused history and physical examination
  Laboratory data
    CBC with platelet count
    Coagulation studies (PT/aPTT)[2]
    Liver enzymes
    Chemistries
  Radiographic (if perforation suspected)
    Upright chest x-ray
    Abdominal x-ray
  Electrocardiogram
  Localization of bleeding site (upper GI vs lower GI[3] vs small bowel)
  Surgery consultation
  Gastroenterology consultation for upper panendoscopy
    Diagnostic
      Localize source of bleeding
      Determine status of bleeding
      Risk stratification for further or recurrent bleeding
    Therapeutic
      Stop active bleeding
      Decrease the risk of recurrent bleeding
Long-term management
  Treatment of recurrent bleeding
    Repeat diagnostic and therapeutic endoscopy
    Angiography
    Surgery
  Preventive measures for peptic ulcer disease bleeding
    Maintenance antisecretory therapy
    Helicobacter pylori eradication
    Strict avoidance of ASA[4]/NSAIDs[5]
    Misoprostol
    Surgery
  Preventive measures for variceal bleeding
    Beta-blockers
    Obliterative endoscopic therapy
    Shunting
    Liver transplatation

[1]ABCs = airway, breathing, circulation.
[2]PT and aPTT = prothrombin time/activated partial thromboplastin time.
[3]GI = gastrointestinal.
[4]ASA = acetylsalicylic acid (aspirin).
[5]NSAIDs = nonsteroidal anti-inflammatory drugs.

ASSESSMENT OF ONSET & SEVERITY OF BLEEDING

The onset of bleeding refers to acute versus chronic blood loss. Symptoms and signs suggestive of chronic bleeding include weakness, lethargy, occult gastrointestinal bleeding with occult-blood-positive stool, and iron deficiency anemia (hypochromic, microcytic). In contrast, acute upper gastrointestinal blood loss is usually overt, demonstrated by **hematemesis** (vomiting of fresh blood or clots), coffee ground emesis (vomiting of coffee-ground-like blood), **melena** (dark, tarry-appearing stool), or **hematochezia** (fresh blood or clot per rectum). Acute upper gastrointestinal bleeding causes tachycardia, orthostatic hypotension, or syncope. Massive bleeding may lead to hypotensive shock, myocardial infarction, and cardiopulmonary arrest.

DETERMINATION OF THE BLEEDING SITE

Once the patient has been adequately stabilized, the next step is to determine the site of bleeding (upper gastrointestinal versus lower gastrointestinal versus small bowel) to guide the diagnostic workup. Emergent upper panendoscopy is indicated for patients with suspected acute upper gastrointestinal bleeding. Patient history, signs of upper gastrointestinal hemorrhage, and passage of a nasogastric tube will help distinguish upper gastrointestinal from lower gastrointestinal bleeding.

DETERMINATION OF THE CAUSE OF BLEEDING

The clinical history can yield useful information suggesting the site of gastrointestinal bleeding as well as the specific lesion. The medical history should include questions about prior episodes of upper gastrointestinal bleeding (ulcers or varices), liver disease, intestinal polyps or cancer, and blood transfusions. Pertinent symptoms include abdominal pain, nausea, vomiting, hematemesis, early satiety, anorexia, or weight loss. Medication history should include aspirin, nonsteroidal anti-inflammatory drugs (NSAIDs), and anticoagulation therapy (warfarin or heparin). Social history should focus on intravenous drug use, alcohol abuse, and sexual partners.

Physical examination should include a rectal examination, a nasogastric tube aspiration, assessment of stigmata of chronic liver disease (jaundice, spider telangiectasias, ascites). Melena is suggestive of upper gastrointestinal bleeding though it may be seen with small bowel bleeding or right-sided colonic lesions. Bright red blood per rectum or clot suggests a lower gastrointestinal bleeding source, though massive upper gastrointestinal bleeding may also present in this manner. A positive nasogastric aspirate yielding coffee ground material, clots, or bright red blood is highly suggestive of a recent upper gastrointestinal bleed. A negative nasogastric aspirate yielding clear fluid without bile will not exclude duodenal lesions, such as an ulcer.

For example, a patient with a history of peptic ulcer disease and aspirin use who presents with nausea, coffee ground emesis, and abdominal pain is suggestive of acute upper gastrointestinal bleeding resulting from recurrent peptic ulcer disease. A patient with a history of alcohol abuse presenting with massive hematemesis and signs of cirrhosis (eg, jaundice, tense ascites, and encephalopathy) should be suspected of having a variceal hemorrhage.

Laboratory data can be useful for assessing the degree of bleeding, determining possible sources of bleeding, and guiding therapy. Laboratory studies should include a complete blood count (CBC), an automated chemistry panel that includes liver function studies (alanine aminotransferase [ALT], aspartate aminotransferase [AST], bilirubin, albumin, total protein), and coagulation studies (prothrombin time [PT], partial thromboplastin time [PTT], bleeding time). It is important to keep in mind that the hematocrit may significantly underestimate the amount of blood loss during an acute bleed.

For example, abnormal liver enzymes may lead the clinician to suspect undiagnosed liver disease, and this abnormality may suggest varices as the source of acute bleeding. Laboratory studies such as serial hematocrits may be an indicator of ongoing bleeding or rebleeding and can help guide transfusions with packed red blood cells, fresh frozen plasma, and platelets. An electrocardiogram should be obtained for all patients with significant cardiac risk factors. An upright chest and abdominal x-ray should be performed in patients with suspected intestinal perforation, obstruction, or pulmonary aspiration.

PREPARATION FOR EMERGENT UPPER PANENDOSCOPY

Both a gastroenterologist and a surgeon should be notified promptly of all patients with severe acute upper gastrointestinal bleeding. Patients with hemodynamic instability (shock, orthostatic hypotension, decrease in hematocrit of *at least* 6%, or transfusion requirement over 2 units of packed red blood cells) or active bleeding (manifested by hematemesis, bright red blood per nasogastric tube, or hematochezia) should be admitted to an intensive care unit for resuscitation and close observation with automated blood pressure monitoring, ECG monitoring, and pulse oximetry.

Nasogastric tube or orogastric tube lavage should be performed to remove particulate matter, fresh blood, and clots. This will facilitate endoscopy and decrease the risk of massive aspiration.

CONTROL OF ACTIVE BLEEDING OR HIGH-RISK LESIONS

Diagnostic endoscopy can localize the site of acute upper gastrointestinal bleeding and stratify lesions at high risk versus low risk of bleeding. Stigmata of re-

cent ulcer hemorrhage include active bleeding, visible vessel, or adherent clot (Table 3–5). Endoscopic therapy should be limited to these high-risk lesions. Endoscopic treatments include thermal coagulation, injection therapy, and combination therapy. Specific modalities are discussed in further detail (see the following section, "Treatment").

MINIMIZATION OF TREATMENT-RELATED COMPLICATIONS

Complications can arise prior to, during, or after endoscopy. Complications that can occur before endoscopy include aspiration (especially in a sedated, combative, or encephalopathic patient), hypoventilation (related to oversedation), hypotension (due to inadequate volume replacement or transfusions in addition to sedation with narcotics). As previously mentioned, patients must be adequately resuscitated before endoscopy. Elective endotracheal intubation (with or without mechanical ventilation) may facilitate endoscopy and decrease the risk of aspiration.

Endoscopic complications are usually related to endoscopic hemostasis therapy and include precipitation or worsening of bleeding and perforation. Overly aggressive and repeated applications of thermal or injection therapy rarely increase the hemostasis rate but may increase the risk of treatment-induced complications. Therefore, a predetermined limit (amount of injection solution or total energy delivered) should be set and not exceeded.

TREATMENT OF PERSISTENT OR RECURRENT BLEEDING

For active bleeding that is not stopped or slowed down significantly with endoscopic therapy, alternative interventions such as surgery or radiographic modalities are indicated. For rebleeding lesions initially controlled by endoscopic therapy, endoscopy is repeated and the bleeding source is re-treated in the initial manner. If the bleeding persists or if rebleeding occurs after two therapeutic endoscopies, the patient is referred for surgery.

SPECIFIC CAUSES OF ACUTE UPPER GASTROINTESTINAL BLEEDING

This section discusses the diagnosis and management of specific causes of acute upper gastrointestinal bleeding, most common of which are peptic ulcer disease and gastroesophageal varices (Table 3–4).

Table 3–4. Causes of severe upper gastrointestinal bleeding.[1]

Diagnosis	Number of patients (%) (n=948)
Peptic ulcers	524 (55)
Gastroesophageal varices	131 (14)
Angiomas	54 (6)
Mallory-Weiss tear	45 (5)
Tumors	42 (4)
Erosions	41 (4)
Dieulafoy's lesion	6 (1)
Other	105 (11)

[1]Data from Center for Ulcer Research and Education (CURE) Hemostasis Research Group, UCLA School of Medicine and the West Los Angeles VA Medical Center.

ULCERATIVE OR EROSIVE DISEASES

Ulcerative or erosive diseases of the upper gastrointestinal tract that can cause acute upper gastrointestinal bleeding include peptic ulcer disease, Zollinger-Ellison syndrome, esophagitis, erosions of the stomach or duodenum, esophageal ulcers, stress-induced ulcers, infectious ulcers (herpes simplex virus, cytomegalovirus, or *Helicobacter pylori*), and medication-induced ulcers (aspirin, NSAIDs, pills).

1. PEPTIC ULCER DISEASE

Pathophysiology

Mucosal erosions or ulcers develop from an imbalance between aggressive factors and the protective factors of the mucosa. Aggressive factors that can damage normal mucosal integrity include hyperacidity, pepsin, bile salts, ischemia, aspirin and NSAIDs (decrease protective barrier by inhibition of mucosal prostaglandins), and *H pylori* (in duodenal ulcer, although the mechanism is not fully understood). Protective esophageal mechanisms include esophageal motility (clearance of refluxed acid), salivary secretions (bicarbonate), and the lower esophageal sphincter (prevents reflux). Gastric mucosal defenses include mucus, rapid epithelial renewal, and tissue mediators. Acute upper gastrointestinal bleeding occurs when an erosion or ulcer disrupts an underlying vein or artery.

Essentials of Diagnosis

- Abdominal pain, nausea, vomiting, and hematemesis or melena.
- Abdominal discomfort improved with food or antacids.
- History of aspirin or NSAID use, history of peptic ulcer disease and upper gastrointestinal bleeding.
- Epigastric tenderness, succussion splash suggestive of outlet obstruction.

General Considerations

Peptic ulcer disease is the most common cause of severe upper gastrointestinal bleeding, accounting for 30–50% of total cases. Bleeding peptic ulcers account for over 100,000 hospital admissions per year. Approximately 20–25% of ulcer patients with acute upper gastrointestinal bleeding have severe or recurrent bleeding. Their mortality rate is as high as 36%, due mainly to recurrent or persistent bleeding, surgical complications, or their underlying disease.

Clinical Findings

A. Symptoms and Signs: The symptoms of patients with bleeding ulcers are nonspecific and can range from silent disease to severe upper abdominal pain. Classically, ulcer pain is described as gnawing or cramping, lasting up to several hours, and relieved with food or antacids. Symptoms may recur episodically for a few weeks followed by asymptomatic periods for weeks or months. Other symptoms may include early satiety, abdominal distention, anorexia, nausea, or vomiting; these symptoms suggest a mechanical obstruction or altered gastroduodenal motility. Generally, however, only 30–40% of patients with severe ulcer hemorrhage have antecedent ulcer symptoms.

B. Laboratory Findings: Biochemical and hematologic abnormalities seen with upper gastrointestinal bleeding from peptic ulcer disease are nonspecific and may be seen with any cause of acute bleeding. These findings include acute anemia (normocytic, normochromic), elevated blood urea nitrogen (BUN) and creatinine (dehydration and prerenal azotemia), and prolonged bleeding time (due to aspirin or NSAID ingestion). An elevated serum gastrin level suggests Zollinger-Ellison syndrome.

C. Imaging: Endoscopy is the diagnostic method of choice because of high sensitivity and specificity. In addition, endoscopy can be used to collect biopsy specimens as well as to treat acute upper gastrointestinal bleeding (see following section, "Treatment"). Barium x-ray studies are less accurate and should not be performed during acute bleeding or when perforation is suspected. Angiography and radionuclide scans are rarely indicated in acute upper gastrointestinal bleeding, though angiography may be used to control acute bleeding with coil or Gelfoam embolization.

Differential Diagnosis

Benign peptic ulcer disease related to hyperacidity must be differentiated from ulcers caused by a malignant process (gastric or esophageal carcinoma), an infectious process, medications, or ischemia. The clinical history and endoscopic biopsies will help define the underlying cause. Other causes of upper abdominal discomfort include nonulcer dyspepsia, malignancy, cholelithiasis, and pancreatitis. However, most of these conditions are not associated with acute upper gastrointestinal bleeding.

Complications

Complications of bleeding peptic ulcer disease include pain, perforation, and obstruction. The latter are extremely rare in patients with bleeding ulcers. Other complications are related to endoscopy or therapeutic hemostasis. Complications associated with endoscopy include respiratory depression from premedication, aspiration, and perforation. Ulcers may enlarge or become deeper, or bleeding may worsen during or following endoscopic therapy because of tissue damage by the sclerosant or thermal coagulation.

Treatment

The immediate treatment of acute upper gastrointestinal bleeding secondary to peptic ulcer disease includes medical, endoscopic, and surgical interventions. Medical treatments may decrease the risk of recurrent bleeding after hospital discharge but do not alter the hospital course. In the case of ulcer hemorrhage with no stigmata or minor stigmata of recent hemorrhage, there is a very low rebleeding rate on medical therapy (Table 3–5). Early refeeding of these ulcer patients may be beneficial and may decrease hospital stay.

Medical treatments include antacids to neutralize gastric acidity, sucralfate, antisecretory therapy to decrease acid production, thereby accelerating ulcer healing and decreasing the long-term risk of ulcer recurrence and rebleeding, and prostaglandin analogs. Eradication of *H pylori* will decrease the risk of recurrent duodenal ulcer disease and may prevent recurrent bleeding. Antimicrobial treatment regimens include: (1) triple therapy with amoxicillin 500 mg four times daily (substitute tetracycline 500 mg four times daily for penicillin-allergic patients), metronidazole 250 mg three times daily and bismuth subsalicylate 2 tablets or 2 tsp four times daily for 2 weeks, or (2) omeprazole 40 mg daily plus clarithromycin 500 mg two times daily or amoxicillin 1 g two times daily for 2 weeks.

In randomized prospective studies, patients with active bleeding or nonbleeding visible vessels have a better outcome with endoscopic therapy than with medical therapy (Table 3–6). Ulcers with a clean base or a flat pigmented spot are at low risk of rebleeding and should not be treated endoscopically. Adherent clots that are not easily removed endoscopically from the ulcer crater, ie, with irrigation or gentle suctioning, carry a 20–30% risk of rebleeding. These clots should not be routinely treated with endoscopic therapy because randomized studies have not demonstrated a benefit compared to medical therapy.

Endoscopic treatment of gastroduodenal ulcers with active bleeding or nonbleeding visible vessels include injection therapy with absolute alcohol (98%) (total volume less than 1.0 mL) or epinephrine (1:10,000 up to 10 mL); thermal coagulation with a heater probe, multipolar probe or bipolar probe; or laser therapy. Gastric ulcers along the lesser curvature and duodenal bulbar ulcers in the posterior wall are at high risk for massive upper gastrointestinal bleeding because of their proximity to large underlying arteries (left gastric and posterior duodenal arteries, respectively). If endoscopic hemostasis is unsuccessful, emergency surgery may be necessary.

Surgery is usually reserved for complicated peptic ulcer disease, such as persistent or recurrent upper

Table 3–5. Endoscopic stigmata of recent hemorrhage in bleeding ulcers: Prevalence and risk of rebleeding.

Stigmata	Prevalence (%)	Risk of Rebleeding (%)
Active arterial bleeding	10	90
Nonbleeding visible vessel	25	50
Adherent clot	10	25
Oozing without visible vessel	5	<20
Flat spot	15	<10
Clean ulcer base	35	<5

Adapted with permission from Freeman ML: The current endoscopic diagnosis and intensive care unit management of severe ulcer and other nonvariceal upper gastrointestinal hemorrhage. In: Severe Nonvariceal Upper GI Hemorrhage. Jensen DM (editor). Gastrointest Endosc Clin North Am 1991;1:229.

Table 3–6. Rebleeding rates following medical versus endoscopic treatment.[1]

	Rebleeding Rate (%)		
	Medical	Gold Probe	Heater Probe
Peptic ulcers			
Active arterial bleeding	90	35	22
Nonbleeding visible vessel	52	35	23
Nonbleeding adherent clot	30	35	35
Oozing bleeding without clot or visible vessel	10	N/A[2]	N/A
Flat spots	7	N/A	N/A
Clean ulcer base	3	N/A	N/A
Dieulafoy's lesion			
Active arterial bleeding	100	40	40
Nonbleeding visible vessel	70	30	30
Mallory-Weiss tear without portal hypertension			
Active arterial bleeding	80	N/A	N/A
Nonbleeding visible vessel	<20	0	0

[1]Data from the Center for Ulcer Research and Education (CURE) Hemostasis Research Group, UCLA School of Medicine and the West Los Angeles VA Medical Center.
[2]N/A = not applicable.

gastrointestinal bleeding, nonhealing or giant ulcers, perforation, pyloric obstruction, or carcinoma. Emergency surgery for bleeding peptic ulcer disease is oversewing of the ulcer (to ligate the bleeding artery) plus truncal vagotomy (to decrease acid secretion) and pyloroplasty (drainage procedure). For nonemergency anti-ulcer surgery, more time-consuming procedures, such as highly selective vagotomy, can be performed laparoscopically.

Prognosis

The majority of patients with upper gastrointestinal bleeding from peptic ulcer disease will stop bleeding spontaneously and most will not rebleed during the hospitalization. However, a subgroup of patients are at high risk for recurrent bleeding. Clinical features suggestive of severe, recurrent upper gastrointestinal bleeding include hemodynamic instability, need for multiple transfusions, hematemesis of fresh blood or clots, hematochezia, the presence of a coagulopathy, and onset of bleeding during hospitalization. Endoscopic predictors of persistent or recurrent bleeding are active bleeding during endoscopy or a visible vessel. Endoscopic hemostasis should be reserved for these high-risk patients. Once patients are discharged from the hospital, the risk of recurrent ulcer bleeding is approximately 1% per month. This risk may be decreased significantly with maintenance H_2 receptor antagonist therapy. Eradication of *H pylori* in *H pylori*-positive patients with duodenal ulcer and prior upper gastrointestinal bleeding may significantly reduce both ulcer recurrence and rebleeding rates.

Graham DY et al: Treatment of *Helicobacter pylori* reduces the rate of rebleeding in peptic ulcer disease. Scand J Gastroenterol 1993;28:939.

Jensen DM: Endoscopic control of nonvariceal upper gastrointestinal hemorrhage. In: *Textbook of Gastroenterology*. Yamada T et al (editors). Lippincott 1991:2618.

Jensen DM et al: A randomized controlled study of ranitidine for preventing recurrent duodenal ulcer hemorrhage. N Engl J Med 1994;330:382.

Jensen DM (editor): Severe non-variceal upper gastrointestinal hemorrhage. Gastrointest Endosc Clin North Am 1991;1:209.

Kovacs TOG, Jensen DM: Therapeutic endoscopy for upper gastrointestinal bleeding. In:*Gastrointestinal Emergencies*. Taylor MD et al (editors). Williams & Wilkins, 1992.

NIH Consensus Conference: Therapeutic endoscopy and bleeding ulcers. JAMA 1989;262:1369.

2. STRESS ULCERS

Pathophysiology

There are relatively few data regarding critically ill patients hospitalized for a nongastrointestinal bleeding problem who subsequently develop upper gastrointestinal bleeding. Secondary upper gastrointestinal bleeding has been attributed to stress-related mucosal damage or stress ulceration. Despite its clinical importance, the pathogenesis of stress ulceration is not well understood. Some factors implicated in the pathogenesis of stress ulceration include acid hypersecretion in some patients, mucosal ischemia, and alteration in gastric mucus.

Essentials of Diagnosis

- Hematemesis or blood via a nasogastric tube in an ICU patient.
- Concomitant illness (multi-organ failure, sepsis, hypotension), trauma, major surgery, severe burn, prolonged mechanical ventilation.

General Considerations

Stress ulceration implies that various physiologic stresses experienced by critically ill patients predispose them to developing ulcers. Risk factors for the development of stress ulcers include multi-organ failure, prolonged mechanical ventilation, hypotension (septic shock carries a higher risk for stress ulceration than hypovolemic shock), severe trauma, major surgery, severe central nervous system injury, and severe burn involving more than 35% of body surface area (**Curling's ulcer**). Other factors that may play a role in secondary upper gastrointestinal bleeding include prior use of aspirin, NSAIDs, or steroids.

Clinical Findings

Patients with stress ulcer bleeding are often intubated and unable to report any symptoms. Signs of acute upper gastrointestinal bleeding in these patients include a falling hematocrit, a positive nasogastric aspirate of coffee ground material, bright red blood or clots, and melena. The diagnostic procedure of choice is upper panendoscopy.

Complications

The primary complication of stress ulceration is bleeding.

Treatment

Antacids, H_2-receptor antagonists, sucralfate, and omeprazole may be given prophylactically to high-risk patients to decrease acid production in hopes of decreasing the incidence of ulceration and upper gastrointestinal bleeding. However, these prophylactic therapies may not always be necessary, may not be uniformly effective, may increase the risk of nosocomial pneumonia, and can be both time-consuming and expensive. Treatment of acute stress ulcer bleeding should include prompt resuscitation and urgent endoscopic hemostasis as outlined above for peptic ulcer disease. Although patients with stress ulcers may have oozing of blood from multiple foci, severe upper gastrointestinal hemorrhage occurring after admission to an ICU for an unrelated problem is most often due to a single large, deep ulcer with active bleeding or visible vessel. Endoscopic hemostasis is feasible but rebleeding and slow healing are common in this subgroup of patients.

Prognosis

Patients with upper gastrointestinal bleeding beginning or recurring in the hospital do more poorly than those with upper gastrointestinal bleeding after discharge. Patients with stress ulcer hemorrhage are at increased risk for recurrent bleeding and other complications, such as perforation and death, and are more likely to require emergency surgery. This may reflect the severity of their concomitant illnesses.

Bresalier RS: The clinical significance and pathophysiology of stress-related gastric mucosal hemorrhage. J Clin Gastroenterol 1991;13(Suppl 2):S35.

Fusamoto H et al: A clinical study of acute gastrointestinal hemorrhage associated with various shock states. Am J Gastroenterol 1991;86:429.

Tryba M: Prophylaxis of stress ulcer bleeding: A meta-analysis. J Clin Gastroenterol 1991;13(Suppl 2):S44.

Weber FH, Peura DA: Gastrointestinal bleeding in the critical care unit. In: *Gastrointestinal Bleeding*. Sugawa C, Lucas CE, Schuman BM (editors). Igaku-Shoin, 1992.

3. MEDICATION-INDUCED ULCERS

Pathophysiology

Various medications play an important role in the development of peptic ulcer disease and acute upper gastrointestinal bleeding. Most notably, aspirin and NSAIDs can cause gastroduodenal erosions or ulcers, especially in elderly patients. A significant proportion of these patients develop bleeding ulcers. Steroids have also been implicated in ulcerogenesis though this hypothesis has not been well established. Other medications that can cause pill-induced esophageal ulcers and bleeding include various antibiotics (doxycycline, tetracycline, clindamycin), potassium chloride, quinidine, and iron pills. Anticoagulation therapy with heparin or warfarin may exacerbate ongoing upper gastrointestinal bleeding or may precipitate bleeding from a previously nonbleeding lesion.

Clinical Findings

Patients with impaired esophageal motility, eg, scleroderma or esophageal strictures are at increased risk for developing pill-induced ulcers. Patient history and medication history are essential in establishing the diagnosis. A history of dysphagia (difficulty with swallowing) or odynophagia (painful swallowing) after pill ingestion suggests a medication-induced ulcer.

Treatment

Medical treatment consists of discontinuation of the inciting medication. Patients on warfarin who are at risk of developing complications from active bleeding should be transfused with fresh frozen plasma and treated with vitamin K 10 mg subcutaneously daily for 3 days. Rebleeding is uncommon from medication-induced ulcers, thus, endoscopic therapy is rarely indicated except for control of active bleeding.

MALLORY-WEISS TEAR

Pathophysiology

Mallory-Weiss tears occur in the distal esophagus at the gastroesophageal junction, presumably after a bout of retching or vomiting, although often this antecedent is lacking. Bleeding occurs when the tear involves the underlying esophageal venous or arterial plexus. Patients with portal hypertension are at increased risk of massive bleeding from Mallory-Weiss tears compared to nonportal hypertensive patients.

Essentials of Diagnosis

- Antecedent nausea, retching, or vomiting followed by hematemesis.
- History of alcohol ingestion, chemotherapy, or medication ingestion.

General Considerations

In a series of 200 patients at UCLA admitted to the ICU with severe upper gastrointestinal bleeding, Mallory-Weiss tear was the fourth most common diagnosis, accounting for 6% of all cases. Most tears heal uneventfully within 24–48 hours and will not be seen if endoscopy is delayed.

Clinical Findings

A. Symptoms and Signs: The classic patient with acute upper gastrointestinal bleeding from a Mallory-Weiss tear is a young or middle-aged man presenting with hematemesis following an episode of retching or vomiting after drinking alcohol. Other systemic symptoms and signs are usually lacking; if there is concomitant chest or abdominal pain, fever, or shortness of breath, then esophageal perforation must be ruled out.

B. Imaging: Prompt endoscopy is the diagnostic procedure of choice. A Mallory-Weiss tear appears as an elliptical or longitudinal ulcer at the gastroesophageal junction, within a hiatal hernia, or on the gastric side just below the gastroesophageal junction. Upper gastrointestinal x-rays are usually nondiagnostic.

Differential Diagnosis

Mallory-Weiss tears must be distinguished from other ulcerative diseases of the esophagus, such as ulcerative reflux esophagitis, infectious esophagitis, or pill-induced esophageal ulcer. Mallory-Weiss tears are usually focal lesions with normal-appearing adjacent mucosa. In contrast, there is usually diffuse involvement of the distal esophagus with reflux or infectious esophagitis. Pill-induced ulcers are suspected by the history; usually these ulcers are more proximal in the esophagus.

Complications

Rebleeding may occur from the tear site. Perforation can occur spontaneously with repeated vomiting (*Boerhaave's syndrome*) or following endoscopic therapy.

Treatment

Because the majority of Mallory-Weiss tears stop bleeding spontaneously, endoscopic treatment is reserved for tears with active bleeding. Both injection therapy (epinephrine 1:10,000) and thermal coagulation have been used successfully to control active bleeding. The esophagus lacks a serosa and is very thin at the tear site. Therefore, injections or repeated coagulation should be avoided due to the risk of transmural injury and perforation. Thermal coagulation should not be performed in patients with portal hypertension and esophageal varices; sclerotherapy is preferable in such cases. Angiography can be performed to embolize a bleeding vessel. Surgical intervention, such as oversewing of the vessel, is rarely indicated. H_2 blockers, omeprazole, or sucralfate may be given to accelerate ulcer healing though this is not of proven benefit.

Prognosis

The majority of Mallory-Weiss tears heal spontaneously within 24–48 hours. Bleeding usually stops spontaneously and rebleeding occurs rarely.

Kovacs TOG: Endoscopic diagnosis and treatment of bleeding Mallory-Weiss tears. In: *Severe Nonvariceal Upper Gastrointestinal Hemorrhage.* Jensen DM (editor). Gastrointest Endosc Clin North Am 1991;1:387.

VASCULAR LESIONS

1. GASTROESOPHAGEAL VARICES

Pathophysiology

Esophageal and gastric varices are venous collaterals that develop as a result of systemic or segmental portal hypertension. The numerous causes of portal hypertension include prehepatic thrombosis (eg, portal or splenic vein), hepatic disease (eg, cirrhosis), and post-sinusoidal disease (eg, schistosomiasis). Alcoholic liver disease and viral hepatitis (B and C) are the most common causes of intrahepatic portal hypertension in the United States. Isolated gastric varices can develop following splenic vein thrombo-

sis (eg, acute or chronic pancreatitis or pancreatic tumor), causing segmental portal hypertension. Secondary gastric varices can develop after obliteration of esophageal varices with sclerotherapy.

Essentials of Diagnosis

- Massive upper gastrointestinal bleeding (hematemesis, hematochezia, hypotension, tachycardia).
- History of chronic liver disease and cirrhosis.
- Prior episodes of variceal bleeding.
- Jaundice, spider telangiectasias, splenomegaly, ascites, encephalopathy, asterixis.
- Elevated liver enzymes, coagulopathy, thrombocytopenia.

General Considerations

Nonbleeding esophagogastric varices that have never bled in the past should not be treated prophylactically via endoscopy. Active variceal bleeding can be acutely controlled by various endoscopic, radiologic, or surgical modalities. However, the risk of rebleeding remains high unless all distal esophageal varices are obliterated by serial endoscopic treatments or until portal hypertension is alleviated by portosystemic shunting or liver transplantation. Long-term survival is dependent on the severity of underlying liver disease.

Clinical Findings

A. Symptoms and Signs: Nonspecific symptoms of variceal bleeding include hematemesis, melena, hematochezia, and dizziness. Mental confusion secondary to hepatic encephalopathy may be seen in patients with severe liver disease. Skin manifestation of cirrhosis include jaundice, spider telangiectasias, caput medusa, palmar erythema, and Dupuytren's contracture. Signs of portal hypertension include hemorrhoids, ascites, splenomegaly. Patients with encephalopathy will have mental confusion and may develop asterixis and hepatic coma.

B. Laboratory Findings: Elevation of liver enzymes (ALT, AST, lactate dehydrogenase [LDH]) is seen with hepatocellular damage. Hyperbilirubinemia may be seen with decreased hepatic function. Poor liver synthetic function will result in hypoalbuminemia, hypocholesterolemia, and elevated PT. Pancytopenia may be secondary to hypersplenism or primary bone marrow suppression by alcohol. Progressive hypoglycemia and BUN and creatinine are seen with liver failure and hepatorenal syndrome.

C. Imaging: Endoscopy is the diagnostic modality of choice. Endoscopic ultrasound may be useful for differentiating gastric varices from gastric folds. Barium x-rays may image large esophageal varices or large gastric folds suggestive of gastric varices but the technique is not very sensitive. Portal vein angiography or abdominal CT may show venous collaterals and recanalization of the umbilical vein.

Differential Diagnosis

Nonvariceal causes must first be excluded before acute upper gastrointestinal bleeding can be attributed to varices. Peptic ulcer disease, esophagitis, and sclerotherapy induced ulcers are often the source of upper gastrointestinal bleeding in patients with previous variceal hemorrhage.

Complications

Massive variceal bleeding may be uncontrollable, resulting in hemorrhage and death. Variceal bleeding may precipitate hepatic encephalopathy and hepatorenal syndrome. Local complications related to endoscopic therapy include secondary ulcers (ulcers induced by sclerotherapy or band ligation), chest pain, esophageal dysmotility, perforation, rebleeding from secondary ulcers, and strictures. Systemic complications of sclerotherapy include pulmonary or pericardial effusion, sepsis, fever, peritonitis, allergic reactions to the sclerosants, mediastinitis, and portal vein thrombosis.

Treatment

Various modalities are available for the acute hemostasis of bleeding esophagogastric varices. They include various medical, endoscopic, radiologic, and surgical treatments.

A. Medical Therapy: Because the most likely source of acute upper gastrointestinal bleeding is nonvariceal in origin (even in patients with prior variceal bleeding), diagnostic endoscopy should be performed prior to instituting empiric therapies. Medical therapies include intravenous vasopressin (bolus of 20 U over 20 minutes, then an infusion of 0.1–0.5 U/min) plus intravenous nitroglycerin (40 µg/min titrated upward to maintain systolic blood pressure above 90 mm Hg; maximum dose of 400 µg/min), intravenous octreotide (25–50 µg bolus, then 25–50 µg/hr continuous infusion), and balloon tamponade (esophageal, gastric, or both). Tamponade balloons have been associated with many complications, such as aspiration and perforation; all patients must be intubated and adequately sedated and the balloon should not be inflated for over 24 hours. These therapies should not be instituted before endoscopic confirmation of variceal bleeding.

B. Endoscopic Therapy: Endoscopic hemostasis is the treatment of choice for bleeding esophageal varices. The first objective of endoscopy is to identify a definitive source for the bleeding episode. Varices should be examined for stigmata of recent hemorrhage (active bleeding, adherent clot, red wale markings, hematocystic spots, veins on veins). If these stigmata are absent, nonvariceal sources of bleeding, such as ulcers or Mallory-Weiss tears, should be suspected and must be excluded. The vast majority of esophageal varices that bleed are located in the distal 5–10 cm of the esophagus, therefore, endoscopic treatments should be limited to this region. Endoscopic therapies include injection sclerotherapy, variceal band ligation, and combination therapy.

Gastric varices have been considered to be poorly responsive to endoscopic therapy because of high rebleeding rates from sclerotherapy-induced ulcers. Bleeding gastric varices can be technically difficult to treat endoscopically. Therefore, gastric varices should not be treated outside of randomized controlled trials. Recent studies report successful hemostasis and obliteration of gastric varices with intravariceal injections of absolute alcohol and cyanoacrylate, although the latter is not available in the USA.

1. Endoscopic injection sclerotherapy–Endoscopic injection sclerotherapy is the most well-established endoscopic treatment for bleeding esophageal varices. Endoscopic sclerotherapy has many advantages. It has proven safe and effective, it is low in cost and widely available, it is easy to learn and can be performed simply and rapidly, and it can be used in the outpatient setting for elective (obliteration) treatment. Numerous sclerotherapy techniques and various sclerosants have been used successfully for bleeding esophageal varices. A suggested sclerotherapy technique for bleeding esophageal varices is summarized in Table 3–7.

2. Variceal band ligation–Variceal band ligation is a new endoscopic modality for the treatment

Table 3–7. Endoscopic injection sclerotherapy technique for bleeding esophageal varices.

Needle size	25 gauge
Needle length	4–5 mm
Sclerosant	
Agent	Equal volume mixture of 3% sodium tetradecyl sulfate, 98% ethanol, 0.9 normal saline (TES)
Amount/injection	≤ 2–3 mL
Maximum volume	< 50 mL[2]
Injection site	
Initial treatment	Bleeding site
Concomitant treatment	Each varix at GEJ[3] then 2.5 and 5.0 cm above GEJ
Follow-up treatment	Residual esophageal varices in the distal 5 cm
Adjuvant therapy	Ranitidine 150 mg twice daily
Treatment interval	1 week after initial treatment, then once every 2–3 weeks until obliteration of distal esophageal varices

[1]Data from the Center for Ulcer Research and Education (CURE) Hemostasis Research Group, UCLA School of Medicine and the West Los Angeles VA Medical Center.
[2]Maximum volume for esophageal refers to volume to inject into all distal esophageal varices at GEJ, then 2.5 cm and 5 cm above the GEJ during first sclerotherapy session.
[3]GEJ = Gastroesophageal junction.

of bleeding and nonbleeding esophageal varices. The variceal banding technique is similar to hemorrhoid banding and involves placing small elastic bands around varices in the distal 5 cm of the esophagus. Varices are suctioned into the banding device and bands are released around the base of the varix by pulling a trip wire via the biopsy channel. The advantages of band ligation over sclerotherapy include fewer local complications (secondary bleeding from ulcers or strictures), no systemic side effects, and the need for fewer treatments for variceal obliteration. Some of the drawbacks of band ligation include a restricted endoscopic view (due to the banding device and blood pooling within the hood mechanism), difficulty performing treatments in the retroflexed position in the fundus of the stomach, and repeated removal and reinsertion of the endoscope to reload the single-shot banding device.

3. Radiologic therapy–Radiologic therapies include venous embolization and **transjugular intrahepatic portosystemic shunt (TIPS)**. TIPS is a new radiologic method of creating a portosystemic shunt via a transjugular approach to decrease portal pressure. It can control active variceal bleeding in patients who have failed endoscopic treatment and has been used for the treatment of refractory ascites. Some complications of TIPS include worsening of encephalopathy, shunt occlusion and rebleeding, and shunt migration. In addition, the procedure is expensive and is technically difficult to perform. Stenosis or TIPS occlusion occurs in at least 40% of patients followed for 6 months; repeat TIPS or other therapy is required to prevent recurrent variceal hemorrhage. This treatment should be reserved for patients with persistent variceal bleeding despite endoscopic treatments.

4. Surgical therapy–Surgical therapies include portosystemic shunting, esophageal transection and devascularization, and liver transplantation. Portosystemic shunting may decrease the risk of rebleeding; however, encephalopathy may worsen and overall survival is not improved. Esophageal transection and devascularization has been utilized for acute hemostasis and prevention of rebleeding in Europe and Japan, but is not performed in the USA. Splenectomy is the treatment of choice for isolated gastric varices due to splenic vein thrombosis.

Prognosis

Variceal bleeding stops spontaneously in over 50% of patients. In those patients with continued bleeding, mortality approaches 70–80%. Medical treatments are only temporary measures and the patient is at high risk of rebleeding once these treatments are removed or discontinued. Each recurrent episode of bleeding carries a significant risk of mortality. The risk of rebleeding is high (60–70%) until gastroesophageal varices are obliterated by subsequent endoscopic sclerotherapy session to treat resid-

ual varices. Unfortunately, long-term survival is not improved following successful variceal obliteration. Propranolol therapy for patients undergoing elective sclerotherapy can further decrease the risk of rebleeding and may increase survival. The onset of massive upper gastrointestinal bleeding from gastroesophageal varices usually signifies advanced liver disease (Child class B or C). The majority of patients die within 6–12 months because of progressive hepatic decompensation, rebleeding, or other complications. Liver transplantation is the only treatment that significantly improves the long-term prognosis.

Jutabha R, Jensen DM: Endoscopic injection sclerotherapy for bleeding esophageal and gastric varices. In:*Advanced Therapeutic Endoscopy,* 2/e. Barkin JS, O'Phelan CA (editors). Raven Press, 1994.

Laine L et al: Endoscopic ligation compared with sclerotherapy for the treatment of bleeding esophageal varices. Ann Intern Med 1993;119:1.

Sarin SK et al: Prevalence, classification and natural history of gastric varices: A long-term follow-up study in 568 portal hypertension patients. Hepatology 1992;16:1343.

Stiegmann GV et al: Endoscopic sclerotherapy as compared with endoscopic ligation for bleeding esophageal varices. N Engl J Med 1992;326:1527.

Vinel J et al: Propranolol reduces the rebleeding rate during endoscopic sclerotherapy before variceal obliteration. Gastroenterology 1992;102:1760.

2. ANGIODYSPLASIA OF THE UPPER GASTROINTESTINAL TRACT

Pathophysiology

In contrast to colonic angiomas, which are believed to develop from chronic low-grade venous obstruction associated with aging, the cause of upper gastrointestinal angiomas is unknown.

Essentials of Diagnosis

- Chronic or acute recurrent episodes of bleeding.
- Long history of bleeding requiring multiple transfusions prior to diagnosis.
- Multiple nondiagnostic endoscopic procedures performed previously.
- Iron deficiency anemia and occult-blood-positive stools.
- Associated disorders–renal failure, von Willebrand's disease, aortic stenosis, cirrhosis, pulmonary disease.

General Considerations

Other terms used synonymously with angioma include arteriovenous malformation, telangiectasia, vascular ectasia, and angiodysplasia. Upper gastrointestinal angiomas account for 1.2–8.0% of patients with occult-blood-positive stool and iron deficiency anemia. Infrequently, patients with upper gastrointestinal angiomas present with acute bleeding. Small bowel angiomas are the most common cause of gastrointestinal bleeding of obscure origin. Upper gastrointestinal angiomas may be suggestive of angiomas elsewhere in the gastrointestinal tract or may be part of the Osler-Weber-Rendu syndrome or hereditary hemorrhagic telangiectasia.

Clinical Findings

Bleeding from upper gastrointestinal angiomas is usually low-grade and intermittent, causing hemoccult-positive stools and iron deficiency anemia. Video endoscopy and enteroscopy are the diagnostic procedures of choice for evaluating upper gastrointestinal and small bowel angiomas. The classic angiographic features of intestinal angiomas include an early filling vein, a vascular tuft, and a late-draining vein.

Differential Diagnosis

Because upper gastrointestinal angiomas infrequently cause acute gastrointestinal bleeding, it is important to exclude other causes of upper gastrointestinal bleeding such as peptic ulcers, Mallory-Weiss tears, or varices. Incidental angiomas rarely bleed, therefore, treatment is not indicated.

Treatment

Hormonal therapy with combination estrogen and progesterone for bleeding angiomas has yielded conflicting results. Endoscopic therapy with thermal coagulation is the treatment of choice for bleeding upper gastrointestinal angiomas. Thermal coagulation may be performed with contact probes at a low power setting, eg, multipolar electrocoagulation (10–15 watts × 1-second pulses) or heater probe (10–20 joules/pulse). Nd:YAG laser may be used at a low power setting (40–100 watts × 0.2–0.5 seconds). There is limited experience with injection therapy for upper gastrointestinal angiomas.

The endoscopic endpoint for thermal coagulation of angiomas is mucosal whitening and ablation of all visible angiomatous tissue. It is important to avoid excessive bowel distention, high power generator settings, firm probe pressure, and repeated coagulation to the same area to minimize the risk of transmural injury and perforation. Surgical therapy such as intraoperative enteroscopy is reserved for failures of endoscopic and medical therapy.

Prognosis

Over one-half of patients stop bleeding spontaneously without any therapy. For patients with recurrent bleeding, endoscopic therapy can decrease the number of bleeding episodes as well as the transfusion requirement.

Foutch PG: Angiodysplasia of the gastrointestinal tract. Am J Gastroenterol 1993;88:807.

Lewis BS et al: Does hormonal therapy have any benefit for bleeding angiodysplasia? J Clin Gastroenterol 1992;15(2):99.

Machicado GA, Jensen DM: Upper gastrointestinal angiomata. Diagnosis and treatment. In: *Severe Nonvariceal Upper GI Hemorrhage*. Jensen DM (editor). Gastrointest Endosc Clin North Am 1991;1:241.

Van Cutsem E, Rutgeerts P, Vantrappen G: Treatment of bleeding gastrointestinal vascular malformations with oestrogen-progesterone. Lancet 1990;335:953.

3. DIEULAFOY'S LESION

Pathophysiology

Dieulafoy's lesion is a dilated aberrant submucosal vessel that erodes the overlying epithelium and is not associated with a primary ulcer. The cause of Dieulafoy's lesion is unknown but it may be related to ischemia with thinning of the mucosa. Massive arterial bleeding occurs when the submucosal artery erodes through the gastric mucosa.

Essentials of Diagnosis

- Massive upper gastrointestinal bleeding with multiple nondiagnostic upper panendoscopies.
- Endoscopy reveals a visible vessel (actively bleeding or nonbleeding) without an associated ulcer.

Clinical Findings

Bleeding may be self-limited though it is usually recurrent and can be massive. Diagnosis is best made with endoscopy during acute bleeding, which may reveal active arterial pumping from a point without an associated ulcer or mass lesion. In the absence of active bleeding, it may look like a raised nipple or visible vessel without an associated ulcer. The aberrant vessel is often not seen unless there is active bleeding from the site. Dieulafoy's lesions are usually located in the upper stomach along the high lesser curvature within 6 cm of the gastroesophageal junction.

Treatment

Endoscopic hemostasis with multipolar electrocoagulation or heater probe thermal coagulation is the treatment of choice for controlling acute bleeding. The risk of rebleeding after endoscopic therapy remains high because of the unusual size of the underlying artery. Surgical wedge resection, therefore, is recommended when endoscopic therapy fails. Endoscopic tattooing with India ink injections helps to locate the lesion intraoperatively. Recently, Doppler ultrasound has been used to confirm ablation of a Dieulafoy's lesion by documenting the absence of blood flow after injection therapy. There is no further risk of rebleeding from a Dieulafoy's lesion once it is surgically resected.

Jaspersen D: Dieulafoy's disease controlled by Doppler ultrasound endoscopic treatment. Gut 1993;34:857.

Reilly HF, Al-Kawas FH: Dieulafoy's lesion. Diagnosis and management. Dig Dis Sci 1991;36:1702.

4. WATERMELON STOMACH (Gastric Antral Vascular Ectasia)

Clinical Findings

Watermelon stomach, or **gastric antral vascular ectasia** has a characteristic endoscopic appearance of longitudinal rows of erythematous mucosa radiating from the pylorus into the antrum. The red stripes represent ectatic and sacculated mucosal vessels resembling the stripes on a watermelon. Diagnosis is based on the classic endoscopic appearance but may be confirmed with endoscopic biopsy. Bleeding is most often chronic, with patients presenting with occult-blood-positive stools and iron deficiency anemia and requiring repeat transfusions. Occasionally, acute or massive upper gastrointestinal bleeding can occur.

Treatment

Acute bleeding may be controlled with endoscopic coagulation with heater probe, multipolar electrocoagulation, or laser therapy, which decreases transfusion requirement. Antrectomy will prevent recurrent bleeding.

Potamiano S, Carter CR, Anderson JR: Endoscopic laser treatment of diffuse gastric antral vascular ectasia. Gut 1994;35:461.

5. PORTAL HYPERTENSIVE GASTROPATHY

Clinical Findings

Portal hypertensive gastropathy or congestive gastropathy has a characteristic endoscopic appearance described as a fine, white reticular pattern separating areas of pinkish mucosa (snakeskin appearance). Histologically there is extensive edema and capillary and venous dilatation in the submucosa extending into the mucosa. The mucosa is friable and bleeding occurs presumably when the ectatic vessels rupture. It has been postulated but not proven that sclerotherapy increases the likelihood of developing portal hypertensive gastropathy by increasing back pressure; however, there is no correlation between the degree of portal hypertension and portal hypertensive gastropathy.

Bleeding gastroesophageal varices must be excluded before attributing acute upper gastrointestinal hemorrhaging to portal hypertensive gastropathy. Portal hypertensive gastropathy appears to be a rare cause of significant upper gastrointestinal bleeding in cirrhotic patients.

Treatment

Treatments for bleeding from portal hypertensive gastropathy are directed at decreasing portal pressure, such as portocaval shunt surgery, TIPS, or low-dose propranolol (20–40 mg/d, then doubled each day until bleeding stops or diastolic blood pressure falls below 70 mm Hg or encephalopathy develops). Endoscopic thermal coagulation or injection therapy are ineffective for control of active bleeding. H_2 blockers, sucralfate, and surgical resection are also ineffective.

Hosking SW: Portal hypertensive gastropathy. Gastrointest Endosc Clin North Am 1992;2(1):111.

Viggiano TR, Gostout CJ: Portal hypertensive intestinal vasculopathy: A review of the clinical, endoscopic, and histopathologic features. Am J Gastroenterol 1992;87(8):944.

6. AORTOENTERIC FISTULA

Pathophysiology

Aortoenteric fistulas arise from a direct communication between the aorta and the gastrointestinal tract. Prior to 1960 the most common causes of abdominal aortoenteric fistulas were aortic aneurysm and infectious aortitis secondary to syphilis or tuberculosis. Now an infected prosthetic aortic graft eroding into the intestine is a more common cause. Other conditions that can result in an aortoenteric fistula include penetrating ulcer, tumor invasion, trauma, radiation therapy, and foreign body perforation. Pressure necrosis and graft infection have been implicated in the development of a fistula.

Essentials of Diagnosis

• Massive upper gastrointestinal bleeding with a history of aortic prosthetic graft or abdominal aortic aneurysm.
• Endoscopy often nondiagnostic in the absence of active bleeding or protruding prosthetic graft.
• Positive endoscopy may reveal a graft, adherent clot, or extrinsic pulsatile mass in the distal duodenum.

General Considerations

Aortoenteric fistula is a rare cause of acute upper gastrointestinal bleeding but is associated with a very high mortality rate if undiagnosed and left untreated. The third or fourth portion of the duodenum is the most common site for aortoenteric fistulas, followed by the jejunum and ileum.

Clinical Findings

A. Symptoms and Signs: Most patients have an initial herald bleed manifested by hematemesis or hematochezia, or both. This may be followed by a massive bleed resulting in hemorrhagic shock. Intermittent bleeding can be seen if a blood clot temporarily seals the fistula. About one-half of patients have abdominal or back pain, and fewer than 50% have fever or signs of sepsis. Infrequently an abdominal mass may be palpable or an abdominal bruit may be heard.

B. Imaging: A high index of suspicion is needed to exclude this diagnosis. In a stable patient without active bleeding, endoscopy with a colonoscope (ie, enteroscopy) is the procedure of choice to rule out other causes of acute upper gastrointestinal bleeding, such as ulcers. Occasionally, endoscopy shows an aortic graft that has eroded into the bowel lumen. Abdominal CT and aortography can be useful in confirming the diagnosis but may be unreliable. Exploratory laparotomy is indicated for patients with suspected aortoenteric fistula and severe, ongoing bleeding.

Treatment & Prognosis

The treatment for aortoenteric fistula resulting from an infected graft is emergent surgery for graft removal and intravenous antibiotics. The mortality rate of an untreated aortoenteric fistula is nearly 100%.

Nagy SW, Marshall JB: Aortoenteric fistulas. Postgrad Med 1993;93:211.

TUMORS

Pathophysiology

Acute bleeding from upper gastrointestinal tumors usually represents a late stage of disease in which the neoplasm has outgrown its blood supply, resulting in mucosal ulceration. Bleeding can occur from diffuse mucosal ulceration or from erosion into an underlying vessel.

Essentials of Diagnosis

- Anorexia, weight loss, early satiety, or dysphagia.
- Cachexia, hemoccult-positive stools, iron deficiency anemia.
- Upper endoscopy reveals an ulcerated mass with stigmata of recent hemorrhage (oozing, clot, or visible vessel).

General Considerations

Neoplasms of the upper gastrointestinal tract account for less than 3% of cases of acute upper gastrointestinal bleeding. These tumors can be benign or malignant; malignant lesion may be either primary tumors or metastatic lesions. Benign lesions of the upper gastrointestinal tract include leiomyomas, lipomas, polyps, and blue rubber bleb nevus syndrome. Primary malignant tumors include adenocarcinoma, leiomyosarcoma, lymphoma, Kaposi's sarcoma, and carcinoid tumor; metastatic tumors to the upper gastrointestinal tract include melanoma, breast cancer, colon carcinoma, and lung cancer.

Clinical Findings

A. Symptoms and Signs: Esophageal tumors may produce luminal obstruction or ulceration causing **dysphagia** (difficulty swallowing) or **odynophagia** (painful swallowing). Bulky gastric tumors may cause anorexia and early satiety. Duodenal tumors can cause gastric outlet obstruction resulting in chronic nausea, vomiting, and bezoar formation. Ulcerative tumors may cause perforation or fistulas, such as an esophageal-pulmonary fistula, which may present as recurrent aspiration pneumonia. Nonspecific signs of malignancy include cachexia and weight loss.

B. Laboratory Findings: Nonspecific laboratory findings include hypoalbuminemia and hypocholesterolemia (owing to malnutrition) and iron deficiency anemia (as a result of chronic bleeding). Metastatic colon carcinoma to the upper gastrointestinal tract may be associated with an elevated carcinoembryonic antigen (CEA) level.

C. Diagnostic Techniques: The diagnostic modality of choice is upper panendoscopy. Endoscopic findings suggestive of malignancy are irregular ulcer margins, and exophytic or fungating ulcerated mass. Endoscopic biopsy, brushing, or needle aspiration for histologic or cytologic examination are performed for definitive diagnosis. Endoscopic ultrasound is useful for staging local disease. Barium x-rays should be avoided if bleeding, obstruction, or fistulas are suspected because the barium will interfere with endoscopy and may result in barium peritonitis or aspiration. CT is helpful for staging and evaluating distant metastases.

Differential Diagnosis

Mucosal and submucosal upper gastrointestinal tumors must be differentiated from malignant extrinsic masses that erode through the upper gastrointestinal tract. Because such extrinsic masses involve the gut wall transmurally, endoscopic treatment should be conservative due to the high risk of perforation.

Complications

Complications of upper gastrointestinal tumors besides bleeding include cachexia, luminal obstruction (esophageal or duodenal tumors), perforation, and fistula formation.

Treatment

For potentially curable lesions, surgical resection is the treatment of choice. Large upper gastrointestinal tumors, either benign or malignant, that are symptomatic, ie, producing bleeding, obstruction, perforation, or fistulas, should be resected if the patient is a good surgical candidate. Endoscopic treatment for bleeding upper gastrointestinal tumors includes injection therapy, thermal contact probes (tumor probe, multipolar electrocoagulation, heater probe), and laser therapy. Rebleeding frequently occurs, thus, endoscopic hemostasis is a temporizing measure before staging and surgical resection. Medical therapy is most often palliative and consists of chemotherapy, radiation therapy, or both.

Prognosis

Patients with bleeding secondary to malignant upper gastrointestinal tumors have a very dismal prognosis, with the majority of patients dying within 1–3 months. Patients with benign upper gastrointestinal tumors that are successfully resected are cured.

Randall GM, Jensen DM: Diagnosis and management of bleeding from upper gastrointestinal neoplasms. In: *Severe Nonvariceal Upper Gastrointestinal Hemorrhage.* Jensen DM (editor). Gastrointest Endosc Clin North Am 1991;1:401.

MISCELLANEOUS CAUSES OF ACUTE UPPER GASTROINTESTINAL BLEEDING

1. HEMOBILIA

Hemobilia, or bleeding from the biliary system, is a rare cause of acute upper gastrointestinal bleeding. The classic triad of hemobilia includes biliary colic, obstructive jaundice, and occult or acute gastrointestinal bleeding. Some causes of hemobilia include hepatic trauma (eg, after liver biopsy), gallstones, hepatic or bile duct tumors, hepatic artery aneurysm, and hepatic abscess. The diagnosis is often overlooked, but the condition can be identified by endoscopy if there is active bleeding from the ampulla. A side-viewing duodenoscope may be helpful in viewing the ampulla or for performing diagnostic endoscopic retrograde cholangiography. Technetium tagged red blood cell scan or selective hepatic arteriography may reveal the source of hemobilia. Hemobilia may be associated with obstructive jaundice and biliary sepsis. Treatment is directed at the primary cause of bleeding, utilizing surgical resection or arterial embolization.

2. HEMOSUCCUS PANCREATICUS

Bleeding from the pancreatic duct is also a rare cause of upper gastrointestinal bleeding. Pancreatic pseudocysts and pancreatic tumors are the most common causes of hemosuccus pancreaticus. Bleeding occurs when a pseudocyst or tumor erodes into a vessel, forming a direct communication between the pancreatic duct and blood vessel. The diagnosis may be made by endoscopy and a retrograde pancreaticogram, angiography, or abdominal CT. Complications related to the pseudocyst include infection and perforation. Surgical resection with ligation of the bleeding vessel provides definitive treatment. Mesenteric arteriography with coil embolization usually will control acute bleeding and may obviate the need for an operation.

Acute Lower Gastrointestinal Bleeding

4

Thomas J. Savides, MD, & Dennis M. Jensen, MD

Lower gastrointestinal bleeding is generally defined as bleeding from below the ligament of Treitz. In this chapter, lower gastrointestinal bleeding will refer to bleeding from the colon, while bleeding from between the ligament of Treitz and the ileocecal valve will be referred to as **small bowel bleeding.** Bleeding from the esophagus, stomach, or duodenum is **upper gastrointestinal bleeding.**

Patients with lower gastrointestinal bleeding usually present with bright red bleeding per rectum. The majority of patients (approximately 85%) have acute, self-limited, nonhemodynamically significant bleeds, such as occurs with hemorrhoids, colonic polyps, colon cancer, or colitis. Approximately 15% of patients will have severe, ongoing hematochezia, which is hemodynamically significant (Figure 4–1).

Severe bleeding that appears to be from a lower source may actually come from an area proximal to the terminal ileum, as 11% of patients with severe hematochezia actually have an upper gastrointestinal source (proximal to the ligament of Treitz) and 9% have a small bowel source (between the ligament of Treitz and the ileocecal valve) (Figure 4–2). Even with extensive diagnostic evaluation, the source of bleeding is not determined in 6% of patients with severe hematochezia. When severe bleeding is localized to the colon on the basis of colonoscopy or angiography, the bleeding lesion is located in the right colon 75% of the time.

The potential sources of colonic bleeding are shown in Table 4–1. The most common causes of severe lower gastrointestinal bleeding are angiomata and diverticula, as shown in Table 4–2.

CLINICAL CHARACTERISTICS OF LOWER GASTROINTESTINAL BLEEDING

Hematochezia is defined as bright red blood passed per rectum; it is the most common presentation of lower gastrointestinal bleeding. Hematochezia usually suggests a left colon source of bleeding, although it may occur with brisk upper gastrointestinal or small bowel bleeding and rapid transit of blood.

Maroon stools are defined as maroon-colored blood mixed with melena, and are usually indicative of a lower gastrointestinal source (especially the right colon). However, upper gastrointestinal or small bowel bleeding with rapid transit of blood also can cause maroon stools.

Melena is defined as black, tarry, foul-smelling stools, melena occurs when hemoglobin is converted to hematin or other hemochromes by bacterial degradation over a period of at least 14 hours. These degradation products cause the black color of melena. Melena usually indicates an upper gastrointestinal or small bowel site, although melena can occur from a right colon lesion if motility is slow. All black stools are not melena, as bismuth, charcoal, licorice, and iron preparations can turn the stool color black. For this reason it is important to do a guaiac test on all black stool for the presence of hemoglobin degradation products.

Occult bleeding occurs when there is no change in the color of the stool because only small quantities of blood pass into the gastrointestinal tract at any given time. This is detected by testing the stool with a guaiac card test.

INITIAL EVALUATION OF PATIENTS WITH RECTAL BLEEDING

The history should include direct questions, for example:

1. Does the blood coat the outside of formed, hard stool (suggesting internal hemorrhoidal bleeding), or is it mixed in with the stool (internal source)? Is there bloody diarrhea or tenesmus (eg, owing to colitis)?
2. Is this a chronic, intermittent problem, or an acute event?
3. Is there a history of gastrointestinal bleeding, previous gastrointestinal surgery, peptic ulcer, inflammatory bowel disease, ischemic heart disease (suggesting the possibility of ischemic colitis), internal hemorrhoids, rectal trauma, change in bowel habits (cancer), weight loss (cancer), aspirin or nonsteroidal anti-inflamma-

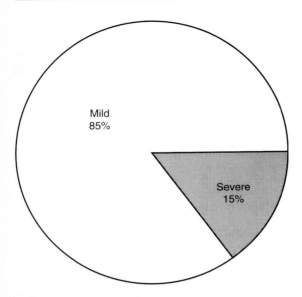

Figure 4–1. Severity of lower gastrointestinal bleeding.

Table 4–1. Potential etiologies of hematochezia from colonic lesions.

Internal hemorrhoids
Angiodysplasia
Diverticula
Cancer
Polyps
Ulcerative colitis
Crohn's colitis
Infectious colitis
Ischemic colitis
Rectal trauma
Rectal varices
Anal fissures
Anal ulcers
Post-polypectomy
External hemorrhoids

tory drug (NSAID) use, alcohol abuse (upper gastrointestinal or rectal varices), abdominal pain (ischemia, inflammatory bowel disease), rectal pain (anal fissure, hemorrhoids, rectal ulcer), constipation (hemorrhoids, mass), lack of pain (hemorrhoids, diverticula, angiodysplasia), recent antibiotics (antibiotic-associated colitis), or recent travel (infectious colitis)?

The following steps should be followed to ensure a complete physical examination:

1. Assess vital signs, particularly for the presence of shock or orthostatic hypotension.
2. Palpate the abdomen to assess for tenderness or masses.
3. Evaluate stool color by rectal examination and perform guaiac card test to determine if blood is in the stool.
4. Perform anoscopy to look for active bleeding from internal hemorrhoids. The presence of a nonbleeding hemorrhoid implies that the bleeding site is probably not hemorrhoidal.
5. Perform nasogastric tube lavage (if bleeding is severe). Even if no blood returns, there is still about a 15% chance that bleeding is from a site proximal to the ligament of Treitz. If bile returns, however, this virtually excludes an active upper gastrointestinal source of bleeding.

Hematocrit, mean cell volume, platelet count, prothrombin time, and partial thromboplastin time should be measured.

INITIAL ASSESSMENT & MANAGEMENT OF SUSPECTED LOWER GASTROINTESTINAL BLEEDING

Severe bleeding is defined as acute bleeding with either postural hypotension or a decrease in hemat-

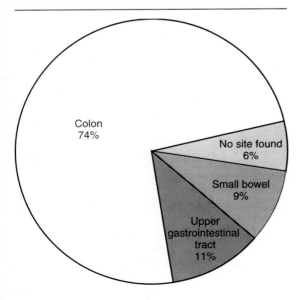

Figure 4–2. Actual bleeding sites in patients with hematochezia.

Table 4–2. Frequency of colonic bleeding sites in patients with severe hematochezia.

Angiomata	40%
Diverticulosis	22%
Polyps or cancer	15%
Colitis	12%
Other	11%

ocrit (or both) of at least 8% from baseline after volume resuscitation. Severity should also account for the higher risk of complications in elderly patients or patients with other significant medical problems.

Patients with **mild** lower gastrointestinal bleeding can be electively evaluated as outpatients. If the patient is younger than 50 years old, has a bleeding history characteristic of internal hemorrhoids, and has a normal hematocrit and mean cell volume, then anoscopy and flexible sigmoidoscopy should be performed to confirm the presence of hemorrhoids and exclude the possibility of a distal rectosigmoid polyp or cancer. An elective air-contrast barium enema is also recommended if a bleeding lesion is not found by flexible sigmoidoscopy and anoscopy. Patients 50 years old or over should undergo a full colonoscopy if they present with new onset hematochezia, even if suggestive of hemorrhoids, because of the increased risk of colonic polyps and tumors (Figure 4–3).

Patients with **severe** lower gastrointestinal bleeding should be hospitalized for resuscitation, diagnosis, and treatment (Figure 4–4). Stabilization involves fluid resuscitation with saline and packed red blood cells, and correction of any coagulopathy or thrombocytopenia. Patients with severe, acute gastrointestinal bleeding should be admitted to an intensive care unit and should be seen by both a gastroenterologist and a surgeon. Once a patient is medically stabilized, a polyethylene glycol purge should be given over 3–4 hours, followed by urgent colonoscopy. Enough polyethylene glycol solution should be given such that the rectal effluent is relatively free of blood clots and debris. The polyethylene glycol may need to be given via a nasogastric tube. If a patient with profuse hematochezia cannot be medically resuscitated because of ongoing bleeding, then that patient should go immediately for surgical exploration and treatment.

Figure 4–5 is a flow chart summarizing the initial assessment of rectal bleeding, as previously described.

DIAGNOSTIC & THERAPEUTIC OPTIONS

Anoscopy

Anoscopy is excellent for diagnosing bleeding lesions in the rectal canal, such as fissures, ulcers, or internal hemorrhoids. Anoscopy should be used in conjunction with flexible sigmoidoscopy or colonoscopy in the evaluation of hematochezia.

Flexible Sigmoidoscopy

Flexible sigmoidoscopy uses a 65-cm instrument (as opposed to the colonoscope measuring 130–160 cm). It is mostly indicated for outpatient examination of patients younger than 50 years old who have mild lower gastrointestinal bleeding with an expected source located distal to the splenic flexure. Turnaround examination in the rectum is necessary to exclude isolated lesions that can be missed by rigid sigmoidoscopy. Sigmoidoscopy is not as reliable as anoscopy for diagnosing internal hemorrhoids.

Colonoscopy

Colonoscopy should be the initial imaging procedure in patients with severe rectal bleeding after medical resuscitation. An oral polyethylene glycol purge over 3–4 hours will clear the gastrointestinal tract of stool and blood. Colonoscopy can generally be performed safely, offering examination of the entire colon, including the cecum and possibly the terminal ileum. Bleeding site is determined by visualizing active bleeding from a lesion, stigmata of a recent bleed (such as a visible vessel or adherent clot), or blood in an area around a lesion without other lesions in that segment of bowel to explain the blood. Flat mucosal lesions, such as angiodysplasia, can be easily seen. Hemostasis can be performed through the colonoscope with electrocautery probes, heater probes, epinephrine injection, or polypectomy snares. Complications from colonoscopy and colonoscopic hemostasis are rare, and include perforation and induced bleeding.

Push Enteroscopy

When no source for the bleeding is seen with colonoscopy or esophagogastroduodenoscopy (standard endoscopy), then repeat upper endoscopy can be performed with a pediatric colonoscope (130 cm long). Using the **push enteroscopy** technique, the endoscope can be passed 40–60 cm beyond the ligament of Treitz. Longer enteroscopes have been developed that measure 200–250 cm and can be advanced 80–120 cm beyond the ligament of Treitz.

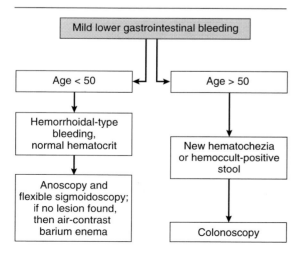

Figure 4–3. Diagnostic and therapeutic approach to mild lower gastrointestinal bleeding.

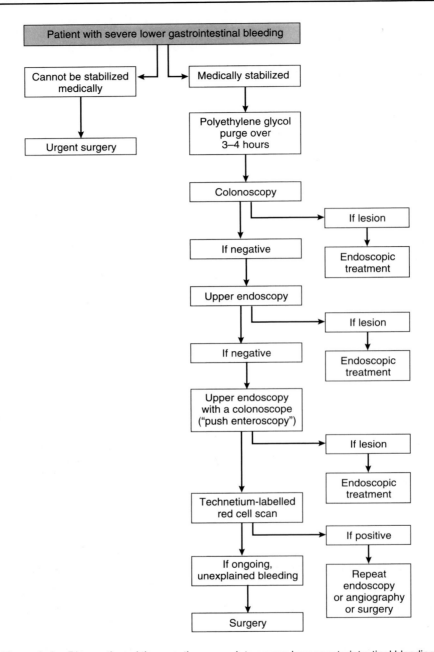

Figure 4–4. Diagnostic and therapeutic approach to severe lower gastrointestinal bleeding.

Forcep biopsies or therapeutic coagulation of bleeding lesions can be performed with these enteroscopes. Other flexible endoscopes are being developed to allow visualization into the ileum.

Barium Enema

There is no role for emergency barium enema in a patient with severe lower gastrointestinal bleeding. This test is rarely diagnostic because it cannot demonstrate vascular lesions and may be misleading if only diverticula are present. Subsequent colonoscopy will be necessary for obtaining biopsies if a suspicious lesion is seen on barium enema, and unlike colonoscopy or angiography, barium enema provides no opportunity for simultaneous therapy. Furthermore, barium enema will delay subsequent colonoscopy or angiography until the barium clears after several days. Nevertheless, air-contrast barium enema is indicated for complete evaluation of young adult outpatients (younger than 50 years old) with

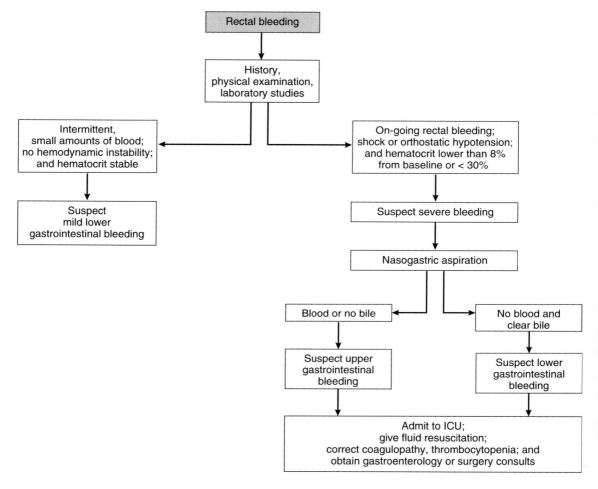

Figure 4–5. Initial assessment of rectal bleeding.

self-limited bright red blood per rectum when flexible sigmoidoscopy and anoscopy are negative.

Angiography

Angiography involves cannulating the femoral artery, then passing catheters into the superior mesenteric artery and inferior mesenteric artery and injecting contrast. Arterial bleeding can only be detected when the rate is 0.5 ml/min or greater. The diagnostic yield depends on patient selection, timing of the procedure, and the skill of the angiographer, with positive yields in 12–69% of cases. An advantage of angiography is that intravascular selective embolization can allow control of some bleeding lesions. The possible complications of angiography include bowel ischemia and infarction, hematomas, arterial embolization, and renal failure induced by contrast dye.

Nuclear Medicine Scintigraphy

Nuclear medicine scintigraphy involves injecting a radio-labelled substance into the patient's bloodstream, then performing serial scintigrams to detect focal collections of radio-labelled material. It has been reported to detect bleeding at a rate as low as 0.1 ml/min. Blood is removed from the patient, the red blood cells are labelled with ^{99m}technetium, and the labelled blood is reinjected into the patient. Scanning is typically performed early (1 and 4 hours after injection) and late (24 hours). An early scan that is positive is often more helpful than a delayed scan for localization of the bleeding site. The labelled red blood cells will circulate for at least 24 hours after injection, therefore, repeated scans can be performed in cases of intermittent bleeding.

In patients with active bleeding, the red blood cell scan demonstrates a bleeding site in approximately 50% of patients with active bleeding, but the detection rate is lower with slower or intermittent bleeding. The most common false positive scan occurs when there is rapid transit of luminal blood, such that labelled blood is detected in the colon although it originated in the upper gastrointestinal tract. There is no therapeutic benefit from nuclear medicine scintigraphy.

Surgical Exploration

Surgical exploration is indicated for those patients with severe, ongoing hematochezia who cannot be medically resuscitated because of active blood loss. Patients with recurrent bleeding from a site previously localized by colonoscopy, angiography, or scintigraphy may also require surgical intervention. Preoperative localization of a lesion by endoscopy lowers the operative mortality risk.

Baum S: Angiography of the gastrointestinal bleeder. Radiology 1982;143:569.

Farrands PA, Taylor I: Management of acute lower gastrointestinal hemorrhage in a surgical unit over a 4-year period. J R Soc Med 1987;80:79.

Jensen DM, Machicado GA: Diagnosis and treatment of severe hemotochezia. Gastroenterology 1988;95:1569.

Jensen DM, Machicado GA: Techniques of hemostasis for lower GI bleeding. In:*Medical Laser Endoscopy.* Jensen DM, Brunetaud JM (editors). Kluwer Academic Publishers, 1990;99.

Lewis BS, Waye JD: Chronic gastrointestinal bleeding of obscure origin: Role of small bowel enteroscopy. Gastroenterology 1988;94:1117.

Nicholson ML et al: Localization of lower gastrointestinal bleeding using in vivo technetium-99m-labelled red blood cell scintigraphy. Br J Surg 1989;78:358.

Rex DK et al: Flexible sigmoidoscopy plus air contrast barium enema versus colonoscopy for suspected lower gastrointestinal bleeding. Gastroenterology 1990;98:855.

Ryan P, Styles CB, Chmiel R: Identification of the site of severe colon bleeding by technetium-labelled red-cell scan. Dis Colon Rectum 1992;35:219.

SPECIFIC DISORDERS CAUSING LOWER GASTROINTESTINAL BLEEDING

1. INTERNAL HEMORRHOIDS

Essentials of Diagnosis

- Intermittent, self-limited bright red blood per rectum.
- Blood often coats outside of stool and is seen on tissue.
- Characteristic findings on anoscopy.

General Considerations

Internal hemorrhoids are a plexus of veins just above the rectal squamocolumnar junction. Symptomatic hemorrhoids are common in adults, mostly associated with prolonged straining during bowel movements, chronic constipation, pregnancy, obesity, and low-fiber diet.

Clinical Findings

A. Symptoms and Signs: Bleeding is usually bright red blood per rectum that coats the outside of the stool. Fresh blood is often present on the tissue paper after wiping and in the toilet water. Bleeding from internal hemorrhoids is usually painless and may be associated with constipation, straining, or hard stool. Patients often have a lifelong history of such intermittent bleeding. Patients may also note nonbleeding symptoms of hemorrhoids, such as prolapse, itching, or mucus discharge.

B. Laboratory Findings: The hematocrit is generally normal, although patients can occasionally loose large amounts of blood from hemorrhoidal bleeding.

C. Imaging: Anoscopy is the best imaging modality for determining the presence of internal hemorrhoids. A slotted, metal anoscope is better than a clear plastic cylindrical anoscope in detecting hemorrhoids. Hemorrhoids should be suspected as the site of bleeding if active bleeding is seen, or if there is a fresh clot overlying a hemorrhoid. Otherwise, all other colonic sources of bleeding should be excluded.

D. Grading: Internal hemorrhoids are graded for severity. Grade 1 are inside the rectal canal and do not prolapse. Grade 2 prolapse with bowel movements, but spontaneously go back into the rectal canal. Grade 3 are prolapsed (outside the rectal canal) but can be manually reduced. Grade 4 remain outside the rectal canal and cannot be reduced. Lower grades of internal hemorrhoids respond to medical therapy. Anoscopic therapy is effective for grades 1–3, and surgery is usually required for grade 4.

Differential Diagnosis

Bright red blood per rectum in a hemodynamically stable patient with a normal hematocrit implies a rectal source of bleeding. Besides internal hemorrhoids, the differential diagnosis includes external hemorrhoids, rectal varices, fissures, ulcers, polyps, tumors, and proctitis. External hemorrhoids that bleed are acutely painful and are located outside the rectal canal.

Complications

Rarely, ongoing bleeding may occur that requires urgent treatment.

Treatment

A. Medical Therapy: Most patients will respond to warm sitz baths, lubricant rectal suppositories (with or without steroids), and increased dietary fiber.

B. Anoscopic Therapy: Injection sclerotherapy, rubber band ligation, cryosurgery, infrared photocoagulation, and bipolar and direct current electrocoagulation have all been successfully used to treat acute and chronic internal hemorrhoidal bleeding.

C. Surgical Hemorrhoidectomy: Surgery is reserved for patients with chronic bleeding or other symptoms that cannot be controlled with medical or anoscopic treatment. Usually, such patients have grade 3 or 4 hemorrhoids, which require manual reduction or are not manually reducible.

Prognosis

Most patients will have resolution of bleeding with medical measures, whereas the patients who fail medical management will almost always respond to anoscopic treatment. Surgical treatment is reserved for patients who fail medical and anoscopic treatment.

Dennison AR, Wherry DC, Morris DL: Hemorrhoids: Nonoperative management. Surg Clin North Am 1988;68: 1401.
Randall GM et al: Prospective randomized comparative study of bipolar versus direct current electrocoagulation for treatment of bleeding internal hemorrhoids. Gastrointest Endosc 1994;40:403.

2. COLONIC ANGIOMAS

Essentials of Diagnosis

- Common cause of lower gastrointestinal bleeding in the elderly.
- Bleeding typically intermittent, mild, and painless, but can cause severe hematochezia.
- Mostly located in the right colon.

General Considerations

Colonic angiomas are also referred to as angiodysplasia, arteriovenous malformations, or vascular ectasias. These lesions, which are acquired with age, represent degeneration of previously normal blood vessels in the cecum and proximal ascending colon. They are not associated with systemic telangiectasias, which are contained and can occur at any age. Histopathology reveals a large, dilated, submucosal vein and, in advanced cases, dilated mucosal veins with small arteriovenous communications. Proposed explanations for angioma formation include the partial obstruction of submucosal veins passing through the colonic muscle layers, with eventual dilation of the submucosal and mucosal veins, and local mucosal ischemia.

By histopathologic injection studies, colonic vascular ectasias may be found in over 25% of asymptomatic persons over the age of 60. However, by colonoscopy the frequency of incidental (asymptomatic) right colonic angiomata is less than 5%. An association between colonic angiomas and aortic stenosis has been reported, as has improvement of recurrent bleeding after aortic valve replacement, although the cause and effect of this relationship is unclear.

Clinical Findings

A. Symptoms and Signs: Elderly patients can present with occult bleeding manifested by iron-deficiency anemia, or intermittent mild or severe episodes or hematochezia. There is no pain associated with angiomas.

B. Laboratory Findings: Acute bleeding causes an acute decrease in hematocrit; chronic bleeding causes microcytic anemia.

C. Imaging: Colonoscopy reveals angiomas as red, spider-like subepithelial lesions in the right colon. The colonoscopic appearance of vascular lesions is influenced by blood pressure and intravascular volume, and lesions may not be evident until after a patient has had adequate fluid resuscitation. Sedation with meperidine hydrochloride during colonoscopy may make vascular lesions difficult to see because of splanchnic vasodilation, resulting in decreased mucosal blood flow; therefore, this drug should be used in minimal doses or reversed with naloxone during the procedure. Colonoscopic biopsy of suspected angiomas demonstrates histologic evidence of these lesions in fewer than 50% of biopsies. This may be related to tissue damage during processing or submucosal location of the lesions.

Angiography can identify the site of active bleeding if contrast material extravasates into the intestinal lumen. Bleeding is usually intermittent, and no active extravasation is found. Angiography can also demonstrate angiodysplasia even without active bleeding. The angiographic signs of angiodysplasia are (1) a densely opacified, slowly emptying dilated tortuous vein seen during the venous phase, (2) a vascular tuft seen during the arterial phase, which represents dilated mucosal venules, and (3) an early-filling vein in the arterial phase, which represents an arteriovenous communication.

Differential Diagnosis

Vascular lesions can also occur as part of systemic diseases. **Osler-Weber-Rendu** disease (hereditary hemorrhagic telangiectasias) is an autosomal dominant condition characterized by telangiectasias that affect mucocutaneous areas as well as internal organs. Patients may have telangiectasias involving the lips, mouth, face, hands, gastrointestinal tract, liver, lungs, and brain. Diffuse vascular lesions can also be seen in uremia, pseudoxanthoma elasticum, Ehlers-Danlos syndrome, and the CREST variant of scleroderma (calcinosis, Raynaud's phenomenon, esophageal dysmotility, sclerodactyly, and telangiectasia).

Trauma during colonoscopy may cause artifacts that resemble colonic angiomata. Therefore, the colonoscopist must look closely for lesions before pressing the colonoscope against an area of mucosa.

Treatment

Endoscopic therapy allows colonic angiomata to be coagulated with either bipolar electrocoagulation, monopolar electrocoagulation, heater probe, or laser. Endoscopic coagulation can control acute bleeding from colonic angiomata in most patients, although at least 20% of patients will have recurrent bleeding and require additional colonoscopic treatment sessions. With long-term follow-up, patients who receive colonoscopic treatment of angiomata will have a significant decrease in frequency of bleeding episodes and number of units of packed red blood cells transfused per year, and an increase in mean hematocrit compared to pretreatment levels.

The main risks of colonoscopic coagulation of angiomata are perforation, postcoagulation syndrome, and delayed bleeding. Perforation occurs in fewer than 1% of patients; **postcoagulation syndrome,** defined by abdominal pain, focal rebound tenderness, fever, and leukocytosis without evidence of perforation, occurs in 2%; and delayed bleeding occurs in 4%.

Actively bleeding angiomata can be treated at the time of angiography with selective embolization of branches of the mesenteric artery using gelfoam or metal coils. Surgery may also be useful in treating active bleeding and bleeding that recurs despite adequate endoscopic treatment.

Prognosis

Patients with bleeding angiodysplasia often have scattered or diffuse lesions in the colon and even other parts of the gastrointestinal tract. Although endoscopy, angiography, or surgery can stop acute bleeding, these patients are likely to have recurrent bleeding in the future. The goal of repeat endoscopic therapy is to reduce, if not totally eliminate, the number of bleeds, hospitalizations, and transfusions.

Boley SJ et al: On the nature and etiology of vascular ectasias of the colon. Degenerative lesions of aging. Gastroenterology 1977;72:650.

Jensen DM, Machicado GA: Endoscopic diagnosis and treatment of bleeding colonic angiomas and radiation telangiectasia. In: *Prospectives in colon and rectal surgery.* Schrock T (editor). Quality Medical Publishing, 1989.

Reinus JF, Brandt LJ: Vascular ectasias and diverticulosis. Gastro Clin North Am 1994;23:1.

3. COLONIC DIVERTICULA

Essentials of Diagnosis

- Painless hematochezia.
- Common cause of lower gastrointestinal bleeding in the elderly.
- Mostly located in the sigmoid colon.

General Considerations

Diverticula are acquired lesions that occur with aging. Diverticula are herniations of colonic mucosa and submucosa through the muscular layers of the colon. What are called diverticula in the colon, are, in fact, pseudodiverticula, as true diverticula contain all layers of the intestinal wall. Colonic diverticula seem to form when colonic tissue is pushed out by intraluminal pressure. They vary in diameter from a few milliliters to several centimeters. The most common location is the left colon. Most colonic diverticula are asymptomatic and remain uncomplicated.

Diverticula are common in Western countries, with a prevalence of 50% in adults. In contrast, fewer than 1% of the African and Asian populations have diverticula. This has lead to the hypothesis that regional differences in prevalence can be explained by the low amounts of dietary fiber in Western diets. Presumably, the low-fiber diet results in less stool content, longer fecal transit time, increased colonic muscle contraction, and, ultimately, increased intraluminal pressure that results in the formation of propulsion diverticula.

Diverticula occur at the point of entry of the small arteries that supply the colon, the **vasa recta.** The entry points of the vasa recta are areas of relative weakness through which the mucosa and submucosa can herniate when under increased intraluminal pressure. Bleeding usually occurs from vessels at the neck of the diverticula, but can occur from vessels at the base as well.

Diverticular bleeding will stop spontaneously in over 80% of patients but will recur in approximately 25% of these persons.

Clinical Findings

A. Symptoms and Signs: Patients generally present with painless hematochezia, although mild left lower quadrant discomfort may be present. Most patients have mild, self-limited bleeding, but occasionally severe bleeding occurs.

B. Laboratory Findings: Patients may have anemia with acute blood loss.

C. Imaging: Colonoscopy after urgent bowel cleansing can identify diverticula as the source of bleeding based on active bleeding or fresh blood in a segment of colon with no other lesions but diverticula. Mesenteric angiography and radionuclide bleeding scans can also demonstrate diverticular bleeding if there is active bleeding and contrast extravasates into the colon lumen.

Differential Diagnosis

The main differential diagnosis in elderly patients is angiodysplasia, once internal hemorrhoids have been excluded. Other causes for painless hematochezia include polyps or tumors.

Complications

Patients with colonic diverticula can also develop diverticulitis (left lower quadrant pain, fever, elevated white blood cell count) or peridiverticular abscess, but these complications are extremely unusual in the presence of diverticular bleeding.

Treatment

Endoscopic treatment of bleeding diverticula has been reported with heater probe coagulation, bipolar probe coagulation, and epinephrine injection. Endoscopic treatment is best directed at the active bleeding site or visible vessel at the neck of the diverticulum, because this area is thicker than the base and therefore at less risk for perforation. Patients treated for bleeding diverticula have reportedly shown no recurrent bleeding during an average follow-up of 1 year.

Mesenteric angiography can demonstrate bleeding diverticula, and selective arterial infusion of vasopressin or selective embolization of mesenteric arterial branches can provide effective initial hemostasis. These patients often undergo subsequent elective surgical resection of the diseased area.

Surgical segmental colectomy is recommended for uncontrollable bleeding in patients who cannot be medically resuscitated or in whom bleeding cannot be stopped with endoscopic or angiographic means. Surgery may be considered in cases of recurrent diverticular bleeding in which the exact location of bleeding is fairly certain.

Prognosis

Most patients will have self-limited bleeding, which requires supportive care and accurate diagnosis. Those patients with profuse bleeding or recurrent bleeding can generally be managed successfully with surgical therapy.

Baum S et al: Selective mesenteric arterial infusions in the management of massive diverticular hemorrhage. N Engl J Med 1973;288:1269.

Bertoni G et al: Endoscopic injection hemostasis of colonic diverticular bleeding: A case report. Endoscopy 1990;22:154.

Goldberger LE, Bookstein JJ: Transcatheter embolization for treatment of diverticular hemorrhage. Radiology 1977;122:613.

Kim YI, Marcon NE: Injection therapy for colonic diverticular bleeding. A case study. J Clin Gastroenterol 1993;17:46.

McGuire HH, Haynes BW: Massive hemorrhage from diverticulosis of the colon: Guidelines for therapy based on bleeding patterns observed in fifty cases. Ann Surg 1972;175:847.

Savides TJ, Jensen DM: Colonoscopic hemostasis for recurrent diverticular hemorrhage associated with a visible vessel: A report of three cases. Gastrointest Endosc 1994;40:70.

4. COLON CANCER

Essentials of Diagnosis

- Weight loss.
- Change in bowel habits.
- Iron-deficiency anemia.

General Considerations

Colon cancer is one of the leading causes of cancer-related morbidity and mortality in the United States. Most patients with colon cancer present with occult gastrointestinal blood loss rather than hematochezia. For adult patients with hematochezia, determining the presence or absence of a colon cancer is imperative, because early diagnosis improves survival. Because a cancer must ulcerate for overt bleeding to occur, most bleeding cancers present at a relatively advanced tumor stage.

Clinical Findings

A. Symptoms and Signs: Patients with left-sided colonic cancers may note a recent change in bowel habits. This can be new constipation owing to an obstructing lesion, or can be diarrhea caused by only liquid stool passing around a distal colonic lesion. Some patients may have weight loss and a palpable mass, either on abdominal or rectal examination. Painless occult or overt rectal bleeding is the most common presentation.

B. Laboratory Findings: Patients often will have had chronic blood loss in addition to acute blood loss and will be found to have a microcytic and iron-deficiency anemia. Patients with suspected colon cancer should not be screened with a carcinoembryonic antigen (CEA) test, as this is useful only after the diagnosis and primary treatment of the colon cancer.

C. Imaging: Colonoscopy is the procedure of choice. Not only will the lesion be imaged, but biopsies can also be obtained at the same time. Flexible sigmoidoscopy combined with air-contrast barium enema has also been used for colorectal cancer screening of patients with hemoccult-positive stools.

Treatment

The most definitive therapy is surgical resection. Surgery is useful for both attempted cure, as well as palliation by preventing colonic obstruction. If the patient is not able to undergo surgery because of other medical problems, then endoscopic therapy (especially in the rectum) can be attempted, using laser coagulation, bipolar probe coagulation, or injection of epinephrine or alcohol.

Eckhauser ML: The neodymium-YAG laser and gastrointestinal malignancy. World J Surg 1992;16:1054.

Randall GM, Jensen DM: Diagnosis and management of bleeding from upper gastrointestinal neoplasms. Gastrointest Endosc Clin North Am 1991;1:401.

5. ISCHEMIC COLITIS

Essentials of Diagnosis

- Sudden-onset, crampy, left lower abdominal pain followed by hematochezia.

- Radiographs show thick wall ("thumb-printing").
- Colonoscopy shows segmental submucosal hemorrhage.

General Considerations

Ischemic colitis, which results from mucosal hypoxia, is caused by hypoperfusion of the intramural vessels of the intestinal wall, rather than by large vessel occlusion. Usually, this hypoperfusion is caused by vascular disorders, such as atherosclerosis or vasculitis, but it can also be caused by increased blood viscosity, such as occurs with polycythemia vera. Acute hypotension may also precipitate local ischemia in patients with vascular disease. Because of collateral circulation, the ischemic involvement is usually segmental and primarily affects the mucosal aspect of the intestine. The colon is mostly affected in the "watershed areas," such as the splenic flexure or rectosigmoid junction, in which there is reduced collateral circulation.

Clinical Findings

A. Symptoms and Signs: Patients usually present with sudden- onset, severe, crampy left lower quadrant abdominal pain with diarrhea and hematochezia. Physical examination should reveal bowel sounds and mild distention and tenderness. If there are peritoneal signs, one must consider transmural damage with perforation.

B. Laboratory Findings: Decreased hematocrit is noted, but transfusion is usually not required.

C. Imaging: Abdominal radiographs typically demonstrate "thumb-printing" or thickening of the colon wall caused by intramural hemorrhage. Usually there is segmental involvement, especially of the splenic flexure or rectosigmoid junction. Colonoscopy will reveal submucosal hemorrhage, ulceration, or necrosis. There is no role for angiography because large mesenteric vessels are not involved.

Differential Diagnosis

This includes acute infectious colitis, ulcerative colitis, Crohn's disease, and *Clostridium difficile*-induced pseudomembranous colitis.

Complications

Patients may develop severe intestinal ischemia or infarction with peritoneal signs, chronic segmental ulcerating colitis, colonic strictures, or fulminant pancolitis.

Treatment

Most patients' symptoms resolve with 24–48 hours, with radiographic or colonoscopic resolution by 2 weeks. Specific therapy is not needed for mild, self-limited disease. Treatment with 5-aminosalicylic acid or steroids may be useful, although effectiveness is not clearly proven. Attention should be paid to cor-

recting any underlying medical conditions which may have contributed to the ischemia, such as cardiac disease, medications, vasculitis, or polycythemia vera. Patients with severe or ongoing bleeding should receive broad-spectrum antibiotics. If uncontrollable bleeding or peritoneal signs are present, surgical resection of the diseased bowel is indicated.

Boley SJ, Brandt LJ: Colonic ischemia. Surg Clin North Am 1992;72:203.
MacDonald PH, Beck IT: Mesenteric ischemia. In: *Current therapy in gastroenterology and liver disease,* 4/e. Bayless TM (editor). Mosby 1994.

6. RADIATION COLITIS

Essentials of Diagnosis

- Symptoms begin weeks to months after radiation treatment.
- Recurrent hematochezia and rectal pain.
- Multiple telangiectasias seen on colonoscopy.

General Considerations

Ionizing radiation can cause acute and chronic damage to the normal colon and rectum after radiation treatment for gynecologic, prostatic, bladder, or rectal tumors. Approximately 75% of patients who receive 4000 rads will develop acute, self-limited diarrhea, tenesmus, abdominal cramping, and rarely bleeding during the first few weeks. Chronic radiation affects occur 6–18 months after completion of treatment. Bowel injury resulting from chronic radiation is related to vascular damage, with subsequent mucosal ischemia, thickening, and ulceration.

Clinical Findings

A. Symptoms and Signs: Recurrent hematochezia and rectal pain are common.

B. Laboratory Findings: Hematocrit is decreased.

C. Imaging: Endoscopy shows telangiectasias, strictures, ulcers, and inflammation. Barium studies reveal flattened mucosa with loss of haustral markings.

Treatment

Endoscopic bipolar coagulation, heater probe, or laser can coagulate the mucosal telangiectasias and result in decreased frequency and transfusion requirements. Steroid or sucralfate enemas have been used with variable success. Patients with chronic blood loss require iron supplementation. Rarely surgery is necessary for difficult-to-manage recurrent hematochezia.

Ahlquist D et al: Laser therapy for severe radiation-induced rectal bleeding. Mayo Clin Proc 1986;61:927.
Kochlar R et al: Radiation-induced proctosigmoiditis. Prospective, randomized, double-blind controlled trial of

oral sulfasalazine plus rectal steroids versus rectal sucralfate. Dig Dis Sci 1991;36:103.

Taylor JG, Disario JA, Buchi KN: Argon laser therapy for hemorrhagic radiation proctitis: Long term results. Gastrointest Endosc 1993;39:641.

7. INFLAMMATORY BOWEL DISEASE

Essentials of Diagnosis
- Painless, bloody diarrhea.
- Hematochezia more common in ulcerative colitis than Crohn's disease.
- Intermittent symptoms.

Clinical Findings
Patients may present with intermittent painless hematochezia. Laboratory findings include low hematocrit, low iron, and low albumin. Inflammatory bowel disease is diagnosed on basis of friable, ulcerated, edematous mucosa seen during colonoscopy. Stool should be evaluated for ova and parasites, as well as *C difficile* to exclude infectious causes.

Treatment
Medical treatment using 5-aminosalicylic acid products, steroids, or immunomodulatory agents. There is no role for endoscopic therapy. In cases of severe ulcerative colitis not responsive to intensive medical management, surgical colectomy may be necessary.

8. INFECTIOUS COLITIS

Essentials of Diagnosis
- Acute onset of bloody diarrhea.
- Abdominal pain, fever, or both are common.
- Stool cultures positive for organism.

Clinical Findings
Lower gastrointestinal bleeding can occur with infection by *Campylobacter jejuni*, *Salmonella*, *Shigella*, invasive *Escherichia coli*, *E coli* 0157, or *C difficile*. Rarely is there significant blood loss. Diagnosis is made by stool cultures and flexible sigmoidoscopy.

Treatment
Depending on the cause and severity, antibiotic treatment may be necessary. There is no role for endoscopic treatment. In severe cases of *C difficile* pseudomembranous colitis with impending perforation, surgical colectomy may be needed.

9. RECTAL VARICES

Essentials of Diagnosis
- Hematochezia in patients with portal hypertension.
- Varices located proximal to internal hemorrhoids.

Clinical Findings
In response to portal hypertension, varices can develop in the rectal mucosa between the superior hemorrhoidal veins (portal circulation) and the middle and inferior hemorrhoidal veins (systemic circulation). With anoscopy or sigmoidoscopy, rectal varices are seen as vascular structures located several centimeters above the dentate line. The incidence of rectal varices increases with the degree of portal hypertension. About 60% of patients with a history of bleeding esophageal varices have rectal varices.

Treatment
Rectal varices can be treated similarly to esophageal varices, with either sclerotherapy or portosystemic shunts.

Hosking SW et al: Anorectal varices, haemorrhoids, and portal hypertension. Lancet 1989;8634:349.

10. MECKEL'S DIVERTICULUM

Essentials of Diagnosis
- Most common cause of gastrointestinal bleeding in children.
- Painless melena or bright red blood per rectum ("currant jelly").
- Diagnosis with technetium scanning.

Clinical Findings
Meckel's diverticula occur in 1–2% of the general population and are the most common cause of gastrointestinal bleeding in children. A **Meckel's diverticulum** is a congenital anomaly of the gastrointestinal tract in which there is incomplete obliteration of the vitelline duct, leaving an ileal diverticulum. It is located on the antimesenteric border of the ileum, within 100 cm of the ileocecal valve and is 1–10 cm long. Approximately one-half of Meckel's diverticula are lined with gastric mucosa. Most bleeding occurs in Meckel's diverticula that contain gastric mucosa because of acid-induced ulceration of adjacent ileal mucosa.

Preoperative diagnosis can be supported by a ^{99m}Tc sodium pertechnetate scan, which demonstrates ectopic gastric mucosa because it binds to parietal cells. This test has a sensitivity of 75–100%, with 15% false-positive and 25% false-negative rates. The accuracy of the Meckel's scan may be improved with the use of pentagastrin or cimetidine, which increase the uptake of pertechnetate by parietal cells. In active bleeding, angiography may also be helpful.

Treatment
The condition is treated by surgical resection of the diverticulum.

OTHER RELATED CONDITIONS

Small bowel angiodysplasias receive evaluation and treatment similar to colonic angiomatas. Small bowel tumors include stromal cell tumors, lymphomas, carcinoids, and metastatic tumors, which are diagnosed by endoscopy or small bowel barium radiographs, and are treated by surgical resection. Small bowel Crohn's disease may be best diagnosed with barium small bowel series or enteroclysis study.

Chronic Gastrointestinal Bleeding   5

Don C. Rockey, MD

Chronic bleeding from the gastrointestinal tract may be apparent or **occult** (hidden or concealed). Each form presents unique challenges for the clinician.

Clinically evident bleeding that is chronic (ie, recurrent) is by definition from an obscure source, rendering this group of patients extremely difficult to diagnose and manage. Occult bleeding is an extremely common problem. Patients may present with blood detected in the stool (**fecal occult blood**), or iron deficiency anemia if the occult bleeding is of great enough quantity over a long time period.

Chronic occult gastrointestinal bleeding is especially problematic because significant amounts of blood may be lost through the gut yet remain undetected by the patient. For example, instillation into the stomach of 150–200 ml of blood is required to consistently produce **melena** (black, tarry stools), and patients with blood loss of up to 100 ml/d may have entirely normal-appearing stools.

RECURRENT GASTROINTESTINAL HEMORRHAGE OF OBSCURE ORIGIN

Essentials of Diagnosis

- History of gastrointestinal hemorrhage.
- History and physical examination.
- Visible signs of bleeding, such as hematemesis, melena, hematochezia.
- Changes in hemoglobin or hematocrit.
- With acute massive blood loss, orthostatic changes in heart rate and blood pressure.

General Considerations

Recurrent gastrointestinal bleeding is particularly troublesome for the clinician. The majority of these patients typically have undergone some form of diagnostic evaluation, usually endoscopic or radiographic examination of the upper or lower gastrointestinal tracts, or both. Readily identifiable causes of gastrointestinal bleeding (for example, duodenal ulcer or colonic carcinoma) have, by definition, been excluded. After recognition that bleeding is recurrent, the major emphasis should be to formulate a differential diagnosis, localize the site, and then determine the origin of bleeding before instituting therapy.

Clinical Findings

The usual clinical findings of gastrointestinal hemorrhage are present. These include visible bleeding consistent with that of the upper (hematemesis, melenemesis, or melenic stools) or lower (hematochezia) gastrointestinal tract. The well-known alterations in vital signs and changes in hemoglobin or hematocrit are present. In patients with acute loss of 10–15% of blood volume, orthostatic changes in heart rate, diastolic blood pressure, and systolic blood pressure are prominent. Tachycardia and hypotension in the supine position signify significant blood loss. The history and physical examination are not only useful to help localize the site of bleeding within the gastrointestinal tract, but can be directed by knowledge of the possible causes of recurrent gastrointestinal bleeding.

Differential Diagnosis

Table 5–1 lists the causes of recurrent obscure gastrointestinal hemorrhage. The most common entities leading to recurrent gastrointestinal bleeding arise from the small intestine. The most frequently encountered small bowel abnormalities are vascular ectasias or mass lesions, the former being more common than the latter.

Vascular ectasias are generally found in older patients (mean age of 69) whereas mass lesions are seen in younger persons (mean age of 51). Generally, vascular ectasias tend to increase in incidence with age, are often multiple, may be found anywhere in the bowel (classically the right colon), and are associated with underlying medical conditions, such as chronic renal insufficiency. Valvular heart disease, particularly aortic stenosis, has been reported to be associated with vascular ectasias, although more rigorous investigation has failed to confirm this. While hemangiomas are much less common than vascular ectasias, bleeding associated with these lesions may be massive. Mass lesions include leiomyoma, leiomyosarcoma, adenocarcinoma, lymphoma, and carcinoid tumors. The former two are most often as-

Table 5–1. Causes of recurrent gastointestinal hemorrhage of obscure origin.

Small Intestine	Other Sites
Vascular ectasias	Vascular ectasia
Mass lesions	Dieulafoy's lesion
Hemobilia	Gastric varices
Aortoenteric fistula	Watermelon stomach
Hemosuccus pancreaticus	Hemangioma
Duodenal or jejunal diverticulum	
Meckel's diverticulum	
Ulceration	
Drug (NSAIDs, 6-MP, potassium)	
Infectious (tuberculosis)	
Other	
Duodenal varices	
Kaposi's sarcoma	
Crohn's disease	
Vasculitis	

MP = mercaptopurine; NSAIDs = nonsteroidal antiinflammatory drugs.

sociated with brisk bleeding, the latter three with low-volume bleeding (and even chronic occult bleeding resulting in iron deficiency anemia). Clues to mass lesions include abdominal pain, weight loss, and obstructive symptoms.

Aortoenteric fistula almost always occurs after previous aortic surgery. The primary form of the disease is extremely rare. Patients with this disorder typically present 1 to 5 years after surgery. Bleeding is often hemodynamically significant, and occurs initially in the form of a "herald" or "sentinel" bleed. Subsequent bleeding is recurrent and may be fatal.

This disease is usually caused by introduction of bacteria, typically *Staphylococcus aureus,* into the graft bed at the time of surgery. The inflammatory response eventually results in perigraft inflammation, necrosis, and erosion into the fourth portion of the duodenum. Therefore, many of these patients manifest subtle symptoms and signs of infection; low-grade fever and leukocytosis are common. Further, since the periaortic infection produces phlegmonous changes or fluid collections in the graft area, computed tomography (CT) is often useful in diagnosis.

Upper endoscopy is usually unremarkable but is important in that it helps exclude other more common causes of upper gastrointestinal hemorrhage. **Extended upper endoscopy** (ie, enteroscopy with a small-caliber colonoscope), while often nondiagnostic may show erosions or defects in the distal duodenum. Rarely, frank evidence of aortoduodenal communication is identified.

The natural history of aortoenteric fistula is one of recurrent and often fatal hemorrhage, and treatment is difficult. Thus, it is important to consider and exclude this process in patients with previous aortic surgery.

Bleeding from **Meckel's diverticula** is caused by ulceration in ileal mucosa adjacent to ectopic gastric mucosa. It represents the most common congenital anomaly of the gastrointestinal tract and the most common cause of gastrointestinal bleeding in children, but should be considered in young adults as well. Preoperative diagnosis is difficult, although technetium-99 radionuclide scanning is diagnostic in some cases.

Hemobilia (bleeding from the biliary tree) is classically characterized by the triad of gastrointestinal hemorrhage, jaundice, and right upper quadrant pain. However, patients rarely present with the "typical" triad. Trauma to the right upper quadrant, either accidental or iatrogenic, is usually a prominent feature in the history and is present in over 50% of the cases. Angiography is required to identify and localize the exact site of the biliary-arterial fistula.

Hemosuccus pancreaticus most often results from erosion of a pseudocyst into a peripancreatic artery, producing recurrent massive hemorrhage. Since there is usually a history of pancreatitis or pancreatic injury, confirming the diagnosis requires a high index of suspicion, which may lead to angiographic demonstration of the bleeding vessel.

Dieulafoy's lesion (exulceratio simplex) refers to a hemorrhage from an abnormally large submucosal vessel. Bleeding is often torrential and may be recurrent. Dieulafoy's lesions are said to account for approximately 5% of all upper gastrointestinal bleeds. Many are discovered during initial endoscopy, but they may be difficult to detect because they are not usually associated with frank ulcerative lesions. They are almost always located in the proximal stomach (within 6 cm of the gastroesophageal junction). Repeated endoscopy, often during active bleeding, is required to detect these lesions. However, once detected, endoscopic therapy is often effective.

Gastric varices and **duodenal varices** are an important and problematic cause of recurrent bleeding. These lesions may bleed briskly and be particularly difficult to detect, especially after an episode of active bleeding (owing to partial decompression of collateral systems resulting in collapse of the varices). This diagnosis should be considered in patients with evidence of chronic liver disease.

Watermelon stomach (gastric antral vascular ectasia) is an unusual vascular lesion of the antrum that consists of tortuous dilated vessels radiating outward from the pylorus. It is associated with both acute recurrent bleeding and occult bleeding (eg, leading to iron deficiency anemia). It should be suspected in elderly women with associated achlorhydria, atrophic gastritis, and cirrhosis. The relationship with cirrhosis (and portal hypertension in many cases) suggests that portal hypertension may be important in the pathogenesis of watermelon stomach in some patients. Familiarity with the endoscopic appearance of this lesion is essential to making the diagnosis.

Approach to Evaluation

A. History and Physical Examination: Patient history and physical examination are critical in the diagnostic process. They should first be directed at localization of the site of bleeding (ie, upper or lower gastrointestinal tract). Melena suggests upper gastrointestinal tract bleeding and hematochezia is most consistent with distal colonic or even anorectal bleeding. Of note, occasional patients with aggressive bleeding from an upper gastrointestinal source present with conspicuous hematochezia. Further, patients with slow oozing from right colonic lesions may have melena.

Nasogastric lavage is a helpful adjunct to the history and physical examination for determining the site of bleeding. Lavage revealing fresh or digested blood documents upper gastrointestinal bleeding (in the absence of nasopharyngeal or pulmonary bleeding), however, return of bile without blood does not exclude this site. At least 25% of patients with upper gastrointestinal hemorrhage have falsely negative nasogastric lavages.

The cause of bleeding must be determined next. Again, the history and physical examination are relevant (Table 5–2). In patients with upper gastrointestinal tract bleeding, nasopharyngeal and pulmonary causes of bleeding must be excluded as these may often be confused with true gastrointestinal bleeding by patients. Likewise, bleeding from the perianal area must be considered in patients with recurrent hematochezia. Symptoms such as midepigastric pain, nausea, and vomiting suggest an upper gastrointestinal abnormality. Lower gastrointestinal symptoms and

signs, particularly localized pain, diarrhea, and a palpable rectal mass may help identify a colonic lesion.

B. Laboratory Tests: A blood urea nitrogen elevated out of proportion to creatinine is consistent with blood in the small bowel and suggests a possible upper gastrointestinal tract source. The hemoglobulin level, while useful to follow ongoing bleeding, must be assessed in context of the overall clinical picture.

C. Invasive Studies: In the absence of specific clinical clues to the diagnosis, evaluation should begin as noted in Figure 5–1. For upper gastrointestinal bleeding, routine upper endoscopy can be useful, especially in the patient with active bleeding. In this setting every effort must be made to lavage the stomach clear of blood. Spurting or obvious bleeding can direct the endoscopist directly to the lesion. In the patient with ongoing bleeding, technetium scanning or angiography should be undertaken. The former has been reported to be 10 times more sensitive than angiography and can detect as little as 3 ml of blood loss per hour.

If bleeding is very active, angiography should be performed. The lower limit of sensitivity for angiography is reported to be approximately 30 ml per hour, although from a practical standpoint, bleeding must approach several hundred milliliters per hour for angiography to be diagnostic. It must be emphasized that technetium scanning and angiography simply localize bleeding; they generally do not delineate a specific cause.

In patients with modest or intermittent bleeding, or both, the small bowel should be evaluated (after esophagogastroduodenoscopy or colonoscopy). **Enteroclysis** (fluoroscopic intubation of the duodenum and instillation of barium and methylcellulose into the small bowel) is excellent for detecting mass lesions of the small intestine, but is inadequate for detecting mucosal lesions, particularly vascular ectasias.

Enteroscopy, either of the "push" or "sonde" variety, has been advocated to evaluate patients with chronic gastrointestinal bleeding of obscure origin. Push enteroscopy, performed either with a standard colonoscope or a push enteroscope, has been reported to identify a cause of bleeding in up to 50% of patients with recurrent bleeding. Its major advantage over small bowel radiography is that it allows ready identification and treatment of mucosal lesions, such as vascular ectasias. A colonoscope or push enteroscope can be passed beyond the ligament of Treitz into the proximal jejunum. It is readily available and relatively safe, although it can be uncomfortable for the patient. Sonde enteroscopy permits examination of the entire small bowel. However, this test is of limited applicability because it requires 4–6 hours of study as well as a specialized and fragile endoscope. Its use is largely limited to those institutions with a special interest in investigation of the small intestine.

In the patient with apparent lower gastrointestinal bleeding, initial evaluation should begin with anoscopy (unless bleeding is massive), followed by an endo-

Table 5–2. Clinical clues in patients with recurrent gastrointesinal bleeding of obscure origin.

History or physical finding	Cause of bleeding
Young adult <25 yrs	Meckel's diverticulum
Childhood epistaxis/family history	Hereditary telangiectasia
Pancreatic injury, history of pancreatitis	Hemosuccus pancreaticus
RUQ injury or surgery	Hemobilia
Abdominal aortic surgery	Aortoenteric fistula
NSAIDs, especially prolonged use	Small or large (or both) bowel ulceration
AIDS, cutaneous Kaposi's sarcoma	Kaposi's sarcoma
Chronic renal failure	Vascular ectasias
Spider angiomata (chronic liver disease)	Gastric, duodenal or stomal varices
Bowel obstruction	Mass lesions (small or large bowel)
Skin telangiectasias (CRST, OWR)	Telangiectasia
Blue raised lesions (blue rubber bleb syndrome)	Hemangiomas

RUQ = right upper quadrant; NSAIDs = nonsteroidal anti-inflammatory drugs; AIDS = acquired immunodeficiency syndrome; CRST = *c*alcinosis, *R*aynaud's, *s*cleroderma, *t*elangiectasia syndrome; OWR = Osler-Weber-Rendu disease.

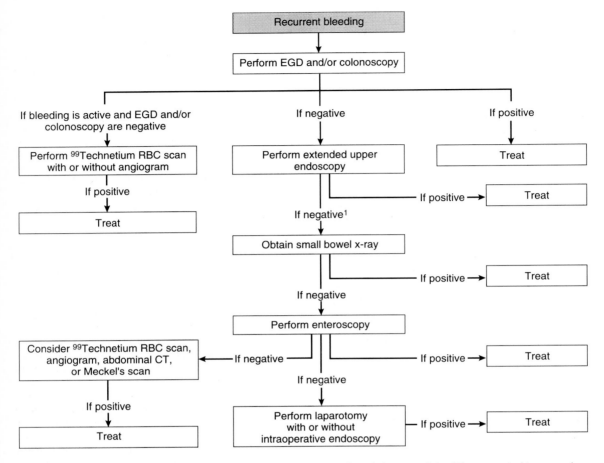

Figure 5–1. Approach to patients with recurrent gastrointestinal bleeding of obscure origin. CT = computed tomography; EGD = esophagogastroduodenscopy; RBC = red blood cell.
[1]The degree of further evaluation varies depending on the amount of recurrent bleeding.

scopic procedure. Sigmoidoscopy can be performed emergently, although the diagnostic yield in a bloody field is low. In patients with massive bleeding and a negative sigmoidoscopy, upper gastrointestinal tract evaluation should be considered because bleeding may originate there in as many as 10–15% of these patients. Colonoscopy, difficult in patients with active bleeding, is useful after thorough cleansing of the colon. If colonoscopy is unrevealing and evidence of bleeding persists, technetium scanning or angiography should be performed. In patients with apparent lower gastrointestinal bleeding and no obvious colonic abnormalities, the small bowel should be considered as a possible source and investigated accordingly.

Occasional patients with documented pandiverticulosis present with recurrent lower gastrointestinal bleeding. These patients are problematic because it may be difficult to document bleeding from diverticula. It is important to exclude other causes of bleeding (especially in the small bowel). If bleeding can be localized to a specific site in the colon, partial re-

section can be undertaken. However, if bleeding cannot be narrowed to a specific locale, pancolectomy may be the only option. These patients can be instructed to present emergently at the first sign of bleeding, whereupon they should undergo emergent technetium scanning, angiography, or both.

D. Surgical Exploration: Surgical exploration as a diagnostic option is generally a last resort, but may identify a cause of bleeding in up to 70% of patients. When a lesion is not identified, intraoperative endoscopy should be considered for inspection of the small bowel, and possibly the colon. Caution must be employed with intraoperative enteroscopy, as complications have been reported. Unfortunately, many patients who have resection of a "correctable" lesion during exploratory surgery continue to bleed. This is particularly true in patients with vascular ectasias of the small intestine (because vascular ectasias are usually multiple and tend to recur).

Patients with recurrent gastrointestinal bleeding of obscure origin are often difficult to manage and require the efforts of a multidisciplinary team, including gastroenterologist, radiologist, and surgeon.

Treatment & Prognosis

Initial treatment of the patient with gastrointestinal hemorrhage centers primarily on assessment of hemodynamic status with adequate fluid resuscitation as needed. Further treatment depends on the specific cause of bleeding. For example, surgical intervention is generally required for mass lesions that bleed recurrently. Polyps and vascular ectasias can be approached endoscopically. Coagulative therapy with multipolar electrodes, heater probe, or laser has been espoused in patients with vascular ectasias. Caution is warranted when using these modalities (particularly in the right colon) because of the risk of perforation.

Unfortunately, most patients with vascular ectasias continue to bleed despite therapy because of the multiplicity of lesions. Hormonal therapy with estrogen or progesterone derivatives (or both) has been used in patients with chronic bleeding from vascular ectasias. Despite early enthusiasm, controlled trials have failed to show significant benefit. Small doses of aminocaproic acid have been recently suggested for patients with hereditary telangiectasias, and may be worth consideration in patients with vascular ectasias in whom other options are not feasible.

The results of surgical intervention in patients with recurrent bleeding have been disappointing; in one series, complete resolution of bleeding occurred in only 41% of patients. Patients with vascular ectasias are especially prone to rebleeding, because ectasias are not all removed at the time of surgery.

Foutch PG, Sawyer R, Sanowski RA: Push-enteroscopy for diagnosis of patients with gastrointestinal bleeding of obscure origin. Gastrointest Endosc 1990;36:337. (An early study demonstrating the potential utility of enteroscopy, and documenting causes of gastrointestinal bleeding of obscure origin.)

Lewis BS, Kornbluth A: Hormonal therapy for bleeding from angiodysplasia: Chronic renal failure, et al? Am J Gastroenterol 1990;85:1649. (A cohort study of hormonal therapy for recurrent bleeding from vascular ectasias. The results demonstrated no benefit for patients treated compared to controls.)

Reilly HF, al-Kawas FH: Dieulafoy's lesion. Diagnosis and management. Dig Dis Sci 1991;36:1702. (Review of a large series of patients with Dieulafoy's lesion.)

Szold A, Katz LB, Lewis BS: Surgical approach to occult gastrointestinal bleeding. Am J Surg 1992;163:90. (An excellent review of the experience at one center, with emphasis on the importance of a multidisciplinary approach.)

IRON DEFICIENCY ANEMIA

General Considerations

Under normal circumstances, iron homeostasis is tightly regulated such that iron absorption in the proximal small bowel is balanced by iron loss (Figure 5–2). The usual Western diet contains 5–15 mg of elemental iron and 1–5 mg of heme-iron, of which about 10% is absorbed. Heme-iron, derived primarily from myoglobin in meat, is preferentially absorbed and accounts for 60–80% of the 1–2 mg of iron absorbed per day.

Microcytosis alone is not sufficient to make the diagnosis of iron deficiency anemia. Other major causes of microcytic anemia include thalassemia, lead poisoning, sideroblastic anemia, and anemia of chronic disease. Thalassemia should be suspected in patients with microcytosis with inappropriately elevated red blood cell counts. Anemia of chronic disease is suggested by a low serum transferrin in the setting of a low serum iron levels.

Pathophysiology

Normally, iron loss of approximately 1 mg[1] (2 ml of blood) iron per day results from occult bleeding in the form of microerosions or microulcerations in the gastrointestinal tract. Additionally, trace amounts of iron are lost via sloughing of gut epithelial cells (which contain iron-containing enzymes).

Normal iron balance can be maintained even in the face of small additional amounts of iron loss. However, while the absorptive capacity of the small bowel can increase two- to threefold during states of iron depletion, if blood loss exceeds the compensatory capacity of the small bowel, depletion of total body iron stores ensues and ultimately leads to iron deficiency anemia. The time required to develop iron deficiency depends on the size of initial iron stores, intestinal iron absorption, and the rate of bleeding. Iron deficiency anemia occurs only after storage iron is exhausted and is thus a late manifestation of the iron-depleted state.

Essentials of Diagnosis

- Mild anemia is generally asymptomatic.
- Severe anemia producing fatigue or other symptoms associated with end-organ compromise.
- Exclusion of other causes of microcytosis.
- Low serum ferritin or low serum iron in the setting of a high serum transferrin level.

Clinical Findings

Patients with mild anemia are usually asymptomatic. Patients with more severe anemia may present with fatigue or any of a number of associated symptoms typical of end-organ compromise (shortness of

---

[1] Amount of iron loss per day in fecal blood: Assuming Hemoglobin (Hgb) = 15 g/dl, then 2 ml blood loss per day = 0.3 g Hgb per day. If stool weight is 150 g, then the Hgb content is 2 mg Hbg per gram of stool. If iron is 0.35% of the total weight of Hgb, then 300 mg Hgb = 1.0 mg iron lost per day in fecal blood.

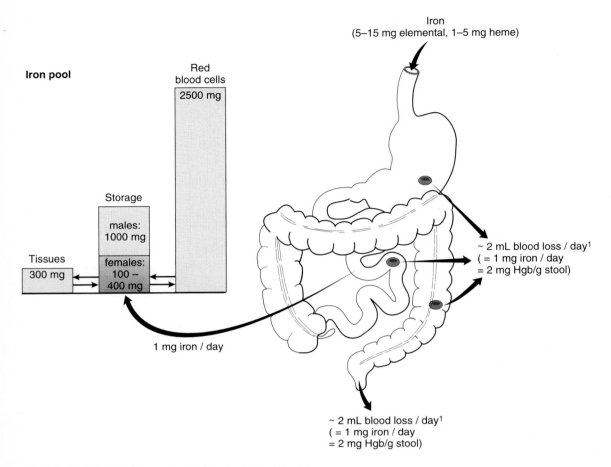

Figure 5–2. Pathophysiology of gastrointestinal blood (iron) loss.
[1]Blood loss occurs through possible microerosion, ulceration; trivial iron loss occurs via intestinal cell cytochromes, ferritin.

breath, chest pain, light-headedness, and cognitive impairment). Physical findings in patients with severe anemia are well known and include pallor, tachycardia, wide pulse pressure, and a hyperdynamic state. A significant number of elderly patients with severe anemia present with serious end-organ injury, such as myocardial infarction and stroke. Some patients with gastrointestinal lesions will have typical symptoms of bleeding (diarrhea, change in stool caliber in colon lesions; epigastric pain, heartburn, early satiety for upper gastrointestinal lesions).

Differential Diagnosis

It is generally well accepted that in men and post-menopausal women with iron deficiency anemia, occult chronic bleeding from the gastrointestinal tract is responsible for iron deficiency. Traditional dogma has held that such bleeding is usually from right-sided colonic malignant neoplasms. However, virtually any lesion in the bowel may bleed chronically in an occult fashion leading to iron deficiency anemia.

Indeed, the list of potential causes of occult gastrointestinal bleeding is protean (Table 5–2). Whatever the source within the bowel, bleeding is almost always due to disrupted gastrointestinal mucosa.

Data suggest that in Western societies, the most common cause of iron deficiency anemia is gastric and duodenal ulceration. While it has been debated whether upper gastrointestinal tract lesions such as duodenal and gastric ulcers could be responsible for iron deficiency anemia, studies have documented up to 20 ml of blood loss per day in patients with such lesions. In addition, a substantial proportion of the gastric and duodenal ulcers identified in patients with iron deficiency anemia have been giant ulcerations, leaving little doubt as to their role in causing iron deficiency anemia.

It has been argued that heme-iron from upper gastrointestinal tract lesions theoretically could be reabsorbed, making the development of iron deficiency anemia less likely in patients with upper gastrointestinal bleeding sites. However, if the daily blood loss from upper gastrointestinal tract lesions exceeds the compensatory absorption of iron in the small bowel, iron deficiency will ensue.

Other upper gastrointestinal lesions that may lead to chronic blood loss resulting in iron deficiency anemia include severe reflux esophagitis, erosive gastritis, and vascular ectasias. Gastric malignancy is a rare cause of iron deficiency anemia in the United States, but should be considered in Asian patients. Trivial gastritis is a common endoscopic finding, and in most cases is probably not consistent with significant blood loss. Esophageal (and gastric) varices have been reported to cause chronic occult blood loss, however, varices are an uncommon cause of iron deficiency anemia. A recently emphasized lesion is watermelon stomach (see previous section), which typically occurs in women of age 50 or more. It has a characteristic endoscopic appearance, may cause recurrent obscure upper gastrointestinal hemorrhage, and is associated with liver disease in up to 50% of patients.

The role of hiatal hernia in iron deficiency anemia is controversial. An association between large hiatal hernia and iron deficiency anemia has been reported, and diaphragmatic hernias are found in up to 10% of patients with iron deficiency anemia. Bleeding occurs not from the hiatal hernia per se, but from associated **Cameron** erosions, characteristic longitudinal mucosal lesions located in gastric mucosa at the level of the diaphragm.

The most common colonic lesion in patients with iron deficiency anemia is colorectal carcinoma. These lesions may be located anywhere within the colon. Right-sided lesions tend to be "silent" more often than left-sided lesions. Most of these lesions are ulcerated, and many are advanced.

Colonic lesions other than malignant neoplasms that may cause chronic blood loss include polyps, vascular ectasias, and ulcerations. Small polyps (which are not ulcerated) probably do not bleed substantially and should not be considered the source of blood loss in patients with iron deficiency anemia. The available data demonstrate that polyps must be at least 1.5–2.0 cm (in the absence of ulceration) to cause significant blood loss. While diverticula have been clearly associated with acute gastrointestinal hemorrhage, bleeding from this lesion generally is not chronic and therefore does not lead to iron deficiency anemia.

In the small bowel, vascular ectasias and mass lesions appear to be the most common causes of chronic blood loss. Important mass lesions include leiomyoma, leiomyosarcoma, adenocarcinoma, lymphoma, and carcinoid tumors. While these mass lesions may cause obstructive symptoms, iron deficiency anemia may be the only sign.

Any cause of severe mucosal injury may also cause malabsorption of iron (ie, Whipple's disease, eosinophilic, gastroenteritis, systemic mastocytosis, celiac sprue). These lesions are often associated with significant inflammation microscopically, though are not always evident endoscopically. Rare patients may present with iron deficiency anemia as the only symptom of celiac disease (so called "monosymptomatic" sprue).

Hookworm infestation, the most common cause of iron deficiency anemia worldwide, is uncommon in the United States. Small endemic areas persist in the southeastern USA. Hookworm should be considered in immigrants arriving from underdeveloped countries. Other nematodes may rarely cause iron deficiency anemia; again these are uncommon in the USA. Amebiasis is a rare cause of chronic blood loss.

Vascular ectasias, acquired or hereditary, may be located anywhere in the gastrointestinal tract and are found in up to 6% of patients with iron deficiency anemia. Identification and control of specific bleeding lesions may be difficult because of their multiplicity. Iron deficiency anemia is typical in patients with hereditary telangiectasia (Osler-Weber-Rendu syndrome).

The role of nonsteroidal anti-inflammatory drugs (NSAIDs), including aspirin, as a cause of chronic gastrointestinal bleeding is yet to be fully elucidated. NSAIDs clearly predispose to duodenal and gastric ulcer (gastric greater than duodenal ulcer), which may cause chronic blood loss. Importantly, patients (especially elderly) taking NSAIDs tend to be less symptomatic from ulcers than are those not taking NSAIDs. Thus, iron deficiency anemia may be the only manifestation of an NSAID-induced ulceration.

NSAIDs are an important cause of ulceration and bleeding in the small or large bowel. These ulcerations tend to be chronic and may eventually lead to stricture formation. Although NSAIDs may cause persistent or recurrent superficial erosions, or both, especially in the upper gastrointestinal tract, whether these superficial lesions are sufficient to cause iron deficiency anemia is unknown. In a recent study of patients with iron deficiency anemia, a significant number of patients taking NSAIDs did not have obvious lesions in the gastrointestinal tract. It is possible that these patients had ulcers that healed by the time of investigation, had ulcers in difficult places to examine (eg, the small intestine), or that superficial lesions contributed to blood loss. Whether aspirin in the doses used for prophylaxis against cardiovascular events can induce substantial chronic bleeding in the absence of ulceration has not been fully investigated.

A subset of patients will have no lesion identified by gastrointestinal evaluation. Iron deficiency in those patients is probably due to nongastrointestinal blood loss, misdiagnosis of the type of anemia, nutritional deficiency, or subtle lesions missed by evaluation.

Approach to Evaluation

Although chronic intestinal blood loss is an important potential cause of iron deficiency anemia in men and postmenopausal women, other sources of chronic blood loss should be considered (eg, menses, epistaxis, hematuria, skin lesions). In the patient with microcytic indices and equivocal iron studies, all potential causes of microcytosis other than iron deficiency anemia should be considered. Ultimately, the diagnosis of iron deficiency anemia should be firmly established before an expensive gastroenterologic evaluation is begun.

Because colonic malignancies are a prominent cause of iron deficiency anemia, early evaluation of the colon, either by colonoscopy or by barium enema, is important. However, while colonic malignant neoplasms are clearly an important consideration, several recent studies have documented the importance of upper gastrointestinal tract lesions as well. For example, in a recent study, approximately two-thirds of all patients with iron deficiency anemia had gastrointestinal lesions consistent with chronic blood loss. In the population with lesions, over 60% of the lesions were identified in the upper gastrointestinal tract. Thus, upper gastrointestinal tract lesions appear to be more common than colonic lesions, in general, and more common than colonic malignant neoplasms in particular.

A. History and Physical Examination: Symptoms in either the lower or upper gastrointestinal tract may help localize the bleeding site and can predict identification of a lesion in the corresponding site. The presence of fecal occult blood appears to increase the likelihood of colonic lesions, however, it does not appear to be particularly helpful in predicting those patients who will have positive upper gastrointestinal tract evaluation. Because the combination of colonic symptoms and fecal occult blood has a high positive predictive value for colonic pathology, these patients should be evaluated expeditiously. The initial investigation should be directed toward locating the source of any specific symptoms (ie, upper or lower gastrointestinal tract). In the absence of symptoms, particularly in elderly patients, it is probably most reasonable to begin evaluation with the colon and proceed to the upper gastrointestinal tract if the colon is normal.

B. Laboratory Tests: Laboratory studies important in the evaluation of iron deficiency anemia include Hgb, MCV, serum ferritin, serum iron, and serum transferrin. While iron deficiency anemia is suspected in patients with a low Hgb and MCV, low serum ferritin or serum iron (with normal or high transferrin) is required to confirm the diagnosis. In patients with equivocal iron studies, other causes of microcytic anemia must be considered.

C. Invasive Studies: Modalities used to evaluate the gastrointestinal tract include both endoscopic (esophagogastroduodenoscopy and colonoscopy) and radiographic (barium enema and upper gastrointestinal series) tests. Radiographic studies generally are excellent for detection of mass and large ulcerative lesions. Their sensitivity for vascular ectasias and other mucosal lesions (such as gastritis, esophagitis, and colitis), however, is less than the sensitivity of endoscopic procedures. A major advantage of endoscopy is that biopsy can be performed and therapy (eg, polypectomy) instituted. The major advantages of radiographic studies over endoscopic studies are ones of reduced cost and complications. Given that patients with iron deficiency anemia have a high pretest probability of disease, much of which is mucosal or will require biopsy, endoscopic investigation is preferable to radiographic study. From a pragmatic standpoint, it is simple to perform both upper and lower endoscopy on the same occasion (this is not possible with barium studies). Whether the lower cost and the reduced risk of complications associated with radiographic studies make them an acceptable alternative to endoscopic studies is unknown.

In those patients with negative examinations of both the colon and upper gastrointestinal tract, evaluation of the small bowel, at least with radiographic studies, has proved to be of limited value. **Enteroclysis** (fluoroscopic intubation of the duodenum and instillation of barium and methylcellulose into the small bowel) is useful for identifying mass lesions of the bowel but is poor at detecting mucosal lesions. Enteroscopy has a much higher sensitivity for mucosal abnormalities and possibly for mass lesions as well. Although small bowel investigation with enteroscopy is likely to have a greater diagnostic yield, whether its attendant time and expense requirements justify its use is unknown. Small bowel investigation should probably be reserved for those patients with persistent symptoms or failure to respond to iron therapy.

Use of other studies, including CT, technetium scanning, and angiography, should be individualized.

An algorithm for evaluation of patients with iron deficiency anemia is presented in Figure 5–3.

Treatment

All patients should be treated with iron. Therapy with ferrous sulfate is inexpensive and generally well tolerated. The initial dosage should be 325 mg two to three times daily. Repletion of iron stores requires prolonged iron therapy, but reticulocytosis should occur within 7–14 days. Side effects associated with iron therapy occur in 10–20% and appear to be dose-related. The most common include constipation and nausea. Parenteral iron is rarely indicated in patients with iron deficiency anemia and its association with anaphylaxis makes this route undesirable.

In addition to iron repletion, all patients should have specific therapy directed at the underlying abnormality—for example, a histamine$_2$ antagonist or antibiotic therapy (or both) for ulcer disease; a histamine$_2$ antagonist or omeprazole for esophagitis; and surgery for carcinoma. Vascular ectasias are particu-

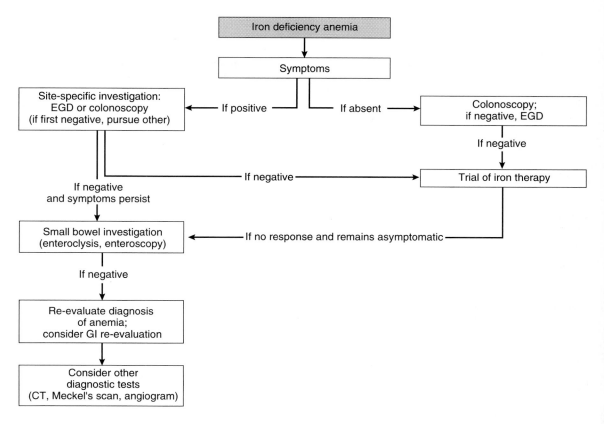

Figure 5–3. Approach to patients with iron deficiency anemia. CT = computed tomography; EGD = esophagogastroduodenoscopy; GI = gastrointestinal.

larly difficult to manage, primarily because they tend to be multiple. Repeated sessions with laser, multipolar electrode, or heater probe in patients with accessible vascular ectasias may be beneficial.

Prognosis

The prognosis for patients with iron deficiency anemia and lesions amenable to medical therapy (eg, duodenal ulcer, esophagitis, colonic polyp) is excellent. The prognosis for patients with iron deficiency anemia who do not have lesions identified during gastrointestinal evaluation is also generally quite good. Very few of these patients are found to have significant gastrointestinal lesions at later times. Additionally, the majority of patients respond to oral iron therapy. In patients who do not respond to iron therapy, the diagnosis of iron deficiency anemia should be questioned. In patients with clear recurrence or persistence of iron deficiency anemia, a search for nongastrointestinal sources of bleeding should ensue. If such a source is not present, repeat gastrointestinal evaluation should be considered. Consideration should also be given to examining and

biopsing the small bowel to exclude occult celiac disease, especially in patients of European origin.

The prognosis for patients with gastric or colonic malignant neoplasms is not as good. By the time carcinomas cause considerable amounts of daily blood loss, they are frequently large and ulcerated. Colonic carcinomas, particularly those on the right side, are often advanced (Dukes stage C or D) by the time of diagnosis.

McIntyre AS, Long RG: Prospective survey of investigations in outpatients referred with iron deficiency anaemia. Gut 1993;34:1102.

Rockey DC, Cello JP: Evaluation of the gastrointestinal tract in patients with iron-deficiency anemia. N Engl J Med 1993;329:1691.

Sahay R, Scott BB: Iron deficiency anaemia—how far to investigate? Gut 1993;34:1427.

Zuckerman G, Benitez J: A prospective study of bidirectional endoscopy (colonoscopy and upper endoscopy) in the evaluation of patients with occult gastrointestinal bleeding. Am J Gastroenterol 1992;87:62.

(These references are recent studies of the gastrointestinal evaluation of iron deficiency anemia.)

FECAL OCCULT BLOOD

General Considerations

Occult gastrointestinal blood loss is common. In cross-sectional studies, over 5% of the population is found to have elevated fecal blood levels. Mean fecal blood levels are between 0.5 and 1.5 ml per day. (Assuming a daily stool weight of 150 g, this is the equivalent of 0.5–1.5 mg hemoglobin per g of stool.)

Pathophysiology

A. Intraluminal Gastrointestinal Hemoglobin Metabolism: An understanding of gastrointestinal hemoglobin metabolism is critical to evaluating patients with fecal occult blood (Figure 5–4). Degradation of hemoglobin in the bowel critically affects interpretation of the various tests used to measure fecal blood loss.

Hemoglobin is cleaved to heme and globin moieties primarily by pancreatic proteases in the proximal small intestine and to a lesser degree by gastric pepsin. Some of the intraluminal heme (generally < 15%)is reabsorbed in the small intestine. The heme not absorbed is converted (presumably) by bacteria to porphyrins and iron via poorly understood mechanisms. The fraction of heme converted to porphyrins by gut bacteria varies greatly. This portion has been termed the **intestinal converted fraction** of heme. Importantly, porphyrins, which do not possess peroxidase-like activity, are not detected by standard guaiac tests.

The globin chains of hemoglobin are digested by pepsin and by pancreatic and intestinal proteases. Globin chains may also be partially catabolized in the colon. Thus, immunoassays for hemoglobin, which use antibodies directed at the globin chain, will be very insensitive for upper gastrointestinal bleeding.

B. Bleeding Sources: Occult bleeding may arise from virtually any lesion shown in Table 5–3. The most common abnormalities of the gastrointestinal tract leading to occult blood loss include neoplasia (especially in the colon) and ulcerative processes (upper gastrointestinal tract).

Gastrointestinal bleeding has been described as a common complication of anticoagulant therapy. Occult bleeding has also been commonly described in patients receiving warfarin and heparin. In fact, the incidence of fecal occult blood in patients receiving anticoagulants has been as high as 12%. Theoretically, bleeding may arise from preexisting lesions (such as carcinoma, polyps, ulcers) or from mucosal bleeding secondary to over-anticoagulation. Available data suggest that the former postulate is most likely, and that a high percentage of anticoagulated patients with fecal occult blood (measured by guaiac stool test) have underlying gastrointestinal pathology.

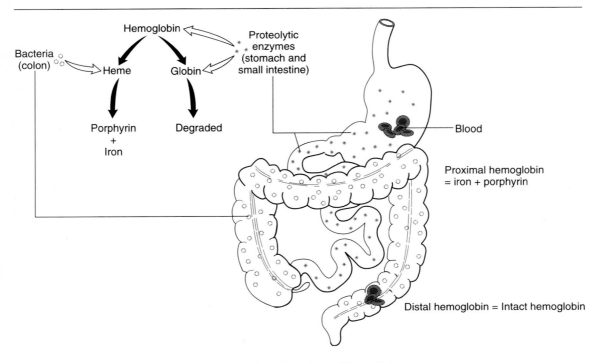

Figure 5–4. Fate of intraluminal hemoglobin.

Table 5–3. Causes of occult gastrointestinal blood loss.

Stomach/Esophagus	Colon
*Reflux esophagitis	Ischemic colitis
*Erosive gastritis	Ulcerative colitis
Cameron lesions (associated with hiatal hernia)	Unspecified colitis
	Amebiasis
Portal hypertensive gastropathy	**Any gastrointestinal location**
Watermelon stomach	Ulceration (*duodenal, *gastric, small intestinal, cecal, rectal)
Small intestine	
Celiac sprue	Carcinoma (esp. *colon)
Whipple's disease	Large polyps (esp. *colon)
Meckel's diverticulum	*Vascular ectasia and telangiectasia
Nematodes (esp. hookworm)	Hemangioma
Tuberculous enterocolitis	**Extra-gastrointestinal**
Crohn's disease	Hemoptysis
Miscellaneous	Nasopharyngeal
Nonsteroidal anti-inflammatory drugs	
Aspirin	
Long-distance running	
Factitious	

* = Common gastrointestinal lesions associated with iron deficiency anemia in the United States.

Screening for Colorectal Neoplasias

Principles of cancer screening for a general population include (1) the disease must have an asymptomatic period during which detection could improve survival, (2) the disease has serious consequences, (3) screening techniques are sensitive enough to detect early lesions, (4) screening tests are specific enough to make further investigation worth the time, risk, and expense, and (5) the prevalence of disease is high enough to justify the costs of screening.

Screening for colorectal carcinoma using fecal blood as a marker has received a great deal of attention. Current data indicate that fecal blood is an imperfect marker for colorectal neoplasia because (1) currently available tests for detection of fecal occult blood inconsistently detect hemoglobin, and (2) the rate of bleeding from colon cancers is variable.

A number of factors determine the amount of bleeding from colorectal neoplasms. Occult bleeding increases with the size and the degree of ulceration, thus, smaller lesions may not bleed and therefore may go undetected. Furthermore, some colon cancers bleed infrequently or not at all. For these reasons, the sensitivity of fecal occult blood tests for detection of colonic neoplasms has been extremely low. Overall, in large screening studies, 1–4% of patients screened have positive tests. Of these patients, fewer than 10% are found to harbor colonic carcinoma. The positive predictive value of a positive fecal occult blood test for colon cancer appears to be about 10%. The value of rehydration of slides before development continues to be debated. This maneuver increases sensitivity but lowers specificity (and thus the positive predictive value).

The use of fecal occult blood tests for detection of bleeding in patients out of the screening context has not been well studied.

Differential Diagnosis

In patients who undergo fecal occult blood testing as a screening modality, colorectal carcinoma and polyps are the major disorders of interest. However, as with occult bleeding leading to iron deficiency anemia, virtually any gastrointestinal lesions can cause bleeding and result in a positive fecal occult blood test. Disorders detected with the currently available fecal occult blood tests will be biased toward the colon, because these tests are better for detecting lower gastrointestinal bleeding than upper gastrointestinal bleeding.

Approach to Evaluation
A. Fecal Occult Blood Tests:
1. Heme-porphyrin tests–The heme-porphyrin test is capable of spectrofluorometrically measuring heme and porphyrin, each derived from hemoglobin. Because it measures both heme and porphyrin, this test allows precise determination of total hemoglobin in the stool. Further, many substances that may interfere or cause false-positive guaiac tests (ie, vegetable peroxidases) do not interfere with this assay. A remaining confounder, however, is myoglobin, an important source of nonhuman heme, found in high abundance in red meats. Unfortunately, the extremely high sensitivity of this test has limited its usefulness, primarily because of decreased specificity for colonic cancer. Finally, it is currently available only from reference laboratories.

2. Guaiac (leuco-dye) tests–Guaiac is a leuco-dye that turns color in the presence of substances such as peroxidases and hydrogen peroxide. Guaiac-based tests take advantage of the fact that hemoglobin possesses pseudoperoxidase activity. Other leuco-dyes include benzidine, O-toluidine, and leuco-malachite. Numerous tests are available and all are simple, inexpensive, and easy to use.

The guaiac test is notoriously unpredictable in its ability to reproducibly detect fecal blood. There does not appear to be a critical level at which fecal blood is reliably detected by guaiac tests. On one hand, fecal hemoglobin levels must exceed 10 mg/g (10 ml daily blood loss) before guaiac tests are positive at least 50% of the time. However, guaiac tests may be positive in stools of patients with less than 1 mg/g hemoglobin (1 ml of blood loss per day). A large part of the variability in guaiac tests may be related to individual differences in intestinal metabolism of hemoglobin.

A number of factors can influence guaiac test results. As previously emphasized, degradation of heme to porphyrin results in decreased sensitivity of guaiac tests for blood because porphyrin derived from hemoglobin is not measured. The sensitivity of guaiac tests can also be reduced by vitamin C, antacids, acid pH, prolonged storage, and erroneous reading of the developing slides.

A major element affecting the reactivity of guaiac is fecal hydration. Fecal hydration before the development of guaiac has been shown to markedly raise its sensitivity, however, this concomitantly lowers its specificity. False-positive tests are caused by a multitude of factors, as shown in Table 5–4. For this reason patients must be carefully instructed regarding diet when testing for occult blood in the stool.

It is commonly assumed that oral iron causes false-positive guaiac tests. In vitro, when iron sulfate is dissolved in water and placed on the test kit cards, ferrous ions are converted to ferric ions by hydrogen peroxide in the developer. Ferric ions acting as electron acceptors oxidize guaiaconic acid, producing a blue color reaction. Thus, an iron salt such as ferrous sulfate in the test tube could produce a false-positive test. However, when the pH of an iron solution rises above 5, the iron precipitates out as the highly insoluble ferrous dihydroxide (the pH of ferrous sulfate dissolved in water is acidic). Because the pH of stool is greater than 5, iron is usually insoluble (ferrous sulfide), and would not be likely to give a positive result. Prospective studies have confirmed that orally administered iron, even in large doses, does not cause false-positive guaiac reactions.

3. Immunochemical tests–Immunochemical tests use antihuman hemoglobin antibodies, directed against globin epitopes, to detect human hemoglobin. In addition to being very sensitive for hemoglobin (they can detect as little as 0.3 mg of blood added to stool), they provide at least a theoretical advantage over guaiac tests in that they detect only human hemoglobin. Digestion or degradation of globin during intestinal transit reduces the sensitivity of these tests. As would be predicted, immunochemical tests are much less likely to detect upper gastrointestinal bleeding than distal colonic lesions. A recent study suggested that immunochemical tests are better at detecting colorectal neoplasias and adenomas than gua-

iac or heme-porphyrin tests, presumably as a result of its high chemical sensitivity for hemoglobin A. In addition, rapid degradation of globin in the upper gastrointestinal tract helps increase the specificity of the test for distal hemoglobin.

B. Imaging: Once a patient is determined to have fecal occult blood, investigative options include either colonoscopy or barium enema. Flexible sigmoidoscopy should be added for patients undergoing barium enema to better evaluate the sigmoid colon (which can sometimes be inadequately examined by barium enema alone). The advantages and disadvantages of colonoscopy and barium enema are important to consider. In short, colonoscopy is more accurate than barium enema, especially for detecting small polyps and mucosal lesions, and it allows for biopsy and therapy at the time of evaluation. Barium enema, however, is less expensive and less uncomfortable to the patient, and carries a lower risk of complications, but these advantages are diminished by the fact that patients who have suspicious lesions identified by barium enema will be required to have colonoscopy anyway. The selection of colonoscopy versus barium enema and flexible sigmoidoscopy for evaluation of fecal occult blood largely depends on individual (patient and physician) familiarity and preference.

Patients with fecal occult blood and a normal colonic examination may harbor upper gastrointestinal abnormalities. In the few available studies addressing this issue, upper endoscopy has detected abnormalities in more than 75% of such patients. This finding is somewhat surprising, given that guaiac tests have a low sensitivity for detection of upper gastrointestinal bleeding. Patients with fecal occult blood and upper gastrointestinal symptoms should probably undergo evaluation of their upper gastrointestinal tract. The advantages and disadvantages of endoscopic versus radiographic procedures are similar to those in the colon. Whether the asymptomatic patient with fecal occult blood and a normal colon should undergo upper gastrointestinal investigation is an open question.

C. Laboratory Measures: All patients with fecal occult blood should have their hemoglobin or hematocrit measured. Patients with fecal occult blood and iron deficiency anemia require careful evaluation of the gastrointestinal tract, as described in previous section and in Figure 5–3. In the setting of iron deficiency anemia, patients with fecal occult blood appear to have a higher incidence of colonic lesions than those without fecal occult blood. No association between fecal occult blood and upper gastrointestinal tract lesions existed.

Treatment & Prognosis

Treatment depends on the specific lesion identified in the gastrointestinal tract and is identical to that for iron deficiency anemia. The prognosis of pa-

Table 5–4. Causes of false positive fecal occult blood tests (guaiac).

Extra-gastrointestinal blood loss
  Epistaxis
  Gingival bleeding
  Hemoptysis
Medications
  Aspirin
  Nonsteroidal anti-inflammatory drugs (NSAIDs)
Exogenous peroxidase activity
  Red meat (non-human hemoglobin)
  Fruits (canteloupe, grapefruit, fig)
  Uncooked vegetables (especially radish,   "Vegetable
    cauliflower, broccoli, turnip; also   peroxidases"
    cucumber, carrot, cabbage, potato,
    pumpkin, parsley, zucchini)

tients with occult bleeding and no obvious gastrointestinal lesion is excellent.

Ahlquist DA et al: Fecal blood levels in health and disease. A study using HemoQuant. N Engl J Med 1985;312:1422. (A classic study examining fecal blood loss in normal subjects and patients with various gastrointestinal disorders.)

Hsia PC, al-Kawas FH: Yield of upper endoscopy in the evaluation of asymptomatic patients with Hemoccult-positive stool after a negative colonoscopy. Am J Gastroenterol 1992;87:1571. (Suggests that many patients with fecal occult blood may have upper gastrointestinal tract pathology.)

Lang CA, Ransohoff DF: Fecal occult blood screening for colorectal cancer. Is mortality reduced by chance selection for screening colonoscopy? JAMA 1994;271:1011. (Review addressing the findings of the Minnesota Colon Cancer Control Study.)

Mandel JS et al: Reducing mortality from colorectal cancer by screening for fecal occult blood. Minnesota Colon Cancer Control Study [published erratum appears in N Engl J Med 1993 Aug 26;329(9):672]. N Engl J Med 1993;328:1365. (Large, prospective national study of fecal occult blood testing.)

St. John DJ et al: Evaluation of new occult blood tests for detection of colorectal neoplasia. Gastroenterology 1993;104:1661. (Recent study examining sensitivity and specificity of tests for fecal occult blood.)

6   Functional Gastrointestinal Disorders

Nicholas J. Talley, MD, PhD

A large group of patients seen by gastroenterologists in clinical practice present with chronic or recurrent gastrointestinal symptoms that continue to defy explanation, despite structural and biochemical studies. These patients are generally labelled as having a **functional gastrointestinal disorder.** Up to 50% of outpatients referred to gastroenterologists, in fact, receive this diagnosis.

The best recognized functional gastrointestinal disorder is the irritable bowel syndrome (IBS), which is marked by chronic or recurrent abdominal pain associated with disturbed defecation and often bloating for at least 3 months. This chapter deals largely with this condition, however, much of the information is pertinent to all functional gastrointestinal disorders.

Essentials of Diagnosis: Irritable Bowel Syndrome

- Abdominal pain associated with disturbed defecation.
- Abdominal pain relieved by defecation.
- Stools looser or more frequent at onset of pain.
- Feeling of incomplete evacuation.
- Mucus per rectum.
- Visible abdominal distension.
- Sigmoidoscopy and routine blood testing necessary to rule out organic disease; further tests dependent upon clinical setting.

General Considerations

While IBS has been considered to be the prototypic functional disorder, a number of other conditions have been identified. A new classification of functional gastrointestinal disorders based on clinical experience and epidemiologic data has been developed by an international group of clinical investigators who met in Rome in 1990, and is referred to as the **Rome criteria.** In this classification, symptom patterns by anatomic location are attributed to disordered function in the oropharynx, esophagus, stomach, small or large bowel, anorectum, or biliary tree (Table 6–1).

The functional gastrointestinal disorders are important because they may be easily misdiagnosed and can cause considerable morbidity. Moreover, they are economically very costly to society, not only in terms of medical expenditures but in time lost from work. Work absenteeism in persons with functional bowel complaints is double that of the general population; the average number of days missed annually in one large household survey was nearly 9 for persons with any functional gastrointestinal complaints and over 13 for those with IBS.

Epidemiology

Functional gastrointestinal disorders are common conditions in otherwise healthy persons. up to two thirds of such persons have one or more symptoms (Table 6–1). The worldwide prevalence of IBS is 10–20%, a rate that tends to be stable from year to year (Figure 6–1). The prevalence is higher in lower socioeconomic groups in the United States, which may reflect unknown environmental factors. While most patients continue to have chronic, recurring symptoms, up to 30% become asymptomatic over time.

For unknown reasons, the reporting of symptoms slightly declines with age, perhaps because older people are less likely to remember minor symptoms. Despite a decline with age, functional bowel symptoms are still common in the elderly. In this age group they are more likely to be misdiagnosed or inappropriately labelled as, for example, "symptomatic diverticulosis."

"Illness behavior" refers to the way people experience and deal with illness; some ignore symptoms while others misinterpret normal sensations as illness and seek medical care. Only a minority with functional gut symptoms—including just 15–50% of adults with IBS—ever consult a physician. Women tend to report more functional gut symptoms than men and are more likely to be diagnosed with IBS in Western nations. It has been postulated that this gender difference is culturally related, since in some countries (eg, India) more men than women present with complaints consistent with IBS.

Table 6–1. The Rome classification of functional gastrointestinal disorders.

Disorder	Approximate percentage prevalence United States
Functional esophageal disorders	
Globus	10
Rumination syndrome	10
Functional chest pain of presumed esophageal origin	12
Functional heartburn (no pathological acid reflux)	29
Functional gastroduodenal disorders	
Functional (nonulcer or idiopathic) dyspepsia	10
Aerophagia	24
Functional bowel disorders	
Irritable bowel syndrome	15
1. Abdominal pain or discomfort, relieved with defecation or associated with a change in the frequency or consistency of stools, and	
2. An irregular pattern of defecation (at least 25% of the time) consisting of 3 or more of the following: altered stool frequency; altered stool form; altered stool passages; mucus; bloating or feeling of distension	
Functional abdominal bloating	32
Functional constipation	3
Functional diarrhea	2
Functional abdominal pain	2
Functional biliary pain (biliary dyskinesia)	<1
Functional anorectal disorders	
Functional incontinence	7
Functional anorectal pain	
Levator syndrome	6
Proctalgia fugax	8
Pelvic floor dyssynergia	13

Illness behavior may be learned; in one study, persons with IBS compared to others with peptic ulcer disease were more likely to have received gifts or remained home from school during childhood when they were unwell. Those with functional bowel symptoms are also more likely to see a physician for nongastrointestinal complaints; this may reflect a general tendency to report symptoms (perhaps related to widespread abnormalities of visceral sensory thresholds or somatization), abnormal behavior in seeking health care (perhaps learned in childhood), or a combination of both.

Pathophysiology

Functional bowel symptoms almost certainly reflect a group of conditions with many causes. Several mechanisms may interact at any one time to induce symptoms (Figure 6–2). The evidence is now clear that physiologic disturbances occur in at least a subset of patients, suggesting that symptoms are neither imagined nor just the product of chronic complaining. However, a plausible disease model that takes into account all of the known abnormalities has yet to be derived, and none of the abnormalities are specific enough to be used as diagnostic criteria. The mechanisms identified to date that may be linked to specific symptoms in IBS are summarized in Table 6–2.

A. Abnormal Visceral Perception: Abnormal visceral perception may represent one of the key physiologic disturbances. Afferent traffic is carried from the gut to the brain by vagal and spinal afferent nerves. In IBS rectal, colonic, or small bowel sensa-

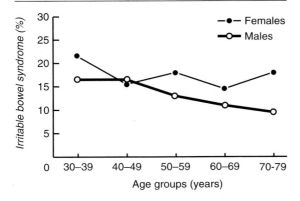

Figure 6–1. Prevalence of irritable bowel syndrome in a random sample of a representative county (Olmsted, Minnesota) in the United States (n=1163).

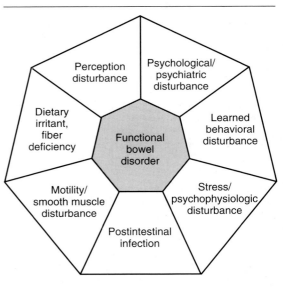

Figure 6–2. Potential mechanisms linked to functional bowel disease, including irritable bowel syndrome. Therapy should ideally be targeted at reversing abnormal pathophysiology but this remains impractical.

Table 6–2. Pathophysiology of the irritable bowel syndrome.

Symptom	Putative abnormalities
Abdominal pain	Increased responsiveness of colon and terminal ileum to meals
	Prolonged propagated contractions in terminal ileum
	Discrete clustered contractions in proximal small intestine
Constipation	Reduced high-amplitude colonic contractions
Diarrhea	Increased high-amplitude colonic contractions
	Increased colonic tone during fasting
	Excess fluid secretion in ileum in response to bile acids
Bloating/distension	Intestinal hypersensitivity (colon, small bowel)
	Decreased ileocolonic transfer of chyme
	Not related to gas retention, voluntary protrusion, lumbar lordosis, depression of diaphragm
Feeling of incomplete evacuation/ urgency	Rectal hypersensitivity

tion may be disturbed; a subset of patients have a more "sensitive" bowel to distension compared with healthy controls. In diarrhea-predominant IBS, for example, increased rectal resistance to stretch as well as increased rectal sensitivity has been found in up to 60% of patients, compared with less than 10% who have constipation-predominant symptoms.

On the other hand, studies show that most functional patients do not have lower thresholds for general bodily discomfort (eg, pain induced by immersion of the hand in ice water), even in the presence of a hypersensitive gut (eg, a gut sensitive to balloon distension). Thus, visceral hypersensitivity in IBS is not explained by a generally low pain threshold. Whether this increased gut perception is due to an end-organ abnormality, increased relay of afferent inputs, or altered central processing is unclear.

B. Altered Gut Motor Function: Altered gut motor function has been theorized to be of major significance. Abnormal colonic myoelectric activity at 3 cycles/minute was reported in the 1970s to be associated with IBS, but is now considered to represent either artifact or an epiphenomenon. Basal colonic motility is not altered in IBS, but the colon may be abnormally responsive to stress, cholinergic drugs, or hormonal factors (eg, cholecystokinin). Colonic and small bowel transit may also be disturbed and has in general correlated with the predominant symptom pattern in IBS (eg, fast transit with diarrhea and slow transit with constipation).

Certain small intestinal motor patterns have been linked to the abdominal pain in IBS. For example, during fasting clusters of jejunal pressure waves occur in some patients with IBS that coincide with abdominal pain and disappear during sleep (Figure 6–3). Ileal propulsive waves associated with pain have also been documented in IBS (Figure 6–4). It has been postulated that abnormalities in sensory perception may induce alterations in local neural reflexes that in turn alter motor function in IBS.

C. Extraintestinal Motor Dysfunction: Extraintestinal motor dysfunction has been observed in the lung, urinary bladder, and gallbladder in IBS. The studies overall suggest that there is a generalized abnormality of either smooth muscle itself or the nervous system innervating the gut and other organs. Extrinsic dysfunction could originate in the central

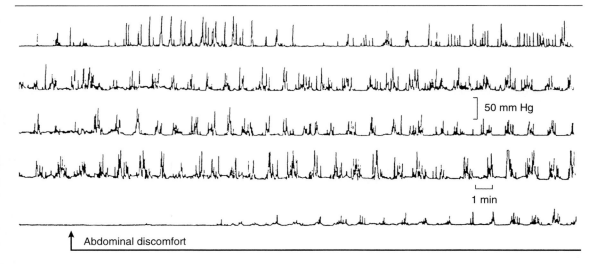

Figure 6–3. Fasting small bowel motility recordings in an irritable bowel patient. Note the clusters of contractions ("minute rhythm") associated with pain; this pattern is more frequently seen in irritable bowel patients than in control subjects. From Phillips SF, Talley NJ, Camilleri M. The irritable bowel syndrome. In: Anuras S. Motility disorders of the gastrointestinal tract. Raven Press, 1992:315.

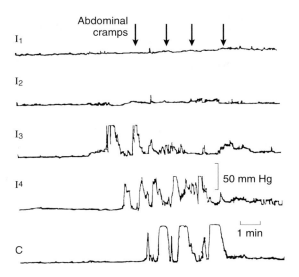

Figure 6–4. Motility recording from the terminal ileum *(I₁-I₄)* and cecum *(C)* in a patient with irritable bowel syndrome. Note the coincidence of abdominal pain with high-pressure peristaltic waves propagated from ileum to colon. From Kellow JE, Phillips SF. Gastroenterology 1987;92:1885.

nervous system or within the vagus nerve (which provides sensory and motor innervation of the stomach, small bowel, and proximal colon).

D. Autonomic Nervous System Abnormalities: Vagal dysfunction and sympathetic adrenergic dysfunction have been documented in a minority of patients with IBS referred to specialist centers.

E. Psychological Factors: Psychological distress may play a role because gut function can be altered in response to acute stress or other emotional factors. Co-existent psychiatric disease and past sexual abuse may contribute to the exacerbation of psychological distress and, hence, bowel dysfunction in predisposed individuals.

It has been reported that 40–100% of patients with IBS have psychiatric disease, but this figure may be unrealistically high since these studies were based on selected patients seen at specialist centers, and psychiatric disease commonly co-exists with organic bowel disease. Sexual or physical abuse is rarely spontaneously reported to physicians. A history of sexual abuse, however, is recognized to be linked to chronic illness and multiple complaints, and an association between abuse and IBS has been found, both in outpatients and in the community. In one study, 30% of female outpatients with IBS had a history of incest or rape. Those with a history of abuse are also more likely to suffer from psychiatric disease.

It is under-recognized that persons who consult for their IBS symptoms differ from IBS sufferers who do not seek health care. Pain and other symptoms alone are poor predictors of consultation behavior. How-

ever, studies have shown that those with IBS who do not consult physicians have psychological profiles very similar to asymptomatic persons; in contrast, those who seek care for their IBS tend to be much more psychologically disturbed. Those with a history of a stressful life event or abuse are also more likely to go to a physician. It has thus been postulated that psychological factors do not cause functional symptoms, but when they coexist they may enhance symptom severity and promote the seeking of health care. One of the reasons an excess of psychiatric disease and psychological distress has been observed in IBS is likely related to health care seeking and not functional gut disease per se.

F. Diet and Infection: Other factors may be relevant. In susceptible patients, luminal contents such as sorbitol, fructose, and bile acids can induce symptoms, including diarrhea and bloating. Other dietary factors have been implicated, including a deficient fiber intake and food intolerance in IBS, but convincing data are still lacking. However, in a United Kingdom trial, dietary exclusions induced symptomatic improvement in 50% of patients with functional diarrhea, providing some support for food sensitivity.

It has also been theorized that infection may prime the gut, resulting in functional disturbances. Historically, a minority of IBS patients postdate the onset of their symptoms to a viral illness or travellers' diarrhea. An excess of mast cells, which occur in close proximity to sensory nerves in the mucosa, has been observed in the terminal ileum of some patients with IBS. It is conceivable that inflammation or other noxious stimuli could sensitize gut receptors that sustain symptoms, even after the initial stimulus has disappeared.

Clinical Findings

A. Symptoms and Signs: A functional gastrointestinal disorder should not be diagnosed only after a battery of expensive and invasive tests has failed to identify organic disease. Rather, the physician should strive to make a positive diagnosis at the initial consultation. After taking a careful history and examining the patient, the experienced clinician can often correctly apply a functional or organic label. The diagnostic tests should then be used to confirm the clinical impression.

Abdominal pain and disturbed defecation are characteristic of IBS, but these symptoms may also occur temporarily in certain conditions (Table 6–3) or chronically with a number of serious diseases (Table 6–4). The pain in IBS is often poorly localized, may migrate around the abdomen, and tends to be variable in nature. It is useful to remember that pain unrelated to defecation or pain induced by activity, menstruation, or urination is very unlikely to be explained by bowel dysfunction as occurs in IBS.

Bowel disturbance may be manifest by constipa-

Table 6–3. Common causes of transient bowel symptoms.

Pregnancy, peri-menstrual
Posthysterectomy
Dietary indiscretion
Travellers' diarrhea or constipation
Food poisoning, gastroenteritis
Bed rest or recent weight loss (constipation)
Nervous diarrhea (job interview, examinations, etc)

Adapted from Heaton KW: Epidemiology of irritable bowel syndrome. Europ J Gastroenterol Hepatol 1994;6:465.

tion or diarrhea, rectal urgency, feelings of incomplete emptying, or passage of mucus. Patients may use the term "constipation" to mean a variety of symptoms, from infrequent stooling to straining or incomplete evacuation. Similarly, "diarrhea" can mean frequent passage of hard stools rather than loose or watery stools.

In IBS, specific symptoms help to discriminate this condition from organic disease. In a classic study from the United Kingdom, 15 symptoms were evaluated for diagnostic value. It was found that four symptoms—relief of pain with bowel movements, more frequent stools with the onset of pain, looser stools at the onset of pain, and visible abdominal distension—were significantly more common in IBS, while two symptoms—a feeling of incomplete rectal evacuation and mucus per rectum—tended to occur more frequently (Table 6–5). Of those with IBS, 94% had two or more of these six symptoms.

These features have become known as the "Manning criteria" (after the first author) and have subsequently been confirmed to be of diagnostic value. The more of these symptoms that are present, the more likely the diagnosis is IBS, especially in

Table 6–4. Differential diagnosis of chronic abdominal pain and bowel dysfunction.

Functional bowel disease
Drugs
  Constipation (eg, calcium channel blockers,
    antidepressants, aluminium-containing antacids)
  Diarrhea (eg, laxatives, antibiotics, magnesium-containing
    antacids)
Neoplasia (may be incidentally found in investigated patients)
Inflammatory bowel disease
Other types of colitis
  Infectious colitis
  Diverticulitis
  Ischemic colitis
  Radiation colitis
Psychiatric disease
  Depression
  Panic disorder
  Somatization
Intestinal parasites
  Giardia
  Strongyloides

Table 6–5. Discriminant value of symptoms in identifying the irritable bowel syndrome (IBS) compared with organic bowel disease.

Manning criteria	Organic (%)[1]	IBS (%)
Pain relief after defecation	30	81*
Looser stools at pain onset	27	81*
More frequent stools at pain onset	30	74*
Abdominal distention	21	53*
Mucus per rectum	21	47#
Feeling of incomplete rectal emptying	33	59#

[1]Percentage of patients with this symptom.
*p<0.05
#Trend towards significance at 0.05<p<0.1
Data from Manning AP, et al. Br Med J 1978;2:653.

younger patients and in women; although these features are not very sensitive, they are the best currently available diagnostic criteria. The exact diagnostic value of symptoms in other functional disorders is less certain; symptom clusters may be least useful in dyspepsia where they cannot reliably differentiate peptic ulcer from functional dyspepsia.

Symptoms of gastroesophageal reflux are reported by one third of patients with IBS. Other complaints frequently reported by patients with IBS include headache, backache, fatigue, sexual dysfunction, and genitourinary symptoms. However, these features are not useful diagnostically.

Accompanying symptoms or the physical examination may, on the other hand, strongly point against a diagnosis of IBS (Table 6–6). The physical examination in IBS and other functional disorders is usually normal, but there may be tenderness or abdominal scars. Localized abdominal tenderness that persists on tensing the abdominal wall muscles suggests abdominal wall pain (eg, from muscle strain, nerve entrapment, or myositis), which should not be misdiagnosed as functional pain. Local perianal dis-

Table 6–6. Clinical features against a diagnosis of a functional gastrointestinal disorder.

First onset in an elderly patient
Symptoms wake the patient from sleep
New symptoms after a prolonged period
Progressive steady worsening of symptoms
Weight loss
Dysphagia
Evidence of bleeding or dehydration
Evidence of steatorrhea
Recurrent vomiting
Fever
Elevated erythrocyte sedimentation rate
Anemia or leukocytosis
Blood, pus, or excess fat in stool
Hypokalemia or persistent diarrhea during fasting
Stool weight > 350g/day

ease or an abdominal mass would argue against a diagnosis of IBS. Gynecologic examination can help to exclude endometriosis.

B. Diagnostic Studies: Selected investigations will help to rule out organic disease (Table 6–7). Laboratory tests are generally unremarkable. Flexible sigmoidoscopy should be routine in all patients who require initial investigation for suspected functional bowel disease; biopsies may also be obtained if the mucosa is normal and the patient has diarrhea, to exclude collagenous or microscopic colitis, but the yield is low. Colonoscopy is preferable, however, if the patient is over 40 years of age or there is a strong family history of colon cancer; alternatively, flexible sigmoidoscopy and double-contrast barium enema can be performed. In patients with diarrhea and bloating, lactase deficiency is a possibility and a 2-week trial of a lactose-free diet is worthwhile; alternatively, a lactose hydrogen breath test can be performed. While lactose intolerance is common in certain racial groups (eg, Asians, blacks, Native Americans, persons of Jewish descent), it frequently co-exists with IBS so that withdrawal of lactose often does not eliminate symptoms.

C. Differential Diagnosis: Occasionally, further tests are helpful to rule out other disorders. With severe constipation, it is important to consider two other possibilities, namely, colonic inertia and outlet delay (pelvic floor dysfunction). Colonic inertia may be simply diagnosed using the radio-opaque marker method (20 markers are ingested on three separate days and a flat plate is obtained on the fourth day to calculate the colonic transit time). Anorectal manometry, balloon expulsion, rectal sensation, and measurement of pelvic floor descent will detect pelvic floor dysfunction.

Severe diarrhea also requires further consideration. A jejunal aspirate to examine for parasites and to exclude bacterial overgrowth may be worthwhile. Assessment of small bowel transit (eg, using breath hydrogen testing) or for bile acid malabsorption (eg, using Se^{75} homocholic acid taurine) is not of great practical use. Remember that the laxative abuser may present with functional diarrhea but deny laxative use.

In patients with intractable pain or bloating, mechanical obstruction and intestinal pseudo-obstruction need to be considered. A small bowel follow-through should be performed in this clinical setting.

Other diseases that should be considered in the differential diagnosis are presented in Table 6–4.

The presence of psychological distress is not helpful diagnostically. Many patients with organic disease also manifest psychological disturbances, probably by chance, in some cases, since both conditions are prevalent. But it is important to screen for psychiatric disease, particularly depression (which may manifest by weight loss in addition to sleep disturbances and mood alterations) and anxiety. Panic attacks may accompany lower gastrointestinal symptoms; characteristically, these are discrete episodes of extreme fear or apprehension often with dyspnea, palpitations, chest pain, a choking or smothering sensation, dizziness, flushes, pins and needles, sweating, or fainting.

Patients with somatoform disorder complain of a panoply of symptoms where gastrointestinal complaints are but one minor component. Chronic pain syndrome patients have unexplained pain all of the time that is unrelated to defecation. These psychiatric diseases should not be misdiagnosed, as appropriate referral and treatment will otherwise not be applied.

Principals of Management

The principals of management that apply to all functional gastrointestinal disorders are listed in Table 6–8. A step-wise approach to treatment is outlined in Table 6–9.

Patients seen in primary care practice will often not require drug or behavioral therapy, but patients referred to gastroenterologists tend to be more psychologically distressed and are usually more difficult to manage.

A. Reassurance and Explanation: This is a key component. The decision to seek health care may be influenced by the severity and type of symptoms, fear of serious disease, and psychosocial factors. Tell the patient you know what the problem is and you understand that the symptoms are real, but explain that they are common in the general population and will not lead to any life-threatening problems, such as cancer. Explore the patient's agenda. Find out why

Table 6–7. Laboratory investigations for suspected functional gastrointestinal disorders.

Representative tests	Conditions being screened for
Recommended for all patients	
Hematology and ESR	Anemia, inflammation
Biochemistry	Liver dysfunction, electrolyte disturbance
Thyroid function testing (optional)	Thyroid dysfunction
Recommended for suspected functional bowel and anorectal disorders	
Stool for blood	
Flexible sigmoidoscopy (+/– biopsy)	Bleeding Colitis, neoplasia
Stool/jejunal studies (microscopy, microbiology)	Infection (if diarrhea)
Colonoscopy or barium enema (>40 years)	Colitis, neoplasia
Lactose tolerance test (optional)	
Colonic transit studies (optional)	Lactose intolerance Colonic inertia (if severe constipation)
Pelvic floor studies (optional)	Outlet obstruction (if severe constipation)
Stool/urine for laxatives (optional)	Surreptitious abuse

Table 6–8. Management principles in functional gastrointestinal disorders.

1. Make a positive clinical diagnosis based on the history and physical.
2. Minimize invasive investigations and avoid giving "mixed messages"; don't perform repeated testing without substantial indication.
3. Determine the patient's agenda; ask why the patient with chronic symptoms has presented now.
4. Provide education and firm reassurance.
5. Try dietary modification.
6. Set realistic treatment goals and center therapy around adjustment to illness and patient-based responsibility for care.
7. Prescribe drugs sparingly, targeting the symptom(s) of most concern to the patient; remember the placebo response.
8. Consider behavioral treatments or psychotherapy for moderate-to-severe cases.
9. Organize a continuing care strategy.

the patient with chronic complaints has come to see you now; unwanted fears (eg, the recent death of a relative with bowel or pancreatic cancer) may explain the behavior and need specific attention from the physician.

It is important to avoid sending "mixed messages." For example, stating that you are not concerned about serious disease, then proceeding with extensive and invasive diagnostic tests with little explanation may be confusing and can undermine patient confidence. Providing an early positive diagnosis, spending time explaining the possible causes of the symptoms, and reassuring the patient about the benign prognosis represents a simple but effective form of supportive psychotherapy.

B. Precipitating Factors: The correction of precipitating factors can be therapeutic. Patients may be helped by changing the diet (eg, lactose intolerance in bloating or diarrhea, or lack of dietary fiber in IBS or functional constipation), avoiding certain drugs (eg, heavy alcohol or caffeine use, or sorbitol-

containing gum), and reducing life stress and daily hassles (where possible).

C. Diet: Dietary recommendations are particularly important in the treatment of IBS patients. A high-fiber diet should be prescribed whatever the predominant bowel habit. A daily intake of 20–30 g of fiber is recommended, which is approximately double the amount in the normal American diet. The fiber content should be increased slowly to avoid increased bloating and flatulence. If patients are unwilling or unable to try such a diet, a bulking agent (commercially available fiber supplement) should be started once daily and increased by one dose every week until symptoms improve, or until a daily consumption of 5–10 g three times daily is achieved. Treatment with high fiber should not be abandoned unless it has failed to control symptoms over a 2- to 3-month period. If excess gas is a major symptom, an anti-gas diet should also be instituted; this involves the avoidance of certain foods—eg, cabbages, beans, legumes, and lentils that are fermented in the colon—and carbonated and sorbitol-containing drinks. With constipation, adequate fluid intake and exercise is also helpful.

D. Drug Therapy: Since the functional gut disorders are a heterogeneous group of conditions, it is not surprising that drug therapy is often found to be unsatisfactory in the long term. The placebo response is impressive in functional gastrointestinal disorders, approaching 70% in some controlled trials. The placebo response occurs even if patients are aware that they are taking an inert pill. The large effect may partly reflect the fluctuating course of the symptoms in many patients. Patients tend to present when symptoms are worse and are then more likely to spontaneously improve. Patients may also be responding to the powerful influence of reassurance. Consequently, placebo-controlled trials are essential for determining whether a drug is truly efficacious in these patients.

Unfortunately, few trials in this field have been

Table 6–9. Treatment of irritable bowel syndrome: A stepped-care approach.

Step	Severity	Clinical picture	Management
1.	Mildly troubled/ primary care	Fear of serious disease, anxious, worried, stress	Positive diagnosis Explanation Reassurance Dietary management Regular follow-up
2.	Complainer/ secondary care	Uncertainty re: diagnosis; disturbed lifestyle	Reinforce above measures Stress management Target drugs to specific complaints
3.	Difficult/tertiary care	Co-existant psychiatric disease, possible secondary gain, disability, chronic pain	Avoid overtesting Low dose antidepressant Treat depression Treat anxiety Pain clinic

Adapted from Drossman DA, Thompson WG: Irritable bowel syndrome: A graduated, multicomponent treatment approach. Ann Intern Med 1992;116:1009.

Table 6–10. Drugs for irritable bowel syndrome.[1]

Predominant symptom	Medication
Constipation	Bulking agent (eg, psyllium)
	Prokinetic (eg, cisapride)
	Lactulose/milk of magnesia
Diarrhea	Bulking agent
	Loperamide
	Cholestyramine
Bloating	Prokinetic agent
	Simethicone
	Charcoal
Flatus	Alpha-D-galactosidase enzyme with vegetable meals
Postprandial pain	Anticholinergic (eg, dicyclomine)
Chronic pain	Antidepressant (Table 6–11)

[1]No drug is established to be truly superior to placebo.

Table 6–11. Commonly used antidepressant drugs in functional gastrointestinal disease.

Generic name	Trade name	Usual daily dose (mg)
Amitryptiline	Elavil	25–100
Desipramine	Norpramin	25–100
Doxepin	Sinequan	25–100
Imipramine	Tofranil	25–100
Nortryptiline	Pamelor	25–100
Trazodone	Desyrel	100–150 (divided doses)
Fluoxetine	Prozac	20–40 (morning)

From Zighelboim J, Talley NJ: Irritable bowel syndrome. In: Rakel RE (ed). *Conn's Current Therapy.* WB Saunders, 1994.

rigorously conducted. A review of IBS studies, for example, concluded that no trial provided convincing evidence of therapeutic efficacy over placebo. Drugs, therefore, should be used sparingly in most cases, and targeted at the major symptom or symptoms. It is useful to inquire whether a patient actually wants drug treatment; not all patients desire or need a drug after receiving firm reassurance, explanation, and general advice. It is also important to ask patients what they perceive as their dominant complaint; sometimes the answer is quite surprising. A bulking agent or a prokinetic drug for constipation, imodium or cholestyramine for diarrhea, and an anticholinergic drug for postprandial IBS pain represent some examples of appropriately targeted drug treatment (Table 6–10). With constipation, stimulant laxatives should be avoided.

Experimental drugs being evaluated for IBS include calcium channel blockers, selective antimuscarinics, serotonin-receptor antagonists, gonadotrophin-releasing hormone analogs, somatostatin agonists, and opioid agonists. However, their efficacy is as yet uncertain.

Antidepressants may be particularly useful in patients with chronic pain, resistant complaints, or impaired daily functioning (Table 6–11). Even those without associated depression may markedly improve. The mechanism of action is unknown, but most effect 5-hydroxytryptamine levels centrally, which may in turn modulate gut sensation and motility. All these drugs should be started at a low dose and, if necessary, titrated upward; benefit is usually not apparent for 3–4 weeks. If successful, this treatment should be continued for 3–6 months before tapering it and observing the clinical outcome. Anxiolytics should generally be avoided, since they are potentially habituating, may interact with other drugs, and can induce a rebound effect on withdrawal.

E. Non-Pharmacological Treatments: Other approaches are of value in patients with persistent symptoms. Useful behavioral treatments include nonspecific relaxation therapy, hypnosis (which may reduce visceral gut perception and in controlled trials is beneficial in IBS) and biofeedback (most valuable in constipation with pelvic floor dysfunction). Psychotherapeutic approaches, such as cognitive-behavioral therapy (which usually includes anxiety management techniques and progressive muscular relaxation) are valuable, particularly in motivated patients whose complaints are exacerbated by environmental stressors or emotional difficulties. Patient support groups for IBS can also be very beneficial.

These approaches can all provide patients with a sense of greater control over their illness, promote healthy behavior patterns, and reduce anxiety. Least likely to respond are patients with unremitting pain and those who are resistant to the concept that psychological factors could be linked to their illness.

Prognosis

Prognostic studies have confirmed that once a diagnosis of IBS has been made, it is unlikely to be altered on follow-up (Table 6–12). The physician

Table 6–12. Prognosis of the irritable bowel syndrome in selected series.

Authors	Year	Follow-up (yrs)	n	Symptomatic (%)	Altered diagnosis
Holmes & Salter	1982	6	77	57	4
Svendsen et al	1985	2	112	N/A	3
Harvey et al	1987	5–8	97	74	0
Owens et al	1995	32	112	N/A	3

N/A = not available

should feel secure in making a diagnosis of functional gastrointestinal disease, which in addition gives the patient the satisfaction of having a diagnostic label. The majority of patients continue to be symptomatic intermittently, but up to 30% will spontaneously become asymptomatic over time for unknown reasons.

Follow-up of patients is therapeutic. Regular but brief visits are of particular help for those with unremitting symptoms. In such cases, it is essential to set realistic goals and help the patient to adjust to his or her illness; cure is not usually feasible but improved quality of life and better functional status can be achieved. If a patient with an established diagnosis returns unexpectedly, it is important to determine the reason (Table 6–13). While the physician must be

Table 6–13. Reasons that patients with a documented functional gastrointestinal disorder seek health care.

1. New exacerbating factor (eg, side effect of treatment, dietary change, concurrent medical disorder)
2. New fear of serious disease (eg, death in the family)
3. Psychological or psychiatric co-morbity (eg, abuse, depression, anxiety)
4. Recent inability to socialize or work (eg, development of incontinence)
5. "Hidden agenda," (eg, laxative or narcotic abuse)

vigilant to a change in symptom status that may indicate the development of new organic disease, the physician should not yield to the patient's demand for testing in the absence of an objective change.

REFERENCES

Camilleri M, Ford MJ: Functional gastrointestinal disease and the autonomic nervous system: A way ahead? Gastroenterology 1994;106:1114.

Camilleri M, Prather CM: The irritable bowel syndrome: Mechanisms and a practical approach to management. Ann Intern Med 1992;116:1001.

Drossman DA et al (editors): *The Functional Gastrointestinal Disorders.* Little Brown, 1994.

Drossman DA, Thompson WG: The irritable bowel syndrome: Review and a graduated multicomponent treatment approach. Ann Intern Med 1992;116:1009.

Harvey RF, Mauad EC, Brown AM: Prognosis in the irritable bowel syndrome. Lancet 1987;i:963.

Klein KB: Controlled treatment trials in the irritable bowel syndrome. Gastroenterology 1988;95:232.

Lynn RB, Friedman LS: Irritable bowel syndrome. N Engl J Med 1993;329:1940.

Mayer EA, Raybould HE: Role of visceral afferent mechanisms in functional bowel disorders. Gastroenterology 1990;99:1688.

McKee DP, Quigley EMM: Intestinal motility in irritable bowel syndrome: Is IBS a motility disorder? Dig Dis Sci 1993;38:1761.

O'Keefe E, Talley NJ: The irritable bowel syndrome in the elderly. Gastroenterol Clin North Am 1991;20:369.

Owens D, Nelson D, Talley NJ: The irritable bowel syndrome: Long-term prognosis and the physician-patient interaction. Ann Intern Med 1995;102:107.

Phillips SF, Talley NJ, Camilleri M: The irritable bowel syndrome. In: *Motility Disorders of the Gastrointestinal Tract.* Anuras S (editor). Raven Press, 1992.

Read NW (editor): Review in depth: Irritable bowel syndrome. Europ J Gastroenterol Hepatol 1994;6:457.

Thompson WG: Irritable bowel syndrome: Pathogenesis and management. Lancet 1993;341:1569.

Zighelboim J, Talley NJ: What are functional bowel disorders? Gastroenterology 1993;104:1196.

Inflammatory Bowel Disease

7

Robert F. Willenbucher, MD

Inflammatory bowel disease encompasses two distinct chronic, idiopathic inflammatory diseases of the gastrointestinal tract: Crohn's disease and ulcerative colitis. Although these two entities are frequently grouped together, it is important to appreciate the marked phenotypic differences between them, because these differences may have a profound impact on medical and surgical management.

The incidence of Crohn's disease and ulcerative colitis in the United States is approximately 5 and 15 per 100,000 persons, respectively. There is evidence that the incidence of Crohn's disease has been increasing worldwide over the past several decades, although this rise appears to have plateaued over the past 10 years. The incidence of ulcerative colitis has remained fairly constant. The prevalence of these diseases, which is a more difficult parameter to measure, has been estimated at 90 per 100,000 persons for Crohn's disease and 200 per 100,000 persons for ulcerative colitis. The annual medical cost for the care of inflammatory bowel disease patients in the United States is considerable and has been estimated to be $1.6 billion (1990 US dollars) ($1.1 billion for Crohn's disease and $0.5 billion for ulcerative colitis). When adjusted for loss of productivity of patients, the total economic cost is estimated to be $2.2 billion. It is interesting to note, however, that approximately 2% of patients with inflammatory bowel disease account for 30–40% of the costs. These economic figures obviously do not address the personal and psychological toll of inflammatory bowel disease, particularly in patients with severe disease. Attention to the personal and psychological impact of this disease should be an important part of any treatment approach.

PATHOPHYSIOLOGY OF INFLAMMATORY BOWEL DISEASE

An in-depth discussion of the pathophysiology of inflammatory bowel disease is beyond the scope of this chapter. It is probably the result of the complex interaction of genetic susceptibility and numerous environmental influences. The pathophysiologic characteristics of Crohn's disease and ulcerative colitis are discussed together in this section for convenience only. The obvious phenotypic heterogeneity that is seen not only between Crohn's disease and ulcerative colitis but also within subgroups of the two disorders (eg, pancolitis versus proctitis) underscores the theory that this is probably a clinically related but genetically diverse group of diseases. This genetic diversity most likely accounts not only for the variable clinical manifestations but also the variable clinical responses to standard medical treatments.

A. Immunologic Mechanisms of Tissue Injury: Inflammatory bowel disease is frequently referred to as an autoimmune disorder, but this appears to be a misnomer, according to currently available information. In fact, there is little convincing evidence that there is an immune response directed against any specific self-antigen that would account for the inflammatory process observed in inflammatory bowel disease. There is, however, a large and growing body of evidence showing that there is an enhanced level of lamina propria T cell activation in patients with this disease. This notion is derived from a variety of observations, including increased expression of surface markers of T cell activation, increased production of T cell cytokines, and increased cytotoxic T cell function. This enhanced T cell activation leads to the recruitment of effector cells such as neutrophils, and the subsequent elaboration of destructive substances such as proteases and reactive oxygen metabolites. It appears that intestinal injury in inflammatory bowel disease is due to an "innocent bystander" mechanism as a consequence of enhanced nonspecific T cell activation rather than a directed attack against self-antigen.

The trigger for T cell activation in inflammatory bowel disease is unknown. There has been enthusiasm in the past for chronic mycobacterial infection as the underlying cause of Crohn's disease, but there has been no substantial support for this hypothesis. It is unlikely that a single trigger for T cell activation exists; it is more likely that mucosal T cells are activated by fairly ubiquitous triggers and that the underlying defect in inflammatory bowel disease results in a state of perpetual T cell activation. The nature of this defect in immune regulation is now the subject of considerable investigation. This defect may be a complex interaction among exogenous antigen, enhanced delivery of antigen (increased intestinal permeability), and a heritable propensity to mucosal immune dysregulation. It is plausible that variation in these factors and their interaction results in the variable expression of disease.

Of special note is the description of antineutrophil cytoplasmic antibodies with a nongranular, perinuclear distribution (p-ANCA) in patients with ulcerative colitis. Their presence has been described in 60–70% of patients with ulcerative colitis and only occasionally in patients with Crohn's disease. While p-ANCA does not appear to be involved in pathogenesis, its presence has been associated with the HLA-DR2 allele, whereas ulcerative colitis patients negative for p-ANCA are more likely to be HLA-DR4 positive. This observation lends support to the notion of genetic heterogeneity within ulcerative colitis patients. p-ANCA has little usefulness in differentiating ulcerative colitis from Crohn's colitis.

B. Genetic Factors: Much of the evidence for genetic factors as a cause of inflammatory bowel disease is derived from family and twin studies. While familial clustering of disease can frequently be explained by common environmental exposures, the finding of increased levels of concordance among monozygotic twins and discordance among spouses speaks for a heritable predisposition. The age-corrected empiric risk of Crohn's disease for a first-degree relative of a Crohn's disease patient is 5–8%, whereas that of a first-degree relative of an ulcerative colitis patient is 2–5%. When rates of disease are compared in Jewish and non-Jewish families, the risk appears higher in Jewish families. An increased incidence of inflammatory bowel disease has long been reported in Jews, primarily in those of Ashkenazi origin. Given that Ashkenazi Jews living throughout the world have higher rates of inflammatory bowel disease than their geographically similar but non-Jewish counterparts, it is likely that Ashkenazi Jews represent a genetically predisposed segment of the population.

Twin studies further support the notion of an inherited susceptibility to inflammatory bowel disease. The concordance rates for monozygotic twins for Crohn's disease and ulcerative colitis are approximately 67% and 20%, respectively, whereas the rates for dizygotic twins are 8% and 0%, respectively. There have been no convincing reports that the risk of inflammatory bowel disease in the spouse of a patient varies from that in the general population.

C. Environmental Factors: Higher rates of inflammatory bowel disease have been reported in urban areas than in rural areas. The disease also appears to be more common in higher socioeconomic classes. It is possible, however, that living in a rural area and lower socioeconomic status are associated with more limited access to health care, and this leads to underreporting of incidence. It is interesting to note that this rural-urban disparity is observed in Sweden, where rural access to health care is excellent.

An increased risk of inflammatory bowel disease among users of oral contraceptives has been reported by several investigators in prospective and case-control studies. The relative risk of Crohn's disease and ulcerative colitis has usually been in the 2–3 range, although some studies have failed to show an increased risk. The mechanism by which oral contraceptive use may cause inflammatory bowel disease is not known.

Another environmental risk factor that deserves special mention is cigarette smoking. There are now numerous studies that have consistently demonstrated a decreased risk of ulcerative colitis among smokers compared with nonsmokers. In addition, these studies usually show an increased risk of ulcerative colitis among former smokers compared with those who have never smoked. Meta-analyses have described a risk of ulcerative colitis among smokers as being 40% of that of nonsmokers. In contrast, cigarette smoking is associated with an increased risk of Crohn's disease. This risk applies to both current and former smokers, with a relative risk of 1.2–3.9 (current smokers) and 0.8–3.2 (former smokers). There is also some evidence that cigarette smoking may increase the likelihood of Crohn's disease recurrence. The mechanism for the effects of smoking on inflammatory bowel disease is unknown. The increased risk of ulcerative colitis in former smokers is particularly interesting and unexpected.

Other potential environmental risk factors include diet and perinatal exposure to an inciting agent. While food is the major source of nonbacterial antigen in the gut, no compelling dietary factor has been identified. The most consistent factor identified is increased consumption of refined sugars in patients with Crohn's disease, although the significance of this may be confounded by socioeconomic status. The occasional finding of clustered birth dates among patients who have subsequently developed inflammatory bowel disease (primarily Crohn's disease) has led several investigators to hypothesize a common perinatal exposure to an inciting agent. There is some limited evidence of a greater than expected number of cases of Crohn's disease in individuals born at the time of a viral epidemic (eg, influenza, measles).

CROHN'S DISEASE

In the overwhelming majority of cases, the diagnosis of Crohn's disease is made on the basis of a constellation of characteristic radiologic, endoscopic, and histologic findings in the appropriate clinical setting. The combined radiologic and endoscopic appearances as well as the anatomic pattern of involvement form the basis of diagnosis. Histologic examination of biopsy specimens is useful in that it strengthens the diagnosis when the expected lesions are found and helps exclude other entities (see following section, "Differential Diagnosis"). The diagnosis is rarely made solely on the basis of a biopsy.

The pattern of anatomic involvement in Crohn's disease is important and deserves special consideration. Crohn's disease may affect any portion of the gastrointestinal tract, but a few characteristic patterns of involvement account for most cases (Table 7–1). Approximately 40–50% of patients have involvement of both the terminal ileum and the cecum. About one-third have small bowel disease alone (usually of the terminal ileum), and approximately 20% have disease confined to the colon. Typically, the rectum is spared, and the pattern of involvement is often discontinuous, with intervening normal regions. The finding of discontinuous or "skip" lesions on colonoscopy or barium studies is characteristic. Overall, 75% of patients have small bowel involvement and about 90% of these have terminal ileal involvement. Crohn's disease may also involve the cryptoglandular structures of the anal canal (crypts of Morgagni) in up to one-third of patients, although this is especially common in patients with colonic involvement. Perineal disease alone is unusual. Involvement of the upper gastrointestinal tract (mouth, esophagus, stomach, and duodenum) is rare and almost always occurs in association with disease elsewhere.

Pathology

In Crohn's disease patients, gross examination of the involved portion of bowel and its associated mesentery shows that they are thickened and edematous. Adipose tissue from the mesentery may be seen to spread over the serosal surface of the bowel, giving rise to the classic description of "creeping fat." Bowel loops are frequently adhered together or to adjacent structures. The gross mucosal lesion typically begins as an aphthous ulcer. As the disease process advances, these ulcers enlarge, deepen, and eventually coalesce to form transverse and longitudinal linear ulcers, giving rise to a cobblestone appearance. The base of these linear ulcerations may penetrate deeply, forming fissures in the underlying muscularis

Table 7–1. Patterns of involvement in Crohn's disease.

Pattern	Proportion at Presentation
Ileocecal disease	40–50%
Small bowel disease only	30–40%
Colon disease only	20%

propria. This transmural penetration is the underlying mechanism leading to the abscess and fistula formation that frequently complicates Crohn's disease. Healing and fibrosis of these penetrating lesions may lead to stricture formation, another characteristic complication.

Histologically, transmural inflammation is the characteristic finding in Crohn's disease, as is a patchiness of the inflammatory infiltrate. Nonnecrotizing granulomas are another characteristic but frequently absent lesion; thus, their absence is not helpful in excluding the disease. Although the presence of granulomas is probably a function of the diligence exercised in searching for them, they are probably not present in more than 60% of surgical specimens and 20% of endoscopic biopsy specimens. Even when granulomas are found on biopsy, their presence must be interpreted in the appropriate clinical context, as they may also be seen in association with gastrointestinal tuberculosis and sarcoid, *Yersinia* infection, and even disrupted crypts in severe crypt abscesses in ulcerative colitis. These granulomas in association with entities other than Crohn's disease frequently have a different appearance, and their specificity should be addressed by a gastrointestinal pathologist in cases where the diagnosis of Crohn's disease is in doubt.

Clinical Findings

In most patients, Crohn's disease is characterized by intermittent exacerbations of disease separated by periods of complete or relative remission. A subset of patients have ongoing, persistent symptoms. As might be expected, the clinical presentation and findings are a function of not only the pattern of involvement but also the presence or absence of complications (see following discussion). In addition, the clinical presentation can be divided into three general patterns that are usually independent of anatomic location, including inflammatory, fibrostenotic (stricturing), and perforating (fistulizing) forms. Recognition of these patterns is valuable in that flare-ups and postoperative recurrences of disease tend to fit the same pattern for each individual patient, and the appreciation of these patterns provides a basis for a rational approach to treatment.

There are a variety of rating scales combining clinical and laboratory data that are used to assess disease severity. These scales are cumbersome to use and serve primarily a research purpose. An overall assessment of severity is derived from the patient's complaints, impact of the disease on daily function, pertinent physical examination findings (eg, fever, mass), and the presence of abnormal laboratory parameters (eg, anemia, hypoalbuminemia). Attention to these parameters usually allows the clinician to categorize the patient as mildly, moderately, or severely ill.

A. Symptoms and Signs: The classic presentation of Crohn's disease is that of colicky right lower quadrant pain and diarrhea. Low-grade fever and weight loss are frequently present as well. High fever should alert one to a possible infectious complication (ie, abscess). Hematochezia occurs in a minority of patients, most often in those with colonic involvement. Patients with distal colonic involvement typically have more "colitic" symptoms, including frequent bowel movements, fecal urgency, and tenesmus.

Findings on physical examination may include evidence of chronic illness and weight loss (eg, bitemporal wasting). The abdomen may be tender, most frequently in the right lower quadrant. A palpable right lower quadrant fullness or mass may be present; this typically corresponds to thickened and adherent loops of bowel but may also be the manifestation of an intra-abdominal abscess. A careful rectal examination may reveal evidence of a perirectal abscess, a fistula, or prominent skin tags representing healed perianal lesions.

As has been stated previously, the symptoms and signs of Crohn's disease are a function of the disease pattern. Patients with more diffuse inflammatory disease of the small bowel may have a more indolent presentation, with a prominent component of malabsorption and consequent weight loss and a less prominent complaint of abdominal pain. Patients with fibrostenotic disease may present primarily with complaints compatible with a partial small bowel obstruction, including diffuse abdominal pain, nausea, vomiting, and bloating. Physical examination may reveal distention and tympany. Patients with fistulizing disease may present with a sudden onset of profuse diarrhea (due to an enteroenteric fistula), signs and symptoms of an intra-abdominal abscess (eg, fever, localized tenderness), or a more dramatic example of fistulizing disease such as an enterocutaneous fistula. Patients with enterovesicular fistulas may have a primary presentation of pneumaturia and recurrent urinary tract infections.

B. Laboratory Findings: In general, laboratory findings are nonspecific. Mild leukocytosis and thrombocytosis are frequently present. Anemia may be found. Marked leukocytosis should prompt one to suspect a suppurative complication. The erythrocyte sedimentation rate (ESR) is usually elevated. Hypoalbuminemia indicates disease severity and chronicity. Iron studies may reveal iron deficiency or an anemia of chronic disease. Serum vitamin B_{12} levels may be low owing to ileal disease or resection. Stool studies may reveal leukocytes but no enteric pathogens. Qualitative or preferably quantitative measurements of fecal fat may reveal steatorrhea as a manifestation of malabsorption.

C. Imaging Studies: Contrast radiography of the gastrointestinal tract provides valuable information in the diagnosis and management of Crohn's disease. Contrast studies of the small bowel allow docu-

mentation and delineation of the extent of small bowel disease. Characteristic findings of small bowel disease include "skip lesions," cobblestoning (owing to the intersection of transverse and longitudinal linear ulcers), and luminal narrowing ("string sign") and separation of bowel loops as a result of bowel wall thickening and edema. Small bowel images can be obtained by a standard barium small bowel follow-through or by enteroclysis. Enteroclysis provides much improved mucosal detail but requires duodenal intubation for injection of contrast medium and air, with the inherent problems of patient tolerability. Anterograde contrast studies are also extremely useful in demonstrating and defining strictures and fistulas. Barium enema is inferior to colonoscopy in evaluating the extent of mucosal involvement of the colon. It is useful in demonstrating fistulas and strictures involving the colon. Reflux of barium into the terminal ileum may provide documentation of ileal disease, which is particularly useful in differentiating Crohn's disease from ulcerative colitis. CT of the abdomen and pelvis is not a useful primary diagnostic tool in Crohn's disease but is crucial in the evaluation of complications related to the disease. It is the procedure of choice in determining if an intra-abdominal abscess is present and may be useful in demonstrating enterovesicular fistulas and ureteral involvement by inflammatory masses.

Colonoscopy is the procedure of choice for evaluating the presence and extent of Crohn's disease involvement of the colon. Characteristic colonoscopic findings include aphthae (small shallow ulcers with a red halo), round or linear serpiginous ulcers juxtaposed to normal-appearing mucosa, "skip lesions," and rectal sparing. Biopsies of both affected and normal-appearing areas (particularly the rectum) confirm the variable and discontinuous nature of Crohn's disease. Colonoscopy also allows for intubation of the terminal ileum, so that ileal disease can be documented directly.

Differential Diagnosis

The differential diagnosis of Crohn's disease is summarized in Table 7–2.

A. Small Bowel and Ileocecal Disease: Two entities frequently confused are ileocecal Crohn's disease and acute appendicitis. Frequently, patients with Crohn's disease have a relatively rapid onset of right lower quadrant pain, tenderness, and fever. The diagnosis is often made at laparotomy. Patients often will report having had antecedent symptoms of pain and diarrhea before the onset of more acute symptoms. In acutely ill patients in whom the diagnosis of Crohn's disease versus appendicitis or periappendiceal abscess is in doubt, abdominal CT scanning is often useful in differentiating the two. Other entities that must be considered in the more acutely symptomatic patient include cecal diverticulitis, pelvic inflammatory disease (including tubo-ovarian abscess),

Table 7–2. Differential diagnosis of Crohn's disease.

Ileocecal small bowel disease
  Infectious disease
    Acute appendicitis
    Cecal diverticulitis
    Pelvic inflammatory disease
    Ileocecal tuberculosis
    Yersinia enterocolitica infection
    Celiac disease
    Cytomegalovirus (immunosuppressed)
  Noninfectious disease
    Ectopic pregnancy
    Cecal carcinoma
    Vasculitis (including Behçet's disease)
    Radiation enteritis
    Lymphoma or lymphosarcoma
    Eosinophilic gastroenteritis
    Chronic nongranulomatous ulcerative jejunoileitis
Colonic disease
  Infectious disease
    Acute bacterial colitis (*Salmonella, Shigella,*
      Campylobacter)
    Amebic colitis
    Antibiotic-associated colitis (including *Clostridium difficile*
      toxin)
    Cytomegalovirus (immunosuppressed)
  Noninfectious disease
    Ulcerative colitis
    Radiation colitis
    Ischemic colitis

and ectopic pregnancy. Menstrual and gynecologic symptoms, a pregnancy test, and pelvic ultrasound studies (using both the cutaneous and transvaginal views) aid in excluding gynecologic disorders.

Two infectious entities that may be confused with Crohn's disease are *Yersinia enterocolitica* and ileocecal tuberculosis. *Yersinia* may cause an acute self-limited ileitis. Diagnosis may be made by stool culture or serologic studies. Tuberculosis may cause ileocecal disease that is difficult to distinguish from Crohn's disease. In the United States, ileocecal tuberculosis is rare and is frequently but not always associated with active pulmonary disease. In immunosuppressed patients, particularly patients with acquired immunodeficiency syndrome (AIDS), cytomegalovirus may lead to ileocecal disease similar to that seen in Crohn's disease. It should be noted that active Crohn's disease is unusual in immunosuppressed patients.

Other entities to consider include cecal carcinoma and gynecologic malignant tumors, particularly when there is a palpable mass. Celiac disease should be considered when diarrhea and weight loss are prominent symptoms.

Ischemic disease of the small bowel may resemble Crohn's disease and may be a result of oral contraceptives, radiation enteritis, or systemic vasculitis. A particularly interesting vasculitis is Behçet's disease, which may be associated with ileocecal disease that is virtually indistinguishable from Crohn's disease. Behçet's disease is usually differentiated by the presence of painful oral and genital ulcers.

Other rare entities included in the differential diagnosis of small bowel and ileocecal Crohn's disease include lymphoma, lymphosarcoma, eosinophilic gastroenteritis, and chronic nongranulomatous ulcerative jejunoileitis.

B. Colonic Disease: In a small number of cases of Crohn's disease limited to the colon, differentiation from ulcerative colitis can be difficult (see following section). Other entities included in the differential diagnosis of colonic Crohn's disease include acute colitis caused by bacterial infection with *Salmonella, Shigella,* or *Campylobacter,* colitis caused by cytomegalovirus or ameba, ischemic colitis, colitis associated with use of antibiotics (including *Clostridium difficile* colitis), or colitis resulting from radiation therapy.

Complications

A. Perforating Disease: The consequence of the penetrating transmural disease characteristic of the subgroup of patients with perforating disease is abscess and fistula formation. Free intra-abdominal perforation is rare, owing to the fact that the serosal surface of involved bowel usually adheres to adjacent structures.

Abscesses occur in up to 20% of Crohn's disease patients and may be of an intra-abdominal or extra-abdominal type. The intra-abdominal type is more common and may be located within the mesentery or between loops of bowel or the abdominal wall. Examples of extra-abdominal abscesses include retroperitoneal and abdominal wall abscesses.

Fistulas result from the penetration of a sinus tract (presumably beginning in a penetrating ulcer) into an adjacent structure, which may be a viscus or may extend externally to the skin. Fistulas complicate the course of Crohn's disease in up to 40% of patients. They may be symptomatic or asymptomatic, depending on their course and physiologic consequences.

Enteroenteric fistulas are fairly common and may be asymptomatic or associated with high-output diarrhea, depending on the amount of gastrointestinal tract that is bypassed. Enterovesicular fistulas may present with pneumaturia and recurrent urinary tract infections. These fistulas may be well tolerated or associated with urinary sepsis. Enterocutaneous fistulas frequently arise from anastomotic sites after surgical resection or may occur de novo. Depending on size and location, enterocutaneous fistulas may have a low output or a high output associated with metabolic sequelae. Rectovaginal fistulas are usually the result of rectal or anal disease. Occasionally, enterovaginal fistulas occur, but these are seen most frequently in women who have had hysterectomies.

B. Strictures: Stricture formation is another relatively common complication of Crohn's disease. Obstructive symptoms may be secondary to acute inflammation and edema, compression owing to the mass effect of an abscess, or formation of adhesions, but most often they result from the formation of a fibrostenotic stricture. Formation of recurrent strictures is the hallmark of the fibrostenotic variant of Crohn's disease. The typical clinical presentation of a stricture is one of partial obstruction, which resolves rapidly with conservative management. Strictures are best demonstrated with barium studies and usually reveal a narrowed segment of variable length, with evidence of dilatation of bowel proximal to the affected segment. Patients with strictures are at increased risk of developing bacterial overgrowth. A patient with a radiologically demonstrable stricture, diarrhea, and minimal obstructive symptoms should alert one to the possibility of bacterial overgrowth.

C. Perirectal Disease: Perirectal Crohn's disease may result in anorectal fistulas and abscesses. Typically, the initial lesion is an abscess involving an anorectal gland located in the intersphincteric space. This abscess may extend along different tissue planes leading to cryptoglandular, perianal, ischiorectal, or supralevator abscesses or fistulas.

D. Nutritional Deficiencies: Malnutrition may complicate Crohn's disease, and its basis is frequently multifactorial. Patients often have poor caloric intake due to food avoidance so as not to precipitate symptoms of nausea, vomiting, abdominal pain, and diarrhea. Extensive ileal disease or surgical resection may lead to bile salt depletion and subsequent fat malabsorption. Fat malabsorption may further lead to deficiencies of fat-soluble vitamins. In addition, colonic fatty acids compete for the calcium of dietary calcium oxalate, resulting in enhanced colonic oxalate absorption and possible oxalate nephrolithiasis. Vitamin B_{12} deficiency is common in patients with ileal disease. In a small subgroup of patients, extensive jejunoileal disease results in a significant loss of absorptive surface and malabsorption of carbohydrates, proteins, and water-soluble vitamins. Of course, multiple and extensive surgical resections may result in a true short-gut syndrome.

E. Other Causes of Diarrhea: Diarrhea in Crohn's disease is not only caused by active intestinal inflammation but may also be the result of a structural consequence of Crohn's disease. Resection of the distal ileum (< 100 cm) often results in moderate bile acid malabsorption and interruption of the normal bile salt enterohepatic circulation. Bile acids passing onto the colon cause electrolyte and water secretion. More extensive ileal resections (> 100 cm) result in severe bile acid malabsorption that exceeds the hepatic synthetic capabilities of maintaining an adequate bile acid pool. This results in fatty acid malabsorption with diarrhea, which is further aggravated by bacterially hydroxylated long-chain fatty acids, which also induce water and electrolyte malabsorption. Patients with strictures and fistulas are predisposed to small bowel bacterial overgrowth, which appears to cause diarrhea by disrupting bile acid enterohepatic circulation. Patients with fistulas may

also have increased diarrhea if the fistula serves to bypass a significant portion of the gastrointestinal tract.

F. Cancer: There is a clearly increased risk of small bowel adenocarcinoma in patients with Crohn's disease. Typically, these cancers arise in areas of long-term active disease. Segments of bypassed bowel may be particularly at risk. Although it has been estimated that the risk of small bowel cancer is 100-fold higher than in the general population, it should be noted that this type of cancer is rare in the general population, so the absolute risk is quite low. While colon cancer risk in patients with colonic Crohn's disease is still controversial, there is increasing evidence of a higher risk in these patients, particularly when the extent of disease is taken into account (see following section, "Ulcerative colitis").

Treatment

The goal of treatment in Crohn's disease is to restore well-being and an active lifestyle while minimizing the side effects related to medications. The side effects and potential consequences of glucocorticoids and immunosuppressives should not be underestimated. Treatment of complications of this disease usually requires a concerted effort by a gastroenterologist and a colorectal surgeon skilled in the management of inflammatory bowel disease.

Special attention should be given to the psychological impact of Crohn's disease. While psychological factors have never been clearly shown to affect disease activity, they certainly have an impact on a patient's sense of well-being. Inflammatory bowel disease can be an isolating disease in that patients frequently feel uncomfortable discussing their illness and symptoms even with close friends and family. Support groups and psychological therapies are an important adjunct to medical therapy (see following discussion).

A. General Approach to Treatment:

1. 5-aminosalicylic acid–Sulfasalazine has been the mainstay of treatment for both mild to moderately active Crohn's disease and ulcerative colitis for more than 30 years. 5-aminosalicylic acid (5-ASA, or mesalamine) appears to account for most of the therapeutic effect of this agent. Sulfasalazine is actually 5-aminosalicylic acid that is diazo-bonded to sulfapyridine. When taken orally, 5-aminosalicylic acid is released primarily in the colon by the action of bacterial azoreductase (Figure 7–1). 5-aminosalicylic acid acts topically by a variety of mechanisms, including inhibition of synthesis of leukotriene B_4 (a potent chemotactic compound), impairment of phagocytosis, inhibition of interleukin-1 production, and scavenging of free oxygen radicals. At a dose of 4 g/d, sulfasalazine is moderately effective in the treatment of mild to moderate colonic and ileocecal Crohn's disease. Given its colonic release site, it is not surprising that this agent has limited efficacy in

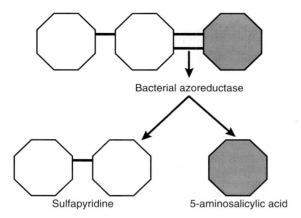

Figure 7–1. When taken orally, intact sulfasalazine is delivered to the colon, where bacterially derived azoreductase cleaves sulfasalazine's diazo bond, resulting in the release of the active 5-aminosalicylic acid moiety and the sulfapyridine carrier moiety.

Table 7–3. Mesalamine preparations.

Medication	Preparation	Release
Delayed release		
Asacol	Eudragit-S, coated	Release at pH > 7
Claversal or Salofalk	Eudragit-L, coated	Release at pH > 6
Rowasa	Eudragit-L100	Release at pH > 5
Sustained release		
Pentasa	Ethylcellulose microgranules	Time-dependent release

small bowel Crohn's disease. Side effects limit its use in a large proportion of patients (approximately 25%). Common side effects include nausea, vomiting, headache, rash, and fever. Some of these may be mitigated to some extent by gradually building up to the full therapeutic dose of 1 g orally four times a day over the course of a week. Less common side effects include anemia, hemolysis, epidermolysis, pancreatitis, pulmonary fibrosis, and sperm motility disorders. Patients undergoing long-term sulfasalazine therapy should also be given folate, 1 mg/d orally, to avoid folate deficiency.

Nearly all of the side effects of sulfasalazine have been attributed to the sulfapyridine moiety. This has led to the introduction and ongoing development of a variety of compounds containing mesalamine (5-aminosalicylic acid). If mesalamine is taken in its native form, it is systemically absorbed in the proximal gastrointestinal tract and therefore is not topically active in the distal gastrointestinal tract. Delayed-release forms of mesalamine are coated in pH-sensitive methylacrylate (Eudragit). By varying the pH of dissolution, the level of release in the gastrointestinal tract also varies. Methylacrylate adjusted to dissolve at a lower pH releases 5-aminosalicylic acid more proximally. Another type of delivery is mesalamine packaged in ethylcellulose microgranules, resulting in a time-dependent sustained release. Examples of delayed-release and sustained-release preparations are shown in Table 7–2. Asacol and Pentasa are available in the United States, while Claversal, Salofalk, and oral Rowasa (Table 7–3) are available in Europe. Two additional compounds containing 5-aminosalicylic acid include olsalazine (available in the USA) and balsalazide (under development in the USA). Both are diazo-bonded and therefore have the

same delivery characteristics as sulfasalazine. Olsalazine is a 5-aminosalicylic acid dimer, and balsalazide is 5-aminosalicylic acid that is diazo-bonded to an inert carrier (Figure 7–2).

Although Asacol and Pentasa are approved only for the treatment of acute ulcerative colitis, it can be readily seen from Figure 7–3 that their release characteristics have potential usefulness in the treatment of small bowel Crohn's disease. A variety of studies have suggested that these mesalamine preparations do have efficacy in small bowel and ileocecal Crohn's disease, particularly when they are used at high dosages. In this manner, selection of 5-aminosalicylic acid drugs can be guided by the release characteristics of the drug and the distribution of disease in the patient. Olsalazine is only approved for maintenance of remission in ulcerative colitis. A side effect unique to this agent is a secretory diarrhea in a small but significant minority of patients; this limits its usefulness in active Crohn's disease and ulcerative colitis. In general, these sulfasalazine analogs are well tolerated, with minimal side effects. Rare side

Azo compounds

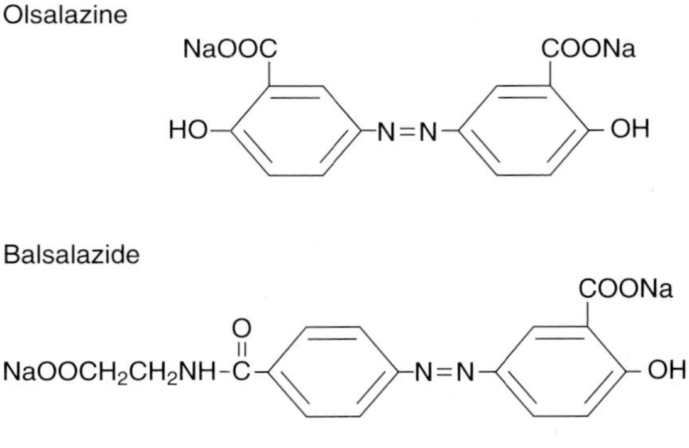

Olsalazine

Balsalazide

Figure 7–2. Olsalazine and balsalazide are also diazo-bonded and require degradation by bacterial azoreductase for the release of 5-aminosalicylic acid. Olsalazine is a 5-aminosalicylic acid dimer currently available in the United States. Balsalazide is 5-aminosalicylic acid diazo-bonded to an inert carrier molecule and is currently under development in the United States.

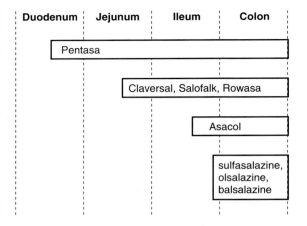

Duodenum	Jejunum	Ileum	Colon

Pentasa

Claversal, Salofalk, Rowasa

Asacol

sulfasalazine, olsalazine, balsalazine

Figure 7–3. A schematic representation of approximate release and distribution sites in the gastrointestinal tract for a variety of 5-aminosalicylic acid agents that are either currently available or under development in the United States or Europe.

effects include pancreatitis, nephrotoxicity, hair loss, and pericarditis.

Mesalamine is also available in enema and suppository preparations. Mesalamine enemas may be useful in the treatment of distal colonic Crohn's disease. Suppositories are helpful in the treatment of disease limited to the rectum and may be useful in some patients with perirectal disease.

2. Corticosteroids–Corticosteroids are the mainstay of treatment of moderate to severe Crohn's disease. Their efficacy has been demonstrated in large cooperative trials performed in both the USA and Europe. Corticosteroids appear to act through a variety of mechanisms, including impairment of T cell function, impairment of chemotaxis and phagocytosis, and reduction of cytokine and eicosanoid synthesis. Most patients with moderate exacerbations of Crohn's disease will achieve fairly prompt remission with oral prednisone at doses of 40–60 mg/d. Severely ill patients with Crohn's disease should be hospitalized for exclusion of suppurative complications and treatment with intravenous methylprednisolone at doses of 60–100 mg/d. Once remission is achieved, corticosteroids should be tapered over the next several weeks (ie, 8–12 weeks, sometimes with alternate-day tapering at lower doses). A significant proportion of patients (perhaps up to one-third) will have flare-ups during the tapering period and be dependent on corticosteroids to maintain remission. Every effort should be made to avoid the long-term use of corticosteroids, however, because of their potentially devastating side effects. These include, but are not limited to, the typical cushingoid appearance, osteoporosis, hypertension, diabetes, psychosis, aseptic necrosis of bone, neuropathy, and myopathy.

Crohn's disease patients should be treated with 5-aminosalicylic acid (high-dosage) compounds in an effort to achieve some corticosteroid-sparing effect. Alternate-day tapering may be useful in some patients and may minimize side effects. Patients with aggressive and difficult-to-control disease should be given immunosuppressives early rather than after a prolonged course of high-dosage corticosteroids.

A potentially exciting class of corticosteroids is those that are topically active but have an extensive first-pass hepatic metabolism such that there is diminished systemic effect. These agents include tixocortol pivalate, fluticasone propionate, beclomethasone dipropionate, and budesonide. These are available in Europe as enema preparations. Of particular promise is an oral preparation being developed in which budesonide is delivered via a delayed-release system similar to that in delayed-release mesalamine preparations. Recent studies suggest that oral budesonide may be as effective as prednisolone in active Crohn's disease, may decrease the frequency of relapse, and is associated with less corticosteroid toxicity.

3. Immunosuppressive drugs–The purine analogs, 6-mercaptopurine and azathioprine, have an important place in the treatment of Crohn's disease. They are the drugs of choice in the management of disease that is dependent on or resistant to corticosteroids. 6-mercaptopurine and azathioprine, a prodrug of 6-mercaptopurine, can be used interchangeably, with the choice usually based on previous experience. Purine analogs inhibit nucleotide synthesis. Their mechanism of action in inflammatory bowel disease is unclear but may be related to inhibition of T cell clonal expansion.

While the dose of 6-mercaptopurine is frequently stated to be 1.5 mg/kg/d orally, most patients seem to respond to 50 mg/d, and many physicians now prescribe this dose from the beginning. The main downside to the purine analogs is their slow onset of action. The mean time to clinical response is 3 months, with full clinical response in some patients taking 6–9 months. In patients who have failed to respond to 50 mg/d at 3 months, the dose may be adjusted upward in 25-mg increments to a maximum of 1.5 mg/kg, until the desired clinical effect is achieved. Patients should be fully informed of the toxicities, which include marrow suppression, pancreatitis, hepatitis, and infections. Because of the potential for marrow suppression, complete blood counts should be monitored weekly initially for the first month, then biweekly for 2 months, and finally monthly during long-term treatment. Pancreatitis occurs in 3–5% of patients, usually within the first month of therapy. Infections may occur in 5–10% of patients, but severe infections occur in less than 2%. Of special concern is the theoretic risk of cancer in patients taking purine analogs. Lymphoma has been reported in renal transplantation patients taking azathioprine; however, there is little convincing evidence of an excessive risk of malignant tumors in inflammatory bowel disease patients taking purine analogs. Patients should be made aware of this theoretic concern. Teratogenicity is also a theoretic concern, although no birth defects have been reported in children of inflammatory bowel disease patients taking purine analogs. Of course, it is prudent to avoid the use of these drugs in pregnant women and in women of child-bearing age who fail to use adequate birth control.

Approximately 75% of patients treated with 6-mercaptopurine are able to taper off or significantly reduce their steroid dose. In addition, up to one-third of fistulas may close over a 2-year period of treatment. Because of their slow onset of action and the clinical setting in which they are used (for disease dependent on or resistant to corticosteroids), the purine analogs are usually used as long-term agents. There is little rationale for using them for less than 4–5 years, as the limited available information suggests that the relapse rate associated with stopping the drug before this time is unacceptably high.

Other immunosuppressives have been investigated in the treatment of Crohn's disease, including cyclosporine and methotrexate. To date, there have been reports of only modest efficacy, and given the unfavorable side effect profile compared with that of 6-mercaptopurine, their use should only be considered in patients who have failed 6-mercaptopurine therapy and then preferably in the context of a clinical trial. Preliminary reports suggest that cyclosporine may be useful in the treatment of fistulas, although the relapse rate may be high.

4. Antibiotics—Metronidazole is the only antibiotic that has been used extensively in the treatment of Crohn's disease. It appears to have reasonable efficacy in some subgroups of colonic and ileocolonic Crohn's disease, although there is little controlled supporting data. Metronidazole is a widely accepted treatment of perianal Crohn's disease. Other antibiotics and antibiotic regimens have been espoused in the treatment of Crohn's disease, although there is no convincing data to support their use.

5. Nutrition—Aggressive nutritional support is an important adjunct in the treatment of Crohn's disease. Wherever possible, an enteral route should be used. Of special note, there is a large body of evidence in the pediatric and adult literature that suggests elemental enteral diets may be as effective as prednisone (particularly in small bowel disease). Because elemental solutions have an unpleasant taste, they usually have to be given via some type of feeding tube, and this makes them an infeasible form of treatment in most cases. Elemental diets may be useful in treating small bowel disease that is refractory to corticosteroids and providing nutritional support in patients with borderline short-gut syndrome. Total parenteral nutrition should be reserved for patients in whom an enteral route is not feasible, as in high-output fistula or obstructive disease.

Despite the fact that food is a major source of intraluminal antigen, there is no consistent evidence that elimination or highly restrictive diets have a role in the treatment of Crohn's disease. Lactose restriction may be helpful in some patients but is not mandatory in all patients. Patients with symptomatic fibrostenotic disease frequently benefit from a low-residue diet.

6. Education, group support, and psychological therapy—As has been mentioned previously, the psychological impact of a chronic illness, especially one associated with disordered bowel function, should not be ignored. As is the case with most chronic illness, fears surrounding the loss of well-being, risk of cancer, treatment, future complications, and possibility of death are common. These fears are best addressed through education by the physician, nurse, and patient-based materials. The Crohn's and Colitis Foundation of America is an excellent source of patient-based educational materials. Social support is also an extremely important factor leading to successful adjustment to a chronic disease. The foundation provides a fairly extensive network of peer support groups, which have proved to be invaluable to many patients. In a large proportion of patients, disease exacerbations impose limitations on personal and professional activities, resulting in significant psychological stress. In some patients, psychotherapy may aid in the management of psychological stress and result in an enhanced sense of well-being.

B. Approach to Specific Problems and Complications:

1. Perforating disease—Patients with abscesses will usually require surgery. When an abscess is suspected, broad-spectrum antibiotics should be instituted and the abscess should be localized by CT scanning. If possible, the abscess should be drained and a catheter placed percutaneously under CT guidance. After catheter drainage has slowed, the patient may be fed orally, with careful monitoring of catheter output, and if the output is high, a course of total parenteral nutrition is required. Definitive surgery may then be delayed (for up to several weeks) until the abscess is fully drained and the underlying Crohn's disease is brought under medical control. This approach allows for a technically easier, more limited resection of the segment of involved bowel. Catheter drainage without subsequent surgery usually results in a persistent enterocutaneous fistula. If drainage guided by CT scanning is not feasible or if there is evidence of peritonitis, immediate surgical intervention is required.

Fistulas associated with significant symptoms also usually require surgery. Incidentally identified enteroenteric fistulas without significant metabolic consequences need no particular therapy. In the case of moderately symptomatic enterovesicular, enterocutaneous, and enteroenteric fistulas, treatment may be undertaken surgically or medically. Definitive surgery must be weighed against the modest success (at best, one-third of patients are successfully treated) and long duration of medical therapy (with 6-mercaptopurine), with the ultimate decision being based on symptoms and patient preference. Before surgery is undertaken, bowel disease should be under good control. Fistulas causing severe symptoms and especially complex fistulas associated with abscesses require surgical management.

2. Fibrostenotic disease—Patients with Crohn's disease presenting with obstructive symptoms as a result of stricture formation typically improve within the first 2–3 days of hospitalization, with conservation therapy consisting of bowel rest, nasogastric suction, and intravenous hydration. It is reasonable to treat patients with evidence of active disease (on colonoscopy or contrast x-ray) with aggressive medical therapy, in that there may be a significant inflammatory component to their partial obstruction. A low-residue diet may reduce the incidence of subsequent episodes of partial bowel obstruction. Patients with recurrent bouts of partial obstruction and patients who fail to respond to conservative therapy require surgery. Patients with complete bowel obstruction require urgent surgery. Surgery for stricturing disease may take the form of limited resection and primary anastomosis or a stricturoplasty (technically similar to a pyloroplasty).

3. Perirectal disease—Treatment of perirectal disease requires a team approach with a gastroenterologist and an experienced colorectal surgeon. Draining fistulas may close with prolonged treatment with metronidazole. More severe disease may require corticosteroids and 6-mercaptopurine. Abscesses require surgical drainage. Severe perianal disease sometimes requires bowel rest, with total parenteral nutrition or fecal diversion. In truly refractory cases, especially when there has been significant destruction of the anal sphincters, proctectomy may be required. Rectovaginal fistulas commonly complicate perianal disease. They may close with intensive treatment with metronidazole or 6-mercaptopurine. Surgery may be undertaken for persistent fistulas, but the success of repair is based on adequate control of the rectal or perianal disease.

4. Other causes of diarrhea—As has been discussed previously, diarrhea may be the result of bacterial overgrowth or bile acid wasting or depletion. In patients with strictures or fistulas, bacterial overgrowth may be contributing to or responsible for the diarrhea. This should be considered especially when there is little evidence of ongoing active disease. While a hydrogen breath test may be used to document bacterial overgrowth (although it may be difficult to interpret in patients with fistulas), it is more practical to treat empirically with a course of broad-spectrum antibiotics. Patients with ileal resections of

less than 100 cm may be treated empirically with bile acid-binding resins (eg, cholestyramine, 4 g orally two or three times daily). Diarrhea in patients with more extensive ileal resections will worsen following treatment with bile acid-binding resins because of the further depletion of their bile acid pool. After documentation of steatorrhea, treatment requires a low-fat diet supplemented with medium-chain triglycerides, which are more readily absorbed without micelle formation.

5. Prevention of relapse and postoperative recurrence—There is no drug that has definitively been shown to prevent Crohn's disease relapse. This is particularly true of patients with quiescent disease who are receiving no current therapy. Patients with more aggressive disease requiring immunosuppressives are more likely to stay in remission if they continue to take the drugs. There is a fine distinction between suppression of ongoing active disease and prevention of relapse in the setting of a true remission. Some recent data appear to suggest that prolongation of remission may be achieved with delayed-release or sustained-release mesalamine preparations in patients who were recently brought into remission. There is also some evidence that metronidazole and mesalamine preparations may delay postoperative recurrences. Studies of a variety of agents are ongoing.

Prognosis

It is important to remember that in placebo-controlled trials, 30–40% of patients assigned to placebo achieve a remission during the course of the study. In addition, 10–20% of Crohn's disease patients have prolonged remissions after the initial episode of disease. Over the course of their disease, 60–70% of patients will require surgery, and of these, approximately 50% will require subsequent surgery at some point. Mortality rates from Crohn's disease have declined over the past several decades because of the improved management of suppurative and metabolic complications. Currently, mortality rates appear to be slightly higher in Crohn's disease patients compared with age-matched controls; this may be due to cancer associated with Crohn's disease.

ULCERATIVE COLITIS

Ulcerative colitis is characterized by intermittent exacerbations and remissions of typical symptoms. The first attack of ulcerative colitis has a broad differential diagnosis, however (see following discussion), and the diagnosis is made by exclusion of other causes (particularly infectious causes) and the typical findings seen on sigmoidoscopy or colonoscopy with biopsy. A first attack of ulcerative colitis typically has a longer prodrome of symptoms than acute infectious disorders. Supportive evidence of the diagnosis of ulcerative colitis is the absence of small bowel involvement or complications more typical of Crohn's disease.

Pathology

The gross appearance of a colon involved with ulcerative colitis varies with the extent and severity of disease. In mild disease, there may be mucosal erythema and edema and perhaps small erosions. The inflammation always begins distally in the rectum and spreads proximally for variable distances. There is usually a sharp demarcation between involved colon and more proximal uninvolved colon. Inflammatory polyps or pseudopolyps may be present. Chronically involved colons lose their normal haustral folds and take on a flat appearance. Severely involved colons may exhibit large areas of ulceration and hemorrhage. In extremely ill patients manifesting "toxic megacolon," the inflammatory process is transmural.

Histologically, the characteristic lesion of ulcerative colitis is the crypt abscess, which in its fully developed form is characterized by neutrophils within the crypt as well as in the crypt wall and the adjacent lamina propria. While crypt abscesses are characteristic of ulcerative colitis, they may also be seen in acute self-limited colitis as well as in Crohn's disease. The lamina propria in ulcerative colitis is frequently infiltrated with increased numbers of mononuclear cells, indicating chronicity. This would be unusual in acute self-limited colitis but is common in Crohn's colitis. One of the helpful histologic findings in differentiating ulcerative colitis from acute self-limited colitis is crypt architectural distortion (frequently referred to as chronic colitis, as opposed to chronic inflammation), which is characterized by gland branching, shortening (not reaching the muscularis mucosa), and loss of the normal parallel arrangement of glands. There may also be Paneth cell metaplasia (these cells are typically seen only in the right colon), which is another sign of chronicity. Many of these features may be seen in Crohn's colitis as well. The inflammatory process in ulcerative colitis does not usually disrupt the muscularis mucosa, but in more severe cases, there may be extension into the submucosa.

Clinical Findings

The clinical presentation of ulcerative colitis is to some extent based on the severity of disease as well as the extent of colonic involvement. Ulcerative colitis may involve only the rectum (ulcerative proctitis), the entire colon (universal colitis or pancolitis), or parts of each in varying degree. The hallmark of ulcerative colitis is that the rectum is always involved and disease extends proximally in a continuous fashion, without skip areas. In rare circumstances, there is rectal sparing, but this is most often due to previous topical treatment (enema or suppository). Biopsies of the "spared" rectum usually reveal typical histologic changes of ulcerative colitis. Ulcerative colitis is categorized by the extent of involvement, however there are no standard terms to describe this involvement. The terms most frequently used are ulcerative proctitis (usually limited to the distal 10–20 cm), pancolitis (universal involvement or at least involvement beyond the hepatic flexure), or left-sided colitis (which is variably defined but indicates intermediate involvement). Because of the variability in the definitions used to describe the extent of disease and the relatively recent introduction of fiberoptic (now video) colonoscopy, it is difficult to quantify the percentage of patients who fall into each category at the time of presentation. A best guess is that about one-third of patients have pancolitis, 30–40% have disease limited to the rectosigmoid, and the remainder have some intermediate form.

For the purposes of this chapter, the extent of disease will be divided into two categories. Limited disease is defined as ulcerative colitis confined to the rectosigmoid and extensive disease extends beyond the rectosigmoid. The value of this classification is that the determination can be made by flexible sigmoidoscopy, and it has implications for therapy and cancer screening. Extensive disease usually would not be expected to respond to rectal therapies alone. Patients with this type of disease include those with a substantially higher risk of developing colon cancer.

As in Crohn's disease, there are a variety of scales that can be used to assess disease severity in ulcerative colitis. An overall assessment of severity is derived from the patient's complaints, impact of the disease on daily function, pertinent physical examination findings (eg, fever, tenderness) and the presence of abnormal laboratory parameters (eg, anemia, hypoalbuminemia). Attention to these parameters usually allows the clinician to categorize the patient as mildly, moderately, or severely ill. In addition, there are numerous endoscopic scales to grade the severity of colitis. Therapeutic decisions should be based primarily on clinical status and not endoscopic appearance, however.

A. Symptoms and Signs: Most patients with ulcerative colitis complain of bloody diarrhea, crampy abdominal pain, and tenesmus. A small percentage of patients either complain of bleeding alone or diarrhea alone. Fever and weight loss are present in approximately one-third of patients, and up to 15–25% have some extracolonic manifestation of ulcerative colitis (eg, eye, joint, and skin complaints). In general, patients with ulcerative colitis will have had some symptoms for weeks to months prior to presentation, whereas patients with acute self-limited colitis typically have an abrupt onset of symptoms.

The physical examination in patients with acute ulcerative colitis may range from completely normal or mild left lower quadrant tenderness to signs of systemic toxicity (eg, fever, tachycardia, and orthostasis), depending on the severity and extent of disease.

Patients with **toxic megacolon** (a life-threatening form of ulcerative colitis) manifest signs of toxic colitis (fever > 101°F, heart rate > 120 beats/min, abdominal distention, and signs of localized or generalized peritonitis), with leukocytosis (white blood cell count usually > 11,000/μL) and dilated colon on plain abdominal x-ray.

B. Laboratory Findings: Abnormal laboratory parameters in ulcerative colitis patients are not specific to ulcerative colitis but represent the degree of systemic impact. Patients with more severe disease may exhibit leukocytosis, thrombocytosis, anemia, and hypoalbuminemia. The ESR is usually elevated. Stool studies for culture, ova, and parasites and *Clostridium difficile* toxin are negative.

C. Imaging Studies: Contrast radiography of the colon has limited clinical usefulness in the diagnosis and management of ulcerative colitis given the availability of flexible endoscopy. Double-contrast barium enema in mild ulcerative colitis reveals a fine granular-appearing mucosa. With increased disease severity, discrete ulcers are seen. In more long-standing disease, there is loss of haustral markings, shortening of the colon, and, frequently, a tubular appearance of the colon. Typical filling defects representing pseudopolyps may be seen. Of course, atypical masses or strictures may represent a neoplasm.

The endoscopic appearance of mild ulcerative colitis is characterized by erythema, granularity, loss of vascularity, and contact bleeding (friability). With increasing severity, there is pinpoint ulceration, spontaneous bleeding, and extensive frank ulceration. As has been previously stated, ulcerative colitis begins in the rectum and extends proximally in a continuous fashion. The most severe disease tends to be seen distally, unless there has been ongoing therapy per rectum. Random biopsies should be taken throughout the affected area (labeled by location). Separately labeled biopsies should always be taken in the rectum, particularly when there is some question of endoscopic sparing. In the acute setting of moderate to severe colitis, it is wise to perform only a limited inspection of the rectosigmoid for fear of perforating an acutely diseased colon. Rectal biopsies should be taken to aid in the diagnosis. A more complete endoscopic examination to assess the extent of involvement can be performed at a later date, after the disease has been adequately controlled.

Differential Diagnosis

The differential diagnosis of ulcerative colitis is summarized in Table 7–4.

There are a variety of infectious entities that must be considered. Acute self-limited colitis is most commonly caused by *Campylobacter, Salmonella, Shigella, Yersinia,* and *Escherichia coli* 0157:H7, although stool cultures are only positive 50% of the time. Rectal biopsies frequently aid in differentiating acute self-limited colitis from ulcerative colitis.

Table 7–4. Differential diagnosis of ulcerative colitis.

Infectious disease
  Acute bacterial colitis (acute self-limited colitis)
    Campylobacter
    Salmonella
    Shigella
    Yersinia
    Escherichia coli 0157:H7
  Antibiotic-associated diarrhea (including *Clostridium difficile*)
  Amebic colitis
  Immunocompromised host
    Cytomegalovirus
    Herpes simplex virus
    Neisseria gonorrhoeae
    Blastocystis hominis
    Chlamydia
Noninfectious disease
  Crohn's colitis
  Ischemic colitis
  Radiation colitis
  Collagenous or microscopic colitis

Amebiasis may cause a chronic colitis that can be confused with ulcerative colitis. Amebiasis should be excluded by mucosal biopsy and ova and parasite examination in patients who have traveled to endemic areas or are in contact with others from such areas. *Clostridium difficile* and antibiotic-associated diarrhea should be considered in patients who have taken antibiotics recently.

Of the noninfectious colitides, Crohn's colitis and ischemic colitis are usually differentiated from ulcerative colitis by their pattern of distribution. Radiation-induced and diversion colitis are usually readily identified based on historical information. Collagenous and microscopic colitis are typically only diagnosed histologically and are readily differentiated from ulcerative colitis.

In the immunocompromised patient, a variety of pathogens may cause proctitis or colitis, including cytomegalovirus, herpes simplex virus, gonorrhea, *Blastocystis hominis,* and *Chlamydia.* It is also noteworthy that there are reports of persistent ulcerative colitis activity in ulcerative colitis patients who have subsequently developed AIDS.

Complications

A. Toxic Megacolon: Toxic megacolon usually occurs in patients with pancolitis but has been reported in more limited disease. The true frequency of toxic megacolon in ulcerative colitis is unknown, but it is probably seen in less than 5% of patients. It may occur at any time during the disease course but is more likely early in the course. In some patients, the initial presentation of ulcerative colitis may be toxic megacolon. Reported mortality rates vary from 15 to 50%. Not unexpectedly, perforation at presentation is associated with a high mortality rate.

B. Perforation: Colonic perforation complicating severe colitis in the absence of toxic megacolon has been reported. Perforation of this type tends to occur during an initial episode of ulcerative colitis, and the sigmoid is the most common site of perforation. Free perforation is associated with a high mortality rate.

C. Stricture: Strictures are uncommon in ulcerative colitis, and the presence of a stricture should raise serious concern for an underlying malignant tumor. Colectomy should be strongly considered in a patient with long-standing ulcerative colitis and a stricture, even if mucosal biopsies are unrevealing. Dysplasia found in biopsies of a stricture is an absolute indication for colectomy. When benign strictures occur in ulcerative colitis, they are usually seen in patients with extensive, chronically active disease.

D. Massive Hemorrhage: Massive colonic hemorrhage requiring urgent colectomy is a rare complication of ulcerative colitis.

E. Cancer: The extent of colonic involvement and the duration of disease are positively correlated with cancer risk. Reports of long-term risk vary and are significantly higher than in age-matched controls. Studies done at tertiary referral centers report a cancer risk of 13% after 20 years and 34% after 30 years of ulcerative colitis, while population-based studies report risks of 5.5% and 13% for 20 and 30 years, respectively. It is usually accepted that pancolitis carries the highest risk, whereas ulcerative proctitis is associated with little risk above that of age-matched controls. Left-sided colitis is thought to have an intermediate risk. Because of the variability in the definition of left-sided colitis in available studies, it is virtually impossible to determine whether the risk is significantly different than that of pancolitis. Therefore, it is probably more reasonable to characterize patients as having limited or extensive colitis.

Cancer in ulcerative colitis patients does not develop from a colonoscopically recognizable adenomatous polyp like that in sporadic colon cancer but rather arises from flat dysplastic epithelium, which is not colonoscopically distinguishable from adjacent nondysplastic mucosa. Because of this increased cancer risk, it is common practice to have patients with extensive ulcerative colitis for more than 7 years undergo yearly surveillance colonoscopic examination. At each examination, between two and four biopsies are taken at 10-cm intervals throughout the colon and evaluated for the presence of dysplasia. If dysplasia is present, it is categorized as either low grade or high grade. The finding of dysplasia (confirmed by a gastrointestinal pathologist) should prompt a recommendation for colectomy. Others have recommended following patients with low-grade dysplasia (surveillance examinations at more frequent intervals), but given the large sampling error associated with random biopsies, it seems prudent to recommend colectomy for confirmed low-grade dysplasia. Low-grade or high-grade dysplasia may also be associated with an endoscopically suspicious lesion or mass called a **dysplasia-associated lesion or mass**. It is associated with a high rate of underlying neoplasm (approximately 50%) and is therefore a clear indication for colectomy. Prophylactic colectomy is an alternative to a program of colonoscopic surveillance (see following section, "Surgery Treatment").

Treatment

The reader is directed to the treatment section on Crohn's disease for a more complete discussion of mechanism of action and side effects of the following classes of medications. In this section, they are discussed primarily in the context of ulcerative colitis. The comments and section on group support, education, and psychological therapy appearing in the Crohn's disease section are equally relevant to the treatment of ulcerative colitis.

A. General Approach to Treatment:

1. 5-aminosalicylic acid–Sulfasalazine remains the drug of choice for the treatment of mild to moderately active ulcerative colitis. There is little evidence to suggest that the newer preparations of this agent are any more efficacious than sulfasalazine in controlling inflammation. Twenty to 30% of patients will either be intolerant of sulfasalazine or have a sulfa allergy. Therefore, given their substantially higher cost, the main role of these newer 5-aminosalicylic acid preparations is in the treatment of sulfasalazine-intolerant patients. It is also important to note that the pH- and time-dependent preparations have a more variable delivery of 5-aminosalicylic acid to the colon than diazo-bonded compounds. Both types of newer preparations usually have substantial release of 5-aminosalicylic acid in the small bowel (especially the time-dependent preparation), although pH-dependent preparations may fail to adequately release active drug in the colon. One possible explanation for this is the reduced intraluminal colonic pH during an acute flare-up. This variability in release should be considered when patients fail to respond to treatment, but despite this factor, these newer 5-aminosalicylic acid preparations (particularly Asacol) are capable of delivering higher concentrations of 5-aminosalicylic acid than sulfasalazine, with minimal side effects when used in high dosages. This will be especially true of the new diazo compounds under development. In patients failing to respond to sulfasalazine or standard dosages of alternative 5-aminosalicylic acid compounds, some will respond favorably to high-dose Asacol (up to 4.8 g/d). Renal function should be monitored periodically in patients treated with high-dose 5-aminosalicylic acid compounds. Given the possibility of diarrhea as a side effect, use of olsalazine should be avoided in the treatment of acute colitis.

Patients with more limited disease are good candidates for medication applied per rectum once or twice daily. Patients with disease limited to the rectum (the distal 10 cm) may be treated with 5-amino-salicylic acid (mesalamine) suppositories. Patients with disease beyond the rectum but not beyond the descending colon may be treated with 5-aminosali-cylic acid retention enemas. It is important to con-sider that some patients with acute colitis will have difficulty retaining enemas. If this is the case, they should be treated with oral medications until their disease is brought under better control.

2. Corticosteroids—Prednisone, at doses of 40–60 mg/d orally, induces remissions in 75–90% of patients with ulcerative colitis. As with Crohn's dis-ease, their long-term use should be avoided. Patients treated with corticosteroids should be treated con-comitantly with 5-aminosalicylic acid preparations to take advantage of their potential "steroid sparing" ef-fects. After induction of remission, corticosteroids are tapered slowly over a 6- to 8-week period.

Patients with limited disease who fail to respond to 5-aminosalicylic acid may be treated with hydro-cortisone enemas (100 mg) once or twice daily. Cor-ticosteroid foam and suppositories can be used for the treatment of ulcerative proctitis. There is signifi-cant systemic absorption of these preparations, which may lead to full-blown Cushing's syndrome with long-term use. Topically active but rapidly metabo-lized corticosteroids will avoid many of these long-term toxicities.

3. Immunosuppressive drugs—There is sub-stantial evidence (primarily uncontrolled data) sup-porting the efficacy of the purine analogs, 6-mercap-topurine and azathioprine, in the treatment of ulcerative colitis. As with Crohn's disease, they are indicated when a patient is refractory to or dependent on corticosteroids. The dosages, potential toxicities, and guidelines are the same as those described for Crohn's disease. Use of these agents in the treatment of ulcerative colitis has increased over the past sev-eral years because of their successful and largely safe use in Crohn's disease. It must be appreciated, how-ever, that ulcerative colitis is a surgically curable dis-ease. The risks and benefits of these drugs must be weighed against the risks and benefits of surgery. The decision in each case must be individualized and should only be made after the patient is fully in-formed. The process of educating the patient should include addressing any misconceptions about surgi-cal treatment. While it may be reasonable to use 6-mercaptopurine in some selected patients early in the course of disease, it is less reasonable to use the drug to delay surgery in a patient with long-term extensive disease, who is therefore a substantial cancer risk.

Recently, there has been some enthusiasm for the use of cyclosporine in the treatment of severe ulcera-tive colitis refractory to intravenous corticosteroids. In this patient group, intravenous cyclosporine ap-pears to induce a rapid remission in up to 80% of pa-tients. Short-term follow-up of these responders re-veals that up to 30–50% ultimately require colectomy

within the first 6 months for persistent symptoms or drug intolerance. The toxicities associated with cy-closporine appear to be substantial in the inflamma-tory bowel disease population. Seizures, hyperten-sion, and nephrotoxicity as well as severe and opportunistic infections have been reported. The use of cyclosporine may be considered in highly se-lected, fully informed patients as a bridge to the slower-acting purine analogs. Given the side effect profile of cyclosporine, one would have to question its long-term use in patients who have failed treat-ment with 6-mercaptopurine. There has also been some recent investigation into the use of methotrex-ate in the treatment of refractory ulcerative colitis. It is crucial that when the use of these newer immuno-suppressives in the treatment of ulcerative colitis is being considered, their efficacy and toxicities must be weighed against a surgical outcome.

4. Surgical treatment—In general, the indica-tions for surgical treatment of ulcerative colitis in-clude perforation, severe hemorrhage, dysplasia or cancer, and disease refractory to medical therapy. The role of prophylactic proctocolectomy in patients with long-standing extensive disease is controversial. It is usually held that the risk of cancer is too high to ignore but not high enough to warrant prophylactic proctocolectomy. It has not been definitively demon-strated, however, that currently available surveillance techniques are adequate to reliably diminish the risk of a cancer-related death. Patients should be in-formed of the probable limitations of colonoscopic surveillance and given the option of prophylactic proctocolectomy.

In the past, the standard ulcerative colitis opera-tion was a proctocolectomy with either a standard (Brooke) ileostomy or a technically more difficult continent (Koch) ileostomy. In the past 15 years, ma-jor surgical advances have been made in restorative proctocolectomy. In this procedure, an abdominal colectomy is performed and a pouch fashioned from the distal ileum. Rectal mucosa is stripped from the cuff of the distal rectum, and the pouch is anasto-mosed to this cuff. Typically, a diverting ileostomy is performed to allow the pouch and anastomosis to heal for several months, after which the ileostomy is taken down at a second operation. This operation is frequently termed an ileoanal pullthrough or ileal pouch-anal anastomosis. A more recent modification of this operation omits the rectal mucosectomy and instead anastomoses the ileal pouch to the distal rec-tum in close proximity to the dentate line (1–4 cm). This ileal pouch-distal rectal anastomosis is techni-cally easier to perform, is thought by some to have less risk for incontinence, and in some hands can be performed as a single-stage operation without a di-verting ileostomy. The controversy around the ileal pouch-distal rectal anastomosis is related to the fact that some "transitional" epithelium is left intact that may be a source of future cancer risk. In experienced hands, both operations have excellent outcomes. After 1 year, patients typically report having approximately six bowel movements per day (one at night). Incontinence, impotence, and the need for pouch removal all appear to occur in less than 5% of patients. The most common late postoperative complication is pouchitis. Pouchitis is characterized by increased stool frequency, urgency, cramps, and malaise. It is probably related to stasis within the pouch and responds well to metronidazole in most cases.

B. Specific Treatment Recommendations:

1. Limited disease—In mild to moderate disease, mesalamine (5-aminosalicylic acid) suppositories (500 mg) or enemas (4 g), depending on extent of disease, can be administered once or twice daily. If symptoms worsen or fail to improve over 2 weeks, hydrocortisone enemas (100 mg) may be substituted for or alternated with the 5-aminosalicylic acid preparation.

In patients who fail to respond to this regimen or who present with more severe disease, oral prednisone should be administered in doses of 40–60 mg/d. It is best to start at high doses to rapidly induce remission and then to taper the dose, rather than starting at low doses and increasing them. In patients who have relapsed and failed to respond to their previously successful rectal regimen, it is important to consider the possibility of the proximal extension of disease. This can be evaluated with a flexible sigmoidoscopy or colonoscopy after their disease has been brought under better control. Severely ill patients should be hospitalized for bed rest, intravenous hydration, intravenous methylprednisolone (60–100 mg/d), and nutritional support. Treatment with immunosuppressives may be considered in patients who are refractory to or dependent on corticosteroids (see preceding section, "Immunosuppressive Drugs").

2. Extensive disease—In mild to moderate disease, sulfasalazine may be started at an oral dose of 500 mg twice per day, and then gradually increased to a dose of 3–4 g/d over 1 week. If the patient is allergic to or intolerant of sulfa, an alternative oral 5-aminosalicylic acid drug should be used (Asacol, 2.4–4.8 g/d, or Pentasa, 4 g/d). Patients taking sulfasalazine should be supplemented with folate, 1 mg/d orally.

In patients who fail to respond to this regimen or who present with more severe disease, oral prednisone should be administered in doses of 40–60 mg/d. It is best to start at high doses to rapidly induce remission and then to taper them, rather than starting at low doses and then increasing them. Severely ill patients should be hospitalized for bed rest, intravenous hydration, intravenous methylprednisolone (60–100 mg/d), and nutritional support. Treatment with immunosuppressives may be considered in patients who are refractory to or dependent on corticosteroids (see preceding section, "Immunosuppressives Drugs").

3. Toxic megacolon—Toxic megacolon is a life-threatening complication of ulcerative colitis that requires an intensive team approach by a gastroenterologist and surgeon. Care is best provided in the intensive care unit setting. Management consists of aggressive fluid and electrolyte replacement, intravenous methylprednisolone (100 mg/d), broad-spectrum intravenous antibiotics, and placement of nasogastric and rectal tubes. Total parenteral nutrition should be started initially, as it is unlikely that an enteral route will be a viable option until much later in the hospitalization. Frequent abdominal examination and daily or twice-daily abdominal and upright chest x-rays should be performed. Indications for surgical intervention include free intra-abdominal air, colonic intramural pneumatosis, peritoneal signs on abdominal examination, and failure to improve within 24–48 hours. Patients who fail to improve within 48 hours are unlikely to improve and risk a poorer outcome if surgery is delayed.

4. Prevention of relapse—Patients who have achieved remission should be placed on 5-aminosalicylic acid maintenance therapy, as there is convincing evidence that this substantially reduces the incidence of relapse. For extensive disease, sulfasalazine (1 g orally twice daily) or olsalazine (500 mg to 1 g twice daily) is reasonable. While maintenance dosages have not been clearly determined for the other compounds, Asacol, 800 mg to 2.4 g/d, and Pentasa, 2–4 g/d, have been shown to reduce relapse rates. Patients with limited disease may be treated with rectal preparations on an every-other-day or every-third-day regimen. The optimal dosing regimen for all patients must be individualized.

Prognosis

There are few population-based studies that have examined the course of this disease. Many previous reports of poor outcome were derived from tertiary care centers, whose population is not representative of all patients. There have also been dramatic advances in both medical and surgical therapies over the past several decades. In general, the severity of disease at presentation is somewhat predictive of the future course and probability of requiring a colectomy. A recent Danish study suggests that the overall likelihood of being in remission at any given time is 50%. The overall colectomy rate was 24% at 10 years and 30% at 25 years. The probability of colectomy was related to disease extent. At 5 years, the colectomy rate was 9% in proctosigmoiditis, 19% in "substantial" colitis, and 35% in pancolitis. The probability of maintaining capacity for work was 93% after 10 years of disease.

The risk of progression from limited to extensive disease is also difficult to assess. The limited available population studies appear to put this risk at 30–50% after about 10 years of follow-up.

Whether ulcerative colitis is associated with an increased mortality rate compared with that of the general population is controversial. In the past, a high mortality rate was seen early in the course of patients presenting with severe disease. Given improved medical and surgical therapies, it is not clear whether this high rate still exists. Some recent population-based studies have failed to show increased mortality rates in ulcerative colitis patients. In the future, any higher rates of death will most likely be related to colon cancer.

DIFFERENTIATING CROHN'S DISEASE FROM ULCERATIVE COLITIS

In approximately 75% of patients with Crohn's disease, there is characteristic involvement of the ileum seen on contrast x-ray. Occasionally, Crohn's disease limited to the colon is difficult to differentiate from ulcerative colitis. In most cases, ulcerative colitis and Crohn's disease limited to the colon can be differentiated using the criteria summarized in Table 7–5. In 10–15% of cases of chronic colitis, a clear differentiation of ulcerative colitis and Crohn's disease cannot be made. This subgroup is usually referred to as "indeterminate" colitis.

EXTRAINTESTINAL MANIFESTATIONS OF INFLAMMATORY BOWEL DISEASE

Extraintestinal manifestations of inflammatory bowel disease are common (up to 25% of patients in some series). These manifestations can be divided into two types: those which flare up during periods of active inflammatory bowel disease and those which may occur at any time in a patient with inflammatory bowel disease. While these categories are useful for the purpose of discussion, there are numerous examples of overlapping between them.

Extraintestinal Manifestations Occurring During Active Inflammatory Bowel Disease

A. Reactive Arthropathy: An acute synovitis is seen in up to 20% of patients with inflammatory bowel disease, primarily in patients with colitis. Its incidence is strongly correlated with the extent of colonic involvement, and because of this, it is frequently referred to as "colitic" arthritis. It is asymmetric and migratory, typically involving fewer than six large joints. The arthritis usually resolves with treatment of the underlying bowel disease. In approximately 15% of patients, the arthritis persists, and a subset of these patients may develop a deforming arthritis. A subset of patients with reactive arthropathy will also have uveitis and erythema nodosum. There is clear overlapping of this subgroup with those that manifest the related seronegative spondyloarthropathies such as postinfectious arthritis, Reiter's syndrome, and psoriasis-associated arthritis. This subgroup is more likely to be HLA-B27 positive.

B. Ocular Manifestations: Episcleritis is the most common ocular manifestation of inflammatory bowel disease. It is characterized by a tender area of dilated blood vessels. Episcleritis occurs more commonly in patients with colitis or ileocolitis, and its course closely follows the activity of the bowel disease. It is more commonly seen in the setting of Crohn's disease.

C. Dermatologic Manifestations: Erythema nodosum is the most common dermatologic manifestation of inflammatory bowel disease. It is associated with both Crohn's disease and ulcerative colitis but appears to occur more commonly in Crohn's disease. Erythema nodosum parallels the activity of the bowel disease in most, but not all, cases. It is frequently associated with reactive arthritis and uveitis.

Pyoderma gangrenosum is a serious dermatologic complication of inflammatory bowel disease. It is more frequently associated with ulcerative colitis but

Table 7–5. Differentiating ulcerative and Crohn's colitis.

	Ulcerative Colitis	Crohn's Colitis
Clinical findings		
Perianal disease	Rare	Common (1/3 of patients)
Fistulas	Rare	Common (up to 40% of patients)
Abscess	Rare	20% of patients
Stricture	Rare	Common
Colonoscopic findings		
Rectal involvement	Always	Usually spared
Pattern	Continuous, proximal extension from rectum	Usually skip lesions
Radiologic findings		
Ileal involvement	Rare, nonspecific "backwash ileitis"	75% of patients with Crohn's disease
Histologic findings		
Depth of inflammation	Usually limited to mucosa or submucosa, except in fulminant cases	Typically transmural
Granulomas	Only associated with crypts in severe colitis	20% of endoscopic biopsies

may also be seen with Crohn's disease. The relationship of pyoderma gangrenosum to the activity of bowel disease is not always clear. Patients with extensive and severe colonic involvement are more likely to develop pyoderma gangrenosum. In many patients, the pyoderma recedes with treatment of the underlying bowel disease, but there are many instances in which pyoderma persists even after colectomy.

Extraintestinal Manifestations That May Occur at Any Time in a Patient With Inflammatory Bowel Disease

A. Axial Arthropathy: Sacroiliitis is the most common axial abnormality associated with inflammatory bowel disease. It is seen in approximately 10% of inflammatory bowel disease patients by plain x-ray but may be detected in most patients (two-thirds) by MRI. Most cases are asymptomatic.

Ankylosing spondylitis has been estimated to be 30 times more common in inflammatory bowel disease patients than in the general population and may complicate the course of disease in up to 5% of patients. There appears to be two subsets of patients who develop ankylosing spondylitis. Patients who are HLA-B27 positive have a high incidence of ankylosing spondylitis, typically with an accelerated course, whereas patients who develop ankylosing spondylitis and are HLA-B27 negative tend to have a benign course.

B. Ocular Manifestations: Scleritis and uveitis are two serious ocular complications associated with inflammatory bowel disease. They are serious in that they may result in impairment or loss of eyesight. Neither entity appears to parallel the bowel disease activity. As stated previously, uveitis (particularly anterior uveitis) is seen in association with reactive arthritis and erythema nodosum. This clustering has a strong association with HLA-B27.

C. Hepatobiliary Manifestations: Primary sclerosing cholangitis complicates the course of inflammatory bowel disease in 2–5% of patients. The overwhelming majority of cases are associated with ulcerative colitis. Primary sclerosing cholangitis is not associated with bowel disease activity, and its incidence is unaffected by colectomy. Pericholangitis is a term that has been used to describe a variety of different hepatobiliary abnormalities associated with inflammatory bowel disease. Pericholangitis has been used to describe nonspecific elevations in alkaline phosphatase and transaminase levels, nonspecific portal inflammation, and chronic hepatitis in patients with inflammatory bowel disease, as well as early histologic lesions of primary sclerosing cholangitis. Because of its lack of specificity, the term pericholangitis should be abandoned.

Cholesterol gallstones occur with increased incidence in patients with ileal disease or resection. This is primarily due to a decrease in the bile salt pool.

INFLAMMATORY BOWEL DISEASE & PREGNANCY

Early reports suggested that women with inflammatory bowel disease were less fertile than their age-matched control population. More recent studies fail to show any difference in fertility for ulcerative colitis patients, however. For women with Crohn's disease, there is conflicting information. Overall, the success of pregnancy in women with inflammatory bowel disease does not differ from that of the general population. For both ulcerative colitis and Crohn's disease, active disease at conception and during the course of pregnancy is associated with an increase in spontaneous abortions and prematurity.

The effect of pregnancy on the course of inflammatory bowel disease appears to be similar for Crohn's disease and ulcerative colitis. Most patients (two-thirds to three-fourths) with inactive disease at conception will remain inactive. Patients with active disease at conception are likely to remain active during the course of the pregnancy. Crohn's disease may flare up during the postpartum period, ulcerative colitis is unlikely to do so.

Treatment and management of inflammatory bowel disease during pregnancy can be particularly challenging. Gastrointestinal symptoms associated with a normal pregnancy can be confused with those associated with inflammatory bowel disease. Management is also made more difficult by the limitation pregnancy imposes on the usual repertoire of diagnostic tests. Flexible sigmoidoscopy may be performed safely during pregnancy, but colonoscopy and x-rays should be avoided. Potentially life-threatening complications do require the use of radiologic and surgical interventions, however. Ultrasound (cutaneous and transvaginal) can be extremely helpful in some cases. Management in these situations is best accomplished by a team approach involving a gastroenterologist, colorectal surgeon, and high-risk obstetrician.

Drug treatment during pregnancy should follow the same approach as that in the nonpregnant patient. Untreated or undertreated inflammatory bowel disease usually poses a substantially greater risk to mother and fetus than the appropriate drug therapies. There is a great deal of experience with sulfasalazine during pregnancy, and its use has not been shown to have any untoward effects on the fetus. It appears to be safe during breast-feeding as well. Folate supplements should be given when sulfasalazine is being used. Although there is a general suspicion that oral 5-aminosalicylic acid analogs are safe during pregnancy, there are no adequate confirmatory studies. Many of these preparations are associated with measurable serum levels of 5-aminosalicylic acid, particularly when used at high doses. The safety of 5-aminosalicylic acid during breast-feeding is unknown.

Corticosteroids are usually safe during pregnancy. Dosages are the same as for the nonpregnant patient (ie, high doses are given to rapidly gain control of symptoms and then are tapered to the lowest effective dose). Despite reports of successful use of the purine analogs during pregnancy, they should be avoided, because the long-term effects on children born to these mothers is unknown. It appears prudent to stop purine analogs in women who have accidently become pregnant while taking them. Metronidazole is also contraindicated during pregnancy.

Both total parenteral nutrition and elemental diets have been used successfully to support the nutritional needs of pregnant women with inflammatory bowel disease. Elemental diets may be a reasonable firstline therapy in pregnant patients with small bowel Crohn's disease and may be especially useful in patients with small bowel disease that is refractory to or dependent on high-dosage steroids.

REFERENCES

Ekbom A et al: Ulcerative colitis and colorectal cancer: A population-based study. N Engl J Med 1990;323:1228.

Greenberg GR et al: Oral budesonide for active Crohn's disease: Canadian Inflammatory Bowel Disease Study Group [see comments]. N Engl J Med 1994;331:836.

Hay JW, Hay AR: Inflammatory bowel disease: Costs-of-illness. J Clin Gastroenterol 1992;14:309.

Langholz E et al: Course of ulcerative colitis: Analysis of changes in disease activity over years [see comments]. Gastroenterology 1994;107:3.

Lichtiger S et al: Cyclosporine in severe ulcerative colitis refractory to steroid therapy [see comments]. N Engl J Med 1994;330:1841.

Rutgeerts P et al: A comparison of budesonide with prednisolone for active Crohn's disease [see comments]. N Engl J Med 1994;331:842.

Sandborn WJ: Pouchitis following ileal pouch-anal anasto-
mosis: Definition, pathogenesis, and treatment. Gastroenterology 1994;107:1856.

Singleton JW et al: Mesalamine capsules for the treatment of active Crohn's disease: Results of a 16-week trial. Pentasa Crohn's Disease Study Group. Gastroenterology 1993;104:1293.

Sutherland LR, May GR, Shaffer EA: Sulfasalazine revisited: A meta-analysis of 5-aminosalicylic acid in the treatment of ulcerative colitis. Ann Intern Med 1993;118:540.

Targan SR: The lamina propria: A dynamic, complex mucosal compartment: An overview. Ann NY Acad Sci 1992;664:61.

Yang H et al: Familial empirical risks for inflammatory bowel disease: Differences between Jews and non-Jews. Gut 1993;34:517.

Acute Diarrheal Diseases

8

Anne H. Wang, MD

Acute diarrhea is a sudden alteration in normal bowel habits whereby normally formed stool passed daily or every few days changes to frequent, multiple loose-to-watery stools. Diarrhea may be associated with increased frequency of defecation or increased liquidity of stools, or both, and often is accompanied by an abnormal increase in daily stool weight (> 200 g/d).

Pathophysiology of Diarrhea

A. Normal Fluid and Electrolyte Absorption and Secretion: The small intestine and colon are normally involved in the absorption and secretion of fluid and ions. Absorption of nutrients and fluids far exceeds secretion, with most of the absorption occurring in the small bowel. The small intestine will receive up to 10 L/d of fluid consisting of oral intake and salivary, gastric, biliary, and pancreatic secretions. Fluid absorption by the small intestine and colon is exceedingly efficient, with 9.9 L absorbed and only 100 mL passed into the stool. The maximal absorptive capacity of the colon is 4–5 L every 24 hours, whereas that of the small intestine remains undefined.

B. Mechanisms of Acute Diarrhea: Acute diarrhea may be classified clinically and pathophysiologically as either noninflammatory or inflammatory (Table 8–1).

1. Noninflammatory diarrhea–Noninflammatory diarrheas are caused by organisms or substances that do not result in disruption or damage to the intestinal epithelium. Enterotoxins produced by infecting organisms stimulate excessive intestinal secretion of ions and water. Poorly absorbed substances, which are osmotically active, cause net fluid secretion into the intestinal lumen. The clinical hallmarks of infectious noninflammatory diarrhea are watery stools with minimal or no blood, and the absence of fecal leukocytes on stool examination. The small intestine is more likely to be affected.

2. Inflammatory diarrhea–Inflammatory diarrheas are caused by organisms or substances that disrupt the intestinal mucosal barrier through direct invasion or elaboration of cytotoxin. Disruption of the mucosa results in exudation of inflammatory cells, blood, and sera into the lumen. Clinical findings of inflammatory diarrheas are characterized by bloody, small-volume stools, often with associated lower abdominal cramping or urgency. Occasionally, symptoms including fever or shock may be present. The preferential intestinal site of involvement is the colon, and examination of a stool sample will reveal numerous fecal leukocytes and red blood cells.

Classification of Acute Diarrhea

Acute diarrhea may be classified according to clinical data obtained through the patient history, physical examination, and laboratory findings (Table 8–2). Once this has been done, any necessary diagnostic testing can be focused and reduced significantly.

Clinical Approach to the Evaluation of Acute Diarrhea

The objective in evaluating acute diarrhea is to identify patients with medically important diarrhea and provide appropriate triage. It is paramount to distinguish the patient with potentially life-threatening diarrhea from one with benign, self-limited disease, in order to expedite delivery of specific therapy. This cannot be done on the basis of clinical findings alone and requires integration of data obtained from the patient history, physical examination, and laboratory tests (Figure 8–1).

A. Patient History: A careful, thorough history is the most important tool for uncovering the origin of diarrhea. The focus should be on the following areas:

1. Possible causative factors–The setting in which the diarrhea developed is useful in suggesting an origin. Questions should focus on the following factors:

1. Travel history, including international, domestic, and wilderness travel
2. Foods eaten, including types of foods or liquids ingested and locations at which food was eaten
3. Recent hospitalizations or closed community confinements, ie, nursing home, boot camp, dormitory

Table 8–1. Inflammatory and noninflammatory diarrhea.

	Inflammatory Diarrhea	Noninflammatory Diarrhea
Clinical presentation	Small-volume, bloody diarrhea; lower abdominal cramping or pain; fecal urgency; tenesmus; sometimes, fever	Large-volume, watery diarrhea; upper or paraumbilical abdominal pain or cramping; possible nausea or vomiting
Presence of fecal leukocytes	Yes	No
Common causes	*Shigella, Campylobacter, Salmonella, E histolytica, Yersinia*, enteroinvasive *E coli, C difficile*	*Vibrio, Giardia, Cryptosporidia*, enterotoxigenic *E coli*, rotavirus, Norwalk virus, toxigenic food poisoning (*S aureus, C perfringens, B cereus*)

4. Recent use of antibiotic or new medication
5. Exposure to other similarly affected individuals
6. Sexual history, including homosexual activities
7. History of shellfish ingestion
8. Exposure to farm animals
9. Presence of systemic disease.

Table 8–2. Classification of acute diarrhea.

Noninflammatory diarrhea
  Viral disease
    Rotavirus
    Norwalk virus
    Cytomegalovirus
    Herpesvirus
  Bacterial disease (toxin-mediated)
    Nontyphoidal *Salmonella*
    S aureus
    B cereus
    C perfringens
    Listeria
  Protozoal disease
    G lamblia
    C parvum
  Medication-induced diarrhea
    Antacids (containing magnesium)
    Antibiotics
    Laxatives
    Miscellaneous drugs (colchicine, lactulose)
  Irritable bowel syndrome
  Dietary intolerance
    Disaccharidase deficiency (eg, lactase)
    Altered diet, with diarrhea induced by osmotic agent (eg, due to sorbitol ingestion)
Inflammatory diarrhea
  Bacterial disease
    Invasive disease
      Shigella
      Salmonella
      Campylobacter
      Yersinia
      Vibrio
      C difficile
      Enteropathogenic *E coli* (enteroinvasive)
    Toxin-mediated disease
      Enterohemorrhagic *E coli* (O157)
  Protozoal disease
    E histolytica
    Strongyloides stercoralis
  Mesenteric ischemia
  Radiation colitis
  Inflammatory bowel disease

2. Severity of illness–The severity of the illness is determined through the interview and direct examination of the patient. It is important to elicit the following information:(1) appearance of stools, including the presence of blood; (2) frequency of bowel movements; and (3) presence of other symptoms, including fever, abdominal pain, or volume depletion.

Physical examination may reveal signs consistent with systemic illness or volume depletion.

3. Duration of illness–Most infectious causes of diarrhea have a self-limited course. Prolonged diarrhea (more than 5 days' duration) may indicate the presence of a more severe illness or a systemic illness with gastrointestinal manifestations.

B. Physical Examination: Examination of the patient may aid in determining the need for more aggressive therapy or hospitalization. Careful assessment should include the following:

- Overall appearance of the patient, including mental status (ie, toxic appearance)
- Vital signs, including high fever or hypotension
- Skin turgor and mucous membrane examination, to determine volume status
- Abdominal examination for tenderness or peritoneal signs
- Rectal examination for tenderness and for stool collection.

C. Diagnostic Studies: A variety of diagnostic tests are available, including stool cultures for enteric pathogens and tests for fecal parasitic or viral agents and fecal leukocytes. Flexible sigmoidoscopy with biopsy may also be helpful. Tests should be used to help define a specific cause that has been suggested by the history and physical examination. They should not be considered the initial step but rather a supplemental step to support the clinician's suspicions of the cause. Despite the multitude of tests available, the cause cannot be determined in 20–40% of cases of acute diarrheal illness.

The most frequently used tests are fecal leukocyte determination, stool culture for enteric pathogens, stool examination for parasites, *Clostridium difficile* toxin testing, and flexible sigmoidoscopy with biopsy.

1. Fecal leukocyte determination–Fecal leu-

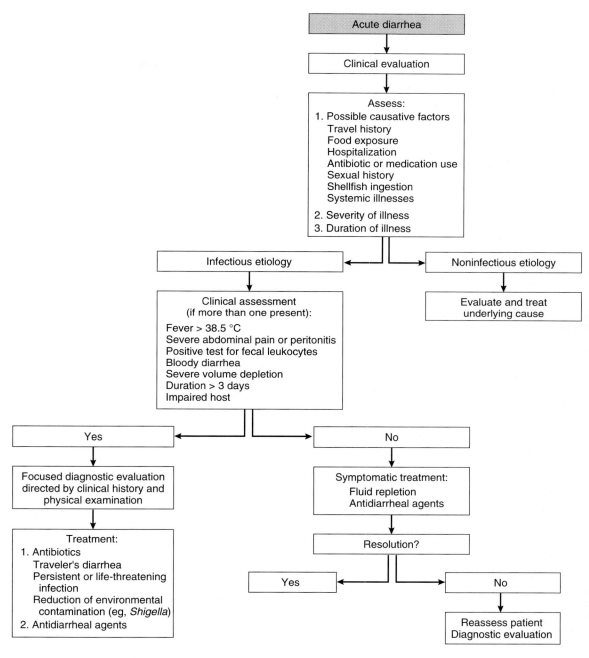

Figure 8–1. Clinical approach to the evaluation of acute diarrhea.

kocyte determination should be made in all patients with acute diarrhea. The presence of leukocytes distinguishes inflammatory from noninflammatory diarrhea and allows the clinician to focus the search for the causative agent. Stool obtained from a specimen or by digital examination is smeared on a glass slide and diluted with a small amount of saline to thin the consistency. Several drops of methylene blue are added, and a coverslip is placed over the mixture. After 2–3 minutes, the slide is examined under a high-power microscope. The presence of three or more polymorphonuclear cells per high-power field in four or more fields is considered a positive examination. This examination is not specific for an infectious disorder. Other inflammatory conditions of the bowel (eg, inflammatory bowel disease, radiation colitis) may also yield a positive test.

2. Stool culture for enteric pathogens–In the patient with a high likelihood of an enteric pathogen as the cause of diarrhea, stool cultures may be useful to focus therapy. Careful specimen collection is vital, because many enteric organisms are fastidious and stool specimens left at room temperature for a prolonged period may result in a false-negative culture. In most microbiology laboratories, a stool culture is routinely processed for the presence of only three enteric pathogens: *Shigella, Salmonella,* and *Campylobacter.* If high suspicion exists for the presence of other organisms (eg, *Yersinia, Vibrio,* and *Escherichia coli* O157:H7), the laboratory should be alerted, so that the appropriate tests can be arranged.

3. Stool examination for parasites–If a patient has a high pretest likelihood of parasitic infestation, stool should be obtained for ova and parasite examination. At least three stool specimens are needed to accommodate for the sporadic passage of parasites and ova in the stool.

4. *C difficile* toxin testing–In the patient with recent or remote antibiotic usage, hospitalization, closed-community living arrangement (eg, nursing home), or recent chemotherapy exposure, a stool sample should be obtained for *C difficile* toxin determination.

5. Flexible sigmoidoscopy–Flexible sigmoidoscopy may be useful in the patient with signs and symptoms of proctitis (ie, tenesmus, rectal pain, and rectal discharge). Patients with moderate to severe illness suspected of *C difficile*-induced diarrhea should be considered for sigmoidoscopic examination, because the presence of pseudomembranes is highly suggestive of the diagnosis. In addition, flexible sigmoidoscopy may assist in distinguishing patients with other causes of bloody diarrhea (eg, inflammatory bowel disease, ischemic colitis) from those with infectious causes. Examination of the mucosa, including the distribution and endoscopic appearance of colitis, may be diagnostic, although infectious colitis may have an identical endoscopic appearance. Mucosal biopsies may be helpful in distinguishing inflammatory bowel disease from infectious colitis.

D. Empiric Therapy: Specific antibiotic therapy is rarely indicated for the treatment of acute infectious diarrhea, despite the clinical evidence for inflammation and invasion. Most cases are effectively resolved by the host's cellular and humoral defense mechanisms. Antibiotic therapy may result in prolonged duration of fecal excretion of the enteric pathogen, drug-related side effects (including *C difficile* diarrhea), and the development of bacteria resistant to multiple antibiotics. Antibiotic therapy is indicated, however, in these selected circumstances: (1) to reduce fecal excretion and environmental contamination by a highly infectious agent (eg, *Shigella*); (2) for persistent or life-threatening diarrheal infections (eg, cholera); or (3) for traveler's diarrhea, to accelerate resolution of symptoms in individuals who cannot afford to be indisposed by illness (eg, politician, concert pianist).

INFECTIOUS CAUSES OF ACUTE DIARRHEA

VIRAL INFECTIONS

Although viral diarrhea is a major cause of gastroenteritis in the United States and the world (accounting for up to 40% of acute episodes), it accounts for few episodes of traveler's diarrhea. Rotavirus and Norwalk virus are the two most common agents in viral diarrhea in children and adults, respectively.

Rotavirus

The disease occurs primarily in children age 3–15 months, with infections less common after 2 years of age. Adults can develop mild infection but rarely with the magnitude of diarrhea seen in the pediatric population. Typically, a child develops vomiting, followed by profuse, watery diarrhea. The average duration of illness is 5–7 days. Dehydration may develop rapidly in children and contributes significantly to the severity of the illness.

Rapid diagnosis can be achieved by detection of rotavirus antigen in feces by commercially available kits. In clinical practice, however, this usually is unnecessary.

Symptomatic treatment is the mainstay of therapy. Rehydration is imperative and can be accomplished through oral rehydration solutions available commercially or through home preparation.

Norwalk Virus

Norwalk viruses have been implicated in up to 40% of nonbacterial diarrheal epidemics in the USA. Its role in traveler's diarrhea is not well defined.

The small intestine is the affected region during invasion by Norwalk virus. The exact mechanism of injury is unclear due to difficulty imaging the virus, even by electron microscopy. Morphologic and physiologic abnormalities appear to reverse within 1–2 weeks after infection.

The clinical spectrum of disease is varied, although all cases are mild. Diarrhea is the most prominent symptom, noted in up to 92% of patients. Abdominal pain, nausea, and vomiting are noted in up to 75% of patients. The duration of illness is usually 24–48 hours.

At this time, the virus cannot be cultured and stool viral antigen identification is not offered routinely. Diagnosis may be established by identification of viral antigen in the stool, when this is deemed necessary.

No specific treatment is available or required. Volume repletion for dehydrated patients is indicated.

Cytomegalovirus

Cytomegalovirus infection of the gastrointestinal tract can occur in the course of HIV infection when the CD4 lymphocyte count falls below 100/μL (see Chapter 2). Cytomegalovirus colitis accounts for up to 25% of cases of diarrhea in HIV patients.

The clinical spectrum of presentation is varied, ranging from abdominal pain, weight loss, fever, and watery diarrhea to hemorrhagic colitis with perforation. Cytomegalovirus colitis has been implicated in cases of appendicitis in AIDS patients.

Frequently, the CD4 lymphocyte count will be less than 100/μL. The demonstration of characteristic intranuclear cytomegalovirus inclusions on tissue biopsy is diagnostic. Immunohistochemical staining of tissue may be required to demonstrate the presence of the virus. Culture of cytomegalovirus from tissue biopsies is not helpful.

Colonoscopy with biopsy may be useful in determining the presence of cytomegalovirus colitis. Endoscopic appearances range from diffuse colitis to hemorrhagic colitis with deep, irregular ulcerations.

Ganciclovir, an acyclovir derivative, has been shown to be effective in most cases of cytomegalovirus colitis. For patients with neutropenia or ganciclovir resistance, foscarnet, a pyrophosphate analog, has been used for treatment.

BACTERIAL INFECTIONS

1. NONINVASIVE INFECTIONS

Foodborne Gastroenteritis

Food poisoning is a frequently overlooked cause of diarrhea. Important clues to diagnosis can be found in the food history, the geographic location, the season of the year, and the order and timing of onset of symptoms.

Nontyphoidal *Salmonella*

Nontyphoidal salmonellosis is the leading cause of food poisoning in the USA. Animals are a natural reservoir for nontyphoidal salmonellosis and, consequently, animal products derived from contaminated animals are the source of infection. Commonly implicated foods include eggs, poultry, milk, and beef.

The onset of illness is characterized by fever, chills, and diarrhea, followed by the variable presence of nausea, vomiting, and abdominal cramping. Grossly bloody diarrhea is uncommon. The duration of illness is usually less than 7 days.

Stool smears reveal moderate red and white blood cells. Blood cultures are positive in 5–10% of cases and are more common in HIV-infected patients.

The treatment in uncomplicated nontyphoidal salmonellosis is supportive care, with adequate hydration being paramount. Routine use of antibiotics is not recommended, because of increased incidence of resistant strains and prolongation of bacterial shedding. Patients who are immunocompromised or have evidence of bacteremia should receive antibiotics. The antibiotic of choice is a fluoroquinolone such as ciprofloxacin or norfloxacin by mouth or a third-generation cephalosporin given intravenously in patients unable to tolerate oral medications.

Staphylococcus aureus

Staphylococcal food poisoning is caused by ingestion of preformed staphylococcal toxin, which accumulates in protein-rich foods that have been inadequately refrigerated. It is the third most common cause of foodborne illnesses. The most commonly implicated foods are cream-filled cakes, potato and macaroni salads, and ham. Staphylococcal enterotoxins are heat stable and cause symptoms through their effects on enteric autonomic sensory neurons and intestinal cell permeability.

Symptoms occur within 1–6 hours after ingestion of contaminated food. Approximately 75% of patients have nausea, vomiting, and abdominal pain, which are followed by diarrhea in 68%. Fever is exceedingly rare. The duration of illness is less than 24 hours.

Definitive diagnosis can be made by culturing *S aureus* from the contaminated food, or from the stools and vomitus of the patient. This may be considered in large outbreaks of presumptive food poisoning. Peripheral leukocytosis is rare, and white blood cells are absent on fecal smears.

Treatment is supportive, including adequate oral hydration and antiemetics. No role exists for antibiotics for eradication of ingested staphylococci.

Bacillus cereus

B cereus is a gram-positive, aerobic, spore-forming rod. Two separate enterotoxins are responsible for the distinct phases of illness, the emetic syndrome and the diarrheal syndrome, with the emetic syndrome being more common.

The onset of symptoms is 1–6 hours after ingestion of contaminated food, and the duration of illness is less than 24 hours. Acute symptoms include nausea, vomiting, and abdominal pain, which usually resolve within 10 hours. The emetic syndrome is more commonly associated with ingestion of fried rice, while the diarrheal syndrome is associated with ingestion of inadequately refrigerated prepared foods.

The diarrheal syndrome occurs 8–16 hours after ingestion of contaminated food and produces a syndrome of profuse watery diarrhea and abdominal cramping. Nausea and vomiting are rare.

Treatment is supportive, with oral rehydration and antiemetics.

Clostridium perfringens

C perfringens is an anaerobic, spore-forming, gram-positive rod. It is the fourth most common cause of documented foodborne disease. It has been implicated in several distinct syndromes of food poisoning, with the most common type being a self-limited illness characterized by ingestion of organisms, with in vivo production of enterotoxin. Clostridial food poisoning is common in the setting of delayed serving of cooked meat and poultry products. When meat products are stored at room temperature, clostridial spores may germinate and be ingested, and elaboration of the enterotoxin may ensue.

The self-limited syndrome is characterized by onset of symptoms 6–24 hours after ingestion of the meat product. The onset of watery diarrhea and significant epigastric pain occurs, and this may be followed by nausea, vomiting, and fever, rarely. The symptoms resolve within 24 hours.

Microbiologic examination of the suspected food, with isolation of more than 10^5 organisms per gram of food, confirms the diagnosis of clostridial food poisoning. Fecal smears reveal no polymorphonuclear cells, and other laboratory testing is not indicated.

Treatment is supportive, with oral rehydration and antiemetics as needed.

2. INVASIVE INFECTIONS

Shigella

Shigella account for many cases of diarrheal illness (up to 8% of travelers to Latin America). *Shigella* organisms cause bacillary dysentery and produce an intense inflammatory response in the colon via elaborated enterotoxin and invasion.

Classically, shigellosis presents with crampy abdominal pain, fever, and multiple small-volume bloody, mucoid stools. Initial symptoms may consist of fever, abdominal pain, and watery diarrhea without gross blood, with a second stage with bloody stools occurring 3–5 days later. The average length of symptoms in adults is 7 days, with more severe cases persisting for 3–4 weeks. Chronic shigellosis can mimic ulcerative colitis, and a chronic carrier state is possible.

Fecal smears reveal multiple polymorphonuclear and red blood cells. Stool culture may be used for isolation and identification of antibiotic sensitivity.

Sigmoidoscopy can be used to confirm the presence of colitis, although the endoscopic presence of colitis is not specific for shigellosis. In addition, sigmoidoscopy in the face of acute inflammation may prove extremely uncomfortable for the patient.

Extraintestinal manifestations of shigellosis may occur, including respiratory symptoms, neurologic symptoms such as meningismus, and hemolytic-uremic syndrome. An asymmetric oligoarticular arthritis may occur up to 3 weeks after onset of dysentery, mimicking Reiter's syndrome.

The mainstay of treatment is adequate rehydration by oral or intravenous methods, depending on the severity of illness. Opiate derivatives should be avoided. In moderate and severe cases of dysentery, antibiotics should be given. For drug-sensitive strains, ampicillin, 500 mg orally 4 times a day or 1 g intravenously every 6 hours, is the drug of choice. For drug-resistant strains, trimethroprim-sulfamethoxazole is the treatment of choice.

Salmonella typhi

Typhoid fever is characterized by a prolonged febrile illness with associated splenomegaly, delirium, abdominal pain, and other systemic manifestations. Typhoidal disease is a systemic disease and has few primary symptoms relating to the gastrointestinal tract.

After the initial bacteremia, the organism is sequestered in the reticuloendothelial system, resulting in hyperplasia of the system, including lymph nodes and Peyer's patches within the small intestine. Progressive enlargement and ulceration of nodes may result in perforation of the small bowel or gastrointestinal hemorrhage.

The classic form of typhoid fever involves a 4-week cycle. The incubation period is 7–14 days. The first week is characterized by high fever, headaches, and abdominal pain. A pulse-temperature dissociation can be found. Approximately 50% of patients describe normal bowel habits. During the second week, splenomegaly and an evanescent rash are evident. The third week is characterized by decreasing mentation and increasing toxemia. Intestinal involvement, with greenish diarrhea and potential intestinal perforation, occurs during this period. The fourth week is characterized by defervescence and improved clinical status.

The diagnosis is established by isolation of the organism. Blood cultures are positive in up to 90% of patients within the first week of clinically apparent illness. Stool cultures become positive during the second and third weeks.

Intestinal perforation and gastrointestinal hemorrhage can occur during the course of the illness. Altered mental status and acute cholecystitis are less common; however, chronic infection of gallstones may attribute to a carrier state once the patient has recovered from the acute illness.

The traditional drug of choice is chloramphenicol, 500 mg orally four times a day for 2 weeks. Third-generation cephalosporins have demonstrated excellent efficacy against *S typhi* and should be administered intravenously for 7–10 days. Quinolones, such as ciprofloxacin, 500 mg twice daily by mouth for 14 days, has demonstrated high efficacy and a low resultant carrier state.

Campylobacter

Campylobacter species found in human infection include *Campylobacter jejuni* and *Campylobacter fetus,* more commonly found in immunocompromised hosts. Approximately 5–10% of all cases of bacterial diarrhea in the USA are caused by *C jejuni.* It accounts for up to 15% of traveler diarrhea cases from Asia. The most common route of transmission is from infected animals and their food products to humans, with chickens being the main source. Pathogenesis of disease is by toxin elaboration and mucosal invasion.

The clinical manifestations of *Campylobacter* infection vary widely, from asymptomatic disease to dysentery. The incubation period is 24–72 hours after ingestion of organisms. Diarrhea and fever are present in 90% of patients, and abdominal pain and bloody stools in 50–70%. Other constitutional symptoms such as fever, nausea, vomiting, and malaise may also be present. The duration of illness is less than 7 days. Relapses can occur in as many as 25% of patients.

Fecal smears demonstrate numerous fecal leukocytes and the presence of red blood cells. Stool for culture will yield the presence of *Campylobacter.*

Campylobacter is sensitive to erythromycin and quinolones; however, debate has occurred regarding the need for antibiotic administration. Studies have revealed that inception of treatment after 4 days of onset of symptoms yielded no clinical benefit, except for decreased fecal excretion of organisms. Antibiotics are indicated in the severely ill patient or the patient with frank dysentery. As with all diarrheal illnesses, volume repletion and correction of electrolyte derangements is paramount.

Vibrio cholerae

V cholerae is a gram-negative, comma-shaped rod that produces a severe diarrheal disorder leading to profound dehydration; death may result within 3–4 hours in an untreated patient. Cholera toxin affects small intestinal fluid transport by increasing cyclic AMP, promoting secretion, and inhibiting absorption of fluid. The major vehicle of spread of cholera is contaminated food and water, particularly shellfish.

The initial presentation is abdominal distention and vomiting, followed rapidly by diarrhea. The diarrhea is frequent, large in volume, and has the appearance of rice water. Patients may present with profound electrolyte abnormalities and volume depletion. Mild fever may be present.

Blood chemistries may be compatible with pro-

found volume and electrolyte depletion and should be replaced accordingly. Bicarbonate and potassium are lost in significant quantities, and scrupulous replacement is warranted. Fecal cultures may be appropriate in the patient in whom a diagnosis of cholera is suspected and a lack of endemic exposure demonstrated.

Treatment is primarily targeted at aggressive volume and electrolyte replacement by intravenous and oral methods. Commercially available oral rehydration solutions can be given in conjunction with intravenous fluids. Antibiotics are useful as ancillary measures. Tetracycline, 40 mg/kg/d in four divided doses for 2 days, is recommended. Aggressive management of volume status results in low mortality rates (usually < 1%).

Pathogenic Escherichia coli

Pathogenic *E coli* is the major causative agent for traveler's diarrhea. The pathogenic mechanisms employed by this agent include elaboration of enterotoxin and diffuse mucosal adherence. There are several important agents:

1. Enterotoxigenic *E coli* (ETEC) accounts for approximately one-half of all *E coli* diarrhea cases and is the most common cause of traveler's diarrhea.
2. Enteropathogenic *E coli* (EPEC) causes a large proportion of the remaining cases of traveler's diarrhea.
3. Enteroadherent *E coli* (EAEC) appears to account for 15% of cases of traveler's diarrhea.
4. Enterohemorrhagic *E coli* (EHEC) is a rare cause of traveler's diarrhea but a major cause of sporadic and epidemic cases of infectious bloody diarrhea (discussed separately following).

Most patients with ETEC, EPEC, or EAEC have mild symptoms consisting of watery diarrhea, nausea, and abdominal cramping. The diarrhea is rarely severe, with most patients having five or fewer stools within 24 hours. The average length of illness is 5 days. Fever is present in fewer than a third of patients. Stools can be mucoid but rarely contain blood or white blood cells. Leukocytosis is uncommon. ETEC, EAEC, and EPEC are self-limited, with no significant sequelae.

Laboratory findings are nonspecific for *E coli* diarrhea, including rare fecal leukocytes, absence of other pathogens on stool culture, and occasional peripheral leukocytosis. EPEC and EHEC can be isolated in culture, and a latex agglutination assay specific for EHEC type O157 is available. However, other immunologic assays for ETEC are laborious and not widely available commercially.

Treatment is supportive, with the mainstay being adequate rehydration. Bismuth subsalicylate and antimotility agents are effective in reducing the frequency of stools. Antimotility agents should be avoided in severe illness.

Enterohemorrhagic *Escherichia coli* (subtype O157)

Enterohemorrhagic *E coli* (EHEC) has become well-recognized for its role in outbreaks of hemorrhagic colitis. Many cases can be traced to ingestion of contaminated hamburger that has been improperly cooked. Other outbreaks have been attributed to contaminated swimming water. Most cases occur within 7–10 days of ingestion of contaminated meat or water. Secondary infections may occur via a fecal-oral route among household contacts or children and personnel in daycare centers. EHEC may be the most common cause of infectious bloody diarrhea. Subtype O157:H7 may be associated with the development of hemolytic-uremic syndrome in up to 10% of cases, especially in children. EHEC is noninvasive but produces cytotoxin closely related to Shiga's toxin, which produces endothelial damage, microangiopathic hemolysis, and renal damage.

The onset of illness is characterized by moderate to severe diarrhea (up to 10–12 liquid stools per day). Initial diarrhea is nonbloody but frequently progresses to grossly bloody stools. Severe abdominal pain and cramping are common, and nausea and vomiting is present in about two-thirds of patients. Abdominal examination may reveal marked abdominal distention and diffuse abdominal or focal right lower quadrant tenderness. Fever occurs in fewer than one-third of patients and is of short duration. Up to one-third of patients require hospitalization.

Peripheral leukocytosis with a left shift is frequently present. Urinalysis may reveal hematuria or proteinuria or leukocyte casts. Evidence of microangiopathic hemolytic anemia (hematocrit < 30%), thrombocytopenia (< 150×10^9/L), and renal insufficiency (blood urea nitrogen > 20 mg/dL) is diagnostic of hemolytic-uremic syndrome.

When EHEC is suspected, the laboratory must be alerted to culture stool specimens for *E coli* on sorbitol-McConkey agar. Specific serotyping usually is performed in special laboratories.

Colonoscopic examination may reveal colonic edema, friability, and microulceration of the mucosa but is nonspecific. Roentgenogram of the abdomen may demonstrate a paralytic ileus or, rarely, toxic megacolon. Colonoscopic biopsies rarely reveal adherent bacteria and show nonspecific colitis.

Toxic megacolon with intestinal perforation or intussusception may occur as a result of EHEC infection. Hemolytic-uremic syndrome, characterized by renal failure, and microangiopathic anemia occur in 5–10% of patients, particularly children and adults over age 60 years. Thrombotic thrombocytopenic purpura can occur but is less common than hemolytic-uremic syndrome. Central nervous system complications of thrombotic thrombocytopenic purpura, manifested by confusion, myoclonic jerking, and sensorimotor deficits, occur variably.

Treatment is supportive, with scrupulous attention to volume status and treatment of renal and vascular complications. Antibiotics have not been effective in reducing symptoms or the risk of complications of EHEC infection.

Death occurs in less than 1% of patients; however, in a nursing-home outbreak in Michigan, 19 of 55 patients died.

PROTOZOAL INFECTIONS

Entamoeba histolytica

E histolytica is the causative agent of amebiasis, which is characterized as both an acute and a chronic illness. A worldwide prevalence of amebiasis has been estimated at 10%, with up to 80% of citizens infected in endemic regions. It accounts for less than 3% of cases of traveler's diarrhea. A wide range of clinical states can be seen in amebiasis, from the asymptomatic carrier to the patient with frank dysentery or amebic hepatic abscess. Asymptomatic carriers have evidence of cysts in their stools but no clinical evidence of enteroinvasion. Patients with amebic dysentery demonstrate evidence of trophozoite and cyst passage into the stool.

E histolytica is directly invasive and is capable of mucosal invasion, with potential widespread distal dissemination. Histologically, colonic lesions demonstrate diffuse inflammation, with a dense cell infiltrate into the lamina propria. As the disease advances, ulceration occurs, eventually producing classic flask-shaped ulcers with undermined edges.

The clinical spectrum of disease varies widely, from asymptomatic carrier to frank dysentery. In the patient with evidence of colitis, the presenting symptoms include diffuse lower abdominal pain, intermittent bloody, mucoid stools, anorexia, and malaise. The stool frequency may be 7–10 bowel movements within 24 hours. Physical examination may reveal diffuse or focal abdominal tenderness. In extremely ill patients, there may be signs of peritonitis and evidence of ileus suggested by abdominal distention.

Stool samples for ova and parasites may reveal the presence of trophozoites and establish the diagnosis in 90% of patients. Serologic testing by indirect hemagglutination or ELISA may detect elevated ameba serologies consistent with invasive disease. A warm saline wet mount of stool may reveal Charcot-Leyden crystals, which, although not specific for amebic colitis, raise suspicion for amebiasis.

Sigmoidoscopy may reveal discrete, small, flat, shallow-based ulcers, with overlying yellowish exudate. Frequently, the intervening mucosa is normal in appearance, in contradistinction to inflammatory bowel disease or other infectious colitides.

Untreated amebic dysentery may result in intestinal perforation or widespread dissemination of disease, with abscess formation.

Metronidazole is the drug of choice. For active disease, metronidazole, 750 mg three times daily for 10 days, should be followed by an intraluminally active agent such as iodoquinol, 650 mg three times daily for 20 days. In asymptomatic carriers, only a luminally active agent is required.

Giardia lamblia

G lamblia is an internationally distributed protozoan that accounts for up to 5% of traveler's diarrhea. It exists in both an encysted form and as a trophozoite. The parasite is common in freshwater streams and lakes in the western United States, as well as in eastern Europe. Animal vectors, particularly beavers, have been felt to be the source of contamination of waters in Rocky Mountain regions. Here, infection may occur in campers who drink contaminated lake or stream water or in international travelers. *Giardia* is also a common cause of diarrhea in daycare centers.

The pathogenesis of diarrhea and steatorrhea is usually unknown. Possible factors include inhibition of nutrient passage secondary to massive numbers of adherent parasites within the small bowel, epithelial damage, competition of the parasite and the host for nutrients, and mucosal invasion.

Patients with symptomatic giardiasis complain frequently of diarrhea, which may be acute in onset and loose to watery in consistency, with associated flatulence. Mucus may be present, but blood is absent from the stools. Steatorrheic stools may be described by patients, as well as symptoms of abdominal bloating, weight loss, and fatigue.

Stool ova and parasites may reveal the presence of *G lamblia.* If steatorrhea is suspected, a Sudan stain may reveal the presence of fat in the stool. Laboratory evidence of malabsorption, with low carotene, vitamin B_{12}, or folate may be rarely present. Although duodenal aspiration may reveal the presence of *G lamblia,* this is a cumbersome test that is done infrequently.

Several excellent treatments exist for giardiasis. Quinacrine, 100 mg orally three times daily for 7 days, will cure 90–95% of patients. Alternatively, metronidazole, 250 mg three times daily for 7 days, will achieve similar cure rates. Because *Giardia* may be difficult to identify from stool samples alone, empiric therapy may be given in patients with chronic watery diarrhea who have traveled to an endemic region.

Cryptosporidium parvum

C parvum is a coccidian protozoan that has been recognized as a common cause of bovine diarrhea. It has become more widely recognized as an important cause of chronic diarrhea in HIV-infected patients and in health care workers. In Latin America, *Crypt-sporidium* causes up to 5% of cases of diarrhea in children and has occurred in daycare centers in the USA. Waterborne outbreaks have occurred in the midwestern United States in normal hosts.

Cryptosporidia trophozoites attach firmly to intestinal epithelial cells, thereby destroying microvilli. Histologically, villi are blunted, with evidence of increased inflammatory cell infiltrate in the lamina propria.

Common presentation for acute cryptosporidial infection includes nausea, abdominal cramping, and low-grade fever, followed by a profuse, watery diarrhea. Nausea and vomiting may occur but are less common. Significant volume depletion may result from the profuse diarrhea. Physical examination may be remarkable for dehydration and mild diffuse abdominal tenderness.

A modified acid-fast stain of fecal smears may demonstrate cryptosporidial oocysts. Biopsy of the small intestine may reveal oocysts embedded in the microvillous border. Sigmoidoscopy may reveal hyperemic mucosa without frank ulceration or colitis.

Treatment is supportive, with volume repletion and correction of electrolyte derangements. In patients with intact immunologic status, the infection is self-limited and will resolve in approximately 14 days. To date, no effective antimicrobial agents have been identified for eradication of cryptosporidia.

SPECIAL CLINICAL SITUATIONS

1. TRAVELER'S DIARRHEA

Traveler's diarrhea is defined as the passage of three unformed stools within a 24-hour period, in conjunction with other gastrointestinal symptoms of nausea, vomiting, abdominal pain, tenesmus, or passage of blood or mucus with the stool. It typically occurs in a person who resides in an industrialized region and travels to a developing country. Up to 50% of travelers to developing countries are affected with diarrhea within the first 2 weeks of travel. After returning home, 10–20% of travelers will have the onset of diarrhea, which may last for longer than 1 week in 10% of patients and longer than 1 month in 2%.

Bacterial enteric pathogens are the causative agents in 80% of cases of traveler's diarrhea. The principal agents in most high-risk areas are enterotoxigenic *E coli, C jejuni,* various species of *Shigella, Salmonella,* and *Aeromonas,* and *Vibrio* species other than *Vibrio cholerae.* Viral agents such as rotavirus and Norwalk virus are responsible for up to 10% of cases. Protozoa such as *G lamblia* and *E histolytica* are less common causes, despite their importance as pathogens within the developing country.

Clinical Findings

Symptoms associated with traveler's diarrhea are

variable. Most patients have a mild, self-limited clinical course consisting of 1–3 days of watery, non-bloody diarrhea, minimal other gastrointestinal complaints, and a lack of dehydration or fever. More severe illness may be also seen, with high fever, frequent bloody stools, abdominal pain, nausea and vomiting, and leukocytosis. Although clinical features on presentation may suggest the causative agent, severely ill patients warrant thorough assessment and close observation.

Treatment

The treatment of traveler's diarrhea is outlined in Table 8–3.

A. Fluid Repletion and Food Precautions: Assessment and treatment of dehydration is imperative in all patients with diarrhea. Because patients have mild, self-limited disease, oral repletion of fluid is adequate. Flavored mineral water taken with saltine crackers or a commercially available oral rehydration solution is frequently sufficient for replacement of ion and water losses. The repletion fluid should contain, at a minimum, glucose (which allows absorption via the small intestinal Na^+-glucose-amino acid cotransport mechanism, which remains intact in diarrheal illnesses), and should be caffeine free. Dairy products should be avoided because infectious diarrhea often results in transient lactase deficiency. Low-residue foods such as toast, rice, bananas, potatoes, boiled chicken, and applesauce may be added back into the diet as diarrheal symptoms improve. High-fiber foods, raw fruits, and vegetables should be avoided, as they may exacerbate diarrhea.

B. Antibiotics: Antibiotics have been demonstrated to decrease the severity and duration of symptoms associated with a particular bacterial organism. Treatment with antibiotics decreases the duration of diarrhea from 59–93 hours to 16–30 hours. However, antibiotic use has been associated with prolonged fe-

cal excretion of the pathogen, adverse side effects such as *C difficile* diarrhea, and development of multiply resistant bacteria. Specific antibiotic therapy is seldom indicated in acute infectious diarrhea, despite the presence of inflammation or invasion. Host immunity defenses are adequate to resolve most cases. Antibiotics are indicated for patients with severe, life-threatening illness, certain infectious agents to reduce environmental contamination (shigellosis, salmonellosis), and prolonged diarrhea.

C. Antidiarrheal Agents: Symptomatic treatment to reduce the frequency of unformed stool can be achieved with various antidiarrheal agents. Their mechanisms of action are as adsorbent, antimotility agent, or direct bactericidal. Adsorbents such as kaolin and pectin add bulk and thus decrease the liquidity of the stool without decreasing the stool quantity. Bismuth subsalicylate appears to have a variety of actions, including direct bactericidal effects via the bismuth moiety, and antisecretory and anti-inflammatory effects via the salicylate moiety. Given its safety, efficacy, and low cost, bismuth subsalicylate should be the first-line agent for treatment of acute infectious diarrhea. Opiate derivatives such as loperamide and diphenoxylate-atropine decrease intestinal motility, thus allowing increased intestinal contact time for absorption of salt and water. By inhibiting intestinal motility, these agents decrease the frequency of bowel movements and alleviate abdominal cramping. Opiate derivatives should be used with caution in patients with clinical toxicity or significant bloody diarrhea because they may precipitate toxic megacolon or clinical deterioration.

Precautions for Travelers to High-Risk Areas

A. Food and Water Precautions: Since infectious agents of traveler's diarrhea are transmitted by the fecal-oral route, travelers should be advised about safe water and food practices. All travelers should be

Table 8–3. Management of traveler's diarrhea.

Clinical Syndrome	Fluid Replacement Therapy	Antimotility Agents	Antibiotic Therapy
Dysentery (bloody diarrhea) with or without fever (> 37.8 °C)	Bottled carbonated beverages; boiled water; commercial oral rehydrating solution; mixture of 1 L water + 1 cup fruit juice + 4 tablespoons sugar or honey + 1 teaspoon baking powder + 3/4 teaspoon salt; for severe dehydration, intravenous fluid replacement	Bismuth subsalicylate, loperamide, diphenoxylate-atropine—use with caution in severely ill patient	Trimethroprim, 160 mg, and sulfamethoxazole, 800 mg, twice a day for 5 days OR Fluoroquinolone (ciprofloxacin, 500 mg, norfloxacin, 400 mg, ofloxacin, 300 mg) twice a day for 5 days
Watery diarrhea (no blood)	As above; for severe dehydration, consider intravenous fluid replacement	Bismuth subsalicylate; loperamide; diphenoxylate-atropine	Not indicated unless diarrhea persists or progresses to bloody diarrhea; then, treat with trimethoprim-sulfamethoxazole or fluoroquinolone

counseled to refrain from drinking tap water, iced drinks (including alcoholic beverages with ice), unpasteurized milk, and noncarbonated bottled water. Carbonated beverages and carbonated bottled water are bactericidal because of their low pH. Travelers should be cautious when showering or brushing their teeth, as ingestion of pathogens can occur. If carbonated beverages are unavailable, travelers may achieve disinfection by boiling water at 100 °C for 5–10 minutes, halogenation using commercially available iodine or chlorine solutions, or filtration via sediment filtration or resin contact devices.

Food may become contaminated at the source, as fertilization with human excreta is a common practice in developing countries. Additionally, food may become contaminated during preparation, or as a result of manipulation by a contaminated handler. Travelers should eat only foods that are served piping hot, and should avoid raw vegetables and fruits that cannot be peeled. Foods requiring elaborate preparation or containing dairy products should be avoided. Only thoroughly cooked shellfish should be eaten.

B. Chemoprophylaxis: Despite the demonstrated efficacy of antibiotic and bismuth subsalicylate in preventing traveler's diarrhea, chemoprophylaxis is not recommended uniformly for all travelers. Arguments against prophylaxis include the high cost of antibiotics, particularly the quinolones; potential adverse side effects, such as Stevens-Johnson syndrome and anaphylaxis (which occurs in 1 in 10,000 patients taking antibiotics); development of antibiotic resistance; and promotion of a false sense of security in the traveler, who may become less vigilant about what is eaten or drunk. The efficacy of antibiotics in reducing the duration of diarrhea if it develops raises the question of whether antibiotic prophylaxis or early self-treatment of diarrhea should be recommended.

Prophylaxis may be indicated in some travelers because of circumstances or inherent risk factors that would make a bout of diarrhea potentially dangerous. The following groups of travelers should be considered for chemoprophylaxis:

1. Travelers unable to tolerate any inactivity (eg, professional athlete, performing artist, politician).
2. Travelers with an underlying medical disorder in whom diarrhea may be poorly tolerated (eg, patients with diabetes mellitus, acquired immunodeficiency syndrome (AIDS), inflammatory bowel disease, chronic renal failure, significant cardiac disease, or gastric pH that has been altered via surgical or medical means (eg, omeprazole).
3. Travelers with a history of repeated bouts of traveler's diarrhea and known poor compliance with general food and water precautions.

The drug should be started on the day of arrival in the country and continued for 1–2 days after leaving the country. Prophylaxis should not be continued beyond 3 weeks, and if the traveler is to remain in the country for a longer time, prophylaxis should not be given because of its cost, potential side effects, and eventual acquisition of natural immunity over time. Recommended prophylactic regimens are outlined in Table 8–4.

NOSOCOMIAL DIARRHEA

Nosocomial diarrhea is defined as the onset of a change in normal bowel habits at least 72 hours after hospital admission for the purpose of clinical investigation. There must be at least 2–3 watery stools per day for more than 2 days. The incidence of nosocomial diarrhea in the USA has increased steadily over the past 15 years, with the most recent reported incidence of up to 31.3 per 100 admissions. Patients over 70 years of age have the highest incidence (17–31 per 100 admission) and experience the highest mortality rates (21–83%). Increasing length of hospital stay has been identified as a significant risk factor for nosocomial infection in adult patients, with an incidence of almost 50% for hospital stays exceeding 21 days. Multivariate models have demonstrated other risk factors, including enteral feeding, the use of antacids, the presence of nasogastric tubes, and the presence of *Candida* in the stool. The most common causative infectious agent identified in adults is *C difficile* (21–52%), followed by *Salmonella* (3–11.8%). Immunosuppressed patients, including transplantation patients, are at risk for various pathogens, including viruses, protozoa, and fungi.

1. MEDICATION-INDUCED DIARRHEA

Medication-induced diarrhea is a common cause of nosocomial diarrhea in the elderly patient. Medications implicated may include parasympathomimetic agents, cardiovascular medications, an-

Table 8–4. Prophylaxis for traveler's diarrhea.

Agent	Indicated Usage	Dosage and Duration
Bismuth subsalicylate	Adult or postpubertal child	2 tablets or 30 mL with meals and at bedtime
Trimethoprim-sulfamethoxazole	Adult traveling to interior Mexico	1 tablet (trimethoprim, 160 mg, and sulfamethoxazole, 800 mg) once daily
Fluoroquinolone, ciprofloxacin, norfloxacin, ofloxacin	All areas of travel, excluding interior of Mexico; adults only	1 tablet (ciprofloxacin, 500 mg; norfloxacin, 400 mg; ofloxacin, 300 mg) once daily

timetabolites, antibiotics, colchicine, antacids, or medications suspended in sorbitol. Enteral feeding preparations may also be a cause. A careful review of a patient's medication list is imperative before embarking on a costly, extensive diarrhea evaluation. A thorough history may implicate a temporal relationship to the inception of medication usage and the onset of diarrhea. A prolonged hospital stay with no change in medication usage may suggest a nosocomial pathogen as the source of diarrhea rather than a medication.

2. ANTIBIOTIC-ASSOCIATED DIARRHEA

Diarrhea may occur during (more commonly) or after a course of antibiotics; there is usually no obvious pathogen. The disorder is dose related, and symptoms resolve promptly after discontinuation of the offending agent. The course is benign, with little evidence of systemic illness. Stool examination is negative for fecal leukocytes, and sigmoidoscopic examination is normal, with no evidence of inflammation on biopsy. The basis for diarrhea in these cases is unclear.

3. *CLOSTRIDIUM DIFFICILE* DIARRHEA & ENTEROCOLITIS

C difficile is the single most important infectious cause of nosocomial diarrhea, accounting for 50–70% of cases of antibiotic-associated colitis. Outbreak clusters have occurred in hospitals and chronic care facilities. Current or prior use of antibiotics (within 6 weeks) is the most significant risk factor. It is unusual for *C difficile* colitis to develop in the absence of antibiotics, but this does occur. The most commonly implicated antibiotics include ampicillin, clindamycin, aminoglycosides, and cephalosporins. *C difficile* is a gram-positive, spore-forming anaerobic bacillus with a tendency to colonize the human intestinal tract when the normal enteric flora have been altered, particularly by antibiotic therapy. *C difficile* is able to survive for long periods of time in a hospital or chronic care facility setting in the form of heat-resistant spores. Asymptomatic carrier states are common in the elderly and serve as potential reservoirs for future outbreaks.

C difficile colitis is a toxin-mediated disease. Toxin A is capable of binding directly to the epithelium, eliciting a severe inflammatory reaction, which involves exudation of protein-rich materials which contain neutrophils, monocytes, and sloughed enterocytes and contributes to the formation of endoscopically apparent pseudomembranes. Histologic studies show that pseudomembranes are made up of necrotic debri, mucus, and inflammatory cells that appear to well out over the surface epithelium in a "volcano" formation.

Clinical Findings

A. Symptoms and Signs: A wide spectrum of clinical states are seen with *C difficile* infection, ranging from the asymptomatic carrier state to mild, self-limited diarrhea to fulminant pseudomembranous colitis with megacolon. In the patient with *C difficile* colitis, the onset of watery diarrhea and crampy lower abdominal pain may occur several days and up to 6 weeks after inception of antibiotic treatment. Approximately one-third of cases develop after discontinuation of antibiotics. The patient may pass up to 10–12 watery, occasionally blood-streaked stools per day. Grossly bloody stools are rarely seen. Patients may complain of abdominal distention, and fever may be present. The average duration of diarrhea is 1–2 weeks. Physical examination may reveal a distended abdomen with diffuse tenderness. In the extremely ill patient, evidence of peritoneal signs, including rebound tenderness and abdominal wall rigidity, may be present. In milder cases, patients may complain only of infrequent loose stools and mild, crampy lower abdominal pain. Fever is uncommon.

In the severely ill patient, megacolon with perforation may develop and is associated with a high mortality rate. Volume depletion and resultant electrolyte disturbances may contribute to the morbidity of the illness and should be monitored closely. Extensive ulceration may result in a protein-losing enteropathy with profound hypoalbuminemia, especially in patients who have had diarrhea for several weeks.

B. Laboratory Testing: In *C difficile* colitis, patients may have a mild peripheral leukocytosis. Fecal stool specimens may reveal leukocytes in up to 50% of patients. A positive *C difficile* cytotoxin assay is necessary for the diagnosis; however, a turnaround time of 24–48 hours is required. Stool cultures for *C difficile* are difficult to perform, require several days to complete, and are not specific, because asymptomatic colonization occurs commonly in the hospital setting. Hence, they are not useful.

C. Endoscopy: Endoscopy is useful in a subset of patients with antibiotic-associated colitis. In patients with mild to moderate symptoms, the diagnosis of *C difficile* colitis is usually established by *C difficile* toxin assay alone. Endoscopy in such cases is unnecessary. When performed, it may show a spectrum of findings ranging from nonspecific colitis with edema, erythema, friability, and erosions, to the more classic pseudomembranous colitis.

In patients with more severe symptoms, it may be desirable to establish a diagnosis of *C difficile* colitis emergently, before the results of the toxin assay are available. Endoscopy can quickly establish the diagnosis of pseudomembranous colitis and helps to distinguish it from other clinical entities such as ischemic colitis or inflammatory bowel disease. The typical features of pseudomembranous colitis are colitis with white or yellow fluffy, loosely adherent plaques and copious mucopus. These changes are evident in the rectum and sigmoid in most patients.

D. Other Studies: Up to one-third of patients have exclusive right colonic involvement; hence, flexible sigmoidoscopy cannot reliably exclude the diagnosis. In the extremely ill patient, a roentgenogram of the abdomen may demonstrate ileus or megacolon, with edema of the colon. CT scanning may demonstrate a markedly thickened colon.

Treatment

Two highly effective treatments exist for *C difficile* colitis: metronidazole and vancomycin. Both are effective when taken orally. Vancomycin has high luminal activity, with minimal absorption. Metronidazole is the drug of choice, however, due to lower cost and absence of metronidazole-resistant strains. Metronidazole, 250 mg orally four times daily for 10 days, is equally as effective as vancomycin, 500 mg four times daily for 10 days, with cure rates of up to 95%.

In the severely ill *C difficile* colitis patient, intravenous metronidazole, 250 mg every 6 hours, plus vancomycin, 500 mg every 6 hours by nasogastric tube or rectal tube, should be administered. Narcotics and antidiarrheal agents should be avoided. In the patient with progressive deterioration despite medical therapy, surgical options, including a subtotal colectomy with ileostomy, should be considered.

Approximately 10–20% of patients relapse and require a second course of antibiotics; the response rate is excellent, nearly 95%. The optimal approach for patients with multiple relapses is unclear. Some authorities advocate prolonged treatment regimens with vancomycin, with gradual tapering of the dose to 125 mg every other day. Alternatively, combined regimens of vancomycin, 125 mg four times a day, and rifampin, 600 mg twice a day, may be used. Use of lactobacilli, 1–2 g four times a day, or cholestyramine, 4 g three times a day, are also expected to be effective.

4. AIDS-RELATED ACUTE DIARRHEA

Diarrhea is one of the most frequent symptoms in HIV-infected patients. As CD4 lymphocyte counts decrease below 200/μL, patients are at increased risk for opportunistic enteric infections, in addition to routine infectious agents. Although acute diarrhea may be seen with bacterial enteric pathogens, chronic diarrhea secondary to fungal, viral, and parasitic infections is much more prevalent (see Chapter 2).

5. PROCTITIS

Proctitis is defined as anorectal symptoms associated with sigmoidoscopic findings limited to the distal 15 cm of the rectum. It encompasses a broad group of clinical disorders with causative mechanisms, including infection, trauma, inflammatory bowel disease, and chemical injury.

Clinical Findings

A. Symptoms and Signs: Typically, patients complain of lower gastrointestinal symptoms, including tenesmus, fecal urgency, and frequent small-volume stools associated with mucoid or mucosanguineous discharge. Although rectal bleeding may be present, large-volume gastrointestinal bleeding is exceedingly rare. True diarrhea is uncommon, and symptoms of fever, weight loss, and malaise are usually absent.

A variety of disease processes may cause inflammation confined to the rectum (Table 8–5). A thorough, careful history should be taken, with close attention to the sexual history, concurrent medical illnesses, duration of illness, travel history, rectal trauma, and history of pelvic irradiation.

B. Diagnostic Studies: Stool culture for enteric pathogens may be useful. Rectal swabbing for specific bacterial and viral cultures may assist in determining the cause. Fecal leukocyte determination is usually positive, indicating active inflammation associated with proctitis.

Proctosigmoidoscopy is the examination of choice and may be accomplished with a rigid or flexible instrument. The endoscopic appearance of the rectal mucosa may aid in narrowing the cause; however, no findings are pathognomonic. Viral proctitis may be associated with discrete ulcerations or vesicles, with surrounding mucosal inflammatory changes. Characteristic endoscopic findings of inflammatory bowel disease may be seen within the distal rectum. Biopsies should be obtained for appropriate cultures and histologic examination.

Table 8–5. Differential diagnosis of proctitis.

Infectious causes	Traumatic proctitis
Bacteria	Foreign bodies
Aeromonas	Solitary rectal ulcer
Campylobacter	syndrome
Salmonella	Radiation proctitis
Shigella	Chemical- or drug-induced
Chlamydia	proctitis
Syphilis	Nonsteroidal anti-
Gonorrhea	inflammatory agents
Enteropathogenic *E coli*	Soap
C difficile	Hydrogen peroxide
Viruses	Fluorouracil
Herpesvirus	Gold and heavy metals
Cytomegalovirus	Miscellaneous causes
Parasites	Behçet's syndrome
Amebiasis	Amyloidosis
Schistosomiasis	Lymphoma
Inflammatory bowel disease	Fecal stream diversion
Crohn's disease	Connective tissue
Ulcerative colitis	disorders
	Vasculitis

Treatment

Therapy should be targeted toward the causative agent. For nonspecific ulcerative proctitis, topical corticosteroids, 5-aminosalicylic acid suppositories, or enemas may be beneficial, with response rates of 70–90% after 4–8 weeks of treatment. Rarely, oral sulfasalazine may be required to ameliorate symptoms.

6. DIARRHEA IN ELDERLY PATIENTS

Diarrheal illnesses may be particularly debilitating for elderly patients. In a report from the Centers for Disease Control, adults over age 74 years accounted for up to 51% of deaths due to diarrhea reviewed from 1979–1987. Age per se is not a risk factor; however, it is a predictor of concomitant medical conditions that may predispose an elderly patient to development of diarrhea. Two important risk factors are nursing home residence and hospitalization. Individuals are at increased risk of fecal-oral contamination from other nursing home residents or supervising personnel. In addition, antibiotic administration during hospitalization is a significant risk factor for *C difficile* diarrhea in the elderly.

Elderly patients are at risk for routine bacterial, viral, and parasitic agents of diarrhea; however, noninfectious causes should be routinely considered. Iatrogenesis is an important cause of diarrhea in the elderly and should always be considered (Table 8–6).

Table 8–6. Noninfectious causes of diarrhea in elderly patients.

Iatrogenesis
  Antibiotics
  Antacids and acid-suppressing drugs
  Osmotically active laxatives (eg, milk of magnesia, lactulose)
  Enteral dietary supplements
  Miscellaneous drugs (eg, quinidine, digoxin, colchicine)
Systemic illness
  Diabetes mellitus
  Thyrotoxicosis
  Amyloidosis
  Scleroderma
  Uremia
Gastrointestinal disease
  Mesenteric ischemia
  Fecal impaction with overflow diarrhea
  Inflammatory bowel disease
  Obstructive lesions
  Malabsorption
  Chronic pancreatic insufficiency
Neoplasia
  Obstructive lesions
  Hormone-secreting tumors

REFERENCES

Behrens RH: Diarrhoael disease: Current concepts and future challenges. Trans Royal Soc Trop Med Hygiene 1993;87(Suppl 3):S35.

Bennett RG, Greenough WB: Approach to acute diarrhea in the elderly. Gastro Clin North Am 1993;22:517.

Bishai WR, Sears CL: Food poisoning syndromes. Gastro Clin North Am 1993;22:579.

Blake PA: Epidemiology of cholera in the Americas. Gastro Clin of North Am 1993;22:639.

Cantey JR: *Escherichia coli* diarrhea. Gastro Clin North Am 1993;22:609.

Chak A, Banwell JG: Traveler's diarrhea. Gastro Clin North Am 1993;22:549.

DuPont HL: Diarrhoeal disease: Current concepts and future challenges: Antimicrobial therapy and prophylaxis. Trans Royal Soc Trop Med Hygiene 1993;87(Suppl 3):31.

DuPont HL: Prevention and treatment of traveler's diarrhea. N Engl J Med 1993;328:1821.

Fine KD, Guenter JK, Fordtran JS: Diarrhea. In: *Gastrointestinal Disease,* 5/e. Sleisenger MH et al (editors). Saunders, 1993.

Gorbach SL: Bismuth therapy in gastrointestinal diseases. Gastroenterology 1990;99:863.

Gorbach SL: Infectious diarrhea and bacterial food poisoning. In: *Gastrointestinal Disease,* 5/e. Sleisenger MH et al (editors). Saunders, 1993.

Keene WE et al: A swimming-associated outbreak of hemorrhagic colitis caused by *Escherichia coli* O157:H7 and *Shigella sonnei.* N Engl J Med 1994;331:579.

Kelly C, Pothoulakis C, LaMont JT: *Clostridium difficile* colitis. N Engl J Med 1994;330:257.

Kelsall BL, Guerrant RL: Evaluation of diarrhea in the returning traveler. Infect Dis Clin North Am 1992;6:413.

Lew JF et al: Diarrheal deaths in the United States: 1979 through 1987. JAMA 1991;265:3280.

McFarland LV: Diarrhea acquired in the hospital. Gastro Clin North Am 1993;22:563.

Owen RL: Parasitic diseases. In: *Gastrointestinal Disease,* 5/e. Sleisenger MH et al (editors). Saunders, 1993.

Park SI, Giannella RA: Approach to the adult patient with acute diarrhea. Gastro Clin North Am 1993;22:483.

Powell DW: Approach to the patient with diarrhea. In: *Textbook of Gastroenterology.* Yamada T et al (editors). Lippincott, 1991.

Powell DW, Szauter KE: Nonantibiotic therapy and pharmacotherapy of acute infectious diarrhea. Gastro Clin North Am 1993;22:683.

Savarino SJ, Bourgeois AL: Diarrhoeal disease: Current concepts and future challenges: Epidemiology of diarrhoeal disease in developing countries. Trans Royal Soc Trop Med Hygiene 1993;87(Suppl 3):S7.

Tellier R, Keystone JS: Prevention of traveler's diarrhea. Infect Dis Clin North Am 1992;6:333.

Viral agents of gastroenteritis: Public health importance and outbreak management. MMWR 1990;39(Suppl RR-5):S1.

Wistrom J et al and the Swedish Study Group: Empiric treatment of acute diarrheal disease with norfloxacin: A randomized, placebo-controlled study. Ann Intern Med 1992;117:202.

Mesenteric Vascular Disease 9

David J. Ellis, MD, & Lawrence J. Brandt, MD

The gastrointestinal system performs a variety of energy-dependent processes, among which are motility, digestion, secretion, absorption, and cellular regeneration. Each of these vital functions relies on the adequate delivery of essential nutrients and oxygen, without which they cannot be performed properly. When the metabolic demands of the intestine outweigh its energy supply, ischemic injury may ensue. Intestinal ischemia produces a broad spectrum of disorders, the clinical presentation of which depends on many variables, including the onset and duration of the injury (acute or chronic), the distribution and the length of bowel affected (small bowel or colon), the type of vessel involved (artery or vein), the mechanism of ischemia (embolus, thrombus, or systemic hypoperfusion), and the degree of collateral flow.

The types of intestinal ischemia and their approximate incidences include colonic ischemia (60%), acute mesenteric ischemia (30%), focal segmental ischemia (5%), and chronic mesenteric ischemia (5%). Acute mesenteric ischemia involves that part of the intestinal tract supplied by the superior mesenteric artery and its branches. Arterial causes of acute mesenteric ischemia are more common than venous, and emboli are more often responsible than thromboses.

Patients with acute mesenteric ischemia usually present during the ischemic episode, but because the amount of intestine involved is frequently extensive and the diagnosis is commonly made late (ie, after infarction has occurred) patients with acute mesenteric ischemia are more ill than those with colonic ischemia and have higher morbidity and mortality rates. In contrast, patients with colonic ischemia present after the ischemic episode, their complaints are mild, their physical examination findings minimal, and their risk of mortality lower than patients with acute mesenteric ischemia. Clinical presentations do overlap, however, and patients who present a diagnostic problem should be considered to have acute mesenteric ischemia until proven otherwise.

Angiography has a minor role in the evaluation of suspected colonic ischemia because on presentation colonic blood flow usually has returned to normal. Colonoscopy or serial barium enemas are used to confirm the diagnosis of colonic ischemia. On the other hand, angiography is an integral part of the diagnosis and management of suspected acute mesenteric ischemia as well as chronic mesenteric ischemia.

ANATOMY OF THE SPLANCHNIC CIRCULATION

The vascular supply to the abdominal viscera is via the three main branches of the abdominal aorta, namely, the celiac, the superior mesenteric artery, and the inferior mesenteric artery. Whereas some consistent patterns have been established, anatomic and angiographic studies have demonstrated a marked variability of these vessels. In many respects, the architecture of this vascular system appears to have been designed to protect itself from ischemic events. For example, anastomoses exist between branches of the major vessels, and as a result, if one artery is occluded, some flow may be maintained via the patent collateral. Furthermore, in certain areas a network of anastomosing arcades is present, which further reinforces this defense against ischemia; the anastomoses in the duodenum and rectum are quite rich, and ischemia is rare in these locations. On the other hand, the vascular supply is less redundant in areas like the splenic flexure and sigmoid colon where ischemic damage, therefore, is more commonly observed.

The celiac artery rises from the anterior aorta at the level of the twelfth thoracic vertebra or the first lumbar vertebra between the diaphragmatic crura. This vessel supplies the foregut structures extending from the distal esophagus to the second portion of the duodenum. The usual branches of the celiac artery are the hepatic, splenic, and left gastric arteries. The splenic artery travels along the superior aspect of the pancreas above the splenic vein and terminates in the spleen. Branches of this artery, particularly the dorsal pancreatic artery, supply the pancreas while the left gastroepiploic artery and the short gastric artery supply the greater curve, fundus, and cardia of the stomach.

The common hepatic artery, variable in its origin and branches, travels along the superior aspect of the head of the pancreas, and before coursing superiorly toward the liver gives off the gastroduodenal artery, which runs inferiorly behind the first part of the duodenum. This latter vessel branches into the right gastroepiploic artery and superior pancreaticoduodenal artery, which anastomoses with the inferior pancreaticoduodenal artery, a branch of the superior mesenteric artery. The anastomosis between these two vessels provides a rich blood supply to the duodenum, and as mentioned previously, safeguards it against ischemic insult.

The left gastric artery runs along the lesser curvature of the stomach toward the pylorus, supplying these areas as well as the anterior aspect of the stomach.

The superior mesenteric artery arises from the anterior aspect of the abdominal aorta at the level of the first lumbar vertebra and about 5–10 mm inferior to the celiac axis. The superior mesenteric artery originates behind the body of the pancreas and, as it travels inferiorly, crosses the third portion of the duodenum anteriorly. Under certain conditions, this part of the duodenum may become trapped between the superior mesenteric artery and the aorta, giving rise to the superior mesenteric artery syndrome. The superior mesenteric artery provides blood flow to the midgut structures, extending from the second portion of the duodenum to the distal transverse colon. The major branches of the superior mesenteric artery include the inferior pancreaticoduodenal artery; the right, middle, and ileocolic arteries; and several separate jejunal and ileal branches. The jejunal and ileal vessels are connected through abundant primary, secondary, and tertiary anastomosing arcades that ultimately give rise to the vasa recta. As mentioned above, the inferior pancreaticoduodenal artery forms an important anastomosis with the celiac artery. The ileocolic artery travels to the right lower quadrant and there divides into ileal and colic arteries, which supply the terminal ileum, cecum, and proximal ascending colon. The ileal artery eventually anastomoses with the distal-most superior mesenteric artery, forming a loop. The right and middle colic arteries usually arise from a common trunk; the right colic artery branches and supplies the ascending colon, while the middle colic travels in the transverse mesocolon and supplies the transverse colon. The marginal artery of Drummond is an anastomosing network that lies close to the bowel wall and involves the right and middle colic arteries as well as the ascending branch of the left colic artery, which originates from the inferior mesenteric artery.

The arc of Riolan is another anastomotic channel that travels in the mesentery and connects the proximal middle celiac artery to the junction of the middle and left colic arteries. The central anatomic artery travels in between the marginal artery and the arc of Riolan.

The inferior mesenteric artery originates at the level of the third lumbar vertebra, 3–5 cm above the aortic bifurcation. Its major branches are the left colic artery, the superior rectal artery, and a series of sigmoid arteries that form an anastomosing arcade around the sigmoid colon. The left colic artery supplies the distal transverse colon, the splenic flexure, and the descending colon and also forms an anastomosis with the middle colic artery. The superior rectal artery descends to provide blood to the rectum and forms anastomoses with the middle and inferior rectal arteries, each a branch of the internal iliac artery.

In regard to the intestinal microcirculation, the vasa recta enter from the mesentery, penetrate the wall of the intestine, and give off branches to the serosa, the external muscular plexus, and the submucosal vascular plexus. From the submucosa, arterioles ascend into each villus and arborize into a dense capillary network. Blood returns via subepithelial venules, which are in close proximity to the arterioles, creating a countercurrent system that has important implications during periods of ischemia. Specifically, an oxygen gradient exists from the base to the tip of the villus, and when oxygen delivery is compromised, the villus tip is the first area to sustain ischemic damage.

PATHOPHYSIOLOGY OF MESENTERIC ISCHEMIA

Ischemic injury of the intestine occurs when there is inadequate delivery of oxygen and other nutrients to meet the intestine's various metabolic demands. Intestinal blood flow is controlled by a variety of factors—autonomic, humoral, and local—and relies on a rich anastomotic vascular network, both extraluminal and intraluminal. Each of these may influence and contribute to the generation of ischemic damage. Attention has also focused on the effects of postischemic reperfusion in this pathophysiologic process. Regardless of the cause, intestinal ischemia produces a spectrum of injury ranging from reversible function alterations to transmural necrosis of the bowel wall. Villus tips are the most sensitive to ischemia, and injury progresses from the intestinal luminal border toward the serosa.

Intestinal blood flow is controlled primarily by resistance arterioles and to a lesser degree by precapillary sphincters. A variety of vasoactive substances participate in the control of intestinal perfusion, either directly or indirectly; and specific substances may exert different effects in different regions of the intestine as well as in different layers of the bowel wall in the same segment.

The sympathetic nervous system via stimulation of α-adrenergic receptors causes arteriolar vasoconstriction that reduces mesenteric blood flow. However, blood flow ultimately returns to normal in the face of continued sympathetic stimulation, a process referred to as **autoregulatory escape.** The role of the sympathetic nervous system in the pathogenesis of mesenteric ischemia is unresolved at present. Angiotensin-II also causes mesenteric vasoconstriction, an effect more pronounced in the colon than small bowel and more pronounced in the muscularis than the mucosa. Vasopressin, released in states of volume depletion, results in a vasoconstrictive effect that is greater in the splanchnic circulation than the systemic circulation. A variety of arachidonic acid metabolites has been evaluated for its effects on mesenteric blood flow; several metabolites result in vasoconstriction while others cause vasodilation. Several products of ischemia also exert vasodilatory effects, including hyperkalemia, acidosis, hyperosmolarity, and hypoxemia. Vasoactive intestinal peptide has been shown to cause vasodilation; however, the role of other gastrointestinal hormones in the regulation of intestinal blood flow is less certain. Recently, short chain fatty acids have been demonstrated to result in dilation of colonic resistance arterioles.

Boley demonstrated that when a major vessel is occluded, collateral pathways open immediately in response to a fall in arterial pressure distal to the obstruction. This compensatory mechanism augments blood flow to those areas beyond the obstruction, thereby preventing ischemic injury. If the obstruction is relieved early, blood flow returns to baseline values in the obstructed artery as well as the collateral vessels. If, however, the obstruction persists, vasoconstriction develops in the distal vascular bed, resulting in elevated arterial pressure and diminished flow through the collateral pathways. Failure to relieve the obstruction promptly has been demonstrated to result in persistent vasoconstriction, which continues even if the obstruction is eventually corrected. If given before or soon after the onset of vasoconstriction, papaverine, a vasodilator, has proven to prevent or reverse this vasospasm. Persistent vasoconstriction helps explain the progression of ischemic injury despite the relief of the obstruction in occlusive ischemia or correction of under-perfusion in nonocclusive disease.

Relief of an arterial obstruction with subsequent reperfusion of ischemic tissue with oxygenated blood has been observed to aggravate tissue injury. Thus, the tissue damage produced by 3 hours of ischemia and 1 hour of reperfusion has been shown to be more severe than that of 4 hours of pure ischemia. There is evidence to suggest that reactive oxygen metabolites generated during ischemia with reperfusion mediate this enhanced injury. These metabolites are generated by the sequential reduction of molecular oxygen to produce superoxide and hydroxyl radicals in addition to hydrogen peroxide. The mechanism by which these metabolites cause injury involves damage to a variety of biomolecules, including nucleic acids, enzymes, and receptors. Hydroxyl radicals attack membrane-bound fatty acids resulting in lipid peroxidation, a process that alters membrane integrity and ultimately causes cellular swelling, lysis, and death.

ACUTE MESENTERIC ISCHEMIA

Essentials of Diagnosis
- High index of clinical suspicion.
- Patient is usually older than 50 years with chronic cardiovascular disease.
- Early in course, abdominal pain is typically out of proportion to findings on physical examination.
- Angiography: diagnostic and potentially therapeutic.

General Considerations
Acute mesenteric ischemia is a medical and surgical emergency that demands a timely diagnosis and a coordinated and deliberate multidisciplinary approach, if death or the short bowel syndrome are to be averted. Acute mesenteric ischemia accounts for approximately one-third of episodes of intestinal ischemia but is responsible for most ischemia-related deaths. In contradistinction to the chronic forms of intestinal ischemia, in which blood flow is adequate under basal conditions and symptoms such as pain are precipitated by eating, basal blood flow in acute mesenteric ischemia is severely compromised and bowel viability is threatened. Mortality rates of 70–90%, once intestinal infarction has occurred, attest to the lethal nature of this disease if acute mesenteric ischemia is not recognized and treated promptly. A high index of clinical suspicion for acute mesenteric ischemia must be maintained; if combined with the early and liberal use of angiography in the correct clinical setting, this can improve the usual and excessive fatal outcome.

The various causes of acute mesenteric ischemia and their approximate incidences include superior mesenteric artery embolus (50%), nonocclusive mesenteric ischemia (25%), superior mesenteric artery thrombosis (10%), mesenteric venous thrombosis (10%), and focal segmental ischemia (5%). The incidence of acute mesenteric ischemia has increased over the past 25 years owing to a longer life expectancy, an expansion of the elderly, and a heightened awareness of the various ischemic syndromes. The salvage of critically ill patients in intensive care units, who are subsequently prone to develop acute mesenteric ischemia, has also contributed to this increased incidence.

In the early part of this century, mesenteric venous thrombosis was considered the most common cause of acute mesenteric ischemia, but it is likely that most cases of mesenteric ischemia believed to be mesenteric venous thrombosis were actually caused by vasospasm secondary to nonocclusive mesenteric ischemia (NOMI). Today, superior mesenteric artery embolus is the most common cause of acute mesenteric ischemia, with the decreased incidence of NOMI reflecting improved ICU monitoring with rapid correction of volume deficits, shock, hemorrhage, congestive heart failure, and arrhythmias, each of which may result in reactive mesenteric vasoconstriction and NOMI if not treated promptly.

Arterial forms of Acute Mesenteric Ischemia:

1. Superior mesenteric artery emboli (SMAE)– Emboli usually originate from a left atrial or ventricular mural thrombus, but can also arise from abnormal cardiac valves as well as from a left atrial myxoma. Many patients with SMAE have had previous peripheral emboli and approximately 20% have synchronous emboli to other arteries. Emboli tend to lodge at points of normal anatomic narrowing, usually just distal to the origin of a major branch.

2. Nonocclusive mesenteric ischemia (NOMI)– NOMI is caused by diffuse splanchnic vasoconstriction, which results from an extensive variety of conditions, each of which has in common splanchnic hypoperfusion. These conditions include a decrease in cardiac output with hypotension secondary to acute myocardial infarction, congestive heart failure, arrhythmias, and valvular heart disease; other shock states secondary to hemorrhage or sepsis; and renal failure, particularly in those requiring hemodialysis. Those undergoing major cardiac or intra-abdominal operations are also susceptible. Localized forms of NOMI can attend SMAE, especially when the plan of management does not include intra-arterial papaverine.

3. Superior mesenteric artery thrombosis (SMAT)– SMAT occurs at areas of severe atherosclerotic narrowing, most commonly at the origin of the superior mesenteric artery. The acute ischemic episode is commonly superimposed on chronic mesenteric ischemia, and 20–50% of these patients have a history suggesting intestinal angina in the weeks to months preceding the acute event. A history of coronary, cerebral, or peripheral artery ischemia is frequent.

Clinical Findings

A. Symptoms and Signs: Acute mesenteric ischemia is associated with abdominal pain in 75–98% of cases. The pain usually develops suddenly and varies in character, intensity, and location. Classically, early in the course of acute mesenteric ischemia, the pain experienced by the patient is markedly out of proportion to objective physical findings. Although the patient may complain of severe abdominal pain, the abdomen is soft, flat, and nontender. A history of postprandial pain in the

weeks to months preceding the onset of severe pain is associated only with SMAT. Pain may be absent in up to 25% of patients with NOMI.

In patients in whom pain is absent, other signs and symptoms—such as unexplained abdominal distention or intestinal hemorrhage—may be the only manifestation of acute mesenteric ischemia. Bacteremia and diarrhea following cardiopulmonary resuscitation suggests NOMI.

Occult blood may be found in the stool in up to 75% of patients with acute mesenteric ischemia. Right-sided abdominal pain associated with the passage of maroon or bright red blood in the stool, although characteristic of colonic ischemia, also suggests the possibility of acute mesenteric ischemia, since the blood supply to the colon proximal to the distal two-thirds of the transverse colon emanates from the superior mesenteric artery. Acute occlusion of the superior mesenteric artery initially results in increased bowel activity, and this heightened motor activity can result in rapid and forceful bowel evacuation early in acute mesenteric ischemia.

Whereas a paucity of physical findings is found early in the course of acute mesenteric ischemia, abdominal tenderness, rebound tenderness, and muscle guarding are all ominous signs, suggesting transmural necrosis and intestinal infarction. Nausea, vomiting, gastrointestinal bleeding, shock, and abdominal distention are also late features in acute mesenteric ischemia.

B. Laboratory Findings: Early in the course of acute mesenteric ischemia, there are no specific laboratory findings. On admission to the hospital, approximately 75% of patients with acute mesenteric ischemia have a leukocytosis above 15,000 cell/μL and about 50% have metabolic acidemia. Elevations of serum phosphate, amylase, lactate dehydrogenase, CPK, and intestinal alkaline phosphatase have been described, but the sensitivity and specificity of these and other markers of intestinal ischemia have not been established.

C. Imaging: Early in acute mesenteric ischemia, plain films of the abdomen are usually normal. Conversely, about 25% of patients with intestinal infarction also have normal plain films; plain films of the abdomen are not especially sensitive in detecting mesenteric ischemia or infarction. Nonspecific plain film findings may include a gasless abdomen, adynamic ileus, or a small bowel pseudo-obstruction pattern. Formless loops of small intestine and thumbprinting, the latter reflecting submucosal edema or hemorrhage, are more suggestive findings. Pneumatosis intestinalis or portal vein gas are late findings, usually associated with transmural necrosis and infarction and each portends a poor prognosis. The role of plain films in acute mesenteric ischemia is not in its diagnosis, but rather to rule out the presence of other entities that produce abdominal pain and mimic acute mesenteric ischemia.

Just as with plain films, findings on computed tomography (CT) may be normal or nonspecific in cases of ischemia or infarction. Nonspecific findings on CT in acute mesenteric ischemia include focal or diffuse bowel wall thickening, focally dilated fluid-filled loops of bowel, mesenteric edema, engorgement of mesenteric veins, and ascites. More suggestive findings include air in the bowel wall or mesenteric or portal venous gas. Intravenous contrast may demonstrate an arterial occlusion, which appears as a filling defect in the vessel lumen.

Angiography plays a critical role in both the diagnosis and management of patients with acute mesenteric ischemia. Angiography is performed only after a patient is adequately resuscitated, because the angiographic findings are similar in patients with NOMI and in those who are hypotensive or on pressors. In the latter instance, mesenteric vasoconstriction is a normal and expected physiologic response, while in the former circumstance it is pathologic. The angiographic criteria for NOMI include narrowing of the origins of multiple branches of the superior mesenteric artery, irregularities in the intestinal branches, spasm of the arcades, and impaired filling of the intramural vessels. Superior mesenteric artery emboli appear as well delineated filling defects in the contrast column associated with obstruction to distal flow. Emboli tend to lodge in areas of vessel narrowing, usually just distal to the origins of major branches. Superior mesenteric artery thrombosis usually occurs in a chronically atherosclerotic vessel. The diagnosis of SMAT is most often made on a flush aortogram, with the thrombosis located either at the origin of the superior mesenteric artery or within its proximal 2 centimeters. If angiographic criteria for NOMI, SMAE, or SMAT are met, intra-arterial infusion of a vasodilator, specifically papaverine, may be indicated.

Treatment

The goals of treatment of acute mesenteric ischemia are early diagnosis by angiography, relief of persistent vasoconstriction by intra-arterial administration of a vasodilator, and resection of any frankly necrotic bowel. Given the excessive mortality rate if ischemia is permitted to progress to infarction, broad selection criteria must be used in addition to early angiography if prompt diagnosis and successful treatment are to be achieved (Figure 9–1).

Initial treatment is directed toward correcting any precipitating causes of acute mesenteric ischemia. Treatment of acute congestive heart failure, stabilization of cardiac arrhythmias, and correction of blood volume or red cell deficits must precede any diagnostic studies. Given the physiologic redistribution of blood flow from the splanchnic to the systemic circulation in states of intravascular volume depletion, efforts at increasing intestinal blood flow will be futile if low cardiac output, hypotension, or hypovolemia

persist. Shock is a contraindication to angiography because mesenteric vasoconstriction, as seen in NOMI, normally accompanies the shock state. Furthermore, intra-arterial vasodilators should not be used to treat shock; they will increase the size of the mesenteric vascular bed and further reduce systemic blood pressure. If needed, placement of a pulmonary arterial catheter may be used to guide fluid management.

After volume resuscitation, patients are sent for plain films of the abdomen. These studies are obtained primarily to exclude other causes of abdominal pain such as perforated viscus or intestinal obstruction and not to establish the diagnosis of acute mesenteric ischemia. Plain films have a low sensitivity and specificity for mesenteric ischemia and infarction.

If the cause of the patient's abdominal pain cannot be elicited from the plain film, visceral angiography is performed. Appropriate management depends on the angiographic findings (SMAT, SMAE, or NOMI) and the presence or absence of peritoneal findings.

Even when the decision to operate has been made based on clinical grounds, a preoperative angiogram should be obtained to help manage the patient before, during, and after laparotomy. Relief of mesenteric vasoconstriction, which may persist after the correction of the underlying cause, is essential in the treatment of emboli, thromboses, and the nonocclusive low flow states. For this purpose, papaverine should be infused at a rate of 30–60 mg/hr through the superior mesenteric artery catheter. The complication rate of mesenteric angiography is usually acceptable and includes an approximately 6% incidence of transient acute tubular necrosis secondary to the contrast medium, an incidence of embolization of less than 1% (possibly resulting from the arterial catheter), and occasional catheter dislodgment with systemic infusion of papaverine and resultant hypotension.

Laparotomy is performed in acute mesenteric ischemia to restore arterial flow after an embolus or thrombus or to resect irreparably damaged bowel. Embolectomy, thrombectomy, or arterial bypass precedes the evaluation of intestinal viability, because bowel that initially appears infarcted may show surprising recovery after blood flow is restored. Short segments of bowel that are nonviable or of questionable viability after revascularization are resected and a primary anastomosis is performed. If extensive portions of bowel are of questionable viability, only the clearly necrotic bowel is resected and a planned reexploration or "second look" is performed within 12–24 hours. The interval between the first and second operations is used to allow better demarcation of viable and nonviable bowel and to attempt to improve intestinal blood flow with intra-arterial papaverine or by maximizing cardiac output.

Use of anticoagulants in the management of acute mesenteric ischemia is controversial. Heparin may

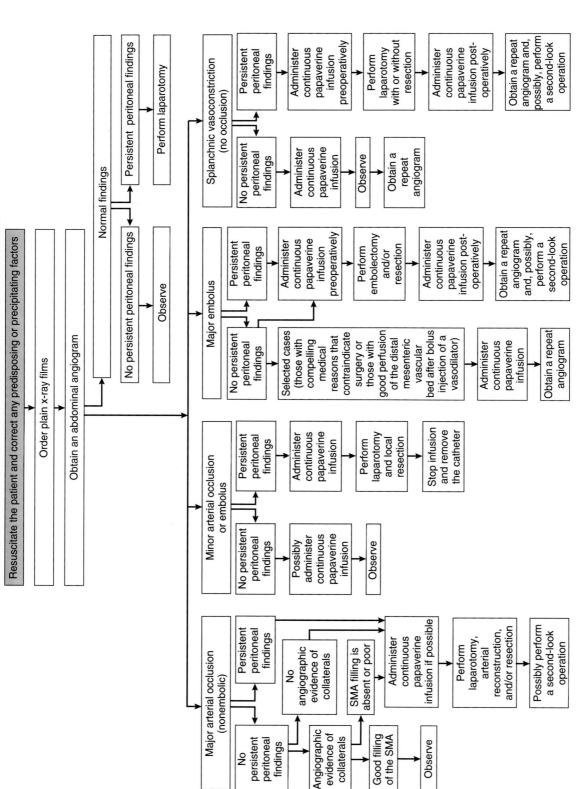

Figure 9–1. Management of patients with suspected acute mesenteric ischemia. SMA= superior mesenteric artery.

cause intestinal or intraperitoneal hemorrhage, and except in the case of mesenteric venous thrombosis, should not be given in the immediate postoperative period. Late thrombosis following embolectomy or arterial reconstruction occurs frequently enough that anticoagulation 48 hours postoperatively seems advisable. Given the high incidence of positive blood cultures in patients with acute mesenteric ischemia, broad-spectrum antibiotics are administered early and continued in the postoperative period.

Prognosis

If acute mesenteric ischemia is not diagnosed early and intestinal gangrene occurs, mortality rates are approximately 70–90%. Approached aggressively as outlined above, survival can be improved to about 55%. In those patients with angiographically proven acute mesenteric ischemia without peritonitis, survival rates approach 90%. Furthermore, if treated aggressively, the length of bowel requiring resection is diminished, allowing the patient a better chance of surviving with a functioning gastrointestinal tract.

MESENTERIC VENOUS THROMBOSIS

Essentials of Diagnosis

- Acute form: abdominal pain associated with a predisposing condition (eg, a hypercoagulable state).
- Chronic form: usually asymptomatic.
- Diagnosed by contrast CT or angiography.

General Considerations

Our understanding of the incidence, pathogenesis, and manifestations of mesenteric venous thrombosis has evolved since its initial description in the late 19th century. Initially, mesenteric venous thrombosis was believed to account for most cases of acute mesenteric ischemia. NOMI was described in the 1950s, and it is likely that those patients felt to have mesenteric venous thrombosis before that time in fact were suffering from NOMI. Since that time, the incidence of mesenteric venous thrombosis has steadily declined, and today mesenteric venous thrombosis accounts for less than 5% of cases of acute mesenteric ischemia. Male-to-female ratios have been variable, ranging from 1.5:1 to 1:1, and the mean age of 48–60 years is lower than that of other forms of mesenteric ischemia.

Formerly an underlying cause of mesenteric venous thrombosis was identified in less than 50% of patients. However, the condition responsible for the development of mesenteric venous thrombosis can be identified in over 80% of patients with the description of various hypercoagulable states (eg, deficiencies of antithrombin III, protein S, and protein C) and other prothrombotic conditions, including a variety of neoplasms and the myeloproliferative disorders. Other conditions associated with mesenteric venous

thrombosis include pregnancy, oral contraceptive use, portal hypertension, and a variety of intra-abdominal processes, eg, pancreatitis, peritonitis, and inflammatory bowel disease. Rarely, nonthrombotic occlusion of the mesenteric veins secondary to venulitis or venous myointimal hyperplasia can simulate mesenteric venous thrombosis.

With the advent of a variety of imaging modalities, the variability of clinical expressions of mesenteric venous thrombosis became evident. Mesenteric venous thrombosis can be categorized into acute, subacute, and chronic forms, each of which will be further described in this section.

Pathophysiology

Ligation of the superior mesenteric vein in canines is associated with a variety of consequences, including dilation of the mesenteric vein, bleeding into the mesentery, cyanosis of the bowel with congestion and spasm, paralytic ileus, and the weeping of serosanguinous fluid from the bowel and mesentery into the peritoneal cavity. Hypovolemia, hemoconcentration, acidosis, and decreased flow in the superior mesenteric artery are also seen resulting in death between 1 and 4 hours secondary to cardiovascular collapse. Release of the superior mesenteric vein ligature may be associated with residual arterial spasm. In animals pretreated with heparin prior to superior mesenteric vein occlusion, death is prevented.

The propagation of the thrombus differs for different disease processes. For example, in mesenteric venous thrombosis secondary to hypercoagulable states, the thrombus is believed to begin in small venous branches and extend toward the major trunks, whereas the opposite is felt to occur in mesenteric venous thrombosis associated with portal hypertension or neoplasia. Intestinal infarction is rare unless the branches of the peripheral arcades and the vasa recta are involved. The extent of the venous collateral circulation also has a significant impact on the course of the disease after thrombus formation.

Clinical Findings

Mesenteric venous thrombosis can have an acute, subacute (weeks to months), or chronic onset. A previous history of deep venous thrombosis in the extremities may be elicited in up to 60% of patients.

A. Symptoms and Signs: The signs and symptoms of acute mesenteric venous thrombosis are highly variable and nonspecific. Abdominal pain is present in more than 90% of patients and usually is out of proportion to physical findings. As with arterial forms of acute mesenteric ischemia, however, the pain is variable in its location, duration, character, and severity. Pain usually begins 1 to 2 weeks before admission, but may be present up to 1 month before admission. Nausea, vomiting, and occult blood in the stool are found in more than one-half of the patients with acute mesenteric venous thrombosis. Hematemesis and hematochezia each are present in 15% of patients and indicate intestinal infarction. Physical findings of mesenteric venous thrombosis include abdominal tenderness in almost all patients, and abdominal distention and hypoactive bowel sounds in about 80%. Temperature greater than 38°C is found in almost 50% of patients and hypotension with a systolic blood pressure less than 90 mm Hg is noted about 25% of the time. Guarding and rebound tenderness occur later in the course and may reflect intestinal infarction.

In the subacute form of mesenteric venous thrombosis, abdominal pain is present for weeks to months in the absence of intestinal infarction. Abdominal pain, again highly variable and nonspecific, is the most common complaint; nausea and diarrhea occur only occasionally. Physical examination is usually normal.

Those patients with chronic mesenteric venous thrombosis experience no symptoms at the time the thrombosis initially develops. They may either continue to remain asymptomatic or develop gastrointestinal hemorrhage secondary to esophageal or intestinal varices. Physical findings are those of portal hypertension, eg, splenomegaly if the portal vein is involved; however, there may be no abnormal findings with only superior mesenteric vein occlusion.

B. Laboratory Findings: In all forms of mesenteric venous thrombosis, the laboratory findings are neither sensitive nor specific and therefore are not useful in confirming or excluding the diagnosis. The white blood cell count may be elevated above 12,000/μL in two-thirds of patients. Thrombocytopenia or pancytopenia secondary to hypersplenism may be seen in the chronic form.

C. Imaging: Abdominal plain film findings of mesenteric venous thrombosis are nonspecific. While 75% of patients with acute mesenteric venous thrombosis may have an abnormal abdominal roentgenogram, 50% reveal a nonspecific ileus pattern. Portal venous air, air in the wall of the small bowel, and free intraperitoneal air are all ominous signs of intestinal infarction. Small bowel series typically reveals luminal narrowing from congested and edematous bowel wall; separation of loops due to mesenteric thickening; and thumbprinting secondary to submucosal edema and hemorrhage.

Selective mesenteric angiography can establish a definitive diagnosis before bowel infarction, can differentiate venous thrombosis from arterial forms of ischemia, and can provide access for vasodilators if persistent arterial vasospasm is present. Angiographic findings in mesenteric venous thrombosis include: demonstration of a thrombus in the superior mesenteric vein with partial or complete occlusion; failure to visualize the superior mesenteric vein or portal vein; slow or absent filling of the mesenteric veins; presence of arterial spasm; failure of arterial arcades to empty; reflux of contrast into the artery;

and prolonged blush in the involved segment of bowel.

Computed tomography is capable of diagnosing mesenteric venous thrombosis in more than 90% of patients. Specific findings using this modality include thickening and persistent enhancement of the bowel wall, an enlarged superior mesenteric vein with a central lucency representing thrombus formation, a sharply defined vein wall with a rim of increased density, and dilated collateral vessels in a thickened mesentery. CT may be used as the initial diagnostic modality in certain clinical settings, for example, a patient with abdominal pain, no peritoneal signs, and a history of a deep venous thrombosis or an inherited coagulation defect (Figure 9–2). If, on the other hand, the history does not suggest mesenteric venous thrombosis but rather an arterial form of acute mesenteric ischemia, superior mesenteric artery angiography is indicated.

Treatment

The treatment of acute mesenteric venous thrombosis has changed over the years and now depends in part whether the presence of intestinal infarction is suspected; several nonoperative approaches are proving to be successful in the subgroup of patients without bowel infarction (Figure 9–3). In patients who have radiologic evidence of mesenteric venous thrombosis and no signs of intestinal infarction, a trial of anticoagulation with heparin or thrombolysis with streptokinase has been successful. However, should signs of intestinal infarction develop, such as muscle guarding and rebound tenderness, laparotomy is mandated. Patients with peritoneal signs should undergo prompt laparotomy and resection of frankly

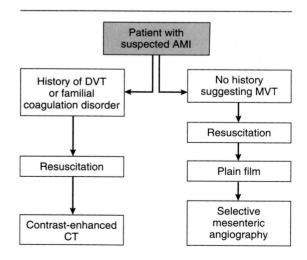

Figure 9–2. Evaluation of the patient with suspected acute mesenteric ischemia. AMI= acute mesenteric ischemia; DVT= deep vein thrombosis; MVT= mesenteric venous thrombosis.

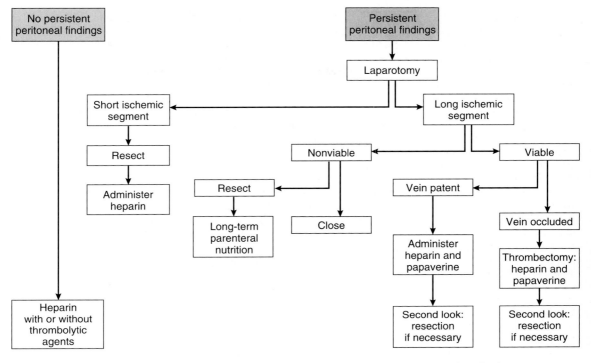

Figure 9–3. Management of the patient with documented mesenteric venous thrombosis.

necrotic bowel, followed by the administration of heparin. In patients anticoagulated with heparin, the recurrence of the disease has decreased from about 25% to 13%, and the mortality rate has improved from 50% in patients who did not receive postoperative heparin to 13% in those who did.

In patients with long segments of bowel involved, the preoperative angiogram will help dictate whether thrombectomy is advisable. When blood flow is adequate through the major trunks or collaterals, only the portions of bowel believed to be irreversibly necrotic are removed; this is followed by the postoperative administration of heparin and transcatheter intra-arterial papaverine to reduce the mesenteric venous thrombosis-associated arterial vasospasm. A second look operation is performed 12–18 hours later to assess bowel viability. Venous thrombectomy is indicated when there is complete thrombosis of the superior mesenteric vein at its junction with the portal vein.

In chronic mesenteric venous thrombosis, treatment is directed at controlling symptoms, which usually consist of bleeding secondary to portal hypertension. Patients who are asymptomatic do not require treatment, as it is felt that venous collaterals are adequate to prevent portal hypertension. The natural history of asymptomatic chronic mesenteric venous thrombosis is not well known. The treatment of those patients with variceal bleeding is directed initially at control of the hemorrhage followed by treatment of

the varices by endoscopy, portosystemic shunting, or surgical devascularization.

FOCAL SEGMENTAL ISCHEMIA

Essentials of Diagnosis
- In acute form: simulates appendicitis.
- In chronic form: simulates Crohn's disease, symptomatically and radiologically.
- Most commonly presents as small bowel obstruction with abdominal pain, distention, vomiting.

Pathophysiology
Briefly, vascular insults to short segments of the bowel produce a broad spectrum of clinical features without the life-threatening complications associated with more extensive ischemia. The causes of focal segmental ischemia include atheromatous emboli, strangulated hernias, immune complex disorders, vasculitis, blunt abdominal trauma, radiation, and oral contraceptive use. With focal segmental ischemia there is usually adequate collateral circulation to prevent transmural infarction; perforation and peritonitis are uncommon. Limited necrosis may result in complete healing, a chronic enteritis simulating Crohn's disease, or a stricture. As a result, patients present with one of three clinical patterns: acute enteritis, chronic enteritis, or obstruction.

Clinical Findings

In the acute pattern, abdominal pain often stimulates acute appendicitis. Physical findings are those of an acute abdomen, and an inflammatory mass may be palpated. Plain films of the abdomen early in the course are usually normal, but later may reveal a "sentinel loop" or a nonspecific ileus pattern. The chronic enteritis pattern may be indistinguishable from that of Crohn's disease, with symptoms including crampy abdominal pain, weight loss, fever, and diarrhea. Radiologically the diseases may be similar as well; however, Crohn's enteritis usually involves the terminal ileum, whereas focal segmental ischemia may occur anywhere in the small bowel. The most common presentation is of chronic small bowel obstruction with symptoms of abdominal pain, distention, and vomiting. Bacterial overgrowth in the dilated loop proximal to the obstruction may produce a blind loop syndrome and manifest with diarrhea. Radiologic studies reveal a smooth tapered stricture of varying length.

Treatment

Treatment of focal segmental ischemia is resection of the involved bowel.

COLONIC ISCHEMIA

Essentials of Diagnosis

- Typically, left lower quadrant pain, followed by the passage of blood per rectum within 24 hours in an elderly patient
- Diagnosed by serial lower endoscopy or barium enemas

General Considerations

Ischemic injury to the large intestine is a common disease in the elderly. Among those organs in the gastrointestinal tract susceptible to ischemia, the colon is the most commonly involved. A spectrum of ischemic injury to the colon is recognized, including reversible colonopathy (30–40%), transient colitis (15–20%), chronic ulcerating colitis (20–25%), stricture formation (10–15%), gangrene (15–20%), and fulminant universal colitis (< 5%). Regardless of the ultimate clinical expression of colonic ischemia, the initial presentation may be identical and is not predictive of the disease course. Exceptions to this rule do exist, however, particularly when the right colon is affected as part of a more extensive process that also involves the small bowel; both are supplied by the superior mesenteric artery. This particular pattern of ischemia within the distribution of the superior mesenteric artery usually reflects an SMAE, SMAT, or NOMI; if not diagnosed and treated appropriately, it is associated with a mortality rate of 70–90%, as described earlier.

The true incidence of colonic ischemia is difficult to determine for a variety of reasons. Many cases of transient or reversible ischemic damage are probably missed, either because the condition resolves before medical attention is sought, or barium enema or colonoscopy is not performed early enough to establish the diagnosis. Furthermore, the diagnosis of colonic ischemia is not frequently considered, and many cases are misdiagnosed as infectious colitis or idiopathic inflammatory bowel disease.

More than 90% of patients with non-iatrogenic causes of colonic ischemia are older than 60 years and have evidence of systemic atherosclerosis. There does not appear to be a significant sex predilection. Colonic ischemia in younger persons has been attributed to vasculitis, especially systemic lupus erythematosis, sickle cell disease, hypercoagulable states, medications (estrogens, danazol, vasopressin, gold, psychotropic drugs), cocaine abuse, and long-distance running.

Two special clinical situations associated with colonic ischemia are its occurrence in patients with carcinoma of the colon and other potentially obstructing lesions and its association with aortic surgery. About 15–20% of patients may have a related disorder, especially colon carcinoma, diverticulitis, volvulus, fecal impaction, postoperative stricture, or radiation stricture. Typically, the associated lesion is distal and there is a segment of normal-appearing colon between the distal lesion and the proximal colitis. Radiologists and gastroenterologists must be careful not to overlook associated lesions in patients with colonic ischemia. Surgeons must examine specimens of colon removed for carcinoma for evidence of ischemia near the anastomosis, because such involvement may lead to postoperative leaks or strictures. Colonic ischemia is a complication of elective aortic surgery in 1–7% of cases, but following surgery for ruptured abdominal aortic aneurysm its incidence may be as high as 60%. Colonic ischemia is responsible for approximately 10% of deaths after aortic grafting.

Pathophysiology

The precise etiology and pathogenesis of colonic ischemia remains ill-defined in most cases. In some instances, however, a cause can be identified, for example, ligation of the inferior mesenteric artery during repair of an abdominal aortic aneurysm. Indeed, ischemic injury to the colon may result from a variety of causes, both iatrogenic and noniatrogenic, occlusive and nonocclusive, systemic and local. Most cases are considered to occur spontaneously and are believed to represent localized forms of nonocclusive ischemia, perhaps in conjunction with small vessel disease. While a systemic low-flow state may be present, as in congestive heart failure or cardiac arrhythmias, in most instances, no such condition exists to explain the ischemic episode.

Given that colonic ischemia most often occurs in

the elderly, age-related acquired abnormalities in the colonic vasculature have been sought. Postmortem angiographic studies of the mesenteric arteries have revealed a distinct age-related tortuosity of the long colic arteries, which may contribute to the development of ischemia by increasing resistance to colonic blood flow. Also noted in pathologic specimens of the rectum of elderly patients are abnormalities of the musculature of the vessel wall.

The ultimate process resulting in colonic ischemia remains speculative. However, colonic blood flow is lower than that of any other intestinal segment, decreases with functional motor activity, and is greatly affected by autonomic stimulation. This combination, in addition to the acquired abnormalities previously mentioned, may predispose the colon to ischemic injury.

Clinical Findings

A. Symptoms and Signs: Most instances of colonic ischemia occur spontaneously, in contrast to acute mesenteric ischemia, in which a major vascular occlusion or period of systemic hypoperfusion usually can be identified. Typically, colonic ischemia presents with the sudden onset of mild, crampy, left-sided lower abdominal pain accompanied by an urgent desire to defecate. This is followed by the passage of either bright red or maroon blood mixed with stool over the ensuing 24 hours. The bleeding is not massive and blood loss requiring transfusion is so unusual as to suggest another diagnosis. Physical examination usually reveals only mild to moderate abdominal tenderness over the involved segment of bowel. The presence of peritoneal signs suggests colonic necrosis, gangrene, and perforation. Any part of the colon may be affected; however, the watershed areas, namely the splenic flexure and rectosigmoid, are the segments most commonly involved.

B. Imaging: Plain films of the abdomen are usually nondiagnostic in patients with colonic ischemia, but radiologic findings suggestive of colonic

ischemia include thumbprinting, transverse ridging, and a tubular appearance of the bowel. Thumbprinting of the colon may be seen in up to 20% of patients with colonic ischemia and represents submucosal hemorrhage and edema. While thumbprinting may be reflective of colonic ischemia, especially in the correct clinical setting, other diseases—including inflammatory bowel disease, infectious colitis, pseudomembranous colitis, and certain malignant lesions—may produce this change as well. Gas in abnormal locations, such as the bowel wall, peritoneum, and portal vein, are indicative of colonic infarction.

If colonic ischemia is suspected in a patient with no signs of peritonitis and an unremarkable abdominal plain film, colonoscopy or the combination of flexible sigmoidoscopy and a gentle barium enema should be performed within 48 hours of the onset of symptoms (Figure 9–4). Whichever test is selected, it should be performed early in the course, as the disease may evolve rapidly. If evaluation is delayed, initial characteristic lesions may be missed. If the patient is studied with serial examinations, which is sometimes the only way to suggest the correct diagnosis, the colon should show progression to a segmental ulcerative colitis within 1 week or reversion to normal within a similar time period. Colonoscopy is preferable to barium studies because it is more sensitive in diagnosing mucosal abnormalities and biopsy specimens may be obtained at the time of examination. Hemorrhagic nodules may be seen on colonoscopy and correspond to the thumbprinting seen on radiologic evaluation. Other findings on colonoscopic inspection may include an erythematous and congested mucosa, ischemic ulcerations, and mucosal gangrene. In cases in which the inflammatory response is excessive, lesions simulating strictures, polypoid neoplasms, or submucosal tumors may be seen. During colonoscopy, particular care must be taken to avoid overdistention with air, since pressures greater than 30 mm Hg, which may

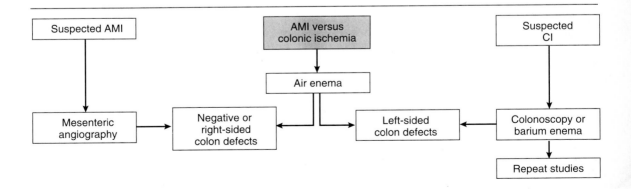

Figure 9–4. Management of suspected ischemic bowel disease. AMI= acute mesenteric ischemia; CI= colon ischemia.

be attained on routine examinations, diminish colonic blood flow and cause a shunting of blood from the mucosa to the serosa.

Although histologic evaluation of biopsy specimens obtained during colonoscopy often reveals a variety of nonspecific inflammatory changes seen in other types of colitides, certain findings are more characteristic of ischemia. These include the preservation of cellular outlines referred to as "ghost" cells and hemosiderin-laden macrophages in the submucosa.

Barium enema is also highly sensitive in the diagnosis of colonic ischemia. The most characteristic early finding of colonic ischemia is the presence of thumbprinting, seen in up to 75% of cases. Thumbprinting is not pathognomonic of colonic ischemia, and if the diagnosis of colonic ischemia is suspected, serial studies should be performed to demonstrate the evolution characteristic of this disease. Other findings may include transverse ridging, segmental ulcerations, and luminal narrowing, which may simulate colonic carcinoma. Up to 20% of patients with colonic ischemia have a potentially obstructing lesion distal to the ischemic segment. One-half of these are due to colonic carcinoma, while the other 50% are due to a variety of other lesions, eg, diverticulitis, stricture, or fecalith.

Mesenteric angiography is usually not indicated in the management of colonic ischemia, as colonic blood flow has usually returned to normal by the time of presentation. Hence, angiography rarely shows any significant occlusions. Angiography may be indicated however, if acute mesenteric ischemia is a consideration, either because only the right side of the colon is affected or the clinical presentation does not allow a clear distinction between colonic ischemia and acute mesenteric ischemia. In the latter situation, if the plain films of the abdomen do not show the thumbprinting pattern characteristic of colonic ischemia, an air enema is performed by gently insufflating air into the colon, either by using a hand bulb or during flexible sigmoidoscopy. On fluoroscopy, the submucosal edema and hemorrhage that produce the thumbprinting pattern of colonic ischemia can be accentuated by the column of air. If thumbprinting is not seen or is identified in the ascending colon only, mesenteric angiography is indicated. Since untreated acute mesenteric ischemia rapidly becomes irreversible, and optimal management requires angiography, acute mesenteric ischemia must be excluded prior to barium studies are performed.

Treatment

Since the outcome of colonic ischemia usually cannot be predicted, serial examinations are necessary to determine the ultimate course of disease. When the physical examination does not suggest gangrene or perforation, the patient is treated expectantly. Parenteral fluids are administered, the bowel is placed at rest, and broad-spectrum antibiotics are given. Cardiac function is optimized and medications that cause mesenteric vasoconstriction, such as digitalis and vasopressors, are withdrawn if possible. Colonic distention is treated with rectal tube decompression and nasogastric aspiration. Serial evaluations of the colon and continuous monitoring of the hemoglobin, white blood cell count, and electrolytes are performed. Increasing abdominal tenderness, guarding, rising temperature, and paralytic ileus indicate colonic infarction and mandate laparotomy and colon resection.

If, as usual, colonic ischemia resolves within several weeks, no further therapy is indicated. When segmental colitis develops, corticosteroid therapy does not appear to be beneficial and may predispose to perforation. Patients who are asymptomatic, but with roentgenographic or endoscopic evident of persistent disease should have frequent follow-up examinations to determine whether the colon is healing, has persisting colitis, or is developing a stricture. Recurrent fevers, leukocytosis, and septicemia in otherwise asymptomatic patients with unhealed segmental colitis are usually caused by the diseased bowel and are an indication for elective resection. In patients with diarrhea, rectal bleeding, or protein-losing colonopathy for more than 2 weeks, colonic perforation is likely and early resection is suggested.

Colonic ischemia may not manifest symptoms during the acute insult but still may produce a chronic colitis frequently misdiagnosed as inflammatory bowel disease. Involvement is segmental, resection is not followed by recurrence, and the response to corticosteroid therapy is usually poor. Local steroid enemas may be helpful, but parenteral steroids should be avoided. In those whose symptoms cannot be controlled by medications, resection of the diseased segment is indicated.

If the ischemic process involves the muscularis propria with subsequent healing and fibrosis, an ischemic stricture may result. Strictures that produce no symptoms should be observed, as some of these will resolve over the next 12–24 months without specific therapy. Strictures that cause obstructive symptoms will require either dilation or resection.

A rare form of fulminating colonic ischemia involving all or most of the colon and rectum has been identified. The clinical course is typically rapid and progressive and management is similar to other forms of fulminant colitides, ie, total colectomy and ileostomy.

Prognosis

Usually symptoms of colonic ischemia subside within 24–48 hours and healing is seen within 2 weeks. Two-thirds of patients with reversible disease exhibit intramural and submucosal hemorrhage or a reversible colonopathy, while one-third manifest a transient colitis. More severe reversible damage may take 1–6 months to resolve. In almost 50% of patients with colonic ischemia, irreversible damage results. Approximately two-thirds of these patients develop segmental colitis or stricture and one-third develop gangrene with or without perforation.

The prognosis of patients with colonic ischemia-complicating shock, congestive heart failure, myocardial infarction, or severe dehydration is poor. One series reported these factors precipitating colonic ischemia in 25% of patients, and 92% of patients who presented in shock died.

CHRONIC MESENTERIC ISCHEMIA

Essentials of Diagnosis
- Postprandial abdominal pain, sitophobia, and weight loss.
- Diagnosed by angiography, which must show involvement of at least two of the three main splanchnic vessels.

General Considerations
Chronic mesenteric ischemia, or intestinal angina, is uncommon, accounting for less than 5% of all ischemic disease. The pathophysiology of this disease is most often related to atherosclerotic narrowing of the mesenteric vessels. These lesions are located proximally and at least two major vessels must be involved in order for ischemia to ensue. As these atherosclerotic narrowings develop over a period of time, usually an adequate collateral circulation has developed to prevent intestinal infarction, although this disastrous complication may occur if thrombosis suddenly develops in the involved artery. Similar to angina pectoris or intermittent claudication, in which blood flow is insufficient to meet the metabolic demands of exercise, the pain of chronic mesenteric ischemia has been attributed to insufficient blood flow to satisfy the increased postprandial demands of motility, secretion, digestion, and absorption. The pain produced by intestinal angina typically occurs soon after eating, prior to food entering the small bowel, and is felt to be secondary to an increased demand for gastric blood flow as food enters the stomach. This requirement is satisfied by a "steal" of blood flow from the small intestine, depriving this segment of its oxygen and nutrients.

Clinical Findings
A. Symptoms and Signs: The cardinal feature of chronic mesenteric ischemia is abdominal discomfort or pain that usually occurs within 30 minutes after eating, gradually increases in severity, and then slowly abates over 1–3 hours. The pain is usually dull, gnawing, or cramping and is located in the periumbilical region or in the epigastrium. Pain is initially precipitated by large meals, however, as the

disease progresses, the amount of food necessary to produce pain gradually diminishes until the patient ultimately becomes afraid to eat (sitophobia) and sustains weight loss. Malabsorption is seen in one-half of the patients, and gastrointestinal dysmotility manifested by bloating, nausea, episodic diarrhea, or constipation also occurs.

Physical findings are usually limited and nonspecific, however, patients with advanced disease may appear cachectic with marked weight loss. The abdomen typically remains soft and nontender, even during painful episodes, although significant distention may be present. An abdominal bruit is common but nonspecific.

Many patients have evidence of systemic atherosclerosis involving the heart, central nervous system, or the peripheral vasculature.

B. Diagnostic Studies: Diagnosis is often difficult because of the vague nature of the complaints and the lack of a specific diagnostic test. Studies of malabsorption may reveal an elevated fecal fat excretion or decreased level of urinary D-xylose excretion, however, these are nonspecific tests and can be caused by a variety of diseases. Barium studies may be normal or reveal nonspecific evidence of either malabsorption or a motility disturbance. Doppler ultrasound and computed tomography are also limited by their lack of specificity.

Angiography in selected patients is quite helpful in the diagnosis of chronic mesenteric ischemia, although all three major arterial vessels have been found occluded in asymptomatic patients. Single-vessel disease does not result in intestinal angina since the intestine within the distribution of the diseased vessel usually will be supplied by collateral vessels. At least two vessels need to be involved before the diagnosis can be considered. Angiographic views are taken anteroposteriorly to demonstrate the extent of the collateral circulation and laterally to show the proximal origins of the splanchnic vessels, especially the celiac axis.

Balloon tonometry, which can directly measure small intestine intramural pH, may be a more specific test of chronic mesenteric ischemia. This test is performed by placing an orally inserted tonometer into the small bowel and measuring the changes in calculated pH before and after the administration of a provocative test meal consisting of cream. As the cream enters the stomach and blood flow is shunted away from the small bowel due to the vascular "steal" mentioned earlier, there is a fall in intramural small bowel pH. Successful corrective surgical revascularization relieves symptoms and diminishes this change in intramural pH; tonometry, thus, can be used to determine the success of the operation.

Treatment
While chronic mesenteric ischemia does not require urgent therapy, surgery may be indicated if

acute complete occlusion of the blood supply occurs, ie, if thrombosis is superimposed on preexisting arterial narrowing. Surgical revascularization should be performed on a patient with the typical pain of abdominal angina and unexplained weight loss, whose diagnostic evaluation has excluded other gastrointestinal diseases and whose angiogram shows occlusive involvement of at least two of the three major arteries. A variety of such surgical procedures exist, including aortovisceral bypass and transaortic visceral endarterectomy, each of which is associated with a reasonable operative risk and a good long-term prognosis. Aside from improving symptoms, the infrequency of fatal acute mesenteric ischemia after a successful revascularization procedure suggests that such operations may prevent a major intestinal ischemic episode.

REFERENCES

Bakal CW, Sprayregen S, Wolf EL: Radiology in intestinal ischemia: Angiographic diagnosis and management. Surg Clin North Am 1992;72:125.

Boley SJ et al: A new provocative test for chronic mesenteric ischemia. Am J Gastroenterol 1991;86:888.

Boley SJ, Kaleya RN: Acute mesenteric ischemia: An aggressive diagnostic and therapeutic approach. Can J Surg 1992;35:613.

Brandt LJ, Boley SJ: Colonic ischemia. Surg Clin North Am 1992;72:203.

Brandt LJ, Boley SJ: Nonocclusive mesenteric ischemia. Annual Review of Med 1991;42:107.

Cunningham CG, Reilly LM, Stoney R: Chronic visceral ischemia. Surg Clin North Am 1992;72:231.

Genta RM, Haggitt RC: Idiopathic myointimal hyperplasia of mesenteric veins. Gastroenterology 1991;101:533.

Harward TR et al: Multiple organ dysfunction after mesenteric artery revascularization. J Vasc Surg 1993;18:459.

Kaleya RN, Boley SJ, Brandt LJ: Mesenteric venous thrombosis. Surg Clin North Am 1992;72:183.

Kaleya RN, Sammartano RJ, Boley SJ: Aggressive approach to acute mesenteric ischemia. Surg Clin North Am 1992;72:157.

Kornblith PL, Boley SJ, Whitehouse BS: Anatomy of the splanchnic circulation. Surg Clin North Am 1992;72:1.

Kubes P: Ischemia-reperfusion in feline small intestine: A role for nitric oxide. Am J Physiol 1993;264:G143.

MacDonald PH, Dinda PK, Beck IT: The role of angiotensin in the intestinal vascular response to hypotension in a canine model. Gastroenterology 1992;103:57.

Patel A, Kaleya RN, Sammartano RJ: Pathophysiology of mesenteric ischemia. Surg Clin North Am 1992;72:31.

Wolf EL, Sprayregen S, Bakal CW: Radiology in intestinal ischemia: Plain film, contrast, and other imaging studies. Surg Clin North Am 1992;72:107.

Zimmerman BJ, Granger DN: Reperfusion injury. Surg Clin North Am 1992;72:65.

Miscellaneous Diseases of the Peritoneum & Mesentery

10

Kip D. Lyche, MD

GENERAL APPROACH TO ASCITES & PERITONEAL DISEASE

The peritoneum consists of a single layer of mesothelium and a thin basement membrane lining the peritoneal cavity. A well-developed microvillus border adds to the total surface area, which approximates that of the skin ($1–2$ m^2). The peritoneal cavity is a closed sac, with the parietal surface extending anteriorly and the visceral peritoneum covering the organs posteriorly. In men, there is normally only a small amount of intraperitoneal fluid, but in women, there may be up to 20 mL of fluid, depending on which phase of the menstrual cycle is occurring. The mesothelium is delicate and easily damaged but heals rapidly. New mesothelial cells arise from subperitoneal fibroblasts. Chronic injury may result in scar tissue formation **(adhesions).** Inflammation of the peritoneum is usually associated with the development of ascites.

The causes of fluid in the peritoneal cavity can be divided into two broad categories, based upon the serum-ascites albumin gradient (SAAG). An SAAG of more than 1.1 g/dL strongly suggests that the ascites is attributable to portal hypertension, whereas an SAAG of less than 1.1 g/dL implies another cause, including cancer, nephrotic syndrome, tuberculous peritonitis, pancreatic disease, biliary disease, or connective tissue disease. The SAAG has been found to be more accurate than the transudate-exudate model for determining the presence of portal hypertension. This chapter will discuss the approach to the patient with ascites and a low SAAG; ascites due to portal hypertension is discussed elsewhere.

The evaluation of a patient with suspected peritoneal disease focuses on careful history taking, physical examination, abdominal paracentesis, limited radiologic evaluation, and, often, laparoscopy. The history is usually one of abdominal pain that is diffuse and constant and occurs in association with increasing abdominal girth. Systemic complaints of fatigue, jaundice, and fevers may guide the clinician in determining the cause. At least 1500 mL of ascitic fluid usually must be present before it can be de-

tected on physical examination. The most sensitive method of determining whether fluid is present is percussion of the flanks to detect dullness; if it is present, percussion should be repeated with the patient in a partial decubitus position ("shifting dullness"). The presence of palmar erythema and spider angiomas on the skin is highly suggestive of liver disease and helps the examiner greatly in determining the cause of ascites.

Abdominal paracentesis is the most critical study in the evaluation of the patient with ascites. The procedure should be performed in a sterile fashion using standard technique in the suprapubic or left lower quadrant position. Fluid should be inspected visually and a description documented in the patient record. Cloudy fluid may suggest an infection, but, often, when the white blood cell count is less than 1000/µL, the fluid will be a clear yellow color. Milky fluid is seen with chylous ascites and is due to the presence of high triglyceride levels. Bloody fluid most commonly suggests traumatic paracentesis, but a malignant tumor must also be considered.

The fluid should be sent for routine studies (Table 10–1). A cell count is the most useful test, and if only a small amount of fluid is available for evaluation, then a cell count should be requested. The fluid should always be sent in a "purple top" tube containing ethylenediamine tetra-acetic acid (EDTA), to prevent clotting of the cells. Normally, ascitic fluid contains fewer than 500 white blood cells per milliliter and fewer than 250 neutrophils per milliliter. Data regarding the normal red cell count of ascitic fluid are not available, but most bloody ascites is due to traumatic paracentesis. Any inflammatory cause of ascites (by definition, "peritonitis") can lead to an elevation of the white blood cell count. A gram-stained smear of ascitic fluid may be helpful in quickly establishing the diagnosis of secondary bacterial peritonitis due to a perforated viscus in a patient with preexisting portal hypertensive ascites. Usually, the gram-stained smear will be negative in spontaneous bacterial peritonitis, whereas it is often positive when there is a perforated viscus. Cultures should be performed by inoculating blood culture bottles with the

Table 10–1. Tests for ascitic fluid that should be routinely ordered.

Test	Purpose
Cell count and differential	To exclude bacterial infection, fungal infection, tuberculosis, atypical mesothelial cell suggesting tumor.
Gram-stained smear	To exclude secondary infection.
Culture	Multiple organisms are rare with spontaneous bacterial peritonitis.
Albumin	To calculate the SAAG.

ascitic fluid at the patient's bedside. Milky turbid fluid should be sent for triglyceride measurement.

The clinical situation will dictate whether AFB smear and culture, fungal smear and culture, and cytologic studies should be requested (Table 10–2). Cytologic studies should be ordered if lymphocytosis is evident in the ascitic fluid or if the patient has a history of a solid organ tumor (eg, breast or colon carcinoma). Cirrhotics with recurrent or poorly responding spontaneous bacterial peritonitis should be suspected of having tuberculosis. Patients undergoing chronic ambulatory peritoneal dialysis are at the highest risk for fungal peritonitis. The glucose concentration in the ascitic fluid will be decreased in bacterial and, especially, mycobacterial infection, but this measurement is seldom helpful in guiding therapy. The ascitic fluid lactate dehydrogenase level may be elevated in secondary bacterial peritonitis, as seen in a cirrhotic patient with ascites and concomitant perforated viscus.

The serum albumin level should be determined at the same time as the above measurements, so that the SAAG may be calculated. This gradient is the difference between the levels of serum albumin and ascitic fluid albumin (eg, 3 g/dL − 1 g/dL = 2 g/dL). Because the SAAG is dependent on the presence of portal hypertension, ascites due to portal hypertension and having a high protein content can be distinguished from ascites due to cancer, which may have a low protein content because of depressed serum protein levels.

Table 10–2. Ancillary tests that may be ordered in selected cases of ascites.

Test	Purpose
Cytologic studies	To detect most malignant tumors, but not mesothelioma.
Fungal smear and culture	To evaluate immunocompromised patients or those on chronic ambulatory peritoneal dialysis who are at risk for fungal peritonitis.
AFB smear and culture	To exclude tuberculosis. The smear is positive in only 5%, and the culture is positive in only 20% of patients with tuberculosis peritonitis.

The diagnosis of "mixed ascites" can raise a diagnostic dilemma in some patients who have both portal hypertension and another cause of ascites. Approximately 4% of patients will have more than one cause. Eleven percent of patients with peritoneal carcinomatosis will also have cirrhosis, and almost half of patients with tuberculous ascites will have underlying cirrhosis. Thus, a high SAAG does not necessarily exclude the possibility of either tumor or infection. Often, the ascitic fluid cell count will help the clinician in this situation. Patients with carcinomatosis and tuberculosis will often have lymphocytosis.

Ultrasound and CT scanning aid in the evaluation of peritoneal disease by allowing distinction between solid masses, cystic masses, and infiltrative processes affecting the peritoneum and mesentery. Associated lymphadenopathy may be detected, and masses affecting the solid organs or mesentery may be noted. Radiologic-guided needle biopsy of masses discovered with these modalities has become a useful "minimally invasive technique" that is safe in experienced hands.

Laparoscopy is another important diagnostic test in the evaluation of patients with ascites and a low SAAG. It is a relatively simple, well-tolerated, safe procedure that can be performed with local anesthesia and mild sedation on an outpatient basis. Peritoneal diseases such as tuberculosis and cancer are best evaluated by this modality. The role of laparoscopy in the evaluation of patients with negative CT scans and suspected hepatic or peritoneal cancer was examined in a recent review. Half the patients were found to have cancer documented by biopsy at laparoscopy. Three-quarters of patients with exudative ascites (even with negative cytologic examinations) had peritoneal metastases. Laparoscopy may provide direct visualization of peritoneal disease and allow biopsy of lesions. In cases associated with intermittent small bowel obstruction, therapeutic lysis of adhesions may be performed as well.

With the combination of these various diagnostic modalities, a cause for ascites may be determined in nearly all patients.

Brady PG, Peebles M, Goldschmid S: Role of laparoscopy in the evaluation of patients with suspected hepatic or peritoneal malignancy. Gastrointest Endosc 1991;37:27.

Hamrick-Turner JE et al: Neoplastic and inflammatory processes of the peritoneum, omentum, and mesentery: Diagnosis with CT. Radiographic 1992;12:1051.

Runyon BA: Care of patients with ascites. N Engl J Med 1994;330:337.

Runyon BA et al: The serum-ascites albumin gradient is superior to the exudate-transudate concept in the differential diagnosis of ascites. Ann Intern Med 1992;117:215.

ASCITES RESULTING FROM CAUSES OTHER THAN PORTAL HYPERTENSION

MALIGNANT ASCITES

About two-thirds of patients with malignant ascites have peritoneal carcinomatosis. The remaining one-third have ascites due to massive liver metastases or hepatocellular carcinoma, or chylous ascites due to lymphatic involvement; cytologic studies of ascitic fluid will typically be negative in these patients.

Peritoneal involvement by spreading cancer from a primary neoplasm ("peritoneal carcinomatosis") is a common peritoneal disease that usually carries a poor prognosis. Patients usually present with nonspecific abdominal discomfort associated with increasing abdominal girth. Physical examination and imaging studies may show evidence of ascites and may indicate the site of the primary tumor. More than 75% of cases are adenocarcinomas. Intra-abdominal primary sites predominate, with ovarian, pancreatic, and colonic tumors the most common, followed by lymphomas and gastric, uterine, lung, and breast tumors. Alterations in the permeability of the peritoneum and infiltration of the abdominal lymphatics play a role in the formation of ascitic fluid.

The diagnostic evaluation should begin with paracentesis. Cytologic studies of the ascitic fluid should be obtained if the SAAG is less than 1.1 mg/dL. Most experts recommend sending at least 1 L for examination. The fluid will be positive for cancer in 50–80% of cases with documented carcinomatosis. Other tests of ascitic fluid such as measurements of cholesterol, fibronectin, α_1-antitrypsin, and carcinoembryonic antigen have also been useful in differentiating malignant ascites from nonmalignant causes. If the cholesterol level is more than 45 mg/dL, 82% of patients will have positive cytologic studies, but if the level is less than 45 mg/dL, then nearly 100% will have negative studies. Focal masses found on noninvasive imaging studies may be examined with radiologic-guided percutaneous needle biopsy for diagnosis. Because of the possibility of peritoneal carcinomatosis, unexplained ascites with a low SAAG should be evaluated by laparoscopy if no cause is determined after the evaluation outlined above. Tuberculous peritonitis and mesotheliomas represent the major alternative considerations in the differential diagnosis.

The prognosis for most patients with peritoneal carcinomatosis is quite poor. The median survival rate after the diagnosis of malignant ascites for all patients is less than 20 weeks. Ovarian carcinomas with malignant ascites may represent an exception to this rule. With new treatment regimens that include intraperitoneal chemotherapy and surgical debulking, prolonged survival times may be expected in a significant proportion of patients.

Treatment of malignant ascites is often difficult. Therapy is directed toward relief of symptoms and improvement in the quality of life. In the absence of portal hypertension, salt restriction and diuretic therapy are not helpful. Large-volume therapeutic paracentesis is often useful, but palliation is of short duration. For patients who have a reasonable life expectancy and rapidly reaccumulating ascites, a peritoneovenous shunt may be a useful palliative modality and has been successful in up to 75% of patients. Shunt occlusion occurs in 25% of patients followed over a long period, but other shunt complications occur less often than in patients with cirrhosis and portal hypertensive ascites. Overall survival rates are similar in patients treated with and without peritoneovenous shunts, but those treated with successful shunts may spend less time in a hospital setting. Experts agree that peritoneovenous shunts should be avoided in patients with grossly bloody peritoneal fluid or those with pseudomyxoma peritonei.

Gerbes AL et al: Ascitic fluid analysis for the differentiation of malignancy-related and nonmalignant ascites. Cancer 1991;68:1808.

Gough IR, Balderson GA: Malignant ascites: A comparison of peritoneovenous shunting and nonoperative management. Cancer 1993;71:2377.

Karp SJ, Shareef D: Ascites as a presenting feature of multiple myeloma. J Royal Soc Med 1987;80:182.

CHYLOUS ASCITES

The peritoneal lymphatic vessels, and especially the diaphragmatic lymphatics, play a major role in the removal of fluid and particulate matter from the peritoneal cavity. The accumulation of lipid-rich lymph in the peritoneal cavity is termed chylous ascites. The usual cause is lymphatic obstruction or leakage resulting in accumulation of fluid with a high concentration of chylomicrons. Patients usually present with abdominal distention and malnutrition. Diarrhea may arise from either a protein-losing enteropathy or steatorrhea due to blocked small bowel lymphatics.

The diagnosis of chylous ascites is made when paracentesis reveals turbid milky fluid that separates into layers upon standing. The triglyceride level in the fluid is often more than 1000 mg/dL but always exceeds the plasma level. The possible causes of the ascites vary, depending on the age of the patient and the acuteness of onset of the illness.

In children, up to 60% of cases are associated with a congenital lymphatic anomaly such as a lymphocele, lymphangiectasia, or lymphatic atresia. Other cases include a variety of disorders, but neoplasms are rare in this age-group. The most common cause in adults is cancer, which is present in 87% of patients. In contrast, congenital lymphatic abnormalities are rare in adults. Intra-abdominal lymphoma that obstructs lymphatic outflow accounts for over half of cases of chylous ascites in adults. Inflammatory conditions that involve the lymphatics such as tuberculosis, pancreatitis, portal vein thrombosis, and mesenteric adenitis make up another large group of causes of chylous ascites. These entities lead to ascites by infiltrating lymph nodes, with resulting obstruction.

Postoperative chylous ascites occurs rarely. It has been reported most commonly following extensive abdominal or retroperitoneal dissection, as may occur during creation of a portacaval shunt, repair of an abdominal aortic aneurysm, or dissection of retroperitoneal lymph nodes. Lymphangiography is useful in this setting, to identify the site of lymphatic leakage for surgical repair.

Chylous ascites has also been reported rarely in uncomplicated cirrhosis with portal hypertension (0.5% of cases). The pathophysiology of this problem is poorly understood. No gross lymphatic obstruction or leak can be demonstrated. In some patients, no discernible cause for chylous ascites can be determined.

Once chylous ascites has been documented, a CT scan of the abdomen should be obtained to evaluate for possible cancer. Lymphangiography is performed in some centers to document the site of obstruction, leakage, or dysplasia. Exploratory laparotomy may be necessary to exclude the possibility of lymphoma with certainty.

Treatment is aimed at the underlying process. Diuretics and salt restriction do not work well, and large-volume paracentesis gives only short-term relief. A low-fat diet supplemented with medium-chain triglycerides will decrease lymph flow and may be useful. Total parenteral nutrition and complete bowel rest has been shown to decrease the lymph flow by up to 43% and may allow small postsurgical leaks to heal in some cases. Surgery has been effectively employed to repair lymphatic leaks in some patients. Placement of a peritoneovenous shunt has also met with modest success.

The prognosis depends on the underlying diagnosis and, for this reason, is better in children. The 1-year survival rate in children is 88% but only 23% in adults.

Ablan CG, Littooy FN, Freeark RJ: Postoperative chylous ascites: Diagnosis and treatment. Arch Surg 1990;125:270.

Browse NL et al: Aetiology and treatment of chylous ascites. Br J Surg 1992;79:1145.

Ohri SK et al: The management of postoperative chylous ascites. J Clin Gastroenterol 1990;12(6):693.

TUBERCULOUS PERITONITIS

Abdominal involvement occurs in only 2% of patients with tuberculosis. This rate is increased in patients coinfected with human immunodeficiency virus (HIV), who have a 50% incidence of extrapulmonary infection compared with only 15% in persons not infected with HIV. Other populations at risk for tuberculous peritonitis include immigrants from underdeveloped countries, the urban poor, prisoners, and nursing home residents. Abdominal tuberculosis can involve the omentum, intestinal tract, liver, spleen, female genital tract, and peritoneum. The onset of disease usually is insidious, with symptoms present for several months before diagnosis. Identification of tuberculous peritonitis is especially difficult in the 20% of patients who also have cirrhosis and portal hypertensive ascites. Most patients are 20–45 years of age, with a slight preponderance of women. Eighty percent of patients will present with abdominal swelling and have clinically apparent ascites, while 97% will have ascites documented by ultrasound or laparoscopy. Other important clinical features include fevers, anorexia, and abdominal tenderness, which are seen in 75% of patients. Weight loss and mild anemia are both seen in 60%. Chest radiographs are abnormal in about half of patients, but active pulmonary tuberculosis is evident in only 14%; skin tests are positive in 70%.

Paracentesis is the most important initial diagnostic test. The ascitic fluid protein exceeds 2.5 g/dL in more than 85% of cases; however, the SAAG should be less than 1.1 g/dL. The white blood cell count will be 150–4000/μL, with a predominance of lymphocytes. AFB smears are positive on ascitic fluid in 5% of patients, and cultures are positive in 20%; therefore, negative AFB smears and cultures are not helpful in excluding tuberculous peritonitis. Laparoscopy is the optimal method for establishing the diagnosis, allowing a presumptive visual diagnosis in more than 85% of cases. Suggestive findings include scattered whitish nodules (< 5 mm) over the visceral and parietal peritoneum and adhesions between adjacent organs. The differential diagnosis includes Crohn's disease and cancer. Biopsies will document the presence of caseating granulomas in more than 85% of cases. Due to the increased prevalence of multiple drug-resistant strains of tuberculosis, especially in HIV-infected patients, culture and sensitivity studies of peritoneal biopsy specimens are imperative. Approximately 3% of patients with peritoneal tuberculosis will not have ascites and may require laparotomy for diagnosis.

Treatment of tuberculous peritonitis is nonsurgical, with a prolonged course of multiple antituberculous antibiotics.

Aguado JM et al: Tuberculous peritonitis: A study comparing cirrhotic and noncirrhotic patients. J Clin Gastroenterol 1990;12(5):550.

Lingenfelser T et al: Abdominal tuberculosis: Still a potentially lethal disease. Am J Gastroenterol 1993;88(5):744.

Manohar A et al: Symptoms and investigative findings in 145 patients with tuberculous peritonitis diagnosed by peritoneoscopy and biopsy over a five-year period. Gut 1990;31:1130.

Marshall JB: Tuberculosis of the gastrointestinal tract and peritoneum. Am J Gastroenterol 1993;88(7):989.

Mimica M: Usefulness and limitations of laparoscopy in the diagnosis of tuberculous peritonitis. Endoscopy 1992;24:588.

PANCREATIC ASCITES

Pancreatic ascites is a distinct clinical entity that is usually seen in patients with chronic pancreatic disease. It is characterized by a massive amount of ascites rich in pancreatic enzymes that is caused by rupture of a pancreatic pseudocyst or disruption of a pancreatic duct. The exact incidence is unknown, but it may occur in up to 3% of patients with acute pancreatitis admitted to Veteran's Affairs Medical Centers in the United States. Patients commonly present with increasing abdominal girth and weight loss. Pain is variable. There may be a history of heavy alcohol intake or recent abdominal trauma. Signs of chronic pancreatitis such as steatorrhea, diabetes, or calcification on CT scanning are variably present. Serum amylase and lipase levels usually are elevated modestly, but ascitic fluid amylase levels are in excess of 10,000 units/mL. Because these enzymes are not active, the ascites usually is painless. The ascitic fluid total protein level is high due to leakage of enzyme-rich pancreatic fluid and exudate from the inflamed pancreas; however, the SAAG is less than 1.1 g/dL, consistent with a cause other than portal hypertension.

Treatment depends on the cause of the pancreatic ascites. After pancreatic trauma, early surgical repair of the duct or drainage of the pseudocyst may be the best initial management. In contrast, in the alcoholic patient with chronic pancreatitis, one may wish to be more conservative, given the increased severity of illness in this patient population and the possibility of recurrent problems. "Resting the pancreas" with bowel rest and total parenteral nutrition has met with success in up to 40% of such cases. Octreotide, the long-acting somatostatin analog, has been used in some uncontrolled series with apparent efficacy in decreasing pancreatic secretion and closing pancreatic leaks. Endoscopic retrograde cholangiopancreatography (ERCP) can be helpful preoperatively to define the location of ductal leaks and detect pancreatic strictures distal to the site of duct disruption. Endoscopic placement of pancreatic stents across the site of duct leakage may allow healing of a leak and thus avoid the need for surgery. The optimal approach to these patients often requires the expertise of radiologists, endoscopists, and surgeons.

Kuo Y-C, Wu C-S: Role of endoscopic retrograde pancreatography in pancreatic ascites. Dig Dis Sci 1994; 39(5):1143.

BILIARY ASCITES

Extravasated bile may lead to acute or chronic peritoneal fluid accumulation. The most common causes of bile leaks are complications of biliary tract surgery and trauma to the abdomen. The incidence of bile duct injuries has increased since the advent of laparoscopic cholecystectomy, with a rate of 0.5% in one large series, compared with a rate of 0.2% with open cholecystectomy. Less commonly, bile leaks are seen following percutaneous liver biopsy or percutaneous transhepatic cholangiography. Rarely, they are due to spontaneous perforation of the gallbladder, as in acute gangrenous cholecystitis.

The signs and symptoms of bile ascites are quite variable, depending on the degree of bacterial contamination of the extravasated bile. Although patients may present acutely with evidence of peritonitis, more often they present without fever, leukocytosis, or abdominal pain. Paracentesis is diagnostic, revealing dark yellow fluid, with a bilirubin level higher than 6 mg/dL and a ratio of ascites bilirubin to serum bilirubin of more than 1.

Treatment depends on the location and rate of bile leakage as well as the sterility of the ascites. Surgery is usually necessary to repair major biliary duct injuries. Localized collections of extravasated bile ("bilomas") can sometimes be drained percutaneously, with spontaneous resolution of a small leak. Endoscopic therapy has been quite useful in dealing with cystic duct leaks following cholecystectomy. By performing a sphincterotomy or placing a stent across the sphincter of Oddi, intraductal pressures are diminished and preferential drainage of hepatic bile into the duodenum occurs, with subsequent healing of the bile duct leak. Successful management of biliary ascites involves close cooperation among skilled interventional radiologists, biliary endoscopists, and hepatobiliary surgeons.

Branum G et al: Management of major biliary complications after laparoscopic cholecystectomy. Ann Surg 1993;217(5):532.

Hartle RJ, McGarrity TJ, Conter RL: Treatment of a giant biloma and bile leak by ERCP stent replacement. Am J Gastroenterol 1993;88(12):2117.

Kozarek RA et al: Endoscopic treatment of biliary injury in the era of laparoscopic cholecystectomy. Gastrointest Endosc 1994;40:10.

ASCITES ASSOCIATED WITH MYXEDEMA

Myxedema is an unusual but treatable cause of clinically significant ascites (affecting approximately 4% of patients). The diagnosis should be suspected in patients with systemic evidence of hypothyroidism or in noncompliant patients with a known history of thyroid disease. The mental status is usually impaired and the liver enlarged. The ascitic fluid has a high total protein level but also an elevated SAAG. The latter finding points to liver dysfunction as the cause of ascites, but the pathophysiology is poorly understood. The ascites usually does not respond well to diuretic therapy but rapidly resolves within a few weeks after thyroid replacement has been initiated.

de Castro F et al: Myxedema ascites. J Clin Gastroenterol 1991;13(4):411.

PERITONITIS ASSOCIATED WITH CHRONIC AMBULATORY PERITONEAL DIALYSIS

Current estimates suggest that 17% of dialysis patients in the United States use ambulatory peritoneal dialysis. Peritonitis remains a potentially life-threatening complication of this treatment and limits its widespread use. Peritonitis affects more than 50% of patients, with a frequency of approximately 1.7 episodes per year. The pathogenesis is completely different from that of suppurative peritonitis, as are the clinical manifestations and management. The pathway of contamination is clearly the dialysis system, usually the connection tubing. Strict aseptic technique decreases the incidence of these infections. Peritonitis occurs to some extent because of the depletion of host defenses of active phagocytic cells and opsonins by continual dilution and removal of peritoneal fluid.

Clinical findings are mild, with fever, abdominal pain, and a cloudy dialysate drainage. The white blood cell count of the peritoneal fluid will be more than 300/μL, with more than 75% polymorphonuclear leukocytes. These white blood cell changes may precede the development of cloudy fluid by 1 week. Gram-stained smears are positive in only 10% of samples. Organisms that commonly account for positive cultures are *Staphylococcus epidermidis* (30%), *Staphylococcus aureus* (23%), gram-negative organisms (16%), and *Streptococcus* (6%). Additional pathogens may include other gram-positive organisms, *Candida albicans,* and *Candida tropicalis.*

Treatment consists of prompt administration of antibiotics (usually on an outpatient basis) and elimination of the local infectious source. An increased frequency of exchanges will also help to resolve the infection. A primary tunnel infection must be excluded, especially if peritonitis fails to resolve promptly. Approximately 15–30% of clinical episodes are sterile and may either be due to a chemical constituent of the dialysate or an endotoxin.

Eosinophilic peritonitis may occur in up to 20% of patients within a few weeks of beginning chronic ambulatory peritoneal dialysis. This is not an infectious disease, and its pathophysiology is poorly understood. Cloudy sterile fluid will be present in asymptomatic individuals. No treatment is necessary, as the syndrome resolves spontaneously in most cases.

Holley JL, Bernarini J, Piraino B: Infecting organisms in continuous ambulatory peritoneal dialysis patients on the Y-set. Am J Kidney Dis 1994;23(4):569.

PERITONITIS ASSOCIATED WITH CHRONIC HEMODIALYSIS

Ascites may become a severe problem in up to 10% of patients undergoing chronic hemodialysis. The pathophysiology of this entity is unclear, but many patients have previously undergone peritoneal dialysis and have developed peritonitis. A decrease in peritoneal fluid drainage through damaged lymphatics is a leading hypothesis. These patients may have no evidence of cardiac failure or fluid overload and have normal serum albumin levels, and attempts to remove fluid during hemodialysis often result in the development of hypotension. The ascitic fluid is characterized by a high protein content and a low SAAG. The peritoneum is normal. Because this is a diagnosis of exclusion, these patients require paracentesis and possibly laparoscopy to determine whether tuberculosis or metastatic cancer may be present.

Treatment may be difficult. Sodium and fluid restriction coupled with adequate intake of protein and calories has met with only mild success. Nephrectomy has been advocated by some, but ascites often reaccumulates. Renal transplantation has had the best results but unfortunately cannot be offered to all patients.

ASCITES ASSOCIATED WITH OVARIAN DISEASE

Multiple benign diseases of the ovary can be associated with the development of ascites. The combination of ascites and hydrothorax associated with ovarian fibromas or cystadenomas is termed **Meig's syndrome**; the pathophysiology of ascites formation is unclear. Torsion of the ovaries or uterine leiomyomas may also be associated with ascites. One-third of patients with the rare ovarian teratoma containing thyroid tissue **(struma ovarii)** will have ascites, especially those with tumors larger than 6 cm in diameter. A florid reaction with diffuse peritoneal fibrosis has been reported to occur in response to the presence of ovarian thecomas.

CHEMICAL PERITONITIS

Chemical causes of peritonitis range from talc or starch from surgical gloves to barium introduced for bowel contrast studies. Talc, glove lubricants, cornstarch glove powder, lint, cotton from sponges and drapes, and cellulose fibers from disposable gowns and drapes have all been associated with granulomatous peritonitis. Clinical manifestations become evident 2–9 weeks after laparotomy in 0.15% of abdominal operations, with the onset of abdominal pain, fevers, tenderness, distention, and ascites. The signs and symptoms are suggestive of either bowel obstruction or peritonitis. Peripheral eosinophilia may be present, and birefringent crystals may be found in the ascitic fluid. Most often, patients will undergo repeat exploratory laparotomy, which will reveal miliary peritoneal nodules, adhesions, and ascites. Pathologic examination reveals granulomas and possible starch granules.

The prognosis is excellent, with no progression to chronic disease. Fortunately, this entity is rare and may be prevented with glove washing and avoidance of "custom cutting" drapes in the operating room.

Barium causes an intense peritoneal reaction when introduced through a perforated viscus and will often cause profound systemic effects. Treatment consists of prompt laparotomy, with rinsing of the peritoneal cavity and repair of the perforated bowel. Long-term complications of adhesion formation are more common in this situation. Water-soluble contrast agents should always be used when the possibility of intraperitoneal perforation exists, as these have been shown (in animal studies) to be less toxic to the peritoneum.

DISEASES OF THE PERITONEUM & MESENTERY ASSOCIATED WITH HIV INFECTION

The approach to the patient with acquired immunodeficiency syndrome (AIDS) who has evidence of peritonitis or mesenteric disease is similar to that for individuals who are not infected with HIV. The patient presenting with "acute abdomen" and evidence of a perforated viscus should undergo emergency laparotomy. The most common cause of perforation in AIDS patients is ileal or colonic cytomegalovirus infection. *Mycobacterium tuberculosis* has also been associated with multiple perforations of the small bowel and can be the presenting complication of AIDS.

Paracentesis is the diagnostic test of choice for evaluation of ascitic fluid. A high SAAG should prompt evaluation for causes of liver disease and portal hypertension such as chronic hepatitis B or C. A high suspicion for infections with mycobacteria (ie, *M tuberculosis, Mycobacterium avium* complex), fungi (ie, cryptococcosis, coccidiomycosis, histoplasmosis) and parasites (ie, *Toxoplasma gondii, Pneumocystis carinii*) must be present when dealing with these immunocompromised patients. Along with the cultures and special stains for organisms, cytologic studies of ascitic fluid may sometimes be useful in documenting the presence of cancer.

Abdominal and pelvic CT scanning play a key role in the evaluation of abdominal pain and persistent fevers in patients with AIDS. Peritoneal inflammation will usually be associated with ascites. Mesenteric disease will often be manifested as lymphadenopathy (which can be massive), tumor masses, or abscesses. The cause of the adenopathy often is attributed to *M avium* complex when blood cultures are positive for the organism. Patients with disseminated cutaneous Kaposi's sarcoma may have intra-abdominal involvement with the tumor as well. Abscesses may be due to bacterial, fungal, or parasitic causes and should be drained. Peritoneal involvement with lymphoma is rare, but abdominal involvement, including mesenteric, periportal, and retroperitoneal lymphadenopathy, is relatively common. This may be an important distinction to make because some AIDS patients may have relief of symptoms and prolonged survival times when treated with chemotherapy for non-Hodgkin's lymphoma.

Two other important diagnostic modalities in the evaluation of HIV-associated ascites or mesenteric disease deserve mention. Percutaneous biopsy and abscess drainage guided by either ultrasound or CT scanning have allowed many diagnoses to be made without surgical intervention, so that these very ill patients can receive appropriate medical therapy in an expeditious manner. Laparoscopy is the most useful modality in the evaluation of unexplained ascites with a low SAAG, for exclusion of infection or cancer. Even with this extensive evaluation, in a few patients there will be no clear explanation for illness affecting the peritoneum or mesentery. Some authors suggest that new, as-yet-unidentified organisms may be the culprits, or, possibly, the HIV infection itself may be the cause of the disease.

Berkowitz FE, Nesheim S: Chylous ascites caused by *Mycobacterium avium* complex and mesenteric lymphadenitis in a child with the acquired immunodeficiency syndrome. Pediatr Infect Dis J 1993;12(1):99.

Fife KM et al: Chylous ascites in Kaposi's sarcoma: A case report. Br J Dermatol 1992;126:378.

Friedenberg KA et al: Intestinal perforation due to *Mycobacterium tuberculosis* in HIV-infected individuals: Report of two cases. Am J Gastroenterol 1993;88(4):604.

Wilcox CM et al: Cytomegalovirus peritonitis in a patient with the acquired immunodeficiency syndrome. Dig Dis Sci 1992;38(8):1288.

Wilcox CM et al: High-protein ascites in patients with the acquired immunodeficiency syndrome. Gastroenterology 1991;100:745.

OTHER MESENTERIC & OMENTAL DISEASES

FAMILIAL MEDITERRANEAN FEVER

Many names have been attached to this rare clinical entity, such as familial paroxysmal polyserositis, periodic peritonitis, and familial Mediterranean fever. The illness almost exclusively affects those of Mediterranean ancestry. Sephardic Jews account for 50% of cases, Armenians 22%, and Arabs, Turks, and Ashkenazi Jews the remainder. The disease is inherited in an autosomal recessive manner. It is associated with episodic acute peritonitis in 95% of patients at some point during its course.

Patients usually present in the first or second decade of life; only 20% present after age 20 years. A sudden attack of serositis involving the peritoneum (55%), joints (25%), or pleura (5%) will be the first manifestation of the disease. Peritoneal attacks are marked by the sudden onset of fever, severe abdominal pain that may be diffuse or localized, and abdominal tenderness with guarding and rebound. Most patients will have some leukocytosis. Plain abdominal x-rays will show dilated loops of small bowel, with air-fluid levels consistent with ileus. If left untreated, the attack will improve within 6–12 hours and end with full recovery within 24–48 hours. Because patients have features of classic "acute surgical abdomen," initial attacks are often treated with exploratory laparotomy. Operative findings may show evidence of acute peritoneal inflammation with serous ascites that contains many polymorphonuclear leukocytes. Smears and cultures of the fluid are always sterile. To avoid confusion, an appendectomy is usually performed at the time of initial exploratory operation. The correct diagnosis is based on the ethnic background of the patient, the family history, a characteristic clinical history with fevers, serositis, and amyloidosis, and the exclusion of other causes of peritonitis.

Attacks of disease occur at unpredictable and irregular intervals. The associated arthritis may be prolonged, is usually oligoarticular, and may be associated with sacroiliitis. Amyloidosis with resultant renal failure is a potentially fatal complication that occurs in 25% of patients. Preliminary investigations have implicated catecholamine metabolism defects and a complement cofactor deficiency in the pathophysiology of the illness; however, the cause of the disease remains unknown.

Colchicine, 0.6 mg given two or three times a day, has been shown to decrease the frequency and severity of attacks. This treatment has little long-term toxicity and should be prescribed to most patients. Colchicine has been documented to decrease the incidence of nephropathy by 67% but is not useful once proteinuria (indicating nephrosis) is present. In patients with infrequent attacks, colchicine taken at the first signs of illness has been shown to ameliorate or even abort the attack. The full mechanism of action of colchicine is unknown, but it appears to alter leukocyte activity by interfering with microtubule function and neutrophil degranulation.

The prognosis is excellent, although attacks may sometimes increase in frequency with age. Most patients will have prolonged symptom free periods.

Barakat M et al: Familial Mediterranean fever (recurrent hereditary polyserositis) in Arabs: A study of 175 patients and review of the literature. Q J Med 1986;60:837.

Zemer D et al: Colchicine in the prevention and treatment of the amyloidosis of familial Mediterranean fever. N Engl J Med 1986;314:1001.

PSEUDOMYXOMA PERITONEI

This is a rare clinical condition that occurs predominantly in women (80%) 45–55 years of age. The peritoneal cavity becomes filled with pale, translucent mucinous ascites due to either a mucinous cystadenoma or cystadenocarcinoma of the ovary (45%), the appendix (29%), or an undetermined source (26%). Only 1–2% of patients with ovarian cancer will develop pseudomyxoma peritonei. The entity must be distinguished from benign mucocele of the appendix, which may have a few local mucinous deposits but carries a more favorable prognosis. Many experts believe that only true adenocarcinomas are associated with the condition.

Patients present with increasing abdominal girth but otherwise feel well. Abdominal pain due to intermittent or chronic small bowel obstruction may be present. Plain films of the abdomen may rarely reveal calcification. Ultrasound or CT scanning of the abdomen often shows ascites with multiple septations and semisolid masses along the peritoneal surfaces. The diagnosis is difficult to establish by imaging or biopsy and is usually made at the time of laparotomy.

Treatment consists of omentectomy and removal of as much of the primary lesion and the mucin as possible. If no primary tumor is apparent, appendectomy and bilateral oophorectomy are performed. In most cases, there is no local tumor invasion and distant metastases are rare. Postoperative adjunctive chemotherapy is useful, especially for ovarian carcinomas. Reexploration with debulking is a reasonable approach to treat recurrences or bowel obstruction. Although two-thirds of patients will eventually succumb to the disease, prolonged survival times have been described. Survival rates of 50% at 5 years and 20% at 10 years are usually reported.

MESOTHELIOMA

Primary malignant peritoneal mesothelioma is a rare tumor arising from the epithelial lining of cells and the mesenchymal elements of the peritoneum. The association of the disease with asbestos was first described in 1960, and more than 70% of cases have a history of prior exposure. Although pleural mesotheliomas occur at least four times as often, a history of extensive asbestos exposure increases the likelihood of peritoneal involvement. The latency period between asbestos exposure and tumor diagnosis typically is more than 30 years, with a median age at diagnosis of 54 years. Risk factors for mesothelioma are the type of asbestos fiber and the duration and concentration of exposure.

Patients present with recent onset of abdominal pain and increasing abdominal girth. Chest x-ray reveals evidence of asbestosis in approximately 50% of cases. More than 90% of patients have ascites, but the amount of fluid may be small. It is characteristically hemorrhagic, with a low SAAG. Cytologic studies may be negative or mistakenly interpreted as consistent with adenocarcinoma. Ultrasound and abdominal CT scanning will reveal ascites and often demonstrate sheetlike masses involving the omentum, mesentery, and peritoneum that may suggest the diagnosis. Laparoscopy usually is necessary and reveals extensive studding of all peritoneal surfaces with hard whitish nodules and plaques. On gross examination, the findings are indistinguishable from secondary carcinomatosis. Laparotomy may be required in some patients because of bowel obstruction or inconclusive findings on laparoscopy. The histologic findings are quite variable. About one-third of patients will have asbestos fibers present in peritoneal tissue. In difficult cases, electron microscopy can allow distinction from other tumors.

The prognosis for patients with peritoneal mesothelioma is poor, and worse than that for pleural tumors. Local tumor invasion and regional lymph node metastases are common and often lead to bowel obstruction that eventually becomes inoperable. Long-term survivors have been described who have undergone aggressive surgical debulking combined with chemotherapy and whole-abdomen irradiation. In general, however, the survival time is less than 1 year from the initial diagnosis, due to extensive disease at the time of presentation.

MESENTERIC PANNICULITIS & RETRACTILE MESENTERITIS

Mesenteric panniculitis is a thickening of the mesentery of the small intestine and colon, resulting from infiltration by lipid-filled macrophages and varying amounts of fibrosis. An alternative name, **mesenteric lipodystrophy,** may be more appropriate because little inflammation is present in this disorder, making the term "panniculitis" incorrect. Retractile mesenteritis is a clinical entity associated with fibrotic thickening and shortening of the mesentery. Patients with this disorder usually present with bowel obstruction. These two disorders may represent different stages of the same pathologic state, as is suggested by rare reports of their coexistence in a patient. Their pathogenesis is unknown. Trauma and infection may play a role in the initiation of damage to the mesenteric fat, with subsequent excessive lipid infiltration and fibrosis. Animal models have documented the propensity for the mesentery to scar following injection of bacteria into the peritoneal cavity. In addition, some patients have a clear temporal relationship of symptomatic disease following abdominal trauma.

The diagnosis of both disorders usually is made during laparotomy, which is performed for the treatment of bowel obstruction or evaluation of an abdominal mass. Alternatively, CT scanning may identify fat-filled mesenteric masses. Laparoscopy has established the diagnosis by providing access for visualization and biopsy. The major problem in the differential diagnosis is distinguishing these entities from neoplastic processes. Up to 30% of patients may have an associated tumor such as a lymphoma. Patients with mesenteric panniculitis may have diffuse mesenteric fatty infiltration (42%), a single discrete mass (32%), or multiple discrete masses of fat throughout the mesentery (26%). The histologic picture reveals lipid-filled macrophages, with a varying degree of inflammatory cells and fibrosis. Patients with retractile mesenteritis have a thickened, firm mesentery that has caused retraction of the small bowel down to the mesenteric root. Adhesions and acute angulations of the small bowel are often seen and clearly add to the propensity for intermittent small bowel obstruction present in this disease state.

The prognosis for patients with mesenteric panniculitis and retractile mesenteritis is good. If a patient has concomitant lymphoma or other neoplasm, the course depends on the outcome of the tumor. Once a diagnosis of mesenteric panniculitis is made, surgical resection is not indicated. Any obstruction related to retractile mesenteritis should be treated with a bypass procedure. Recurrent symptoms are uncommon but most often are related to adhesions. Rare cases of both of these disorders with progressive symptoms have been reported, and a response to corticosteroids and immunosuppressive therapy has been seen.

Cooper CJ et al: Abdominal case of the day: Mesenteric panniculitis. Am J Roentgenol 1990;154(6):1328.

Hamrick-Turner JE et al: Neoplastic and inflammatory processes of the peritoneum, omentum, and mesentery: Diagnosis with CT. Radiographic 1992;12(6):1051.

Weisner J et al: Laparoscopic diagnosis of retractile mesenteritis. Gastrointest Endosc 1992;38(5):615.

RETROPERITONEAL FIBROSIS

Retroperitoneal fibrosis is an uncommon chronic inflammatory disorder associated with slowly progressive fibrosis of fat and connective tissue in the retroperitoneum. Some pathologists have characterized the disorder as a benign neoplasm. The natural history of the disease is one of relentless compression of surrounding structures such as the ureters, nerves, and blood vessels. The cause is unknown in most cases. The pathogenesis of idiopathic retroperitoneal fibrosis is poorly understood. The nature of early pathologic findings, which include macrophage, lymphocyte, and plasma cell infiltration, suggest an immune-mediated process. Cases of secondary retroperitoneal fibrosis have been reported in patients treated with the serotonin blockers methysergide and bromocriptine. Other associated conditions include mediastinal or mesenteric fibrosis, carcinoid tumors, a history of retroperitoneal infection or radiation therapy, and paraneoplastic syndromes in rare patients with sarcomas or lymphomas.

Most patients who develop symptoms from retroperitoneal fibrosis present with flank and abdominal pain associated with fatigue, weight loss, and fevers. Patients are usually men over age 50 years. Medial deviation of both ureters and ureteral obstruction with resultant renal failure are common. Many patients have hypertension. The fibrotic reaction may involve the aorta or iliac arteries or, more rarely, obstruct major veins, with resultant deep venous thrombosis or lower extremity edema. A hydrocele is a relatively common finding due to increased pressure in the retroperitoneal vessels. This diffuse fibrotic process may also extend anteriorly to obstruct the duodenum, common bile duct, or colon. Rare cases of a systemic fibrosing disorder have been reported in patients with retroperitoneal fibrosis. Associated conditions include Riedel's thyroiditis, primary sclerosing cholangitis, mesenteric fibrosis, and mediastinal fibrosis.

The diagnosis of retroperitoneal fibrosis is often established by CT scanning of the abdomen. Pyelography will demonstrate medial deviation of the ureters, with obstruction and resultant hydronephrosis. Ultrasound may suggest a mass in the retroperitoneum and reveals evidence of hydronephrosis and hydroureter. The erythrocyte sedimentation rate is routinely elevated and is useful in following the response to subsequent therapies. The question as to whether all patients require tissue diagnosis before therapy is a difficult one. The noninvasive evaluation will often be helpful in suggesting whether a malignant neoplasm such as lymphoma or sarcoma is present. Many clinicians feel that a trial at medical therapy is justified, given the relatively low incidence of cancers in the large reported series (only 8% of 480 cases).

Previously, treatment of retroperitoneal fibrosis was surgical, with bypass or lysis the mainstay. Corticosteroids have been shown to be useful in almost all patients in the published literature. Prednisone is usually started at doses of 30–60 mg/d, which are then tapered over a period of weeks to 5–10 mg/d as tolerated, to maintain a good response, as evidenced by diminished clinical findings and radiographic studies. Due to reported complications associated with long-term prednisone therapy in these patients, azathioprine and cyclophosphamide have been used as corticosteroid-sparing agents. The most exciting new therapy for retroperitoneal fibrosis is probably tamoxifen. Preliminary reports have shown that doses of 20–40 mg/d have resulted in marked improvement in symptoms and regression of the fibrotic reaction as seen on radiographic studies. The mechanism of tamoxifen's efficacy is unknown but does not appear to be related to its estrogen-receptor blocking ability.

Bonnet C et al: Idiopathic retroperitoneal fibrosis with systemic manifestations. J Rheumatol 1994;21:360.

Clark CP, Vanderpool D, Preskitt JT: The response of retroperitoneal fibrosis to tamoxifen. Surgery 1991;109:502.

Duffy TP: Clinical problem solving: An anatomy lesson. N Engl J Med 1994;331:318.

Higgins PM et al: Nonoperative management of retroperitoneal fibrosis. Br J Surg 1988;75:573.

Rhee RY et al: Iliocaval complications of retroperitoneal fibrosis. Am J Surg 1994;168:179.

Gastrointestinal Complications of Pregnancy

11

Thomas L. Abell, MD, & Said I. Nabhan, MD*

This chapter focuses on the effects of pregnancy on the gastrointestinal tract. There are two sections: (1) gastrointestinal diseases that occur coincidentally with pregnancy and (2) gastrointestinal disorders that are unique to pregnancy. The goal is to emphasize the common disorders that come to the attention of primary care physicians, obstetricians, and gastroenterologists.

The physiologic effects of pregnancy include neurohormonal changes and a general slowing of gastrointestinal motility, which may lead to the development of a number of symptoms. Many "symptoms" that occur during pregnancy may be attributed inappropriately to pregnancy itself rather than to an underlying disease process, and this may result in a serious delay in diagnosis.

This chapter will use the current classification for drug therapy during pregnancy:

Category A: No evidence of damage to the fetus in animal or human studies.

Category B: Some evidence of possible damage to the fetus in animal studies but no evidence in human studies.

Category C: No data available from either animal or human studies.

Category D: Data show that the drug may harm the fetus, but the possible benefit of the drug has to be weighed against this risk.

Category X: Drugs contraindicated in pregnancy.

Few drugs used in gastrointestinal disease have undergone prospective testing in pregnant women, and, hence, there are few category A drugs. Animal safety data often cannot be applied to human pregnancies. The general rule is that the decision to use a drug during pregnancy needs to be individualized, with the physician and patient both aware of the potential risks and benefits. All drugs should usually be avoided during the first trimester. Organogenesis

takes place in the first 8–10 weeks of gestation and is largely completed by 16 weeks (Table 11–1). Drug therapy is usually believed to be safer in the second and third trimesters.

Recommendations for drug treatment of certain disorders in pregnancy are based on the best available information. Anyone treating pregnant patients is referred to one of the excellent texts or handbooks available regarding the latest information on the safety of drug therapy during pregnancy.

GASTROINTESTINAL DISEASES OCCURRING COINCIDENTALLY WITH PREGNANCY

PEPTIC ULCER DISEASE

Peptic ulcer disease is described only rarely during pregnancy, but this generalization is confusing because both peptic ulcer disease and pregnancy are common conditions. Dyspeptic symptoms such as nausea, vomiting, epigastric pain, bloating, and heartburn are common complaints during pregnancy. In most cases, these symptoms are treated empirically with antiulcer therapies by clinicians, and specific diagnostic studies such as upper endoscopy are avoided. Hence, the true prevalence of peptic ulcer disease, as opposed to dyspepsia from causes other than ulcers or gastroesophageal reflux, is unclear. Peptic ulcer disease is assumed to be at least as common in pregnant women as in the general population.

Pathophysiology

The pathophysiology of peptic ulcer disease in pregnancy has not been studied sufficiently, but it is presumed to be the same as in nonpregnant adults (see Chapter 21). In general, the risk factors for acid peptic disease are the same, including use of nonsteroidal drugs, cigarette smoking, and, possibly, use

*The author would like thank Dr. Barbara Kupyer for editorial assistance, Dr. Caroline Riely for manuscript review, and Ms. Becky Potter for assistance with manuscript preparation.

Table 11–1. Critical stages of organogenesis.[1]

Organ	Days (from conception)[2]	
	Started	**Completed**
Central nervous system	18	38
Heart	18	49
Ears	22	59
Limbs	24	49
Eyes	24	40
Gonads	37	46
Palate	41	58
External genitalia	44	62

[1]Reproduced, with permission, from Kousen M: Treatment of Nausea and Vomiting in Pregnancy. Amer Family Phys 1993;48:1283.

[2]For days since last menstrual period (ie, for gestational age), add 14.

of alcohol. Few data are currently available on the role of *Helicobacter pylori* in ulcer disease during pregnancy, but it is assumed to be a significant cofactor.

There are conflicting data about whether acid secretion is increased or decreased in pregnancy. There are reports of lower gastric acid output and increased mucus production secondary to increased prostaglandin production. Histaminase, secreted by the placenta, inactivates histamine, further reducing acid production. In theory, a reduction in acid secretion may lessen the symptoms and severity of peptic ulcer disease during pregnancy. Some studies suggest that up to 90% of patients with a history of peptic ulcer disease are asymptomatic during pregnancy, possibly due to these alterations in acid physiology.

Clinical Findings

The symptoms of peptic ulcer disease are the same in pregnant and nonpregnant patients. Patients most commonly complain of intermittent epigastric pain (dyspepsia), which may be relieved by eating meals or taking antacids. There may be associated complaints of heartburn, early satiety, nausea, and vomiting. In uncomplicated peptic ulcer disease, the physical examination is unremarkable. Significant tenderness or a positive fecal occult blood test warrants careful observation.

In most pregnant patients with dyspepsia, empiric therapy is begun without further diagnostic studies. Further studies are reserved for patients with significant symptoms that fail to respond to conservative measures or those with complications. Although published reports are limited, upper endoscopy with light conscious sedation appears to be safe for both mother and fetus and should be used when deemed necessary and when the findings of such a study might significantly alter therapy. In contrast, a radiologic upper gastrointestinal series should not be performed, due to the risk of radiation to the fetus. Upper endoscopy is indicated and safe in patients with significant upper gastrointestinal bleeding.

The differential diagnosis of dyspepsia in pregnancy includes a number of other conditions, including gastroesophageal reflux, nonulcer dyspepsia, and biliary tract disease. In clinical practice, it is often impossible to distinguish among these entities. In the first trimester, ulcer disease may be confused with hyperemesis gravidarum. With all these conditions, presumptive, empiric therapy usually is begun and the patient followed closely for expected improvement. Patients in whom symptoms worsen or fail to improve require investigation.

Treatment

Practitioners should stress to pregnant patients the importance of abstaining from alcohol, tobacco, and nonsteroidal anti-inflammatory agents. The mainstays of the initial treatment of dyspepsia during pregnancy are life-style changes and antacids. Patients should be encouraged to eat frequent small meals, avoid late-night meals or snacks, and avoid foods that may precipitate esophageal reflux, such as caffeine, alcohol, chocolate, and fatty foods. Antacids are the firstline therapy for dyspepsia and appear to be safe, particularly in the second and third trimesters. They are used by up to two-thirds of women during pregnancy. Aluminum- and magnesium-containing antacids also appear to be safe in nursing mothers.

In patients with persistent dyspepsia, H_2-receptor blockers are believed to be safe during the second and third trimesters and are listed as category B drugs (Table 11–2). Their efficacy, above and beyond the acid-inhibitory effects of progesterone, is unclear, however. These drugs are excreted in small amounts in breast milk, and should therefore not be given to lactating mothers. Sucralfate, which is not absorbed and has no known fetal toxicity, may be used preferentially to H_2-receptor antagonists by some obstetricians.

Omeprazole has demonstrated fetal toxicity in some animal studies (category C drug) and, in general, should be avoided during pregnancy. Misoprostol is an abortifacient and therefore is contraindicated (category X drug). Phenothiazine and related drugs also are category C drugs.

The treatment of *H pylori* infection should be deferred until after delivery. Several of the agents used for *H pylori* eradication, such as bismuth subsalicylate (category C drug), tetracycline (category X drug), and metronidazole, should not be used during pregnancy.

Complications are the same in pregnant and nonpregnant patients (ie, bleeding, perforation, and obstruction) and should be treated in the same manner. Delays in diagnosis or treatment of complications pose an increased risk to the mother and fetus.

Table 11–2. Recommendations for use of antiulcer drugs during pregnancy and lactation.[1,2]

Antiulcer Drug	FDA Pregnancy Category	First Trimester	Second or Third Trimester	Nursing Mother
Antacids	B	R vs B ?	B > R	II
Cimetidine	B	R vs B ?	B > R	IV
Ranitidine	B	R vs B ?	B > R	IV
Sucralfate	B	B > R	B > R	III A
Famotidine	B	B vs R ?	B > R	IV
Nizatidine	C	B vs R ?	B ? R	IV
Omeprazole	C	B vs R ?		IV
Gaviscon	C_2	B > R	B > R	III A
Misoprostol	X	R > B	R > B	IV
Phenothiazines	C_1	R vs B	R vs B	IV
Antihistamines	C_1	R vs B	R vs B	IV
Pepto-Bismol	C_1	R vs B	R vs B	III-B
Simethicone	C_2	R vs B	R vs B	III-A

[1]Reproduced, with permission, from Michaletz-Onody PA: Peptic Ulcer Disease in Pregnancy. Gastroenterol Clin North Am 1992;21:822.
[2]Recommendations are defined as follows:
R vs B: Implies risk; benefit profile has not been determined, and caution is advised for systemically active drugs. R > B: Implies that potential risks outweigh potential benefits, and use of the drug is not recommended. B > R: Implies that the potential benefits outweight the potential risks.
Breast-feeding categories are defined as follows: Group I: Drug does not enter breast milk. Group II: Drug enters breast milk but is not thought to offset the noenate when used in therapeutic doses. Group III: Not known whether the drug enters breast milk. A: No adverse neonatal effects are expected. B: Breast feeding is not recommended, because the drug is systemically absorbed. Group IV: Drug enters breast milk and is not recommended for nursing mother because of potential risk to neonate.

ACUTE PANCREATITIS

Pathophysiology

Little is known about pancreatic exocrine function during pregnancy. Limited data suggest that pregnancy may lead to increased enzyme and bicarbonate secretion and volume output, but the importance of this is unknown. Pregnancy causes a threefold rise in serum triglyceride levels, especially in the third trimester, due to estrogen-induced increases in triglyceride synthesis and very low density lipoprotein secretion. This could result in pancreatitis in a minority of patients. Finally, increased cholelithiasis owing to pregnancy-induced alterations in biliary motility could lead to an increased incidence of gallstone pancreatitis.

These factors notwithstanding, the incidence of acute pancreatitis does not appear to be increased during pregnancy. Because of the nonspecific nature of the associated symptoms, the diagnosis can be easily overlooked, however, and the disorder may be underdiagnosed. Gallstones appear to be the most common cause of pancreatitis during pregnancy. Alcoholic pancreatitis is uncommon, possibly because of the younger age of patients and the general admonishments to avoid alcohol. Drug-induced pancreatitis should be excluded. Hypertriglyceridemia can be missed unless checked on admission. Idiopathic pancreatitis may be due to the passage of microliths or biliary sludge, or, possibly, to the hormonal effects of pregnancy.

Clinical Findings

The symptoms of acute pancreatitis are nonspecific. They include midepigastric or periumbilical pain that may radiate to the back. Nausea and vomiting are usually present. Because of the nonspecific nature of these symptoms, the diagnosis can be easily missed and the symptoms erroneously attributed to pregnancy or other diseases (Table 11–3).

The diagnosis of acute pancreatitis relies on the measurement of serum amylase and lipase levels. Serum amylase values tend to be lower during pregnancy because of increased renal clearance of amylase, and this may obscure the diagnosis. A rapid rise

Table 11–3. Differential diagnosis of pancreatitis in pregnancy.[1,2]

Acute cholecystitis
Penetrating duodenal ulcer
Ruptured spleen
Perinephric abscess
Acute cardiopulmonary events (embolus, infarction)
Acute appendicitis
Ruptured ectopic pregnancy
Hyperemesis gravidarum
Preeclampsia

[1]Reproduced, with permission, from Scott LD: Gallstone Disease and Pancreatitis in Pregnancy. Gastroenterol Clin North Am 1992;21:811.
[2]This list also is expanded because of pregnancy-related conditions (preeclampsia, hyperemesis, ectopic pregnancy) and the effects of the enlarging uterus (appendicitis).

and fall in serum aspartate aminotransferase (AST) and alanine aminotransferase (ALT) levels, often with a rise in the serum bilirubin level, implicates gallstone-induced pancreatitis. A serum triglyceride level of more than 1000 mg/dL suggests hypertriglyceridemia as the causative factor.

Ultrasonography is a safe and useful study in the pregnant patient with suspected pancreatitis. Unfortunately, the fetus or intestinal gas, or both may obscure much of the pancreas. Features that are suspicious for pancreatitis are pancreatic edema and peripancreatic fluid collections. In addition, ultrasound provides useful information about the presence of cholelithiasis or biliary sludge. The presence of dilated intrahepatic or extrahepatic ducts suggests biliary stasis, possibly due to choledocholithiasis. Abdominal radiography or CT imaging should be avoided during pregnancy when possible.

Treatment

Treatment of pancreatitis in pregnant patients is the same as in nonpregnant patients. The mainstay is conservative management, including increasing fluid intake and prescribing medication to relieve symptoms (ie, pain and nausea), being careful to avoid medications that are harmful to pregnancy. Acute pancreatitis is associated with a higher risk to mother and fetus because of a delay in diagnosis and an unjustified reluctance to consider surgical therapy, when appropriate.

In most patients with gallstone-induced pancreatitis, elective cholecystectomy can be deferred until after delivery. When necessary, however, cholecystectomy appears to be safe after the first trimester. In contrast, a common bile duct exploration carries a high rate of fetal death. Hence, endoscopic retrograde cholangiopancreatography (ERCP) with sphincterotomy and stone extraction is indicated in patients with acute pancreatitis and choledocholithiasis who fail to improve with medical management or who have cholangitis.

INFLAMMATORY BOWEL DISEASE

Pathophysiology

Inflammatory bowel disease, which is usually classified as either ulcerative colitis or Crohn's disease, has a unique series of interactions with pregnancy. The pathophysiology is unknown in both pregnant and nonpregnant patients. Pregnancy may have an impact upon its course, and, in turn, the disease may affect the course of pregnancy.

A. Effects of Inflammatory Bowel Disease on Pregnancy: For patients with inactive ulcerative colitis or Crohn's disease, there appears to be no increased risk of prematurity, spontaneous abortion, stillbirth, or congenital anomalies over that of the general population. In contrast, active Crohn's disease and, to a lesser extent, ulcerative colitis, cause a higher incidence of fetal complications, including spontaneous abortion and stillbirth. Activity of the disease, rather than drug treatment, appears to be responsible for the increased incidence of fetal demise. Hence, every effort should be made to induce remission of inflammatory bowel disease before pregnancy. Inflammatory bowel disease does not require cesarean section.

B. Effects of Pregnancy on Inflammatory Bowel Disease: The effects of pregnancy on the course of inflammatory bowel disease depend on the activity of the disease at the time of conception. In both ulcerative colitis and Crohn's disease, if the disease is quiescent at the beginning of pregnancy, it is likely to remain so throughout pregnancy; however, if the disease is active at the time of conception, it is likely to remain so or even worsen during pregnancy. Ulcerative colitis may be likely to flare up during the first trimester, and Crohn's disease may flare up during the third trimester or the postpartum period.

C. Effects of Inflammatory Bowel Disease on Fertility: Fertility appears to be normal in patients with ulcerative colitis. Patients with Crohn's disease may have reduced fertility, which is possibly attributable to poor nutrition, abdominal pain, dyspareunia, or adjacent scarring of the ovaries or fallopian tubes.

Clinical Findings

The clinical features of inflammatory bowel disease during pregnancy are similar to those in the nonpregnant patient. Signs and symptoms such as bleeding, pain, and diarrhea may occur. If a patient is known to have the disease before pregnancy, it usually is considered as part of the differential diagnosis, but in patients without a history of the disease (which is rare), the diagnosis may be obscured and the symptoms attributed to the effects of pregnancy.

Management also is made difficult by limitations on the use of endoscopic or radiologic tests during pregnancy. In patients with known or suspected ulcerative colitis, flexible sigmoidoscopy can be safely performed during pregnancy to confirm disease activity before initiating therapy. In patients with known Crohn's disease, colonoscopy and barium radiography should be avoided, unless absolutely essential for management. In patients without a history of inflammatory bowel disease and severe illness, these procedures are sometimes necessary to establish a diagnosis.

Complications of inflammatory bowel disease are the same in pregnant and nonpregnant patients and have been thoroughly discussed in Chapter 7. There is an increased risk of spontaneous abortion, but this is probably related to disease activity rather than drug treatment.

Treatment

Management of inflammatory bowel disease during pregnancy may best be approached by a team including a gastroenterologist, high-risk obstetrician, and colorectal surgeon. A number of drugs used for this disease have been given safely during pregnancy. Sulfasalazine is safe during all stages of pregnancy. Although it may displace bilirubin from fetal albumin during the third trimester, the risk of fetal kernicterus is considered negligible. Pregnant patients taking sulfasalazine should receive folate to prevent folate deficiency. Corticosteroids appear to be safe, although an increased incidence of placental insufficiency and prematurity is reported. Whether this relates to disease activity or the effects of corticosteroids is unclear. Metronidazole is not believed to be safe, at least in the first trimester, because of known teratogenic effects, and probably is best avoided throughout pregnancy. Azathioprine and mercaptopurine have also been associated with some birth defects, although recent series report a low incidence. Nevertheless, patients taking these agents should be advised not to become pregnant until they are discontinued.

When possible, remission of active inflammatory bowel disease should be achieved before conception. For patients in remission who are taking sulfasalazine or aminosalicylic acid (5-ASA), the drug should be continued throughout pregnancy to maintain remission. Corticosteroids should be withdrawn or maintained at the lowest effective dosage. Flareups of disease during pregnancy should be treated with sulfasalazine, 5-ASA, or corticosteroids, or with one of the first two drugs plus a corticosteroid, as deemed necessary. While surgery is associated with a significant risk of spontaneous abortion, it should be employed in cases of severe bleeding, perforation, and toxic megacolon not responsive to medical therapy.

The prognosis of inflammatory bowel disease during pregnancy is once again determined by the course of the disease before or at the onset of pregnancy and requires close follow-up. Nicotine, which usually should be avoided during pregnancy, does appear to have some positive effects on certain types of inflammatory bowel disease. There is currently no evidence that nicotine should be used during pregnancy, however, and, in fact, it is contraindicated for obvious reasons.

SURGICAL DISORDERS

Appendicitis

The pathophysiology of appendicitis and other surgical disorders in pregnancy is no different from that in nonpregnant patients. Figure 11–1 shows the changes in location and direction of the appendix during pregnancy.

Clinical features are nausea, vomiting, abdominal pain, and bloating, which may be attributed to pregnancy, hyperemesis gravidarum, or infectious diarrhea. The gravid uterus may shift the pain from the lower right to the upper right quadrant, further confusing the diagnostic picture. Thus, the diagnosis

may be delayed until after perforation has occurred in up to 25% of cases. This complication is associated with high maternal and fetal mortality rates (19% and 43%, respectively), compared with 5% and 15% without perforation.

Appendectomy is the mainstay of treatment. Recently, laparoscopic appendectomy has been performed during pregnancy, resulting in less trauma than conventional surgery.

Acute appendicitis may be confused with other obstetric emergencies, including placental abruption, ectopic pregnancy, and ovarian torsion, as well as nonobstetric conditions such as acute cholecystitis, intestinal volvulus, and acute pancreatitis.

Acute Cholecystitis

Pregnancy appears to increase the rate of gallstone formation. Contributing factors include an increase in the bile acid pool and cholesterol synthesis, a change in the ratio of chenodeoxycholic acid to cholic acid (resulting in increased lithogenicity), slowing of the enterohepatic circulation, and a decrease in gallbladder contractility due to the effects of progesterone on smooth muscle. Nevertheless, acute cholecystitis requiring surgery does not appear to be a common problem during pregnancy, occurring in less than 0.1% of pregnancies.

The symptoms of gallstone disease in pregnancy resemble biliary colic in nonpregnant patients (ie, episodic epigastric or right upper quadrant pain lasting up to several hours). The presence of persistent pain, nausea, vomiting, fever, and leukocytosis indicates acute cholecystitis. The diagnosis usually is confirmed by abdominal ultrasound studies demonstrating echogenic gallstones and findings consistent with acute cholecystitis. Other differential considerations include acute appendicitis, peptic ulcer disease, and liver diseases related to pregnancy such as acute fatty liver of pregnancy and HELLP syndrome (Table 11–4) (see also Chapter 47).

Abdominal surgery such as cholecystectomy is associated with an increased risk of fetal death, especially during the first trimester. The risks during the second and third trimesters appear to be minimal. Nonetheless, most surgeons prefer to perform cholecystectomy electively in the postpartum period. For patients with recurrent or worsening symptoms, however, surgery should be undertaken.

Volvulus

Sigmoid volvulus may occur during the third trimester or the puerperium, owing to the effects of the enlarged uterus. The symptoms of abdominal pain, nausea, vomiting, and constipation are nonspecific. The diagnosis usually is established by abdominal radiographic studies, but a general reluctance to perform these studies during pregnancy may delay the diagnosis. Conservative treatment with sigmoidoscopic decompression should be attempted. Surgical

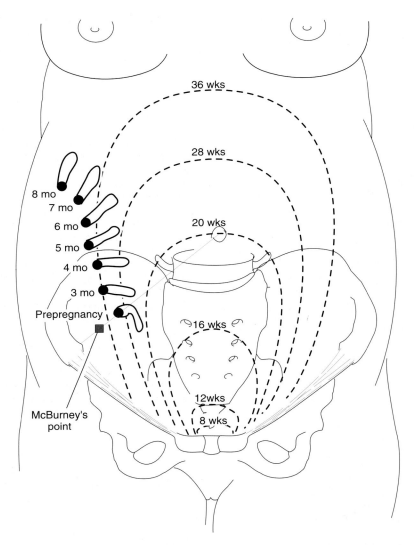

Figure 11–1. Changes in location and direction of the appendix during pregnancy in relationship to McBurney's point and the height of the fundus at various weeks of gestation. (Adapted, with permission, from Mahmoodian S: Appendicitis complicating pregnancy. South Med J 1992;85(1):19.)

intervention should be undertaken when endoscopic therapy is unsuccessful.

GASTROINTESTINAL DISEASES UNIQUE TO PREGNANCY

The clinician is commonly consulted for a host of gastrointestinal symptoms that occur during pregnancy. These symptoms may be directly attributable to the effects of pregnancy or may be indicative of the more serious conditions outlined previously. The wary clinician must be careful to consider all diagnostic possibilities and further diagnostic testing when patients fail to respond to conservative treatment measures. Four disorders unique to pregnancy will be discussed here: gastroesophageal reflux, nausea and vomiting (hyperemesis gravidarum), constipation, and diarrhea or fecal incontinence.

GASTROESOPHAGEAL REFLUX

Pathophysiology

Gastroesophageal reflux is extremely common, occurring in at least 50% of pregnancies. The patho-

Table 11–4. Differential diagnosis of acute cholecystitis in pregnancy.[1]

Acute viral hepatitis
Acute alcoholic hepatitis
Duodenal ulcer
Acute pancreatitis
Pulmonary embolus
Right lower lobe pneumonia
Acute myocardial infarction
Acute appendicitis
Acute fatty liver of pregnancy
Preeclampsia
HELLP syndrome

[1]Reproduced, with permission, from Scott LD: Gallstone Disease and Pancreatitis in Pregnancy. Gastroenterol Clin North Am 1992;21:807.

physiology is related to several factors. First, there is decreased lower esophageal sphincter pressure due to progesterone or other circulating hormones. This explains the occurrence of reflux early in pregnancy, often before pregnancy is otherwise suspected. Female patients who present with otherwise unexplained gastroesophageal reflux should be investigated for possible pregnancy. Later in pregnancy, increased intra-abdominal pressure and compression of the stomach by the enlarging uterus may contribute to gastric reflux.

Clinical Findings

The clinical features of gastroesophageal reflux are the same as in nonpregnant patients. Heartburn is extremely common in pregnancy (> 50% of patients in the first trimester) and may be potentiated by recumbency. Symptoms resolve in almost 100% of patients after delivery. Severe gastroesophageal reflux resulting in peptic stricture with dysphagia or bleeding is rare in pregnancy.

Treatment

Treatment is based primarily on modifications in life-style, for example, elevating the head of the bed; avoiding fats, chocolate, and alcohol; and avoiding smoking. Antacids or sucralfate are safe (see earlier discussion) and may be given for intermittent symptoms. The overwhelming majority of patients will respond to these simple measures. For patients with more refractory symptoms, H_2-receptor antagonists may be given in the second or third trimester; these agents should be avoided in the first trimester (see Table 11–2). The use of proton pump inhibitors or promotility agents is not recommended during pregnancy, although promotility agents have been used in the second and third trimesters in refractory cases. For patients with refractory, disabling symptoms despite H_2-receptor blockers, investigation with esophagogastroduodenoscopy should be considered to document the severity of esophagitis.

NAUSEA & VOMITING OF PREGNANCY

Nausea and vomiting occur in the first trimester in 50–90% of pregnancies. The symptoms may vary from mild to severe. Mild to moderate symptoms are often referred to as "morning sickness." More severe, intractable symptoms are known as **hyperemesis gravidarum,** which is characterized by severe vomiting that results in dehydration, ketosis, electrolyte imbalance, and, in some cases, the need for hospitalization. Hyperemesis gravidarum may complicate 0.3–1% of pregnancies.

Pathophysiology

This discussion of pathophysiology is devoted primarily to hyperemesis gravidarum, recognizing that it represents an extreme end of the spectrum of chronic nausea and vomiting during pregnancy. The pathophysiology has been attributed to a number of factors, including psychological factors, hormonal factors (eg, hyperthyroidism, hyperparathyroidism, effects of gestational hormones), liver abnormalities, abnormal gastric electrical activity, autonomic nervous system function, abnormal lipid metabolism, and nutritional deficiencies (Figures 11–2 to 11–5). All theories have some supporting data, but none fully explain the pathophysiology. Hyperemesis gravidarum is more common in nulliparous patients, twin pregnancies, and women younger than 35 years of age (Table 11–5).

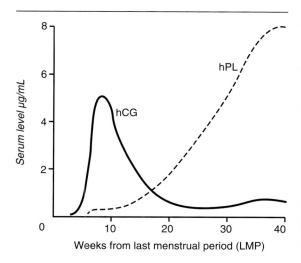

Figure 11–2. Changes in the serum levels of human chorionic gonadotropin (hCG) and human placental lactogen (hPL) over the course of normal pregnancy. The peak of human chorionic goandotropin concentration occurs at week 9 of gestation. (Reproduced, with permission, from Yen SCC: Endocrine and other evaluations of the fetal environment: The endocrinology of pregnancy. In: *Maternal-Fetal Medicine: Principles and Practice.* Creasy RK, Resnik R (editors). Saunders, 1984.)

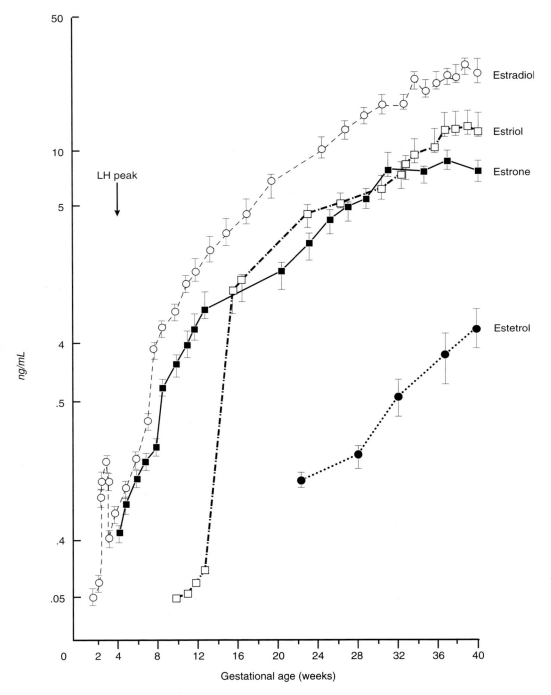

Figure 11–3. Estrogens (estradiol, estriol, estrone, estetrol). (Courtesy of John R. Marshall, MD.)

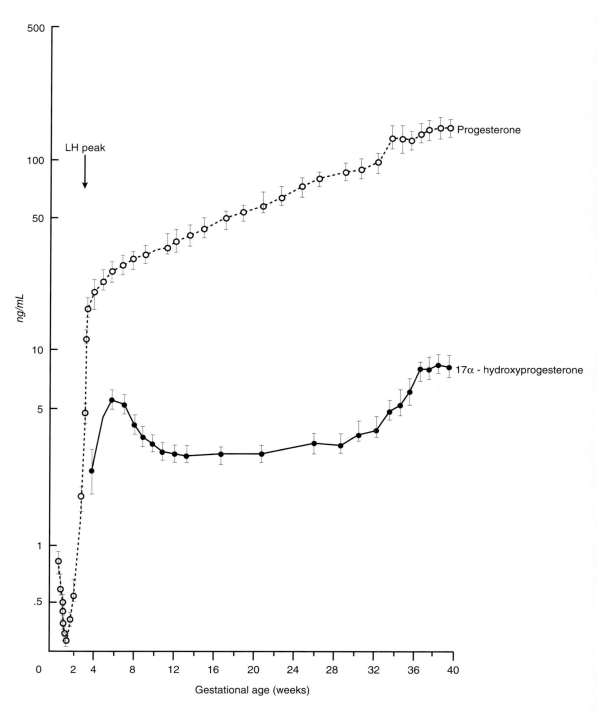

Figure 11–4. Changes over the course of normal pregnancy in serum levels of gestational hormones: progestins (progesterone and 17α-hydroxyprogesterone). (Reproduced, with permission, from Abell TL, Riely CA: Hyperemesis gravidarum. Gastroenterol Clin North Am 1992;21:844.)

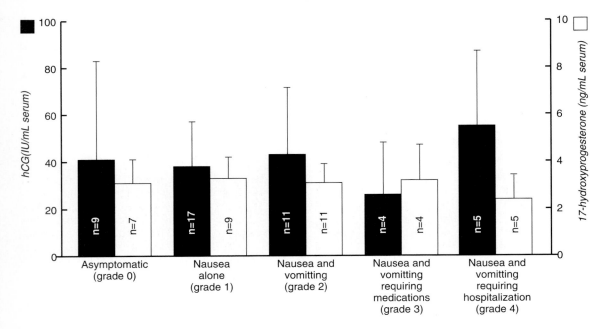

Figure 11–5. Levels of gestational hormones in pregnant patients, from those without nausea through those with hyperemesis gravidarum. No consistent abnormality in either human chorionic gonadotropin *(black bars)* or 17α-hydroxy-progesterone *(open bars)* was demonstrated in patients with severe vomiting. (Reproduced, with permission, from Soules MR et al: Nausea and vomiting of pregnancy: Role of human chorionic gonadotropin and 17-hydroxyprogesterone. Obstet Gynecol 1980;55:696. Reproduced with permission of The American College of Obstetricians and Gynecologists.)

Clinical Findings

Symptoms typically start in the first trimester and resolve by the twentieth week of gestation. They include nausea, vomiting, bloating, distention, anorexia, early satiety, and abdominal pain, but nausea and vomiting predominate. Unfortunately, these are nonspecific symptoms, and the differential diagnosis should therefore include other disorders, including peptic ulcer disease, pancreatitis, hepatitis, hyperthyroidism, and cholecystitis. Physical examination is remarkable in severe cases for signs of dehydration. Fetal distress and demise can occur in severe cases.

Treatment

In most patients with pregnancy-associated nausea and vomiting, reassurance and dietary modifications are all that is needed. Patients should be instructed to eat frequent small meals and avoid offensive food odors. For patients with more refractory symptoms, the stepwise approach outlined in Figure 11–6 is recommended. A number of medications have been used, including the components of Bendectin, which is now no longer available as a formulation but is available in a component form of doxylamine succinate and pyridoxine. Other symptomatic treatments have been used, including phenothiazine and prokinetic drugs. As with all disorders of pregnancy, the benefits of drug therapy must outweigh the risks of treatment.

For patients with dehydration or ketosis, hospitalization and treatment with intravenous fluids is necessary. Rarely, hyperalimentation for hyperemesis gravidarum is required in patients who cannot tolerate enteral feedings. In patients with severe symptoms, other diagnostic entities should be excluded with tests of thyroid, renal, and hepatic function and measurements of amylase, lipase, and calcium. Upper endoscopy may be performed if peptic ulcer dis-

Table 11–5. Factors associated with hyperemesis gravidarum.[1]

Factor	Odds Ratio
Maternal age > 35 years	0.6
High body weight	1.4
Nulliparity	1.4
Cigarette smoker	0.7
Twin gestation	1.5
Fetal loss	0.7

[1]Reproduced, with permission, from Abell T, Riely CA: Hyperemesis Gravidarum. Gastroenterol Clin North Am 1992; 21:836. Klebanoff MA et al: Epidemiology of vomiting in early pregnancy. Obstet Gynecol 66;612:1985.

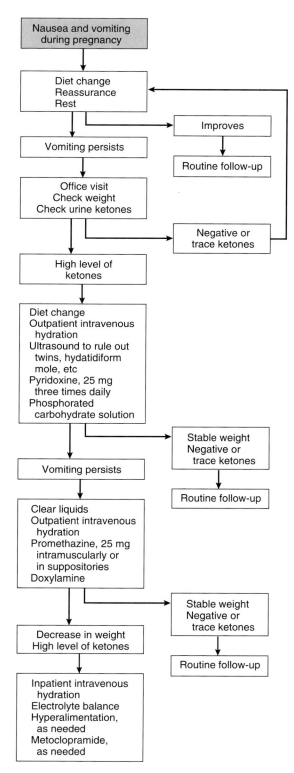

Figure 11–6. Algorithm for the management of nausea and vomiting in pregnancy. (Reproduced, with permission, from Kousen M: Treatment of nausea and vomiting in pregnancy. Am Fam Physician 1993;48:1279.)

ease is suspected. Ultrasonography is useful to detect twin or molar gestations.

The prognosis for hyperemesis gravidarum is good. In fact, pregnancies with nausea and vomiting carry a lower rate of fetal wastage than asymptomatic pregnancies.

CONSTIPATION

Pathophysiology

Constipation, or a change in bowel habits, is extremely common during pregnancy, with 30–50% of patients complaining of altered bowel habits. Constipation is attributed to progesterone-mediated reduction in intestinal motility. However, other factors such as changes in diet, alterations in fluid intake, reduction in exercise, ingestion of supplemental iron, and mechanical factors such as an enlarging uterus and weakening of the pelvic floor all may play a role.

Clinical Findings

The complaint of constipation may refer to a decrease in the frequency of bowel movements, hardness of stools, or a decreased ability to move the bowels. It is important to determine from the patient what she means by "constipation," so that appropriate treatment can be given. The physical examination in benign constipation should be normal.

For the most part, constipation of pregnancy is an annoying problem but seldom poses a serious threat to the mother or fetus. It should be kept in mind, however, that the differential diagnosis includes a host of other organic disorders, including obstruction, endocrine disorders, and other systemic illness (see Chapter 1). Endoscopic evaluation is warranted if organic disease is suspected because of weight loss, iron deficiency anemia, or gastrointestinal bleeding (Table 11–6).

Treatment

Treatment of constipation during pregnancy primarily involves symptomatic measures, including increasing fluids and fiber to at least 25 g/d. Stool softeners (docusate sodium) or hyperosmolar agents (sorbitol, milk of magnesia) may be given as necessary. As with all disorders of pregnancy, any medication that may be harmful to the pregnancy should be avoided. Hemorrhoids may occur commonly during or after pregnancy and may exacerbate the tendency toward constipation due to perianal discomfort. Hemorrhoids should be treated with sitz baths and suppositories.

DIARRHEA

Pathophysiology

Diarrhea should be investigated in the pregnant patient just as in the nonpregnant patient. There is no

Table 11–6. Constipation assessment in pregnancy.[1]

History
  Acute or long-standing problem
  Diet
  Laxative use
  Frequency of bowel movements
  Completeness of evacuation
  Rectal pain, spasm
  Pregnancies
  Drug use
Treatment
  High-fiber diet
  Fluids
  Exercise
  Education
Behavioral considerations
  Regular time daily
  Pelvic floor exercises (biofeedback assisted when possible)
Medication
  Processed hydrophilic stool-bulking agents
  Emollient laxatives
  Lactulose
  Laxative (short-term use)

[1]Reproduced, with permission, from West L, Warren J et al: Diagnosis and Management. Gastroenterol Clin North Am 1992;21:800.

reported increase in the incidence of infectious diarrhea during pregnancy, but infection is still the most common cause of acute diarrhea during pregnancy and must be excluded. Diarrhea may be the first sign of preterm labor. Relaxin, secreted by the placenta during uterine contraction, may be the responsible agent.

Clinical Findings

Diarrhea that persists for more than 48–72 hours or diarrhea associated with signs of inflammation (eg, fever, hematochezia) warrants investigation with stool culture and testing for fecal leukocytes, ova and parasites, and *Clostridium difficile* toxin. Empiric antibiotics should be restricted because of concerns about teratogenicity.

The differential diagnosis of acute diarrhea in pregnancy includes the usual infectious agents (ie, viral, bacterial, and protozoal agents), inflammatory bowel disease, and use of new medications. Chronic diarrhea is unusual, but may be caused by irritable bowel syndrome, inflammatory bowel disease, malabsorption syndromes, and use of osmotic agents (see Chapter 1). Complications of severe diarrhea include dehydration and the threat of fetal death, and hospitalization may be required.

Treatment

Treatment of diarrhea in pregnancy is directed at the underlying cause. Antibiotics that appear to be safe are erythromycin and ampicillin. Metronidazole, sulfa drugs, tetracycline, and the quinolones are best avoided.

FECAL INCONTINENCE

In recent years, special attention has been focused on the fact that fecal incontinence may be a complication of vaginal delivery. A third- or fourth-degree tear may complicate 0.7% of deliveries. Significant damage to the external sphincter can result in gross fecal incontinence, unless the defect is repaired immediately. An even more common cause of fecal incontinence may be damage during childbirth to the pudendal nerve as it passes through the sacrospinous ligament. This neurogenic trauma may lead to denervation of the pelvic floor muscles and external sphincter, resulting in fecal incontinence. It is apparent from recent literature that the incidence of fecal incontinence of pregnancy has been vastly underestimated, and many cases of "idiopathic" neurogenic fecal incontinence in elderly women may be attributable to obstetric trauma. Recognition of fecal incontinence by primary care physicians, obstetricians, and gastroenterologists is important, particularly because it can be treated.

Clinical Findings

Physical examination may reveal evidence of external sphincter damage, with scarring, deformity, or a patulous appearance. Perineal sensation should be tested for sharp and dull sensation and the anal wink elicited. Absence of the anal wink may indicate the presence of pudendal neuropathy or a cauda equina lesion. Digital examination may reveal anatomic defects in the anomuscular ring. Strictures, scars, and gross resting and squeezing pressures can be assessed. Anal electromyography and manometry are useful in detecting defects in the external and internal sphincters, determining the presence or absence of nervous innervation, and localizing the neurologic deficit.

Treatment

A bowel management program is the first element of therapy in most patients. A high-fiber diet is prescribed, with patients encouraged to sit on the toilet

Table 11–7. Sample plan for doing Kegel exercises.[1]

Week 1: 3 repetitions, 10 times a day
Week 2: 3 repetitions, 15 times a day
Week 3: 3 repetitions, 20 times a day, or 6 repetitions, 10 times a day
Week 4: 3 repetitions, 25 times a day, or 6 repetitions, 12 times a day
Week 5: 3 repetitions, 30 times a day, or 6 repetitions, 15 times a day
Week 6: 3 repetitions, 34 times a day, or 6 repetitions, 17 times a day

[1]Reproduced, with permission, from West L, Warren J et al: Diagnosis and Management of Irritable Bowel Syndrome, Constipation, and Diarrhea in Pregnancy. Gastroenterol Clin North Am 1992;21:802.

for 20–30 minutes after eating, at the same time each day. Cotton balls tucked next to the anal opening may absorb small amounts of fecal soilage. Successful treatment is achieved in many mild cases with Kegel exercises (Table 11–7). Motivated patients with more severe symptoms who have some degree

of neurologic impairment but intact rectal sensation and some external sphincter function may benefit from biofeedback therapy and pelvic floor retraining. Discrete muscular injury to the external sphincter with intact innervation may be amenable to surgical repair.

REFERENCES

Abell TL, Riely CA: Hyperemesis gravidarum. Gastroenterol Clin North Am 1992;21:835.

Baron TH, Richter JE: Gastroesophageal reflux disease in pregnancy. Gastroenterol Clin North Am 1992:21:777.

Boyce RA: Enteral nutrition in hyperemesis gravidarum: A new development. J Am Diet Assoc 1992;92:733.

Calhoun BC: Gastrointestinal disorders in pregnancy. Obstet Gynecol Clin North Am 1992;19:733.

Chamberlain G: Abdominal pain in pregnancy. ABC Antenat Care 1991;302:1390.

Crump WJ, Aten LA: Hyperemesis, hyperthyroidism, or both? J Fam Pract 1992;35:450.

DeLancey JOL: Childbirth, continence, and the pelvic floor. (Article review.) N Engl J Med 1993;329:1956.

Hanan IM: Inflammatory bowel disease in the pregnant woman. Compr Ther 1993;19(3):91.

Heise RH et al: Colonic cancer during pregnancy: Case report and review of the literature. Mayo Clin Proc 1992;67:1180.

Heres P et al: Colon carcinoma during pregnancy: A lethal coincidence. Eur J Obstet Gynecol Reprod Biol 1993;48:149.

Hordnes K, Bergsjo P: Severe lacerations after childbirth. Acta Obstet Scand 1993;72:413.

Korelitz BI: Inflammatory bowel disease in pregnancy. Gastroenterol Clin North Am 1992;21:827.

Kousen M: Treatment of nausea and vomiting in pregnancy. Am Fam Physician 1993;48:1279.

Liang CC et al: Cancer of the colon during pregnancy: Report of a case and review of the literature. J Formos Med Assoc 1992;91:1024.

Mabie WC: Obstetric management of gastroenterologic complications of pregnancy. Gastroenterol Clin North Am 1992;21:923.

Mahmoodian S: Appendicitis complicating pregnancy. South Med J 1992;85(1):19.

Michaletz-Onody PA: Peptic ulcer disease in pregnancy. Gastroenterol Clin North Am 1992;21:817.

Morton M: Inflammatory bowel disease presenting in pregnancy. Aust N Z J Obstet Gynaecol 1992;32(1):40.

Perdue PW, Johnson HW, Stafford PW: Intestinal obstruction complicating pregnancy. Am J Surg 1992;164:384.

Sagraves R, Anderson DC: Therapy consultation: Transdermal scopolamine for hyperemesis gravidarum. Clin Pharm 1992;11:832.

Scott LD: Gallstone disease and pancreatitis in pregnancy. Gastroenterol Clin North Am 1992;21:803.

Shoda Y et al: Intussusception caused by a carcinoma of the cecum during pregnancy: Report of a case and review of the literature. Jpn J Surg 1992;223:556.

Shushan A et al: Carcinoma of the colon during pregnancy. Obstet Gynecol Surv 1992;47:222.

Singer AJ, Brandt LJ: Pathophysiology of the gastrointestinal tract during pregnancy. Am J Gastroenterol 1991;86:1695.

Smoleniec JS, James DK: Gastrointestinal crises during pregnancy. Dig Dis Sci 1993;11:313.

Sultan AH et al: Anal-sphincter disruption during vaginal delivery. N Engl J Med 1993;329:1905.

West L, Warren J, Cutts T: Diagnosis and management of irritable bowel syndrome. Gastroenterol Clin North Am 1992;21:793.

Woods JB et al: Pregnancy complicated by carcinoma of the colon above the rectum. Am J Perinatol 1992;9(2):102.

12

Gastrointestinal Problems of the Elderly

Roderick C. Rapier, MD

Epidemiology

The world population has been changing steadily over the last several decades. Significant population growth and shifts in demography are occurring across the world. In the USA, according to the US Bureau of the Census, more people are living longer. Given the current trends in birth and death rates and life expectancy, the total United States population is expected to exceed 300 million by the year 2010. Life expectancy at birth is projected to be approximately 78 years in 2010, compared with 70 years in 1970. The proportion of people older than 65 years also has been steadily increasing. By the year 2000, there will be over 35 million people over the age of 65 in the USA. Of these, over 12% will be older than 85 years—the fastest growing segment of the population.

Currently, more than 1.7 million people reside in nursing homes. More than 75% of these residents are older than 65 years. This, however, represents only 4% of the total population over the age of 65. Nevertheless, the care of these elderly in nursing homes costs over $60 billion annually.

US Bureau of the Census: Statistical Abstract of the United States, 114th ed. 1994.

Gastrointestinal Physiology

The exact details of gastrointestinal physiology in the elderly is unknown; while many assumptions are made about the physiology and pathophysiology, there has been little investigation. In fact, many clinical research projects specifically exclude patients older than 65 years. Hence, most knowledge of disease processes in the elderly has been extrapolated from research in younger individuals. Arbitrary extrapolation to the elderly ignores the likelihood that elderly patients are more likely to have multiple co-existing diseases and may be affected differently by gastrointestinal processes.

The *aging process* should not be blamed for patient's gastrointestinal complaints. In fact, there is little evidence that the gastrointestinal system significantly deteriorates with age. Gastrointestinal diseases may present differently in the elderly, however, than in younger patients. Certain gastrointestinal diseases occur more frequently and some may present more subtly in the elderly. Mental impairment resulting from cerebrovascular accidents or the progressive effects of Alzheimer's dementia can interfere with the patient's ability to adequately describe symptoms. This can hamper the clinician's ability to identify the problem and to make a diagnosis.

Biopsychosocial Problems

A thorough psychosocial evaluation of the elderly patient with gastrointestinal complaints is important. Psychosocial stressors can impact dramatically on the elderly patient, perhaps leading to depression. Sometimes, the presenting gastrointestinal complaints are a somatization of such problems. Notable psychosocial problems include loss of friends and spouse, loss of independence, financial insecurity, decline in health, and waning mental capacity.

The extent of evaluation and therapy of gastrointestinal complaints should take into consideration co-existing illnesses as well as the impact of the gastrointestinal complaints on the patient's quality of life. The goals of therapy must be placed in the appropriate context of all aspects of patients' psychosocial situation and medical care. For example, the patient with terminal illness or other serious medical illness may benefit more from a limited diagnostic evaluation and therapy directed towards an improvement in quality and comfort of life, rather than from invasive procedures that are unlikely to reveal a treatable entity.

OROPHARYNGEAL DYSPHAGIA

Essentials of Diagnosis
- Higher prevalence in the elderly.
- Poor dentition and improperly fitted dentures are often the cause.
- Deficits in neurologic function often contribute.

Pathophysiology

Dysphagia is a common complaint among the elderly. Swallowing is a highly synchronized process that can be separated into: (1) the oropharyngeal phase, and (2) the esophageal phase. Oropharyngeal dysphagia is more frequently encountered in elderly patients than in younger patients.

The oropharyngeal phase of swallowing is further divided into three parts. Part one is preparatory—masticating and sizing the food bolus. This requires adequate salivary and mucus secretion to lubricate and begin the digestive process. Salivary gland output gradually decreases with age and is dramatically decreased in certain chronic inflammatory disorders like Sjögren's syndrome with xerostomia, seen in middle-aged to elderly females. Certain medications can also decrease salivary and mucus flow into the mouth. Another important factor that affects this preparatory phase is neuromuscular dysfunction. The muscles of mastication (ie, masseter, temporalis, lateral pterygoid, and medial pterygoid), the tongue, and the soft palate all function synchronously during proper mastication and food bolus preparation before swallowing. These muscles can be affected by neurologic dysfunction often seen in the elderly—pseudobulbar palsy, Parkinson's disease, amyotrophic lateral sclerosis, brain stem strokes, multiple sclerosis, tabes dorsalis, or myasthenia gravis. Elderly patients are also more likely to have problems with the other tool of mastication—the teeth. Dentures may fit poorly owing to osteoporotis with shrinkage of the mandible. Loose or missing teeth also may affect mastication.

Part two requires the tongue to move the food bolus from the oral cavity to the pharynx. Adequate neurologic function is essential for this phase. The neurologic diseases previously listed can interfere with this phase of swallowing. Parkinson's disease can cause significant tremor of the tongue and delay in the initiation of the swallow, leading to oropharyngeal dysphagia.

The third part protects the respiratory tract from the food bolus while transferring it into the esophagus. In the elderly, structural abnormalities are more likely to block this coordinated sequence. Common abnormalities in the elderly include head and neck tumors, especially in those who have smoked and used significant amounts of alcohol. Cervical osteophytes or hypertrophic osteodystrophy and goiters can impede this phase by pressing on the pharynx and the upper esophagus. Subtle presentations of hyperthyroidism in the elderly include pharyngeal muscle weakness with dysphagia. Upper esophageal sphincter dysfunction can cause a relative obstruction of the upper esophagus. Sphincter dysfunction may be idiopathic or caused by tumor infiltration or neurologic deficits. **Zenker's diverticulum** is a posterior outpouching above the upper esophageal sphincter that may be related to long-standing sphincter dysfunction. Patients with Zenker's diverticula may complain of intermittent dysphagia, aspiration, halitosis, and regurgitation of undigested food. These diverticula are likely to be larger and more symptomatic in the elderly person.

Clinical Findings

History: The clinician should attempt to differentiate between oropharyngeal and esophageal dysphagia. Symptoms of oropharyngeal dysphagia include difficulty initiating a swallow, food sticking in the mouth, nasal regurgitation, or coughing while swallowing. It is important to determine whether these symptoms recently started and are progressive. New onset and rapidly progressing symptoms may suggest an underlying malignant process. Determine if these symptoms occur intermittently and only in certain body positions like lying flat in bed while attempting to eat. Does this only occur with certain consistencies of food (liquid, solid, soft, dry). Symptoms that occur only with solids suggest an obstructive lesion. Dysphagia with liquids alone or with both liquids and solids suggest a motility or neuromuscular disorder. Associated neurologic deficits, such as dysarthria, are important clues to the diagnosis.

The observation by caregivers that food remains in the mouth may be due to severe cognitive impairment that results in the patient simply not remembering how to swallow.

Physical Findings

It is important to observe patients while they attempt to swallow. Particular attention is paid to the neuromuscular examination (particularly the cranial nerves), and evidence of other neuromuscular dysfunction such as brain stem strokes or Parkinson's disease should be sought. Significant dementia or psychiatric abnormalities may result in inability or unwillingness to attempt swallowing. The oral cavity must be examined carefully, paying particular attention to dentition, the presence of dental caries, and evidence of ill-fitting dentures.

Further evaluation of the patient with oropharyngeal dysphagia and associated neuromuscular disease should include videofluoroscopy deglutition study. Thin slurries, thick pastes, or a barium-soaked marshmallow can be used to replicate the particular food consistency for which a problem exists. This study can delineate the extent and the severity of the problem and the risk of aspiration. Osteophytes impeding proper passage of the food bolus into the esophagus can be identified.

Patients with new onset and progressive oropharyngeal dysphagia and associated pharyngeal pain or hoarseness should have laryngoscopy. Upper endoscopy is rarely helpful to identify lesions above the upper esophageal sphincter.

Treatment

Appropriate therapy depends on the cause of dysfunction. The correction of dental problems may improve chewing and swallowing in some patients. Although many neurologic disorders are irreversible, swallowing therapy by a speech pathologist can help motivated patients who are not severely demented. After an acute neurologic event such as a cerebrovascular accident, some patients require interim placement of a nasogastric feeding tube or a percutaneous endoscopic gastrostomy tube to facilitate adequate enteral nutrition until swallowing function improves. Some patients with neurologic dysfunction are helped tremendously by changing the consistency of their foods. Thin liquids can be readily aspirated, hence thicker pureed foods or solids are preferable. Proper upright positioning of the patient during slow assisted feeding is important to facilitate adequate oral intake. In patients with cricopharyngeal dysfunction, myotomy is sometimes recommended. In some patients with severe neuromuscular dysfunction or mental deterioration, adequate oral nutrition cannot be safely provided due to the risk of aspiration. Nutrition may be provided by long-term enteral feedings via nasoenteric tubes or percutaneous gastrostomy. The decision to provide this nutritional support should be guided by the patient's quality of life, the prognosis for recovery, and the wishes of the family.

Mendez L, Friedman LS, Castell DO: Swallowing disorders in the elderly. Clin Geriatr Med 1991;7(2):215.

Ren J et al: Effect of age and bolus variables on the coordination of the glottis and the upper esophageal sphincter during swallowing. Am J Gastroenterol 1993;88(5):665.

ESOPHAGEAL DYSFUNCTION

Essentials of Diagnosis

- Distinguish obstructive from motility disorders.
- Distinguish solid from liquid dysphagia.
- Determine duration of complaint.
- Distinguish intermittent versus progressive dysphagia.
- Pill esophagitis common.

Pathophysiology

Abnormal oropharyngeal function in the elderly can cause difficulty in the normal esophagus. A poorly prepared food bolus can become impacted in the esophagus because it is too large or too dry, because of inadequate chewing, or because of inadequate amounts of saliva and mucus in the bolus.

Esophageal dysphagia may be caused by **motility or structural disorders.** There are conflicting reports about the effect of aging on esophageal motility. Some studies have shown diminished force of esophageal peristalsis, significant tertiary (non-peristaltic) contractions and incomplete lower esophageal sphincter relaxation. Other studies suggest that these changes occur mainly in elderly patients with multi-

ple medical problems of another origin that affect neuromuscular function, eg, diabetes, thyroid disease, and cerebrovascular accidents. It appears that age alone has very little effect on esophageal function; thus, diseases like "presbyesophagus" may actually reflect coexisting metabolic and neuromuscular diseases. Other motility disorders seen in elderly patients include scleroderma and progressive diffuse esophageal spasm (see Chapter 18).

The mechanical lesions of the esophagus that are most common in the elderly are esophageal malignancies and proximal gastric malignancies. Esophageal rings and webs (eg, Schatzki's ring), which are seen in younger patients, are also encountered in the elderly. Gastroesophageal reflux with erosive esophagitis or a peptic stricture are commonly found in the elderly.

A mechanical process specific to the elderly population is compression of the esophagus between a firm atherosclerotic aorta posteriorly and the heart anteriorly, known as "dysphagia aortica."

Clinical Findings

A. Types of Food: A key point in the evaluation of the elderly patient with esophageal dysphagia is whether the problem occurs only with certain types of foods, eg, solids, liquids, or both. Dysphagia that started simultaneously with both solids and liquids is most likely the result of neuromuscular abnormalities or motility disorders. Dysphagia only associated with solids is more likely to be due to a mechanical obstruction.

B. Duration of Symptoms: The duration of symptoms is also important. Recent and progressive symptoms with solids is suspicious for malignancy of the esophagus or the proximal stomach. Progressive symptoms also can result from peptic strictures, especially in patients with a history of heartburn. Achalasia usually presents with slowly progressive dysphagia to both liquids and solids with associated chest pain, halitosis, chest fullness, and nocturnal coughing due to the enlarged, food- and fluid-filled esophagus. Although achalasia can occur at any age, the elderly patient is more likely to have secondary or "pseudochalasia" than idiopathic primary achalasia. Secondary achalasia may be caused by invasion of the lower esophageal sphincter with gastric adenocarcinoma, lymphoma or metastatic tumors, amyloidosis, or paraneoplastic syndromes. Therefore, in the elderly patient with a clinical appearance of achalasia, secondary causes must be excluded. Intermittent dysphagia over a long period can be due to motility disorders, Schatzki's rings, webs, or recurrent food impaction that results from inadequate chewing or oral phase food preparation.

Odynophagia is most commonly associated with pill esophagitis in the elderly. The elderly patient is at high risk because of the increased number of medications that can damage the esophagus, because of decreased salivary output, and because of the increased prevalence of an anatomic disorder (such as peptic strictures) or abnormal motility. Elderly patients also are predisposed because they are more likely to be administered pills while lying in bed and with insufficient water. The elderly should take pills in an upright position with at least one glass of water. Medications that have the greatest potential to damage the esophagus include potassium chloride, quinidine, tetracycline, doxycycline, clindamycin, ciprofloxacin, nonsteroidal anti-inflammatory drugs (NSAIDs), and iron supplements.

A careful history and physical examination facilitate a focused evaluation. If after the history and physical the diagnosis is unclear, barium esophagram is an appropriate screening study. If the patient has solid dysphagia, the esophagram should include a solid phase study with a marshmallow if the liquid phase showed no abnormalities. If an obstructing mass lesion of the esophagus is suspected from the clinical evaluation, one should proceed directly with upper endoscopy. After exclusion of a mechanical cause of dysphagia, esophageal manometry may be considered in selected patients, especially those with suspected achalasia or scleroderma. In other patients with suspected motility abnormalities, the usefulness of a manometric diagnosis in guiding treatment is questionable. As mentioned above, achalasia in the elderly should be thoroughly investigated with upper endoscopy and, in some cases, endoscopic ultrasound to exclude secondary achalasia resulting from a malignant tumor.

Treatment

The specific treatment depends on the diagnosis. Aggressive surgical treatment of esophageal neoplastic lesions depends on the stage of the tumor and the general medical condition of the patient. If esophageal tumors are unresectable, the elderly patients should be considered for palliation with endoscopic laser therapy or endoscopic esophageal stent placement.

The same dilatation therapy offered to younger patients with esophageal webs and strictures is also well-tolerated by most elderly patients. The elderly patient with achalasia has been shown more likely to tolerate pneumatic dilatation than thoracotomy with distal esophageal myotomy. In fact, the treatment of choice for the elderly patient with achalasia is pneumatic dilatation with a small or medium balloon. Elderly patients usually tolerate these endoscopic procedures without difficulty. After endoscopic dilation of peptic strictures, their gastroesophageal reflux disease should be aggressively treated with either H$_2$-receptor antagonists or with the proton pump inhibitors.

Pill esophagitis can be prevented by ensuring that all pills are ingested in an upright position with adequate amounts of water. Where possible, liquid formulations of offending drugs should be used.

Castell DO: Esophageal disorders in the elderly. Gastroenterol Clin North Am 1990;19(2):235.

Kikendall JW: Pill-induced Esophageal Injury. Gastroenterol Clin North Am 1991;20(4):835.

GASTROESOPHAGEAL REFLUX DISEASE

Essentials of Diagnosis

- Rule out coronary artery disease early in the evaluation.
- Associated Barrett's esophagitis should be suspected.
- Look for esophageal malignancy.
- Much longer duration of disease than in younger individuals.
- Recurrent pneumonia and asthma can be the main complaint.

Pathophysiology

Several factors promote symptomatic gastroesophageal reflux disease (GERD) in the elderly. Salivary flow is usually diminished. Saliva is an important protectant of the esophagus from acidic refluxate because it has a high bicarbonate and mucus content. There is also an age related decrease in esophageal motility and gastric emptying which can promote GERD. There is also diminished lower esophageal sphincter tone in the elderly. These alterations may be secondary to the physiology of the aging process, the associated medical illnesses likely to be seen in the elderly population, or the side-effects of the multiple medications taken by some individuals. Elderly individuals with diabetes and neurologic diseases are more likely to have abnormalities in these esophageal manometric functions.

Clinical Findings

The symptoms of GERD are similar to those in younger patients, particularly heartburn, mid-epigastric pain, substernal burning chest pain, sour taste, and nocturnal regurgitation. Recurrent pneumonia in the elderly patient, however, may be due to repeat reflux and aspiration of gastric contents. Recurrent substernal chest pain in the elderly must be carefully investigated as a possible sign of either reflux disease, esophageal dysmotility, or cardiac disease.

Progressive solid dysphagia can be the initial symptom in some patients with long-standing asymptomatic GERD. This may be due to either a benign distal esophageal peptic stricture or the development of an esophageal adenocarcinoma in an area of Barrett's metaplasia.

A clinical diagnosis can be made in most patients with typical signs and symptoms. In the elderly patient with multiple risk factors for cardiac disease, atypical angina must be considered. Reflux disease typically is not worsened by physical exertion or associated with diaphoresis or shortness of breath. If the history and physical examination are suspicious, further cardiac evaluation must be completed before an extensive gastrointestinal evaluation. These two illnesses may coexist; hence, diagnosis of one should not discourage the consideration of the other.

Patients with classic symptoms of reflux disease who have no symptoms or signs of complications (such as dysphagia, weight loss, or anemia) can be given empiric therapy with H_2-receptor antagonist as a therapeutic trial. Elderly patients with the new onset of typical reflux symptoms can be approached in the same way as other patients with long-standing typical symptoms. If no improvement is observed or if signs of complications develop after an adequate trial of empiric therapy, upper endoscopy should be performed to confirm the diagnosis and to exclude complications.

This procedure facilitates the direct visualization of the esophagogastroduodenal mucosa and allows for direct sampling of any mucosal abnormalities. Areas of Barrett's esophagus or erosive esophagitis or other esophageal and gastroduodenal diseases can be identified. Esophagitis is found in 50–75% of elderly patients with GERD. Older patients are also more likely to have Barrett's epithelium, which may give rise to dysplasia and adenocarcinoma. The use of endoscopy to screen elderly patients with long standing uncomplicated reflux symptoms for Barrett's metaplasm is controversial. Screening of younger patients with known Barrett's esophagus often is recommended to screen for the development of high grade dysplasia or early carcinoma. Because elderly GERD patients with multiple, other medical illnesses are not candidates for aggressive surgical therapy if high grade dysplasia is found, screening is not recommended in this group. The 24-hour pH esophageal monitoring is helpful in elderly patients with atypical reflux symptoms and normal endoscopy, especially chest pain, cough, asthma, and recurrent aspiration.

Treatment

The principles of treatment of GERD in the elderly is the same as with younger patients. Therapy should be directed at preventing gastroesophageal reflux, decreasing the acidity of the gastric refluxate, and removing the precipitating factors. The usual non-medical antireflux measures should also be strongly recommended—no late meals, weight loss, head of the bed elevation, avoidance of caffeine, no smoking, avoidance of chocolates and other foods that aggravate symptoms. In the hospitalized or bed-bound elderly it is critical to always keep the head of the bed elevated. This also applies to elderly patients receiving enteral feeds via nasogastric feeding tubes or percutaneous endoscopic gastrostomy tubes. Smaller boluses or a constant slower drip into the jejunum is usually well-tolerated and results in fewer episodes of reflux. Reflux symptoms may be treated with histamine H_2-receptor antagonists or the proton

pump inhibitors. The doses of these acid-lowering medications should not be changed because of age. Medications that decrease the lower esophageal sphincter or delay gastric emptying should be eliminated, when possible. In the elderly patient with diabetic gastroparesis, the prokinetic agent cisapride can be quite useful. Metalclopramide should be avoided in the elderly due to a high incidence of neuropsychiatric side effects. In a small number of elderly patients with intractable reflux symptoms and esophagitis, antireflux surgery may be required. The newer laparoscopic techniques make this a more attractive option for elderly patients who previously tolerated poorly standard surgical procedures through large thoracotomy or laparotomy incisions.

Mold JW et al: Prevalence of gastroesophageal reflux in elderly patients in a primary care setting. Am J Gastroenterol 1991;86(8):965.

Raiha I et al: Determinants of symptoms suggestive of gastroesophageal reflux disease in the elderly. Scand J Gastroenterol 1993;28:1011.

Zhu H et al: Features of symptomatic gastroesophageal reflux in elderly patients. Scand J Gastroenterol 1993;28:235.

PEPTIC ULCER DISEASE

Essentials of Diagnosis

- Incidence increases with age.
- Signs and symptoms are frequently atypical.
- Complication and mortality rates are higher.
- *Helicobacter pylori* plays an important role.
- NSAIDs dramatically increase disease incidence, complication and death rates.

General Considerations

Peptic ulcer disease is a serious problem in the elderly. Almost 20% of gastrointestinal problems in the elderly is related to peptic ulcer disease—the incidence of which increases with age. Elderly patients often present with atypical symptoms and are more likely to present with complications of peptic ulcers. The rates of hospitalization and mortality from peptic ulcers continue to remain high among older people even as these rates decrease in younger individuals. Recurrent bleeding rates are as high as 40%, versus 18% in younger patients. Bleeding ulcers require more blood transfusions and longer hospitalizations. The peptic ulcer disease mortality rate of 20–40% in hospitalized elderly patients is approximately 5–10 times greater than in younger patients. Over 80% of all peptic ulcer-related deaths occur in individuals older than 65 years.

Pathophysiology

The gastroduodenum shows very little variation solely as a result of age. Gastric acid secretion and duodenal mucosal bicarbonate secretion in healthy adults and patients with duodenal ulcer disease show no consistent age related changes. Elderly patients with diminished gastric acid secretion usually have associated chronic gastritis and gastric atrophy. Gastric secretory functions show few significant changes with age independent of these diseases.

Reasons for the higher mortality of peptic ulcer disease include coexisting cardiopulmonary diseases, a delay in diagnosis, and the presence of larger bleeding ulcers. In addition, the elderly are more likely to be infected with *Helicobacter pylori,* and to be using NSAIDs.

H pylori plays a crucial role in the pathogenesis of peptic ulcer disease. In the United States and in other developed countries, the prevalence of *H pylori* is much higher in older age groups. Individuals older than 65 years have more than a 60% chance of having gastric antral *H pylori* infection. In certain susceptible individuals, this antral *H pylori* infection is thought to lead to peptic ulcers. Up to 100% of patients with duodenal ulcers and over 80% of patients with gastric ulcers have antral *H pylori* infection. Multiple clinical trials show that the rate of ulcer recurrence is dramatically lower after *H pylori* eradication.

Another important cause of peptic ulcers in the elderly, especially gastric ulcers, is the use of NSAIDs. All NSAIDs inhibit prostaglandin synthesis and thus can decrease gastroduodenal mucosal cytoprotection. This alteration results in an imbalance in the normal homeostasis of the gastroduodenal mucosa in favor of the aggressive factors. Peptic ulcers occur in 10–20% of patients on chronic NSAID therapy. Approximately 2–3% of chronic NSAID users per year develop a significant NSAID-induced complication. Almost one-half of all NSAIDs are ingested by individuals over the age of 60 years.

Clinical Findings

In the elderly, the presenting symptoms and signs of ulcer disease are usually atypical and poorly defined. Elderly patients tend to have minimal or no epigastric discomfort. In many patients the first manifestation of an ulcer is a complication. This scenario is especially true for elderly patients taking NSAIDs. Up to one-third have no dyspeptic pain and one-half may present with intestinal hemorrhage, obstruction, or perforation as their first sign of gastroduodenal disease. Ulcer disease is more likely to be associated with weight loss, decreased appetite, early satiety, and vague abdominal discomfort. Sometimes, in the absence of any abdominal symptoms, elderly patients can present primarily with the cardiac and neurologic complications of severe anemia due to chronic blood loss from peptic ulcerations. One should suspect the presence of peptic ulcer disease in the elderly when they fall into pertinent risk categories or present with vague upper intestinal symptoms or signs of upper gastro-intestinal bleeding.

Diagnosis

Upper endoscopy is the procedure of choice for diagnosing gastric and duodenal ulcers and is much more sensitive and specific than upper gastrointestinal series with barium. Elderly patients tolerate endoscopy well. Although extra care should be taken in the presence of coexisting cardiopulmonary diseases, little sedation is required in most elderly patients. Giant ulcers may be present in patients over the age of 60. These large ulcers (> 3 cm) are found most often in the lesser curvature and have over 10% chance of malignancy. Most gastric ulcers must be biopsied to exclude malignancy, which is present in 2–3% of affected patients. Repeat endoscopic evaluation should be performed in all patients within 8–12 weeks to assess ulcer healing. Residual ulcerations should be biopsied to exclude malignancy.

Determination of *H pylori* status is important, especially in ulcers not associated with the use of NSAIDs. *H pylori* infection can be detected by multiple methods including serologic determination of IgG antibodies, histologic identification of the bacteria from mucosal biopsy, determination of urease activity in biopsy specimens, or the ^{13}C or ^{14}C-urea breath test.

Treatment

The same general guidelines for therapy of peptic ulcer disease applies to older patients; they respond just as well to acid-lowering therapy. The same doses and duration of anti-ulcer medications are used as in younger patients. Doses should never be adjusted solely because of age. Age is also not an independent predictor for anti-ulcer drug intolerance.

Eradication of *H pylori* from patients with peptic ulcer disease results in a significantly decreased ulcer recurrence rate. Studies are in progress to determine whether the ulcer complication rates are also affected by *H pylori* eradication. All patients with peptic ulcer disease with evidence of *H pylori* infection should undergo treatment. Multiple regimens are available for the treatment of *H pylori* infection (see Chapter 21).

Unless NSAIDs and aspirin are essential, they should not be used by elderly patients who have a history of peptic ulcer disease. If NSAIDs cannot be stopped, the lowest effect doses should be prescribed. Alternatively, newer formulations of NSAIDs, such as nabumetone or etodolac, may have less damaging effects on the gastroduodenal mucosa. Prophylactic therapy with misoprostol is recommended in elderly patients taking NSAIDs who have a prior history of peptic ulcer disease, or who are taking concomitant corticosteroids. All patients should be strongly encouraged to stop smoking, because this facilitates ulcer healing and probably decreases ulcer recurrence and complication.

The treatment of peptic ulcer disease complications is similar in the elderly as in younger patients.

Complications of peptic ulcer disease, however, are associated with a much higher morbidity and mortality rate in the elderly.

Bellary SV, Isaacs PE, Lee FI: Upper gastrointestinal lesions in elderly patients presenting for endoscopy: relevance of NSAID usage. Am J Gastroenterol 1991;86(8):961.
Gilinsky NH: Peptic Ulcer Disease in the Elderly. Gastroenterol Clin North Am 1990;19(2):255.

UPPER GASTROINTESTINAL BLEEDING

Essentials of Diagnosis

- Mortality rates are higher than in younger adults.
- The presenting sign may be worsening of a coexisting illness.
- Early diagnosis and aggressive therapy is important.
- Bleeding can be the first sign of a gastroduodenal disease.

General Considerations

Upper gastrointestinal bleeding usually presents similarly in all age groups. The initial approach to the elderly patient should be the same as with the younger patient. The first step must always be to establish a normal hemodynamics status and to determine whether the bleeding is massive or occult.

Pathophysiology

The most likely origins of upper gastrointestinal bleeding in the elderly include peptic ulcers, gastritis, erosive distal esophagitis, vascular anomalies, Mallory-Weiss tears and malignant neoplasms. Approximately 50% of upper gastrointestinal hemorrhage in the elderly is due to bleeding from peptic ulcer disease. The most likely type of ulcer found in these elderly patients with upper gastrointestinal hemorrhage is the giant gastric ulcer (> 3 cm), which has a very high propensity for bleeding. Elderly patients with upper gastrointestinal bleeding are more likely to be using NSAIDs than would be a younger patient. NSAIDs can cause direct mucosal damage, indirect damage by inhibiting prostaglandin production, and also interfere with proper functioning of platelets. These factors increase the risk of peptic ulcer disease complications and potential bleeding from other upper gastrointestinal lesions.

Other sources of upper gastrointestinal hemorrhage in the elderly include gastritis, due to NSAIDs or alcohol, and esophagitis. Esophagitis is usually due to severe gastroesophageal reflux disease. Esophageal damage can also result from the direct effect of certain medications, eg, potassium, quinidine, and tetracycline.

Clinical Findings

Upper gastrointestinal bleeding can present with either massive hemorrhage or with chronic occult blood loss. Elderly patients who present with evidence of a significant ongoing hemorrhage are at significantly increased risk of dying during that hospitalization. A large national survey by Silverstein showed that patients above the age of 60 have a mortality rate of 13–14% compared to 3–4% in patients younger than 30-years old. Elderly patients with bleeding peptic ulcers are at greatest risk.

Chronic occult blood loss and iron deficiency anemia may arise from a chronic bleeding source anywhere in the gastrointestinal tract. The most common causes are gastrointestinal malignant growths, angiodysplasias, and erosive esophagitis.

The elderly patient with gastrointestinal bleeding may present in atypical fashion with complaints of shortness of breath, chest pain, or signs of a myocardial infarction. Others may present with evidence of transient ischemic attacks or cerebrovascular accidents or syncope. Because of impaired vision or neurologic impairment, the patient may not be able to give a history of melena or hematochezia. Hence, it is important to perform a thorough physical examination that includes testing of the stool for occult or frank blood to identify gastrointestinal bleeding.

Associated medical illnesses may supply clues to the correct diagnosis. Recurrence of upper gastrointestinal symptoms consistent with previous episodes of peptic ulcer disease can be helpful. The patient with hematemesis and a history of cirrhosis and portal hypertension is likely to be bleeding from either esophageal or gastric varices. Gastric malignant tumors commonly result in iron deficiency anemia. Of note, most cases of gastric adenocarcinoma occur in the elderly population. They are often associated with vague nonspecific symptoms such as early satiety, nausea and weight loss. Prior episodes of nonbloody vomiting with significant retching can lead to Mallory-Weiss tears of the lower esophagus. Vascular anomalies like Dieulafoy lesions and angiodysplastic lesions are seen more commonly in the elderly.

Treatment

After appropriate hemodynamic resuscitation of the patient with massive upper gastrointestinal bleeding, standard endoscopic hemostatic therapy is the next step. Elderly patients tolerate this procedure well. All the endoscopic therapeutic maneuvers are equally effective in the elderly. If these maneuvers are not successful or if the bleeding lesion is not identified, angiography, nuclear scintigraphy, or both can be diagnostic. As with younger patients, surgical therapy to halt upper intestinal bleeding remains a final alternative.

The evaluation of the elderly patient with evidence of occult intestinal blood loss and iron deficiency anemia has to be tailored to the individual patient. The patient with associated upper intestinal symptoms (eg, epigastric discomfort, dyspepsia, nausea, early satiety) should be evaluated first with upper endoscopy. Also, patients currently taking NSAIDs and aspirin should have upper endoscopy. If that is completely normal, then the colon should be inspected with colonoscopy. Should the patient not be affected by any of these factors, it is reasonable to evaluate the colon first, followed by upper endoscopy if the colon is normal.

Miller DK et al: Acute upper gastrointestinal bleeding in elderly persons. J Am Geriatr Soc 1991;39(4):409.

Papp JP: Management of upper gastrointestinal bleeding. Clin Geriatr Med 1991;7(2):255.

CONSTIPATION & FECAL IMPACTION

Essentials of Diagnosis
- Common problem in the hospitalized elderly.
- The cause is often multifactorial.
- Duration of constipation is important.
- Adequate fluids, fiber, and physical activity are essential.

General Considerations
Common problems of the hospitalized or institutionalized elderly population include constipation and fecal impaction. Fecal impaction is a complication of constipation. The true prevalence of constipation is difficult to assess in the healthy ambulatory elderly population. It seems, however, that more elderly patients suffer with constipation than do younger adults. The percentage of patients visiting the physician for constipation is approximately 30% in patients over the age of 60 years.

Constipation is a highly subjective complaint, which can be defined in terms of the frequency of bowel movements, the consistency of stool, a sense of incomplete evacuation, and the need to strain to have a bowel movement. Infrequent bowel movements occur in up to 50% of patients with constipation; up to one-third have all these complaints.

Pathophysiology
The pathogenesis of constipation is multifactorial. Various coexisting medical conditions and medications can alter the proper functioning of the colon. Therefore, the hospitalized and institutionalized elderly are particularly prone to developing these colonic problems. There is no known age-related decrease in human colonic motility as measured by transit time. There are, however, some age-related changes—eg, decrease in the muscle mass—in the anorectum.

In the elderly, multiple factors can combine to result in significant constipation. In the hospitalized elderly patient, immobility and bedrest can markedly increase colonic transit time. The normal sitting posture on a toilet facilitates defecation, and patients confined to a bed may find it very difficult to defecate in the bed pan. Depression, altered mental status, and restricted access to a commode may all interfere with timely regular defecation. Inadequate fluid and fiber intake result in dehydration that leads to hard stools which are difficulty to evacuate. Various medical illnesses can exacerbate constipation. For example, hypothyroidism, hyperparathyroidism, or the various neuromuscular disorders can result in constipation. The neuropathy associated with diabetes mellitus also results in significant constipation. Various medications cause constipation, including opioids, anticholinergics, certain antidepressants, iron supplements, calcium channel blockers, and aluminum containing antacids. Finally, colonic obstruction from chronic strictures due to colonic ischemia or radiation-induced colitis must be considered. The elderly may also have obstruction because of colonic tumors or acute diverticulitis.

Clinical Findings
The duration of the symptoms is very important. Any recent change in the bowel habits of the elderly patient should be promptly evaluated. The recent onset of constipation with associated abdominal distention and pain could result from a luminal obstructing lesion such as carcinoma. On the other hand, the patient with several years of the same stool consistency and frequency can be evaluated less urgently. The abdomen and the rectal area must be carefully examined. Rectal prolapse and hemorrhoids can occur because of the excessive straining associated with constipation. The presence of severe rectal pain due to fissures, infections (herpes simplex), or inflamed or thrombosed hemorrhoids can lead to avoidance of defecation and thus constipation.

The use of medications that can alter bowel function should be determined. The patient's diet and activity/exercise schedule must be reviewed. Immobility and bedrest can also slow bowel activity. This is particularly important in the debilitated bed-bound nursing home elderly patient. Thyroid function tests and serum electrolytes, including calcium, potassium, and phosphorous, must be checked.

For the patient with abdominal distention and pain, a plain abdominal radiograph is obtained to look for dilated loops of bowel suggesting intestinal obstruction. Also, it can demonstrate the presence of large amounts of stool in the large bowel proximal to the location of the luminal abnormality. If there has been no recent endoscopic or radiographic evaluation of the colonic lumen, either colonoscopy or flexible sigmoidoscopy and barium enema should be done to exclude a partially obstructing luminal lesion. In the constipated elderly patient with associated iron deficiency anemia, colonoscopy is the appropriate first mode of evaluation of the colon.

If the evaluation to this point is unrevealing,

colonic transit time can be assessed with radiopaque markers. This radiographic procedure can differentiate between generalized decrease in colonic contents (colonic inertia) versus impaired defecation due to pelvic floor dysfunction. In the elderly, many causes of dysfunction are located in the anorectum. Rectocele, intussusception, rectal prolapse, and inadequate relaxation of the puborectalis muscle can prevent easy passage of stool.

Patients with suspected pelvic floor dysfunction may benefit from evaluation of a gastroenterologist. Further evaluation of the anorectum can be accomplished with defecography to assess the mechanism of defecation. Anorectal manometry is another useful tool to assess the relaxation of the pelvic floor. Manometry can document any abnormal functioning of the anal sphincters and the rectum.

Complications of constipation includes fecal impaction, which can lead to painful pressure sores (stercoral ulcers) in the anorectum, and bowel obstruction, which can lead to ischemia and perforation. In addition, the straining and valsalva maneuvers performed by some constipated elderly patients with atherosclerotic disease can lead to syncopal episodes.

Therapy

Therapy should be geared towards the particular findings of the evaluation. Any metabolic or electrochemical disorders must be corrected. Medications that can result in constipation should be stopped. In ambulatory elderly patients, increasing dietary fiber and fluid intake is usually quite effective in increasing stool bulk and decreasing colonic transit times. Daily intake of approximately 2 tablespoons of wheat bran in cereal or in juices is effective. Another bulk-forming agent is psyllium. On average, the gradual increase to a dose of approximately two scoops of psyllium in 6–8 ounces of fluid two or three times per day is effective. This regimen can be continued as maintenance therapy to prevent recurrence of constipation. Also, sedentary patients should be encouraged to increase their physical activity. In debilitated bed-bound elderly patients, the use of large doses of fiber without adequate hydration can lead to a worsening of this problem. In the ambulatory elderly patient who does not respond to increased colonic roughage, the use of gentle tap water enemas or bisacodyl 10 mg suppositories are usually effective within one hour. Other oral osmotic cathartics like sorbitol or lactulose are quite effective but may produce significant flatulence. In the patient without renal disease, oral magnesium citrate solution (200 ml) or Milk of Magnesia (15–30 ml) are usually effective in relieving constipation.

If fecal impaction is present, tap water enemas and careful manual disimpaction should be used. Enemas containing caustic salts, soap suds, or tepid water should be avoided since they can damage the colonic mucosa. Once successful disimpaction is achieved, complete cleansing of the entire colon with a non-absorbable laxative like polyethylene glycol should be performed. This is necessary because the rectal distention associated with fecal impaction can render the distal colon temporarily atonic. Evaluation of colonic transit time with the radiopaque markers should not be done too soon after relieving fecal impaction.

Chronic maintenance laxative therapy may be necessary for some patients. This should be constantly re-evaluated and weaned as patients comply with more natural methods for staying on a regular bowel schedule. High-fiber foods should eventually replace the expensive fiber supplements. Periodic gentle luminal acting laxatives like sorbitol, lactulose, or Milk of Magnesia once or twice per week are helpful. Mineral oil should be avoided in the debilitated elderly because of the much higher risk of aspiration and resultant severe pulmonary complications. If taken on a regular basis, it can also interfere with the absorption of fat-soluble vitamins (A, D, E, K), which can get suspended in the oil and carried out of the colon before adequate absorption. Gentle enemas can be useful, given the caveats mentioned above. The emollient laxatives (docusate sodium or docusate calcium) provide only minimal utility and should not be the only mode of therapy.

Merkel IS et al: Physiologic and psychologic characteristics of an elderly population with chronic constipation. Am J Gastroenterol 1993;88(11):1854.

Wald A et al: Contributions of evacuation proctography and anorectal manometry to evaluation of adults with constipation and defecatory difficulty. Dig Dis Sci 1990;35:481.

FECAL INCONTINENCE

Essentials of Diagnosis

- High prevalence in the hospitalized elderly.
- Higher prevalence in demented and functionally impaired patients.
- Impaired anorectal function.
- Decreased rectal sensation and compliance.

General Considerations

Fecal incontinence is the involuntary loss of stool. Fecal incontinence can either be minor or major. Minor incontinence is the release of small amounts of stool, especially liquid stool. Major incontinence is the involuntary release of an entire liquid or solid bowel movement. This is a more serious and difficult problem to treat. Incontinence is rare in the general population, including the ambulatory elderly individuals. It is a significant problem, however, in the institutionalized elderly patient. Up to 25% of hospitalized elderly patients and up to 50% of residents of nursing homes are incontinent of feces. Approximately 10% of nursing home residents have fecal incontinence every week. Nursing homes with more severely demented patients have a higher rate of incontinence.

Pathophysiology

Fecal continence is maintained by the interaction of several mechanisms. To maintain continence, the patient must be able to sense and distinguish various types of rectal contents—solid versus liquid versus gas. The anal canal has a very dense array of nerves that can sample the contents of the rectum. The distal colon and the rectum must be compliant, to store and act as reservoir for fecal contents until the appropriate time for release. Any disease processes that can alter rectal sensation and distensibility can lead to incontinence. For example, colonic ischemia, radiation proctitis, or inflammatory bowel disease can decrease the storage capacity of the rectum and thus cause urgency and fecal incontinence. The internal and external sphincters must be able to contract to prevent inappropriate extrusion of contents. The autonomic nervous system controls the internal sphincter. The pudendal nerve innervates the striated muscles of the external sphincter. Hence, diseases of the central and peripheral nervous system can cause incontinence. Cerebrovascular accidents, spinal cord injuries, cauda equina lesions, and neuropathies due to diabetes mellitus can all cause incontinence. Various surgical procedures can alter the function of the anal canal. After obstetric surgical mishaps or post-hemorrhoidectomy, there can be damage to the anal canal resulting in incontinence. The pelvic floor muscles and the puborectalis muscle maintain the acute anorectal angle, which also helps to allow stool to be stored in the rectosigmoid colon until the appropriate time for defecation. During diarrheal illnesses, the large volumes of liquid stool entering the rectum can cause urgency and fecal soiling even in patients with completely normal anorectal function.

Cognitive awareness to control the urge to defecate until the appropriate time and place is a major part of the voluntary control of defecation. Severely demented and cognitively impaired elderly persons often suffer from fecal incontinence because they "voluntarily" release stool at inappropriate times and places. Rectosigmoid mass lesions—cancers and polyps—can also interfere with the maintenance of fecal continence by altering proper anorectal function. Fecal soiling can also result from enterocutaneous fistulae, especially in patients with inflammatory bowel disease.

Clinical Findings

A careful perineal and rectal examination is essential. A neurologic examination should note the perianal sensation, the presence of an anal wink reflex, and the anal sphincter tone at rest and with squeezing. The presence of any rectal masses on digital rectal examination should be excluded. The identifica-

tion of surgical scars or fistulous tracts in the perineum may be extremely important. Prolapsed hemorrhoids or skin tags can sometimes result in leakage of small amounts of mucus or liquid stool. Fecal impaction can present with soiling when liquid stool overflows around a solid stool mass.

Flexible proctosigmoidoscopy should be performed to exclude distal colonic carcinoma or colitis. In the ambulatory elderly patient, anorectal manometry is performed to assess the internal and external anal sphincters, the degree of rectal compliance, and the ability of the rectum to sense distention. Patients with diminished rectal sensation may have incontinence because the threshold for sensation exceeds the threshold for internal sphincter relaxation. Thus, the patient is not aware of rectal fullness until leakage occurs. This ambulatory patient with normal cognitive function and decreased rectal sensation may be a good candidate for biofeedback therapy to lower the threshold of rectal perception. For the demented bed-bound nursing home resident, the goal is to maintain good perineal hygiene and to avoid skin breakdown and infection.

Secondary problems of fecal incontinence should also be identified. They include perineal cutaneous maceration, fungal dermatitis, and bacterial cellulitis, which can occur after prolonged periods of moisture and contamination of the perineum.

Treatment

Therapy should be directed towards the specific findings obtained during the evaluation. If the incontinent stool is always liquid and only occurs while there is severe diarrhea, then treating the diarrhea or the colitis can usually improve the symptoms quite dramatically. In some patients, the addition of dietary fiber to increase stool bulk is beneficial. Decreasing the stool frequency with an anti-diarrheal agent is sometimes helpful. Patients with minimal amounts of post-defecatory leakage should be told to tuck a cotton ball near the anal opening. This will absorb small amounts of leakage, reducing staining of undergarments and enhancing perianal hygiene. The perianal area should be cleansed with glycerin wipes (baby wipes). Soaps and harsh cleansing should be avoided.

Especially in the bed-bound, frail elderly, care should be taken to avoid the perianal cutaneous breakdown and infections that occurs when there is fecal incontinence. Good perineal hygiene and nursing is very important. Careful attention to dermatitis and fungal rashes is important.

In highly motivated patients without cognitive impairment and with reduced degree of rectal sensation, remarkable benefit can be obtained from biofeedback or retraining therapy. Success rates approach 70%.

In a few selected patients who are otherwise healthy, surgical repair should be considered. Patients with rectal prolapse and with an abnormal anorectal angle can benefit from surgical repair. If the fecal soiling is via enterocutaneous fistulae, specific medical or surgical therapy should be recommended depending on the underlying reason for such lesions. In severe cases of persistent fecal incontinence, in which all other therapies have failed, surgical diversion via a colostomy is sometimes a drastic but advisable option since the management of a colostomy may be easier than anal incontinence and may improve the quality of life.

Barnett JL, Raper SE: Anorectal Diseases. In: *Textbook of Gastroenterology.* Yamada T (editor). Lippincott, 1991.

Read NW, Celik AF, Katsinelos P: Constipation and incontinence in the elderly. In: *The Aging Gut.* Holt PR (editor). J Clin Gastroenterol 1995;20(1):61.

Schiller LR: Faecal incontinence. Clin Gastroenterol 1986;15(3):687.

VASCULAR ECTASIA

Essentials of Diagnosis

- Age-related vascular degeneration.
- Can be diffusely scattered throughout the gastrointestinal tract.
- Most colonic lesions are on the right side.
- Can cause occult or massive blood loss.

General Considerations

Vascular lesions of the gastrointestinal tract have multiple names, such as arteriovascular malformations, vascular ectasias, or angiodysplasias. These vascular anomalies are often identified in the gastrointestinal tract of elderly patients.

Pathophysiology

Angiodysplastic lesions are thought to result from an age-related degenerative process resulting in ectasia and abnormal communications between mucosal capillaries and submucosal veins. An alternative theory describes vascular anomalies arising after recurrent mucosal ischemia. The majority of patients with these vascular ectasia are above the age of 60. The prevalence of these vascular ectasia in patients in this age group is approximately 25%. Lesions can be found in the stomach, the duodenum and throughout the small and large bowel and are usually in multiple sites. The colonic lesions are most often found in the cecum and ascending colon.

An association between these vascular lesions and aortic stenosis has been made but is controversial. Very few patients with these vascular ectasias had severe aortic stenosis. Other cardiac diseases (eg, mitral stenosis) are not associated with these lesions. Nevertheless, patients have reduced bleeding from these angiodysplastic lesions after aortic valve repair.

Patients with end stage renal disease on dialysis have a high prevalence of angiodysplasias when they are evaluated for upper gastrointestinal bleeding. It is currently believed that the associated coagulopathies in patients with renal disease potentiate bleeding from angiodysplasias, resulting in a higher rate of identification. Thus, any process that alters coagulation may precipitate angiodysplastic bleeding and therefore result in subsequent identification of these lesions.

Clinical Findings

Though recurrent low-level bleeding is typical, most lesions are asymptomatic and are found incidentally. Approximately 15% of patients with bleeding from ectasias present with iron deficiency anemia. Some patients present with melena, maroon stools or hematochezia. When elderly patients with lower intestinal bleeding are examined angiographically, up to 60% have vascular ectasia. It is quite rare, however, that an actively bleeding lesion is seen angiographically. Hence, it is difficult to determine when the search should continue for alternate causes of intestinal bleeding.

The initial evaluation of patients presenting with melena or hematemesis should be with upper endoscopy. The patient with hematochezia and bilious gastric lavage can be evaluated with colonoscopy after appropriate colonic cleansing with a laxative. If the colonic output is persistently bloody, colonoscopy may be non-diagnostic because of the inability to see the colonic mucosa clearly; the diagnostic procedure of choice then becomes angiography. For a small, self-limited bleed in an elderly patient, the initial evaluation can end after a negative endoscopy and colonoscopy. Further evaluation with push enteroscopy and possibly intraoperative enteroscopy to look for small intestine angiodysplasias should only be done if the patient has recurrent significant bleeding requiring transfusion.

Treatment

Angiodysplasias are difficult to treat because they are usually in multiple locations. After ablative therapy, they can recur at different sites in the mucosa. Gastroduodenal and colonic lesions can usually be identified by endoscopic procedures. Effective endoscopic treatments include injection with sclerosants, electrocautery, and Nd:YAG laser therapy. Recurrent bleeding, however, can occur in up to half of these patients because of either new or unrecognized lesions. For significant bleeding, angiography with embolization of these lesions is also effective but is also limited by the same problems with recurrent bleeding. Surgical resection is effective when a definitive bleeding lesion is identified. Coexisting lesions in other parts of the bowels, however, may bleed later. Elderly patients with slow and intermittently bleeding inaccessible lesions (eg, in the small bowel) which do not require blood transfusions to maintain a stable hematocrit do not require specific therapy. These patients can be followed closely and kept on supplemental iron therapy.

Elderly patients with significant and symptomatic aortic stenosis can be considered for valve repair. In some patients, this has been shown to decrease the incidence of recurrent bleeding. It is still controversial, however, to replace the aortic valve solely for treatment of angiodysplasias.

The correction of any coagulopathy also results in less recurrent bleeding. Long-term therapy with synthetic estrogen and progesterone combinations has shown significantly less recurrent angiodysplastic bleeding, especially in elderly patients with chronic renal failure. A double-blind trial with 0.05 mg ethinyl estradiol and 1 mg norethisterone daily resulted in less bleeding and reduced requirements for blood transfusions.

Richter JM et al: Angiodysplasia: Natural history and efficacy of therapeutic interventions. Dig Dis Sci 1989;34:1542.

ISCHEMIC COLITIS

Essentials of Diagnosis
- Coexisting cardiovascular and atherosclerotic disease is common.
- Frequently affects the left colon but spares the rectum.
- Initial therapy is to maintain hemodynamic stability.
- A significant complication is bowel infarction with peritonitis.

Pathophysiology
The majority of patients with colonic ischemia are older than 60 years. In most cases, this process is believed to be related to the degeneration of the vascular system that occurs with age. It may also be indirectly related to the atherosclerotic disease seen in older patients. It is most often due to nonocclusive reduction of blood flow to the intestines. It can also occur after aortoiliac vascular surgical reconstruction, abdominal aortic aneurysm repair, or abdominoperineal resection due to sacrifice of the inferior mesenteric artery. After these operations, ischemic colitis occurs in up to 5% of patients. In patients with severe congestive heart failure, shock, or recent myocardial infarction, there can be significant hypoperfusion of the intestines. Older patients with cardiac arrhythmias are at high risk for embolic events into the vascular supply of the colon.

The most frequently affected areas are the vascular watershed regions of the colon. Thus, the watershed between the inferior mesenteric artery and iliac circulation in the superior rectum, and between the superior mesenteric artery and inferior mesenteric artery in the transverse colon or left colon are most commonly involved. The lower rectum is usually spared because of its dual blood supply. The diagnosis is usually based upon the clinical and colonoscopic information.

Clinical Findings
The most frequent presenting complaint is bloody stools without abdominal pain. The majority of cases are self-limiting and completely resolve and heal within a few weeks. A subset of patients are much sicker and present with abdominal pain and rectal bleeding. They usually have fevers and an elevated white blood cell count. They may proceed to a fulminant ischemic colitis with transmural infarction, perforation, and peritonitis. Both sets of patients can have thumb-printing on their abdominal radiographs which represents mucosal edema.

Approximately 15% of patients have evidence of transmural ischemia with perforation and peritonitis. Another 15% develop a chronic, persistent colitis which is sometimes difficult to differentiate from inflammatory bowel disease. Approximately 50% of patients make a complete recovery without any residual effects. In some patients, scarring results at the site of ischemia, resulting in significant strictures.

Patients must be monitored closely. Vital signs and abdominal examination must be carefully followed, with attention to signs of fever, increasing tenderness, or leukocytosis that suggest necrotic bowel. Daily abdominal radiographs assess for signs of perforation or bowel obstruction.

In the absence of significant tenderness or peritoneal findings, flexible sigmoidoscopy or colonoscopy should be performed to establish the diagnosis and to differentiate for other causes of hematochezia, such as inflammatory bowel disease, infectious colitis, or the presence of a colonic malignancy.

Treatment
The basis of therapy is to establish adequate perfusion and oxygenation of the colonic mucosa. Hence, the mainstay of therapy is supportive. The hemodynamic profile should be adequately maintained. Supplemental intravenous hydration is usually recommended. Optimal cardiac function is very important to adequately perfuse and oxygenate the colon. If possible, medications that decrease intestinal blood flow should be avoided as they would facilitate further colonic ischemia. Patients should be kept without any oral intake to rest the bowels.

In most severe cases, prophylactic antibiotic therapy is recommended, including broad spectrum antibiotic coverage for intestinal flora. The surgical team should be aware of these patients since transmural infarction and peritonitis can occur, requiring bowel resection.

Brandt LJ, Boley SJ: Colonic ischemia. Surg Clin North Am 1992;72(1):203.
Levy PJ, Guernsey JM: Mesenteric ischemia. Med Clin North Am 1988;72:1091.

INFLAMMATORY BOWEL DISEASE

Essentials of Diagnosis

- Second peak incidence between age 55 and 65.
- Differentiate from ischemic colitis or diverticulitis.
- Early diagnosis is the key to a better prognosis.
- Medical therapy is associated with more frequent side effects.

Pathophysiology

There is a bimodal peak incidence of inflammatory bowel disease. The first occurs between ages 15 and 30, and the second, accounting for approximately 10% of all new cases, occurs between ages 55 and 65. Presenting signs and symptoms of inflammatory bowel disease are exactly as in younger patients; the correct diagnosis, however, is usually made after approximately 2 years of symptoms, versus less than 1 year for younger patients. In elderly patients, inflammatory bowel disease can be mistaken for other processes such as diverticulitis, segmental ischemic colitis, carcinoma, and acute infectious colitis. Hence, this entity should be kept in mind to prevent the increased morbidity and mortality associated with making this diagnosis too late.

Clinical Findings

For ulcerative colitis, most patients present with bloody, loose stools mixed with mucus. When there is extensive colitis, there is usually associated diffuse abdominal pain, fevers, and anemia. More distal disease is usually associated with tenesmus, mucus, and blood mixed in formed stools, and less generalized symptoms. Most studies report that approximately 50% of elderly patients present with pancolitis versus approximately 20% of younger patients. Most elderly patients with Crohn's disease have involvement only of the colon—Crohn's colitis.

Presenting signs and symptoms can be mistaken for other illnesses seen frequently in the elderly. For example, segmental ischemic colitis and diverticulitis can both be confused with inflammatory bowel disease. Radiologic, endoscopic, and pathologic evidence may not be enough to differentiate between these processes. Sometimes, coexisting illnesses may not be helpful diagnostic clues. For instance, diffuse diverticulosis occurs in up to 50% of elderly patients with Crohn's disease. Significant atherosclerosis can exist in patients with Crohn's or ulcerative colitis. The presence of megacolon can also be a sign of an acute infectious colitis, paralytic ileus, ischemic colitis, or a distal obstruction like a volvulus. The presence of extraintestinal manifestations of inflammatory bowel disease can be very helpful in clinching the correct diagnosis. Hence, it is important to look for these processes when considering the diagnosis of inflammatory bowel disease.

Treatment

Standard medical therapies are equally effective in both age groups. These medications, however, should be used carefully in the elderly. Older patients are sometimes more susceptible to the untoward effects of, and possible interactions between, medications. Corticosteroids can induce mental status changes that can be mistaken for dementia or other psychological disturbances. Corticosteroids can also accelerate the progression of osteoporosis or the development of subcapsular cataracts in the elderly. For these reasons, 6-mercaptopurine is a good alternative to corticosteroids for elderly patients with Crohn's disease. Anticholinergics may precipitate deterioration of mental status in older patients, leading to increased morbidity. Sulfasalazine can lead to reduced absorption of folic acid and interfere with the other medications they are likely to be taking, eg, digoxin. Hence, folic acid supplementation is recommended. If the patient is on digoxin, then digoxin levels should be monitored closely. Other medications for inflammatory bowel disease like metronidazole can interact with warfarin leading to over-anticoagulation.

The surgical options are well-tolerated by the elderly. Decisions should be made on an individual basis, however. For example, a total colectomy with ileostomy rather than a rectal preserving procedure would be much more appropriate for a demented elderly patient with ulcerative colitis confined to a bed or wheelchair than an ambulatory elderly person with normal anal sphincter function. Coexisting medical illnesses and the patient's general condition should also be carefully considered before recommending any complicated surgical procedures.

Prognosis

Early diagnosis of inflammatory bowel disease is the key for a good prognosis. Elderly patients can do well with appropriate therapy. In ulcerative colitis, most of the elderly patients are without symptoms in the first year. Mortality rates must be adjusted for the time since disease appearance. Patients with inflammatory bowel disease are living longer and so the prevalence in the elderly population is increasing. Hence, screening for colonic carcinoma, a very late complication of inflammatory bowel disease, should be done in the elderly with long-standing active disease.

Lashner BA, Kirsner JB: Inflammatory bowel disease in older people. Clin Geriatr Med 1991;7:287.

Woolrich AJ, Korelitz BI: Ulcerative colitis in older age. Am J Gastroenterol 1988;83:1060.

COLONIC NEOPLASIA

Essentials of Diagnosis

- Increased risk in the elderly.
- Early detection is the key to survival.

General Considerations

Colonic carcinoma is the most common gastrointestinal cancer. The risk of developing this cancer increases dramatically in the elderly and peaks at about age 80. At age 80, there is more than a 500 in 100,000 chance of acquiring colonic carcinoma. Most of these cancers are sporadic and are thought to develop from adenomatous polyps. A family history of colon cancer is of unclear significance in the patient over age 70.

Screening

Colonic screening for early detection of colon carcinoma should always take into consideration the general medical health status of the patient. For example, the severely ill, demented elderly patient without intestinal complaints will probably not benefit from screening with a prolongation of a good quality of life. One should always ask whether the patient could safely undergo subsequent procedures and therapies and would benefit from them if the screening test is positive.

Hence, the recommendations for yearly fecal occult blood testing and the periodic flexible sigmoidoscopic examinations to identify early colonic lesions should be applied to elderly patients who will benefit from such intervention. In the appropriate elderly patients with a high risk of colonic carcinoma and a positive fecal occult blood test, the most cost-effective procedure is a colonoscopy. Repeat procedures can then be performed every 5 years.

Clinical Findings

Colonic malignancies should be suspected in any elderly person presenting with recent changes in their bowel habits—especially diarrhea or constipation. Also, elderly patients with iron deficiency anemia, weight loss, intestinal bleeding, either occult or massive, should be suspected of having colonic carcinoma. In addition, patients can present with bowel obstruction. A careful physical examination sometimes reveals abdominal masses. Digital rectal examination can find palpable masses. The diagnostic procedure of choice, which can also obtain tissue samples, is colonoscopy.

Treatment

Malignant tissues confined to polyps can be safely removed with the colonoscope. Surgical resection is the procedure of choice for early stages of cancer. The more advanced tumors can be treated with surgical resection and adjuvant chemotherapy and radiation therapy. These surgical procedures are usually well-tolerated by the elderly. The key to a low operative and postoperative mortality rate is to have elective surgery after the patient has had a complete preoperative evaluation focusing on a thorough cardiopulmonary assessment. In addition, the tumor must be properly staged before surgery to avoid operations for unresectable cancers.

Adjuvant chemotherapy with 5-FU and levamisole hydrochloride in patients with resected tumors has been shown to reduce death rate and to decrease the rate of recurrence. The use of adjuvant therapy should always take into consideration the general health status of the elderly patient.

Rectal cancers should also be approached in the same manner. The elderly patients with good performance status and early stage cancer should have the tumor resected by low abdominal resection or abdominoperineal resection, followed by chemotherapy and radiation therapy as necessary. By contrast, patients with contraindications to surgery or extensive cancer should be given palliative treatment. Palliation can either be with a diverting colostomy, radiation therapy, or endoscopic laser therapy.

Fleshner P, Slater G, Aufses AH: Age and sex distribution of patients with colorectal cancer. Dis Colon Rectum 1989;32:107.

Mandel JS et al: Reducing mortality from colorectal cancer by screening for fecal occult blood. N Engl J Med 1993;328:1365.

Wallach CB, Kurtz RC: Gastrointestinal Cancer in the Elderly. Gastroenterol Clin North Am 1990;19(2):419.

HEPATOBILIARY DISEASES

Hepatitis

Age has very little effect on the serum levels of the various liver function tests and the hepatic enzymes. The symptoms associated with hepatobiliary diseases are usually blunted in the elderly. Elderly patients do not have a significantly increased risk of complications from the acute infectious hepatitides. Viral infections are associated with lower serum aminotransferase than in younger patients. Hepatitis B is more likely to become chronic in the elderly than in young adults. Also, the hepatitis B vaccine response is less in the elderly.

Hemochromatosis in elderly men often has significant involvement of the heart, pancreas, and liver. Hence, they often have diabetes mellitus and a high risk of hepatocellular carcinoma.

As a result of a higher prevalence of cardiovascular diseases and decreased hepatic blood flow, the elderly are prone to hepatic ischemic damage whenever there are episodes of significant hypotension. Also, congestive heart failure can cause hepatic congestion. The hepatitis associated with ischemic damage is centrilobular necrosis which typically results in very high aminotransferase levels that rapidly fall within 2 to 3 days to near normal if the cardiac dysfunction was corrected and there was no significant underlying hepatic diseases. Hepatic congestion from congestive failure may be manifested by a rise in the serum protime and minor increases in alkaline phosphatase or bilirubin.

Elderly patients are also more susceptible to the

hepatotoxicity of many medications. This is likely due to the altered hepatic metabolism and to interactions of multiple medications. Several of the NSAIDs, sulfa containing drugs, phenothiazines, estrogens, and macrolide antibiotics can cause significant hepatic dysfunction. The infiltrative disorders such as amyloidosis and sarcoidosis occur more frequently. The elderly are also more susceptible to the cholestatic complications of certain infections, such as pneumococcal sepsis.

Cholelithiasis

The prevalence of cholelithiasis increases with age. The prevalence of gallstones vary widely between studies. Between 30% and 50% of people above the age of 70 will have gallstones. Most will be completely asymptomatic. Even in the healthy elderly and the elderly diabetic, asymptomatic gallstones should not be prophylactically removed. Only 10% of stones will become symptomatic, and only a minority of these will present with a biliary complication as their first symptom. Complications usually are preceded by episodes of biliary pain and transient biochemical abnormalities. Symptomatic patients should have elective cholecystectomy. Laparoscopic cholecystectomy is usually better tolerated than standard cholecystectomy by the elderly, even though they both require general anesthesia.

For certain high-risk elderly patients with symptomatic cholelithiasis, another procedure that is only available in certain institutions is percutaneous dissolution of small non-calcified (cholesterol) gallstones with methyl tert-butyl ether (MTBE) and other similar solvents. Oral dissolution therapy with ursodeoxycholic acid is another option in debilitated elderly patients with small cholesterol gallstones and a patent cystic duct.

Choledocholithiasis

Approximately 50% of elderly patients with cholangitis and cholecystitis or choledocholithiasis present with the typical triad of pain, fever, and jaundice. Elderly patients have a higher incidence of malignant obstruction of the biliary system. They are also more likely to have choledocholithiasis and bacteremia. The mortality rate for laparotomy with common duct stone removal in elderly patients is relatively high (up to approximately 19%) but varies from center to center. Hence, the best approach for the elderly patient with cholangitis due to common

duct stones is to undergo endoscopic retrograde cholangiopancreatography (ERCP) with sphincterotomy and stone extraction. In the absence of cholecystitis, a cholecystectomy may not be necessary, since subsequent complicated cholecystitis occurs in only 10% of patients with gallbladder in situ after sphincterotomy.

In elderly patients with acute cholecystitis who are poor operative candidates, a temporizing modality is the placement of a percutaneous drainage (catheter cholecystostomy) into the gallbladder by the interventional radiologist. This can decompress the biliary system until such time that the patient can safely undergo a definitive procedure.

Acalculous Cholecystitis

Approximately 10% of patients with acute necrotic cholecystitis have no associated gallstones—acalculous cholecystitis. The typical patient is the severely ill elderly person with trauma, postoperative complications, sepsis, or hypotension in the intensive care unit (ICU). This can occur especially in elderly men with underlying significant vascular disease. The underlying etiological factor is believed to be non occlusive ischemia.

The signs and symptoms may be overlooked in the ICU patient with multiple medical problems. There is usually an acute worsening in the clinical course with associated leukocytosis and elevated temperatures without an obvious source. Mild elevations in aminotransferase and alkaline phosphatase may occur. There is usually a Murphy's sign present, though this may not be obvious in a sedated or obtunded patient. Abdominal ultrasound reveals a thickened gallbladder wall with pericholecystic fluid but no gallstones. Treatment of acalculous cholecystitis is prompt cholecystectomy or perhaps cholecystostomy. The mortality rate with this aggressive therapy is less than 15%. Other conservative therapies can allow further necrosis to occur resulting in peritonitis, which has a much higher mortality.

Croker JR: Biliary tract disease in the elderly. Clin Gastroenterol 1985;14:773.

Krasman ML, Gracie WA, Strasius SR: Biliary tract disease in the aged. Clin Geriatr Med 1991;7(2):347.

Levinson JR, Gordon SC: Liver diseases in the elderly. Clin Geriatr Med 1991;7(2):3371.

Williamson RCN: Acalculous disease of the gallbladder. Gut 1988;29:860.

Nutritional Disorders & Their Treatment in Diseases of the Gastrointestinal Tract*

13

Siamak A. Adibi, MD, PhD

While the incidence of undernutrition is low in the general population of the United States, several surveys have shown that 25–45% of patients develop undernutrition after admission to hospitals. The cause appears to be inadequate attention to the dietary intake of hospitalized patients.

Undernutrition in ambulatory patients is usually caused by intestinal malabsorption, anorexia, dysphagia, or chronic nausea and vomiting. Intestinal lesions, such as those in patients with acquired immunodeficiency syndrome (AIDS) or celiac sprue, reduce food assimilation. Chronic diseases (eg, cirrhosis) or drug treatment (eg, chemotherapy for cancer) may cause anorexia that results in inadequate food intake. Head and neck cancers or esophageal lesions may interfere with the passage of food. Diseases affecting gastric motility (eg, diabetes) or diseases causing gastric obstruction (eg, peptic ulcer) may cause chronic nausea and vomiting that results in loss of ingested food.

Whatever the cause, undernutrition needs to be recognized and treated. Otherwise, like a systemic disease, it may cause deleterious effects on all organs. The consequences of undernutrition include intestinal malabsorption, hepatic dysfunction, pancreatic insufficiency, anemia, and, most importantly, reduced immunocompetence. Reduced immunocompetence compromises the ability to resist infection, which is often the cause of death in malnutrition.

NUTRITIONAL ASSESSMENT

Nutritional assessment is used to characterize the nutritional state of the patient and to diagnose nutritional problems. It is also used to monitor the response to nutritional intervention. Although there are a variety of techniques for nutritional assessment, some are only available in certain research laboratories, for example, the technique for measurement of whole body rate of protein degradation. The nutritional assessment techniques generally available are listed in Table 13–1.

History & Physical Examination

The medical history is used to elicit information regarding the presence or absence of symptoms of malnutrition and the composition of the patient's diet. Adequacy of the diet can then be estimated from tables of food composition. In physical examination, particular attention is paid to anthropometric measurements and the presence or absence of certain physical signs that are characteristics of nutrient deficiency. For example, muscle wasting may indicate protein-calorie undernutrition, and loss of vibratory and position sense may indicate Vitamin B_{12} deficiency.

Laboratory Tests

The blood tests most commonly employed in nutritional assessment are listed in Table 13–1. However, it should be noted that none of these tests are specific for the diagnosis of undernutrition, because they all could be affected by a variety of other conditions. Their use as nutritional parameters, therefore, is contingent on ruling out the presence of non-nutritional conditions that might affect them.

Body composition can be studied by a variety of techniques, such as the determination of the total body water or the total body potassium (^{40}K). However, these techniques are expensive and require specialized research laboratories. Recently, a technique that is inexpensive and easy to perform has become available for the measurement of body composition. The technique, called **bioelectrical impedance,** is based on the application of a low-frequency electrical current to an extremity and the measurement of the resistance to the flow of current. Because bioelectrical conduction is related to the distribution of water and electrolytes in the body, the bioelectrical imped-

*This chapter is based on the author's contribution to the Gastroenterology & Hepatology syllabus of: Medical Knowledge Self-Awareness Program (MKSAP) 10. American College of Physicians, 1995.

Table 13–1. Nutritional Assessment.

Medical history:
   Acute or chronic change in body weight
   Change in appetite
   Change in bowel habits
   Intake of drugs and alcohol
   Usual daily dietary intake
   Usual daily physical activity
Physical examination:
   Height
   Weight
   Mid-arm circumference (index of muscle mass)
   Skin-fold thickness (index of fat reserve)
Blood levels:
   Albumin
   Folate
   Vitamin B_{12}
   Calcium and phosphorus
   Iron
   Hemoglobin and hematocrit
Body composition:
   Lean body mass
   Total body fat
Nitrogen balance
Energy expenditure

ance technique may not be reliable in situations of disturbed distribution of water and electrolytes.

Nitrogen Balance

Nitrogen balance is used to determine the adequacy of protein intake. The nitrogen balance is the difference between dietary intake and losses in urine, stool, and sweat. In pathologic states, there could be other sources of nitrogen loss, for example, draining gastrointestinal fistula. However, the major loss of nitrogen normally occurs through the urine, and 85% is in the form of urea. The Kjeldahl technique, which is used to measure total nitrogen, is not always available. In this case, the following formula may be used as a crude estimate of nitrogen balance:

$$NB = \frac{\text{Protein intake (g/24 h)}}{6.25} - UUN \text{ (g/24 h)} + 4$$

where NB = nitrogen balance; UUN = urinary urea nitrogen excretion; 4 represents an estimate of nonmeasured nitrogen losses in stool and sweat; and 6.25 represents the percentage of nitrogen in protein. Protein intake is calculated from tables of food composition.

Energy Expenditure

The measurement of energy expenditure is used to assess the adequacy of caloric intake. The resting energy expenditure is measured by indirect calorimetry, which is based on the rates of oxygen consumption and CO_2 production by the body. If indirect calorimetry is not possible, the resting energy expenditure can be calculated from the Harris-Benedict equations:

For males:

Resting energy expenditure (kcal/day) =
$66 + (13.7 \times W) + (5 \times H) - (6.8 \times A)$

For females:

Resting energy expenditure (kcal/day) =
$65.5 (9.6 \times W) + (1.7 \times H) - (4.7 \times A)$

where W = weight in kilograms; H = height in centimeters; and A = age in years.

The energy expenditure of the entire day is influenced by the patient's level of physical activity and physical condition. In hospitalized patients, the daily energy expenditure is calculated as 1.0–1.5 (usually 1.3) × resting energy expenditure. In very catabolic patients, such as those with burns, this could be as much as 2.0 × resting energy expenditure.

DESIGN OF DIET

Calorie Requirement

There are three steps in designing any diet, whether it is planned for oral feeding or for enteral or parenteral nutrition. The first step is to decide the daily total caloric requirement for the patient. The caloric requirement is either measured by indirect calorimetry, calculated using the Harris-Benedict equations or from body weight. The calculation by body weight is based on the Recommended Dietary Allowances (Table 13–2). The energy requirement of hospitalized patients, between the ages of 25 and 50, is usually 30–35 kcal/kg body weight.

Protein Requirement

The second step is to decide the daily protein requirement. The protein requirement is influenced by age, weight, and whether there is wound healing or an abnormal loss of protein, such as from burns or drainage of gastrointestinal contents. The protein requirement is either determined by nitrogen balance or is based on the Recommended Dietary Allowances (Table 13–2). For example, the daily protein requirement of 0.8 g/kg body weight is recommended for healthy subjects. In conditions of increased protein catabolism, such as sepsis or need for weight gain, the daily protein intake is usually 1.2–1.5 g/kg body weight.

Composition of Calories

The third step is to decide on the composition of the non-protein calories of the diet. There is uncertainty regarding the optimal proportion of carbohydrate and fat in the diet. Generally, a ratio of 60% carbohydrate and 40% fat is used. This issue is further discussed under the section on nutrition in critical illness.

Table 13–2. Recommended energy and protein intake for healthy people.[1]

Category	Age (years)	Energy (kcal/kg)	Protein (g/kg)
Infants	0.0–0.5	108	2.2
	0.5–1.0	98	1.6
Children	1–3	102	1.2
	4–6	90	1.2
	7–10	70	1.0
Males	11–14	55	1.0
	15–18	45	0.9
	19–24	40	0.8
	25–50	37	0.8
	51 +	30	0.8
Females	11–14	47	1.0
	15–18	40	0.8
	19–24	38	0.8
	25–50	36	0.8
	51 +	30	0.8

[1]This table is derived from the *Recommended Dietary Allowances,* 10th Edition, National Research Council, National Academy Press, Washington, DC, 1989. This reference also provides recommendations for daily intakes of vitamins, minerals, and electrolytes.

Noncalorie Nutrients

Finally, the diet should include vitamins, minerals, and electrolytes. Vitamins and minerals are usually added according to the Recommended Dietary Allowances (see Table 13–2). The amounts of sodium and potassium are varied according to the state of the patient; the presence of diarrhea or hepatic failure, for example, will influence the prescribed levels.

Efficacy Criteria

The success of dietary design could be monitored by the techniques of nutritional assessment listed in Table 13–1. However, the ultimate criteria for the adequacy of any diet is that it promotes weight gain in patients with weight loss, maintains weight in adult patients with normal body weight, and promotes normal growth in children.

NUTRITION SUPPORT

Patients who are unable to take adequate oral nourishment, maintain body weight or growth, or recover from malnutrition need nutrition support. Nutrition support can be provided either enterally or parenterally.

Enteral Nutrition

Enteral nutrition is preferred over parenteral nutrition because it is more physiologic, less invasive, and much less expensive. Furthermore, complications are less serious with enteral than parenteral nutrition. The prerequisite for enteral nutrition is an adequately functioning gastrointestinal tract. Enteral nutrition is contraindicated in gastrointestinal obstruction.

Intubation, for enteral nutrition, is made through the nose, the stomach, or jejunum. Administration of enteral nutrition through a nasal tube is the least invasive procedure and is the usual route for short-term nutrition support (a few days to a few weeks). For longer nutrition support, enteral nutrition is usually administered through a gastrostomy or jejunostomy. Gastrostomy may be performed by a surgical technique or, more simply, by a percutaneous endoscopic technique (PEG). The latter procedure, which avoids the trauma of surgery, has become more preferred. The jejunostomy for enteral nutrition is usually performed in patients undergoing gastrointestinal surgery or laparoscopy.

A wide variety of diets are currently available for enteral nutrition. The products are designated as polymeric or chemically-defined diets. In **polymeric diets,** the nitrogen source is intact protein and the carbohydrate source is corn starch or dextrin. In **chemically-defined diets,** the nitrogen source is either a protein hydrolysate (a mixture of oligopeptides and amino acids) or a mixture of free amino acids. A protein hydrolysate is superior to a mixture of amino acids as the nitrogen source for enteral nutrition because it is more efficiently absorbed and is less hypertonic. However, all protein hydrolysates must be assured of having a balanced mix of essential and nonessential amino acids. The carbohydrate source is usually a mixture of polysaccharides and oligosaccharides. Both polymeric and chemically-defined diets have a vegetable oil, such as safflower, as the lipid source. In addition, chemically-defined diets may contain medium-chain triglycerides, which are more efficiently absorbed than long-chain triglycerides.

Polymeric diets are used for gastric infusion and in patients who have no impairment of digestion and absorption. Chemically-defined diets are used when rapid absorption in the upper intestine is desired, for example, in patients with inflammatory diseases of the ileum or colon. Chemically-defined diets are also used in situations of impaired digestion or absorption. The superiority of protein hydrolysates over intact protein as a source of nitrogen for enteral nutrition has been shown in patients with pancreatic insufficiency.

Although a number of complications have been reported with enteral nutrition, the most significant ones are diarrhea and pulmonary aspiration. There are many causes of diarrhea. It may be related to the composition of the formula, hypertonicity of the diet, rate of infusion, intake of drugs, or intestinal infection with *Clostridium difficile.* Usually, a step-by-step investigation of each of the above causes is necessary to stop the diarrhea.

It is not yet clear whether oropharyngeal secretion or regurgitation of infused solution is responsible for pulmonary aspiration. Nevertheless, if the patient is prone to aspiration owing to decreased level of consciousness, endotracheal intubation, delayed gastric emptying, or gastroesophageal reflux, enteral nutrition through a jejunostomy should be tried.

Parenteral Nutrition

If enteral nutrition is not possible or desirable, parenteral nutrition can be used to support the patient. Except for the carbohydrate, the same nutrient sources that are used in enteral nutrition can be used in parenteral. When infused intravenously, oligosaccharides and polysaccharides are poorly utilized. Therefore, the carbohydrate source must be a monosaccharide, such as glucose. As in enteral nutrition, the protein source could be amino acids, dipeptides, or tripeptides and the lipid source could be long- and medium-chain triglycerides.

Currently, mixtures of essential and nonessential amino acids, in a proportion to stimulate the composition of proteins of high biologic value, are used as protein sources. However, for technical reasons, these mixtures lack certain amino acids, such as glutamine and tyrosine, which are found in protein. Glutamine is unstable in solution and tyrosine is poorly soluble in water. There is some evidence that the absence of these amino acids from parenteral nutrition may be undesirable. For example, total parenteral nutrition results in hypoplasia of the intestinal mucosa; this appears to be prevented by the addition of stable forms of glutamine (eg, a glutamine-containing dipeptide) to the parenteral solutions. Therefore, it is likely that future amino acid solutions will include glutamine and tyrosine as dipeptides, resolving the problems of stability and solubility.

Parenteral nutrition is administered through a catheter placed either in a central or a peripheral vein. The central vein technique is used in patients who require long-term nutrition support or have to be given hypertonic solutions, which cause phlebitis in peripheral veins. In parenteral nutrition via a peripheral vein, lipid emulsions serve as the main source of calories. This is because provision of adequate calories in the form of glucose requires administration of hypertonic solutions.

A wide range of complications have been reported with the use of parenteral nutrition. These can be categorized as either catheter-related or metabolic. The most frequent catheter-related complications are infections, thrombosis, and pneumothorax. The most common metabolic complications, such as hyperglycemia, hyperlipidemia, and fluid overload, occur as a result of overzealous administration of parenteral nutrition. However, the cause of some metabolic complications, such as liver abnormalities and bone disease, remains uncertain.

NUTRITION AFTER GASTRECTOMY

The chief functions of the stomach are to mix, reduce the size of solid particles to less than 2 mm in diameter, adjust the osmolality of ingested foods, and deliver the resulting gastric chyme to the small intestine at rates that are optimal for digestion and absorption. The impairment of this function by removal of the pyloric sphincter results in the development of dumping syndrome in some patients. The **dumping syndrome** is a consequence of rapid emptying of hyperosmolar gastric contents into the small intestine. Patients with dumping syndrome may benefit from nutritional intervention. The dietary requirement should be given in the form of 5–6 small solid meals per day. Fluid intake should be restricted at the time of meals and delayed for 1–2 hours after meals. Pectin (a water soluble fiber) may be used to slow gastric emptying.

Intestinal absorption of vitamin B_{12} requires the intrinsic factor which is secreted by the stomach. Therefore, a nutritional complication of gastrectomy is vitamin B_{12} deficiency, which can be adequately treated by a monthly injection of 100 µg of vitamin B_{12}.

Although some patients maintain adequate nutrition status after gastrectomy, others may have nutritional problems, such as weight loss, iron deficiency, anemia, and metabolic bone disease. The pathogenesis of these nutritional problems is not fully understood, but probably includes reduced food intake and malabsorption. Treatment may include the use of nutrition support and the addition of extra amounts of iron, calcium, and vitamin D to the diet.

NUTRITION IN PANCREATIC INSUFFICIENCY

Pancreatic insufficiency, whether caused by chronic pancreatitis or pancreatic resection, impairs the assimilation of foodstuffs. Digestion is a necessary first step in this process, and the pancreas is the major source of enzymes for intraluminal digestion of protein, fat, and carbohydrate. It is estimated that when pancreatic secretion of its digestive enzymes falls to about 10% of normal, intestinal assimilation of foodstuffs is greatly impaired. This impairment appears to be greater for fat than for either protein or carbohydrate. Although there is digestion of lipid by lingual and gastric lipases, this digestion does not seem as efficient as the digestion of protein and carbohydrate by the nonpancreatic enzymes.

Another consequence of pancreatic insufficiency is inadequate insulin secretion, leading to the development of diabetes mellitus. Fortunately, exocrine and endocrine pancreatic insufficiencies can be well treated with pancreatic enzyme replacement therapy and insulin injection, respectively. However, if a patient is either noncompliant or refractory to enzyme therapy, a formula diet may be used. The composition of the formula diet may include a protein hydrolysate as the nitrogen source, polysaccharides as the carbohydrate source, and medium-chain triglycerides as a component of the lipid source.

The most common cause of pancreatic insufficiency in children is cystic fibrosis. Malnutrition and growth failure are common findings in these patients. These appear to be due to inadequate food intake as well as to pancreatic insufficiency. A serious consequence of malnutrition in these patients is further insult to the already-compromised lung function. In view of the serious prognosis of malnutrition in cystic fibrosis, patients who fail to respond to conservative nutrition therapy may be considered for nocturnal enteral-tube feeding. There are reports of improvement of nutritional status and lung function after long-term nocturnal feeding.

Therapy for pancreatitis includes "pancreatic rest." Because food ingestion is a powerful stimulus of pancreatic secretion, oral feeding is usually withheld during an acute attack. In most cases, eating can be resumed after a few days. However, if pancreatitis persists beyond a few days, such as in the case of necrotizing pancreatitis, patients may require total parenteral nutrition. Parenteral nutrition has a much less stimulatory effect on pancreatic secretion than does enteral nutrition. The dietary requirements of patients with necrotizing pancreatitis are discussed in a following section, "Nutrition in Critical Illnesses."

NUTRITION IN SHORT BOWEL SYNDROME

The small intestine plays a critical role in digestion and absorption of foodstuffs, while the colon plays an important role in absorption of water and electrolytes. Diseases that damage or necessitate resection of the small intestine impair food assimilation. An example is the occlusion of either the mesenteric artery or vein. This vascular occlusion necessitates resection of the intestine, often from midtransverse colon to upper jejunum. Before the advent of parenteral nutrition, these patients commonly died from undernutrition, but now they have a near-normal life expectancy.

Initially, all patients with short bowel syndrome should receive parenteral nutrition at home. Because of the need for long-term nutritional support, a central vein is used for administration of parenteral nutrition. Patients with short bowel syndrome can take oral feeding in the amount of several hundred calories per day without causing troublesome diarrhea. Furthermore, this food tolerance increases with time owing to the intestine's adaptation to reduced digestive and absorptive surface. Studies in animal and human intestine have shown that, after resection, the remaining intestine undergoes mucosal hyperplasia. The intestinal villi enlarge with an increase in height and the number of surface villus epithelial cells. As a result, absorption is increased in the intestinal remnant.

There is considerable evidence that nutrients in the gut lumen are important for adaptation of the intestine after resection. It has been shown, for example, that parenteral nutrition without oral feeding impairs the development of mucosal hyperplasia that normally occurs after resection. Therefore, it is important that patients with short bowel syndrome be encouraged to eat as much as possible while not exceeding the capacity of intestine for food assimilation.

Several dietary restrictions are beneficial in patients with short bowel syndrome. Because of the limited capacity for absorption, large meals should be replaced with frequent, small meals. Among the disaccharides, the hydrolysis of lactose is most rate-limiting. Since unabsorbed lactose causes diarrhea, milk products should be used with caution. A major effect of high-fiber diets on the gastrointestinal tract is to shorten the transit time. Although this effect appears to be beneficial in healthy people, it may not be desirable in patients with short bowel syndrome. Therefore, a low-fiber diet may be tried. Lastly, some patients with short bowel syndrome may have an increased incidence of oxalate stones in the kidney, as a result of increased oxalate absorption from the colon. Normally, calcium in the gut lumen binds to oxalate to form insoluble calcium oxalate. In patients with short bowel syndrome, calcium is no longer available for binding to oxalate because it is already bound to unabsorbed fatty acids. This results in increased solubility of oxalate and, consequently, increased absorption. Therefore, patients with evidence of hyperoxaluria should avoid foods with high oxalate content (eg, spinach, tea, chocolate) and should increase the amount of calcium in the diet.

NUTRITION IN INFLAMMATORY BOWEL DISEASE

Patients with either Crohn's disease or ulcerative colitis commonly have protein calorie undernutrition or vitamin and mineral deficiencies, or both. Growth retardation is common in children with Crohn's disease. Two major factors in the pathogenesis of malnutrition in these patients are inadequate food intake and malabsorption.

Fecal loss of nutrients, particularly fat, is of much greater importance in patients with Crohn's disease than in ulcerative colitis. This is because the ileum is the only site for the active transport of conjugated bile acids and, furthermore, the ileum is the most common site affected by Crohn's disease. Ileal disease or resection reduces absorption and, consequently, the body pool of bile acids, leading to a decrease in their intraluminal concentration, which is necessary for lipid absorption.

Resection of the ileocecal valve, as a part of the surgery for Crohn's disease, may further aggravate the steatorrhea. Normally, the ileocecal valve prevents proliferation of colonic bacteria in the small intestine. A consequence of the proliferation of bacteria in the small intestine is the increased deconjugation of bile salts. This results in lowering of the critical concentration of conjugated bile salts necessary for efficient lipid absorption. Bacterial overgrowth further enhances the problem of diarrhea by increasing hydroxylation of fatty acids. The hydroxylated fatty acids, like unabsorbed bile acids, stimulate secretion of water and electrolytes.

The objectives of nutritional intervention in inflammatory bowel disease are twofold. One objective is to allow "bowel rest," and the other is to replenish nutritional deficiencies. The concept of bowel rest with total parenteral nutrition emerged from the observation that ileostomy significantly contributes to remission of colitis in Crohn's disease. Furthermore, it has been proposed that Crohn's disease represents an inappropriate immunologic response to antigens contained in food or produced by bacteria in the gut lumen. Therefore, it has been reasoned that total parenteral nutrition allows maintenance of an adequate state of nutrition while eliminating antigens from food and possibly decreasing the bacterial population in the gut lumen. Although the rationale for the use of bowel rest appears reasonable, the evidence is controversial. On occasion, the severity of abdominal symptoms and diarrhea necessitates a trial of total parenteral nutrition.

It is the general consensus that nutritional deficiencies and growth retardation of patients with inflammatory bowel disease should be treated with either parenteral or enteral nutrition. Currently, enteral nutrition, in the absence of any significant obstruction or fistula problem, is preferred over parenteral nutrition. An unsettled controversy concerns the source of nitrogen for enteral nutrition in patients with Crohn's disease. Due to lesser problems with either antigenicity, hypertonicity, or absorption, protein hydrolysates appear superior to both intact proteins and amino acids.

Another controversial issue is whether enteral nutrition or drug therapy should be used for inducing a remission in Crohn's disease. An argument against drug therapy is that it may have serious side effects. An argument against enteral nutrition is that it is not as effective as drug therapy. However, a recent study has shown that enteral nutrition alone reduces intestinal permeability and inflammation in patients with Crohn's disease. A hallmark of Crohn's disease appears to be increased intestinal permeability, whether the patient is symptomatic or asymptomatic. Therefore, if the above results are confirmed by other studies, enteral nutrition may be considered as one of the primary treatments for Crohn's disease.

Finally, patients with Crohn's disease are prone to develop vitamin B_{12} deficiency. This is because ileum is the site of vitamin B_{12} absorption. There-fore, patients with a diseased ileum should receive a monthly injection of 100 μg of vitamin B_{12}.

NUTRITION IN LIVER DISEASE

The liver plays a central, and, sometimes, a unique role in regulating various metabolic processes. For example, the liver has either the dominant or exclusive role in the regulation of glucose homeostasis, synthesis of urea and plasma proteins, storage of fat-soluble vitamins, and activation of vitamins, such as folic acid and thiamine. These roles need to be considered in the treatment of patients with liver disease.

For example, whether hypoalbuminemia or elevated blood prothrombin level is due to protein and vitamin deficiency, respectively, or whether they are due to impaired liver synthesis of these proteins is an issue that must be considered. In the former case, hypoalbuminemia can be improved with an adequate protein diet, and the elevated prothrombin time can be reduced with the administration of vitamin K. In the latter case, nutritional intervention will not be useful because the restoration of hepatic protein synthesis requires improvement in hepatic function.

Undernutrition is quite prevalent in patients with chronic liver disease, particularly those with alcoholic cirrhosis. This is usually evidenced by muscle wasting, anemia, and low blood levels of vitamins and trace elements. The causes of malnutrition include reduced or inappropriate dietary intake, malabsorption, and, in alcoholics, the toxic effects of ethanol on gastrointestinal tract and skeletal muscle.

It is the general consensus that the treatment of malnutrition will be beneficial to patients with liver disease. In fact, recent studies have shown an improvement in liver function through the use of enteral nutrition in such patients. In the absence of hepatic encephalopathy, the treatment of malnutrition is generally similar to treatment in patients without liver disease. The only notable exception is the use of carbohydrates in patients with cirrhosis, who have a high incidence of glucose intolerance. The mechanism appears to be insulin resistance. Therefore, if feeding results in symptomatic hyperglycemia, a greater emphasis should be placed on lipid rather than carbohydrate as the caloric source.

Patients with advanced liver disease may be intolerant to dietary protein. In other words, they may develop hepatic encephalopathy after a high-protein meal. Although the mechanism of protein intolerance in cirrhotic patients is still not fully understood, it is believed to be related to impaired capacity of the liver to convert ammonia to urea. This impairment results in a rise in blood ammonia level, and, consequently, a greater amount of ammonia may reach the brain. In fact, some patients show an elevation in plasma ammonia concentration after a protein meal.

Currently, the main strategy of treatment of protein-induced hepatic encephalopathy is a reduction in ammonia production in the body. This is accomplished by restriction or elimination of protein in the diet, by administration of a high amount of carbohydrate to suppress proteolysis, and by treatment with nonabsorbable antibiotics to suppress bacterial population in the colon. The catabolism of protein and its metabolic products by colonic bacteria is a major source of ammonia in the body. Patients may also be fed lactulose, which is a nonabsorbable disaccharide. Lactulose is metabolized by bacteria, resulting in increased production of hydrogen ions in the colon; this converts ammonia to ammonium, which is less absorbed from the colon.

Even without protein intake, cirrhotic patients may develop hepatic encephalopathy. Among the causative factors implicated is the decreased concentrations of branched-chain amino acids in plasma. It is suggested that a consequence of decreased plasma concentrations of branched-chain amino acids is the increased entry of amino acids (eg, tyrosine, which is normally inhibited by branched-chain amino acids) into the brain. Increased entry of aromatic amino acids results in increased synthesis of false neurotransmitters, which cause hepatic encephalopathy.

The proponents of the above theory have formulated amino acid mixtures with high concentrations of branched-chain amino acids to serve as the nitrogen source for enteral and parenteral nutrition. Although there have been a number of clinical trials of parenteral nutrition with high concentrations of branched-chain amino acids in patients with chronic liver disease, the evidence supporting the use of such solutions remains controversial.

NUTRITION IN CRITICAL ILLNESSES

Patients with critical illnesses, such as necrotizing pancreatitis, burns, or trauma, may develop a hypermetabolic state with profound alterations in the metabolism of protein, carbohydrate, and fat. The intensity of these alterations usually depends on the severity of the illness. Initially, the protein degradation exceeds protein synthesis, resulting in a negative nitrogen balance. The increased protein degradation, which appears to be largely in the skeletal muscle, serves to provide amino acids for gluconeogenesis and the synthesis of acute-phase proteins in the liver. The hyperglycemia that is commonly observed is the result of increased glucose synthesis in the liver and reduced glucose uptake by peripheral tissues. Both of these processes become less sensitive to the action of insulin because of the development of insulin resistance in these tissues. The increased lipolysis is evidenced by the increased mobilization of fatty acids and glycerol. These metabolic alterations appear to be mediated by increased secretion of glucagon, glucocorticoids, catecholamines, and cytokines.

It is generally believed that the treatment of critically ill patients should include nutritional support. This belief is based on the evidence that immune and repair processes are impaired in malnutrition, and starvation may not be well tolerated by patients who are already fighting for their survival.

A key objective of the nutritional support in critically ill patients is to reduce protein catabolism. The reversal of negative nitrogen balance is usually resistant to nutritional intervention and may not occur until the hypermetabolic state has receded. In hypermetabolic critically ill patients, the amounts of calories and protein that are considered adequate are 1.2–1.5 × resting energy expenditure (usually 35–40 kcal/kg) and 1.2–1.5 g protein/kg, respectively.

The composition of nonprotein calories considered appropriate for the nutritional support of critically ill patients is the same as for those not critically ill, 60% carbohydrate and 40% fat. The reason for the use of carbohydrate is that it reduces the enhanced gluconeogenesis, and it is more efficient than fat in sparing body protein. The reason for the use of fat is that it provides essential fatty acids and prevents the reliance on glucose as the sole source of calories.

Administration of all nonprotein calories as glucose exceeds the capacity for utilization and may cause problems, such as hyperglycemia and respiratory failure. On a molar basis, CO_2 production is much greater with glucose than with fat as a source of calories. Increased CO_2 production necessitates increased respiratory ventilation, which may not be desirable in critically ill patients with compromised pulmonary function. On the other hand, the administration of all nonprotein calories as fat may also exceed the capacity for utilization and may cause problems, such as reduced immune function, which is undesirable in septic patients. These considerations underscore the importance of using a mixture of glucose and fat as the caloric source in critically ill patients.

A major concern in the use of nutritional support in critically ill patients is the prevention of fluid overload, which may burden the cardiovascular system. Although the enteral route of administration is preferred in the nutritional support of these patients, it is sometimes necessary for a period of time to use the parenteral route.

Critically ill patients may also require intravenous fluid infusion for administration of therapeutic agents, such as antibiotics. To deal with this problem, a central rather than a peripheral vein should be used for infusion of parenteral solutions with high concentrations of nutrients. The stock solutions with the highest concentrations of nutrients are 15% amino acids, 20% fat, and 70% glucose. Lastly, if critically ill patients develop either hepatic or renal failure, the amount of amino acids infused should be reduced to the **level of tolerance,** which is defined as avoidance of encephalopathy in hepatic failure and azotemia in renal failure.

REFERENCES

Abrams CK et al: Role of nonpancreatic lipolytic activity in exocrine pancreatic insufficiency. Gastroenterology 1987;92:125.

Cabre E et al: Effect of total enteral nutrition on the short-term outcome of severely malnourished cirrhotics. A randomized controlled trial. Gastroenterology 1990; 98:715.

Driscoll DF, Blackburn GL: Total parenteral nutrition 1990. A review of its current status in hospitalised patients, and the need for patient-specific feeding. Drugs 1990;40:346.

Eriksson LS, Conn HO: Branched-chain amino acids in the management of hepatic encephalopathy: An analysis of variants. Hepatology 1989;10:228.

Goldstein SA, Elwyn DH: The effects of injury and sepsis on fuel utilization. Annu Rev Nutr 1989;9:445.

Grunfeld C, Feingold KR: Metabolic disturbances and wasting in the acquired immunodeficiency syndrome. N Engl J Med 1992;327:329.

Kearns PJ et al: Accelerated improvement of alcoholic liver disease with enteral nutrition. Gastroenterology 1992;102:200.

Lochs H et al: Comparison of enteral nutrition and drug treatment in active Crohn's disease. Results of the EUROPEAN COOPERATIVE CROHN'S DISEASE STUDY IV. Gastroenterology 1991;101:881.

Lukaski HC: Methods for the assessment of human body composition: Traditional and new. Am J Clin Nutr 1987;46:537.

Miholic J et al: Nutritional consequences of total gastrectomy: The relationship between mode of reconstruction, postprandial symptoms, and body composition. Surgery 1990;108:488.

Moore MC et al: Enteral-tube feeding as adjunct therapy in malnourished patients with cystic fibrosis: A clinical study and literature review. Am J Clin Nutr 1986;44:33.

Naylor CD et al: Parenteral nutrition with branched-chain amino acids in hepatic encephalopathy. A meta-analysis. Gastroenterology 1989;97:1033.

Purdum PP, III, Kirby DF: Short-bowel syndrome: A review of the role of nutrition support. Journal of Parenteral and Enteral Nutrition 1991;15:93.

Rosenberg IR, Bengoa JM, Sitrin MD: Nutritional aspects of inflammatory bowel disease. Annu Rev Nutr 1985;5:463.

Schulz LO: Methods of body composition analysis. The status of the gold standard. Trends Endocrinol Metab 1993;4:318.

Silk DBA, Grimble GK: Relevance of physiology of nutrient absorption to formulation of enteral diets. Nutrition 1992;8:1.

Sitzmann JV, Converse RL, Jr., Bayless TM: Favorable response to parenteral nutrition and medical therapy in Crohn's colitis. A report of 38 patients comparing severe Crohn's and ulcerative colitis. Gastroenterology 1990;99:1647.

Steinhardt HJ et al: Nitrogen absorption in pancreatectomized patients: Protein versus protein hydrolysate as substrate. J Lab Clin Med 1989;113:162.

Steinkamp G, von der Hardt H: Improvement of nutritional status and lung function after long-term nocturnal gastrostomy feedings in cystic fibrosis. J Pediatr 1994;124:244.

Teahon K et al: The effect of elemental diet on intestinal permeability and inflammation in Crohn's disease. Gastroenterology 1991;101:84.

Vanderhoof JA et al: Short bowel syndrome. J Pediatr Gastroenterol Nutr 1992;14:359.

Vazquez JA, Daniel H, Adibi SA: Dipeptides in parenteral nutrition: From basic science to clinical applications. Nutr Clin Prac 1993;8:95.

The Veterans Affairs Total Parenteral Nutrition Cooperative Study Group. Perioperative total parenteral nutrition in surgical patients. N Engl J Med 1991;325:525.

Minimally Invasive Surgery for Gastrointestinal Diseases

14

Laurence F. Yee, MD, & Sean J. Mulvihill, MD

Beginning with the introduction of laparoscopic cholecystectomy in 1987, gastrointestinal surgery has undergone revolutionary changes. New technology now allows many surgical procedures to be performed with "minimal access" to the thoracic or abdominal cavities, obviating the need for large, painful, and morbid incisions. In the minimal access approach, the operative visual field is provided by telescopes attached to miniaturized video cameras, with the image projected on television monitors. New instruments have been designed for use within the constraints of small incisions. General surgeons have been retrained to adapt to a new two-dimensional visual field. The technical limitations as compared with traditional surgery—including loss of tactile sensation and sensory feedback—are partially offset by improved resolution of anatomic detail through the magnification provided by the operating telescopes.

The initial driving force behind the rapid development of the minimally invasive approach was patient demand. The intuitive benefits of minimal access surgery, including minimal scarring, reduced pain, and quicker return to work, offer clear-cut advantages in many operations. In other operations, however, the advantages are less clear. The challenge for general surgeons today is to evaluate the outcome and costs of the minimally invasive approaches to gastrointestinal disorders, and compare these results to those obtained with traditional open surgical techniques.

DIAGNOSTIC LAPAROSCOPY

General Considerations

Diagnostic laparoscopy refers to the visual examination of the intra-abdominal contents with a telescope or endoscope. Diagnostic laparoscopy is useful in three general clinical scenarios: (1) evaluation of abdominal pain, (2) staging of abdominal tumors, and (3) evaluation of abdominal trauma.

Technical Considerations

Diagnostic laparoscopy is usually performed with the patient under general anesthesia, however, it is possible under local anesthesia. After adequate muscle relaxation, nasogastric and bladder catheters are placed to decompress the stomach and urinary bladder, respectively. The first goal is to create a working space (**pneumoperitoneum**) within the abdomen by insufflation of gas (usually CO_2) through a specially designed Verres needle. The **Verres needle** is a sharp hollow needle with a spring-loaded blunt tipped core designed to penetrate the abdominal wall with minimal risk of intra-abdominal organ injury. If proper Verres needle placement is difficult or if the patient has had prior abdominal surgery, safe access to the abdominal cavity can be achieved through a small fascial and peritoneal incision for direct visual placement of a Hasson cannula. This method avoids the "blind" puncture of the Verres needle, reducing the risk of misplacement or accidental puncture of intra-abdominal organs. Once the surgeon is confident of the Verres needle or Hasson cannula placement, CO_2 is insufflated to a maximum intraperitoneal pressure of 15 mm Hg.

After creation of the pneumoperitoneum, the second step is to place hollow ports or cannulas for telescope and instrument access through the abdominal wall. These ports must be strategically situated for ideal surgical exposure and instrument access. The telescope, which has a fiberoptic light source for illumination, is connected to television monitors for projection of the intra-abdominal image and visualization of the abdominal contents. If the diagnosis is not readily apparent after the initial inspection, a more thorough examination can be performed by placing additional ports to facilitate exposure. Satisfactory evaluation of the visceral and parietal peritoneal surfaces, liver, stomach, small bowel, colon, and pelvic organs can be achieved during routine diagnostic laparoscopy. If necessary, access to the retroperitoneum can be achieved to visualize the pancreas or retroperitoneal masses.

Prognosis

Refinements in video and instrument technology have helped make diagnostic laparoscopy an accepted procedure for the evaluation of abdominal pain, staging of malignant tumors, and evaluation of abdominal trauma. The overall accuracy of diagnostic laparoscopy in the evaluation of chronic or acute abdominal pain is reported to be 80–99%, reducing the need for exploratory laparotomy. When evaluating a patient for a malignant neoplasm, laparoscopy has proved useful in detecting small tumors (< 2 cm) that are undetectable by conventional radiographic modalities (eg, computed tomography and ultrasound). Up to 40% of patients with pancreatic or gastric malignancies have unsuspected peritoneal or liver metastases discovered by diagnostic laparoscopy.

In trauma, diagnostic laparoscopy may be superior to peritoneal lavage in the evaluation of abdominal injury. Although both laparoscopy and peritoneal lavage have 100% sensitivity in detecting major intra-abdominal injuries, the positive predictive value for therapeutic exploratory laparotomy has been reported to be 92% for laparoscopy compared with 72% for peritoneal lavage. Overall, the increased use of diagnostic laparoscopy has reduced the rate of unnecessary laparotomy, decreased morbidity, shortened hospital stays, decreased periods of disability, and lowered overall hospital costs.

MINIMALLY INVASIVE APPROACHES TO ESOPHAGEAL MOTILITY DISORDERS

General Considerations

Esophageal motility disorders represent a spectrum of disease states that range from absent peristalsis (**achalasia**) to hyperperistalsis (**diffuse esophageal spasm**). This array of disease processes can be further classified using a combination of clinical, radiographic, and manometric studies. Achalasia is the esophageal motility disorder most amenable to surgical treatment. It is a neuromuscular disorder of the esophagus associated with absence of the ganglion cells of Auerbach's plexus and characterized by the classic triad of dysphagia, regurgitation, and weight loss.

The distinguishing radiographic feature of achalasia on barium esophagogram is a dilated esophagus with a "bird's beak" taper at the esophagogastric junction. Typically, esophageal manometry studies reveal (1) lack of progressive peristalsis throughout the distal body of the esophagus, (2) a high-pressure lower esophageal sphincter, and (3) failure of the lower esophageal sphincter to relax with swallowing.

Thoracoscopic and Laparoscopic Heller Myotomy

Thoracoscopic Heller myotomy is an important new option in the treatment of achalasia. After the induction of general endotracheal anesthesia and double-lumen tracheal intubation, a fiberoptic endoscope is positioned in the esophagus transorally. The

esophageal endoscope serves three purposes in the operation. It allows: (1) rapid identification of the esophagus by transmural illumination, (2) accurate identification of the muscular and mucosal layers during the myotomy, and (3) accurate assessment of the length of the myotomy.

With the patient positioned in the right lateral decubitus position, five ports are introduced into the left chest. The left lung is retracted cephalad and the inferior pulmonary ligament is divided. Under transmural illumination by the endoscope, the esophagus is identified in the groove between the pericardium and the aorta. A longitudinal esophageal myotomy is created through the longitudinal and circular muscle layers (Figure 14–1). The caudad extension of the myotomy to the gastroesophageal junction must be accurately defined to relieve dysphagia, but not induce gastroesophageal reflux. The edges of the myotomy are separated by blunt dissection, so that approximately 40% of the circumference of the esophageal mucosa is visible. Lastly, a chest tube is placed through the lowest trocar site for overnight reexpansion of the left lung.

The laparoscopic Heller myotomy is an alternative to the thoracoscopic approach. In this technique, the patient is positioned supine with the legs extended on stirrups, allowing the surgeon to stand between them. After creation of the pneumoperitoneum, operating ports are placed into the upper abdomen. The left lobe of the liver is retracted anteriorly and the esophagus is exposed by division of the phrenoesophageal membrane. The esophageal Heller myotomy is performed similarly to that described for the thoracoscopic approach. Because of the improved visualization of the gastroesophageal junction with this approach, intraluminal endoscopy is usually not required. If necessary, an antireflux procedure, such as a partial fundoplication, can be performed in conjunction with the myotomy.

Postoperatively, relief of dysphagia is usually immediate, and oral feedings are started the day after surgery. Patients are typically discharged from the hospital within 2 days. In general, patients are pain-free at the time of discharge and are able to return to work within 1 week.

Prognosis

The minimally invasive approach to achalasia is equivalent to open surgery in terms of relief of dysphagia and postoperative manometry results. Significant benefits of the minimally invasive approach include shortened hospital stay and reduced disability time. The thoracoscopic esophageal myotomy is now the preferred initial approach in many patients with achalasia over other options, such as medical therapy, balloon dilatation, or open surgery. Currently, the thoracoscopic and laparoscopic treatments of other esophageal diseases—including diffuse esophageal spasm, nutcracker esophagus, epiphrenic diver-

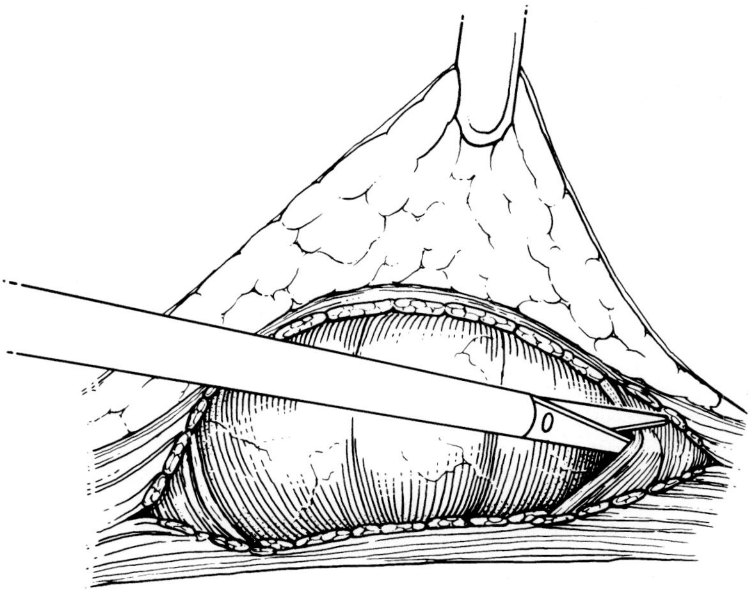

Figure 14–1. Thoracoscopic Heller myotomy. Through the left chest, the longitudinal and circular muscle fibers of the distal esophagus are divided, exposing the esophageal mucosa. The myotomy is carried distally 5 mm beyond the gastroesophageal junction.

ticula, and esophageal carcinoma—are under evaluation.

LAPAROSCOPIC TREATMENT FOR GASTROESOPHAGEAL REFLUX

General Considerations

Gastroesophageal reflux results from the abnormal entry of gastric contents into the esophagus, causing the classic symptoms of heartburn and regurgitation. This abnormal reflux is often due to an incompetent lower esophageal sphincter. Although symptoms of gastroesophageal reflux can be improved with H_2-receptor antagonists or, in more severe cases, omeprazole, the underlying pathophysiology is not corrected. Untreated gastroesophageal reflux can lead to serious complications, including esophagitis, stricture, bleeding, and aspiration. An important consideration is the pathophysiologic role of gastroesophageal reflux in the development of Barrett's metaplasia.

Advances in diagnostic techniques, including fiberoptic endoscopy, esophageal manometry, and 24-hour esophageal pH monitoring, allow selection of patients most likely to benefit from surgery. In addition, a recent large, controlled trial showed that surgery is more effective than medical therapy for control of symptoms, endoscopically detected esophagitis, and acid reflux, as measured by pH monitoring.

Laparoscopic Nissen Fundoplication

The primary goal of gastroesophageal reflux surgery is to reestablish the competency of the lower esophageal sphincter. The Nissen fundoplication is

the most commonly performed antireflux operation, and the laparoscopic Nissen results in an anatomic equivalent to the open operation.

After induction of general anesthesia and creation of the pneumoperitoneum, four abdominal ports are placed in the upper abdomen. The procedure begins with dissection of the diaphragmatic crura, followed by exposure of the gastric cardia and the lower esophagus. After repair of the crural defect, a 2-cm-long, 360-degree wrap of the upper stomach is made around the intra-abdominal segment of the esophagus (Figure 14–2). The wrap is loosely constructed over a 56-French bougie to avoid postoperative dysphagia or gas bloat syndrome.

Although this "floppy" Nissen fundoplication is the standard approach, the operation is tailored to the severity of reflux and the presence of associated pathology, such as defects in esophageal peristalsis or gastric emptying. In patients with defective peristalsis, a 270-degree wrap is more appropriate to prevent dysphagia. Patients with delayed gastric emptying benefit from concomitant pyloromyotomy.

Prognosis

Results of laparoscopic Nissen fundoplication, in terms of postoperative manometry and 24-hour pH monitoring, are equivalent to those achieved after traditional open Nissen fundoplication. Relief of heartburn is achieved in 80–90% of patients. Objective improvement in lower esophageal sphincter pressure and acid reflux, as measured by 24-hour pH monitoring, has been documented at the University of California, San Francisco (Figure 14–3). Postoperative recovery of patients undergoing laparoscopic Nissen fundoplication is dramatically rapid compared

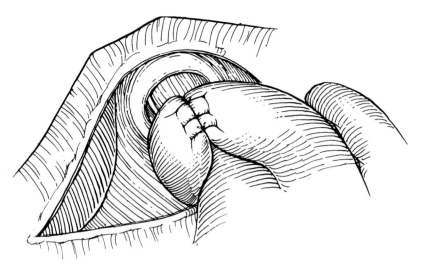

Figure 14–2. Laparoscopic Nissen fundoplication for gastroesophageal reflux. The hiatal hernia is repaired using crural sutures, and a 2-cm-long floppy, 360-degree wrap is constructed around the distal esophagus.

with those undergoing open fundoplication, with typical hospital stays of 1–2 days and resumption of full physical activity within 1 week.

LAPAROSCOPIC TREATMENT OF PEPTIC ULCER DISEASE

General Considerations

Peptic ulcer disease has traditionally been viewed as an imbalance between acid-pepsin secretion and mucosal defense. However, the management of pa-

tients with peptic ulcer disease is currently changing because of the increasing evidence of the pathogenic role of the novel organism, *Helicobacter pylori.* Today, surgery is reserved for the unusual patient refractory to antisecretory medications and eradication of *H pylori,* as well as those with complicated ulcer disease, including bleeding, perforation, and pyloric obstruction.

Laparoscopic Proximal Gastric Vagotomy

For the rare patient requiring elective surgery, lap-

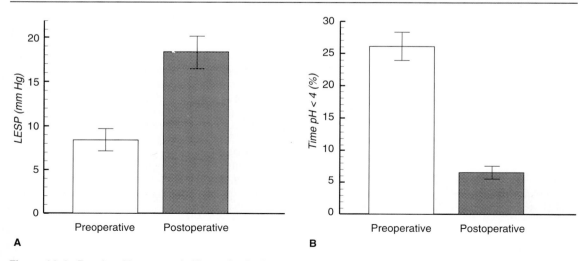

Figure 14–3. Results of laparoscopic Nissen fundoplication. In panel A, laparoscopic Nissen fundoplication results in a significant increase in lower esophageal sphincter pressure compared to preoperative values. In panel B, laparoscopic Nissen fundoplication results in a significant decrease in the percentage of time the esophagus has a pH less than 4, compared to preoperative values.

aroscopic proximal gastric vagotomy is recommended. This operation is anatomically equivalent to that performed during open surgery. The crucial elements include denervation of the distal 5 centimeters of the esophagus and proximal lesser curvature of the stomach, with preservation of the nerves to the pylorus and distal 6–7 centimeters of antrum (Figure 14–4). This procedure inhibits basal and vagally-mediated acid and pepsin secretion but preserves normal gastric emptying.

An alternative approach is the laparoscopic Taylor procedure, which includes a posterior truncal vagotomy and an anterior seromyotomy over the portion of the stomach containing the acid-secreting parietal cells.

Perforated duodenal ulcers are also amenable to laparoscopic treatment. The most common approach has been to combine simple closure of the perforation and placement of an omental patch. The laparoscopic approach allows a thorough lavage of the soiled peritoneal cavity. Some selected, stable patients with perforations are candidates for simultaneous proximal gastric vagotomy. Selected patients with gastric outlet obstruction due to peptic ulcer disease are candidates for laparoscopic truncal vagotomy and gastrojejunostomy. In this case, both vagal trunks are divided at the diaphragm and gastric drainage is achieved by a gastrojejunal anastomosis. The latter can be constructed with an endoscopic stapling device or by endoscopic suturing techniques.

Prognosis

The role of laparoscopic vagotomy in the management of patients with refractory ulcer disease is still under evaluation, however, the early results are encouraging. In two small series of patients treated for chronic duodenal ulcers, laparoscopic vagotomy resulted in appropriate reduction in basal and stimulated acid secretion, and low rates of recurrent ulceration. As with other laparoscopic procedures, recovery is rapid and postoperative disability is generally less than 1 week.

LAPAROSCOPIC APPROACH TO APPENDICITIS

General Considerations

Acute appendicitis remains a challenging clinical problem. Because there is no definitive preoperative diagnostic test, clinical judgement and surgical exploration remain the gold standard for the diagnosis of appendicitis. A number of diseases, however, are commonly mistaken for appendicitis, including gastroenteritis, pelvic inflammatory disease, ectopic pregnancy, urinary tract infection, renal calculi, and mesenteric adenitis. An overall negative exploration rate for suspected appendicitis of approximately 15% is currently accepted; this rate is as high as 34% in women of child-bearing age.

Clearly, an approach that reduces the need for open surgical exploration has merit. Ultrasonography is useful, especially in young women, either in identifying a clearly abnormal appendix or gynecologic pathology. Recent evidence suggests that diagnostic laparoscopy is highly accurate in the diagnosis and treatment of appendicitis. Developments in minimally invasive surgery have made laparoscopic appendectomy feasible.

Laparoscopic Appendectomy

After creation of the pneumoperitoneum, a single port is placed below the umbilicus for insertion of the laparoscope. Usually, the inflamed appendix is immediately evident in the normal anatomic position in the right lower quadrant. Rotational maneuvers and placement of accessory ports facilitate exposure of the difficult or retrocecal appendix. If the appendix is normal, a thorough laparoscopic exploration to identify other pathology is performed. Exposure and visualization of the abdominal cavity is usually superior to that achieved through a small right lower quadrant incision.

The technique for laparoscopic appendectomy is similar to that used in open surgery. The mesoappendix is dissected and the appendiceal artery is controlled with clips. The appendix is ligated near the cecum with loops of absorbable suture material, and then divided. Alternatively, the mesoappendiceal vessels and the appendix may be divided with a laparoscopic stapling device (Figure 14–5). The appendix is then placed into a plastic bag and withdrawn

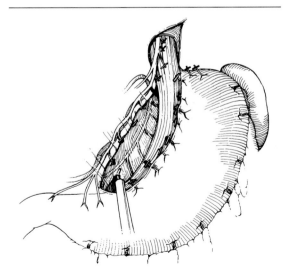

Figure 14–4. Laparoscopic proximal gastric vagotomy. The distal 5 cm of esophagus and the proximal stomach are denervated by dividing the anterior and posterior leaflets of the gastrohepatic ligament. The nerves of Laterjet innervating the antrum and pylorus are preserved.

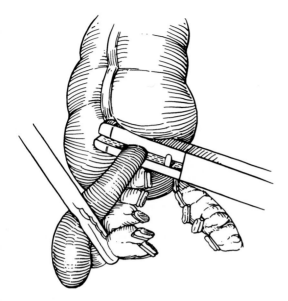

Figure 14–5. Laparoscopic appendectomy using a stapling device. Through a small suprapubic incision, a mechanical device divides the appendix between parallel rows of occluding staples.

through a trocar site, thus preventing contact of the infected appendix with the trocar incision. Postoperatively, patients generally do not require intravenous narcotic medication and are allowed oral feedings when hungry.

Prognosis

Laparoscopic appendectomy appears to have several advantages over open appendectomy. In three of four randomized controlled trials (Table 14–1), the laparoscopic approach to appendectomy resulted in fewer wound infections, and in two of these trials, shortened hospital stay. Although the postoperative results in terms of hospital stay, wound infections, and disability are not dramatically different, many surgeons now prefer the laparoscopic over the open approach because of the improved visualization of the abdomen and potential to diagnose and treat other disorders

that may be confused with appendicitis. Figure 14–6 summarizes an algorithm using this minimally invasive approach to patients with suspected appendicitis.

LAPAROSCOPIC APPROACH TO COLON RESECTION

General Considerations

Large organs, such as the colon, are more difficult to resect laparoscopically than small organs, such as the gallbladder and appendix. Technical problems include identification of the lesion, mobilization of a large organ, assurance of adequate resection margins, production of a watertight anastomosis, and removal of a large intra-abdominal specimen. Laparoscopic colectomy has been performed for cancer, diverticulitis, endometriosis, regional enteritis, villous adenoma, polyposis, and volvulus. Concern has been raised, however, about the adequacy of laparoscopic colon resection for cancer, and this issue is now the subject of a large, randomized, multicenter trial.

Laparoscopic Colon Resection

The first technical issue related to laparoscopic colon resection is identification of the lesion. Because of the limited tactile sensation afforded by minimally invasive techniques, small lesions such as tumors may not be detectable with the laparoscope. Preoperative localization of these lesions by barium enema, or intraoperative confirmation of lesion position via colonoscopy, is required. Once the colonic segment of interest is identified, it is mobilized and suspended for access to its mesentery. Mesenteric transection is accomplished with hemostatic clips, ligatures, or a stapling device.

Following mesenteric division, colonic resection and anastomosis is accomplished in one of two ways. Through a small incision, the colonic segment can be exteriorized, resected, and reanastomosed. This is termed **laparoscopic-assisted colectomy.** Alternatively, the colon can be divided and anastomosed intracorporeally, usually with the aid of mechanical stapling devices. With this technique, the specimen should be placed in a plastic bag to protect the

Table 14–1. Randomized controlled trials of laparoscopic versus open appendectomy.

Group (year)	Surgical Treatment	Number of Patients	Wound Infections (%)	Operating Time (min)	Post-op Stay (days)
Kum, et al (1993)	Laparoscopic	52	0*	43	3.2
	Open	57	9	40	4.2
Tate, et al (1993)	Laparoscopic	70	7	70*	3.5
	Open	70	10	47	3.6
McAnena, et al (1992)	Laparoscopic	29	4*	48	2.2*
	Open	37	11	52	4.8
Attwood, et al (1992)	Laparoscopic	30	0*	61	2.5*
	Open	32	12	51	3.8

*p<0.05 compared to open appendectomy.

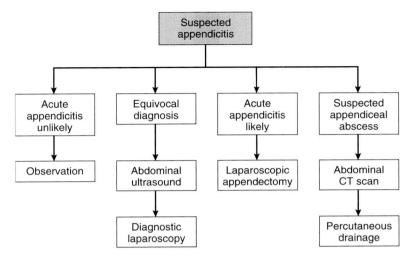

Figure 14–6. An approach to patients with suspected appendicitis.

wound edges during removal. After removal, the specimen must be immediately examined to ensure that adequate resection margins have been achieved. Finally, the anastomosis should be tested for integrity, either via direct inspection colonoscopically, or via instillation of air or fluid intraluminally.

Prognosis

Laparoscopic colectomy is relatively complicated compared with other minimally invasive gastrointestinal operations. Although virtually all colon resections, including right and left colectomy, low anterior resection, and abdominoperineal resection, can be performed with these techniques, at present they have limited practical applicability. For benign disease, the laparoscopic approach is technically difficult, time-consuming, and expensive compared to the equivalent open approach. Current data does not suggest that the morbidity or hospital stay is dramatically improved after laparoscopic colectomy, when compared to open colectomy.

It is not yet clear that an adequate cancer operation can be reliably performed laparoscopically. There have been several troubling reports of cancer recurrence at the trocar site. For now, laparoscopic colectomy is best performed in selected patients with benign disease or in the setting of prospective trials evaluating adequacy of a cancer operation.

LAPAROSCOPIC APPROACH TO CHOLECYSTECTOMY

General Considerations

Until recently, the open cholecystectomy for symptomatic gallstone disease was the treatment of choice, providing excellent results in terms of relief of symptoms and low mortality rates. However, laparoscopic cholecystectomy has emerged as the new standard approach to symptomatic gallstone disease, providing decreased postoperative pain, shorter hospital stays, and an earlier return to work compared to open surgery. With greater experience, it is now clear that patients with previous contraindications to laparoscopic cholecystectomy, including previous abdominal surgery, obesity, acute cholecystitis, and even pregnancy, can be handled safely with these minimally invasive techniques.

Laparoscopic Cholecystectomy

Laparoscopic cholecystectomy is usually performed under general anesthesia with special attention paid to muscle relaxation. After induction of anesthesia, bladder and nasogastric tubes are placed for decompression to prevent inadvertent injury to those organs. With the patient in the supine position, the abdomen is prepared with antiseptics and appropriately draped. Intravenous antibiotics are not routinely required for prophylaxis against wound infection in elective cases. Either sequential compression stockings or low-dose heparin are used in patients at high risk for deep venous thrombosis.

After satisfactory development of the pneumoperitoneum, an umbilical trocar is placed for the laparoscope, and three additional ports are placed in the right upper quadrant for exposure and dissecting instruments. The patient is then placed in reverse Trendelenburg position to improve exposure to the gallbladder. The assistant, standing on the patient's right side, elevates the gallbladder fundus to the diaphragm and retracts the infundibulum laterally, exposing the triangle of Calot. The surgeon, standing at the patient's left side, dissects the cystic artery and duct from the gallbladder wall down towards the porta hepatis. This is a crucial step, and special care must be taken to avoid mistaking the common bile duct for the cystic duct.

Once the anatomy is identified, a clip is placed across the cystic duct at its gallbladder origin and a small incision is made in the cystic duct for placement of a cholangiogram catheter. Cholangiography is performed fluoroscopically and is valuable both in confirming the ductal anatomy and excluding the presence of occult common bile duct stones. After completion of the cholangiogram, the cystic duct and artery are secured with metal clips and divided. The gallbladder is then dissected from the liver bed with electrocautery and delivered out of the umbilical or epigastric trocar site.

Postoperative management is straightforward. The bladder and nasogastric catheters are removed at the end of the procedure. A diet of clear liquids is offered the evening of surgery, and light solid foods are given the next morning. Selected patients may be treated on an outpatient basis. Overall, hospital stay averages 20 hours. Most patients require mild oral analgesics for several days; narcotic injections are rarely necessary to control pain. Patients are allowed to shower the day after surgery, with waterproof dressings in place. Full physical activity is resumed 1 week postoperatively, although patients may return to sedentary employment before this time.

Prognosis

Two recent randomized controlled trials examining hospital stay, pain, and work disability suggest that the laparoscopic approach is superior to open mini-cholecystectomy. A major concern, however, has been whether the incidence of bile duct injury with the laparoscopic approach is unacceptably high. Early in the introduction of laparoscopic cholecystectomy, the rate of bile duct injury appeared to be as much as ten-fold higher than the rate observed during open cholecystectomy. Data now, however, suggests that the average general surgeon can perform this operation with a risk of bile duct injury no greater than 0.2%. This rate does not differ from that observed after open cholecystectomy (Table 14–2). Patients with acute cholecystitis can now usually be managed

safely laparoscopically. In the presence of severe inflammation, however, the judicious surgeon will convert to an open approach.

LAPAROSCOPIC EXPLORATION OF THE COMMON BILE DUCT

General Considerations

Overall, choledocholithiasis is present in 10–15% of patients undergoing cholecystectomy. These stones usually have migrated from the gallbladder, but some form within the bile ducts. Common bile duct stones may cause the presenting symptoms (biliary colic, obstructive jaundice, or cholangitis) in patients with biliary tract disease; they may be silent but discovered at the time of operation for cholelithiasis, or they may become evident following cholecystectomy.

Diagnosis of common bile duct stones can be suggested by liver function tests and ultrasound, but the most accurate method is cholangiography (intraoperative, endoscopic, or percutaneous).

The natural history of asymptomatic common bile duct stones is unknown, but because of their potentially serious sequelae, they should be treated when discovered. Many patients with choledocholithiasis can be managed safely and successfully by endoscopic or percutaneous stone extraction. Surgery is appropriate in a number of clinical scenarios, and treatment must be individualized. New technologies allow extraction of common duct stones during the course of laparoscopic cholecystectomy. The relative safety, cost, and efficacy of this approach compares favorably to alternative treatments.

Laparoscopic Common Bile Duct Exploration

Common bile duct stones may be approached laparoscopically through either the cystic duct (**transcystic access**) or the common bile duct (**choledochotomy**). The first step in transcystic access to the common bile duct is cystic duct dilatation via a balloon-tipped catheter. Direct choledochoscopy is then performed with a miniaturized flexible telescope.

Table 14–2. Comparison of laparoscopic and open cholecystectomy.

Group	Years Encompassed	Number of Patients	Mortality Rate (%)	Common Duct Injury Rate (%)	Conversion Rate (%)	Post-op Stay (days)
Laparoscopic cholecystectomy						
Southern Surgeons	1990–1991	1,518	0.07	0.50	4.7	1.2
European	1989–1991	1,236	0	0.30	3.6	3.0
Louisville	1989–1991	1,983	0.10	0.25	4.5	2.1
Canadian	1990–1991	2,201	0	0.14	4.3	—
Open cholecystectomy						
Roslyn JJ, et al	1989	42,474	0.17	0.20	NA	4
Morgenstern L, et al	1982–1988	1,200	1.80	0.17	NA	5–7
Bredesen J, et al	1977–1981	13,854	1.20	—	NA	—

Stones are entrapped with baskets under direct vision and extracted retrograde through the cystic duct. Larger stones may require mechanical lithotripsy for removal. For proximal biliary stones and larger stones that cannot be removed by the transcystic route, a choledochotomy is made for insertion of a large choledochoscope that can be directed anterograde or retrograde. After stone removal, the choledochotomy is closed over a rubber T-tube with absorbable, monofilament suture using intracorporeal suturing techniques.

Prognosis

Laparoscopic clearance of common bile duct stones can be accomplished, in expert hands, in up to 95% of patients. The postoperative convalescence of patients undergoing laparoscopic transcystic common bile duct exploration is no different from those undergoing laparoscopic cholecystectomy alone. When laparoscopic cholodochotomy and T-tube placement are performed, hospital stay is somewhat longer, and the T-tube must be removed at a later date. Decisions regarding approaches to common duct stones are best based on the clinical scenario, the patient's overall condition, and the expertise of the treating physicians (Figure 14–7). Endoscopic retrograde cholangiopancreatography and endoscopic sphincterotomy offer effective minimally invasive approaches to common bile duct stones in medical centers where expertise in laparoscopic common bile duct exploration is lacking.

LAPAROSCOPIC APPROACH TO PANCREATIC CANCER

Role of Laparoscopy

An important advance in the management of patients with pancreatic cancer is the use of diagnostic laparoscopy for accurate staging of the extent of the disease. Diagnostic laparoscopy allows direct visualization and biopsy of capsular hepatic metastases and peritoneal implants. Diagnostic laparoscopy and computed tomography (CT) are complementary staging procedures. Today, approximately 60% of patients thought to have resectable pancreatic cancer on radiographic grounds are found to have metastases at the time of laparotomy. Minimally invasive surgery is currently playing an important role in the management of patients with pancreatic cancer. The goals of minimally invasive surgery are to accurately identify patients who will not benefit from pancreatectomy, and to effectively palliate those with biliary or pancreatic obstruction.

Patients with pancreatic cancer can be broadly categorized into one of three groups. First, a large number of patients are found, at radiographic staging, to have metastatic disease and are not candidates for cu-

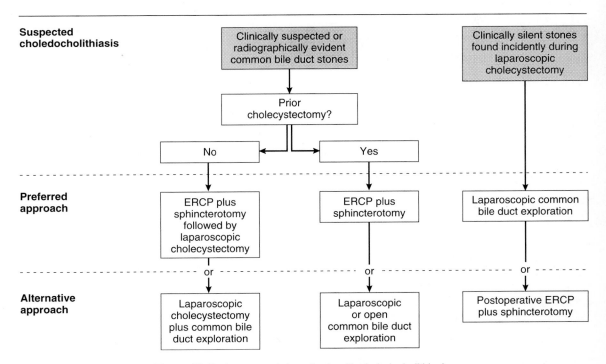

Figure 14–7. An approach to patients with choledocholithiasis.

rative pancreatectomy. These patients, however, may require palliation of bile duct obstruction and, in some cases, gastric outlet obstruction. A second group of patients have no radiographic evidence of metastases by CT, but are found at laparotomy to have small hepatic metastases or peritoneal implants. These patients are not suitable for pancreatectomy, but may benefit from palliative bypass procedures. The third group of patients have cancer limited to the pancreas and are candidates for potentially curative resection. With this staging approach, the morbidity and disability of nontherapeutic exploratory laparotomy is avoided.

Patients with bile duct obstruction from unresectable pancreatic cancer can be palliated in one of three ways. Patients with radiographic evidence of metastatic pancreatic cancer are best treated with endoscopic or percutaneous biliary stenting. A smaller number of patients found to have metastatic disease at the time of laparoscopy benefit from laparoscopic cholecystojejunostomy or choledochojejunostomy. In patients with concomitant duodenal obstruction, laparoscopic gastrojejunostomy is performed. This approach is summarized in Figure 14–8.

Recently, the results of open radical resection of pancreatic cancer have improved, both in terms of decreased operative morbidity and mortality and increased cure rates. Although laparoscopic pancreatectomy has been reported, at present this technique has limited applicability and open radical re-

section of the pancreas is still recommended for curative intent.

LAPAROSCOPIC APPROACHES TO OTHER GASTROINTESTINAL DISEASES

Laparoscopic Approach to Nonparasitic Liver Cysts

Nonparasitic liver cysts are largely asymptomatic and seldom produce functional abnormality of the liver. They can be solitary, multiple, or diffuse in the liver, as in polycystic liver disease. Asymptomatic liver cysts, whether solitary or diffuse, require no treatment. However, some become large, leading to palpable hepatomegaly and abdominal discomfort. These symptomatic patients are candidates for surgical treatment.

Today, laparoscopic fenestration of symptomatic liver cysts is the preferred approach for most patients. After induction of general anesthesia and creation of the pneumoperitoneum, diagnostic laparoscopy is performed and the liver cyst or cysts are identified. The roof of each cyst is widely excised by electrocautery and the excised cyst wall is sent for histologic examination. More than 90% of patients with solitary cysts have improved symptoms after this procedure. Patients with multiple, small cysts throughout the liver have a much higher rate of recurrence of symptoms after surgery. Laparoscopic

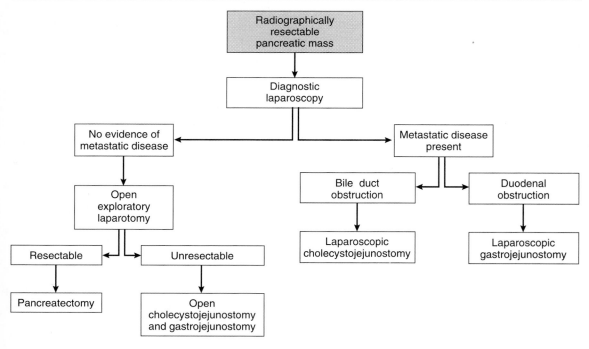

Figure 14–8. An approach to patients with pancreatic cancer.

treatment of liver cysts should be reserved for patients with symptomatic large or solitary cysts.

Laparoscopic Approach to Pancreatic Pseudocysts

Patients who are candidates for internal drainage of pancreatic pseudocysts, particularly those in whom cystogastrostomy is considered, are candidates for a novel, minimally invasive approach. In this operation, ports are placed percutaneously into the stomach, which is distended with gas, exposing the pseudocyst behind the posterior gastric wall. A cystogastrostomy is then created under direct vision with débridement of the pseudocyst cavity and, if necessary, biopsy of the cyst wall to exclude neoplasm. Only a small number of these procedures have been performed to date, however, the preliminary results are promising.

LAPAROSCOPIC APPROACHES TO OTHER ABDOMINAL CONDITIONS

Laparoscopic Splenectomy

A laparoscopic approach to diseases related to solid organs, such as the spleen and liver, has lagged behind operations on hollow organs because of problems related to hemostasis and extraction of the specimen. Recent experience suggests that these problems may not be insurmountable. Laparoscopic splenectomy, for example, is feasible for indications such as immune thrombocytopenic purpura (ITP). Splenectomy appears to increase platelet survival in these patients by removing both a potential source of antibody production and the major organ of platelet sequestration and destruction.

Technically, the laparoscopic splenectomy is performed with the patient in low lithotomy position with the surgeon standing between the patient's legs. Children may be approached supine with the surgeon on the patient's right. A 30-degree telescope provides excellent visualization of the operative field. Fan retractors and Babcock clamps aid in retraction of the liver, stomach, and omentum. The hilar vessels are most expeditiously controlled with an endoscopic vascular stapler, however, division between laparoscopic ties and suture ligatures is possible. Short gastric vessels are controlled with clips. Extraction of the spleen is accomplished by morcellation within a plastic bag. Special care must be taken to avoid intraabdominal spillage of splenocytes because splenosis or recurrent ITP may develop.

It is not yet clear that laparoscopic splenectomy will supplant the open approach for the average patient with ITP, but early results are encouraging. As with other minimally invasive operations, the main advantages of the laparoscopic approach to splenectomy are reduced patient discomfort, reduced postoperative disability, and minimal scarring.

Laparoscopic Inguinal Hernia Repair

Laparoscopic inguinal hernia repair is performed with the use of general anesthesia and three laparoscopic ports. After the hernia is visualized, the peritoneum overlying the inguinal floor is incised and, along with the peritoneal sac, is elevated from the underlying structures. A large sheet of prosthetic mesh is placed over the entire myopectineal orifice and secured with sutures or staples. The peritoneum is then closed to reduce the frequency of postoperative adhesions to the mesh. Alternatively, an extraperitoneal approach is feasible, confining the CO_2 insufflation and port placement to the preperitoneal space. Although this approach is technically more difficult, this method avoids the risks associated with laparoscopy, including intestinal perforation and adhesion formation.

Recent studies suggest that patients undergoing laparoscopic hernia repair have decreased postoperative pain and an earlier return to full activity compared with those undergoing standard open repair. However, since most hernia recurrences develop after 5 years, the long-term integrity of the laparoscopic hernia repair will not be known for some time. Other pertinent factors concerning the efficacy of the laparoscopic hernia repair include the risks of general anesthesia, the risks of laparoscopy, and the potential increase in cost. Whether the improvements in postoperative pain and earlier return to full activity offset the potential risks and costs of laparoscopic hernia repair is unknown at this time. Laparoscopic hernia repair should probably remain limited, at this time, to patients with bilateral hernias or recurrent unilateral hernias.

Laparoscopic Approach to Gastrostomy and Feeding Jejunostomy

For patients requiring access for enteral feeding, the preferred initial approach is percutaneous endoscopic gastrostomy (PEG). Some patients, however, do not tolerate gastrostomy feedings secondary to aspiration, and in others the procedure cannot be performed safely due to technical reasons. These patients are candidates for laparoscopic placement of gastrostomy or feeding jejunostomy catheters.

With minimally invasive techniques, feeding catheters are introduced into the gut lumen through the gastric or jejunal wall. Laparoscopic T-fasteners aid in the placement and security of the feeding catheters. These laparoscopic procedures are equivalent to their open surgical counterparts, except that the painful, disabling laparotomy incision is avoided. For patients with neurologic impairment and severe gastroesophageal reflux, a fundoplication procedure can be added to reduce the risk of aspiration.

REFERENCES

Alexander RJT, Jaques BC, Mitchell KG: Laparoscopic assisted colectomy and wound recurrence. Lancet 1993;341:249.

Attwood SEA et al: A prospective randomized trial of laparoscopic versus open appendectomy. Surgery 1992; 112:497.

Bailey RW, Zucker KA: Laparoscopic management of peptic ulcer disease. In: *Surgical Laparoscopy Update.* Zucker KA (editor). Quality Medical, 1993.

Barkun JS, Barkun AN, Meakins JL: Laparoscopic versus open cholecystomy: The Canadian experience. Am J Surg 1993;165:455.

Bittner HB, Pappas TN: Laparoscopic approaches to symptomatic gastroesophageal reflux. Seminars in Gastrointestinal Disease 1994;5:113.

Bredesen J et al: Early postoperative mortality following cholecystectomy in the entire female population of Denmark, 1977-1981. World J Surg 1992;16:530.

Cuschieri A et al: Diagnosis of significant abdominal trauma after road accidents: Preliminary results of a multicentre clinical trial comparing minilaparoscopy with peritoneal lavage. Ann R Coll Surg Engl 1988;70:153.

Cuschieri A et al: The European experience with laparoscopic cholecystectomy. Am J Surg 1991;161:385.

Deziel DJ et al: Complications of laparoscopic cholecystectomy: A national survey of 4,292 hospitals and an analysis of 77,604 cases. Am J Surg 1993;165:9.

Duh QY, Way LW: Laparoscopic jejunostomy using T-fasteners as retractors and anchors. Arch Surg 1993;128:105.

Fusco MA, Paluzzi MW: Abdominal wall recurrence after laparoscopic-assisted colectomy for adenocarcinoma of the colon: report of a case. Dis Colon Rectum 1993;36:858.

Gross E, Bancewicz J, Ingram G: Assessment of gastric cancer by laparoscopy. Br Med J 1984;288:1577.

Hunter JG, Soper NJ: Laparoscopic management of common bile duct stones. Surg Clin North Am 1992;72:1077.

Katkhouda N, Mouiel J: A new technique of surgical treatment of chronic duodenal ulcer without laparotomy by videocoelioscopy. Am J Surg 1991;161:361.

Kum CK et al: Randomized controlled trial comparing laparoscopic and open appendicectomy. Br J Surg 1993;80:1599.

Larson GM et al: Multipractice analysis of laparoscopic cholecystectomy in 1983 patients. Am J Surg 1992;163:221.

Lefor AT et al: Laparoscopic splenectomy in the management of immune thrombocytopenia purpura. Surgery 1992;114:613.

Litwin DE et al: Laparoscopic cholecystectomy: Trans-Canada experience with 2201 cases. Can J Surg 1992;35:291.

McAnena OJ et al: Laparoscopic versus open appendicectomy: A prospective evaluation. Br J Surg 1992;79:818.

McKernan JB, Laws HL: Laparoscopic repair of inguinal hernias using a totally extraperitoneal prosthetic approach. Surg Endosc 1993;7:26.

McMahon AJ et al: Laparoscopic versus minilaparotomy cholecystectomy: a randomised trial. Lancet 1994;343: 135.

Monson JRT et al: Prospective evaluation of laparoscopic-assisted colectomy in an unselected group of patients. Lancet 1992;340:831.

Morgenstern L, Wong L, Berci G: Twelve hundred open cholecystectomies before the laparoscopic era. A standard for comparison. Arch Surg 1992;127:400.

Morino M et al: Laparoscopic management of symptomatic nonparasitic cysts of the liver. Ann Surg 1994;219:157.

Mulvihill SJ: Laparoscopic management of gallstone disease. Seminars in Gastrointestinal Diseases 1994;5:120.

Nagy AG, James D: Diagnostic laparoscopy. Am J Surg 1989;157:490.

Patti MG, Pellegrini CA: Minimally invasive approaches to achalasia. Seminars in Gastrointestinal Diseases 1994;5: 108.

Pellegrini C et al: Thoracoscopic esophagomyotomy: Initial experience with a new approach for the treatment of achalasia. Ann Surg 1992;216:291.

Petelin JB: Laparoscopic approach to common duct pathology. Am J Surg 1993;165:487.

Phillips EH et al: Laparoscopic colectomy. Ann Surg 1992;216:703.

Poulin E et al: Laparoscopic splenectomy: Clinical experience and the role of preoperative splenic artery embolization. Surg Laparosc Endosc 1993;3:445.

Reddick EJ, Olsen DO: Laparoscopic laser cholecystectomy: A comparison with mini-lap cholecystectomy. Surg Endosc 1989;3:131.

Roslyn JJ et al: Open cholecystectomy. A contemporary analysis of 42,474 patients. Ann Surg 1993;218:129.

Shima S, Banting S, Cuschieri A: Laparoscopy in the management of pancreatic cancer: Endoscopic cholecystojejunostomy for advanced disease. Br J Surg 1992;79:317.

Soper NJ, Brunt LM, Kerbl K: Laparoscopic general surgery. N Engl J Med 1994;330:409.

Spechler SJ, and the Department of Veteran Affairs Gastroesophageal Reflux Disease Study Group: Comparison of medical and surgical therapy for complicated gastroesophageal reflux disease in veterans. N Engl J Med 1992;326:786.

Stoker DL et al: Laparoscopic versus open inguinal hernia repair: Randomized prospective trial. Lancet 1994;343: 1243.

Tate JJJ et al: Laparoscopic versus open appendicectomy: Prospective randomised trial. Lancet 1993;342:633.

Taylor TV et al: Anterior lesser curve seromyotomy with posterior truncal vagotomy in the treatment of chronic duodenal ulcer. Lancet 1982;2:846.

The Southern Surgeons Club: A prospective analysis of 1518 laparoscopic cholecystectomies. N Engl J Med 1991;324:1073.

Warshaw AL, Gu ZY, Wittenberg AC: Preoperative staging and assessment of resectability of pancreatic cancer. Arch Surg 1990;125:230.

Zucker KA, Bailey RW: Laparoscopic truncal and selective vagotomy for intractable ulcer disease. Seminars in Gastrointestinal Disease 1994;5:128.

Imaging Studies in Gastrointestinal & Liver Diseases

15

Judy Yee, MD

There have been important technological advances in the field of radiology in the past 5 years that have impacted significantly on imaging of gastrointestinal and liver diseases. This is a review of the various conventional and state-of-the-art imaging modalities available for gastroenterologic diagnosis. There is an initial presentation of the contrast media available for fluoroscopic gastrointestinal examinations along with their practical applications.

CONTRAST MEDIA FOR GASTROINTESTINAL EXAMINATIONS

Barium sulfate is the most commonly used contrast media for opacification of the gastrointestinal tract during fluoroscopy. The selected agent should allow for maximal diagnostic information while posing the least risk to the patient. The clinical history and condition of each patient will determine the appropriate selection of a contrast agent.

BARIUM SULFATE

Barium sulfate is an inert substance that is mixed with water to form a suspension. The weight-to-weight (w/w) and weight-to-volume (w/v) systems are used to describe the dilution. In general, high-density barium (85% w/w or 250% w/v) is used for double-contrast studies and low-density barium (50% w/w or 80% w/v) is used for single-contrast examinations. Barium sulfate provides the best contrast and anatomic detail during fluoroscopy and therefore yields the most diagnostic information.

Risks

If barium leaks into the peritoneal cavity, barium peritonitis occurs. Patients will exhibit signs of acute peritonitis; eventually, granulomas and scarring with adhesions will form. If barium leaks into the mediastinum, an inflammatory reaction occurs that may evolve into scarring and fibrosis; this process is less pronounced than in the peritoneal cavity.

Aspiration of barium into the lungs is usually of minimal clinical significance unless the quantity is large or the patient has significant lung disease. Barium itself is inert and nonirritating to the lungs. Barium has been used in the past for bronchography without complications.

Oral barium should never be given above a colonic obstruction because inspissation will occur. If colonic obstruction is a possibility, a single-contrast barium enema must be performed first.

IODINATED (WATER-SOLUBLE) CONTRAST AGENTS

Iodinated contrast agents used for opacification of the gastrointestinal tract—meglumine diatrizoate and diatrizoate sodium—are water-soluble. These agents provide less contrast and reduced anatomic detail compared to barium and are therefore the second choice as contrast agents, based on diagnostic criteria. Iodinated contrast agents may be ionic (less expensive) or non-ionic (more expensive).

Risks

There is no risk of chemical peritonitis if iodinated contrast material is spilled into the peritoneal cavity, because it will be absorbed. There may be risk of infection when there is contamination from the gastrointestinal tract.

The ionic iodinated contrast material that is most

often used in clinical practice is hyperosmolar; its aspiration into the lungs causes a significant risk of chemical pneumonitis and pulmonary edema that may be intractable. Newer non-ionic iodinated contrast agents are more iso-osmolar and pose less of a risk when aspirated. However, these agents are more expensive than ionic iodinated contrast material and are not routinely used for opacification of the gastrointestinal tract.

Hyperosmolar iodinated contrast agents may also cause intraluminal movement of fluid, resulting in hypovolemia in children, debilitated patients, or patients with electrolyte imbalances.

PRACTICAL APPLICATIONS

- If a study is being obtained to evaluate for an esophageal perforation, then the study should be initially performed with a small amount of water-soluble contrast media. If no perforation is identified, the study is then repeated with barium.
- If a patient has signs, symptoms, or a history suggestive of an abdominal gastrointestinal tract perforation, water-soluble contrast should be used. (Examples: perforated duodenal ulcer, perforated colon, anastomotic leak in the immediate postoperative period.)
- If a patient's condition or history suggests a risk of aspiration* or esophago-respiratory fistula, barium should be used. Alternatively, at some institutions non-ionic iodinated agents are administered. (Examples: patients with (1) depressed mental status who cannot reliably protect their airway, (2) dysfunction of oropharyngeal swallowing mechanism, (3) upper esophageal injury with edema, (4) esophageal obstruction, or (5) gastric outlet obstruction.)
- In patients at risk for aspiration in whom a perforated ulcer is suspected, contrast should not be given unless exceptional circumstances exist. In select cases, water-soluble contrast may be carefully administered under fluoroscopic guidance into the stomach via nasogastric tube. At the end of the study, the remaining contrast should be removed from the stomach via nasogastric tube to prevent aspiration.
- Most radiologists prefer to wait at least 24 hours following endoscopic biopsy before performing a contrast study of the gastrointestinal tract.
- If there is clinical suspicion of bowel perforation following colonoscopy, CT of the abdomen and pelvis with the administration of diluted water-soluble contrast per rectum may be more sensitive than conventional enema with diatrizoate sodium.

---

*A patient's aspiration risk may be assessed by initially giving a small sip of water to see if this induces coughing or choking.

IMAGING MODALITIES

PLAIN FILM

Chest X-ray

An erect chest x-ray should be obtained in the setting of acute abdomen. This is the plain film study of choice for detection of pneumoperitoneum and can also be used to evaluate for chest pathology—such as basilar pneumonias—as the cause of abdominal pain.
Cost: $135–$170

Plain Film of the Abdomen (kidney, ureter, bladder [KUB])

The symptom of abdominal pain does not mandate an abdominal film. Clinical judgment and suspected diagnoses in each case should determine if a patient will benefit from an abdominal film. Each film should be examined for abnormal air collections, calcifications, fluid, organomegaly, masses, and foreign bodies, and the bowel gas pattern should be evaluated. The most commonly obtained abdominal film is the supine view. An upright view of the abdomen may be helpful in cases of intestinal obstruction. The left lateral decubitus view may be used for suspected pneumoperitoneum in acutely ill patients when the upright view cannot be obtained.

Pneumoperitoneum is most commonly due to recent abdominal surgery. Persistent or increasing amounts of free air after 3–7 days suggests the possibility of a leaking surgical anastomosis. Perforated peptic ulcer is the second most common cause of pneumoperitoneum. Approximately 80% of perforated ulcers are located in the duodenum, and about 80% of perforated ulcers will result in sufficient free air that is detectable by plain film.

Other causes of pneumoperitoneum include perforation of an abdominal gastrointestinal tract neoplasm or diverticulum (Meckel's or sigmoid diverticulitis), perforated appendix, and traumatic or iatrogenic perforation following an endoscopy or enema. Extension of air from the chest or retroperitoneum, or through the female genital tract, are other sources of free intraperitoneal air. Rarely, abscess rupture can result in pneumoperitoneum. In addition to the presence of air under the diaphragm, other radiographic evidence of pneumoperitoneum includes (1) **Rigler's sign** (outline of the inner and outer intestinal wall), (2) **football sign** (large ovoid air collection), (3) outline of the falciform ligament, (4) triangle of air seen between bowel loops, (5) perihepatic air, (6) **urachus sign** (outline of the middle umbilical ligament), and (7) **inverted V sign** (outline of the lateral umbilical ligaments).

Pneumoretroperitoneum may be seen as air outlining the kidneys or as streaks of air following the course of the psoas muscles. Causes include perforated duodenal ulcer or traumatic duodenal rupture, dissection of mediastinal air, or trauma or infection of the urinary tract.

Pneumatosis intestinalis, or gas within the bowel wall, may be primary or secondary. Primary or idiopathic pneumatosis is usually benign and most often involves the descending colon and sigmoid. About 85% of cases are secondary and may be due to intestinal ischemia (mesenteric arterial or venous thrombosis or decreased flow), bowel obstruction, trauma, infection, inflammatory bowel disease, connective tissue disorders, and chronic obstructive pulmonary disease. Primary pneumatosis appears radiographically as clusters of radiolucent cysts along the contour of the bowel wall. More linear collections of gas paralleling the wall of the bowel are seen with secondary pneumatosis. Small bowel involvement is more common with the secondary form.

Abnormal gas collections may also be contained within abscesses. Common locations of intra-abdominal abscesses include the subphrenic space, lesser sac, Morison's pouch, and pouch of Douglas. Hepatic, splenic, and pancreatic abscesses may also contain air. Necrotic tumor containing air may suggest a fistulous tract to the bowel. Emphysematous cholecystitis can be diagnosed if gas is seen outlining the gallbladder wall or within the gallbladder lumen. It occurs more commonly in diabetics and is thought to be due to ischemic changes of the gallbladder initiated by obstruction of the cystic duct by a stone.

Gas in the portal venous system is an ominous sign and is usually associated with mesenteric vascular thrombosis with associated intestinal ischemia and necrosis. This leads to the development of intramural gas and subsequent extension of gas through mesenteric veins to the portal vein. Gas in the portal venous system follows centrifugal portal venous flow and will appear as branching tubular lucencies extending into the liver periphery.

Gas in the biliary system may result from prior sphincterotomy or surgery, eg, choledochoenterostomy. It may also be seen with biliary-enteric fistula as a result of penetrating duodenal ulcer. Scarring of the ampulla owing to Crohn's disease, parasitic infection, or malignancy are other causes of pneumobilia. Rarely, biliary sepsis resulting from gas-producing bacteria can cause biliary tract gas. Biliary gas appears as centrally located tubular lucencies as it follows biliary drainage into the larger bile ducts.

Abnormal calcifications may also be detected on the abdominal film. Lamellated calcifications in the right upper quadrant are typical for gallstones. Only 10% of gallstones are radiopaque whereas 90% of urinary tract calculi are radiopaque. Porcelain gallbladder describes sheet-like wall calcifications of the gallbladder and is associated with a high incidence of gallbladder carcinoma, for which prophylactic chole-

cystectomy is recommended. A focal calcification in the right lower abdomen may represent an appendicolith, which is seen in 10–15% of patients with acute appendicitis. Mucocele of the appendix may appear as circular or rim calcification in the same location. Enteroliths may also be found in small or large bowel diverticula. Infections such as tuberculosis or *Pneumocystis carinii* can cause visceral or nodal calcifications. Alternatively, calcified lymph nodes may represent metastatic tumoral involvement. Certain tumors more commonly calcify. Mucinous adenocarcinoma of the stomach, colon, and ovary can cause mottled or punctate calcifications in the primary tumor as well as in metastatic foci. Gastrointestinal tract leiomyomas and lipomas may also calcify. Pancreatic calcifications more commonly occur in association with chronic pancreatitis or pancreatic pseudocyst. Pancreatic tumors that calcify include the rare serous cystadenoma and mucinous cystic neoplasm.

Ascitic fluid initially accumulates in the pelvis, where symmetric bulges of increased density ("dog ears") may be seen on either side of the bladder. Thickening of the peritoneal flank stripe and increased distance (> 3 mm) between the properitoneal fat and ascending colon are seen. With increased ascites, the right inferolateral margin of the liver becomes obscured and there is medial displacement of the liver and of the ascending and descending colon. With marked ascites there is diffuse haziness or ground-glass appearance of the abdomen, and bowel loops may appear to separate or float centrally.

The **pattern of bowel dilatation** on the abdominal film can suggest adynamic ileus versus mechanical bowel obstruction. The radiographic pattern of **adynamic ileus** is uniform dilatation of both small and large bowel with gas present in the rectum. Clinically, the abdomen is distended and bowel sounds are decreased or absent. Adynamic ileus is common after abdominal surgery but may also be caused by peritonitis, hypokalemia, metabolic disorders, trauma, mesenteric ischemia, and various medications, such as morphine and barbiturates. Localized ileus in which there is an isolated loop of dilated bowel (**sentinel loop**) is due to an adjacent acute inflammatory process. Pancreatitis can cause dilatation of the proximal small bowel and transverse colon whereas appendicitis will cause dilatation of the cecum and distal ileum.

Mechanical small or large bowel obstruction will cause dilatation of bowel proximal to the level of obstruction. The contour of dilated bowel is also examined for evidence of thickening or of thumbprinting, which is suggestive of ischemia. Bowel obstruction at two different sites produces a closed loop obstruction. The appearance of air-fluid levels at the same level suggests an ileus, whereas air-fluid levels of different heights is compatible with mechanical obstruction (Figure 15–1).

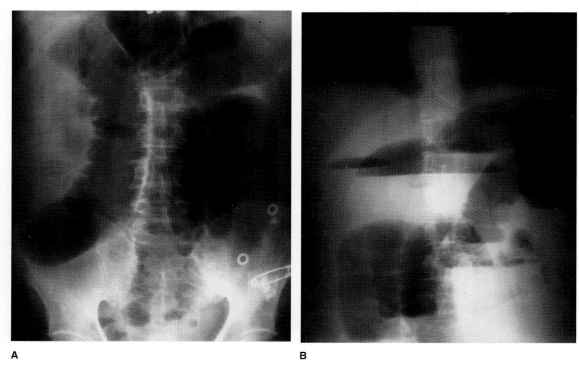

A   B

Figure 15–1. **A:** Supine plain film of the abdomen demonstrates multiple air-filled, markedly dilated small bowel loops with relative paucity of colonic air. **B:** Upright film of the abdomen in the same patient demonstrates air-fluid levels of different heights, consistent with mechanical small bowel obstruction. At surgery, adhesions were found in the distal ileum, causing obstruction.

Adhesions, incarcerated hernia, tumor, and inflammatory bowel disease are common causes of small bowel obstruction. Colon carcinoma and diverticulitis are the most common causes of large bowel obstruction. Occasionally it may be unclear as to whether an obstruction is at the level of the distal small bowel or ascending colon. A barium enema should be the initial study before administering barium orally. Obstruction from a sigmoid volvulus produces a distinctive inverted U-shaped dilated sigmoid, which is a type of closed loop obstruction (Figure 15–2). A contrast enema typically reveals a beak-like tapering of the contrast column at the site of mesenteric twist.

Cost: $160–$210.

DEGLUTITION STUDY

The **deglutition study** is an assessment of swallowing function. The oropharyngeal phase of swallowing is a complex but organized series of events that transports a bolus from the oral cavity to the upper esophageal sphincter (cricopharyngeus). After relaxation of the cricopharyngeus, the bolus passes into the cervical esophagus and is propelled by peristalsis down the thoracic esophagus and into the stomach.

Regulation of the swallowing mechanism is mediated by cranial nerves: (V) trigeminal, (VII) facial, (IX) glossopharyngeal, (X) vagus, and (XII) hypoglossal, all of which are involved with innervation of the intrinsic pharyngeal muscles. Support muscles are innervated by the accessory (XI) nerve and the first three cervical nerves.

The ingested bolus is transported from the mouth posteriorly into the oropharynx as swallowing starts. Pharyngeal peristalsis continues propulsion of the bolus through the hypopharynx. The larynx closes and elevates as the epiglottis deflects.

A. Indications: Impairment of the oropharyngeal swallowing mechanism can produce symptoms such as coughing, choking, dysphagia, regurgitation, and hoarseness. Aspiration pneumonia may be the initial sign of swallowing dysfunction. Symptoms often are nonspecific, and the patient may complain of a symptom distant from the actual location of a lesion. Patients with mid or distal esophageal mechanical obstruction may present with referred pharyngeal or cervical dysphagia.

Oropharyngeal dysphagia may be caused by structural lesions (head and neck tumors, webs, diverticula), diseases of the central nervous system (cerebrovascular accident [CVA], neoplasms, poliomyelitis, extrapyramidal disease), muscle disor-

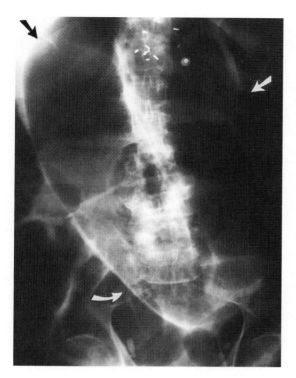

Figure 15–2. Large bowel obstruction due to a sigmoid volvulus. Air-filled dilated sigmoid has a distinctive inverted U-shaped appearance *(arrows)*. This is a type of closed loop obstruction. Beak-like tapering is typically seen on contrast enema.

ders (polymyositis, dermatomyositis), and myasthenia gravis.

The deglutition study is a cooperative study performed by the radiologist and speech pathologist. During the study, patients are instructed to ingest barium liquids of various consistencies as well as barium-coated solids. If the patient demonstrates swallowing difficulty, various compensatory maneuvers may be attempted to relieve symptoms. The entire study is performed under fluoroscopy and is videotaped. This provides a dynamic recording of each phase of swallowing that can be reviewed frame-by-frame for complete evaluation.

B. Cost: $500 (combined fee).

ESOPHAGRAM (BARIUM SWALLOW)

A complete esophagram consists of an evaluation of the oral cavity, pharynx, and esophagus. Although more extensive radiographic evaluation of oropharyngeal function is usually performed in a formal deglutition study, gross imaging of this area during the esophagram can detect significant motility abnormalities. Mass lesions of the oral cavity, however,

are not easily identified on barium study unless they are large.

Biphasic barium radiography of the esophagus using both single- and double-contrast techniques is the preferred method for evaluation of the esophagus. The advantages of each technique are discussed in the following sections.

Single Contrast

A. Indications: The single-contrast technique is used to study both the pharynx and the esophagus. Pharyngeal contour and distensibility are well demonstrated and webs, pharyngeal pouches, and Zenker's diverticulum can be detected. The single-contrast phase of the esophagram provides information on esophageal motility as well as esophageal contour and distension. Primary peristalsis is stimulated by the swallowing process and propels the bolus down the esophagus into the stomach. Secondary peristalsis is stimulated by focal distension, such as that due to residual bolus or reflux, and can start anywhere in the esophagus. Tertiary contractions are nonpropulsive segmental contractions that may occur in many asymptomatic patients and with increasing frequency in the elderly. Motility disorders of the esophagus, such as achalasia and diffuse esophageal spasm, are well demonstrated with the single-contrast technique. Esophageal motility disorders are optimally evaluated by videotape recording, although rapid filming by cine provides a more permanent hard copy of the examination.

Significant esophageal contour abnormalities, such as benign or malignant strictures, are evaluated with the single-contrast technique (Figure 15–3). More subtle strictures may be detected by the delayed passage of an administered barium pill. Extrinsic processes impressing on or displacing the esophagus are also well visualized on single-contrast images.

Varices will cause a scalloped or serpiginous contour of the esophagus with a changeable configuration depending on peristalsis, respiration, and the degree of distension. They are best seen on partially collapsed single-contrast views of the esophagus (Figure 15–4). Overdistension and peristalsis tend to obliterate these dilated submucosal veins. Traditionally, endoscopy has been more reliable than the esophagram in the detection of varices.

A single contrast esophagram has limited usefulness in the diagnosis of gastroesophageal reflux. Spontaneous gastroesophageal reflux may occur during the single-contrast portion of the examination; however, this may not be clinically significant, since spontaneous reflux is observed fluoroscopically in 40% of asymptomatic individuals. On the other hand, fluoroscopic demonstration of reflux is found in only 40% of patients who have endoscopic evidence of reflux esophagitis. Although various provocative maneuvers, such as increasing intra-abdominal pressure, have been used by radiologists to elicit reflux during

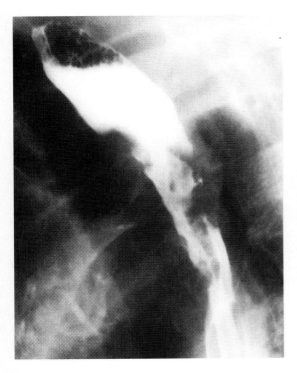

Figure 15–3. Single-contrast image of a typical malignant stricture due to squamous cell carcinoma located in the proximal esophagus with nodularity, fold thickening, and evidence of abrupt narrowing due to concentric mass. Contour abnormalities, such as benign or malignant esophageal strictures, are evaluated with the single-contrast technique.

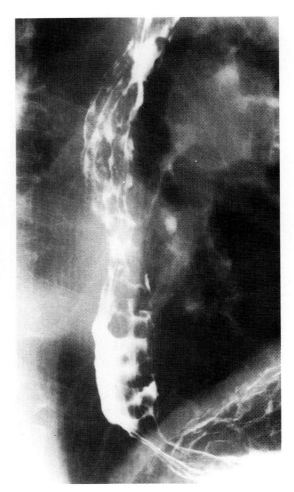

Figure 15–4. Multiple esophageal varices representing dilated submucosal veins. Varices are best visualized on partially collapsed single-contrast views. A scalloped contour of the esophagus with a changeable configuration is observed. Overdistension will obliterate the varices.

the esophagram, the significance of the results obtained is controversial.

B. Contraindications: Single contrast barium swallow is contraindicated in patients with esophageal perforation. In these patients, water-soluble contrast media may be administered. If no perforation is identified, a barium swallow may then be performed.

C. Patient Preparation: Patients should fast for at least 1 hour before the study.

D. Cost: $235–$285.

Double Contrast

A. Indications: Double-contrast imaging of the pharynx and esophagus is obtained as part of a standard biphasic esophagram. Mucosal lesions of the pharynx, such as lymphoid hyperplasia, ulcerations, and masses, are best seen with this technique. Most pharyngeal masses are malignant epithelial neoplasms (squamous cell carcinoma), although lymphomas, sarcomas, and benign tumors can occur in this location. An intraluminal mass or mucosal irreg-

ularity accompanied by asymmetric decreased distensibility are suggestive findings.

Double-contrast views may also show extension of tumor into the valleculae, base of tongue, inferior hypopharynx, and pharyngoesophageal segment, which are areas that are difficult to evaluate by endoscopy. In addition, this technique can play a complementary role to endoscopy by allowing evaluation of areas distal to strictures or bulky masses. In patients in whom a pharyngeal carcinoma is detected, the esophagram may also demonstrate a second site of carcinoma in either the pharynx or esophagus. A second primary tumor develops in approximately 10% of patients with squamous cell carcinoma of the head and neck. About 1% of patients will develop synchronous or metachronous esophageal carcinoma.

Double-contrast esophagography allows significantly improved evaluation of the mucosa of the esophagus as compared to single- contrast images. The esophageal lumen is distended by administered effervescent granules and the esophagus is coated by high-density barium. This technique is best for identification of superficial esophageal carcinomas and for evaluation of malignant neoplasms in general (Figure 15–5). In cases of high-grade malignant esophageal strictures, double-contrast views may be difficult to obtain and the single-contrast technique is employed.

Double-contrast technique is the preferred method

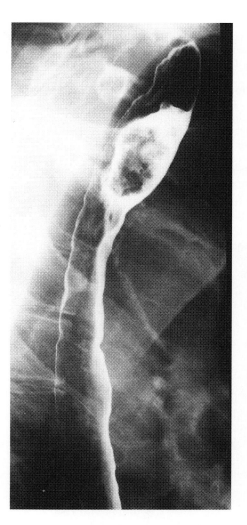

Figure 15–5. Double-contrast view from an esophagram demonstrating a large intraluminal mass of the proximal esophagus that represents squamous cell carcinoma. This technique is preferred for evaluating malignancy in general as well as for demonstrating mucosal lesions, such as those associated with esophagitis.

for demonstrating mucosal ulcerations, plaques, and nodular lesions associated with esophagitis. A granular or mildly nodular mucosal pattern with ulcerations involving the distal esophagus is typical for reflux esophagitis, especially if associated with a hiatal hernia or fluoroscopic evidence of gastroesophageal reflux.

More defined mucosal nodules with plaque formation, cobblestoning, or a shaggy-appearing esophagus are findings of *Candida* esophagitis. Recent studies have shown that the double-contrast technique is up to 90% sensitive in diagnosing esophageal candidiasis. Focal, shallow, midesophageal ulcerations may suggest herpes simplex, esophagitis, or drug-induced esophagitis. One or more giant superficial ulcers (> 2 cm) is suggestive of cytomegalovirus (CMV) esophagitis, especially in AIDS patients.

The advantages of an esophagram are its low relative cost and low risk compared with endoscopy. Esophagoscopy, however, has the advantage of allowing biopsy samples or brushings to be taken for histology and culture.

B. Contraindications: Double contrast barium swallow is contraindicated in patients with esophageal perforation. In these patients water-soluble contrast media may be administered. If no perforation is identified, a barium swallow may then be performed.

C. Patient Preparation: Patients should fast for at least 1 hour before the study.

D. Cost: $235–$285.

UPPER GASTROINTESTINAL STUDY

Biphasic barium evaluation is the radiologic study of choice for the stomach. This method takes advantage of the complementary information that can be obtained by the use of both the single- and double-contrast techniques.

The routine upper gastrointestinal study (UGI) series consists of double-contrast views of the esophagus, stomach, and proximal small bowel followed by single-contrast images of these areas in the prone or upright positions.

Single Contrast

A. Indications: Single-contrast images are obtained following the administration of low-density barium. Spot compression of portions of the lumen filled with barium will demonstrate filling defects due to thickened folds, large ulcerations, or masses (Figure 15–6). Abnormalities of motility and contour are well depicted, such as linitis plastica due to scirrhous adenocarcinoma of the stomach (Figure 15–7). Gastric varices are best seen on single-contrast or partially collapsed double-contrast images.

A single-contrast examination alone is performed in certain clinical settings. This includes patients who

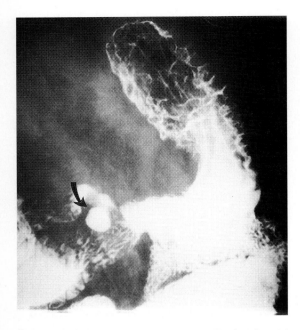

Figure 15–6. Large, rounded barium collection **(arrow)** representing a duodenal bulb ulcer crater seen with single-contrast technique on UGI series.

are obtunded, debilitated, or with limited mobility, in whom a double-contrast study is not possible. Patients who have had recent abdominal surgery often cannot tolerate a double-contrast examination. In patients with suspected gastric outlet obstruction or gastric motility disorders, the single-contrast technique also is used. The primary cause of gastric outlet obstruction in adults is peptic ulcer disease involving the duodenal bulb or pyloric channel. These patients often have large amounts of residual fluid and debris in the stomach, making a double-contrast study impossible to perform.

B. Contraindications: Suspected gastric or bowel perforation (in which case water-soluble contrast material is used).

C. Patient Preparation: An overnight fast prior to study. Patients are asked to refrain from smoking on the day of the study to minimize gastric secretions.

D. Cost: $400–$500.

Double Contrast

A. Indications: Double-contrast images are obtained following administration of an effervescent agent and high-density barium. This technique is best for demonstrating mucosal detail and is more sensitive for detecting erosions, ulcerations, and polyps. A double-contrast UGI series can define changes due to infectious gastritis, such as CMV or cryptosporidiosis, presenting as mucosal nodularity, ulceration, fold

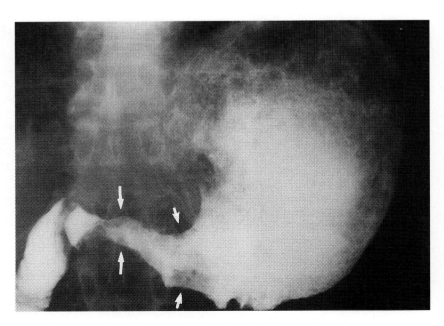

Figure 15–7. Single-contrast image from UGI series demonstrating markedly distended proximal stomach. Stomach shows retained fluid and debris with fixed rigid narrowing of the antrum **(arrows)** due to scirrhous adenocarcinoma (linitis plastica or leather bottle stomach). Double-contrast technique is not performed due to residual material in the stomach.

thickening, or antral narrowing. *Helicobacter pylori* gastritis may cause nonspecific fold thickening. However, endoscopy with biopsies and culture is required for the diagnosis of infectious gastritis.

Double-contrast study of mucosal abnormalities surrounding an ulcer is helpful in distinguishing benign versus malignant ulcers. Most gastric ulcers and almost all duodenal ulcers are benign. Features of a benign gastric ulcer include a round ulcer crater with a smooth mound of edema or regular mucosal folds that radiate to the rim of the crater. Benign ulcers tend to project outside the expected line of the gastric lumen when viewed in profile. Malignant gastric ulcers have an irregular eccentric ulcer crater with distortion of the surrounding mucosa. Radiating folds are nodular, thickened, and fused and do not extend to the crater edge. Malignant ulcers do not project beyond the gastric lumen when viewed in profile. Unequivocally benign gastric ulcers may be followed with a repeat radiographic study in 2–3 months until healing is complete. However, equivocal or suspicious ulcers, or ulcers that do not heal after 2–3 months require endoscopy with biopsy to exclude gastric malignancy. Mucosal lesions such as polyps or nodules (Figure 15–8) and submucosal lesions such as leiomyomas are best imaged by double-contrast technique (Figure 15–8).

B. Contraindications: Double-contrast studies are contraindicated in patients who have complete gastric outlet obstruction, large amounts of retained gastric fluid, or suspected perforation, in which case water-soluble contrast material is used. They are un-

feasible in patients who are unable to cooperate for the study or have limited mobility.

C. Patient Preparation: An overnight fast is required before the study. Patients are asked to refrain from smoking on the day of study to minimize gastric secretions.

D. Cost: $400–$500.

SMALL BOWEL FOLLOW-THROUGH EXAMINATION

The primary imaging modality for small bowel disease is the barium study. The small bowel follow-through (SBFT) is the most commonly employed technique, although the use of enteroclysis has increased over the past 10 years. A plain film of the abdomen is routinely obtained before contrast administration. SBFT is most often performed immediately following a double-contrast UGI series, for which the patient has already ingested an effervescent agent and high-density barium. Additional low-density barium is administered for the SBFT so as to completely fill the small bowel. Overhead radiographs and compression spot films of small bowel loops are obtained at sequential time intervals. Careful compression under fluoroscopy is essential to separate overlapping bowel loops. The terminal ileum and a portion of the cecum or ascending colon must be imaged before the study is complete. Normal transit of contrast through the small bowel into the colon is variable, most often spanning 1–2 hours. Accelerating agents such as

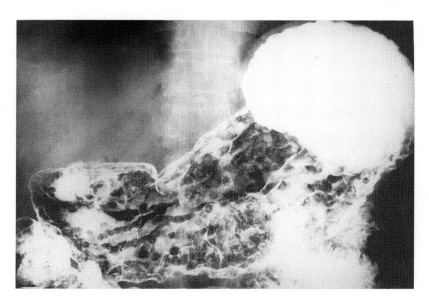

Figure 15–8. Multiple small nodular filling defects scattered diffusely throughout the stomach with central ulceration, causing bulls-eye appearance seen on this double-contrast UGI series. This is typical of hematogenous metastases to the stomach due to metastatic melanoma.

metoclopromide or meglumine diatrizoate mixed with barium can be given in cases of slow transit.

The **dedicated SBFT** is a study performed independently of a UGI series. The patient ingests only low-density barium so that there is more uniform opacification of the small bowel. More accurate evaluation is possible, since artifacts from mixing of gas and barium suspensions of different density are avoided.

A. Indications: SBFT should be the initial study performed in patients with nonspecific symptoms (Figure 15–9) who elicit low clinical suspicion for small bowel pathology. These patients often have had negative findings on upper and lower endoscopy. Therefore, in most of these patients a dedicated SBFT is preferred. SBFT is also indicated for further evaluation of high-grade small bowel obstruction located proximally within the first few feet of the jejunum (Figure 15–10).

SBFT is technically less difficult and less expensive, and requires a smaller radiation dose than enteroclysis. It is the preferred study in female patients of child-bearing age with possible small bowel disease. A small percentage of patients who refuse tube placement or who have unsuccessful tube placement for enteroclysis will require SBFT.

B. Contraindications: Small bowel follow-through is contraindicated in patients with bowel perforation.

C. Patient Preparation: An overnight fast is required before the study.

D. Cost: $300–$350 (dedicated SBFT); $450–$550 (UGI with SBFT).

ENTEROCLYSIS (SMALL BOWEL ENEMA)

Enteroclysis is the optimal method for establishing small bowel as normal. After the administration of 10–20 mg of metaclopramide intravenously and topical anesthesia for the nostril and throat, a special balloon-tipped enteroclysis catheter containing a guidewire is inserted from the nose into the stomach and guided fluoroscopically into the proximal jejunum. Once the tip of the catheter is about 5 cm distal to the ligament of Treitz, the balloon is inflated. Barium followed by methylcellulose is infused at high rates via a pump into the jejunum. Careful compression spot films of each quadrant and overhead films are obtained. Difficulty in tube placement is encountered in patients with pyloric or duodenal scarring. Large sliding hiatal hernias or prior surgery, such as gastroduodenostomy and gastrojejunostomy, also may preclude tube placement.

Enteroclysis demonstrates excellent mucosal detail, fold pattern, and bowel distension (Figure 15–11). Through the adjustment of infusion rates, adequate distension of the entire small bowel can be achieved. This makes it easier to recognize areas of

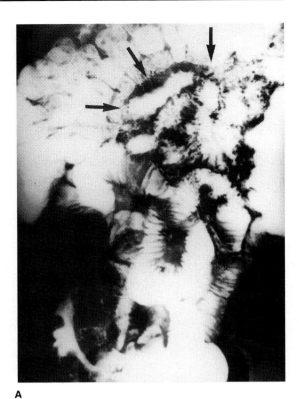

A

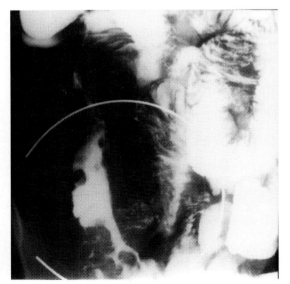

B

Figure 15–9. **A:** Overhead film from a small bowel follow-through examination with barium filling entire small bowel and proximal colon in a patient with nonspecific abdominal complaints. Fold thickening and nodularity are present, involving the jejunum **(arrow).** The terminal ileum is straightened, rigid, and narrowed. **B:** Spot compression view of the terminal ileum from the same patient showing "string sign," nodularity, and ulcerations typical of Crohn's disease.

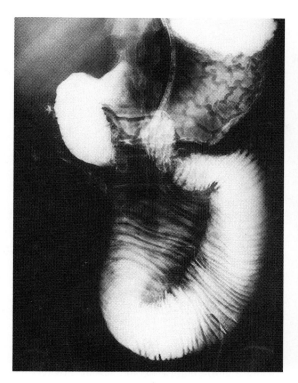

Figure 15–10. Small bowel follow-through examination in a patient with high-grade proximal jejunal obstruction due to an adhesion. The significantly dilated loop of proximal jejunum demonstrates a coiled appearance representing a closed loop construction.

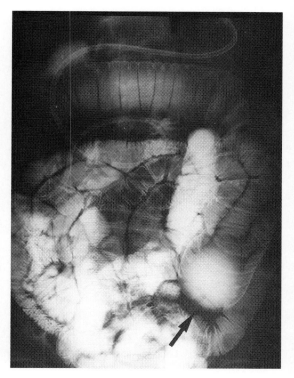

Figure 15–11. Enteroclysis or small bowel enema study that optimally demonstrates mucosal detail, fold pattern, and distension. This is the optimal study for evaluating partial small bowel obstruction. This patient has a dilated jejunal loop with a transition point to decompressed bowel, which is easily identified *(arrow)*. An adhesion found at surgery correlated exactly to this level in the jejunum.

subtle narrowing that may not be detected on conventional SBFT. An increasing number of institutions are using enteroclysis as the radiologic technique of choice for evaluating disorders of the small intestine. However, controversy does exist, since no large prospective controlled trial has compared SBFT with enteroclysis. Enteroclysis is more invasive, requiring either nasal- or oral-jejunal catheter placement. Enteroclysis is also approximately twice as expensive as a dedicated SBFT, and delivers a higher radiation dose to the patient (one and one-half times > UGI with SBFT and three times > dedicated SBFT). However, enteroclysis has a shorter total examination completion time, approximately 30 minutes. Many studies demonstrate a high sensitivity (93–100%), specificity (89–99%), and accuracy (96–99%) of enteroclysis for evaluation of the small bowel.

A. Indications: Enteroclysis is particularly helpful in patients with partial small bowel obstruction, a history of radiation or pelvic surgery, suspected primary or secondary small bowel tumor,

Meckel's diverticulum, malabsorption, and chronic unexplained gastrointestinal bleeding. (Arteriovenous malformations of the small bowel are a common cause of occult gastrointestinal bleeding but cannot be demonstrated by enteroclysis.) Enteroclysis is the best examination for demonstrating the features of early Crohn's disease, such as a granular mucosal pattern, distorted folds, and small nodules. It is also the best study for evaluating the extent of involvement of Crohn's disease, especially if surgical management is being considered. This technique can help distinguish areas of fibrotic stricture due to Crohn's disease from spasm by demonstrating the degree of distensibility. Ulcerations, cobblestoning, and fistulae are particularly well demonstrated. Enteroclysis should also be performed if conventional SBFT is negative but there is high clinical suspicion of small bowel abnormality.

B. Contraindications: Patients with complete small bowel obstruction or possible perforation should be excluded.

C. Patient Preparation: This is the same as for

barium enema (to prevent artifacts and slow intestinal flow due to a filled ascending colon or ileum).

D. Cost: $625–$700.

PERORAL PNEUMOCOLON

The peroral pneumocolon may be performed either as an individual examination or following SBFT. The patient ingests low-density barium, after which sequential films are obtained. When the oral contrast reaches the ascending colon to mid-transverse colon, air is insufflated through a rectal tube until the cecum is distended. This air then refluxes into the terminal ileum, providing a double-contrast appearance. Compression spot films are obtained. Occasionally, glucagon is administered to relax the ileocecal valve and to facilitate reflux.

A. Indications: The peroral pneumocolon is used to specifically evaluate the terminal ileum. The peroral pneumocolon is more sensitive for disease of the terminal ileum than is the SBFT alone. The SBFT with peroral pneumocolon is often useful for patients with known terminal ileal disease, however, it is not as accurate as enteroclysis for proximal disease. It can also be used for evaluation of the ascending colon or cecum when a barium enema is unsuccessful or equivocal.

B. Contraindications: It is contraindicated in cases of toxic megacolon.

C. Patient Preparation: This is the same as for barium enema (see following section).

D. Cost: $50–$75 added to cost of UGI series.

CONTRAST ENEMA

Thorough patient preparation for a barium enema, as described below, is essential for accurate interpretation of the study. In acute situations, such as obstruction or inflammatory bowel disease, colonic preparation may be unfeasible or limited. A plain film of the abdomen is obtained immediately before beginning a contrast enema. Residual contrast material from prior radiology study or retained fecal material may be detected, which may preclude the current examination. The bowel gas pattern is reviewed to evaluate for obstruction or pneumatosis. If toxic megacolon is suspected, contrast enema is contraindicated. Glucagon may be given intravenously to reduce colonic spasm during the study.

Single Contrast

About 15% of barium enemas are performed as single-contrast studies. Low-density barium is administered per rectum, and the leading edge of the contrast column is followed under fluoroscopy. Careful graded compression is applied as films are taken. The single-contrast examination is able to demonstrate bowel distensibility, contour deformities, larger filling defects, bowel obstruction, and fistulae or sinus tracts.

A. Indications: The single-contrast barium enema is performed in specific situations only. It is used for suspected large bowel obstruction and diverticulitis, in the very young or elderly, and in those who are debilitated or unable to cooperate for a double-contrast enema. Fistulae and sinus tracts involving the colon, such as in Crohn's disease, are particularly well demonstrated with the single-contrast technique. A good rule to remember is that a poor double-contrast enema is worse than a poor single-contrast enema.

B. Contraindications: Single-contrast barium enema should not be performed in patients with toxic megacolon, suspected severe acute ulcerative colitis, or possible colonic perforation, or immediately after endoscopic biopsy (wait 24 hours). Also, it should not be used if a double-contrast examination is needed to evaluate the mucosa and to detect small lesions.

C. Patient preparation: See following section.

D. Cost: $375–$425.

Double Contrast

The double-contrast barium enema involves the administration of high-density barium into the colon per rectum followed by air insufflation. It is also called **air-contrast barium enema (ACBE)** or **pneumocolon**.

A. Indications: ACBE is the recommended radiographic study for routine examination of the colon because it allows optimal evaluation of mucosal detail. It is the best imaging technique for detecting polyps or tumors and for demonstrating early inflammatory disease of the colon, such as fine ulcerations and mucosal granularity (Figures 15–12 and 15–13).

The role of the double-contrast barium enema versus colonoscopy in the screening and detection of colorectal carcinoma remains controversial. Screening strategies are still evolving and being evaluated. In the workup of the individual patient, the clinician must consider a given method's cost-effectiveness and proven efficacy in reducing mortality. Colonic lesions such as polyps or carcinomas greater than 1 cm are detected by barium enema with an accuracy of 90–95%, which is similar to the accuracy of colonoscopy. Colonoscopy is more sensitive than barium enema for detecting polyps less than 7 mm, however, these diminutive polyps are rarely malignant, are often hyperplastic, and their clinical importance is unclear. In general, colonoscopy is about three times higher in cost than a barium enema and has up to a five times higher complication rate. Colonoscopy may be technically difficult in certain individuals and visualization of the whole colon may not be possible. In about 5% of patients, the cecum is not reached, and an estimated 10–20% of colonic le-

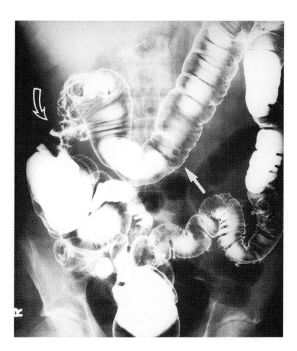

Figure 15–12. Typical "apple-core" annular carcinoma involving the ascending colon and hepatic flexure. Lesion is well demonstrated on this double-contrast barium enema *(open arrow)*. In addition, a small sessile polyp is present in the transverse colon *(arrow)* and there are small sigmoid diverticula.

sions can be missed. Barium enema is the diagnostic tool for such situations and can offer evaluation of the right colon.

B. Contraindications: These include the previously mentioned contraindications to single-contrast barium enema. Any patient with suspected colonic perforation requires a water-soluble contrast enema if the exact site of perforation needs to be demonstrated. Toxic megacolon is also a contraindication to barium enema. Colonic obstruction (eg, volvulus), diverticulitis, and colonic fistulae, are better evaluated by the single-contrast technique.

C. Patient Preparation: A typical colonic cleansing preparation for contrast enema includes: (1) 24-hour clear liquid diet and no breakfast on the day of the study, (2) 350 ml magnesium citrate at lunch and 4 bisacodyl tablets in the evening before the study, (3) 1 bisacodyl suppository in the morning of study.

D. Cost: $525–$575.

Water-Soluble Contrast Enema

A. Indications: The water-soluble contrast enema is primarily used in patients with suspected colonic perforation. This includes patients who have had recent instrumentation, surgery, or trauma. Water-soluble enemas can be used with caution in patients with the potential for perforation (such as those with colonic distension) when further anatomic delineation is necessary. Water-soluble contrast also is preferred for evaluation of possible colo-vesical fistula. Finally, the administration of water-soluble hyperosmolar contrast can also be used as a therapeutic

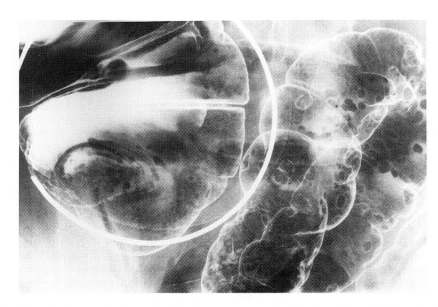

Figure 15–13. Spot view from a double-contrast barium enema revealing innumerable small polyps in a patient with familial adenomatous polyposis.

maneuver to evacuate stool in cases of severe fecal impaction.

B. Contraindications: Patients with toxic megacolon should be excluded.

C. Patient Preparation: Although a bowel preparation is preferred, water-soluble enemas are often obtained in situations in which colonic cleansing is not possible.

D. Cost: $400–$425.

BILIARY IMAGING

Ultrasound

Real-time ultrasound is the imaging modality of choice for evaluation of the gallbladder and biliary ducts. The liver and pancreas are also routinely imaged when evaluating for biliary tract disease. Ultrasound is noninvasive and does not use ionizing radiation. Scanning units are portable and bedside examinations are possible. This modality can also be used to guide fine-needle biopsy, percutaneous transhepatic cholangiography, and biliary drainage procedures. **Intravenous cholangiography (IVC)**, which is associated with significant toxic reactions to the contrast material and poor opacification of the bile ducts in patients with a bilirubin greater than 2 mg/dl, has largely been replaced by sonography.

Relative limitations of ultrasound include the dependence of diagnostic accuracy on the skill of the operator performing the study, the patient cooperation, and body habitus. Obese patients image poorly. Bowel gas or recently administered barium also will interfere with image quality.

A. Indications: Ultrasound has a 95% sensitivity for the detection of cholelithiasis. A gallstone can be diagnosed unequivocally when a mobile hyperechoic intraluminal mass is present with acoustic shadowing. Sonography has been demonstrated to be 15–20% more sensitive than oral cholecystography (OCG) and has a lower false-positive rate. Hence, it has largely supplanted the OCG in most circumstances. Ultrasound is the initial examination of choice in cases of suspected acute cholecystitis because it is noninvasive, is readily available, and has excellent sensitivity for this entity. Sonographic findings supporting this diagnosis include the presence of gallstones, gallbladder wall thickening (greater than 3 mm), and pericholecystic fluid, and the detection of maximum tenderness directly over the gallbladder (sonographic **Murphy's sign**). When these findings are present there is a high (> 90%) sensitivity in the diagnosis of acute cholecystitis (Figure 15–14). Ultrasound is less useful in the diagnosis of acalculous cholecystitis, demonstrating a 60–70% sensitivity for detection of this condition. The presence of gallbladder wall thickening is suggestive but not specific. Radionuclide imaging has a similar diagnostic sensitivity to ultrasound for acalculous cholecystitis.

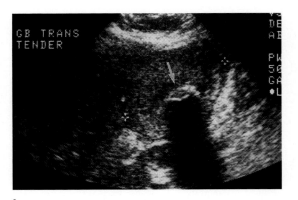

A

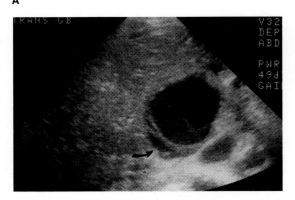

B

Figure 15–14. **A:** Ultrasound in a patient with acute cholecystitis, demonstrating a sludge-filled, thick-walled gallbladder containing a hyperechoic stone with acoustic shadowing **(arrow)**. A sonographic Murphy's sign was also present. Ultrasound has a high sensitivity for acute cholecystitis when these findings are present. **B:** Ultrasound of the gallbladder in another patient with acute cholecystitis demonstrating sludge and a small amount of pericholecystic fluid **(arrow)** but no stones. This patient had a sonographic Murphy's sign.

Ultrasound is less capable of detecting choledocholithiasis than gallstones, with reported sensitivity ranging from as low as 13% to as high as 75%. The true sensitivity likely falls between these two figures. The difficulty arises in visualizing an intraductal stone, particularly if it is located in the distal common bile duct. These stones often do not demonstrate acoustic shadowing. Although dilated extrahepatic ducts are commonly seen in patients with choledocholithiasis, non-dilated ducts are present in up to 30%, making sonographic diagnosis even more difficult. Therefore, a "negative" ultrasound does not reliably exclude choledocholithiasis. ERCP is the definitive diagnostic study.

Ultrasound is very valuable in the evaluation of the jaundiced patient with biliary obstruction. It is 95% accurate in the detection of biliary ductal dilatation although it may not be able to determine whether the obstruction is due to a stone, tumor, or stricture. Direct visualization of the bile ducts by ERCP or PTC is required to define the cause, at which time brushings and biopsies may also be obtained. CT has a sensitivity comparable to ultrasound for the diagnosis of bile duct obstruction and is more likely than sonography to demonstrate the cause. A CT using thin sections through the pancreas and portal region should be obtained if tumor is suspected as the cause of biliary obstruction.

B. Contraindications: There are none.

C. Patient Preparation: A fasting period of 6 hours is required to distend the gallbladder and decrease bowel gas.

D. Cost: $250–$300; $375–$425 for complete abdominal examination.

Oral Cholecystogram

Contrast agents used for oral cholecystography (OCG) are absorbed through the intestinal mucosa into the bloodstream and are transported to the liver, where they are conjugated and excreted into the bile. If the cystic duct is patent, the conjugated contrast enters the gallbladder. The gallbladder mucosa resorbs water, thereby concentrating the contrast and opacifying the gallbladder. Iopanoic acid is the most commonly used OCG agent. It is the most lipid-soluble agent and requires bile salts and fat in the diet for absorption. Peak opacification occurs 17 hours after ingestion. Tyropanoate sodium is a newer agent that is more water-soluble and produces gallbladder opacification in about 10 hours. It does not require bile salts for absorption and is not affected by lack of fat in the diet.

Nonvisualization of the gallbladder on OCG after administration of two consecutive doses of contrast agent is reliable evidence of gallbladder disease, if other causes can be excluded. Intrinsic gallbladder disease causing nonvisualization includes: cystic duct obstruction, chronic cholecystitis, cholecystectomy, and anomalous gallbladder position. Extrabiliary causes of failure to view the gallbladder on OCG include: fasting, failure to ingest contrast, vomiting, esophageal disorders (such as diverticula, obstruction, or hiatal hernia), gastric outlet obstruction, gastrocolic fistula, malabsorption states, diarrhea, ileus, acute pancreatitis or peritonitis, and deficiency of bile salts resulting from Crohn's disease or severe liver disease.

A. Indications: OCG is used as an adjunctive examination to ultrasound. It is obtained when the clinical symptoms are highly suggestive of cholelithiasis but the ultrasound either is normal or equivocal. OCG plays a role in helping to determine the eligibility of patients for nonsurgical treatment of gallstones. Chemical stone dissolution and biliary lithotripsy require knowledge of cystic duct patency as well as stone number, size, and composition: bile salt therapy requires small stones (< 5 mm) whereas lithotripsy is most effective on a solitary stone less than 2 cm. Ultrasound can be used to measure stones smaller than 2 cm, but OCG is superior to ultrasound for sizing larger stones and for counting multiple stones. Noncalcified cholesterol stones are required for nonoperative therapy. Buoyancy is a sign of cholesterol stones on OCG (Figure 15–15). Gallbladder opacification on OCG establishes cystic duct patency.

Large doses of OCG contrast agent can cause renal failure. It will also cause the gallbladder to become very dense, which decreases the procedure's sensitivity for detecting small stones. Other side effects include diarrhea (25%), dysuria (14%), nausea (6%), and vomiting (0.5%).

B. Contraindications: OCG cannot be performed in patients with bilirubin greater than 3 mg/dl or in pregnant patients.

C. Patient Preparation: The recommended dose of OCG agent is 3.0 g. For outpatients, a 2-day consecutive dosage schedule is used, with 3.0 g of iopanoic acid administered each day. The patient fasts overnight of the second day and radiographs are obtained the morning of the third day. For inpatients, a single dose of 3.0 g of iopanoic acid or other OCG agent is administered. If there is no image or a faint image of the gallbladder, a second dose of 3.0 g of contrast agent is given that evening and repeat radiographs are performed the next morning.

D. Cost: $275–$325.

Percutaneous Transhepatic Cholangiogram

Percutaneous transhepatic cholangiography (PTC) is a technique that permits direct visualization of the biliary tree and may be extended during the same examination to include interventional biliary procedures. PTC is performed by percutaneous placement of a fine needle through the chest wall and the hepatic parenchyma and into a branch of either the right or left bile duct. A cholangiogram is then obtained by injection of water-soluble contrast directly into the biliary tree. Ultrasound, CT, or fluoroscopy may be used for guidance of the needle. The success of injecting a bile duct increases when the ducts are dilated. There is a 90–100% success rate for obtaining a diagnostic cholangiogram when intrahepatic ducts are dilated. This drops to 70–85%, however, in patients with nondilated ducts.

Complications of PTC occur in about 5% of patients, including cholangitis, sepsis, hemorrhage, bile peritonitis, and pneumothorax.

A. Indications: Transhepatic cholangiography is obtained in the following situations:

- In patients with evidence of obstructive jaundice by noninvasive imaging in whom determination of the cause of obstruction is required for planning treatment. PTC is particularly helpful if there is a need to see the extent of a lesion located in the proximal biliary tree.

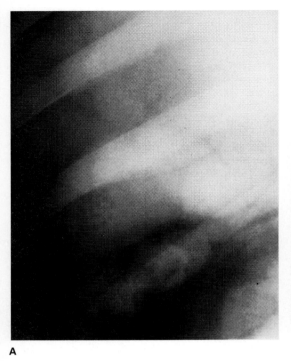
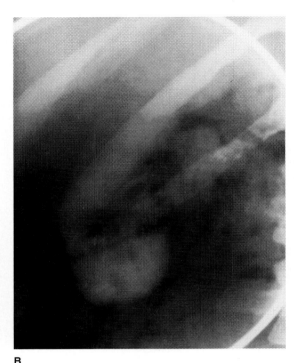

A   **B**

Figure 15–15. **A:** Supine view of an opacified gallbladder from an oral cholecystogram that contains multiple small noncalcified gallstones. **B:** Upright view of the same patient demonstrating buoyant stones that layer. Buoyancy on oral cholecystogram is a characteristic of cholesterol stones. These stones would be amenable to nonoperative therapy.

- For decompression of the biliary ree in patients with biliary obstruction. Drainage is achieved through the use of percutaneous catheter drainage or by the placement of stents in patients with unresectable malignant obstructions or benign strictures of the bile duct. Retrieval of stones and dilatation of strictures can also be performed.
- Following a failed attempt at endoscopic retrograde cholangiography or for complications of endoscopic stent placement.

B. Contraindications: Patients with abnormal clotting parameters, massive ascites, or diffuse hepatic metastases are excluded. Caution in patients with renal insufficiency to avoid excessive intravascular administration of contrast medium.

C. Patient Preparation: All patients are premedicated with broad-spectrum antibiotics.

D. Cost: $450–$550.

Endoscopic Retrograde Cholangiopancreatography

Endoscopic retrograde cholangiopancreatography (ERCP) is a procedure allowing for direct retrograde opacification of the biliary tree and pancreatic duct with a side-viewing duodenoscope. The patient is sedated and glucagon is given to induce atony of the duodenum. In the left lateral decubitus or prone posi-

tion the endoscope is introduced orally and directed into the duodenum. Following cannulation of the papilla of Vater, water-soluble contrast is injected under fluoroscopy into either the pancreatic duct or common bile duct.

A. Indications: The most important indication for ERCP is obstructive jaundice. ERCP can demonstrate the cause as well as the extent of biliary obstruction. It is the preferred examination in patients with possible choledocholithiasis because stones can be extracted with balloons or gaskets after sphincterotomy. In patients with suspected periampullary tumor, ERCP permits direct visualization and biopsy of the papilla and duodenum (Figure 15–16). ERCP can identify intra- and extrahepatic strictures. It is the best modality for imaging primary sclerosing cholangitis and AIDS cholangiopathy. Alternate areas of narrowing and dilatation involving the intra- and extrahepatic biliary tree is the appearance of sclerosing cholangitis. The intrahepatic tree may also appear pruned. AIDS cholangiopathy is due to opportunistic infection of the biliary system with *Cryptosporidium* or CMV. It can mimic sclerosing cholangitis radiographically. Shaggy irregularity of the common duct contour may also be seen. A distinguishing feature of AIDS-related cholangitis is the presence of papillary stenosis in many patients. Isolated papillary stenosis

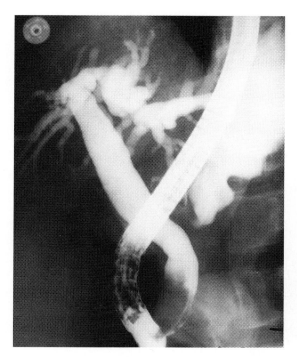

Figure 15–16. Film from an endoscopic retrograde cholangiopancreatogram (ERCP) of a jaundiced patient, showing dilatation of the intrahepatic and extrahepatic bile ducts. In the distal common bile duct there is a large irregular intraluminal filling defect due to a periampullary cholangiocarcinoma.

pancreatic head. Findings of chronic pancreatitis also include dilatation of the pancreatic duct, often resulting in a tortuous, beaded, or "chain of lakes" appearance. Debris or calculi within the pancreatic duct may cause focal filling defects. Secondary branches of the pancreatic duct are enlarged and clubbed. Pancreatic parenchymal calcifications may be present and are diagnostic of chronic pancreatitis. Pseudocysts communicating with the duct may fill with contrast.

The success rate of ERCP is greater than 90% and is not dependent on the presence of ductal dilatation (unlike PTC). Failure to cannulate the papilla of Vater occurs in the following settings: papillary stenosis, severe duodenal inflammation or scarring, prior gastric surgery (particularly Billroth II), choledochocele, or juxtapapillary diverticulum.

The overall incidence of complications resulting from ERCP is about 2%. ERCP may cause injection-related pancreatitis, cholangitis, sepsis, duodenal perforation, and hemorrhage, particularly if a sphincterotomy is performed.

B. Contraindications: Caution is advised in patients with concurrent or recent acute pancreatitis, who are at a higher risk for developing procedure-related pancreatitis, and when pancreatic pseudocyst is present, since there is risk of developing abscess.

C. Cost: $750–$800.

Hepatobiliary Scan

The radiopharmaceutical used for the hepatobiliary scan is ^{99m}Tc N-substituted iminodiacetic acid (IDA). The most common analog is ^{99m}Tc diisopropyl-IDA (DISIDA) because it allows visualization of the hepatobiliary system at serum bilirubin levels up to 20 mg/dl. Following intravenous injection of DISIDA, there is rapid uptake by hepatocytes with subsequent conjugation and excretion into the biliary ducts. The liver is visualized within 5 minutes. The gallbladder, common bile duct, and duodenum are normally seen within 30–40 minutes. Diseases that affect liver perfusion, cause hepatocyte dysfunction, or cause cystic or common duct obstruction will result in an abnormal scan.

A. Indications: Hepatobiliary scan is indicated in the following situations:

• Cholecystitis: Cystic duct obstruction is present in the majority of patients with acute cholecystitis. In the correct clinical setting, acute cholecystitis can be diagnosed accurately if there is failure to see the gallbladder within 4 hours of injection and the patient demonstrates hepatic excretion into the common duct and small bowel (Figure 15–18). If there is delayed visualization of the gallbladder at 1-hour to 4-hours and cholecystokinin (CCK) or morphine has been administered, then the diagnosis is chronic cholecystitis. CCK stimulates gallbladder contraction and enhances biliary excretion,

or a long common duct stricture may occasionally be seen without the intrahepatic findings in AIDS cholangiopathy.

Malignant stricture due to cholangiocarcinoma is well demonstrated by ERCP, typically appearing as an area of abrupt cutoff. Other causes of biliary ductal narrowing include postinflammatory or postsurgical strictures. Extrinsic compression of the biliary tree can occur secondary to hepatocellular carcinoma, portal adenopathy, or duodenal and pancreatic carcinoma. Decompression of the biliary system by endoscopic stent placement or balloon dilatation of benign or malignant biliary strictures involving the extrahepatic biliary tree can be achieved in more than 90% of cases. Intrahepatic strictures may be better approached by transhepatic cholangiography.

Opacification of the pancreatic duct is useful for diagnosing pancreatic carcinoma, pancreatitis, or identifying a fistula extending from the pancreatic duct to a pseudocyst. Carcinoma of the pancreas head is often the cause of distal common bile duct stricture as well as stricture of the pancreatic duct in this region, producing the "double duct" sign (Figure 15–17). However, this appearance may also be seen with chronic pancreatitis due to stricturing within the

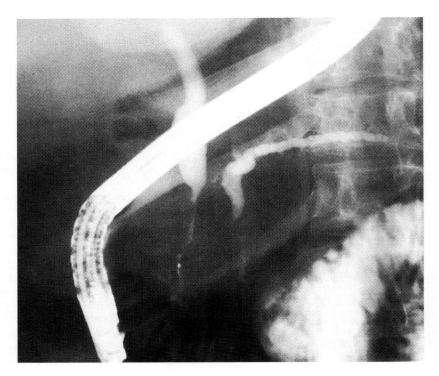

Figure 15–17. Film from an ERCP in a patient with pancreatic head carcinoma. Opacification of both the common bile duct and pancreatic duct reveals biductal strictures causing obstruction ("double duct" sign). This appearance is most commonly associated with pancreatic carcinoma but also may be seen with chronic pancreatitis.

promoting gallbladder visualization in chronic cholecystitis. Intravenous morphine causes constriction of the sphincter of Oddi and increases the flow of radiopharmaceutical into the gallbladder.

The overall accuracy of hepatobiliary scintigraphy for acute cholecystitis is 95%. Normal visualization of the gallbladder reliably excludes acute cholecystitis. Nonvisualization or delayed visualization of the gallbladder (false-positive study) can be caused by nonfasting or prolonged fasting, hyperalimentation, acute pancreatitis, and hepatocellular dysfunction. False-negative studies may occur in patients with acalculous cholecystitis. Duodenal diverticulum, simulating the gallbladder or an accessory cystic duct, may also result in a false-negative study.

• Cholestasis: If there is hepatic uptake but nonvisualization of the gallbladder, common duct, and small bowel, then common bile duct obstruction is suggested. Rarely, severe hepatocellular disease can produce a similar appearance. Findings on the hepatobiliary scan can help differentiate between intrahepatic cholestasis owing to hepatocellular dysfunction and extrahepatic cholestasis resulting from common duct obstruction. While both will cause a decrease in hepatic uptake, this is usually more impaired by hepatocellular disease than by

mechanical obstruction. Hepatocellular disease is also characterized by normal or delayed visualization of bowel activity but lack of biliary dilatation. A partial common duct obstruction will cause delayed bowel visualization associated with a dilated bile duct.

• Postsurgical complications: Complications of hepatobiliary surgery that result in abnormal biliary flow and biliary leakage can be easily identified with scintigraphy. Ductal obstruction resulting from retained stone or stricture is suggested by dilated ducts and delayed bowel visualization.

B. Patient Preparation: A fasting period of 6 hours is required before the study.

C. Cost: $500–$600.

CROSS-SECTIONAL IMAGING

Modalities

A. Computed Tomography: Recent advances in computed tomography (CT) include faster scan times and higher spatial resolution, allowing for more accurate evaluation. The administration of intravenous contrast material with the rapid bolus technique permits improved detection and characterization of many lesions. CT is also used as guidance for

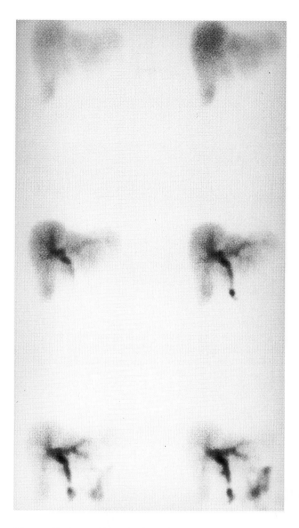

Figure 15–18. Acute cholecystitis. Activity is present in the common duct and small bowel within 30 minutes (images were taken at 5-minute intervals from 5–30 minutes). This study was continued for 4 hours and the gallbladder was not visualized.

percutaneous fine-needle aspiration biopsy and drainage catheter placement. The recent advent of spiral CT eliminates respiratory motion artifacts and decreases the required amount of intravenous contrast. Spiral CT requires a slip-ring scanner, which permits continuous imaging so that a large area of the body can be scanned quickly—in about 30 seconds compared with 2–3 minutes for conventional CT.

1. Contraindications–CT is contraindicated in pregnancy. Renal insufficiency (creatinine > 1.5–2.0 mg/dl) is a contraindication to the administration of intravenous contrast. The use of intravenous contrast also is associated with the risk of allergic reaction and, rarely, death.

2. Patient preparation–A fasting period of 4–6

hours is required before the study. Opacification of the gastrointestinal tract is necessary for abdominal-pelvic CT. Patients receive oral contrast approximately 1 hour before scanning. Some centers also administer rectal contrast before imaging the pelvis. A recent serum creatinine is necessary if intravenous contrast is to be given.

3. Cost–$900–$1250; add $275–$350 for nonionic contrast.

B. Ultrasound: Ultrasound of the abdomen and pelvis is noninvasive, requires no ionizing radiation or iodinated contrast material, and is relatively inexpensive. In addition, units are portable so that bedside studies may be performed. Ultrasound is the best modality for determining cystic versus solid nature of lesions, and it remains the primary modality for biliary imaging. Ultrasound is often used for following lesions such as pancreatic pseudocyst and drained fluid collections. Ultrasound guidance for percutaneous fine-needle biopsy or catheter placement is less expensive than CT. Endoscopic and intraoperative ultrasound are now more widely employed with the development of small high-resolution transducers and improved operator expertise.

1. Contraindications–There are none.

2. Patient preparation–A fasting period of 6 hours is required before the study.

3. Cost–$375–$425 for complete abdomen examination.

C. Magnetic Resonance Imaging: Magnetic resonance imaging (MRI) provides better tissue contrast than other radiographic modalities. It is noninvasive and does not require ionizing radiation or iodinated contrast material. Imaging can be performed in multiple planes (transaxial, coronal, sagittal, nonorthogonal). MRI can be used to clarify areas surrounding surgical clips that are not seen on CT because of induced artifacts. MRI is useful for evaluation of vascular patency without the need for contrast material. Intravenous contrast material (gadopentetate dimeglumine) can be given to evaluate enhancement patterns and offer complementary information to that obtained by CT or ultrasound.

1. Contraindications–Patients with pacemakers, intraocular metallic fragments, intracranial aneurysm clips, cochlear implants, some artificial heart valves, some implanted metallic hardware.

2. Patient preparation–A fasting period of 6 hours is required. Glucagon is administered intramuscularly to inhibit peristalsis for abdominal-pelvic MRI.

3. Cost–$1400–$2000.

Esophagus

The most commonly used cross-sectional technique for evaluation of the esophagus is CT. CT is useful for evaluation of esophageal trauma, permitting detection of involvement of the mediastinum, lung, and pleural space. CT allows delineation of the extraluminal extent of disease.

CT is the best noninvasive method for staging esophageal carcinoma. It is limited in its ability to evaluate the actual depth of invasion in the layers of the esophageal wall. However, wall thickening or mass may suggest direct invasion of adjacent structures by causing a mass effect and loss of fat planes (Figure 15–19). Tumors demonstrating aortic or tracheobronchial invasion are considered unresectable. Pericardial and vertebral involvement may also be demonstrated on CT. Aortic invasion is suspected when there is obliteration of the triangular fat space between the esophagus, aorta, and spine or if there is contact of the esophagus involving more than 90 degrees of the aortic circumference.

The ability of CT to detect local tumor involvement is controversial. Published studies indicate that CT has a relatively high sensitivity and specificity for predicting mediastinal invasion with an accuracy of over 90% for staging esophageal carcinoma. However, most of these series consisted of patients with advanced disease. Local esophageal tumor involvement and mediastinal lymph nodes are more accurately assessed by endoscopic ultrasound (EUS). Thus, EUS is a superior technique for the preoperative evaluation of early esophageal cancer. Mediastinal lymph nodes are considered suspicious for malignancy when they are greater than 1 cm. However, the absence of enlarged nodes is not a reliable finding since CT cannot detect metastases in normal-sized nodes. Thus, CT has a low sensitivity but a high specificity for detection of malignant nodes.

MRI offers an alternative to CT for evaluating esophageal tumors although it has not been accepted widely for the staging of esophageal carcinoma. MRI of the esophagus may be limited by motion artifacts, long imaging times, cost, and availability. However, studies indicate that MRI is as accurate as CT for staging esophageal carcinoma.

EUS is the newest modality for evaluation of the esophagus. It plays a complementary role to CT and MRI in the staging of esophageal carcinoma. EUS allows visualization of the individual layers of the esophageal wall and can assess depth of invasion. Five alternating hyperechoic and hypoechoic layers are seen: mucosa (hyperechoic), deep mucosa (hypoechoic), submucosa (hyperechoic), muscularis propria (hypoechoic), and adventitia (hyperechoic). Esophageal carcinoma appears as a hypoechoic lesion with disruption of the normal layers. EUS is 73–92% accurate in the T-staging of esophageal cancer. It has proven most useful for earlier stage tumors and gastroesophageal junction tumors, which are often difficult to evaluate by CT and MRI.

The accuracy of EUS for diagnosing periesophageal nodal metastasis ranges from 70–81%. Findings suggestive of malignant nodal involvement include well-circumscribed hypoechoic nodes with a rounded shape. Mediastinal and perigastric nodal involvement are considered regional disease whereas celiac axis nodal involvement, which can also be detected by EUS, is indicative of distant metastasis. A limitation of EUS is the poor depth of penetration of the high-frequency transducers (7.5 or 12 MHz) so that CT or MRI is still required to detect distant

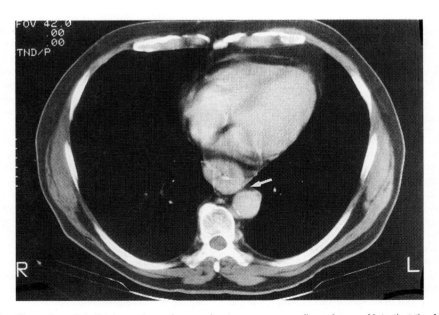

Figure 15–19. Circumferential distal esophageal mass due to squamous cell carcinoma. Note that the fat surrounding the mass is not infiltrated. There is a clear fat plane between the esophageal mass and the aorta *(arrow)*. This mass was subsequently resected.

metastases, such as those to the liver. In addition, in about 25% of patients the transducer is unable to pass beyond a malignant stricture.

Stomach

The primary modalities for diagnosing gastric lesions are barium UGI series and endoscopy, both of which allow evaluation of the mucosa. CT allows evaluation of extraluminal malignancy, including distant metastases. Gastric carcinoma can appear as wall thickening or polypoid or ulcerative masses on CT. In addition to hematogenous and nodal metastases, direct tumor extension and peritoneal implants may also be detected. The role of CT in the preoperative staging of gastric carcinoma remains controversial. Earlier reports were favorable, but more recent series have better defined the limitations of CT. CT has not proven reliable for detection of malignant adenopathy or pancreatic invasion. The overall accuracy of CT staging of gastric carcinoma is about 75%. At centers where all patients with gastric carcinoma undergo curative resection or palliative bypass, CT is not required preoperatively. However, if surgery is not always performed, preoperative CT may obviate laparotomy if diffuse metastatic disease is detected in patients who are asymptomatic or poor surgical candidates. Some surgeons request CT preoperatively to help in planning surgery. CT remains valuable in detecting distant metastases, particularly to the liver and lung. CT has proven more useful in the workup of patients with gastric lymphoma and leimyosarcoma where it is able to show tumor extent, identify metastases, and localize for percutaneous biopsy. CT has also been used in planning radiation ports, evaluating response to therapy, and detecting recurrence.

MRI of the stomach and the gastrointestinal tract is still being developed. The advantages of MRI include multiplanar imaging (transaxial, coronal, sagittal), the lack of ionizing radiation or need for iodinated contrast, and fewer surgical clip artifacts. However, there are technical problems, such as motion artifact from respiration or peristalsis and the lack of an adequate oral contrast agent for luminal opacification. With the development of phased array surface coils with faster imaging sequences and echo-planar imaging, MRI may prove useful in the future for delineating gastric abnormalities, including staging of gastric carcinoma.

EUS is superior to CT in determining the depth of wall invasion by gastric carcinoma. It can also detect perigastric spread and local adenopathy that may not be apparent on CT. Gastric carcinoma appears as a hypoechoic, vertically oriented mass disrupting the five normal wall layers. EUS is 73–80% accurate in staging gastric carcinoma and 68–80% accurate in diagnosing nodal metastasis. Limitations include the poor depth of penetration and the inability to pass the EUS transducer beyond some obstructing lesions.

EUS can often distinguish lymphoma from carcinoma. Gastric lymphoma appears as an extensive horizontal infiltration of the wall involving predominantly the second and third layers with focal ulceration. Other indications for EUS include evaluation of submucosal lesions such as leiomyoma, leiomyosarcoma, lipoma, and gastric varices (Figure 15–20).

Bowel

CT is useful for evaluation of small and large bowel obstruction, tumor, ischemia, and inflammatory disease. Bowel dilatation, wall thickening, mesenteric involvement, and intramural air are easily demonstrated. CT can be used to characterize bowel disease as focal or diffuse, to determine the degree, symmetry, and contour of wall thickening, to demonstrate the pattern of enhancement, as well as to delineate extraluminal disease such as inflammatory changes, abscesses, ascites, adenopathy, and metastases.

Whereas benign diseases of the bowel causes circumferential and symmetric wall thickening, malignancy presents as an eccentric wall thickening or mass with luminal narrowing and an irregular outer contour. Bowel wall hemorrhage as a result of trauma, coagulopathy, or ischemia may be seen as high-density wall thickening. Findings of ischemic bowel are often nonspecific and include wall thickening and bowel dilatation. In addition, CT may identify thrombus within the mesenteric vessels or portal vein and is more accurate than plain films for identifying intramural air and portal venous gas owing to bowel infarction.

In the evaluation of Crohn's disease, CT can delineate the distribution of bowel wall thickening and is useful for identifying "creeping" mesenteric fat as well as complications of Crohn's, such as intra-abdominal abscess, obstruction, and fistula. These findings are often helpful for differentiating between ulcerative colitis and Crohn's disease.

Infectious enteritis often produces nonspecific findings consisting of benign-appearing wall thickening with dilatation and increased intraluminal fluid. CT is slightly more sensitive than barium enema in detecting diverticulitis and is better able to demonstrate the extent of extraluminal disease. Thickened bowel wall, diverticula, and pericolonic involvement such as infiltration of the fat, abscess, and fistulae may be identified.

CT has been demonstrated to have a high sensitivity for diagnosing small bowel obstruction (SBO) as well as determining the location and cause. When clinical and plain film evaluation are equivocal, CT should be obtained. CT can help to distinguish SBO from other conditions causing small bowel dilatation, such as ileus. In both small and large bowel obstruction, CT can demonstrate the level of obstruction by identifying a transition zone from dilated to decompressed bowel, and in some cases it can determine the cause of obstruction (Figure 15–21). For partial

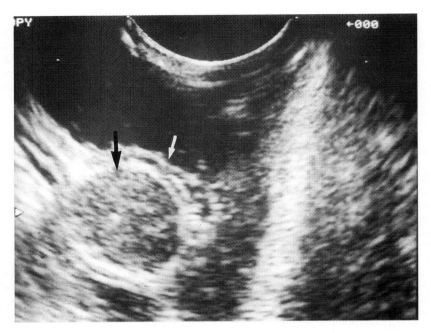

Figure 15–20. Endoscopic ultrasound (EUS) of a gastric leiomyoma *(black arrow)* arising in the submucosa. Note that the hyperechoic mucosa *(white arrow)* is intact and not thickened.

bowel obstruction, contrast studies often prove more helpful than CT in diagnosis and clinical management.

MRI of the bowel is still under investigation and is not used widely except in evaluation of the rectosigmoid region. Colonic cleansing and rectal air insufflation aid in obtaining diagnostic images. In addition to the use of T1- and T2-weighted images, intravenous contrast (gadopentetate dimeglumine) may be used with T1 imaging to help stage rectal carcinoma and to detect recurrent tumor. A recurrent tumor is often of low signal (dark) on T1 images, but of mixed or high signal (brighter) on T2 images. Postsurgical fibrosis has a low signal (dark) on T1 and T2 images. Scar enhancement may normally occur for about 1–1.5 years following surgery.

CT and MRI are comparable in their ability to stage rectosigmoid tumors. Both modalities can also identify metastatic disease and adenopathy, although neither can distinguish malignant adenopathy from benign hyperplasia. MRI of the rectum using endorectal coil is a newer technique which in initial studies appears promising in its ability to distinguish rectal wall layers and to detect perirectal adenopathy.

Transabdominal ultrasound is of limited use in the evaluation of bowel abnormalities. Ultrasound is able to detect distended fluid-filled bowel loops in cases of obstruction. However, air within the bowel will deflect the ultrasound beam and limit further evaluation of the abdomen. Ultrasound can also demon-strate bowel wall thickening resulting from tumor infiltration, inflammation, or hemorrhage.

Transrectal ultrasound (TRUS) permits excellent imaging of the lower two-thirds of the rectum and allows identification of the various layers of the wall. Studies performed so far indicate that TRUS is particularly useful in staging rectal tumors. Direct tumor extension and perirectal nodes that may be difficult to identify by CT and MRI are seen easily on TRUS.

Appendix

Plain film findings are often nonspecific in patients with appendicitis and may demonstrate an ileus pattern. Although seldom required to establish the diagnosis, single-contrast barium enema (SCBE) may reveal nonfilling of the appendix owing to extrinsic mass effect on the cecum or terminal ileum. Although complete filling of the appendix on SCBE excludes the diagnosis of appendicitis, nonfilling or incomplete filling can occur in patients with a normal appendix and therefore is not specific for the diagnosis.

CT and ultrasound have been employed in diagnosing acute appendicitis. However, more recently CT is preferred over ultrasound because of its slightly higher diagnostic accuracy. CT has a high sensitivity (87–89%), specificity (83–97%), and accuracy (93%) for the diagnosis of appendicitis. Findings include a thickened appendix (which may contain an appendicolith) and associated pericecal inflammation, fluid, or abscess (Figure 15–22).

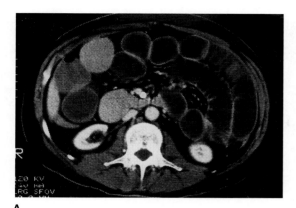

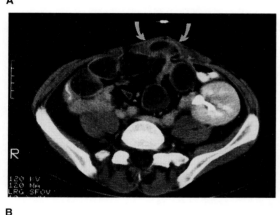

Figure 15–21. **A:** Patient with markedly dilated fluid-filled small bowel loops on CT who recently underwent pancreatic-renal transplant. Native kidneys are small. **B:** In same patient, note decompressed small bowel loop located anteriorly in the abdominal wall **(arrows)**, representing an incarcerated incisional hernia causing small bowel obstruction diagnosed by CT. (Note: transplanted pancreas in the right pelvis and transplanted kidney in the left pelvis).

CT has the ability to identify non-appendiceal disease that clinically may be confused for appendicitis. The extent of extraluminal disease is optimally demonstrated by CT, and it is particularly useful in patients with (1) a suspected appendiceal perforation (eg, debilitated or immunosuppressed patients), (2) severe clinical signs, or (3) palpable right lower abdominal mass. CT is the best modality for distinguishing a periappendiceal phlegmonous (inflammatory) mass from an abscess. CT-guided percutaneous catheter drainage, when clinically indicated, may be performed during the same examination if a periappendiceal abscess is identified.

Ultrasound has been shown to have a sensitivity of 77–89% and specificity and accuracy of over 90% for the diagnosis of acute appendicitis. The sonographic criteria used are an aperistaltic, noncom-

pressible, thickened appendix (diameter > 7 mm) (Figure 15–22).

The advantages of ultrasound include its lower cost compared to CT and the lack of ionizing radiation. Ultrasound should be the initial study performed in children as well as in young women of child-bearing age. Ultrasound (and transvaginal ultrasound) also has the ability to distinguish gynecologic disease from appendicitis. However, ultrasound is a more operator dependent diagnostic modality and it may not be useful in obese or uncooperative patients. Ultrasound also is less useful than CT in identifying other intra-abdominal causes of a patient's symptoms.

Liver

CT continues to be the preferred modality for the

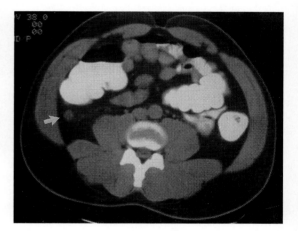

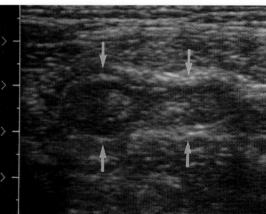

Figure 15–22. **A:** Patient with appendicitis found on CT to have a thickened appendix with mild periappendiceal stranding of the fat **(arrow)**. **B:** Different patient who underwent ultrasound for abdominal pain, found to have a thickened appendix that was peristaltic and noncompressible, consistent with appendicitis **(arrows)**.

evaluation of focal hepatic abnormalities, including tumor, infection, and trauma. CT also can be used for identification of diffuse liver diseases, such as fatty infiltration, cirrhosis, iron deposition (hemosiderosis, hemochromatosis), as well as infiltrative neoplasms. Technical advances have resulted in improved detection and characterization of mass lesions. Dynamic CT scanning of the abdomen that takes place during a rapid power-injected intravenous contrast bolus is the established screening modality for liver lesions. With this technique, scanning of the liver occurs within 2 minutes of intravenous contrast administration, allowing optimal demonstration of mass lesions. Delayed scanning at 4–6 hours can be performed to further increase sensitivity for lesions, due to iodine contrast uptake by normal tissue but not tumors.

CT arteriography (CTA) involves scanning of the liver during contrast injection directly into the hepatic or celiac artery via a catheter so that hepatic lesions are optimally enhanced and more easily detected. Most hepatic lesions derive their blood supply from the hepatic artery, whereas normal liver parenchyma receives 75–80% of its blood supply from the portal vein.

CT arterial portography (CTAP) is performed by scanning the liver during injection of contrast into the superior mesenteric artery. As contrast passes through the mesenteric artery and into the portal venous system, hepatic lesions may be seen as hypovascular compared with surrounding normal hepatic parenchyma, which enhances intensely. CTAP is the most sensitive technique (approximately 90%) for detecting hepatic metastases preoperatively and can accurately detail the precise hepatic segmental location of the metastatic deposits. Some studies indicate that CTAP can detect more than twice as many metastases as standard CT. However, because this technique is more invasive, it is used selectively for staging cancer or planning surgical resection. One drawback of CTAP is the high false-positive rate resulting from perfusion defects in up to 30% of cases.

Spiral CT is the newest modality for rapid scanning the liver. The entire liver can be imaged within 32 seconds. Scanning occurs during peak vascular enhancement when there is the maximum difference in density between hepatic lesions and normal parenchyma. Spiral CT with arterial portography, image reconstruction using thinner slices, and 3D analysis can be performed to further enhance detection of smaller lesions.

Ultrasound is often the initial examination in the evaluation of nonspecific abdominal clinical signs and symptoms and in patients with suspected biliary disease. State-of-the-art equipment permits real-time scanning with duplex Doppler or color flow Doppler capabilities. This allows differentiation between blood vessels and bile ducts and can demonstrate vascular occlusion, flow in collateral vessels, and flow within liver tumors. Ultrasound is not employed as a screening modality if liver disease is suspected because small lesions (< 1 cm) may not be detected. Hepatic sonography is useful for (1) distinguishing cystic versus solid liver lesions, (2) assessing the patient preoperatively or staging of tumors by evaluating lesion location and vascular invasion, (3) evaluating for inferior vena cava, hepatic and portal venous thrombosis, and (4) evaluating liver transplant patients pre- and postoperatively.

The use of intraoperative ultrasound has increased with the improvement of small high-resolution transducers. Small linear array transducers can fit into small incision sites, and fingertip probes can be used to help locate small lesions. Intraoperative ultrasound is used to determine whether small lesions identified preoperatively are cystic or solid. It can demonstrate additional lesions that may be unsuspected preoperatively. This modality can be used to help plan surgical resection and to monitor hepatic cryotherapy. Intraoperative ultrasound has been shown to effectively detect liver nodules less than 1 cm that may not be visible or palpable during surgery. It is more sensitive than preoperative CT or ultrasound for detecting hepatic metastases and is as sensitive as CTAP.

MRI of the abdomen must include techniques to reduce motion artifacts due to respiration and peristalsis. Fast gradient-echo sequences have been developed in conjunction with the breath-holding technique and are performed in addition to standard T1 and T2 sequences. Dynamic MRI using gradient-echo imaging can be performed after intravenous contrast (gadopentetate dimeglumine) to evaluate the enhancement pattern of liver lesions (Figure 15–23).

The relative strength of MRI versus CT for liver tumor staging is controversial and related to differences in expertise as well as equipment and scanning protocols. At present, both CT and MRI are noninvasive and have high sensitivity and accuracy for lesion detection and characterization. MRI may be particularly helpful in cases of suspected focal fatty infiltration of the liver or for detecting hepatic iron deposition (hemosiderosis, hemochromatosis).

A. Hepatocellular Carcinoma (HCC): CT or ultrasound is usually the initial examination for hepatocellular carcinoma. These modalities may also be used as guidance for percutaneous fine-needle biopsy. CT findings of HCC include a heterogeneously enhancing necrotic mass that may be encapsulated. Vascular invasion can be seen, as can hemoperitoneum due to HCC rupture. HCC may also be identified using ultrasound. MRI can demonstrate fat-containing HCC, pseudocapsules, daughter nodules, and septations. Tumor thrombus in the portal and hepatic veins or inferior vena cava is as reliably demonstrated on both MRI and with color flow Doppler. MRI should be performed in patients with severe cirrhosis when CT or ultrasound is equivocal, because MRI more easily detects and characterizes HCC against a background of abnormal parenchyma.

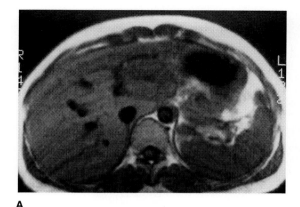

A

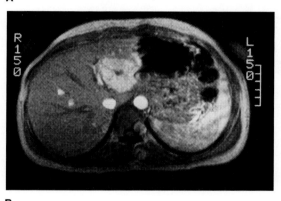

B

Figure 15–23. **A:** MRI of the liver using a T1-weighted sequence demonstrates a rounded lesion located in the left lobe. **B:** Fast gradient-echo image after administration of intravenous contrast (gadopentetate dimeglumine) showing immediate homogeneous enhancement of this lesion with a small central nonenhancing scar. This appearance and enhancement pattern is characteristic of focal nodular hyperplasia.

B. Metastases: CT is the primary modality for the evaluation of hepatic metastatic disease because of its high sensitivity for liver lesions and because it can study the rest of the abdomen and pelvis for a primary malignant neoplasm or other metastatic lesions (Figure 15–24). Liver metastases typically appear on CT as multiple rim-enhancing heterogeneous lesions that may have irregular margins. Although ultrasound can identify hepatic metastases, it provides less information about the rest of the abdomen and pelvis. MRI is preferred if a patient is allergic to iodinated contrast or if the CT findings are nonspecific. CTAP is the most sensitive modality for detection of hepatic metastases and should be performed if surgical resection of isolated hepatic metastases is being considered.

C. Cavernous Hemangioma: CT allows a reliable diagnosis of hemangioma when characteristic features are present. Lesions demonstrating early pe-ripheral, nodular, or globular contrast enhancement, which fills in centrally on delayed images, are typical of hemangiomas. However, these typical CT features are present in only 50–75% of cases. Incomplete fill-in may occur, especially in larger lesions that contain a central fibrous scar. If hemangioma cannot be confidently diagnosed by CT, other imaging studies may be helpful (Figure 15–25).

The typical ultrasound features of hemangiomas—well-defined hyperechoic lesions with increased through-transmission—are seen in about 80% of cases. If such a lesion is identified incidentally during ultrasound imaging, the need for further evaluation is determined by clinical symptoms and liver function tests; follow-up sonogram in 3–6 months often is suggested to reevaluate the lesion. The patient with a known primary tumor, a hepatic tumor that has atypical sonographic features of hemangioma, or abnormal liver function tests should undergo additional imaging (CT, MRI, or ^{99m}Tc-labeled red blood cell [RBC] scan) to evaluate the hepatic lesion.

One of the major applications of abdominal MRI is in the evaluation of hemangiomas. Hemangiomas characteristically demonstrate a marked high signal (very bright) on heavily T2-weighted images and have a similar enhancement pattern as CT. MRI is about 90–95% accurate in the diagnosis of hepatic hemangiomas, but is much more costly than ^{99m}Tc RBC scintigraphy.

^{99m}Tc RBC scintigraphy identifies hepatic hemangioma as a focal area of increased activity on delayed imaging at 1–2 hours. This finding is present in 70–90% of cases on planar imaging and in close to 95% of cases if single photon emission computed tomography (SPECT) is employed. ^{99m}Tc RBC scan with SPECT should be used for lesions greater than 1.5 cm, whereas MRI is preferred for lesions less than 1.5 cm or for lesions adjacent to the heart or major vessels. This modality is safe and relatively inexpensive and is currently the modality of choice at many institutions for diagnosing hepatic hemangiomas.

Angiography once was considered the "gold standard" for diagnosing hemangiomas. It is only rarely performed now when all other noninvasive imaging modalities fail to establish the diagnosis. Fine-needle aspiration biopsies of hemangiomas with 20-gauge or smaller needles have been performed with a low incidence of complications. This may be warranted in some clinical situations to distinguish a lesion that has atypical features of hemangioma from a malignant lesion.

Pancreas

CT is the imaging technique of choice for the diagnosis of acute pancreatitis and for detecting related complications. Acute edematous pancreatitis appears as pancreatic enlargement with peripancreatic fluid and infiltration (Figure 15–26). CT can detect complications such as pseudocyst formation or pancreatic

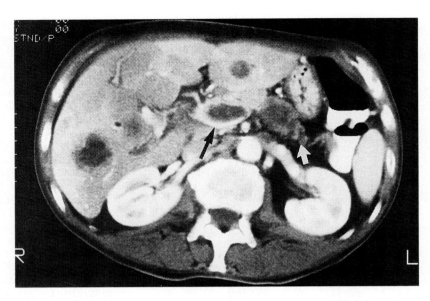

Figure 15–24. Low-density metastases are scattered throughout the liver, some with necrosis and some with rim enhancement. CT was able to demonstrate thrombosis of the main portal vein *(black arrow)* as well as the primary tumor, which was located in the pancreas *(white arrow)*.

abscess, hemorrhage, and necrosis. Large areas of absence of pancreatic enhancement during dynamic contrast-enhanced CT correlates well with pancreatic necrosis and portends a worse prognosis. Associated biliary obstruction and gastrointestinal inflammatory changes may also be identified on CT. Features of chronic pancreatitis on CT include pancreatic atrophy with fatty replacement, calculi, pancreatic and bile duct dilatation, pseudocyst, venous obstruction, and pseudoaneurysm.

CT is considered the best screening and staging modality for pancreatic carcinoma. This tumor typically appears as a low-density mass with associated pancreatic duct obstruction. Rapid dynamic contrast-enhanced CT using thin 5-mm sections is recommended for maintaining a high detection rate. Less commonly a mass is not identified and only biductal (pancreatic and bile ducts) dilatation is present. CT can determine surgical resectability by evaluating for vascular involvement (loss of fat plane around the superior mesenteric artery [SMA]), infiltration of adjacent organs, and distant metastases. A CT-guided fine-needle biopsy of the pancreas is often helpful to confirm the diagnosis of pancreatic carcinoma. If CT or fine-needle biopsy do not confirm the diagnosis of pancreatic carcinoma, ERCP may be required. Spiral CT has been successfully applied to imaging the pancreas. Improved vascular enhancement and the ability to reconstruct images at overlapping intervals may improve detection of small pancreatic carcinomas as well as islet cell tumors.

With the widespread availability of CT, ultrasound is used infrequently for the diagnosis of pancreatic carcinoma. Ultrasound has a reported sensitivity for pancreatic carcinoma of 80–95%. However, the sensitivity decreases when an adequate study is not obtained. Bowel gas may interfere with viewing the body and tail of the pancreas, and an incomplete examination occurs in up to 25% of cases. Sonographic findings include an irregular hypoechoic mass with dilatation of the pancreatic and bile ducts.

EUS has been demonstrated in preliminary studies to be highly accurate in the diagnosis and local staging of pancreatic carcinoma and is particularly useful for small tumors (< 2 cm). CT or MRI for full staging is still necessary to detect distant metastases. The role of endosonography in clinical practice must be evaluated by further studies. Intraoperative ultrasound has proven useful in helping to distinguish between pancreatic carcinoma and inflammatory lesions. It can evaluate the pancreatic duct as well as identify pancreatic cystic lesions. Intraoperative ultrasound is an excellent modality for identifying small islet-cell tumors.

MRI of the pancreas is still being studied and has not gained wide acceptance because of its higher cost and decreased resolution compared with CT. MRI can identify pancreatic carcinomas and can delineate vascular involvement, biliary duct dilatation, and hepatic metastases. Fat suppression technique and contrast enhancement (gadopentetate dimeglumine) can improve detection of carcinoma, which appears as a low-signal (dark) mass with poor enhancement. MRI offers an alternative to CT in those patients who cannot receive intravenous iodinated contrast.

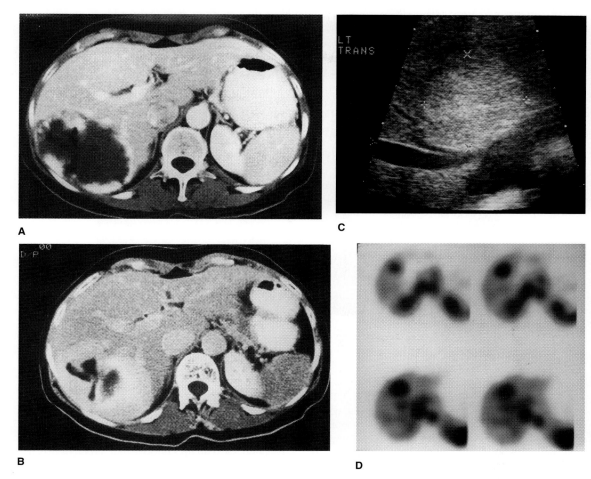

Figure 15–25. *A:* CT of a large cavernous hemangioma of the right lobe of the liver with initial peripheral nodular, globular enhancement. *B:* Delayed image demonstrating central fill-in of enhancement except for central fibrous scar. This appearance is typical of cavernous hemangioma of the liver. *C:* Ultrasound demonstrating a well-defined hyperechoic mass with increased through-transmission characteristic of hepatic hemangioma. *D:* ^{99m}Tc-labeled red blood cell scan with single photon emission computed tomography (SPECT), which should be used for lesions larger than 1.5 cm. These delayed images from a different patient show increased activity compatible with hepatic hemangioma. This modality is currently the modality of choice at many centers for diagnosing hepatic hemangiomas.

INTERVENTIONAL RADIOLOGY

Percutaneous Abscess Drainage

Percutaneous abscess drainage (PAD) has become the procedure of choice for treating many intra-abdominal abscesses and fluid collections. The optimal therapeutic approach depends on the organism and on the cause, location, and appearance of the abscess. CT or ultrasound is used as guidance for percutaneous needle placement into an abscess, which should have a relatively well-defined wall. The abscess contents are aspirated and examined for leukocytes and bacteria. Once this is confirmed, the catheter can be placed. Follow-up care consists of a periodic sinogram or tube check every 3–5 days after tube insertion, until abscess resolution is confirmed.

A. Liver: Most amebic abscesses of the liver are treated with antibiotics alone (metronidazole). Percutaneous drainage is performed in amebic abscesses with impending hepatic rupture, especially of left lobe abscesses, which can rupture into the thorax. PAD has also been performed successfully for large amebic abscesses (over 8–10 cm) and in cases where therapy is desired before serologic results are obtained.

Hydatid cyst was previously a contraindication to PAD because of the potential for anaphylaxis or peritoneal spread. However, PAD has been found to be safe in this situation, and transcatheter sclerosis has been performed. Surgical resection is still the preferred treatment modality for hydatid cyst of the liver in most centers.

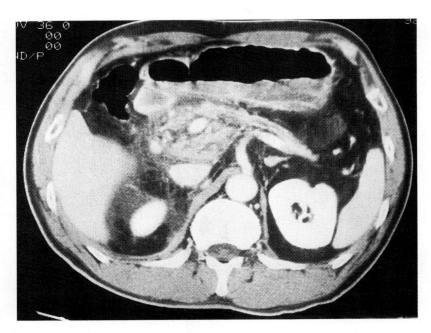

Figure 15–26. CT of the abdomen, demonstrating acute superimposed on chronic pancreatitis. CT is the technique of choice for imaging acute edematous pancreatitis. The pancreatic head is enlarged and there is infiltration of the peripancreatic fat with fluid present. The remainder of the pancreas is atrophied and the pancreatic duct is mildly dilated.

Pyogenic abscesses are treated with a combination of PAD and antibiotic therapy, with cure rates of 70–90%. Pyogenic liver abscess can be due to biliary obstruction or to seeding from the gastrointestinal tract via the portal vein. Diverticulitis and inflammatory bowel disease are common causes that should be searched for and treated. The complication rate of PAD of the liver is low (< 5%). Complications include pleural effusion, pneumothorax, hemorrhage, bacteremia, and peritonitis. Bile duct injury or biliary communication following drainage are uncommon.

B. Spleen: Splenic abscesses are uncommon, usually occurring in the setting of immunosuppression or bacterial endocarditis. Splenectomy has been the standard therapy although PAD has been successful in treating splenic abscesses with low morbidity (Figure 15–27). The most feared complication is hemorrhage. Multiple microabscesses due to hematogenous dissemination are not amenable to PAD.

C. Pancreas: Pancreatic abscesses are optimally treated by surgical drainage and débridement. Percutaneous drainage is particularly difficult because pancreatic abscesses are often septated and poorly defined, and may be associated with necrotic tissue or fistulae. The material within pancreatic abscesses is often viscous and will not drain well through a catheter. In patients with severe necrotizing pancreatitis who are critically ill, PAD may be used as a temporizing therapy with surgery performed after improvement of the patient's clinical

condition. PAD can be performed in patients who develop new pancreatic abscesses following surgery.

Percutaneous drainage of infected pancreatic pseudocysts remains controversial although it is now commonly performed as the initial therapy in many centers. Intravenous antibiotics are given and drainage is continued until the communication closes. If the distal pancreatic duct is obstructed, the fistulous communication may not close with percutaneous treatment and surgery may be required. The issue of surgical drainage versus PAD is still being debated, but PAD is used increasingly at many centers. Pseudocysts should be drained when they are enlarging, greater than 5 cm, painful, or when they are causing biliary or gastric or duodenal obstruction. Complications occur in 5–10% of cases and include infection, fistula, rupture, and hemorrhage. Most noninfected pseudocysts do not require drainage.

D. Bowel: Percutaneous drainage has been used successfully for enteric-related abscesses. This procedure is best performed under CT guidance so as to avoid traversing the adjacent intestine. PAD of periappendiceal abscesses allows drainage of infected inflammatory material, thereby permitting elective interval appendectomy at a later date. Peridiverticular abscesses treated by PAD also can facilitate subsequent surgical management by allowing bowel resection and primary anastomosis to be performed as a one-stage operation. Peridiverticular abscesses and periappendiceal abscesses treated by PAD have a

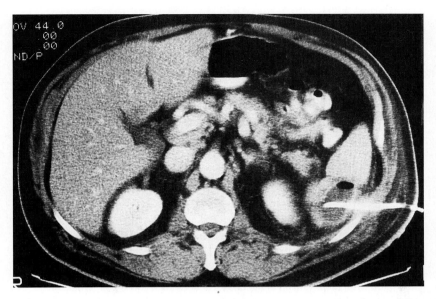

Figure 15–27. Successful CT-guided percutaneous catheter drainage of a splenic abscess in a patient with bacterial endocarditis. Multiple microabscesses of the spleen cannot be drained percutaneously.

success rate of over 90%. The need for interval appendectomy and subsequent bowel resection following PAD of appendiceal and diverticular abscesses is controversial. Most do agree that if surgery is not done, a barium enema should be performed to exclude an undiagnosed perforated tumor. Abscesses related to Crohn's disease may be treated successfully by PAD alone, without the need for surgery. Pelvic abscesses that cannot be drained by an anterior approach because of interfering bowel loops may be drained through transgluteal, transrectal, or transvaginal routes.

Angiography

A. Gastrointestinal Bleeding: Endoscopy is the primary diagnostic tool in patients with upper gastrointestinal hemorrhage. Endoscopy can identify the bleeding site or source as well as provide access for therapeutic intervention. If no source is identified and the patient has continued brisk bleeding, arteriography may be performed. Arteriography can identify and treat many causes of upper gastrointestinal bleeding, including varices, gastritis, ulcers, and Mallory-Weiss tears. Transcatheter treatment with intra-arterial vasopressin (splanchnic vasoconstrictor) or embolotherapy often obviates surgery.

Colonoscopy is often not possible in patients with acute active lower gastrointestinal tract hemorrhage because blood obscures the endoscopic view. In this setting, nuclear scintigraphy or arteriography is performed. **^{99m}Tc sulfur colloid scan** is a sensitive examination and is capable of detecting bleeding rates as low as 0.05–0.1 ml/min, which is one-fifth to one-

tenth of the minimal rate seen by arteriography. However, sulfur colloid imaging will be positive only if bleeding is active within 10–15 minutes of injection. **^{99m}Tc-labeled red blood cell scan** can detect similar rates of blood loss as sulfur colloid scans and has the advantage of allowing imaging up to 24 hours after injection. It is preferred in patients with intermittent bleeding. Causes of false-positive labeled RBC scan include gastric, kidney, and bladder uptake due to poor labeling efficiency. Neither of the scintigraphic studies will be helpful unless hemorrhage is ongoing, and neither can determine the origin of the bleeding.

If nuclear scintigraphy is positive, arteriography is performed. This study is useful for diagnosis as well as therapy (Figure 15–28). Lower gastrointestinal bleeding arteriography can locate the site of bleeding if bleeding exceeds 0.5 ml/min. Arteriography can diagnose angiodysplasia, arteriovenous malformation, vascular tumor, and bleeding diverticulum. In some situations subsequent transcatheter vasopressin or embolotherapy is performed in an attempt to arrest the bleeding. If nuclear scintigraphy or arteriography is negative, further workup should include CT, colonoscopy, and barium studies. Barium studies should never be done in the initial workup of gastrointestinal bleeding, since barium will interfere with subsequent angiography and endoscopy.

B. Mesenteric Ischemia: Early angiography is important in the diagnosis and treatment of mesenteric ischemia. Plain film findings often occur late in the course and include bowel wall thickening (thumbprinting), fixed bowel loops, a gasless ab-

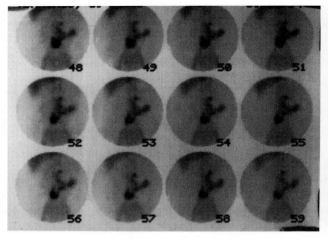
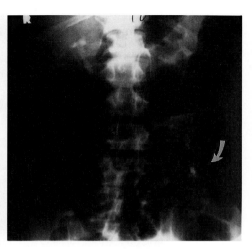

A   B

Figure 15–28. **A:** ^{99m}Tc-labeled red blood cell scan shows increased activity on delayed images in patient with lower gastrointestinal hemorrhage. The configuration of the uptake is consistent with small bowel source. **B:** Superior mesenteric arteriogram shows extravasation of contrast in the region of the ileum with a tumor blush **(arrow)**. At surgery a bleeding carcinoid tumor was found.

domen, small bowel pseudo-obstruction, and bowel distension to the level of the splenic flexure. Pneumatosis and portal vein gas are findings that indicate bowel necrosis and are associated with poor prognosis. CT and ultrasound can detect bowel abnormalities as well as vascular occlusions.

Mesenteric angiography is the diagnostic modality of choice for identification of occlusive disease (SMA embolus or thrombus, superior mesenteric vein [SMV] thrombus) versus nonocclusive disease (mesenteric vasoconstriction). SMA emboli usually occur in the setting of atrial fibrillation. The emboli appear as meniscoid filling defects at major branching points distal to the first 2 cm of the SMA. SMA thrombosis is usually seen in patients with pre-existing atherosclerotic disease. Thrombus typically causes occlusion of the first 2 cm of the SMA.

SMV thrombosis may be idiopathic or occur in association with portal hypertension, hypercoagulable states, sepsis, or trauma. Angiographic findings include diffuse arterial spasm, slow arterial flow and either absent visualization of the SMV or SMV thrombus. Nonocclusive ("low flow") mesenteric ischemia is due to arterial vasoconstriction commonly occurring in patients with underlying severe cardiac disease with low cardiac output or hypovolemic hypotension. During angiography, narrowing of the SMA branches is present with poor visualization of the SMV. In addition, focal or segmental spasm at branch points or diffuse spasm of the SMA system may be seen.

Mesenteric ischemia due to nonocclusive mesenteric ischemia is treated nonoperatively. In contrast, patients with SMA emboli or thrombus often require emergency surgery with embolectomy or thrombectomy with resection of infarcted bowel. A vasodilator such as papaverine may be infused into the SMA both before and after laparotomy and local resection. It may also be beneficial in patients with nonocclusive mesenteric ischemia. Patients with SMV thrombosis may be managed conservatively if collateral veins have formed. If peritoneal signs are present, laparotomy with bowel resection is often necessary.

C. Transjugular Intrahepatic Portosystemic Shunt: Placement of transjugular intrahepatic portosystemic shunt (TIPS) is a nonoperative treatment (which is still undergoing clinical investigation) used for the management of acute variceal bleeding in patients with portal hypertension. In this procedure, the right or middle hepatic vein is accessed by passing a catheter through the right internal jugular vein and into the superior vena cava. A needle is advanced blindly from the hepatic vein out of the catheter and through the hepatic parenchyma into a branch of the portal vein. A wire is passed through the needle catheter into the portal vein system. An expandable metallic stent is then inserted across the tract, thereby creating a portal-systemic shunt.

TIPS is clinically indicated for patients with acute or recurrent variceal bleeding that is unresponsive to sclerotherapy and for patients with variceal bleeding who are awaiting liver transplantation. TIPS is also being evaluated as possible therapy for intractable portal hypertensive ascites. Contraindications for TIPS placement include severe right sided heart failure, severe hepatic failure, polycystic liver disease, hypervascular hepatic masses, portal vein thrombosis and sepsis.

Preliminary studies indicate that TIPS is an effective and safe method of decompressing portal pressure and controlling acute variceal bleeding (apparently as effective as surgical portocaval shunts and more effective than sclerotherapy, according to initial data). TIPS also avoids the need for surgery and general anesthesia and, due to its intrahepatic location, does not interfere with subsequent liver transplantation.

Reported complications of TIPS include intraperitoneal hemorrhage, hemobilia, bacteremia, and contrast-induced renal failure. Long-term complications include encephalopathy (in up to 20% of patients), recurrent variceal bleeding (18–26%), and shunt occlusion (in 10–20%). Shunt patency is usually maintained for up to 1–2 years, with occlusion related to the development of intimal hyperplasia.

RADIONUCLIDE SCANS

Gastroesophageal Reflux Study

The oral administration of ^{99m}Tc sulfur colloid rarely is used to evaluate patients presenting with atypical manifestations of gastroesophageal reflux, especially bilious vomiting or recurrent aspiration pneumonia. This technique is more sensitive than fluoroscopic barium esophagram or endoscopy for detecting reflux.

A. Technique: Following an overnight fast, the patient drinks 300 ml of acidic solution containing a radiotracer. With the patient in the supine position, images are obtained over the chest with an abdominal binder in place.

B. Cost: $500–$675.

Gastric Emptying Scan

This study is used for evaluation of gastric motility. It is most often employed in the evaluation of patients with suspected gastroparesis, especially diabetic gastroparesis or post-vagotomy. The gastric emptying scan should not be the initial study for suspected mechanical gastric outlet obstruction. Although both liquid and solid phase emptying can be assessed, the solid portion of the study is more sensitive for detecting gastroparesis. For the liquid phase of the study, ^{111}In DTPA is used, and ^{99m}Tc sulfur colloid is used as the label for the solid phase (often tagged to egg whites). The normal time for one-half of the activity to leave the stomach is 90 minutes.

A. Technique: Following a fasting period of at least 4–6 hours, the patient consumes the labeled meal. Supine images are obtained every 15 minutes for 3 hours. The patient is required to sit up between each image.

B. Cost: $400–$600.

Liver-Spleen Scan

The liver and spleen both contain reticuloendothe-lial cells that readily take up ^{99m}Tc sulfur colloid from the blood. The pattern of uptake reflects the distribution of functioning reticuloendothelial cells as well as hepatic perfusion. The liver normally phagocytoses 80–90% of the tracer whereas the spleen sequesters 5–10% under normal circumstances. The bone marrow takes in a negligible amount of tracer. Lesions measuring 2–2.5 cm are readily identified. Smaller (1–1.5 cm) deep lesions may be detected by SPECT. Parenchymal defects demonstrated on this scan are nonspecific and cannot distinguish inflammatory from neoplastic lesions. However, the liver-spleen scan can detect some lesions that are missed by CT or ultrasound because of isodensity.

Causes of a solitary "cold" defect in the liver include: hepatocellular carcinoma, metastasis, hemangioma, cyst, abscess, hematoma, and adenoma. Hepatic adenomas typically occur in young women with a history of oral contraceptive use. They usually do not contain a significant number of Kupffer cells and therefore will appear as an intrahepatic "cold" defect. In contrast, focal nodular hyperplasia (FNH) is a benign neoplasm that also occurs often in females. Because FNH contains Kupffer cells that are able to concentrate radiocolloid, it will appear indistinguishable (isodense) from the normal parenchyma or may occasionally appear as "hot" lesions with increased uptake. Multiple focal "cold" intrahepatic defects are commonly due to metastatic disease, multiple cysts, or hemangiomas.

Diffuse liver disease may also be detected on liver-spleen scan. Cirrhosis is manifest by a small right hepatic lobe and an enlarged left lobe. Increased colloid uptake in the spleen and bone marrow typically is present. Causes of hepatomegaly with diffusely decreased colloid activity include infiltrative disorders, such as hepatitis or cirrhosis, fatty infiltration, passive congestion, lymphoma, and hemochromatosis.

Causes of splenic "cold" defects include: cyst, hemangioma, abscess, and malignancy. Splenic infarcts are typically identified by peripheral wedge-shaped defects. Splenomegaly may be due to portal hypertension, hemolytic anemia, lymphoma or leukemia, and infectious causes. The liver-spleen scan also may be used to localize accessory splenic tissue.

A. Technique: No patient preparation is necessary. Following the intravenous administration of ^{99m}Tc sulfur colloid, patients are imaged with multiple views, including anterior, posterior, lateral, and oblique positions.

B. Cost: $600–$800.

Meckel's Scan

Meckel's diverticulum represents the remnant of the omphalomesenteric duct and occurs in approximately 2% of the population. It is usually located within 100 cm of the ileocecal valve along the antimesenteric border of the ileum. There is a strong male preponderance, and the majority cause symptoms in children younger than 10 years. Most Meckel's diverticula patients are asymptomatic; however complications such as bleeding, obstruction, intussusception, and volvulus can occur. Approximately 30% of Meckel's diverticula contain gastric mucosa, which increases the likelihood of complications. The frequency of ectopic gastric mucosa in symptomatic Meckel's diverticula is about 60%. In diverticula complicated by gastrointestinal hemorrhage, the incidence of ectopic gastric mucosa increases to over 95%.

Intravenous ^{99m}Tc pertechnetate is secreted by gastric mucosa into the gastrointestinal tract. Radiopertechnetate also is secreted by the ectopic gastric mucosa located in a Meckel's diverticulum. It will be seen as a solitary focus of increased activity, usually located in the right lower quadrant of the abdomen. Activity in this focus should appear at the same time that activity appears in the stomach. Causes of false-positive results include: inflammatory bowel disease, obstruction, urinary tract uptake (hydronephrosis), and intussusception. The accuracy of radiopertechnetate imaging for symptomatic Meckel's diverticulum is more than 95%.

A. Patient Preparation: Patients should fast for 6 hours to decrease gastric secretions and peristalsis. Patients should also empty bladder and bowel before the imaging procedure.

B. Technique: Following intravenous administration of radiopertechnetate, images are obtained in the supine position at 5-minute intervals up to 1 hour. Lateral views are also obtained. The administration of certain agents will improve localization: Pentagastrin (increases pertechnetate uptake), glucagon (decreases peristalsis), or cimetidine (decreases pertechnetate secretion but not uptake).

C. Cost: $550–$650.

REFERENCES

Balthazar EJ et al: Acute appendicitis: CT and US correlation in 100 patients. Radiology 1994;190:31.

Bluemke DA, Fishman EK: Spiral CT of the liver. Am J Roentgenol 1993;160:787.

Botet JF et al: Preoperative staging of esophageal cancer: Comparison of endoscopic US and dynamic CT. Radiology 1991;181:419.

Botet JF et al: Preoperative staging of gastric cancer: Comparison of endoscopic US and dynamic CT. Radiology 1991;181:426.

DelMaschio A et al: Pancreatic cancer versus chronic pancreatitis: Diagnosis with CA 19-9 assessment, US, CT, and CT-guided fine-needle biopsy. Radiology 1991;178:95.

Dixon PM, Roulston ME, Nolan DJ: The small bowel enema: A ten-year review. Clinical Radiol 1993;47:46.

Ferrucci JT: Liver tumor imaging. Am J Roentgenol 1990;155:473.

Ferrucci JT: Screening for colon cancer: Programs of the American College of Radiology. Am J Roentgenol 1993;160:999.

Frazer D et al: CT of small bowel obstruction: Value in establishing the diagnosis and determining the degree and cause. Am J Roentgenol 1994;162:37.

Gazelle GS et al: Efficacy of CT in distinguishing small bowel obstruction from other causes of small bowel dilatation. Am J Radiol 1994;162:43.

LaBerge JM et al: Creation of transjugular intrahepatic portosystemic shunts with the Wallstent endoprosthesis: Results in 100 patients. Radiology 1993;187:413.

Levine MS, Laufer I: Perspective: The upper gastrointestinal series at a crossroads. Am J Roentgenol 1993;161:1131.

Levine MS, Rubesin SE, Ott DJ: Update on esophageal radiology. Am J Roentgenol 1990;155:933.

Maglinte DT, Torres WE, Laufer I: Oral cholecystography in contemporary gallstone imaging: A review. Radiology 1991;178:49.

Niederau C, Grendell JH: Diagnosis of pancreatic carcinoma: imaging techniques and tumor markers. Pancreas 1992;7:66.

Ott DJ, Pikna LA: Clinical and videofluoroscopic evaluation of swallowing disorders. Am J Roentgenol 1993;161:507.

Philpotts LE et al: Colitis: Use of CT findings in differential diagnosis. Radiology 1994;190:445.

Rosh T et al: Staging of pancreatic and ampullary carcinoma by endoscopic ultrasonography–comparison with conventional sonography, computed tomography, and angiography. Gastroenterology 1992;102:188.

Soyer P et al: Detection of liver metastases from colorectal cancer: Comparison of intraoperative US and CT during arterial portography. Radiology 1992;183:541.

Takishima S et al: Carcinoma of the esophagus: CT versus MR imaging in determining resectability. Am J Roentgenol 1991;156:297.

van Sonnenberg E et al: Percutaneous abscess drainage: Current concepts. Radiology 1991;181:617.

Whitaker SC, Gregson RH: The role of angiography in the investigation of acute or chronic gastrointestinal haemorrhage.Clinical Radiol 1993;47:382.

Zuckerman DA, Bocchini TP, Birnbaum EH: Massive hemorrhage in the lower gastrointestinal tract in adults: Diagnostic imaging and intervention. Am J Roentgenol 1993;161:703.

Endoscopic Management of Biliary & Pancreatic Diseases

16

Richard A. Kozarek, MD

Endoscopic retrograde cholangiopancreatography (ERCP) was originally used to facilitate diagnosis in a variety of benign and malignant pancreaticobiliary disorders. In the past 20 years, however, since the original description of endoscopic sphincterotomy, it has evolved from a purely diagnostic modality to one that entails a therapeutic intervention 50–75% of the time. Thus, the majority of common bile duct calculi can be removed, most malignant biliary strictures can be stented, and a subset of biliary injuries are now amenable to endotherapeutic procedures. Many of the questions that remain are technical: What is the safest way to undertake sphincterotomy? Should a dilating or balloon catheter be used? Should prostheses be conventional or expandable?

By way of contrast, endotherapy directed towards the pancreas is in its infancy. Treatment of pancreatic calculi requires not only technical expertise but also a conviction that these calculi are more than epiphenomena, are not only the consequence of chronic pancreatitis, but also the cause of pain and relapsing attacks of clinical pancreatitis in a subset of patients. Treatment of benign and malignant pancreatic stenoses, in turn, requires a belief that impaired flow of pancreatic secretions causes clinical symptoms related to ductal obstruction. Finally, treatment of ductal disruptions presupposes that techniques used within the biliary tree can be readily adapted to the pancreatic duct with comparable results and an acceptable complication rate. Most of the above assumptions await confirmatory studies before widespread application of these procedures can be recommended.

BILIARY DISEASE

Biliary tree processes amenable to therapeutic ERCP include calculi with or without concomitant jaundice, cholangitis, or pancreatitis; benign and malignant strictures; sphincter of Oddi stenosis or spasm; biliary fistulas; and miscellaneous conditions to include choledochocele, sump syndrome, biliary parasitosis, and AIDS cholangiopathy.

Calculus Disease

Endoscopic biliary sphincterotomy, developed simultaneously in Japan and Germany in the mid-1970s, is now widely applied for treating bile duct stones. Procedures require fluoroscopic monitoring, antibiotic precoverage, and access to a wide range of equipment. Using accessories that have evolved from free-hand to wire-guided, the endoscopist who performs electrocautery incision of the distal bile duct accesses the biliary tree for subsequent calculus extraction using balloon catheters or stone baskets (Figure 16–1). Most series and surveys suggest a success rate of approximately 85–95% for complete stone retrieval. This rate is contingent upon several factors, including stone size (large stones may require mechanical, extracorporeal, or electrohydraulic lithotripsy, dissolution therapy, or endoprosthesis placement). Other factors include concomitant biliary stricture, or the presence of variant anatomy such as juxtampullary diverticula, Billroth II gastric resection, and Roux-en-Y jejunal anastomoses. Complications, in turn, average 7–8% and the mortality rate is approximately 1% in the largest series. The former include bleeding and pancreatitis most frequently, but acute cholecystitis in patients with intact gallbladders, bile duct or intestinal perforation (Figure 16–2), basket entrapment, and more mundane types of complications (drug reaction, aspiration, cardiopulmonary events) are all well-described.

The above-mentioned success and complication rates have led practitioners to accept endoscopic sphincterotomy as the procedure of choice in postcholecystectomy patients who have common bile duct stones or the high-risk patient who has an intact gallbladder. It is also the procedure of choice in most patients with acute cholangitis with or without a gallbladder, and ERCP may be both diagnostic and therapeutic in a significant subset of patients with gallstone pancreatitis. Finally, the introduction of laparoscopic cholecystectomy has radically altered the approach to choledocholithiasis in many centers, even in the young and otherwise surgically fit patient. As such, open common bile duct exploration has been relegated to a small role in the treatment of

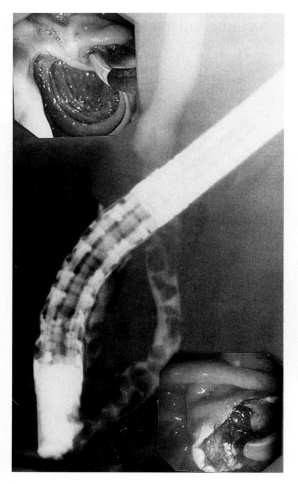

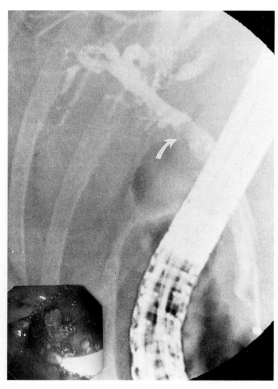

Figure 16–1. *A:* Cholangiogram demonstrating multiple calculi. Inserts depict biliary sphincterotomy. ***B:*** Copious debris retrieved (insert) utilizing extraction balloon *(arrow)*.

choledocholithiasis despite the absence of controlled clinical trials justifying this alteration in practice patterns.

Cholangitis

Pus in the biliary tree, often a consequence of endoprosthesis occlusion, occurs most commonly de novo related to impacted bile duct stones. Presenting clinically with Charcot's triad (fever, jaundice, hepatic pain) or Reynolds pentad (jaundice, pain, fever, change in mental status, shock), bacterial cholangitis has a higher than 80% associated mortality rate when undrained. Open surgical intervention, in turn, carries mortality rates between 7 and 50%. Endoscopic drainage, in turn, uses biliary sphincterotomy and either a large bore endoprosthesis or nasobiliary drain to effect irrigation. Several recent studies document

relative procedural safety and a mortality as low as 5% within 24 hours.

Pancreatitis

Gallstone pancreatitis may be mild and is often associated with calculus passage through the papilla of Vater (Figure 16–3). It may be severe, recurrent, or associated with concomitant cholangitis, however, and be associated with major morbidity. Several studies have prospectively addressed whether urgent endoscopic intervention ameliorates or exacerbates presumptive biliary pancreatitis. For example, in one study conducted by Neoptolemos et al, 121 patients were randomized to conventional medical therapy versus urgent ERCP and stone extraction, if indicated. Findings included: (1) ERCP did not appear to exacerbate the acute pancreatitis; (2) patients under-

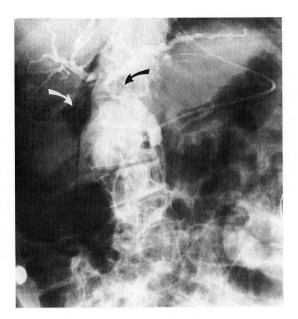

Figure 16–2. Nasobiliary drain **(black arrow)** in cholangitis patient who sustained perforation with sphincterotomy. Note para-psoas air **(white arrow).** Patient did well with conservative therapy.

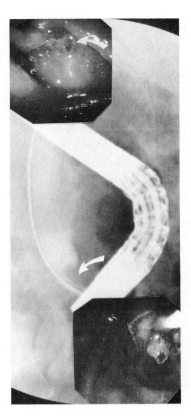

Figure 16–3. Arrows depict impacted calculus in patient with biliary pancreatitis. Lower insert shows stone retrieval following small sphincterotomy.

going urgent ERCP/sphincterotomy had fewer complications (P = 0.03), particularly those with severe disease (P = 0.007) as defined by the Glasgow system for scoring severity; (3) hospitalization for the endoscopically treated group was approximately one-half that of the conservatively managed patients; and (4) there was no statistically significant difference in mortality between the two groups. Data such as the above, as well as additional recent data by Fan et al documenting clinical improvement following sphincterotomy in patients with both mild and moderate biliary pancreatitis, suggest that urgent ERCP should be considered in at least a subset of pancreatitis patients. Current practice in the author's institution is to use ERCP in any patient with severe biliary pancreatitis, patients with persistent liver function test abnormalities, those who develop recurrent biliary colic or exacerbation of their pancreatitis, as well as those patients who appear to have superimposed elements of cholangitis.

Interaction Between ERCP & Laparoscopic Cholecystectomy for Stone Disease

Since the advent of laparoscopic cholecystectomy in this country in 1989, there have been widely disparate practice patterns espoused regarding the treatment of choledocholithiasis. Both universal and selective preoperative ERCP have been espoused, the former as an anatomic "outline," the latter if there is

any suspicion of common bile duct stone (elevated liver function tests, dilated CBC with ultrasound, cholangitis, or pancreatitis). Intraoperative ERCP has been used in a few centers for stones documented with operative cholangiography. Finally, postoperative ERCP has been performed to study patients who become symptomatic after laparoscopic cholecystectomy or those in whom common duct stones cannot be retrieved through the cystic duct or by means of open common bile duct exploration. Currently, approaches to choledocholithiasis are institutionally dependent, contingent on relative skill and confidence levels of both the laparoscopic surgeon and biliary endoscopist. Institutions in which both the endoscopist and surgeon are uncomfortable with their ability to retrieve bile duct stones tend to do more preoperative ERCPs. If a stone cannot be retrieved in this setting, failure of laparoscopic retrieval would result in open exploration.

ERCP is used preoperatively in a small number of cases, restricting its use to the patient with acute cholangitis, significant biliary pancreatitis, or obstructive jaundice. Intraoperative cholangiography is done in all cases, and if stones are found, attempts are made to remove them through the cystic duct. Unsuccessful cases as well as those patients who develop biliary symptoms postoperatively undergo ERCP and sphincterotomy, if indicated. This recommended approach limits the number of ERCPs utilized, the cumulative complications and expense associated with two procedures, and limits the need for, and complications associated with biliary sphincter ablation (bleeding, perforation) in a sizable percentage of patients.

Stone Extraction Without Sphincterotomy

Given the significantly increased application of ERCP since the advent of laparoscopic cholecystectomy, as well as the realization that most of the severe complications of endoscopic stone retrieval are a consequence of sphincter section, a number of endoscopists have been studying stone retrieval without sphincterotomy. Some early studies suggest similar efficacy and complication rates to that seen after sphincterotomy. From some studies currently underway, preliminary data demonstrate equal efficacy and complication rates. Because of previous data, however, that suggest a significant incidence of pancreatitis with sphincter dilation, and because of uncertainty regarding the subsequent incidence of sphincter dysfunction, this approach remains investigational.

BILE DUCT STRICTURES

Benign Strictures

Ampullary Spasm–Papillary Stenosis: Sphincter of Oddi dysfunction may manifest as a papillary stricture and bile duct dilation, probably developing as a consequence of gravel passage and papillitis. Alternatively, the "spastic" subset presents with a non-dilated bile duct and a sphincter mechanism that demonstrates a variety of manometric abnormalities (baseline hypertension, tachyoddia, paradoxical response to cholecystokinin). Either patient subset usually presents with post-cholecystectomy biliary colic with variably fluctuating liver function tests. A wide variety of diagnostic tests have been used to define sphincter dysfunction and have been variably embraced and include the Nardi test, fatty meal ultrasound, biliary nuclear medicine scan, and conventional ERCP. Biliary manometry, however, has been considered the gold standard by most endoscopists. Endoscopic sphincterotomy in patients with a hypertensive sphincter has been associated with sustained relief in 60–90% of such patients contingent upon the presence or absence of additional abnormalities (eg, elevated liver functions, delayed drainage of the common bile duct or biliary tree dilation.

In contrast to sphincterotomy, however, balloon dilation in the setting of biliary dyskinesia is associated with a prohibitive risk of pancreatitis and has had no sustained effect either on sphincter pressure or patient symptoms.

Strictures Associated with Bile Duct Injury

For a variety of reasons, laparoscopic cholecystectomy has been associated with a significant incidence of bile duct injuries (Figure 16–4). When discovered early, these injuries are frequently associated with a bile duct fistula. This problem will be discussed subsequently in this chapter (see "Bile Duct Stents"). When discovered later, a stenosis is often the result. Occurring as a consequence of a misdirected scalpel, scissors, clip, or cautery (Figure 16–4), or as an ischemic injury related to devascularization, bile duct strictures have been traditionally handled surgically, most commonly with Roux-en-Y hepaticojejunostomy. The endoscopic approach requires sphincterotomy, balloon dilation, and passage of 1 or 2 endoprostheses through the stenosis. Stents are exchanged and the stricture redilated every 3–4 months for up to 1 year.

Results of endotherapy for iatrogenic biliary injuries have been encouraging to date, with 70–80% of patients reported to be asymptomatic over follow-up periods of 3–6 1/2 years. Despite the foregoing, long-term follow-up in these patients is mandatory as restenosis may be subtle and has been shown to occur many years after a "successful" surgical repair.

Miscellaneous Benign Strictures

Balloon dilation with or without endoprosthesis placement has been used for a plethora of additional benign biliary stenoses to include the distal bile duct strictures associated with chronic pancreatitis, radiation stenoses, Mirizzi's syndrome, and dominant strictures in the setting of sclerosing cholangitis. In the instance of pancreatic stenoses, stricture improvement is uncommon and endoprosthesis placement often complicated by occlusion or migration. As such, authors of the largest series in which stents have been placed in this setting recommend their application only as a temporary measure. From the standpoint of sclerosing cholangitis, endotherapy of a dominant stenosis has been shown to improve liver function tests, decrease the incidence of secondary bacterial cholangitis, and may delay or preclude the need for liver transplant in the patient subset that responds to treatment.

Malignant Biliary Strictures

Most malignant obstructive jaundice is caused by carcinoma of the pancreatic head. Less common causes include biliary or gallbladder neoplasia, ampullary or duodenal carcinoma, or metastases to the porta hepatis. The vast majority of these neoplasms

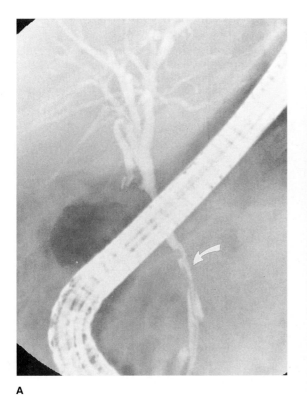

A

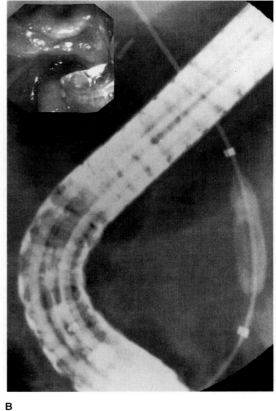

B

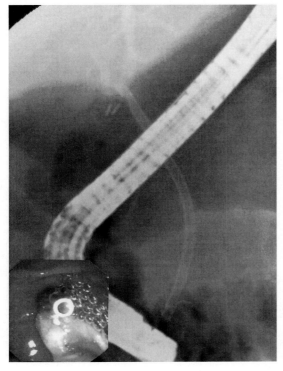

C

Figure 16–4. Asymmetric distal common bile duct stenosis as a consequence of cautery injury during laparoscopic cholecystectomy *(A).* Stricture treated with balloon dilation *(B)* and stent insertion *(C).*

will be unresectable for cure and, as such, patients will be candidates for a variety of surgical, percutaneous, or endoscopic palliative maneuvers (eg, sphincterotomy, stenosis dilation, and endoprosthesis placement).

Plastic Stents

From the endoscopic standpoint, polyethylene prostheses have been inserted through an obstructing stenosis often in conjunction with attempts at brush biopsy or needle aspiration of the tumor. Results of

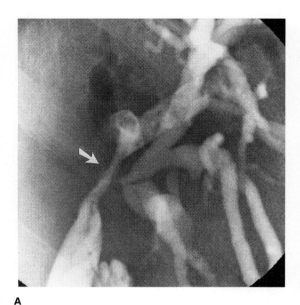

A

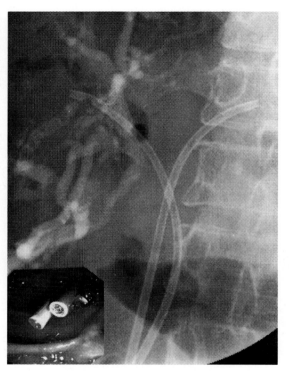

B

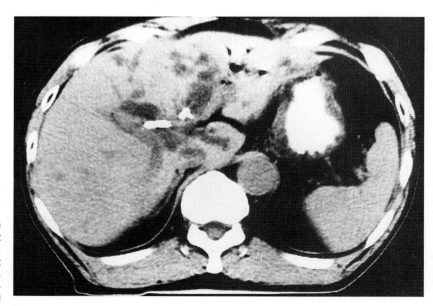

Figure 16–5. Tight bifurcation stenosis *(arrow)* in patient with cholangiocarcinoma *(A).* 10 Fr stents placed into right and left intrahepatic ducts *(B).* Note CT demonstrating adequate placement into dilated intrahepatic ducts *(C).*

C

endotherapy for malignant obstructive jaundice in large numbers of patients have demonstrated successful drainage in 85–90% of patients with a median survival of approximately 5 months (Figure 16–5). About 15–30% of patients developed stent occlusion, making stent replacement necessary.

Randomized prospective studies comparing palliation of malignant obstructive jaundice with either biliary-enteric bypass or surgery have shown that these palliative modalities appear to be equivalent with regard to adequacy of biliary decompression, procedure-related complications, 30-day mortality, and median survival.

Metallic Stents

Despite the abovementioned complications and a defined procedure-related mortality, and despite data documenting that treating patients endoscopically is more cost-effective than surgery (taken from time of diagnosis to death), occlusion of polyethylene prostheses remains problematic. Accordingly, a number of metallic prostheses have been devised in the hopes that large-diameter conduits (8–10 mm) will preclude or minimize plugging with bacterial biofilm. Although a variety of endoprostheses have been used including the Z stent, biliary Endocoil and Stryker stent, most experience to date has accrued with the Wallstent (Figure 16–6). Prospective studies randomizing patients to receive either the latter prosthesis or plastic stents in the setting of malignant obstructive jaundice have confirmed superior stent patency, but no improvement in patient survival. Placement of the metallic prosthesis in the Amsterdam study, for example, resulted in a median stent patency of 273 days as compared to 126 days for a conventional stent. This was associated with a 28% decrease in need for subsequent endoscopic procedures. Despite a 20-fold difference in cost between metallic and polyethylene prostheses, the authors concluded that metal stents were ultimately cost-effective.

Bile Duct Fistulas

Although bile duct fistulas may follow penetrating abdominal trauma, stone erosion, or liver transplantation, the bulk of these fistulas occur in the setting of cholecystectomy. Presenting clinically with variable degrees of abdominal pain, nausea, fever, and abdominal distention, diagnosis is usually made by abdominal ultrasound or CT. Biliary HIDA, while having the capability of defining the leak, does not delineate the presence or extent of bile ascites that may require percutaneous drainage, and as such, should not be used in isolation.

Technically, endotherapy for biliary fistulas depends on the site of the leak (cystic duct, common duct, intrahepatic duct), presence of an associated bile duct stricture, and the presence or absence of biliary calculi or papillary stenosis (Figure 16–7). Most

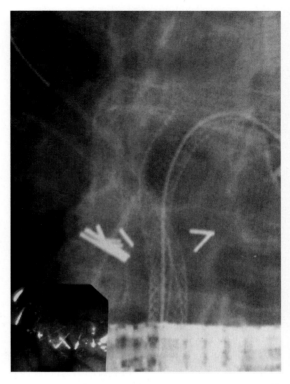

Figure 16–6. Bilateral Wallstents used in patient with bifurcation cholangiocarcinoma. Insert shows transpapillary stent in good position.

cystic duct or intrahepatic duct leaks close rapidly after placing a short 7–10 Fr stent, but will also close after biliary sphincterotomy if stone or sphincter stenosis is present. Bile duct leaks will also usually close, although this may depend on the degree of ductal injury and whether the stent can be placed above associated ductal stenosis.

Successful results of endotherapy for biliary fistulas have been reported by a number of authors. Using sphincterotomy alone or stent replacement (in some cases supplemented by percutaneous drainage), fistula closure has been reported in 67–90% of patients.

Miscellaneous Conditions

ERCP has proven not only useful in the differential diagnosis of a variety of miscellaneous biliary conditions; it has been utilized therapeutically in a subset. Examples include sphincterotomy treatment for biliary ascariasis, choledochocele and sump syndrome, gallbladder decompression in high-risk patients with acute cholecystitis or Mirizzi's syndrome, and gallstone dissolution in poor surgical-risk patients with symptomatic cholelithiasis.

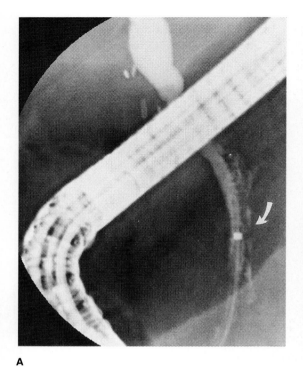

A

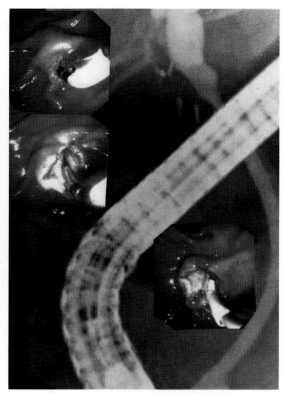

B

Figure 16–7. Irregular distal CBD leak as consequence of cautery injury *(A)* treated with sphincterotomy *(inserts)* and stent insertion.

PANCREATIC DISEASE

Most commonly used in the diagnosis of pancreatitis or pancreatic malignant growths, ERCP has recently been applied therapeutically. When undertaken in the setting of chronic pancreatitis, therapeutic interventions have included major or minor pancreatic duct sphincterotomy; calculus retrieval; transpapillary, transgastric, or transduodenal pseudocyst drainage; and dilation or stenting of pancreatic stenoses. Endoprostheses are also being used for disrupted pancreatic duct and an associated fistula or biliary stenosis as a consequence of chronic pancreatitis-induced bile duct cicatrization.

Sphincter Dysfunction/Sphincterotomy

Whereas pancreatic endoprostheses have been placed in an attempt to relieve chronic pain or relapsing attacks of pancreatitis in some patients with presumed sphincter dysfunction, their use has been associated with induction of focal pancreatitis and even ductal stenoses. Accordingly, pancreatic duct sphincterotomy of either the major or minor papilla may be preferable to treat sphincter dysfunction and has also been used to facilitate other maneuvers within the pancreas (eg, stone extraction or stenosis dilation).

Once considered high-risk, endoscopic sphincterotomy of the major pancreatic duct can be undertaken with conventional sphincterotomy or using a needle-knife over a stent. Undertaking major pancreatic sphincter section in 57 patients (55 with chronic pancreatitis) Kozarek et al (1994) recorded a 9% complication rate, most commonly mild pancreatitis. Grimm et al, in turn, were successful in effecting sphincterotomy in 61 chronic pancreatitis patients. Indications included strictures (6), stones (28), and pseudocysts (17), and 50 of 61 patients had initial improvement in symptoms with a variety of endotherapeutic maneuvers. Ultimately, 35 of 61 (57%) had sustained relief from chronic pain.

Similar data have been noted utilizing minor papilla sphincterotomy. For instance, 19 of 39 pancreas divisum patients treated with endoscopic sphincterotomy at the author's institution had chronic pancreatitis. Clinical complaints included chronic pain and relapsing pancreatitis; other complaints

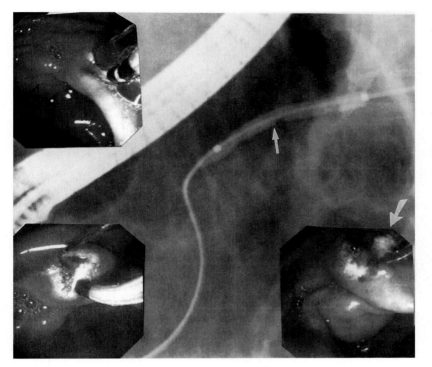

A

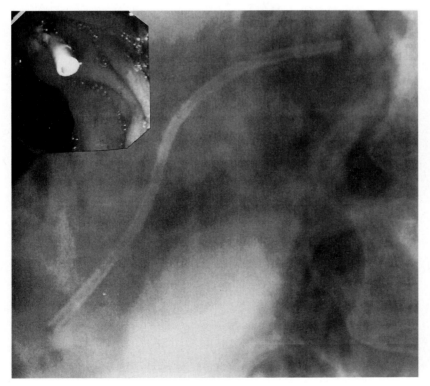

Figure 16–8. Pancreatic divisum patient with chronic pancreatitis, dorsal duct stricture treated with minor sphincterotomy (inserts), balloon dilation *(arrow),* and stone extraction *(arrow) (A).* Open arrow depicts major papilla. Subsequent endoprosthesis insertion *(B).*

B

were a consequence of ductal disruption. Associated with healing of ductal disruption in 80%, approximately one-half of the patients were symptomatically improved. Moreover, 11 of 15 patients with acute relapsing attacks of pancreatitis resolved their attacks. In an additional study by Lehman et al, 17 patients, with acute relapsing pancreatitis treated by minor duct papillotomy were improved. In contrast, 11 patients with chronic pancreatitis were statistically less likely to respond to endotherapy. Procedure-related pancreatitis was noted in approximately 10% of patients.

Ductal Stenoses

Endoprostheses have been inserted beyond pancreatic stenoses both diagnostically and therapeutically. In the latter instance, they have been used in the high surgical-risk patient following catheter or balloon dilation (Figure 16–8). One series reported successful stenting of 75 of 76 patients with chronic pancreatitis and dominant duct strictures (Cremer et al). Most also underwent major or minor duct sphincterotomy and some had extracorporeal shock wave lithotripsy (ESWL) for concomitant calculi. Ninety-four percent

were symptomatically improved and 11 ultimately underwent longitudinal pancreaticojejunostomy. Stent patency in this study was estimated to be 1 year and recurrent symptoms a consequence of endoprosthesis occlusion. Less than 10% of patients in this study had ultimate resolution of their stricture. Because of the low incidence of stricture resolution and the complications associated with endotherapy (eg, pancreatic sepsis, stent migration into duct, cholangitis, pseudocyst development, and hematobilia), endotherapy is not an acceptable long-term treatment in most patients with pancreatic ductal strictures.

Calculi

Usually considered the consequence of chronic pancreatitis as opposed to the cause of pain or relapsing attacks of pancreatitis, calculi can at times be obstructive. For instance, early experience by Kozarek et al (1991) demonstrated successful stone retrieval in 10 of 11 patients utilizing conventional balloon or baskets following a pancreatic sphincterotomy (Figure 16–9). At a mean follow-up of 18 months 8 of 9 patients with relapsing pancreatitis were symptom-free. One of the two chronic pain patients, in turn,

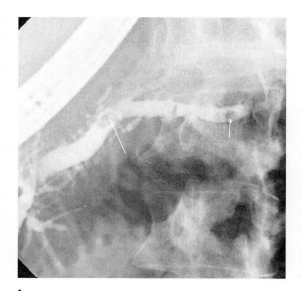

A

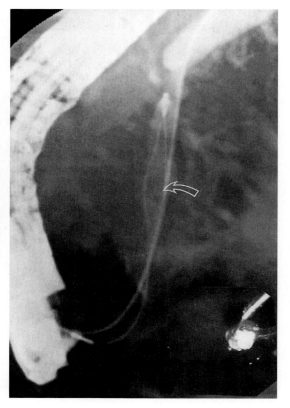

B

Figure 16–9. Arrows depict calculi *(A)* in patient with chronic pancreatitis. Basket retrieval of stones *(B: arrow, insert)* following pancreatic duct sphincterotomy.

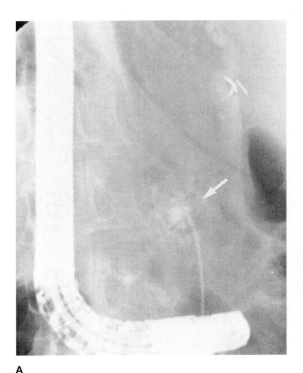

A

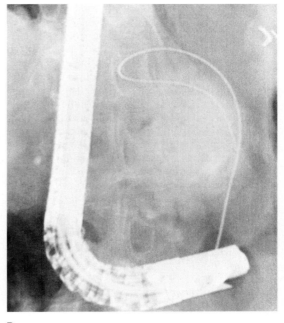

B

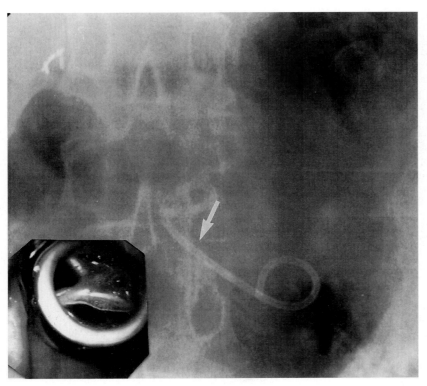

C

Figure 16–10. Transgastric puncture *(arrow)* into lesser sac pseudocyst *(A)* followed by guidewire insertion *(B)* and transgastric endoprosthesis placement *(C, insert).*

was symptomatically improved. Similar data have been noted by Sherman et al, who reported partial or complete stone retrieval was achieved in three-quarters of 31 chronic pancreatitis patients. Two-thirds of patients in this series were clinically improved.

Large, adherent, or impacted calculi must be pre-fragmented for successful retrieval. This has been done most commonly using ESWL. In the largest series reported to date, Delhaye et al treated 123 patients with obstructing pancreatic calculi with the Lithostar lithotriptor after initial pancreatic duct sphincterotomy and nasopancreatic drain insertion. Virtually all stones could be fragmented and one-half of the patients had complete stone retrieval. Complications included mild flare of pancreatitis in approximately one-third. All patients were noted to have initial symptom relief although one-half developed symptom recurrence as a consequence of stone migration or recurrence, ductal stenosis, or stent occlusion.

Ductal Disruption

Ductal disruptions may present in the form of pseudocysts, pancreaticocutaneous fistula, pancreatic ascites, or chronic pleural effusion. Treatment of these disruptions is contingent on both anatomic constraints and competing local expertise (surgical, interventional radiologic).

Kozarek et al (1992–1995) has utilized transpapillary endoprosthesis for both pancreatic ascites and ductal disruptions associated with contained fluid collections including pseudocysts. In the former instance, four patients rapidly resolved their ascites utilizing a combination of stent placement and a single large volume paracentesis. There has been no recurrence at a mean follow-up of 2 years. In the latter instance, transpapillary drains or stents were placed in 17 patients, 14 of whom had ultimate resolution of their fluid collections. Complications were noted in four patients and included mild pancreatitis in two, and stent occlusion with recurrent pseudocyst (1) and cyst infection (1). Both of the latter complications responded to stent exchange.

Pseudocysts can also be drained transgastrically or transduodenally using a needle-knife sphincterotomy in association with chronic catheter placement (Figure 16–10). The initial reports indicate that successful resolution of the pseudocyst is observed in about 75–80% of patients. Side effects include iatrogenic cyst infection, local hemorrhage, and retroperitonitis.

Miscellaneous

Endotherapy to include sclerotherapy or banding of gastric varices has been used to treat bleeding associated with splenic or portal vein thrombosis that may be a consequence of pancreatitis or neoplasia. It has also been used to treat the cholestasis and cholangitis associated with distal bile duct strictures that can be the consequence of pancreatitis. While endoprosthesis placement is technically successful in most patients, stenosis resolution is unusual and therapy is usually undertaken in an attempt to convert a poor risk surgical patient into a good one.

CONCLUSIONS

The endoscopic management of pancreaticobiliary disorders cannot be done in a vacuum. As such, the technical ability to apply a procedure does not imply that this procedure is superior to surgical or radiologic intervention, or even to comfort care in the functional Class IV (bed-ridden, moribund) patient. Clearly, well-controlled data demonstrate that patients with an unresectable pancreatic malignant growth causing obstructive jaundice fare equally well (or poorly) whether surgically bypassed or endoscopically stented. Moreover, data are ample suggesting that endoscopic sphincterotomy is the treatment of choice for most post-cholecystectomy or high-risk patients with choledocholithiasis. Data are accumulating that a subset of biliary injury patients as well as those with diverse causes and consequences of acute or chronic pancreatitis can also be managed endoscopically. In the latter settings, further experience and controlled clinical trials are required before widespread application of this technology can be recommended.

REFERENCES

Barthet M et al: Management of cysts and pseudocysts complicating chronic pancreatitis. Gastroenterol Clin Biol 1993;17:270.

Binmoeller KF, Soehendra N: Endoscopic therapy of chronic pancreatitis. In: *Surgical Disease of the Biliary Tract and Pancreas. Multidisciplinary Management.* JW Braasch, RK Tompkins (editors). Mosby-Year Book, 1994.

Botoman VA et al: Long-term outcome after endoscopic sphincterotomy in patients with biliary colic and sus-pected sphincter of Oddi dysfunction. Gastrointest Endosc 1994;40:165.

Brandabur JJ, Kozarek RA: Biliary tract. In: *Endoscopic Interpretation.* Laine L (editor). Raven, 1994.

Cotton PB et al: Endoscopic sphincterotomy complications and their management: An attempt at consensus. Gastrointest Endosc 1991;37:383.

Cremer M et al: Stenting in severe chronic pancreatitis: Results of medium-term follow-up in 76 patients. Endoscopy 1991;23:171.

Cremer M, Deviére J, Engelholm L: Endoscopic management of cysts and pseudocysts in chronic pancreatitis: Long-term follow-up after 7 years of experience. Gastrointest Endosc 1989;35:1.

Davids PHP et al: Randomized trial of self expanding metal stents versus polyethylene stents for distal malignant biliary obstruction. Lancet 1992;240:1488.

Delhaye H et al: Extracorporeal shock-wave lithotripsy of pancreatic calculi. Gastroenterology 1992;102:610.

Fan S-T et al: Early treatment of acute biliary pancreatitis by endoscopic papillotomy. N Engl J Med 1993;328:228.

Fletcher DR: Laparoscopic cholecystectomy: Role of preoperative and postoperative endoscopic retrograde cholangiopancreatography and endoscopic sphincterotomy. Gastrointest Endosc Clin North Am 1993;3;249.

Huibregtse K: Biliary stenting: Cosmetic or clinical value? Scand J Gastroenterol 1992;27(Suppl 1):77.

Johlin FC, Neil GA: Drainage of the gallbladder in patients with acute acalculous cholecystitis by transpapillary endoscopic cholecystotomy. Gastrointest Endosc 1993;39:645.

Knyrim K et al: A prospective, randomized, controlled trial of metal stents for malignant obstruction of the common bile duct. Endoscopy 1993;25:207.

Kozarek RA: Biliary dyskinesia: Are we any closer to defining the entity? Gastrointest Endosc Clin North Am 1993;3:167.

Kozarek RA: Endoscopic management of pancreatic cancer. In: *The Pancreas. A Clinical Textbook.* Beger HG, Warshaw AC, Carr-Locke P, Russel C, Büchler M, Neoptolemos J, Sarr M (editors). Blackwell Scientific Publications, 1994.

Kozarek RA: Endoscopic therapy in chronic pancreatitis. In: *Alimentary Tract Radiology.* Freeny PG, Stevenson GW (editors). Mosby-Year Book, 1994.

Kozarek RA: Endoscopic therapy of pancreatitis. In: *Current Therapies In Gastroenterology and Liver Diseases.* Bayless TM (editor). Mosby-Year Book, 1994.

Kozarek RA: Expandable stent therapy for GI tract stenoses. Gastrointest Clin North Am 1994;4:279.

Kozarek RA: Pancreatic stents can induce ductal changes consistent with chronic pancreatitis. Gastrointest Endosc 1990;36:93.

Kozarek RA: The role of ERCP in bile duct injuries. Gastrointest Endosc Clin North Am 1993;3:261.

Kozarek RA et al: Bile duct leak after laparoscopic cholecystectomy: diagnostic and therapeutic application of endoscopic retrograde cholangiopancreatography. Arch Intern Med 1992;152:140.

Kozarek RA et al: Endoscopic transpapillary therapy for disrupted pancreatic duct and peripancreatic fluid collections. Gastroenterology 1991;100:1362.

Kozarek RA, Ball TJ, Patterson DJ: Pancreatic duct stone removal in the treatment of chronic pancreatitis. Am J Gastroenterol 1991;87:600.

Kozarek RA, Jiranek G, Traverso LW: Endoscopic management of pancreatic ascites. Am J Surg 1994;168:223.

Lai ECS et al: Endoscopic biliary drainage for severe acute cholangitis. N Engl J Med 1992;326:1582.

Lauri A et al: Endoscopic extraction of bile duct stones: management related to stone size. Gut 1993;34:1718.

Lehman GA et al: Pancreas divisum: results of minor papilla sphincterotomy. Gastrointest Endosc 1993;39:1.

Leung JWC et al: Urgent endoscopic drainage in acute suppurative cholangitis. Lancet 1989;1:1307.

May GR et al: Removal of stones from the bile duct at ERCP without sphincterotomy. Gastrointest Endos 1993;39:749.

Neoptolemos JR, London NJ, Carr-Locke DL: Controlled trial of urgent endoscopic retrograde cholangiopancreatography and endoscopic sphincterotomy versus conservative treatment for acute pancreatitis due to cholelithiasis. Lancet 1988;2:979.

Sherman S et al: Complications of endoscopic sphincterotomy. A prospective series with emphasis on the increased risk with sphincter of Oddi dysfunction and nondilated bile ducts. Gastroenterol 1991;101:1068.

Sherman S et al: Pancreatic ductal stones: Frequency of successful endoscopic removal and improvement in symptoms. Gastrointest Endosc 1991;37:511.

Section II
Esophageal Diseases

Gastroesophageal Reflux Disease & its Complications

17

Stuart Jon Spechler, MD

The reflux of material from the stomach into the esophagus does not invariably result in disease. Indeed, normal individuals every day experience brief, asymptomatic episodes of gastroesophageal reflux that cause no esophageal injury. When the reflux of gastric material into the esophagus causes symptoms, tissue damage, or both, the resulting condition is called **gastroesophageal reflux disease (GERD).** Heartburn and regurgitation are the symptoms most frequently associated with GERD.

Reflux-induced esophageal injury (**reflux esophagitis**) is recognized endoscopically by the presence of erosions and ulcerations in the squamous epithelium of the esophagus. Reflux esophagitis can be complicated further by the development of esophageal strictures and columnar epithelial metaplasia (**Barrett's esophagus**).

Furthermore, the complications of GERD are not limited to the esophagus. In some patients, refluxed gastric material reaches the oropharynx and causes sore throat, burning tongue, and dental erosion. Aspiration of the refluxed material can cause laryngitis and pulmonary problems, including cough, bronchitis, and asthma. Thus, GERD can have protean clinical manifestations.

The development of GERD is a multifactorial process that involves dysfunction of mechanisms that normally prevent excessive gastroesophageal reflux, and of mechanisms that normally clear the esophagus rapidly of noxious material.

Pathophysiology of Gastroesophageal Reflux Disease

A. Antireflux Mechanisms:

1. Lower esophageal sphincter–Normally, there is a positive pressure gradient between the abdomen and the thorax that tends to promote the reflux of material from the stomach into the esophagus. In the absence of effective antireflux mechanisms, this pressure differential would result in virtually continuous gastroesophageal reflux. One of the pri-

mary barriers to reflux is the lower esophageal sphincter, a 1.0- to 3.5-cm segment of specialized circular muscle in the wall of the distal esophagus that prevents reflux by maintaining a resting pressure some 10–40 mm Hg higher than that of the stomach (Figure 17–1).

Although the muscle of the lower esophageal sphincter cannot be distinguished morphologically from the muscle of the esophageal body, the lower esophageal sphincter exhibits a number of distinctive functional characteristics. Unlike muscle of the esophageal body, strips of lower esophageal sphincter muscle develop spontaneous tension on stretching and relax with transmural electrical stimulation. Gastroesophageal reflux can result from any of several types of lower esophageal sphincter dysfunction, including intrinsic weakness of the lower esophageal sphincter muscle that causes feeble resting lower esophageal sphincter pressure (**hypotonic lower esophageal sphincter**), inadequate lower esophageal sphincter response to increased abdominal pressure, and transient episodes of lower esophageal sphincter relaxation (Figure 17–2).

When the resting pressure in the lower esophageal sphincter remains at or near zero (**feeble resting lower esophageal sphincter pressure**), the sphincter does not pose an effective barrier to reflux (Figure 17–2C). Normal individuals uncommonly exhibit such feeble resting lower esophageal sphincter pressures, and few episodes of gastroesophageal reflux in normal subjects are associated with this phenomenon. In patients who have severe GERD, however, approximately one-quarter of all episodes of acid reflux are associated with feeble resting lower esophageal sphincter pressure.

In addition to maintaining resting pressure, the lower esophageal sphincter prevents reflux by rapidly increasing its tone in response to the sudden abdominal pressure elevations that occur during coughing, sneezing, or straining. Through this mechanism, sudden increases in abdominal pressure nor-

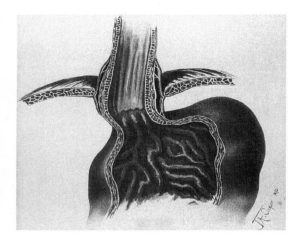

Figure 17–1. Lower esophageal sphincter anatomy. The esophagus passes into the abdomen through the esophageal hiatus, an opening in the right crus of the diaphragm. The distal few centimeters of circular muscle in the esophagus comprise the lower esophageal sphincter. (Reprinted, with permission, from the Clinical Teaching Project of the American Gastroenterological Association.)

mally are accompanied by simultaneous increases in lower esophageal sphincter pressure of similar magnitude. Some patients, particularly those who exhibit feeble resting lower esophageal sphincter pressure, may have an inadequate lower esophageal sphincter response to increased abdominal pressure. If sudden increases in abdominal pressure are not accompanied by a commensurate rise in lower esophageal sphincter pressure, gastric material can be propelled into the esophagus (Figure 17–2B). The precise contribution of this mechanism to GERD is disputed, as is the contribution of the crural diaphragm to the observed lower esophageal sphincter pressure increase.

Transient lower esophageal sphincter relaxation appears to be the most important lower esophageal sphincter mechanism for reflux (Figure 17–2A). During primary peristalsis (**peristalsis induced by swallowing,**) the lower esophageal sphincter normally relaxes for 3–10 seconds to allow the swallowed bolus to enter the stomach. Transient lower esophageal sphincter relaxations, in contrast, are not preceded by a normal peristaltic sequence and last for up to 30 seconds. When lower esophageal sphincter pressure falls to zero during a transient lower esophageal

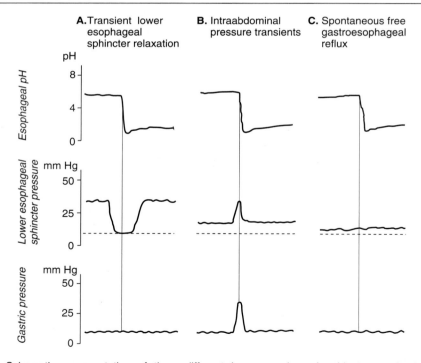

Figure 17–2. Schematic representation of three different lower esophageal sphincter mechanisms for gastroesophageal reflux. Acid reflux (a drop in esophageal pH below 4) is represented by vertical lines. Panel A shows acid reflux associated with a transient lower esophageal sphincter relaxation. Panel B shows acid reflux during an inadequate lower esophageal sphincter response to increased intra-abdominal pressure (note that the rise in lower esophageal sphincter pressure is not as great as the rise in gastric pressure). Panel C shows acid reflux in a patient with feeble resting lower esophageal sphincter pressure. (Reprinted, with permission, from Dodds WJ et al: N Engl J Med 1982;307:1547.)

sphincter relaxation, the sphincter does not function as an antireflux barrier. This phenomenon explains how patients with apparently normal resting lower esophageal sphincter pressures can experience frequent episodes of reflux. Transient lower esophageal sphincter relaxations can be stimulated by gastric distention, and often occur after meals both in normal individuals and in patients with GERD.

Gastroesophageal reflux in normal individuals occurs almost exclusively through this mechanism, and transient lower esophageal sphincter relaxation is the most frequent cause of reflux in patients with GERD. More than two-thirds of all reflux episodes in patients with severe GERD are associated with transient lower esophageal sphincter relaxations.

2. Crural diaphragm–The esophagus passes from the thorax into the abdomen through an opening in the right crus of the diaphragm called the **esophageal hiatus** (Figure 17–1). When the crural diaphragm contracts, as occurs during inspiration, the crurae come together and pinch the distal esophagus. This pinching effect appears to function as an important barrier to reflux during inspiration and during other activities that increase intra-abdominal pressure. In this fashion, the crural diaphragm serves as an external esophageal sphincter that buttresses the antireflux function of the lower esophageal sphincter. As evidence of the efficacy of this external sphincter mechanism, studies in dogs have shown that gastroesophageal reflux does not occur during transient lower esophageal sphincter relaxation unless the relaxation is attended by inhibition of the crural diaphragm. Furthermore, transient lower esophageal sphincter relaxation with inhibition of the crural diaphragm in dogs often is associated with contraction of the costal diaphragm that further promotes reflux. A similar sequence of events is seen in humans during belching, suggesting that gastroesophageal reflux during transient lower esophageal sphincter relaxation may occur through a variant of the belch reflex.

3. Anatomic features–In addition to the lower esophageal sphincter and the crural diaphragm, certain other anatomic features of the distal esophagus may contribute to the antireflux barrier (Figure 17–1). For example, the acute angle formed by the junction of esophagus and stomach (**the angle of His**) may result in a one-way flap valve that prevents reflux. Also, a segment of the distal esophagus ordinarily is located within the abdomen where the segment is subject to external pressure that tends to force the walls together, thereby preventing reflux.

4. Effects of hiatal hernia on the antireflux barrier–Most patients with severe GERD have a sliding hiatal hernia in which both the esophagogastric junction and a portion of the gastric fundus protrude through the hiatus in the crural diaphragm into the chest. The susceptibility to gastroesophageal reflux induced by abrupt elevations of intra-abdominal pressure has been found to correlate significantly with hi-

atal hernia size. Resting lower esophageal sphincter pressure often is low in patients who have large, sliding hiatal hernias, and this lower esophageal sphincter hypotension predisposes to gastroesophageal reflux. Hiatal herniation also predisposes to reflux by disrupting the extrasphincteric antireflux mechanisms. With a large hiatal hernia, the distal esophagus is no longer subject to the external squeeze of abdominal pressure that might prevent reflux. Furthermore, the diaphragmatic crurae no longer pinch the distal esophagus during inspiration. Instead, approximation of the crurae creates a pouch of stomach within the chest that may function as a reservoir of material for reflux.

Although hiatal hernia clearly contributes to GERD in many patients, it is difficult to quantitate the precise contribution. Clinicians should appreciate that hiatal hernia is not always associated with GERD, and vice versa. Finally, one recent study has shown that esophageal acid perfusion in the opossum causes the long axis of the esophagus to shorten, an effect that could promote the development of a sliding hiatal hernia. This observation raises the possibility that hiatal hernia might be an effect rather than a cause of reflux esophagitis, in some cases.

B. Gastric Contents: Gastroesophageal reflux causes esophageal injury only when the refluxed material is caustic to the esophageal mucosa. Potentially caustic agents that can be found in the stomach include acid, pepsin, bile, and pancreatic enzymes. The dramatic efficacy of potent inhibitors of gastric acid secretion, such as omeprazole, in the treatment of GERD underscores the importance of acid and pepsin in the pathogenesis of reflux esophagitis, in most cases. However, occasional patients with severe reflux esophagitis may not heal completely with acid suppression therapy alone, suggesting that refluxed bile or pancreatic secretions may be contributing to the esophageal damage.

Using sensitive radionuclide tests, some investigators have found delayed gastric emptying in more than 50% of patients with GERD. Delayed gastric emptying causes gastric distention that can stimulate gastric acid secretion and trigger transient relaxation of the lower esophageal sphincter. Both of these effects can be harmful for patients with GERD.

C. Esophageal Clearance Mechanisms: If caustic material is cleared quickly from the esophagus, no damage may result. Normally, the esophagus is cleared of acid by four important mechanisms: (1) gravity, (2) peristalsis, (3) salivation, and (4) intrinsic esophageal bicarbonate production. When a bolus of acid enters the esophagus, most of the material is cleared by the combined effects of gravity and peristalsis. The small quantity of residual acidic material that escapes clearance by gravity and peristalsis might cause mucosal damage if it were not neutralized by swallowed saliva, which is highly alkaline, and by bicarbonate produced by the esophageal mucosa itself.

GERD can be associated with conditions that impair esophageal clearance. For example, the severe reflux esophagitis that occurs in patients with scleroderma often is associated with disordered peristalsis that delays esophageal clearance. Reflux that occurs during sleep can be particularly damaging to the esophagus for several reasons relating to esophageal clearance. In recumbency during sleep, gravity retards the clearance of refluxed material. Swallowing and salivation virtually cease during sleep and, therefore, there is no primary peristalsis and little saliva available to clear acid from the esophagus. Cigarette smoking has been shown to increase esophageal acid exposure by increasing the frequency of acid reflux events and, perhaps, by decreasing salivary flow. Finally, hiatal hernia has been shown to interfere with esophageal clearance.

D. Esophageal Epithelial Resistance: Several types of epithelial protective factors enable the esophagus to resist peptic injury. First, there are pre-epithelial protective factors that prevent H^+ ions in the esophageal lumen from coming into direct contact with the squamous epithelial cells. Potential components of the pre-epithelial defenses include the surface mucus layer, the unstirred water layer, and the layer of bicarbonate ions that line the luminal surface of the epithelial cells (Figure 17–3). These pre-epithelial factors are poorly developed in squamous epithelium, and appear to play a minor role in protecting the esophagus from peptic injury. When the pre-epithelial factors are overwhelmed, there are epithelial protective factors that prevent H^+ ions in contact with the cell membrane from entering the cells, and that buffer or eliminate the H^+ ions that do penetrate.

To penetrate the epithelium, H^+ ions either must pass through the cell membrane or through intercellular spaces where ion movement is restricted by tight junctions and by intercellular material such as lipid and mucin. Both the squamous cell membranes and their intercellular junctional complexes pose substantial barriers to the passage of H^+ ions. Nevertheless, exposure to relatively high concentrations of acid can overwhelm these barriers. H^+ ions that enter the epithelial cells are buffered by intracellular proteins, phosphate, and bicarbonate. Also, squamous cell membranes have ion transport systems that can extrude H^+ ions out of the cell. These transport systems include a Na^+/H^+ exchanger and a Cl^-/HCO_3^- exchange mechanism that appears to have both Na-dependent and Na-independent components. Finally, the esophageal blood supply provides post-epithelial protection by removing noxious substances that are extruded by the epithelial cells (eg, CO_2 and H^+ ions), and by supplying bicarbonate that is used for buffering acid in the intercellular space.

Ambulatory esophageal pH monitoring studies have shown that normal individuals experience brief episodes of acid reflux each day. Apparently, the normal epithelial defenses are sufficient to prevent these brief episodes from causing esophagitis. Most patients with reflux esophagitis have an abnormally prolonged duration of esophageal acid exposure that overwhelms the normal epithelial defenses (Figure 17–4). However, some patients have reflux esophagitis even though 24-hour pH monitoring studies demonstrate a normal daily duration of acid reflux. These patients may have yet uncharacterized defects in their pre-epithelial, epithelial, or post-epithelial protective factors.

E. NSAIDs and GERD: Epidemiologic studies suggest that the ingestion of aspirin and other nonsteroidal anti-inflammatory drugs (NSAIDs) can contribute to GERD. Patients with esophageal strictures appear to be especially susceptible to NSAID-induced esophageal injury. Many NSAID preparations

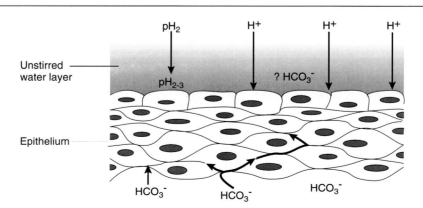

Figure 17–3. Pre-epithelial defenses. The esophageal pre-epithelial defenses against acid include the surface layer of mucus, unstirred water layer, and bicarbonate ions. (Reprinted, with permission, from Orlando RC: Esophageal epithelial defense against injury. J Clin Gastroenterol 1991(Suppl 2);13:S1.)

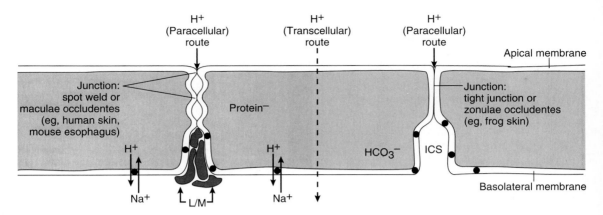

Figure 17–4. Epithelial defenses. The epithelial cell membranes, the intercellular junction complexes, and lipids and mucins (L/M) in the intercellular spaces all limit the penetration of H^+ ions. Once within the cell, H^+ ions are buffered by intracellular proteins and bicarbonate. The H^+ ions also can be extruded by a Na^+/H^+ exchange mechanism. (Reprinted, with permission, from Orlando RC: *Gastroesophageal reflux disease: Pathogenesis, diagnosis, therapy*. Castell DO, Wu WC, Ott DJ (editors). Futura Publishing, 1985.)

are caustic to the mucosa, and severe local injury can result when a stricture impedes passage of the NSAID tablet into the stomach. Esophageal strictures themselves may be the result of NSAID-induced injury. For patients without strictures, the mechanisms whereby NSAIDs contribute to GERD are not clear.

Essentials of Diagnosis

- Heartburn and/or regurgitation.
- Esophagitis (eg, erosions, ulcerations).

General Considerations

GERD can be defined as any symptomatic condition or anatomic alteration caused by the reflux of noxious material from the stomach into the esophagus. It is important to appreciate that, by this definition, patients with GERD can have symptoms without objective evidence of esophagitis. The finding of reflux esophagitis on endoscopic examination confirms the diagnosis of GERD, but a normal esophagoscopy does not rule out GERD as a cause of symptoms.

Clinical Findings

A. Symptoms and Signs: Heartburn, the cardinal symptom of GERD, is an uncomfortable, hot or burning sensation located beneath the sternum. The sensation frequently originates in the epigastrium and radiates up the chest, sometimes into the throat or back. When describing heartburn, patients often wave their open hand vertically over the sternum, in contrast to patients with angina pectoris due to cardiac ischemia who typically hold their clenched fist stationary over the chest while describing their pain.

If refluxed gastric material reaches the orophar-

ynx, the patient may experience the symptom of regurgitation wherein sour or bitter-tasting material appears in the mouth. Patients who have peptic strictures of the esophagus often complain of dysphagia. Even in the absence of a fixed stricture, however, dysphagia may be associated with the esophagitis and motility abnormalities that can accompany GERD. Odynophagia in patients with GERD suggests the presence of esophageal ulceration. Some patients describe the symptom of **water brash,** in which the mouth suddenly fills with saliva as a result of reflex salivary secretion stimulated by acid in the esophagus.

Heartburn associated with GERD can be aggravated by the ingestion of foods that predispose to reflux by decreasing pressure in the lower esophageal sphincter. These include chocolate, onions, peppermint, coffee, and foods that have a high content of fat and sugar. Certain foods have no affect on the lower esophageal sphincter, but can cause the sensation of heartburn in patients with GERD by irritating the esophageal mucosa directly. These include spicy foods, citrus products, and tomato products. Certain practices that predispose to reflux by increasing intra-abdominal pressure also can precipitate heartburn in susceptible patients. For example, many patients experience heartburn when they bend over, lift a heavy object, strain to defecate, or run.

Characteristically, heartburn caused by gastroesophageal reflux is relieved, if only temporarily, by antacids. For most patients with GERD, the symptom of heartburn can be eliminated by the administration of potent acid suppressing agents.

B. Diagnostic Tests: Table 17–1 lists the diagnostic tests that are commonly used to evaluate patients with GERD, and the clinical questions that

Table 17–1. Clinical questions and diagnostic tests for GERD.

	Is there gastroesophageal reflux?	Is there esophagitis (inflammation, ulceration)?	Is there Barrett's esophagus?	Is there an esophageal stricture?	Are symptoms due to acid reflux?
Barium swallow	+	+	+	+++	−
Endoscopy	+	+++	+++	++	−
Esophageal biopsy	−	+++	+++	−	−
Bernstein test	−	−	−	−	++
Ambulatory pH monitoring	+++	−	−	−	+++

Utility of diagnostic test for answering clinical question: −, not useful; +, somewhat useful; ++, useful; +++, very useful.

these tests can answer. Note that the barium swallow, endoscopic examination, and histologic examination of esophageal biopsy specimens are performed primarily to seek the anatomic alterations of reflux esophagitis. As previously noted, GERD is any symptomatic condition or anatomic alteration caused by the reflux of noxious material from the stomach into the esophagus. By this definition, patients can have GERD without anatomic alterations. For patients who have a characteristic history, therefore, diagnostic tests are not necessary merely to establish the diagnosis of GERD. For example, patients who complain of typical heartburn and regurgitation that respond readily to treatment with acid-suppression therapy do not need diagnostic tests merely to make a diagnosis of GERD. An **endoscopic examination** might be performed in such patients to seek evidence of esophagitis that could require more aggressive therapy, or to look for complications, such as Barrett's esophagus, that cannot be diagnosed on the basis of history alone. However, a normal esophagoscopy would not eliminate acid reflux as the cause of symptoms.

Diagnostic tests may be required for patients with atypical signs or symptoms, or for patients with typical signs and symptoms that do not respond well to acid suppression. A **barium swallow** can reveal signs of esophagitis, including thickening of the esophageal folds, erosions, ulcerations, and strictures; it can also demonstrate the gastroesophageal reflux of barium. Radiography is considerably less sensitive than endoscopy for demonstrating esophagitis, however, and endoscopic examination has the added advantage that biopsy specimens can be obtained from any abnormal areas.

How often do patients with typical heartburn have endoscopic evidence of reflux esophagitis? Several studies suggest that esophagitis is present endoscopically in approximately 50–70% of patients with typical, frequent heartburn. **Histologic changes** of esophagitis are found more frequently, with over 90% of patients exhibiting histologic changes characteristic of GERD. The histologic changes of reflux esophagitis include lengthening of the papillae so that they occupy more than two-thirds of the thickness of the squamous mucosa, hyperplasia of cells in the basal zone so that this zone occupies more than 15% of the mucosal thickness, and infiltration of the epithelium

with eosinophils and polymorphonuclear cells. The importance of the histologic changes of GERD are disputed, however, and most authorities hold that the endoscopic findings have more clinical relevance.

Several studies suggest that heartburn severity is not a reliable index of esophagitis. There appears to be no significant correlation between the severity of heartburn reported by the patient and the severity of reflux esophagitis on endoscopic examination. In fact, patients can have severe esophagitis with no heartburn whatsoever. The precise frequency of this situation is not clear, as asymptomatic patients seldom have endoscopic examinations, but a number of reports have described patients who had severe ulcerative esophagitis with no complaints of heartburn. It appears that less than two-thirds of patients with esophagitis complain of frequent heartburn.

Diagnostic tests may be needed for patients who have atypical chest pains with features that are suggestive, but not entirely characteristic, of reflux-induced heartburn. For example, one occasionally encounters patients who complain of a burning sensation in the lower chest that does not radiate, that is unaffected by activities, and that is only partially or unreliably relieved by antacids and antisecretory drugs. This is not typical heartburn, and it is not clear that the symptom is triggered by acid reflux even if endoscopic examination demonstrates esophagitis. The **acid perfusion (Bernstein) test** has been used in this situation to support acid reflux as the cause of symptoms. During this test, the esophagus is perfused with 0.1N hydrochloric acid. Reproduction of the patient's chest pain with acid perfusion implicates GERD as a cause of the chest pain and suggests a role for antireflux therapy. This test has limited sensitivity and specificity, however, and has largely been replaced by ambulatory esophageal pH monitoring.

Ambulatory monitoring of esophageal pH can be used to document the pattern, frequency, and duration of acid reflux, and to seek a correlation between reflux episodes and symptoms. In most ambulatory systems, an episode of acid reflux is defined (somewhat arbitrarily) as a drop in esophageal pH below 4. Standard 24-hour pH monitoring records a number of different variables, such as the total number of reflux episodes, the number longer than 5 minutes in duration, and the duration of the longest episode.

The single most clinically applicable variable appears to be the total percentage of the monitoring period that esophageal pH remains below 4. In normal individuals, esophageal pH remains below 4 for less than 4.5% of the 24-hour monitoring period. Most patients who have both endoscopic signs and symptoms of GERD also have abnormal 24-hour esophageal pH monitoring studies, whereas subjects with no such signs and symptoms usually have normal studies. It is difficult to determine the precise sensitivity and specificity of the test, however, because there is no universally accepted "gold standard" for the diagnosis of GERD.

In theory, protracted esophageal pH monitoring should be very useful to establish that acid reflux is the cause of heartburn in individual patients. In practice, however, the correlation between discrete episodes of acid reflux and heartburn is poor. For example, although normal individuals often experience brief episodes of acid reflux during the day (particularly after meals), these episodes usually are not associated with heartburn. Even in patients with heartburn who have endoscopic evidence of reflux esophagitis, 24-hour esophageal monitoring reveals that fewer than 20% of episodes of acid reflux (defined as a drop in pH of less than 4) are accompanied by heartburn. These observations indicate that most episodes of acid reflux do not trigger the sensation of heartburn.

It is not clear why only the minority of episodes of acid reflux cause heartburn. It appears, however, from experimental studies that provocation of pain is dependent on the pH of the refluxate and the length of time of acid exposure. The duration of acid perfusion required to produce pain is a function of the pH of the perfusion solution; ie, the lower the pH, the shorter the duration of acid perfusion necessary to produce heartburn. The frequency with which acid perfusion induces pain also is related to the pH. In one study all patients experienced heartburn during perfusion with solutions of pH 1, whereas only 50% of patients experienced pain during esophageal perfusion with solutions of pH 2.5–6. Once a subject had experienced pain with an acid solution, subsequent perfusions of the same solution caused pain more rapidly than the first perfusion. During 24-hour pH monitoring, reflux episodes associated with pain were significantly longer than those without pain, and often were preceded by another episode of heartburn. These findings suggest that the reflux of strongly acidic material is more likely to cause heartburn than weakly acidic material. Furthermore, once an episode of reflux has caused pain, the esophagus may become sensitized so that subsequent reflux episodes are more likely to be painful.

Treatment

When planning a management strategy for patients with GERD, it is important to appreciate that the effi-cacy of any antireflux therapy is inversely related to the severity of the underlying reflux esophagitis, ie, the worse the esophagitis, the poorer the healing rate. A treatment that is highly effective for mild esophagitis may be virtually useless for patients with severe disease. This section outlines a step-wise approach to the therapy of GERD. For patients who are found to have severe, ulcerative, reflux esophagitis, it may be appropriate to begin therapy immediately with potent acid-suppression (eg, by administering a proton pump inhibitor) rather than proceeding step-wise through trials of agents less likely to effect healing. Conversely, it may not be appropriate to begin the treatment of very mild GERD with a proton pump inhibitor. The official indications, dosage, and duration of treatment for commonly prescribed antireflux medications are listed in Table 17–2.

A. Life-style Modifications: The management of GERD commonly begins with lifestyle modifications (Table 17–3) that are aimed at reducing acid reflux and minimizing the duration of contact between refluxed material and the esophageal mucosa. The head of the bed is elevated on 4–6 inch blocks to exploit the effect of gravity in clearing the esophagus of noxious material.

Obese patients are advised to lose weight, with the rationale that obesity may contribute to reflux by increasing abdominal pressure; dieting also helps patients avoid fatty foods that promote reflux. Bedtime snacks can stimulate gastric acid production and trigger transient lower esophageal sphincter relaxation. Both of these effects promote the reflux of gastric acid during sleep, a time when swallowing and salivation decrease dramatically. With no swallowing to initiate peristalsis and no saliva to buffer retained acid, reflux during sleep can be especially damaging.

Tobacco and alcohol consumption should be avoided because these agents may decrease lower esophageal sphincter pressure, and because cigarette smoking also decreases salivation. Fatty foods, chocolate, and carminatives (spearmint, peppermint) contribute to GERD by decreasing lower esophageal sphincter pressure and by delaying gastric emptying. Drugs that have anticholinergic effects (eg, phenothiazines, tricyclic antidepressants), theophylline preparations, and calcium channel blocking agents can decrease lower esophageal sphincter pressure and delay gastric emptying; these medications should be avoided if possible. NSAIDs can be caustic to the esophageal mucosa, and these agents also should be avoided.

B. H₂-Receptor Blocking Agents: In some patients who have mild GERD, life-style modifications alone can be very effective therapy and medications may not be necessary. For these patients, antacids with or without alginic acid can be used as necessary for occasional episodes of heartburn. For patients who remain symptomatic despite the implementation of life-style modifications, a histamine H₂-

Table 17–2. Official indications, dosage, and duration of treatment for commonly prescribed antireflux medications.*

Drug	Official Indication	Recommended Dosage	Recommended Duration
Cimetidine	Erosive esophagitis diagnosed by endoscopy	800mg BID or 400 mg QID	12 weeks
Famotidine	Short term treatment of symptoms or esophagitis due to GERD including erosive or ulcerative disease diagnosed by endoscopy	20mg BID symptoms 20mg or 40 mg BID for esophagitis	6 weeks 12 weeks
Nizatidine	Endoscopically diagnosed esophagitis including erosive and ulcerative esophagitis and associated heartburn due to GERD	150mg BID	12 weeks
Ranitidine	Treatment of symptoms and endoscopically diagnosed erosive esophagitis	150mg BID symptoms 150mg QID esophagitis	No limit specified
Metoclopramide	Short term treatment for adults with symptomatic documented gastroesophageal reflux who fail to respond to conventional therapy	10mg to 15mg QID	12 weeks
Cisapride	Symptomatic treatment of patients with nocturnal heartburn due to GERD	10mg to 20mg QID	No limit specified
Omeprazole	Short term treatment of erosive esophagitis which has been diagnosed by endoscopy; short term treatment of symptomatic GERD poorly responsive to customary medical therapy usually including a histamine H_2-receptor antagonist	20mg QID	4 to 8 weeks

*Recommendations as specified in the Physician's Desk Reference 1995; Medical Economics Data Production Co., Montvale, N.J.

receptor blocking agent (eg, cimetidine, famotidine, nizatidine, ranitidine) often is the next step. When administered in conventional doses, H_2-blockers relieve GERD symptoms and heal esophagitis within 12 weeks in approximately one-half to two-thirds of patients. If relief is not complete, the dose of the agent can be increased. Although very high doses of histamine H_2-receptor blockers (up to 8 times the conventional dose) have been used effectively to treat esophagitis in refractory cases, there is little to be gained by prescribing more than a double-dose of these agents. When used in very high doses, H_2-blockers are expensive, and their long-term safety has not been established. For refractory patients, it seems preferable to add another agent or to use a more potent inhibitor of gastric acid secretion, such as a proton pump inhibitor.

C. Prokinetic Agents: Prokinetic agents can decrease gastroesophageal reflux by increasing lower esophageal sphincter pressure, and by enhancing gastric and esophageal emptying. The prokinetic agents presently available for use in the United States include metoclopramide and cisapride. Metoclopramide is a dopamine antagonist that can be effective in treating patients who have relatively mild GERD. Metoclopramide increases pressure in the lower esophageal sphincter, and enhances gastric emptying by coordinating motor activity in the stomach, pylorus, and duodenum. The use of metoclopramide often is limited by its frequent side effects, including agitation, restlessness, somnolence, and extrapyramidal symptoms, that occur in up to 30% of patients.

Cisapride appears to work as a prokinetic agent by increasing the availability of acetylcholine released from enteric neurons. Like metoclopramide, cisapride has been shown to increase lower esophageal sphincter pressure, stimulate esophageal peristalsis, and enhance gastric emptying. Some patients treated with cisapride develop mild abdominal cramps, diarrhea, or constipation, but, unlike metoclopramide, cisapride causes few serious side effects. It appears that cisapride may have a therapeutic role primarily in patients with relatively mild GERD, where its efficacy appears to be comparable to that of the H_2-receptor blockers.

D. Sucralfate: Sucralfate is an exceptionally safe medication that has been found to be effective in the treatment of mild reflux esophagitis. In several studies performed outside of the USA, the efficacy of sucralfate in relieving symptoms and healing esophagitis appeared to be similar to that of the H_2-receptor blockers. Sucralfate can be administered either in tablet form or as a suspension.

E. Proton Pump Inhibitors: The proton pump inhibitors (eg, omeprazole, lansoprazole) are the most effective of the available agents for the treat-

Table 17–3. Lifestyle modifications for GERD.

Elevate the head of the bed
Weight loss for obese patients
Avoid:
  Bedtime snacks
  Chocolate, fatty foods, and carminatives
  Cigarettes and alcohol
  Drugs that decrease LES pressure and delay gastric
    emptying
  NSAIDS

ment of GERD. In patients with mild to moderately severe reflux esophagitis treated with omeprazole 20 mg daily, healing rates of 80–100% can be expected within 8 weeks. Very severe (grade 4) esophagitis may persist, however, despite omeprazole therapy administered in conventional dosage in up to 40% of cases. Recent studies have shown that aggressive acid suppression with proton pump inhibitors improves dysphagia and decreases the need for esophageal dilation in patients who have peptic esophageal strictures.

Proton pump inhibitors are highly effective in healing esophagitis, but they do nothing to correct the underlying diathesis for reflux. Consequently, in the majority of cases, GERD returns shortly after stopping these agents. Presently, omeprazole is approved only for the short-term treatment of erosive esophagitis or GERD that is poorly responsive to other forms of therapy (up to 12 weeks). The concerns about long-term usage of proton pump inhibitors are related primarily to the theoretical carcinogenic effects of profound chronic acid suppression and hypergastrinemia. With profound acid suppression, the stomach may become colonized with bacteria that can convert dietary nitrates to carcinogenic nitrosamines. Gastrin is a hormone that is trophic to the gastric mucosa, and chronic hypergastrinemia conceivably could predispose to neoplasia. Indeed, rats treated chronically with high doses of omeprazole have developed carcinoid tumors. To date, no such carcinogenicity has been documented in humans, and the risks of long-term therapy appear to be small.

A recent study by Klinkenberg-Knol and her colleagues explored the long-term efficacy of omeprazole treatment for GERD. The study spanned more than 5 years, and included 91 patients with severe esophagitis who were refractory to treatment with H_2-blockers. All patients were treated initially with 40 mg of omeprazole each day until there was endoscopic evidence of complete healing, at which time they were switched to a maintenance dose of 20 mg/d. Follow-up endoscopy was done at 3-month intervals in the first year, and at 6-month intervals thereafter. If endoscopy showed a relapse, the omeprazole dose was increased by 20 mg.

During the 5-year follow-up period, esophagitis recurred in 47% of the patients receiving maintenance omeprazole. All of the patients experienced rehealing when the dose was increased by 20 mg. Eighteen percent of patients had a second relapse after a mean interval of 24 months; this relapse also responded to a 20 mg increase in the omeprazole dose. An elevation in the serum gastrin level above 500 was observed in 11% of patients during omeprazole therapy, and the frequency of micronodular argyrophil cell hyperplasia in gastric biopsy specimens increased from 2.5% at baseline to 20% at the last endoscopy. Similarly, the frequency of atrophic gas-

tritis increased from less than 1% to 25%. This study shows that omeprazole is an effective maintenance therapy for GERD for up to 5 years. However, approximately one-half of patients with severe esophagitis will require increasing doses of the drug to maintain remission. Furthermore, hypergastrinemia, micronodular argyrophil cell hyperplasia, and atrophic gastritis develop frequently during omeprazole therapy. Some authorities have suggested that serum gastrin levels should be monitored during chronic omeprazole administration. The utility of this practice is unproved.

F. Combination Therapy: Relatively few investigations have explored the efficacy of combination drug therapy for GERD. Drug combinations that have been studied have included an H_2-blocker plus either sucralfate or a prokinetic agent. Cimetidine (1200 mg/d) combined with sucralfate (5 g/d) was found to be superior to cimetidine alone for relieving daytime heartburn and for improving the endoscopic signs of esophagitis. For patients unresponsive to treatment with cimetidine alone, Lieberman and Keefe found that the addition of metoclopramide resulted in symptomatic improvement significantly more often than the addition of placebo, but side effects of metoclopramide were frequent. A combination of ranitidine (300 mg/d) and cisparide (40 mg/d) was found to be significantly superior to cimetidine alone in effecting endoscopic healing of esophagitis. However, a combination of ranitidine (300 mg/d) plus metoclopramide (40 mg/d) was not as effective as omeprazole alone (20 mg/d) in healing the signs and symptoms of esophagitis. For patients with moderately severe reflux esophagitis, the use of combination therapy may eliminate the need for treatment with a proton pump inhibitor. However, the addition of a second medication increases the cost of therapy substantially and increases the chance for side effects. Furthermore, the long-term benefit of combination therapy has not been demonstrated. For patients who are refractory to single-agent therapy (with an H_2-blocker, sucralfate, or a prokinetic), a change to a proton pump inhibitor generally is less expensive and more likely to effect healing than the addition of a second drug.

G. Antireflex Surgery: Most of the commonly used antireflux operations (eg, Nissen fundoplication, Hill posterior gastropexy, Belsey fundoplication) share several fundamental features. In all these procedures, the surgeon creates an intra-abdominal segment of esophagus, reduces the hiatal hernia, and wraps a portion of the gastric fundus around the distal esophagus. As a result, the surgery narrows the **angle of His** (the angle formed by the junction of esophagus with stomach), which may create an antireflux flap-valve effect. Restoration of the distal esophagus to the positive pressure environment of the abdomen also may prevent reflux. Reduction of the hiatal hernia and approximation of the dia-

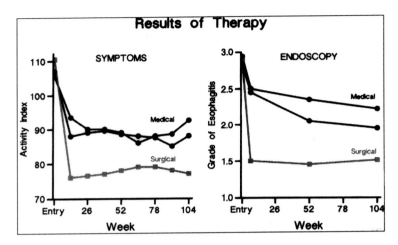

Figure 17–5. Results of the VA Cooperative Study on GERD (Spechler SJ and The Department of Veteran Affairs Gastroesophageal Reflux Disease Study Group. N Engl J Med 1992;326:786–792). Patients were randomly assigned to receive one of three types of treatment: continuous medical therapy, symptomatic medical therapy, or surgical therapy. The left panel shows the effects of therapy on the activity index score, an index of GERD symptom severity [range of scores: 74 (no symptoms) to 172 (worst symptoms)]. The right panel shows the effects of therapy on the endoscopic signs of esophagitis [range of scores: 1.0 (no esophagitis) to 4.0 (esophageal ulceration)]. The points on the graphs represent mean values ± SE. The two medical groups are represented by black lines, and the surgical group by gray lines. (Reprinted, with permission, from the Clinical Teaching Project of the American Gastroenterological Association.)

phragmatic crurae may restore the normal antireflux function of the crural diaphragm. The fundoplication itself may act as a one-way valve, and may prevent distention of the gastric fundus that can trigger transient lower esophageal sphincter relaxations. Finally, lower esophageal sphincter pressures increase after fundoplication for reasons that are not clear. The importance of the latter mechanism is disputed, because the efficacy of antireflux surgery is not directly proportional to the postoperative increase in lower esophageal sphincter pressure.

Recently, a Department of Veterans Affairs cooperative study compared the efficacy of medical and surgical therapies for GERD.[1]

The 247 study subjects all had GERD complicated by Barrett's esophagus, esophageal ulceration, esophageal stricture, or severe erosive esophagitis. Antireflux life-style modifications were prescribed for all study subjects regardless of treatment group. Patients were randomly assigned to receive one of three types of treatment: continuous medical therapy, symptomatic medical therapy, or surgical therapy. Continuous medical therapy included antacid tablets and ranitidine taken on a daily basis regardless of symptoms; metoclopramide and sucralfate were added in a stepwise fashion for patients who remained symptomatic. For patients in the sympto-

matic medical therapy group, drug therapy was used only for control of symptoms. Therapy in these patients began with antacid tablets; ranitidine, metoclopramide, and sucralfate were added in a stepwise fashion for symptoms that could not be controlled with antacids alone. Patients in the surgical therapy group had Nissen fundoplications.

All three therapies resulted in significant improvements in the symptoms and endoscopic signs of GERD for up to 2 years (Figure 17–5). However, surgical therapy was significantly better than either medical therapy for the 2-year duration of the study. Overall satisfaction with therapy also was better for patients in the surgical group. Although this prospective, randomized study predated the availability of proton pump inhibitors, the investigation clearly demonstrates that surgical therapy is superior to medical therapy without omeprazole. Presently, there is no reported study that has compared the efficacy of antireflux surgery with proton pump inhibitors. As previously mentioned, however, proton pump inhibitors are not yet approved for long-term use.

Presently, antireflux surgery should be considered in the following situations:

1. Patients who have esophageal symptoms, ulcerations, or strictures due to GERD that are intractable to medical therapy. In this era of proton pump inhibitors, such intractability is decidedly uncommon.
2. Patients who have aspiration pneumonia resulting from gastroesophageal reflux. This is an un-

[1] Spechler SJ: Comparison of medical and surgical therapy for complicated gastroesophageal reflux disease in veterans. The Department of Veterans Affairs Gastroesophageal Reflex Disease Study Group. N Engl J Med 1992;326:786.

common condition seen most often in patients who have neurologic deficits. Fundoplication may prevent aspiration due to gastroesophageal reflux in this situation, but will not prevent pneumonia due to aspiration of oropharyngeal contents in patients with neurologic disorders.

3. Patients who are unwilling to accept life-long medical therapy.

4. Young patients who require chronic omeprazole or high-dose H_2-blocker therapy for control of symptoms and complications. Although this is by no means an absolute indication for antireflux surgery, the option should at least be considered.

Complications

A. Esophageal Stricture: Peptic strictures form when reflux-induced ulceration stimulates fibrous tissue production and collagen deposition in the esophagus. These strictures develop in approximately 10% of patients who have reflux esophagitis, and typically cause slowly-progressive dysphagia for solid foods, such as meats and breads. Liquids alone do not cause dysphagia unless the stricture is associated with an esophageal motility disorder such as scleroderma. Patients with peptic strictures often modify their diets to avoid the foods that produce dysphagia but, unlike patients with malignant strictures, profound weight loss is uncommon.

The length of peptic strictures varies from fine, focal narrowings to long constrictions that involve virtually the entire esophagus. On barium swallow, peptic esophageal strictures characteristically have a smooth, tapered appearance. Radiography is more sensitive than endoscopy for demonstrating subtle esophageal narrowing, particularly when the radiographic examination includes swallowing of a solid bolus, such as a barium tablet or a barium-soaked marshmallow. Radiography does not reliably distinguish benign and malignant esophageal strictures, however, and endoscopic examination with biopsy and brush cytology of the esophagus is necessary to exclude cancer. Other conditions that can mimic peptic esophageal stricture include esophageal narrowing due to radiation, infectious esophagitis, or the ingestion of caustic substances, such as lye. Also, a variety of medications taken in pill form (eg, tetracycline, NSAIDs) can cause caustic injury with stricture formation if the pills linger in the esophagus. Unlike peptic strictures that usually involve the distal esophagus, however, pill-induced stricture often involves the proximal esophagus at the level of the aortic arch.

Peptic strictures usually are treated by the peroral passage of devices that dilate the esophagus. These devices include fixed-size dilators (eg, mercury-filled rubber bougies, Savary-Gilliard dilators) and balloons that can be inflated within the stricture. For strictures that are neither very tight nor tortuous, the passage of mercury-filled rubber bougies often is effective. Tight or tortuous strictures can be treated with dilators that are passed over a guidewire that is positioned within the stricture using either fluoroscopic or endoscopic guidance. As mentioned above, aggressive acid suppression with proton pump inhibitors both improves dysphagia and decreases the need for esophageal dilation in patients who have peptic esophageal strictures. Strictures can also be dilated surgically, and this procedure can be combined with an antireflux operation. Rarely, intractable strictures require resection. In such cases, the esophagus is reconstructed with a segment of bowel.

B. Barrett's Esophagus: Barrett's esophagus is the condition in which a metaplastic columnar epithelium replaces squamous epithelium in the distal esophagus. The condition is a sequela of reflux esophagitis in most cases, and is the major recognized risk factor for adenocarcinoma of the esophagus and gastroesophageal junction.

1. Histology—Histologic examination of biopsy specimens obtained from patients with Barrett's esophagus can reveal any of three types of columnar epithelia: (1) Gastric fundic-type epithelium that has a pitted surface lined by mucus-secreting cells, and a deeper glandular layer that contains chief and parietal cells; (2) junctional-type epithelium that has a foveolar surface and glands lined almost exclusively by mucus-secreting cells; and (3) specialized intestinal metaplasia (also called specialized columnar epithelium) that has a villiform surface and intestinal-type crypts lined by mucus-secreting columnar cells and goblet cells (Figure 17–6). The former two epithelial types can be morphologically indistinguishable from epithelia normally found in the stomach. Specialized intestinal metaplasia, in contrast, is readily distinguished from normal gastric epithelia. Specialized intestinal metaplasia also is the most common and important of the three epithelial types found in Barrett's esophagus. Dysplasia and carcinoma in this condition invariably are associated with intestinal metaplasia.

2. Diagnosis—On endoscopic examination, columnar epithelium in the esophagus can be identified readily, in most cases, by its characteristic red color and velvet-like texture that contrast sharply with the pale, glossy appearance of the adjacent squamous epithelium. Consequently, endoscopists recognize Barrett's esophagus easily when they see long segments of columnar epithelium extending up the esophagus, well above the junction with the stomach (Figure 17–7). Such segments can be found in 10–15% of patients who have endoscopic examinations for symptoms of GERD. However, diagnostic difficulties arise when patients are found to have short segments of columnar lining in the distal esophagus. This is because some authors have claimed that gastric mucosa normally can extend at least 2 cm into the distal esophagus and, therefore, the finding of gastric-type epithelia in this distal segment does not establish a diagnosis of Barrett's esophagus.

To avoid making false-positive diagnoses, investi-

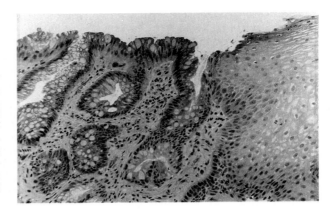

Figure 17–6. This photomicrograph of a biopsy specimen obtained at the squamo-columnar junction in the distal esophagus shows an abrupt transition from stratified squamous epithelium to specialized intestinal metaplasia. Both the surface and the intestinal-type glands of the specialized columnar epithelium are lined by mucus-secreting cells and goblet cells (H&E; original magnification × 200). (Reproduced, with permission, from Spechler SJ: Prevalence of metaplasia at the gastro-oesophageal junction. Lancet 1994;344:1533).

gators who designed studies on Barrett's esophagus often included only those patients whose esophageal columnar lining extended some specified distance (eg, over 3 cm) above the esophagogastric junction. Over the years, gastroenterologists adopted those investigative criteria into their clinical practices. Such diagnostic standards clearly are arbitrary, however. If a clinician chooses 3 cm as the diagnostic criterion for Barrett's esophagus, for example, then patients with 2.5 cm of metaplastic columnar lining (with potential for neoplastic change) will be ignored. Furthermore, criteria based on the extent of esophageal columnar lining are subject to the considerable imprecision both of endoscopic measurement and of endoscopic localization of the anatomic esophagogastric junction.

To avoid the problems inherent in diagnostic criteria based on arbitrary and imprecise endoscopic measurements, some investigators have proposed that the histologic finding of specialized intestinal metaplasia anywhere in the esophagus establishes the diagnosis

of Barrett's esophagus. This approach does not obviate diagnostic difficulties, however. Specialized intestinal metaplasia can be found in the stomach, and inadvertent biopsy of such a stomach (as can occur during attempts to obtain biopsy specimens from the distal esophagus of patients who have large hiatal hernias or whose gastric mucosa transiently prolapses into the esophagus) can result in a false-positive diagnosis of Barrett's esophagus. Furthermore, short segments of specialized intestinal metaplasia will go unrecognized by endoscopists who consider columnar epithelium confined to the distal few centimeters of esophagus a normal finding that does not require biopsy sampling.

Spechler and colleagues recently conducted a prospective study on the frequency, epidemiology, and clinical features of patients who had such short-segments of specialized intestinal metaplasia.[1]

Patients scheduled for elective endoscopic examinations had biopsy specimens obtained at the squamo-columnar junction in the distal esophagus irrespective of its appearance and location. Among 142 patients who had columnar epithelium involving no more than 3 cm of the distal esophagus, 26 (18%) were found to have specialized intestinal metaplasia in biopsy specimens of the squamo-columnar junction. Surprisingly, signs and symptoms of esophagitis were not reliable markers for the presence of intestinal metaplasia. Specific esophageal symptoms (heartburn, regurgitation, dysphagia, and odynophagia) were absent in 42% of cases, and 69% had few or no endoscopic signs of esophagitis. Indeed, the metaplastic epithelium in these patients would have gone unrecognized if the study protocol had not mandated the acquisition of biopsy specimens from a normal-appearing squamo-columnar junction. Furthermore, for 9 of the 26 patients with specialized intestinal metaplasia, the squamo-columnar junction

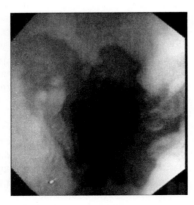

Figure 17–7. This endoscopic photograph of the distal esophagus shows long segments of red, columnar epithelium extending well above the esophago-gastric junction. This is the characteristic endoscopic appearance of Barrett's esophagus.

---

[1] Spechler SJ et al: Prevalence of metaplasia at the gastro-oesophageal junction. Lancet 1994;344:1533.

and the anatomic junction were located at the same level, ie, these patients did not have an appreciable segment of columnar-lined esophagus. For the remaining 17 patients, columnar epithelium extended a variable distance (up to 3 cm) above the esophagogastric junction.

If one requires only the presence of specialized intestinal metaplasia to establish the diagnosis of Barrett's esophagus, then the aforementioned study suggests that the disorder can be found in 18% of patients in a general endoscopy unit (many of whom have no other signs or symptoms of esophageal disease). This finding challenges traditional concepts on the pathogenesis and clinical features of Barrett's esophagus. The lack of universally-accepted and clearly reproducible diagnostic criteria for Barrett's esophagus has resulted in much confusion about the condition. Most of the data are based on studies of patients who had endoscopically-obvious disease with long segments of columnar epithelium lining the esophagus. It is not clear that the conclusions of these studies are applicable to patients who have short segments of specialized intestinal metaplasia in the region of the esophagogastric junction.

To circumvent this diagnostic confusion, it is proposed that whenever columnar epithelium is seen in the esophagus, regardless of extent, the condition is called **columnar-lined esophagus.** In these cases, biopsy specimens are obtained from the esophageal columnar lining to seek specialized intestinal metaplasia. The condition then can be classified as either "columnar-lined esophagus with intestinal metaplasia" or "columnar-lined esophagus without intestinal metaplasia." The term "Barrett's esophagus" can be applied to the subset of patients with columnar-lined esophagus who have long segments of columnar epithelium extending well above the esophagogastric junction. Most of the latter patients are found to have intestinal metaplasia. For practical purposes, endoscopic surveillance appears to be appropriate only for patients who have columnar-lined esophagus with intestinal metaplasia.

3. Clinical features–Columnar-lined esophagus with intestinal metaplasia has been described in children as young as age 5, but Barrett's esophagus usually is discovered in middle-aged and older adults. The average age at diagnosis is approximately 55 years. White males predominate in most series and, for unknown reasons, Barrett's esophagus appears to be uncommon in blacks and Asians.

Most patients are seen initially for symptoms of underlying GERD, such as heartburn, regurgitation, and dysphagia. The Barrett's epithelium causes no symptoms, and even may be more resistant to acid-peptic injury than the native squamous mucosa.

Many patients with endoscopically-apparent Barrett's esophagus have no symptoms of GERD, however, and recent data suggest that the large majority of patients with Barrett's esophagus do not seek medical attention for esophageal symptoms. Among patients identified by physicians, the GERD associated with Barrett's esophagus often is severe and associated with esophageal ulceration, stricture, and hemorrhage.

A variety of physiologic abnormalities have been described that might contribute to the severity of GERD in patients with Barrett's esophagus (see Table 17–1). For patients with these abnormalities, the gastric contents available for reflux are exceptionally caustic because they contain high concentrations of acid, bile, and pancreatic secretions. Patients who have extreme hypotension of the lower esophageal sphincter are exceptionally predisposed to the reflux of their caustic gastric contents. Poor esophageal contractility interferes with clearance of the refluxed material, allowing protracted contact with the esophageal epithelium. With diminished esophageal pain sensitivity, reflux may not induce the symptoms that lead patients to seek medical attention to prevent further damage to the esophagus. Finally, decreased secretion of epidermal growth factor might delay the healing of the reflux-induced injury. With all these abnormalities, it is not surprising that GERD frequently is severe in patients with Barrett's esophagus.

Given the propensity for severe GERD in patients with Barrett's esophagus, it has been assumed that the metaplasia should progress in extent over the years as more and more columnar epithelium replaced reflux-damaged squamous epithelium. Surprisingly, however, recent studies suggest that in most cases Barrett's esophagus develops to its full extent relatively quickly, neither progressing nor regressing substantially with time. The length of esophagus lined by Barrett's epithelium does not differ significantly among various age groups. Furthermore, no significant change in the extent of Barrett's epithelium is found among patients who have had follow-up endoscopic examinations performed after a mean interval of 3 years. It is not clear why Barrett's esophagus usually does not progress in extent, despite ongoing GERD.

4. Cancer risk–Barrett's esophagus is the single most important risk factor for adenocarcinoma of the gastroesophageal junction. Adenocarcinomas develop in Barrett's esophagus at the rate of approximately one cancer per 125 patient-years of follow-up. The frequency of adenocarcinoma of the gastroesophageal junction has been increasing at a rate exceeding that for any other cancer in the USA to the point that adenocarcinomas comprise approximately 50% of all esophageal malignancies in this country.

Carcinogenesis in Barrett's esophagus appears to begin with genetic alterations that activate proto-oncogenes (eg, c-erb-B) and disable tumor suppressor genes (eg, p53). These DNA abnormalities endow the cells with certain growth advantages. The advantaged cells hyperproliferate, and in so doing acquire more genetic changes that result in neoplasia with autonomous cell growth. When enough DNA abnormalities accumulate, clones of malignant cells emerge that have the ability to invade adjacent tissues and to proliferate in unnatural locations. Before the cells acquire enough DNA damage to become frankly malignant, the earlier genetic alterations often cause histologic changes that can be recognized by the pathologist as dysplasia.

Dysplasia in Barrett's epithelium is defined as a neoplastic alteration of columnar cells that remains confined within the basement membranes of the glands from which the cells arose. Dysplasia is the precursor of invasive malignancy, and the finding of dysplasia can provide an opportunity to initiate therapy to interrupt the progression to invasive cancer. Endoscopic surveillance for cancer in Barrett's esophagus is performed primarily to seek high-grade dysplasia, with the rationale that resection of the dysplastic epithelium may prevent the progression to invasive malignancy.

The usefulness of dysplasia as a biomarker for a malignant neoplasm is limited by the problem of biopsy sampling error. For example, patients who have esophageal resections performed for high-grade dysplasia in Barrett's esophagus often are found to have an inapparent malignant neoplasm in the resected specimen. These cancers were missed by the endoscopist preoperatively because of biopsy sampling error, a problem that can be reduced by increasing the number of biopsy specimens obtained during endoscopic examinations. Although it has been reported that clinicians can differentiate high-grade dysplasia from early adenocarcinoma in Barrett's esophagus by rigorously sampling the esophagus extensively, the extensive biopsy protocol required may be too rigorous to be clinically applicable.

Another problem with dysplasia as a biomarker for malignancy is the fact that the natural history of dysplasia is not well defined. Available data suggest, however, that high-grade dysplasia progresses to malignancy often and rapidly. Up to 25% of patients with high-grade dysplasia may progress to invasive cancer during a follow-up period of 2–46 months. This appears to be an alarming rate of progression to malignancy. In some cases, however, high-grade dysplasia has persisted for years with no apparent progression to carcinoma.

Noting the shortcomings of dysplasia as a biomarker for malignancy, investigators have studied alternative biomarkers, such as flow cytometry, ornithine decarboxylase activity, mucus abnormalities, chromosomal abnormalities, oncogenes, tumor suppressor genes, growth regulatory factors, and endosonography findings. None of these biomarkers have been shown to be superior to the histologic finding of dysplasia for predicting the development of malignancy in Barrett's esophagus, however. De-

spite the problems, the finding of dysplasia remains the best biomarker for the clinical evaluation of patients with Barrett's esophagus.

5. Treatment–There is no specific treatment for Barrett's esophagus other than treatment of the underlying reflux esophagitis. Furthermore, neither medical nor surgical therapy for GERD reliably results in the regression of the columnar epithelium. In recent studies, regression has been achieved by laser irradiation of Barrett's epithelium combined with the administration of a proton pump inhibitor. The rationale for this approach is the hypothesis that, in the absence of acid reflux, damaged esophageal tissue should heal normally by regeneration of squamous mucosa.

The largest study involved 10 patients who had argon laser irradiation of their columnar-lined esophagi.[1]

Patients were treated with omeprazole for the duration of the study (6–38 weeks). Squamous mucosa was found to replace photoablated columnar epithelium in 38 of 40 treatment locations in these 10 patients. Most patients required multiple endoscopic laser treatments to achieve ablation of the irradiated segment. Other recent reports describe the use of photodynamic therapy to obliterate dysplasia and early malignancy in Barrett's esophagus. These reports document the feasibility of laser ablation of Barrett's epithelium, but none of them have established the benefit of the technique. Photoablation entails some risk, and has not been shown to reduce the risk of esophageal cancer. Also, it is not clear whether life-long, intensive acid suppression will be necessary to prevent return of the columnar epithelium. Further studies addressing these issues are necessary before laser ablation of Barrett's epithelium can be recommended for clinical application.

6. Management recommendations–The management of patients with Barrett's esophagus is disputed, and will remain so until studies demonstrate the cost-effectiveness of endoscopic surveillance and clarify the natural history of high-grade dysplasia. Clinicians reviewing the available data on these issues might reasonably arrive at different conclusions regarding management. With minor modifications, the following management approach is that recommended by the 1990 Barrett's Esophagus Working Party of the World Congresses of Gastroenterology:[2]

---

[1]Berenson MM et al: Restoration of squamous mucosa after ablation of Barrett's esophageal epithelium. Gastroenterology 1993;104:1686.

[2]Dent J et al: Working party report to the World Congresses of Gastroenterology, Sydney 1990: Barrett's oesophagus. J Gastroenterol Hepatol 1991;6:1.

1. Patients who have Barrett's esophagus are advised to have regular endoscopic surveillance for dysplasia and early carcinoma, unless endoscopy is contraindicated by comorbidity. In the absence of dysplasia or cancer, endoscopic examination (with procurement of biopsy and brush cytology specimens from the Barrett's epithelium) is performed every other year.

2. If dysplasia is detected, the finding should be confirmed by at least one other expert pathologist. If any doubt remains, the endoscopic examination is repeated immediately to obtain more biopsy and cytology specimens for analysis.

3. For otherwise healthy patients confirmed to have multiple foci of high-grade dysplasia, surgery is advised to resect all of the esophagus lined by columnar epithelium. If advanced age or comorbidity precludes surgery for patients found to have high-grade dysplasia, experimental treatments such as photodynamic therapy can be considered.

4. For patients confirmed to have low-grade dysplasia, intensive medical antireflux therapy (including a proton pump inhibitor) should be given for 8–12 weeks, at which time the endoscopic examination is repeated to obtain multiple esophageal biopsy and cytology specimens. For patients whose specimens show histologic improvement, intensive surveillance (eg, endoscopic examinations every 6 months) is recommended until at least two consecutive examinations reveal no dysplastic epithelium. For patients with persistent low-grade dysplasia, continued intensive treatment and surveillance are recommended.

REFERENCES

Baldi F et al: Acid gastroesophageal reflux and symptom occurrence. Analysis of some factors influencing their association. Dig Dis Sci 1989;34:1890.

Behar J, Biancani P, Sheahan DG: Evaluation of esophageal tests in the diagnosis of reflux esophagitis. Gastroenterology 1976; 71:9.

Berenson MM et al: Restoration of squamous mucosa after ablation of Barrett's esophageal epithelium. Gastroenterology 1993;104:1686.

Blot WJ, Devesa SS, Fraumeni JF Jr: Continuing climb in rates of esophageal adenocarcinoma: an update. JAMA 1993;270:1320.

Blot WJ et al: Rising incidence of adenocarcinoma of the esophagus and gastric cardia. JAMA 1991;265:1287.

Blount PL et al: Clonal ordering of 17p and 5q allelic losses in Barrett dysplasia and adenocarcinoma. Proc Natl Acad Sci USA 1993;90:3221.

Cameron AJ et al: Prevalence of columnar-lined (Barrett's) esophagus. Comparison of population-based clinical and autopsy findings. Gastroenterology 1990;99:918.

Cameron AJ, Lomboy CT: Barrett's esophagus: age, prevalence, and extent of columnar epithelium. Gastroenterology 1992;103:1241.

Collen MJ, Johnson DA: Correlation between basal acid output and daily ranitidine dose required for therapy in Barrett's esophagus. Dig Dis Sci 1992;37:570.

Dent J et al: Mechanism of gastroesophageal reflux in recumbent asymptomatic human subjects. J Clin Invest 1980;65:256.

Dent J et al: Mechanisms of lower oesophageal sphincter incompetence in patients with symptomatic gastrooesophageal reflux. Gut 1988;29:1020.

Dent J et al: Working party report to the World Congresses of Gastroenterology, Sydney 1990: Barrett's oesophagus. J Gastroenterol Hepatol 1991;6:1.

DeVault KR, Castell DO: Current diagnosis and treatment of gastroesophageal reflux disease. Mayo Clin Proc 1994;69:867.

Dodds WJ et al: Pathogenesis of reflux esophagitis. Gastroenterology 1981;81:376.

Frierson HF Jr: Histological criteria for the diagnosis of reflux esophagitis. Pathol Annu (Part 1) 1992;27:87.

Gillen P et al: Implication of duodenogastric reflux in the pathogenesis of Barrett's oesophagus. Br J Surg 1988;75:540.

Gray MR, Donnelly RJ, Kingsnorth AN: Role of salivary epidermal growth factor in the pathogenesis of Barrett's columnar lined oesophagus. Br J Surg 1991;78:1461.

Haggitt RC: Adenocarcinoma in Barrett's esophagus: a new epidemic? Hum Pathol 1992;23:475.

Haggitt RC, Dean PJ: Adenocarcinoma in Barrett's epithelium. In: *Barrett's esophagus: Pathophysiology, diagnosis, and management.* Spechler SJ, Goyal RK (editors). Elsevier, 1985.

Hameeteman W: Clinical studies of sucralfate in reflux esophagitis. The European experience. J Clin Gastroenterol 1991;13(Suppl 2):S16.

Hameeteman W et al: Barrett's esophagus: development of dysplasia and adenocarcinoma. Gastroenterology 1989;96:1249.

Hassall E: Barrett's esophagus: new definitions and approaches in children. J Pediatr Gastroenterol Nutr 1993;16:345.

Helm JF et al: Effect of esophageal emptying and saliva on clearance of acid from the esophagus. N Engl J Med 1984;310:284.

Herrera JL et al: Sucralfate used as adjunctive therapy in patients with severe erosive esophagitis resulting from gastroesophageal reflux. Am J Gastroenterol 1990;85:1335.

Hetzel DJ et al: Healing and relapse of severe peptic esophagitis after treatment with omeprazole. Gastroenterology 1988;95:903.

Hewson EG et al: Acid perfusion test: does it have a role in the assessment of noncardiac chest pain? Gut 1989;30:305.

Holloway RH, Dent J: Pathophysiology of gastroesophageal reflux. Lower esophageal sphincter dysfunction in gastroesophageal reflux disease. Gastroenterol Clin North Am 1990;19:517.

Inauen W et al: Effects of ranitidine and cisapride on acid reflux and oesophageal motility in patients with reflux oesophagitis: A 24-hour ambulatory combined pH and manometry study. Gut 1993;34:1025.

Jamieson GG: Anti-reflux operations: how do they work? Br J Surg 1987;74:155.

Johnson DA et al: Esophageal acid sensitivity in Barrett's esophagus. J Clin Gastroenterol 1987;9:23.

Kahrilas PJ: Cigarette smoking and gastroesophageal reflux disease. Dig Dis 1992;10:61.

Kahrilas PJ, Clouse RE, Hogan WJ: American Gastroenterological Association technical review on the clinical use of esophageal manometry. Gastroenterology 1994; 107:1865.

Kitchin LI, Castell DO: Rationale and efficacy of conservative therapy for gastroesophageal reflux disease. Arch Intern Med 1991;151:448.

Klinkenberg-Knol EC, et al: Long-term treatment with omeprazole for refractory reflux esophagitis: efficacy and safety. Ann Intern Med 1994;121:161.

Koufman JA: The otolaryngologic manifestations of gastroesophageal reflux disease (GERD): A clinical investigation of 225 patients using ambulatory 24-hour pH monitoring and an experimental investigation of the role of acid and pepsin in the development of laryngeal injury. Laryngoscope 1991;101:1.

Lanas A, Hirschowitz BI: Significant role of aspirin use in patients with esophagitis. J Clin Gastroenterol 1991;13:622.

Levine DS et al: An endoscopic biopsy protocol can differentiate high-grade dysplasia from early adenocarcinoma in Barrett's esophagus. Gastroenterology 1993;105:40.

Lieberman DA, Keeffe EB: Treatment of severe reflux esophagitis with cimetidine and metoclopramide. Ann Intern Med 1986;104:21.

Mansfield LE: Gastroesophageal reflux and respiratory disorders: A review. Ann Allergy 1989;62:158.

Marks RD et al: Omeprazole versus H_2-receptor antagonists in treating patients with peptic stricture and esophagitis. Gastroenterology 1994;106:907.

Mattox HE III, Richter JE: Prolonged ambulatory esophageal pH monitoring in the evaluation of gastroesophageal reflux disease. Am J Med 1990;89:345.

McCallum RW: Gastric emptying in gastroesophageal reflux and the therapeutic role of prokinetic agents. Gastroenterol Clin North Am 1990;19:551.

McClave SA, Boyce HW Jr., Gottfried MR: Early diagnosis of columnar-lined esophagus: a new endoscopic criterion. Gastrointest Endosc 1987;33:413.

Meyers RL, Orlando RC: In vivo bicarbonate secretion by human esophagus. Gastroenterology 1992;103:1174.

Mittal RK: Current concepts of the antireflux barrier. Gastroenterol Clin North Am 1990;19:501.

Mittal RK, Rochester DF, McCallum RW: Electrical and mechanical activity in the human lower esophageal sphincter during diaphragmatic contraction. J Clin Invest 1988;81:1182.

Orlando RC: Esophageal epithelial defense against acid injury. J Clin Gastroenterol 1991;13(Suppl 2):S1.

Orlando RC: Esophageal epithelial defenses against acid injury. Am J Gastroenterol 1994;89:S48.

O'Sullivan GC et al: Interaction of lower esophageal sphincter pressure and length of sphincter in the abdomen as determinants of gastroesophageal competence. Am J Surg 1982;143:40.

Overholt B et al: Photodynamic therapy for treatment of early adenocarcinoma in Barrett's esophagus. Gastrointest Endosc 1993;39:73.

Paterson WG, Kolyn DM: Esophageal shortening induced by short-term intraluminal acid perfusion in opossum: a cause for hiatal hernia? Gastroenterology 1994;107:1736.

Paull A et al: The histologic spectrum of Barrett's esophagus. N Engl J Med 1976;295:476.

Pope CE II: Acid-reflux disorders. N Engl J Med 1994;331:656.

Reid BJ: Barrett's esophagus and esophageal adenocarcinoma. Gastroenterol Clin N Am 1991;20:817.

Robinson M et al: Omeprazole is superior to ranitidine plus metoclopramide in the short-term treatment of erosive oesophagitis. Aliment Pharmacol Ther 1993;7:67.

Schmidt HG et al: Dysplasia in Barrett's esophagus. J Cancer Res Clin Oncol 1985;110:145.

Sloan S, Rademaker AW, Kahrilas PJ: Determinants of gastroesophageal junction incompetence: hiatal hernia, lower esophageal sphincter, or both? Ann Intern Med 1992;117:977.

Smith JL et al: Sensitivity of the esophageal mucosa to pH in gastroesophageal reflux disease. Gastroenterology 1989;96:683.

Smith PM et al: A comparison of omeprazole and ranitidine in the prevention of recurrence of benign esophageal stricture. Gastroenterology 1994;107:1312.

Sontag SJ: The medical management of reflux esophagitis. Role of antacids and acid inhibition. Gastroenterol Clin North Am 1990;19:683.

Spechler SJ: Barrett's esophagus. Current Opinion in Gastroenterology 1994;10:448.

Spechler SJ: Barrett's esophagus: Diagnosis, clinical presentation, and prevalence. Practical Gastroenterology 1995 (In press).

Spechler SJ: Comparison of medical and surgical therapy for complicated gastroesophageal reflux disease in veterans. The Department of Veterans Affairs Gastroesophageal Reflux Disease Study Group. N Engl J Med 1992;326:786.

Spechler SJ: Complications of gastroesophageal reflux disease. In: The esophagus. Castell DO (editor). Little, Brown and Company, 1992.

Spechler SJ: Epidemiology and natural history of gastrooesophageal reflux disease. Digestion 1992;51(Suppl 1):24.

Spechler SJ: Laser photoablation of Barrett's epithelium: burning issues about burning tissues. Gastroenterology 1993;104:1855.

Spechler SJ: The frequency of esophageal cancer in patients with Barrett's esophagus. Acta Endoscopica 1992;22:541.

Spechler SJ et al: Prevalence of metaplasia at the gastrooesophageal junction. Lancet 1994; 344:1533.

Tytgat GNJ: Dilation therapy of benign esophageal stenoses. World J Surg 1989;13:142.

Vincent ME, Robbins AH: Radiology of Barrett's esophagus. In: Barrett's esophagus: Pathophysiology, diagnosis, and management. Spechler SJ, Goyal RK (editors). Elsevier, 1985.

Esophageal Motility Disorders & Noncardiac Chest Pain

18

Christine B. Dalton, PA-C, & Scott R. Brazer, MD, MHS

The esophagus is a muscular conduit between the oropharynx and the stomach that is bounded by an upper and lower sphincter. The pharynx, upper esophageal sphincter, and upper third of the esophagus are composed of skeletal muscle; the distal two-thirds and the lower esophageal sphincter are composed of smooth muscle. The esophagus has two functions: (1) to propel food from the pharynx to the stomach, and (2) to prevent reflux of gastric contents.

Each swallow begins as a rapid, orderly sequence of peristaltic pharyngeal contractions that propels a bolus into the esophagus through the relaxed upper esophageal sphincter. **Primary esophageal peristalsis,** which is induced by swallowing, begins as the bolus passes through the upper esophageal sphincter, and peristaltic contractions then transport the bolus down the length of the esophagus through the relaxed lower esophageal sphincter and into the stomach. **Secondary esophageal peristalsis** is initiated by esophageal distention from refluxed gastric contents or an incompletely transported bolus; its function is to assist in esophageal clearance.

Esophageal motility disorders may result from any disruption of the normal muscular movements of the sphincters or esophageal body. Patients typically present with dysphagia to solids and liquids; rarely, they present with chest pain. The most common esophageal motility disorder, gastroesophageal reflux disease, is discussed in Chapter 17.

MOTILITY DISORDERS OF THE HYPOPHARYNX & UPPER ESOPHAGEAL SPHINCTER

Essentials of Diagnosis

- Oropharyngeal dysphagia (difficulty in transferring material from the mouth or pharynx into the esophagus); usually most severe with liquids.
- Nasal or oral regurgitation, aspiration, and coughing with swallowing.
- Documentation with cine-esophagogram.

General Considerations

The oropharyngeal phase of swallowing is quite complex, because the nasal cavity and airway must close during a swallow, to convert the oropharynx from an air conduit to a food conduit. There are four phases of oropharyngeal swallowing:

1. Oral-preparatory phase
2. Reflex initiation phase
3. Pharyngeal phase
4. Pharyngeal-esophageal phase

Any condition that affects smooth muscle or innervation is capable of affecting the integrity of the muscular response and therefore coordination of the oropharynx. Oropharyngeal dysphagia results from the uncoordinated, feeble, or absent contractions of the tongue, pharynx, or hypopharynx. It is basically true, although an oversimplification, that neurologic disorders cause oropharyngeal incoordination, and muscular disorders cause weak or absent pharyngeal contractions. Dysphagia is usually the most prominent esophageal symptom but is often only one of a constellation of symptoms of the neuromuscular disorder.

Table 18–1 lists the various disorders that may cause dysphagia, including disorders of the central nervous system, peripheral nervous system, and muscle. Cerebrovascular accidents are the most common central nervous system cause.

During a swallow, the upper esophageal sphincter must both relax and be actively pulled open by surrounding suprahyoid muscles. True abnormalities of upper esophageal sphincter relaxation are extraordinarily rare. More commonly, the sphincter fails to open adequately because of fibrosis of surrounding tissues, which may result in increased intrabolus pressure, development of a cricopharyngeal bar (which can be seen on radiography), or formation of a diverticulum. **Zenker's diverticulum** is an outpouching of the posterior pharyngeal wall that forms in an area of relative weakness, typically between the inferior pharyngeal constrictor and the superior mar-

Table 18–1. Causes of oropharyngeal dysphagia.

Neurologic causes	Muscular causes	Structural causes
Cerebrovascular accident	Muscular dystrophies	Zenker's and other diverticula
Parkinson's disease	Polymyositis	Neoplasms
Wilson's disease	Amyloidosis	Postoperative changes
Amyotrophic lateral sclerosis		Postradiation changes
Myasthenia gravis		Extrinsic compression (eg, cervical osteophytes)
Multiple sclerosis		
Brain stem tumors		
Tabes dorsalis		
Poliomyelitis		
Diphtheria		
Botulism		
Rabies		

gin of the upper esophageal sphincter (**Killian's dehiscence**).

Clinical Findings

A. Symptoms and Signs: Oropharyngeal dysphagia is the major symptom of oropharyngeal motility disorders. Typically, it is more severe with liquids than solids, and, frequently, there is associated nasal regurgitation, cough ("my food goes down the wrong way"), dysarthria (impaired articulation of speech), or dysphonia (impaired quality of the voice). Patients tend to seek immediate medical attention and are often able to localize precisely the level at which food is arrested. Malnourishment may result either from inability to swallow or from cessation of eating because of tracheal aspiration. The inability to swallow food of any consistency with less than 10% aspiration frequently results in cessation of eating.

Patients at risk for aspiration following stroke may be identified by the presence of an abnormal voluntary cough and the absence of a gag reflex.

B. Imaging Studies: Radiologic evaluation is the first study performed in patients with oropharyngeal dysphagia. Plain x-rays of the neck (lateral views) are helpful for locating soft tissue masses or bony or cartilaginous abnormalities. Barium examination must include videotaping or cineradiography, which are the only methods capable of record-

ing the rapid sequence of events that occurs during the oropharyngeal phase of swallowing. Patients are given boluses of different size and texture. Absent or weak contraction or incoordination may be detected in each of the four phases of oropharyngeal function.

C. Manometry: Although upper esophageal manometry may on rare occasion reveal abnormalities in patients with oropharyngeal dysphagia (eg, pharyngeal-cricopharyngeal incoordination), it is less useful than radiologic evaluation. Manometry can be used to provide limited information about the strength (amplitude) and duration of hypopharyngeal contractions, the resting pressure and relaxation of the upper esophageal sphincter, and coordination of pharyngeal contraction with upper esophageal sphincter relaxation. Esophageal manometry is seldom employed in the routine evaluation of oropharyngeal dysphagia.

D. Endoscopy: Upper esophageal endoscopy is not helpful in the evaluation of patients with oropharyngeal dysphagia.

Differential Diagnosis

The differential diagnosis of oropharyngeal dysphagia is listed in Table 18–1.

Oropharyngeal dysphagia should not be confused with globus sensation ("a lump in the throat"), which does not interfere with eating and typically occurs in patients with anxiety disorders.

Complications

Complications of hypopharyngeal or upper sphincter dysfunction include aspiration pneumonia, weight loss, and malnutrition.

Treatment

Whenever possible, the underlying neuromuscular disorder should be treated. When this does not relieve the dysphagia, the patient may benefit from alteration of eating behavior (eg, tucking the chin, turning the head). In patients who are unable to resume oral intake, percutaneous endoscopic gastrostomy is indicated to maintain adequate nutrition. Zenker's diverticula may be treated surgically with diverticulectomy and upper esophageal sphincter myotomy.

Prognosis

The prognosis for patients with motility disorders of the hypopharynx and upper esophageal sphincter depends on that of the underlying neuromuscular disorder, the severity of the dysphagia, and the ability to eat. The patient with dysphagia resulting from an acute, self-limited process may recover completely, while the patient with a progressive disorder (eg, oculopharyngeal muscular dystrophy) may develop recurrent aspiration pneumonia and malnutrition leading to death.

MOTILITY DISORDERS OF THE BODY OF THE ESOPHAGUS

Essentials of Diagnosis

- Dysphagia to solid foods and liquids.
- Chest pain (see following section, "Noncardiac Chest Pain").
- Confirmation of abnormal motility by esophageal manometry.

General Considerations

Esophageal peristalsis is a propulsive process controlled by the enteric nervous system under the influence of the central nervous system (primary peristalsis is abolished by bilateral cervical vagotomy). A peristaltic wave of amplitude greater than 30 mm Hg will propel a bolus down the esophagus. Upon initiation of a swallow, the lower esophageal sphincter relaxes to approximately 10% of its resting baseline pressure (Figure 18–1). Relaxation is probably mediated by vasoactive intestinal peptide and nitric oxide.

Motility disorders of the esophagus include achalasia (failure of the esophageal sphincter to relax), which is the only motility disorder considered a true disease process. Other disorders that have been defined on the basis of abnormal or unusual patterns at esophageal manometry include nutcracker esophagus, diffuse esophageal spasm, hypertensive lower esophageal sphincter, and nonspecific esophageal motility disorder (Table 18–2). Although there have been case reports of progression of nutcracker esophagus or diffuse esophageal spasm to achalasia, it is unlikely that most of these manometrically defined entities are single disease processes. They may represent an epiphenomenon, a variant of normal, or a response to stress. Many of the esophageal motility disorders are evanescent, and follow-up studies on patients with a prior diagnosis of one motility disorder may reveal a different disorder or even normal function.

Motility disorders of the esophageal body are categorized as primary, involving only the esophagus, or secondary, resulting from a larger, systemic disorder. Achalasia is characterized by failure of the lower esophageal sphincter to relax adequately with deglutition, and aperistalsis of the esophageal smooth muscle. The cause of this disease remains unknown, but it probably results from a degenerative process, possibly infectious or autoimmune, that causes denervation of the esophageal smooth muscle. Histologic studies have shown decreased numbers of interneurons in the myenteric plexus as well as abnormalities of the vagus nerve and its dorsal motor nucleus. Furthermore, myenteric neurons containing vasoactive intestinal peptide, a neurotransmitter capable of relaxing the lower esophageal sphincter, are reduced in number in patients with achalasia.

Secondary motility disorders result from conditions that affect the enteric nervous system or esophageal smooth muscle. These conditions include diabetes mellitus, amyloidosis, alcoholic neuropathy, and scleroderma. Chronic infection with *Trypanosoma cruzi* (Chagas' disease) results in reduction of gut submucosal and myenteric neurons and may lead to megacolon, megaduodenum, and megaesophagus, which closely mimics achalasia.

Clinical Findings

The diagnosis of an esophageal motility disorder must be based on two criteria: (1) the patient must have symptoms that suggest esophageal dysfunction. Dysphagia is the most typical symptom, although patients may also note weight loss, regurgitation, and pulmonary or otolaryngologic symptoms; (2) abnormal motility must be documented by esophageal manometry, barium esophagography, or radionuclide transit studies.

The history suggests the correct diagnosis in most patients with esophageal dysphagia. Three questions will help narrow the diagnosis:

1. What type of food causes dysphagia?
2. Is the dysphagia progressive or intermittent?
3. Does the patient have heartburn? (Figure 18–2)

Patients who complain of dysphagia to both solid foods and liquids are likely to have an esophageal motility disorder. Patients with intermittent solid and liquid dysphagia may have diffuse esophageal spasm; those with progressive solid and liquid dysphagia may have achalasia; and those with progressive solid and liquid dysphagia with prominent symptoms of heartburn may have scleroderma. Patients with achalasia may also have pulmonary symptoms (nocturnal cough, recurrent pneumonia) or weight loss. Progressive dysphagia to solids (especially meat and bread) suggests mechanical obstruction by tumor or peptic stricture. Intermittent dysphagia to solids suggests of a Schatzki's ring. Patients with gastroesophageal reflux disease may present with either dysphagia resulting from peptic stricture or gross esophagitis, or a combination. Infectious or radiation-induced esophagitis may cause dysphagia or odynophagia (pain during swallowing). Finally, neoplasms of the esophageal body and gastric cardia may present with dysphagia, which is usually progressive to solids, and weight loss.

A. Symptoms and Signs: Dysphagia resulting from dysfunction of the esophageal body is described as a feeling that the bolus gets "stuck" or "hung up" on the way down. This may be accompanied by pain or discomfort. The patient typically describes difficulty in swallowing both solid foods and liquids. Notably, although most patients feel as though the bolus stops at the level of the suprasternal notch, the area of obstruction may be well below that.

Patients with esophageal motility disorders may also present with chest pain, which may mimic angina pectoris. The pain is often substernal, burn-

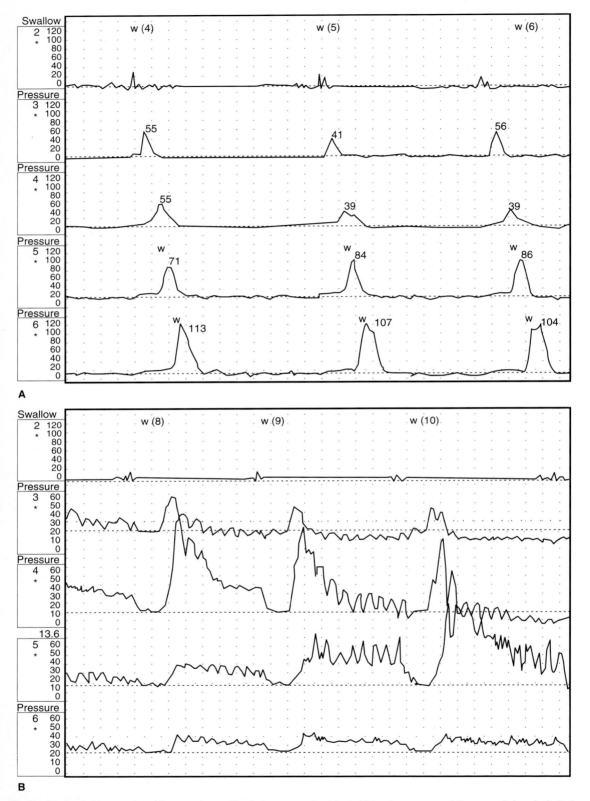

Figure 18–1. **A:** Manometry of the esophageal body in a normal subject. All leads are spaced 5 cm apart. Leads 6, 5, 4, and 3 are positioned in the body of the esophagus, 3, 8, 13, and 18 cm above the lower esophageal sphincter. Lead 2 is in the pharynx. Note that after each wet swallow (w), a peristaltic wave passes through the esophageal body. **B:** Manometry of the lower esophageal sphincter in a normal subject. Leads 3, 4, 5, and 6 are spaced 1 cm apart. Lead 2 is in the pharynx. With a wet swallow (w), the lower esophageal sphincter pressure falls to the level of the gastric baseline pressure **(dotted line)**, and then returns to its tonic level of contraction.

Table 18–2. Manometric criteria for the diagnosis of esophageal motility disorders associated with chest pain.

Diagnosis	Required Manometric Criteria
Achalasia	Aperistalsis of esophageal body Incomplete lower esophageal sphincter relaxation
Nutcracker esophagus	Mean distal esophageal contraction > 180 mmHg Normal peristalsis
Diffuse esophageal spasm	Simultaneous contractions ≥ 20% Intermittent normal peristalsis
Hypertensive lower esophageal sphincter	Lower esophageal sphincter pressure > 45 mmHg
Nonspecific esophageal motility disorder	Abnormal motility not described above (eg, retrograde or triple-peaked contractions, ≥ 20% nontransmitted contractions)

ing, or pressurelike, and may radiate into the neck or down the left arm. Pain may or may not be related to eating or swallowing; it may occur at rest or may awaken the patient from sleep; and it is frequently made worse by stress. The pain may resolve sponta-

neously, or antacids or nitrates may be required for relief. In most cases, the clinical history will not differentiate between cardiac and esophageal chest pain. Patients with esophageal chest pain often report other esophageal symptoms such as heartburn, regurgitation, or dysphagia, which also are common complaints in patients with coronary disease.

B. Manometry: Esophageal manometry can be used to measure the strength (amplitude) and duration of the contractions of the esophageal body as well as the resting pressure and relaxation of the upper and lower esophageal sphincters. This technique involves passage of a small, flexible catheter with pressure sensors through the nose and into the esophagus. The catheter may be water perfused or house miniature solid-state pressure transducers.

Normal esophageal motility consists of orderly, sequential peristaltic contractions of normal amplitude and duration down the body of the esophagus, with no abnormal contractions. Normal values for esophageal manometry (amplitude and duration of contractions, percentage of peristaltic contractions, and percentage of abnormal contractions) have been derived from the study of healthy volunteers. Normal

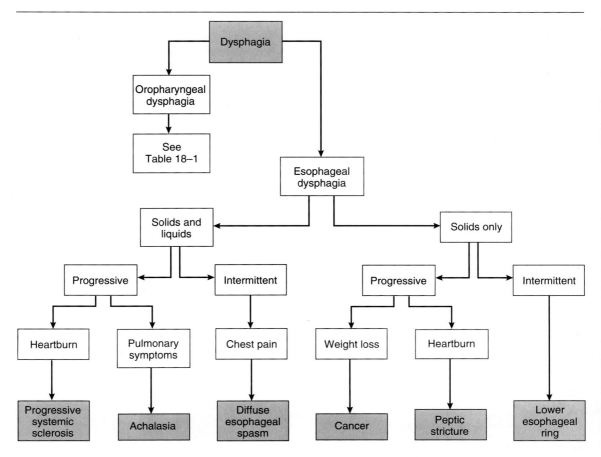

Figure 18–2. Dysphagia algorithm. The cause of dysphagia in most patients can be determined by the history.

lower sphincter function consists of resting pressure within normal ranges and complete relaxation following a wet swallow.

In achalasia, there are two characteristic manometric findings: aperistalsis of the esophageal body, and partial or absent relaxation of the lower sphincter (Figure 18–3).

Nonperistaltic contractions of the esophagus are typically absent during stationary manometry, but up to 5% of contractions are nonperistaltic during 24-hour ambulatory motility testing. A small subset of patients appears to have adequate lower esophageal sphincter relaxation by manometric criteria but abnormal esophageal emptying as measured by more sensitive radionuclide studies. In the past, the terms "classic" and "vigorous" achalasia were used to distinguish patients with low-amplitude simultaneous esophageal contractions (classic) from those with relatively higher amplitude simultaneous contractions (vigorous). These distinctions are not clinically useful and have fallen out of favor.

The most common motility disorder in patients with chest pain is nutcracker esophagus. Other such disorders include diffuse esophageal spasm, hypertensive lower esophageal sphincter, and nonspecific esophageal motility disorder (Table 18–2).

C. Imaging Studies: Radiographic examination of the esophagus should include double-contrast and full-column techniques. The advantage of the double-contrast technique is visualization of the extended esophagus and its mucosal surface; this is helpful in identifying small neoplasms and esophagitis. The full-column technique allows assessment of esophageal motility disorders as well as Schatzki's rings and peptic strictures.

Nuclear medicine studies are sometimes helpful in assessing functional disorders of the esophagus. These studies can detect prolonged esophageal transit time, suggestive of a motility disorder, or high residual fraction or retrograde index, suggestive of gastroesophageal reflux.

D. Endoscopy: Endoscopy is required in all patients with achalasia to rule out **pseudoachalasia,** a syndrome that occurs in certain malignant tumors. Although the syndrome typically involves tumors of the gastric cardia and causes symptoms by compressing the gastroesophageal junction or infiltrating the myenteric plexus, distant tumors occasionally produce similar effects via neurotoxins. Pseudoachalasia may also be seen in patients with amyloidosis, sarcoidosis, or Chagas' disease and in those who have undergone vagotomy.

Differential Diagnosis

The differential diagnosis for esophageal dysphagia is shown in Figure 18–2.

Complications

Complications of achalasia include weight loss,

nocturnal regurgitation, airway obstruction, and the development of squamous cell carcinoma, esophageal diverticula, and pulmonary infections. Squamous cell carcinoma of the esophagus may occur in 2–7% of patients with achalasia, and endoscopic surveillance may therefore be advisable. Complications of scleroderma include peptic stricture and food impaction. Serious complications from other esophageal motility disorders are rare.

Treatment

A. Achalasia: None of the treatments currently available reverse the abnormalities associated with achalasia. All treatments are thus palliative, their aim being to decrease resting lower esophageal sphincter pressure sufficiently to allow gravity and any residual esophageal peristalsis or pharyngeal contraction to empty the esophagus. The five treatments used are bougienage with mercury-weighted dilators, pharmacotherapy, botulinum toxin injection, forceful pneumatic dilation, and surgical myotomy. Of these, only pneumatic dilation and surgical myotomy can permanently decrease the resting pressure of the lower esophageal sphincter and can thus be considered definitive treatment.

1. Bougienage—Three hundred years after Sir Thomas Willis reported the first treatment of achalasia by means of esophageal dilation with a sponge-tipped whale bone, a recent case series suggests that bougienage with mercury-weighted dilators is effective. Until more rigorously designed studies have been undertaken, however, this procedure cannot be recommended as primary or definitive treatment for achalasia. It may be used for a temporary relief of symptoms in patients who are either unwilling or unable to undergo more definitive therapy.

2. Drug therapy—Pharmacotherapy may also be used as a temporary measure in selected patients prior to definitive therapy. These patients include those who are awaiting definitive therapy, are completing their evaluation, or wish to delay their decision about definitive therapy. In addition, pharmacotherapy may be appropriate for patients who refuse definitive therapy, are uncooperative, or are not candidates for definitive therapy because of advanced age or other illnesses.

Calcium channel blockers have been studied the most in a clinical setting. Nifedipine, 10–20 mg sublingually 30 minutes before meals, may be used. Patients must be warned of potential side effects, particularly hypotension. Pharmacologic treatment of achalasia may be effective in 50–75% of selected patients for periods approaching 2 years in duration.

3. Botulinum toxin injection—Botulinum toxin prevents acetylocholine release from nerve terminals. As a result, the toxin decreases lower esophageal sphincter pressure when injected into the sphincter muscle. Although botulinum toxin injection is safe and well-tolerated, its effects are transient. Lower

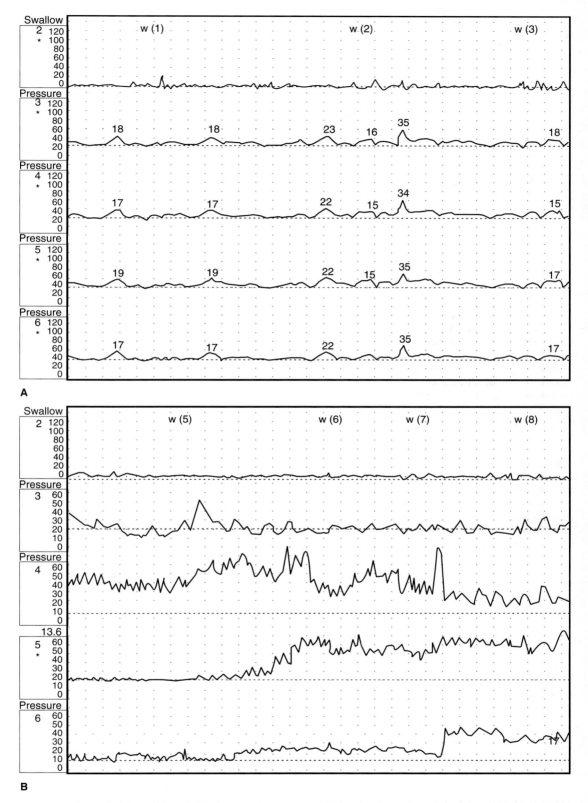

Figure 18–3. A: Manometry of the esophageal body in achalasia. The leads are placed in the same manner as in Figure 18–1A. With a wet swallow (w), simultaneous, low-amplitude, nonperistaltic waves are seen in all leads in the esophageal body. These contractions are virtually identical in all four leads. Note that the baseline esophageal pressure (normally ≤ 0 cm H_2) is elevated to 20 cm H_2, because the esophagus is filled with fluid. **B:** Manometry of the lower esophageal sphincter in achalasia. The leads are placed in the same manner as in Figure 18–1B. The baseline lower esophageal pressure is elevated. With wet swallows, little relaxation in the lower esophageal sphincter pressure occurs, and it remains well above the gastric baseline **(dotted line).**

esophageal sphincter pressure returns to baseline levels within 1–2 years. Botulinum toxin injection may supplant bougienage or drug therapy as the treatment of choice in patients who are not candidates for definitive therapy (pneumatic dilation or surgical myotomy).

4. Pneumatic dilation—In pneumatic dilation, a pneumatic balloon is used to forcefully disrupt the lower esophageal sphincter muscle. The procedure is often done on an outpatient basis. The most widely available balloon is the Microvasive Rigiflex Achalasia Dilator (Microvasive, Watertown, Massachusetts). Pneumatic dilation results in a good or excellent result in 69% of reported cases. Early complications include perforation (3.3%), aspiration pneumonia (0.8%), and death (0.2%). The late complication of gastroesophageal reflux occurs in only 2% of patients treated with pneumatic dilation. Pneumatic dilation is recommended as first-line therapy for achalasia by most gastroenterologists.

5. Esophagomyotomy—Surgical esophagomyotomy is more efficacious than pneumatic dilation in relieving dysphagia. A modified Heller procedure is usually employed, in which myotomy of the circular muscle layers is performed down to the level of the mucosa. The myotomy extends less than 1 cm onto the stomach and up to several centimeters above the lower sphincter.

Csendes and coworkers randomly treated 81 patients with achalasia (11 with Chagas' disease) with surgical myotomy or forceful pneumatic dilation. At a mean follow-up time of 5 years, 95% of patients who had undergone myotomy had a good or excellent result, compared with only 65% of those treated with pneumatic dilation. While surgery is clearly superior to pneumatic dilation for relief of dysphagia, several other factors must be considered in choosing treatment for a specific patient. These include the respective skills of the local surgeon and gastroenterologist (ie, effectiveness versus efficacy and complication rates); the patient's quality of life, health status, and preferences; and costs (surgical myotomy is approximately seven times more expensive than pneumatic dilation).

Recently, several centers have begun to perform myotomy by means of a laparoscopic approach. As this technique is perfected, it may become the desired first-line definitive therapy for most patients.

B. Other Upper Esophageal Motility Disorders: Treatment of the remaining esophageal motility disorders is less straightforward, with mixed success rates reported for a variety of measures attempted. The use of smooth muscle relaxants, including nitrates and calcium channel blockers, has been shown to provide relief in some patients. Because of the concomitant relaxation effect of such agents on the lower sphincter, however, problems associated with gastroesophageal reflux disease may be increased. Psychotropic drugs, bougienage, behav-ioral therapies, and surgical myotomies have been used with success in selected patients.

Prognosis

The prognosis for patients with esophageal motility disorders is generally good. The life expectancy of patients with achalasia is no different from that of patients without the disorder. Surveillance for squamous cell carcinoma may be advisable in these patients.

NONCARDIAC CHEST PAIN

Pathophysiology

Chest pain may occur in patients with cardiac, gastrointestinal, psychiatric, or musculoskeletal disorders. Determining which disorder is truly the cause of the chest pain is difficult, as many purported disorders do not meet strict criteria for causation and may be epiphenomena. The only esophageal motor disorder that is clearly capable of causing chest pain is achalasia. Several studies have demonstrated that multiple disorders may affect a single patient, and it is often difficult to establish which disorder is responsible for the pain.

The mechanism and cause of pain in most patients remain speculative. Abnormal esophageal contractions and distention may cause chest pain in patients with achalasia by stimulating mechanical nociceptors or inducing esophageal ischemia. Stimulation of acid-sensitive esophageal chemoreceptors may cause pain in patients with gastroesophageal reflux. Cardiac ischemia can be demonstrated in patients with microvascular angina when sophisticated tests are performed, although the degree of chest pain seems disproportionate to the severity of ischemia. Provocative testing (see section under "Clinical Findings") induces pain in patients with chest pain of undetermined etiology but not in subjects without the disorder.

Increased visceral sensitivity to normal physiologic or minor noxious stimuli, commonly referred to as **heightened visceral nocioception,** may be the underlying abnormality in many patients with chest pain of undetermined etiology and the common thread linking several disorders in a single patient. This theory is supported by the fact that these patients frequently exhibit an increased sensitivity to visceral stimuli such as distention or acid reflux. The mechanism responsible for this heightened sensitivity is not known, but may involve malfunction of the nociceptor itself, the ascending nociceptive pathway, the central nervous system, the descending antinociceptive pathway, or neurotransmitter release. Several neurotransmitters have been identified that play a role in pain perception and transmission, including substance P, calcitonin gene-related peptide, and serotonin. Specific antagonists of the $5HT_3$ receptor (eg, ondansetron and granisetron) may block visceral pain perception and may be an effective therapy in the future for patients with chest pain of undetermined etiology.

Essentials of Diagnosis

• Exclusion of life-threatening conditions, usually coronary artery disease.
• Search for the two common and treatable conditions that may present with chest pain: gastroesophageal reflux disease and panic disorder.
• Suspicion for unusual causes of chest pain (eg, congenital absence of the pericardium, pneumothorax, dissecting aneurysm).

General Considerations

Noncardiac chest pain, more aptly termed **chest pain of undetermined etiology,** is alarming for both patient and physician because it may herald a potentially life-threatening condition. The first step in the evaluation of all patients with chest pain is to diagnose and treat such conditions, most commonly ischemic heart disease. As many as 20% of cardiac catheterizations in patients with chest pain will reveal normal or insignificantly diseased coronary arteries, however. Although this subset of patients has a low mortality rate (cardiac survival exceeds 98% at 10 years), their quality of life is poor and the yearly cost of their medical care is estimated to be $3500. Once life-threatening conditions have been excluded, the two most important conditions to recognize are gastroesophageal reflux and panic disorder, both of which are common and treatable.

Gastroesophageal reflux is found in 25–50% of all patients with chest pain of undetermined etiology studied with ambulatory pH monitoring. Such monitoring quantifies esophageal acid contact and also establishes the temporal correlation of spontaneous chest pain with reflux episodes (Figure 18–4). A diagnosis of gastroesophageal reflux can lead to relief of chest pain, with effective treatment.

Patients with psychiatric disorders commonly have abnormal esophageal motility. These motility disturbances may be a manometric marker of psychological stress. Panic disorder is present in 30–50% of patients with chest pain of undetermined etiology who undergo psychiatric evaluation. This disorder must be excluded in all patients with disabling chest pain and a history of depression or social phobias. The diagnosis may be suggested by the history or by the score on the Hospital Anxiety and Depression Scale, a brief, well-validated, patient-administered questionnaire (Table 18–3), but should always be confirmed by *Diagnostic Statistical Manual, 4/e (DSM-IV)* criteria. Depression is found in approximately one-third of patients with chest pain of undetermined etiology; it may antedate or coexist with panic disorder. Chest pain is often a symptom of somatization disorder characterized by multiple somatic complaints dating back to childhood or adolescence that defy medical explanation. Chest pain occurs primarily in women in the fifth or sixth decade of life, and a history of panic attacks can often be obtained.

Chest pain may also result from myocardial ischemia, even when coronary arteries are found to be anatomically normal (**microvascular angina**). This diagnosis should be considered in patients with typical anginal symptoms and normal coronary arteries, especially when abnormalities are present on noninvasive tests of cardiac function such as exercise radionuclide angiography or exercise thallium scintigraphy. Although mitral valve prolapse is frequently

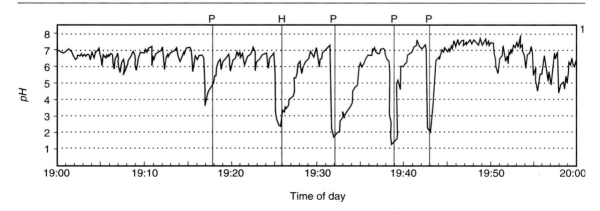

Figure 18–4. Ambulatory pH study in a patient with chest pain of undetermined etiology (time of day on horizontal axis; pH on vertical axis). One hour of the 24-hour record is displayed. The pH probe is placed in the distal esophagus, 5 cm above the lower esophageal sphincter. The normal esophageal pH fluctuates between 5 and 8. A fall in pH below 4 indicates an acid reflux event. In this recording, the chest pain (P) and heartburn (H) occurred during a documented acid reflux episode; this is evidence of reflux-induced chest pain.

Table 18–3. Hospital anxiety and depression scale[1]

Anxiety Questions
1. I feel tense or "wound up":
   (3) Most of the time
   (2) A lot of the time
   (1) From time to time, occasionally
   (0) Not at all
2. Worrying thoughts go through my mind:
   (3) A great deal of the time
   (2) A lot of the time
   (1) From time to time but not too often
   (0) Only occasionally
3. I get a sort of frightened feeling, like "butterflies" in the stomach:
   (0) Not at all
   (1) Occasionally
   (2) Quite often
   (3) Very often
4. I get sudden feelings of panic:
   (3) Very often indeed
   (2) Quite often
   (1) Not very often
   (0) Not at all

Depression Questions
5. I still enjoy the things I used to enjoy:
   (0) Definitely as much
   (1) Not quite as much
   (2) Only a little
   (3) Hardly at all
6. I feel cheerful:
   (3) Not at all
   (2) Not often
   (1) Sometimes
   (0) Most of the time
7. I have lost interest in my appearance:
   (3) Definitely
   (2) I don't take so much care as I should
   (1) I may not take quite as much care
   (0) I take just as much care as ever
8. I can enjoy a good book or TV program:
   (0) Often
   (1) Sometimes
   (2) Not often
   (3) Very seldom

[1]HADS© RP Snaith and AS Zigmond 1983, 1992, 1994. Record form items originally published in Acta Psychiatrica Scandinavica, Volume 67 (1983)© Munksgaard International Publishers Ltd., Copenhagen 1983. Extract reproduced by permission of the publishers NFER-NELSON Publishing Company Ltd, Darville House, 2 Oxford Road East, Windsor, Berkshire, SL4 IDF, UK. All rights reserved.

present in patients with chest pain of undetermined etiology, most investigators agree that it does not cause chest pain or panic disorder.

An array of musculoskeletal disorders may also cause chest pain, including "chest wall" (localized myofascial) pain, ankylosing spondylitis, fibromyalgia, Tietze's syndrome, rheumatoid arthritis, thoracic outlet syndrome, ankylosing spondylitis, fibromyalgia, and "slipping rib" syndrome (via impingement of an intercostal nerve).

The evidence is weak that esophageal motility disorders, with the notable exception of achalasia, cause chest pain for the following reasons:

1. Studies claiming a causal association are not well designed.
2. There is no "dose-response" between the severity of chest pain and the severity of the motility disorder.
3. Abnormal esophageal motility frequently follows rather than precedes chest pain episodes.
4. Treatment of the esophageal motility disorder does not reliably relieve chest pain.

Clinical Findings

A. Symptoms and Signs: The history and physical examination should focus on the patient's description of the chest pain, any associated esophageal symptoms or behavioral disorders, and reproduction of the pain with chest wall palpation.

1. Gastroesophageal reflux–Most patients with gastroesophageal reflux and chest pain complain of typical reflux symptoms (eg, heartburn, regurgitation, water brash, or dysphagia). The chest pain may worsen after meals or when the patient is supine, and may improve with use of antacids. The absence of typical reflux symptoms, however, does not rule out gastroesophageal reflux, because 10–20% of patients who reflux will have chest pain alone.

2. Panic disorder–The diagnosis of panic disorder can be made in patients who have recurrent unexpected panic attacks (Table 18–4) that have been followed by at least 1 month of (1) persistent concern about having further attacks, (2) worry about the implications of the attacks, or (3) change in behavior as a result of the attacks. The panic attacks must not be a result of drugs, other medical conditions, or other psychiatric diagnoses.

3. Musculoskeletal disorders–The diagnosis of a musculoskeletal cause of chest pain rests on the history and physical examination. Patients with tho-

Table 18–4. *DSM-IV* criteria for panic attack.[1]

A discrete period of intense fear or discomfort, in which four (or more) of the following symptoms developed abruptly and reached a peak within 10 minutes:
1. Palpitations, pounding heart, or accelerated heart rate
2. Sweating
3. Trembling or shaking
4. Sensations of shortness of breath or smothering
5. Feeling of choking
6. Chest pain or discomfort
7. Nausea or abdominal distress
8. Feeling dizzy, unsteady, light-headed, or faint
9. Derealization (feelings of unreality) or depersonalization (being detached from oneself)
10. Fear of losing control or going crazy
11. Fear of dying
12. Paresthesias (numbness or tingling sensations)
13. Chills or hot flushes

[1]Reproduced, with permission, from American Psychiatric Association: *Diagnostic and Statistical Manual of Mental Disorders,* 4/e. American Psychiatric Press, 1994.

racic outlet syndrome may complain of chest pain and arm paresthesias due to compression of the brachial plexus and subclavian vessels. The diagnosis of fibromyalgia is based on at least a 3-month history of widespread pain, with more than 10 of 18 sites of tenderness on digital palpation.

B. Diagnostic Studies:

1. Ambulatory pH monitoring–The diagnosis of gastroesophageal reflux should be objectively confirmed in patients who do not respond to empiric treatment, are candidates for long-term treatment, or lack typical reflux symptoms. The "gold standard" for diagnosis is ambulatory pH monitoring, which allows detection of increased esophageal acid contact as well as temporal correlation of chest pain episodes with reflux events. The ratio of chest pain episodes during reflux to total chest pain episodes is referred to as the symptom index. Although gastroesophageal reflux can be diagnosed with barium esophagography, endoscopy, or radionuclide scanning, the sensitivity of these tests is much lower than that of ambulatory pH monitoring.

2. Manometry–The diagnosis of an esophageal motility disorder in patients with central chest pain should be considered in those with complaints of dysphagia to solids and liquids. The diagnosis is confirmed by esophageal manometry.

3. Provocative testing–The diagnosis of heightened visceral nocioception is suggested by the reproduction of chest pain with any positive provocative test. Provocative tests include the acid perfusion test ("Bernstein" test), in which 0.1% hydrochloric acid is perfused by catheter into the distal esophagus; intraesophageal balloon inflation; intravenous edrophonium administration ("Tensilon test"); intravenous sodium lactate infusion; voluntary hyperventilation; rapid atrial pacing; adenosine or ergonovine administration; and chest wall palpation.

4. Noninvasive cardiac testing–The diagnosis of microvascular angina may be confirmed in clinical practice by observing (1) a functional abnormality during noninvasive cardiac testing in patients with normal coronary angiography, (2) a fall in left ventricular ejection fraction or the development of a regional wall motion abnormality with exercise during radionuclide ventriculography, and (3) abnormal uptake or clearance of thallium on exercise scintigraphy. Sophisticated measurement of microvascular coronary resistance during provocative maneuvers such as rapid atrial pacing and ergonovine infusion is the province of specialized cardiac catheterization laboratories.

Differential Diagnosis

It is essential to exclude life-threatening conditions, usually significant coronary artery disease, in any patient who presents with chest pain. This should be accomplished using testing appropriate to the individual patient's probability of significant coronary artery disease. Once this has been done, the differential diagnosis can be expanded to include disorders of the esophagus and upper gastrointestinal tract, psychiatric disorders, cardiovascular disorders other than epicardial coronary artery disease, and musculoskeletal disorders. Clinicians should look for symptoms of achalasia, gastroesophageal reflux, peptic ulcer, biliary colic, anxiety, or depression. Patients with dysphagia should undergo endoscopy, barium swallow, or manometry when appropriate (see preceding section under "Clinical Findings"). A diagnosis of gastroesophageal reflux can be made in those patients with typical reflux symptoms who respond to empiric therapy for gastroesophageal reflux. Patients with affective symptoms should be treated or referred to a psychiatrist or psychologist.

Complications

There are no complications of chest pain of undetermined etiology in the traditional sense. What may be viewed as complications, however, are the poor quality of life and overutilization of health care resources that may result when patients do not receive effective therapy.

Treatment

A. Chest Pain Induced by Gastroesophageal Reflux: Patients with gastroesophageal reflux should be treated in the typical stepwise fashion. This begins with life-style modifications (eg, elevate the head of the bed, avoid fatty foods) and use of an H_2-receptor antagonist (eg, cimetidine, 800 mg twice daily; ranitidine or nizatidine, 150 mg twice daily; or famotidine, 20 mg twice daily). Patients with refractory chest pain and a confirmed diagnosis of gastroesophageal reflux may be treated with omeprazole, 20 mg/d; if there is no response, the dose may be increased to 40 or 60 mg/d. An attempt to discontinue treatment should be made after 8 weeks. Antireflux surgery may be considered for patients with severe chest pain and documented gastroesophageal reflux in whom a proton pump inhibitor has clearly improved chest pain.

B. Esophageal Motility Disorders: Patients with chest pain of undetermined etiology and esophageal motility disorders often have an additional, more treatable condition, such as gastroesophageal reflux or panic disorder. These two disorders should be excluded before treatment directed specifically at the motility disorder is begun. In most cases, the esophageal motility disorder is a manometric epiphenomenon rather than a cause per se of the chest pain. Although it seems logical to presume that drugs relaxing smooth muscle might improve chest pain, only two of five randomized controlled trials concluded that calcium channel blockers were effective. Despite these results, it may be reasonable to try nifedipine, 10–20 mg orally four times daily (30 minutes before meals and at bedtime), in patients in whom an esophageal motility disorder is felt to play a predominant role in causing chest pain. Patients who respond can be switched to long-acting preparations. The antidepressant trazodone (100–150 mg/d), which has no direct effect on esophageal motility, has been effective in decreasing the distress of esophageal symptoms in patients with esophageal motility disorders. This once again suggests that underlying psychiatric problems may play a significant role in patients with esophageal motility abnormalities. Use of trazodone in men is limited by the side effect of priapism. Surgical myotomy has no role in the management of patients with chest pain and esophageal motility disorders other than achalasia.

C. Panic Disorder: The first step in the treatment of panic disorder is patient education. Patients should understand that they suffer from a common disorder which affects approximately 5% of the USA population. Although the cause of panic disorder is unknown, effective treatment exists in the form of antidepressants, anxiolytics, or behavioral cognitive therapy. Antidepressants are the treatment of choice for panic disorder without severe anxiety. Imipramine should be started at a low dose (eg, 10 mg before bedtime) to minimize troubling side effects. The dose should be increased slowly by 10 mg every 2–4 days until the dose is 50 mg. Thereafter, the dose may be increased by 25 mg every 2–4 days to a target dose of 150–200 mg before bedtime (2.5 mg/kg/d). Between six and 24 weeks of therapy may be needed for a response, and treatment should be continued for at least 6 months or as long as there is continued improvement. Unfortunately, up to 25% of patients discontinue therapy because of side effects. The dosage of imipramine should be gradually tapered by 25 mg every 3 days. Despite gradual tapering of the drug, 15–30% of patients will relapse within 2 years.

Patients with a severe anxiety component may benefit from the more rapid effects of an anxiolytic. Alprazolam, begun at 0.25–0.5 mg four times a day, will bring relief of anxiety within 1–2 weeks. The major drawback of the benzodiazepines is the risk for abuse of, or dependence on, the drugs and unpleasant withdrawal symptoms when they are discontinued. Patients with a personal or family history of drug or alcohol abuse should not be given benzodiazepines.

Preliminary reports regarding use of serotonin reuptake inhibitors in panic disorder have been promising. Beta blockers are useful for controlling associated autonomic symptoms. Lastly, behavioral therapy geared toward control of stress and improvement of coping skills brings about a level of improvement comparable to pharmacotherapy. The treatment of depression and somatoform disorder is beyond the scope of this chapter.

D. Heightened Visceral Nocioception: A recent study by Cannon and colleagues suggests that imipramine is effective in patients with chest pain of undetermined etiology, regardless of the underlying diagnosis. Sixty consecutive patients who were referred to the National Institutes of Health for evaluation of chest pain were studied. The following disorders were diagnosed: esophageal motility disorders (41%), panic disorder (43%), and microvascular angina (22%). Eighty-seven percent of patients developed characteristic chest pain during catheterization with right ventricular stimulation or intracoronary adenosine infusion (markers of heightened visceral nocioception). Patients were initially treated with a placebo for 5 weeks and then randomly given imipramine, 50 mg at bedtime; clonidine, 0.1 mg twice daily; or a placebo. Patients treated with imipramine had a 52% reduction in chest pain (p = 0.03) regardless of the underlying diagnosis; this suggests that imipramine was acting as a visceral analgesic. The search continues for other medications, such as the serotonin antagonists, which may act as visceral analgesics.

E. Microvascular Angina: Patients with microvascular angina may respond to treatment with a calcium channel blocker (eg, verapamil, 80 mg four times daily, or nifedipine, 10 mg four times daily).

F. Musculoskeletal Disorders: Patients with musculoskeletal chest pain should be treated with reassurance, local heat application, nonsteroidal antiinflammatory drugs (NSAIDs), and corticosteroid-lidocaine injection when appropriate. Patients with fibromyalgia may benefit from cyclobenzaprine, 2.5–10 mg four times daily, or amitriptyline, 10–50 mg at bedtime. Exercise is beneficial.

Prognosis

Although patients with chest pain of undetermined etiology have an excellent survival rate (cardiac survival exceeds 98% at 10 years), the quality of life and functional status are markedly impaired. Most patients continue to experience chest pain, and up to one-half cannot perform strenuous activities. One retrospective study has suggested that the diagnosis of an esophageal motility disorder may alleviate patient anxiety, leading to improvement in the functional status of patients with chest pain of undetermined etiology. Contradictory results were obtained from a more recent prospective study, in which chest pain improved only in patients *without* an esophageal motility disorder or positive provocative test.

The outlook for patients with chest pain of undetermined etiology may be improved by (1) identification of subsets of patients with treatable causes of chest pain (eg, gastroesophageal reflux, panic disorder, or achalasia), and (2) treatment of the remaining patients with "visceral analgesics" such as imipramine.

An approach based on this strategy is shown in Figure 18–5.

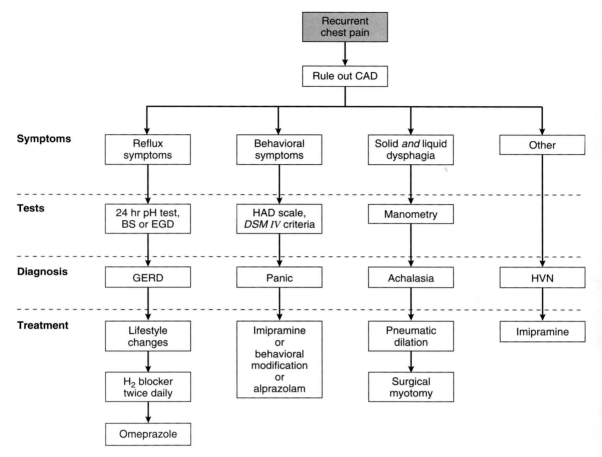

Figure 18–5. Algorithm for chest pain of undetermined etiology. Patients with gastroesophageal reflux disease, panic disorder, and achalasia can be effectively treated as outlined. The remaining patients may respond to a nonspecific visceral analgesic (imipramine). CAD= Coronary artery disease; BS= barium swallow; EGD= esophagogastroduodenoscopy; GERD= gastroesophageal reflux disease; HAD= Hospital anxiety and depression; HVN= Heightened visceral nocioception.

REFERENCES

Cannon RO III et al: Imipramine in patients with chest pain despite normal coronary angiograms. N Engl J Med 1994;330:1411.

Cook IJ et al: Pharyngeal (Zenker's) diverticulum is a disorder of upper esophageal sphincter opening. Gastroenterology 1992;103:1229.

Csendes A et al: Late results of a prospective randomized study comparing forceful dilatation and oesophagomyotomy in patients with achalasia. Gut 1989;30:299.

Eckardt VF, Aignherr C, Bernhard G: Predictors of outcome in patients with achalasia treated by pneumatic dilation. Gastroenterology 1992;103:1732.

Reynolds JC, Parkman HP: Achalasia. Gastroenterol Clin North Am 1989;18:223.

ESOPHAGEAL CANCER

Esophageal cancer is a debilitating disease with an insidious onset and a poor prognosis. Environmental factors and preexisting esophageal disease are important risk factors for esophageal cancer (Table 19–1). The vast majority (90%) of esophageal cancers worldwide are squamous cell carcinomas; the remainder (10%) are adenocarcinoma. In the United States (USA), more recent reports indicate an increasing proportion of adenocarcinoma attributed to Barrett's esophagus. Other malignant tumors of the esophagus are extremely rare.

The incidence of esophageal cancer varies significantly by geographic region, race, and gender. In the USA, esophageal cancer, with over 11,000 new cases per year, is the 24th most common cancer and ranks as the 13th most common cause of cancer- related death. Black men have the highest incidence of squamous cell cancer (16.8/100,000), followed by black women (4.6/100,000), white men (3.0/100,000) and white women (1.2/100,000). The incidence of adenocarcinoma is highest among white men (those with the highest incidence of Barrett's esophagus). The highest incidence of esophageal cancer is in northern China, with 150 cases of squamous cell carcinoma per 100,000.

Pathophysiology

Cigarette smoking and heavy alcohol use are the most important predisposing factors for esophageal cancer in developed countries. In certain regions of the world, exceedingly high rates of esophageal cancer have been attributed to other environmental factors, including the ingestion of hot foods and liquid as well as deficiencies of essential nutrients (eg, vitamin C and E) due to infrequent consumption of fruits and vegetables.

Human papillomavirus has been implicated as a potential cause of esophageal cancer in the Lixian region of China. Long-standing abnormalities or inflammatory lesions of the esophagus also may contribute to the development of esophageal cancer, including achalasia, tylosis, Plummer Vinson syndrome, lye ingestion, and Barrett's esophagus.

Similar to the dysplasia to carcinoma sequence found in colonic neoplasia, esophageal cancers are thought to arise from premalignant lesions, ie, high-grade dysplasia. The most convincing evidence exists in patients with Barrett's esophagus. Adenocarcinoma of the esophagus is nearly always found within Barrett's metaplastic epithelium, specifically the specialized intestinal mucosa form of Barrett's. Barrett's epithelium itself is thought to develop primarily in patients with long-standing reflux esophagitis. The lifetime risk for developing adenocarcinoma in Barrett's epithelium has been estimated to be approximately 5%.

Essentials of Diagnosis
- Progressive dysphagia.
- Barium swallow or endoscopy depict irregular mass in the esophagus.
- Endoscopic biopsy.

General Considerations

Despite the widespread use of endoscopy, significant advances in surgical techniques, and improvements in postoperative care, chemotherapy, and radiation therapy, the overall prognosis for patients with esophageal cancer is poor and remains essentially unchanged for the past 30 years.

In northern China, an area with a high incidence of esophageal cancer, endoscopic screening programs of the general population have been effective at detecting early and curable cancers.

In western countries, population screening is not considered cost-effective, due to the low incidence of disease and the high cost of screening. Patients with Barrett's esophagus, however, have an increased risk of adenocarcinoma that warrants periodic screening. The relative costs and benefits of this strategy remain in question.

Clinical Findings

A. Symptoms and Signs: Progressive dysphagia is the most common presenting complaint, as shown in Table 19–2. The narrowed esophageal lumen leads initially to solid food dysphagia and later with disease progression and further lumen obstruc-

Table 19–1. Predisposing conditions for esophageal cancer.

Squamous cell
Heavy tobacco use
Heavy alcohol use
Previous head and neck squamous cell cancer
Nonreflux esophagitis (most common in Asia & Africa)
Tylosis (palmar and plantar hyperkeratosis)
Achalasia
Adenocarcinoma
Barrett's metaplastic epithelium
Smoking and alcohol in patients with existing Barrett's
syndrome

tion, to liquid dysphagia. Dysphagia usually occurs only with significant luminal obstruction (over 50%). Difficulty in swallowing results in decreased nutritional intake and weight loss.

Approximately 15% of esophageal cancers arise in the upper one-third of the esophagus, 50% in the middle third, and 35% in the lower third and gastroesophageal junction. The presenting symptoms may correlate with the location of the esophageal tumor. Pain may be related to difficulty swallowing or to mediastinal extension of tumor. Food above the obstructing lesion or tumor invasion into the airway may cause regurgitation, coughing, and aspiration. Hoarseness or voice changes may be due to recurrent laryngeal nerve infiltration, recurrent regurgitation, or both. Patients with a long-standing history of reflux symptoms who report a recent onset of progressive dysphagia (at times with abatement of their reflux symptoms) are more likely to have adenocarcinoma in the setting of Barrett's esophagus.

Overt gastrointestinal bleeding manifested by hematemesis or melena is uncommon. Anemia, however, is common at presentation, and chronic, subclinical bleeding is invariably a contributing factor. Massive hemorrhage rarely can occur and may require emergent surgical treatment if endoscopic therapy fails.

Chest x-ray may demonstrate an esophageal air fluid level above the site of obstruction or a pulmonary infiltrate from aspiration. A pleural effusion or mediastinal mass suggests mediastinal tumor extension. Electrocardiogram changes are unusual except in cases of advanced pericardial invasion and impairment of the normal conduction pathways.

B. Laboratory Findings: There are no specific laboratory findings in patients with esophageal cancer. The insidious development of the disease may be

Table 19–2. Signs and symptoms of esophageal cancer.

Dysphagia—initially to solids
Weight loss
Regurgitation
Aspiration, cough
Hoarseness, voice change
Hemorrhage

marked by anemia and low serum albumin. Anemia can be due to bleeding or nutritional deficiency or can be secondary to chronic disease. Serum protein levels (albumin, prealbumin, and transferrin) may be low, reflecting the extent of malnutrition. Abnormal liver function tests may indicate liver metastases. Other evidence of chronic tobacco or alcohol use may be found.

Endoscopic biopsy is the best method for confirming the histopathologic diagnosis. DNA analysis by flow cytometry of esophageal biopsy specimens appears to be a promising method for detecting malignant cells within Barrett's epithelium. Flow cytometry is currently used only in research settings.

C. Diagnostic Studies: The initial diagnostic imaging study for most patients with dysphagia should be a barium esophagram (Figure 19–1). The presence of esophageal narrowing and the location of

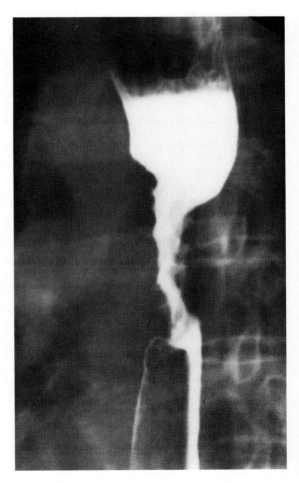

Figure 19–1. Barium swallow, showing mid-esophageal stricture. The abrupt change in caliber, irregular mucosa, and near circumferential narrowing are highly suggestive of an esophageal cancer.

the lesion are readily determined by esophagram. Typical features of malignant obstruction include: irregular mass lesions, irregular mucosal relief, and abrupt angulation of the esophageal contour (so called **tumor shelf**). Benign lesions of the esophagus are associated with smooth outline of the mucosa, symmetric narrowing without angulation, or extrinsic compression.

All patients with abnormal esophagrams should undergo upper endoscopy with biopsy to offer a histologic diagnosis, to assess the patency of the esophageal lumen, and to confirm the extent of the tumor. Endoscopy also offers important information about the feasibility of subsequent therapeutic interventions, including dilation of the narrowed lumen, placement of stents/prostheses, and laser ablation of intraluminal tumor.

Staging Techniques

Once the diagnosis is made, defining the stage of the esophageal cancer is essential to patient management. Esophageal cancer staging by contrast studies and endoscopy alone is often inaccurate. The extent of local invasion and presence of regional lymph nodes and distant metastases cannot be determined, and indirect measures such as tumor length are inaccurate at predicting tumor stage. Therefore, a large number of patients with esophageal cancer have undergone exploratory surgery for staging and possible resection, only to be deemed incurable or inoperable at the time of operation. Historical data indicate that esophageal cancer is not operable in over one-half of patients because of metastasis, extensive local invasion (preventing tumor-free margins), or both.

The advances in imaging techniques have led to more accurate preoperative staging. In 1987, the TNM (*tumor*, *nodes*, *metastasis*) classification was revised to reflect the improved preoperative staging available with computed tomography (CT), magnetic resonance imaging (MRI), and endoscopic ultrasound (EUS) imaging. The older classification system in which tumors were staged based on size, circumferential involvement, and extent of obstruction noted on barium studies or endoscopy was abandoned. The revised classification scheme clearly defines the cancer stage based on the local invasion of the tumor, nodal involvement, and presence of metastases (Table 19–3). The TNM classification is the basis for arranging esophageal cancers in five prognostic stage groups (Table 19–4).

CT imaging is the cornerstone of cancer staging and has provided an important advance for nonoperative staging of esophageal cancer. The standard esophageal cancer CT imaging protocol involves use of oral, rectal, and intravenous contrast, and examination from the neck or upper chest to the upper abdomen, including the entire liver. The advent of EUS offers the most significant advance in preoperative esophageal cancer staging.

Table 19–3. TNM classification system for esophageal cancer.

Tumor infiltration (T)–Depth of primary tumor infiltration
T0   No evidence of primary tumor
Tis Carcinoma *in situ,* intraepithelial tumor
T1   Tumor invades only the mucosa or submucosa
T2   Tumor invades the muscularis propria
T3   Tumor invades the adventitia
T4   Tumor invades adjacent organs
Regional lymph node involvement (N)–Malignant spread to local/regional lymph nodes
N0   Absence of local/regional lymph nodes
N1   Presence of one or more malignant lymph nodes
Nx   Inability to assess nodal involvement
Distant metastasis (M)
M0   Absence of distant metastases (celiac axis nodes are considered metastatic spread for proximal and middle esophageal cancers)
M1   Presence of distant metastases
Mx   Inability to assess metastases (due to esophageal obstruction, for example) and inability to even evaluate from the stomach.

The overall accuracy of CT for staging esophageal cancer is very good for advanced disease. Liver metastasis and findings consistent with adjacent organ invasion can be reliably noted on CT. The sensitivity and specificity for detecting tracheal, bronchial, and pericardial invasion exceed 90–95% in most series. However, CT imaging does not reliably detect local and regional lymph node metastases and "early" (T1–T3) depth of tumor invasion. Hence, other imaging tests should be considered before attempted curative resection.

EUS, the most recent advance in esophageal imaging, is performed with a modified upper endoscope with an ultrasound transducer housed within the endoscope tip. EUS images depict five layers of the esophageal wall, which correspond to distinct histologic layers (Figure 19–2). Malignant tumors are identified as hypoechoic processes with irregular margins that disrupt the normal architecture. The depth of tumor is defined by the outermost margin of the hypoechoic mass (Figure 19–3). Lymph nodes are identified as rounded structures near the esophagus and classified as malignant by their size, shape, and echopattern. Fine needle aspiration biopsies of lymph nodes can also be obtained through some EUS scopes.

Table 19–4. Staging of esophageal cancer based on TNM criteria.

Stage	Depth of tumor infiltration	Nodal involvement	Metastatic disease
Stage 0	Tis	N0	M0
Stage I	T1	N0	M0
Stage IIA	T2/T3	N0	M0
Stage IIB	T1/T2	N1	M0
Stage III	T3	N1	M0
	T4	Any N	M0
Stage IV	Any T	Any N	M1

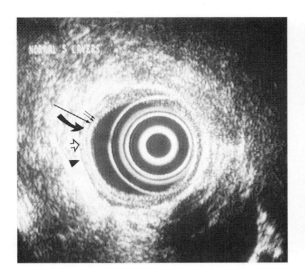

Figure 19–2. Endoscopic ultrasound image of normal five-layered esophagus. ***Two small arrows:*** The inner most layer corresponds to an interface echo and the mucosa. ***Single long arrow:*** The second layer corresponds to the mucosa (including the muscularis mucosa). ***Curved solid arrow:*** The third layer corresponds to the submucosa. ***Open arrow:*** The fourth layer corresponds to the muscularis propria. ***Solid arrowhead:*** The fifth outer-most layer corresponds to an interface echo and the adventitia (serosa equivalent). The five-layered appearance is essentially the same throughout the intestinal tract. The fifth echogenic layer in the esophagus represents the interface echo with the adventitia, since the esophagus lacks a serosa.

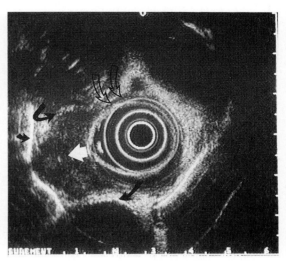

Figure 19–3. T3 esophageal tumor. EUS image of an esophageal cancer in close proximity to mediastinal structures. ***Curved open black arrow:*** Muscularis propria, fourth hypoechoic layer. ***Solid white arrow:*** The tumor extending from mucosa through the muscularis propria (T3). ***Angled arrow:*** Distinct fat plane between tumor and right bronchus, indicating absence of bronchial invasion.***Short curved arrow:*** Hyperechoic (bright white) plane between tumor and right pleura. The tumor mass extends to the pleura but does not definitively invade. ***Curved arrow (bottom of image):*** Intact fat plane between tumor and thoracic aorta.

The overall accuracy of EUS for predicting the extent of esophageal cancers approaches 90% for T and 80% for N classification. EUS can accurately predict early cancers, ie, those classified as T1–T3. The specific EUS criteria for predicting adjacent organ invasion (T4) have not been clearly defined.

EUS is more accurate than CT for both T and N classification when the two modalities are used in the same patient (Table 19–5). The superiority of EUS rests in reliably distinguishing between T2, T3, and T4 lesions and in more accurately detecting local lymph nodes. CT is the best imaging test to detect metastases, although EUS appears superior for defining abdominal lymph node metastases, especially celiac axis nodes (classified as metastases, M1).

Several important limitations of EUS imaging must be noted. The limited depth of penetration offers only incomplete assessment for metastases. Secondly, over 20% of esophageal cancers are obstructing and cannot be traversed with the ultrasound endoscope at the time of presentation. Finally, there are as yet no universally accepted criteria except for biopsy for differentiating benign from malignant lymph nodes or tumor adherence from tumor inva-

sion of adjacent structures. Additional multicenter studies are needed to establish and validate acceptable criteria.

Bronchoscopy is widely used for assessment of bronchial invasion, primarily in mid-esophageal tumors. Although bronchial invasion is common, invasion into the bronchial lumen is rare. Therefore, bronchoscopy generally provides only indirect evidence of bronchial invasion, such as luminal indentation or narrowing.

Table 19–5. Accuracy of endoscopic ultrasound versus computed tomography in esophageal cancer tumor and node classification.[1]

Endoscopic ultrasound Percent of patients accurately classified		Computed tomography Percent of patients accurately classified	
Tumor	Node	Tumor	Node
85%	73%	57%	54%

[1]Data from 227 patients who underwent endoscopic ultrasound and computed tomography before surgical therapy for esophageal cancer (compiled from five studies summarized in review by Koch J, Halvorsen RAJ: Esophageal cancer staging: CT, MR, and EUS. *Semin Roentgenol* 1994;29:364.)

MRI is reportedly more accurate than CT for detecting liver metastases. The usefulness of an MRI is limited, however, by the long imaging time required for a complete mediastinal and liver scan, the lack of a reliable oral contrast agent, and the high cost. Further technologic advances, faster scanners, and spiral CT may improve the accuracy of CT for less advanced tumors.

Differential Diagnosis

The differential diagnosis of patients with dysphagia or odynophagia includes esophageal mucosal diseases, motility disorders, and benign and malignant obstructing lesions. The insidious onset of progressive dysphagia to solids and then to liquids with associated weight loss in patients over 40–50 years of age almost invariably is caused by esophageal cancer.

Patients with benign obstructing lesions of the esophagus may present with features resembling esophageal cancer. Benign peptic strictures, webs and rings, and achalasia are associated with esophageal narrowing and dysphagia. Barium esophagrams offer indirect evidence for benign versus malignant processes, although endoscopy and biopsy invariably are employed to distinguish benign from malignant disease.

Achalasia is a disorder of impaired relaxation of the lower esophageal sphincter and aperistalsis of the esophageal body. The classic appearance on the barium esophagram is a smooth, tapered distal esophagus referred to as having a **bird's beak** appearance. Tumors at the gastroesophageal junction may mimic the signs, symptoms, and manometric findings of achalasia. Hence, endoscopy is required in all patients with suspected achalasia to exclude undiagnosed malignancy.

Malignant tumors of the esophagus (Table 19–6) other than squamous cell and adenocarcinoma are exceedingly rare. These tumors usually cannot be distinguished on clinical grounds and require histologic confirmation. There are case reports of mucoepidermoid carcinomas and cystic adenoid carcinomas. These tumors are extremely aggressive and can elude endoscopic biopsy due to their primarily submucosal growth pattern.

Complications

Most complications from esophageal cancer are attributable to the luminal obstruction and to local tumor extension into the mediastinum. Patients adjust

Table 19–6. Malignant tumors of the esophagus.

Squamous cell cancer
Adenocarcinoma
Sarcoma (eg, leiomyosarcoma, fibrosarcoma)
Mucoepidermoid carcinoma
Adenoid cystic carcinoma

their diets gradually, often subconsciously, to ingest soft or liquid foods to avoid solid food dysphagia. The progressive inability to swallow solids leads to weight loss and nutritional deficiencies. Solid food impaction can result, necessitating emergency endoscopic disimpaction.

Esophageal obstruction may lead to regurgitation of food or oral secretions. Patients may report coughing spells or aspiration, especially on reclining after meals. Pulmonary complications resulting from aspiration include pneumonia and pulmonary abscess. Halitosis may be present due to food stasis and regurgitation.

Blood loss may arise from ulcerated tumors, and chronic, subclinical blood loss is common. Massive bleeding is unusual; when it occurs, however, it can be difficult to control due to the large ulcerated surface area of many tumors. Endoscopy is essential in the evaluation and potential treatment of bleeding esophageal tumors.

Esophageal cancers readily extend through the thin esophageal wall (which lacks a serosa) to invade adjacent organs. The vital mediastinal structures adjacent to the esophagus include the trachea, the right and left bronchi, the aortic arch and descending aorta, the pericardium, the pleura, and the spine. Tumor infiltration into these structures accounts for the most serious, life-threatening complications of esophageal cancer.

Tumor mass may cause compression and obstruction of the bronchial tree, leading to a post-obstructive pneumonia. Invasion into a bronchus can cause a broncho-esophageal fistula. Fistulae are severely disabling and associated with significant mortality owing to the high risk of aspiration, pneumonia, and pulmonary abscess formation. Surgical excision and radiation therapy for esophageal cancers that adhere to or invade the bronchial tree may also be complicated by fistulae. Newer esophageal prostheses may provide important palliative therapy by "sealing off" the fistula.

The aortic arch and descending aorta lie adjacent to the esophagus. Nonetheless, extension into the aortic arch is less frequent than bronchial invasion, for unclear reasons. Erosion through the aortic wall results in hemorrhage. Tumor in-growth of the pericardium has been reported as an infrequent cause of arrhythmias and conduction abnormalities. Infiltration of the recurrent laryngeal nerve can lead to hoarseness. Pleural effusions are usually small, but can predict pleural invasion (T4 disease).

Treatment

Most patients with esophageal cancer present with advanced disease and cannot be cured. The esophageal wall is thin, lacks a serosa, and has extensive lymphatic drainage—factors that facilitate early regional and distant metastases. Over 50% of patients with esophageal cancer are not operative candidates at presentation due either to advanced disease or to significant comorbid disease that would result in prohibitive perioperative mortality. These factors demand that treatment of esophageal cancer be based on a systematic evaluation similar to that outlined in Figure 19–4.

A. Determine Suitability for Operation: The initial step, after diagnosis, is to determine whether a patient is a candidate for major surgery. Extensive medical problems, most commonly severe coronary artery or pulmonary disease, are contraindications to surgery. Cancer staging is generally not required for these nonsurgical candidates.

B. Staging: Patients who are deemed surgical candidates based on their medical condition should undergo thorough staging to determine if they have curable disease, incurable but resectable disease, or unresectable disease, ie, locally advanced or metastatic cancers. Endoscopy, CT, and EUS are complementary tests when used in a coordinated fashion and are highly accurate in predicting the clinical stage of the disease.

Staging will detect the small subset of patients who have potentially curable disease, ie, cancer that has limited local spread (T1–T2) without nodal metastases. Imaging studies define resectable tumors by the absence of extension into mediastinal structures and the absence of nodal or organ metastases. Direct invasion of the aorta, bronchi, pleura, or laryngeal nerve (defined by vocal cord paralysis) or distant organ (liver) metastases are evidence of nonresectable disease. Preoperative radiation with or without chemotherapy can downstage an esophageal cancer to a resectable or potentially curable stage.

C. Surgical Treatment: Surgical therapy has long been the preferred approach and mainstay of therapy, both for cure and palliation in patients with resectable tumors who are able to withstand an operation. Unpredictable preoperative staging had lead to widespread use of intraoperative staging in the past. Today, accurate preoperative imaging techniques have diminished the need for surgical staging. The optimal interventions can now be tailored to the individual patient before potential surgery.

Patients should receive ongoing supportive care to improve the nutritional and functional status and prevent aspiration and other complications (Table 19–7).

1. Curative resection–Esophagectomy with an open thoracotomy and nodal dissection remains the only definitive means of attaining a potential cure, especially of upper and mid-esophagus tumors. This procedure carries significant morbidity and mortality rates, especially in patients with preexisting pulmonary disease. Consequently, it should be restricted to the small subset of patients who appear to have curable tumors on preoperative staging and who are excellent surgical candidates.

2. Palliative resection–Transhiatal esophagectomy is currently the favored surgical approach for palliation of esophageal cancers independent of location. Transhiatal esophagectomy may be a curative procedure in patients with distal esophageal cancer when adequate inspection of the para-esophageal cancer tissue is provided by the abdominal incision. Transhiatal esophagectomy consists of abdominal and cervical incision and a cervical gastroesophageal anastomosis. This procedure does not allow visual inspection of the mediastinal bed, which theoretically is necessary to insure removal of the locally invasive tumor. Esophagectomy without a thoracotomy is the preferred procedure in patients with resectable disease if palliation is the primary goal of surgery.

Locally advanced tumors, ie, tumors classified as T1N1, T2N1, T3N0, and T3N1, are resectable but incurable. These cancers are associated with a high recurrence rate and patients usually die of their disease. The optimal intervention in these patients remains controversial. Several studies are currently underway to examine the effectiveness of surgical resection with or without adjuvant chemotherapy and radiation therapy.

The morbidity and 30-day mortality associated with surgical therapy for esophageal cancer are significant. Transhiatal esophagectomy has lower morbidity and mortality rates compared to thoracotomy. Nonetheless, the reported surgery-related mortality rate exceeds 10% in most centers, with a significant perioperative morbidity rate between 10 and 25%.

Outside of clinical trials, the practice in patients with locally advanced disease varies widely depending on the local surgical expertise and the assessment of the patient's preexisting medical condition. Although surgery offers no survival benefit for the vast majority of patients with esophageal cancer (ie, those with T3 or T4 or N1 disease), thoracic surgeons contend that surgery provides the best means of palliation (restoring swallowing). Therefore, the practice at many university hospitals is to offer palliative transhiatal esophagectomy to all patients without metastases who can undergo an operation.

D. Other Palliative Modalities: Radiation therapy, chemotherapy, and endoscopic therapy are the palliative procedures employed as adjuvants to surgery or for patients who are not candidates for or chose not to have surgery (Table 19–8). The location and extent of the tumor as well as the patient's ability and willingness to undergo repetitive procedures determine the mode of palliation.

1. Radiation therapy–Radiation therapy provides reasonable palliation and 5-year survival curves are similar to surgery for patients with comparable cancer stage. There is virtually no mortality associated with radiation therapy, although high-dose radiation may be associated with complications. Intraluminal irradiation using Cobalt-60 or iridium-192 have been used as adjuncts to radiation therapy.

2. Chemotherapy–Chemotherapy has been of

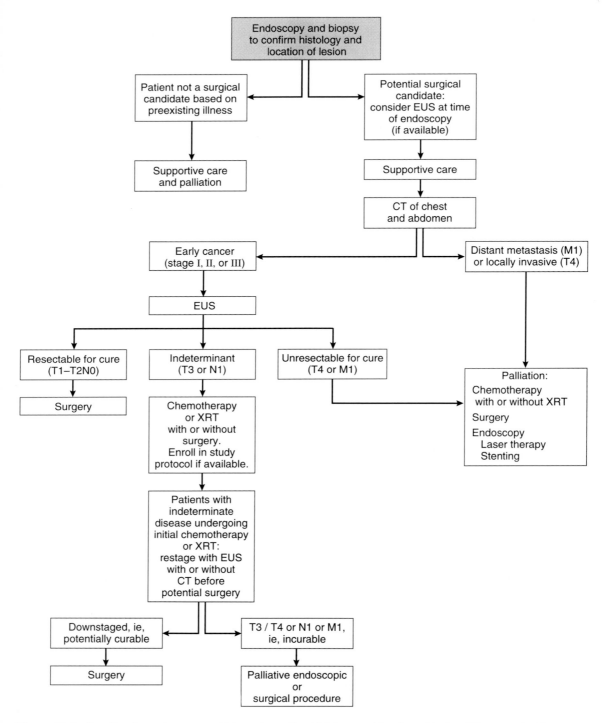

Figure 19–4. Algorithm for endoscopy and biopsy to confirm histology and location of lesion. CT= computed tomography; EUS= endoscopic ultrasound; XRT= radiation therapy.

Table 19–7. Supportive care for patients with esophageal cancer.

Nutritional support and hydration
  Enteral
    Tube feeding
    Percutaneous gastrostomy
Pulmonary toilet
  Prevent or limit aspiration
Stricture dilation
  (Temporary control for nutritional support, hydration, and
    pulmonary toilet)
Pain control
Psychological support

little benefit to patients with esophageal cancer. The most common agents for treating esophageal cancer include 5-fluorouracil, cisplatin, mitomycin, and vincristine. No clear benefit has been shown for adjunctive therapy with chemotherapy, although additional clinical trials are currently underway. Preliminary results from recent trials focusing on the use of chemotherapy with radiation indicate some potential advantage of combined therapy.

3. Endoscopic therapy–Endoscopic therapy includes dilation, tumor ablation, and placement of prostheses. Direct tumor obliteration is achieved with thermal devices, most commonly using the Neodymium-YAG laser. The tumors that are amenable to laser therapy are exophytic or polypoid, and involve a straight segment of the esophagus in the mid-esophagus or lower esophagus, preferably shorter than 5 cm.

Multiple endoscopic laser treatment sessions are generally required to reduce the size of the intraluminal tumor enough to improve swallowing. Periodic follow-up is performed to reduce any recurrent intraluminal tumor growth. Other thermal devices (eg, heater probe) and direct endoscopically-guided tumor injection of sclerosants have been proposed as lower cost and more available alternatives to laser tumor ablation. No definitive trials have compared these methods, and therapy generally is determined by the expertise available at individual centers.

A wide variety of prostheses have been developed to provide a mechanical means of maintaining esophageal patency. Esophageal stents or prostheses can be inserted surgically or endoscopically with fluoroscopic guidance. The traditional polyvinyl prosthesis affords very good palliation in many instances although it is cumbersome to place and can migrate. Recently developed expandable metal stents are currently undergoing clinical investigation. These stents are more easily placed endoscopically and may be used in cancers with significant luminal narrowing.

Photodynamic therapy is a newer, experimental treatment for local esophageal cancer obliteration. Patients are injected with a photosensitizing chemical that is preferentially retained in cancer tissue. Under endoscopic guidance, a diffusing fiber attached to a tunable argon-pump dye laser is placed adjacent to the tumor. Laser activation emits nonthermal light, which at the appropriate wave length causes selective necrosis of the sensitized tumor.

Prognosis

The overall prognosis for patients with esophageal cancer is dismal, reported in most large series to be less than 5–10% at 5 years. As previously noted, this reflects the rapid extension to extra-esophageal structures and relatively large tumor bulk at the time of diagnosis. Patients with earlier stage of disease live longer, with a 5-year survival greater than 40% for patients with T1 or T2 disease and no nodal involvement. On the other hand, patients classified as T3 or T4 are considered to have a 5-year survival of less than 15%. Therefore, preoperative staging is essential in guiding therapy, to prevent unnecessary surgery and to substantiate the prognosis.

Stage 0, I, and II tumors are considered resectable for cure. The 5-year survival for such patients who are sufficiently fit to undergo surgery ranges from greater than 85% for Stage 0, to 50% for Stage I to 40% for Stage II. On the other hand, Stage III tumors are rarely resectable for cure, and Stage IV cancers are considered noncurable and nonresectable by most

Table 19–8. Therapeutic interventions aimed at decreasing cancer mass for palliation or cure.

Palliative Therapies	Clinical Response	Significant intervention-related morbidity	Intervention-related mortality
Surgery	90%	5–10%	5–20%
Chemotherapy	20–60%	*	negligible
Radiation	60–80%	*	negligible
Chemotherapy plus radiation	60–80%	*	negligible
Endoscopic laser	70–85%	*	1%
Stent			
Endoscopic	>90%	10–30%	5–10%
Surgical			15–25%
Other			
Photodynamic			
Peroral dilation	>90% (temporary)		

*Variable. Depends on study and definition of morbidity.

clinicians. The presence or absence of nodal involvement also has a significant prognostic impact. The 5-year survival for N0 disease is over 70% while N1 disease is associated with a survival near 40%, independent of the T classification.

BENIGN ESOPHAGEAL TUMORS

Essentials of Diagnosis
- Incidental finding on esophageal imaging.
- Rarely symptomatic.
- Vague pressure sensation or dysphagia.

General Considerations

A variety of benign mass lesions can arise from different wall layers in the esophagus (Table 19–9). These tumors are usually asymptomatic and noted as incidental findings during radiography or endoscopy or on evaluation for dysphagia or vague chest discomfort. Leiomyomas are the most common benign esophageal tumor. These tumors arise in the muscularis propria, the layer of smooth muscle beyond the submucosa. Leiomyomas are covered by an intact submucosa and mucosa, thereby eluding endoscopic biopsy.

Inflammatory polyps and granulomas arise in the setting of esophagitis and may be confused with malignant lesions. Endoscopic removal is possible, although usually not indicated. Endoscopic biopsy and regression with therapy for esophagitis clearly distinguishes the clinical course of inflammatory polyps and granulomas from cancers.

Clinical Findings

A. Symptoms and Signs: The majority of benign esophageal tumors are clinically silent and go undetected. Occasionally, patients may describe vague fullness or a thoracic pressure sensation. No signs, symptoms, or laboratory tests are specific to these mass lesions. These lesions can be distinguished by further imaging and endoscopic evaluation.

B. Imaging: Endoscopic appearance and biopsy can clarify the cause of some benign esophageal tumors. EUS can suggest the cause in lesions that elude biopsy diagnosis. EUS provides high resolution images that define the individual esophageal wall layers.

Leiomyomas are readily noted as mass lesions within the muscularis propria. Generally, leiomyomas are hypoechoic, an echopattern resembling that of the muscularis layer. Occasionally, the echopattern is more heterogeneous; marked heterogeneity may indicate hemorrhage into the tumor. Cysts appear as hypoechoic structures within the mucosa and submucosa, while inflammatory growths are localized to the mucosa.

Complications

Symptoms of dysphagia or chest discomfort are the most common complication of the benign tumors. Occasionally, hemorrhage into a cyst or from leiomyoma may cause acute symptoms. Leiomyomas can outgrow their blood supply, leading to necrosis and ulceration of the overlying mucosa, leading to overt gastrointestinal hemorrhage.

Treatment

Small, mucosal-based esophageal tumors can be removed endoscopically or obliterated by endoscopic injection of sclerosants. Larger mass lesions, especially leiomyomas, are removed surgically if they are associated with symptoms or other complications. In many instances today, the procedure may be accomplished by minimally invasive techniques.

Table 19–9. Benign esophageal tumors.

Leiomyoma
Congenital cyst
Reduplication cyst
Bronchogenic cyst
Inflammatory polyp
Granuloma
Papilloma
Lipoma
Neurofibroma

REFERENCES

Blot WS et al: Rising incidences of adenocarcinoma of the esophagus and gastric cardia. JAMA 1991;265:1287.

Botet JFC et al: Preoperative staging of esophageal cancer: Comparison of endoscopic US and dynamic CT [see comments]. Radiology 1991;181:419.

Franceschi S: Role of nutrition in the aetiology of oesophageal cancer in developed countries. Endoscopy 1993;25(Suppl): 613.

Greenwald PG et al: Research studies on chemoprevention of esophageal cancer at the United States National Cancer Institute. Endoscopy 1993;25(Suppl.):617.

Halvorsen RAJ, Thompson WM: Primary neoplasms of the hollow organs of the gastrointestinal tract: staging and follow-up. Cancer 1991;67:1181.

Herskovic AMS et al: Combined chemotherapy and radiotherapy compared with radiotherapy alone in patients with cancer of the esophagus. N Engl J Med 1992;326:1593.

Koch J, Halvorsen RAJ: Esophageal cancer staging: CT, MR and EUS. Semin Roentgenol 1994;29:364.

Reid BJ et al: Flow cytometric and histologic progression to malignancy in Barrett's esophagus: Prospective endoscopic surveillance of a cohort. Gastroenterology 1992; 102:1212.

Siewert JR et al: Preoperative staging and risk analysis in esophageal carcinoma. Hepatogastroenterology 1990;37: 382.

Skinner DM et al: Selection of operation for esophageal cancer based on staging. Ann Surg 1986;204:391.

Sugimachi KS et al: Clinicopathologic study of early stage esophageal carcinoma. Surgery 1989;105(6):706.

Takashima SN et al: Carcinoma of the esophagus: CT vs. MR imaging in determining resectability. Am J Roentgenol 1991;156:297.

20 Miscellaneous Disorders of the Esophagus

Wallace C. Wu, MB, BS

ESOPHAGEAL RINGS & WEBS

Lower esophageal ring **(Schatzki's ring)** is the most common cause of intermittent solid food dysphagia. Esophageal webs are uncommon. Both rings and webs are thin diaphragmlike structures that partially interrupt the lumen of the esophagus. Rings occur at the gastroesophageal junction and are covered by squamous epithelium proximally and columnar epithelium distally. A web refers to any ringlike structure along the entire length of the esophagus and is covered entirely by squamous epithelium.

1. CERVICAL ESOPHAGEAL WEB

Cervical esophageal webs are thin diaphragmlike structures usually located anteriorly in the immediate postcricoid area and covered with normal esophageal epithelium. They are more commonly found in females and are often associated with iron deficiency anemia **(Paterson-Kelly syndrome; Plummer-Vinson syndrome).** The pathogenesis is unknown, but it has been associated with thyroid diseases, Zenker's diverticulum, esophageal intramural diverticulosis, and ectopic gastric mucosa in the cervical esophagus. Cervical webs may be part of the syndrome of multiple esophageal webs, which may be idiopathic, associated with bone marrow transplantation, or one component of a dermatologic disorder such as epidermolysis bullosa or benign mucous membrane pemphigoid.

Clinical Findings

A cervical esophageal web may be an incidental finding in an asymptomatic patient. Most symptomatic patients are female and complain of intermittent solid food dysphagia. Signs and symptoms of pulmonary aspiration and iron deficiency anemia may be present.

Endoscopy may easily miss or disrupt webs in the cervical esophagus, and it is therefore less useful in the initial diagnosis than radiographic studies. Endoscopy may be warranted to distinguish cervical webs from other causes of cervical stenosis. Cineesophagography is the study of choice in the diagnosis of this condition. A web is seen as a thin projection anteriorly in the postcricoid esophagus. The differential diagnosis includes extrinsic postcricoid impression, inflammatory stenosis, strictures from various causes, and carcinoma.

Treatment

A cervical web is frequently ruptured during diagnostic endoscopy, so that this procedure may in itself be curative. Esophageal bougienage may be necessary in some patients. Surgery may be indicated if a Zenker's diverticulum is present.

2. LOWER ESOPHAGEAL RING

Lower esophageal ring (ie, lower esophageal mucosal ring; Schatzki's ring) is seen in 6–14% of routine upper gastrointestinal barium studies. It is usually asymptomatic but nevertheless is one of the most common causes of intermittent solid food dysphagia. It is located at the gastroesophageal junction. The pathogenesis of lower esophageal ring is unknown; it is speculated that it may be congenital or developmental in origin. Chronic gastroesophageal reflux may be an important contributing factor, however, particularly in symptomatic patients.

Clinical Findings

Intermittent solid food dysphagia with no dysphagia for liquids is the characteristic history in patients with symptomatic lower esophageal rings. The dysphagia tends to occur particularly when the patient is eating quickly. Inadequate mastication may be an important factor in precipitating symptoms. Daily symptoms are rare, and their presence should raise suspicion for other diagnostic possibilities. Symptoms of gastroesophageal reflux disease may also be present and should raise the possibility of a peptic stricture.

The caliber of the ring is clearly the most important factor in determining whether the patient is symptomatic. Rings with a diameter of 13 mm or less, as measured on radiologic studies, are always symptomatic, whereas rings greater than 20 mm rarely, if ever, produce symptoms. It is speculated that the dysphagia arises from a combination of inadequate ring caliber, a large bolus, inadequate mastication, and ineffective peristalsis.

A properly performed barium esophagogram is the most useful diagnostic tool. The lower esophagus must be fully distended before the ring can be visualized (Figure 20–1). Use of a mashmellow or a barium tablet is helpful in this regard. Barium esophagography is also useful in excluding other diagnostic possibilities such as esophageal motility disorders, peptic strictures, and other esophageal diseases. Endoscopy is of limited usefulness in the initial diagnosis of lower esophageal ring. A small-caliber endoscope can also easily miss a symptomatic ring. In order for the ring to be seen, the lower esophagus must be well distended with air.

Treatment

Esophageal bougienage with a single large dilator (ie, 17 mm or more) is effective in providing initial symptomatic relief. The patient should also be reassured as to the benign nature of this problem and advised to chew properly. Unfortunately, only 35% of patients are free of dysphagia 2 years after the initial dilation. Most of these patients will require repeated bougienage. Gastroesophageal reflux, if present, should be treated aggressively; this may decrease the likelihood of recurrence.

3. MIDESOPHAGEAL WEB

All other ringlike structures in the esophagus are classified as midesophageal webs. These lesions are

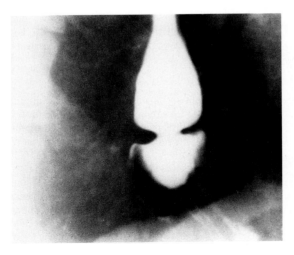

Figure 20–1. Lower esophageal mucosal ring or Schatzki's ring.

uncommon and may be multiple. Diseases that cause desquamation of the esophagus are associated with multiple esophageal webs, including some dermatologic disorders such as epidermolysis bullosa, mucous membrane pemphigoid, psoriasis, and Stevens-Johnson syndrome. Multiple webs may also form after bone marrow transplantation. In many cases, there is no obvious underlying cause.

Esophageal bougienage is effective in the treatment of these patients. Dilation should be done with extreme caution in patients with esophageal webs associated with bone marrow transplantation, since there appears to be a higher incidence of perforation in this group.

PILL-INDUCED ESOPHAGEAL INJURY

Pill-induced esophageal injury was first described in 1970. Since then, it has become common and may occur with a variety of medications. The prevalence is unknown, since most cases are not seen by a physician. The most common medications causing esophageal injury are tetracycline preparations, potassium chloride, quinidine, and nonsteroidal anti-inflammatory agents (NSAIDs). Sustained-release formulations may be more likely to cause injury.

Damage is caused by prolonged contact of the medication with the esophageal mucosa. Pill-induced injury is most common in patients who ingest medications in bed or just prior to reclining, without drinking adequate fluids. Some degree of partial esophageal obstruction such as left atrial enlargement or peptic stricture may also be present, retarding the passage of the pill. The most common area of injury occurs in the midesophagus, although both the proximal and distal esophagus may be affected. Stricture formation may occur as a complication of pill-induced esophageal injury.

Clinical Findings

The diagnosis can be made on the basis of the history alone. In an immunocompetent subject, the sudden onset of severe dysphagia and odynophagia after ingestion of medication is suggestive of pill-induced esophagitis. Many patients may be unable to provide a clear history after prolonged bed rest. In patients with a suggestive history, further diagnostic studies may be necessary.

The diagnosis may be confirmed by upper endoscopic studies, although radiologic studies may also be helpful (Figure 20–2). Endoscopic studies show an area of injury clearly surrounded by normal mucosa. The presence of a midesophageal stricture should always raise the possibility of pill-induced injury. Other diagnostic possibilities include Barrett's esophagus, tumor, and extrinsic compression.

Treatment

The offending medication should be withdrawn; if

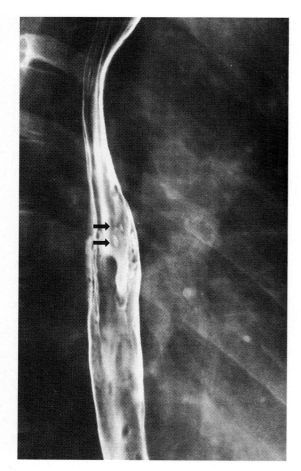

Figure 20–2. Focal erosions (**arrows**) in the midesophagus in a young woman with odynophagia being treated with tetracycline.

this is not possible, liquid formulations should be given. If a liquid preparation is not available, the patient should be instructed to ingest the medication in an upright position, drink plenty of liquids, and remain upright for at least 10 minutes before lying down. Most patients will recover uneventfully after several days or weeks without any specific treatment. If a stricture is present, it can be dilated by bougienage.

CAUSTIC ESOPHAGEAL INJURY

In the United States, caustic injury to the esophagus is usually caused by ingestion of alkali (sodium or potassium hydroxide) contained in drain openers and cleaning preparations. Acids may also be ingested, including hydrochloric, sulfuric, and phosphoric acids, which are marketed in toilet bowl cleaners, battery fluids, and swimming pool cleaners. Of note, sodium hypochlorite (bleach) rarely causes severe esophageal injury. Ingestion is usually accidental in children but intentional in adults. Ingestion of alkali acutely results in a penetrating liquefaction necrosis of the epithelium. This is followed by sloughing of the mucosa, with subsequent fibrosis and reepithelialization. Acids typically produce a more superficial coagulation necrosis. In the acute phase, esophageal perforation and upper airway obstruction are the main causes of complications and death. Esophageal stricture is the most important chronic sequela of caustic ingestion.

Clinical Findings

Clinical features vary widely, and symptoms may not correlate with the extent of esophageal injury. Patients may complain of local pain, dysphagia, odynophagia, chest and abdominal pain, hoarseness, and respiratory difficulties. After the nature of the ingested material has been verified, it is important to assess the extent of injury. Patients with significant lip, mouth, and tongue injury should be monitored closely for the rapid development of airway obstruction. Stridor or other signs of respiratory distress warrant immediate attention to maintenance of airway patency. An initial ear, nose, and throat examination should be performed to exclude significant injury to the pharynx and larynx. If the epiglottis or vocal cords are edematous, endotracheal intubation is contraindicated and cricothyroidectomy is the procedure of choice for airway control. Upper gastrointestinal endoscopy should be done to evaluate the extent of damage to the esophagus and stomach. The presence or absence of oropharyngeal burns is not a reliable indicator of the presence of esophageal burns. If the esophagus and stomach are found to be normal or minimally involved, hospitalization is unnecessary, but the presence of second- or third-degree burns warrants close observation in a hospital setting, preferably in the intensive care unit. Chest and abdominal x-rays may be needed to rule out a perforated viscus.

Treatment

Immediate therapy is mainly supportive. Emetics should not be used, as their use may increase the extent of damage. Burns of the lips, mouth, and tongue can be cleaned with water and all visible granules removed carefully. Neutralization of ingested substances should not be attempted, because damage by the agent is almost instantaneous. Furthermore, neutralization results in exothermic release of heat, which may compound mucosal injury. Patients should be assessed for signs of shock or perforated viscus. When these are present, fluid resuscitation should be initiated and an immediate surgical consultation obtained.

When significant esophageal injury is evident at

endoscopy, antibiotics and steroids previously were given to prevent stricture formation. Recently, a controlled trial has demonstrated no benefit of steroid therapy on the development of stricture formation. Therefore, steroids are not recommended and may increase the risk for infectious complications. Antibiotics are probably not indicated in the absence of proved infection. Chronic strictures are usually treated by esophageal bougienage, but dilation may be extremely difficult, and surgery may be necessary. Barium swallows obtained in the third and fourth weeks following ingestion may detect strictures at a presymptomatic stage that may benefit from repeated dilation.

ESOPHAGEAL FOREIGN BODY

Ingestion of foreign bodies and large food boluses is extremely common, particularly in children. Most ingested foreign bodies pass readily through the gastrointestinal tract, but, occasionally, one will become impacted at an area of physiologic or pathologic narrowing. The esophagus has three areas of physiologic narrowing: (1) the upper esophageal sphincter, (2) the midesophagus at the points where the aortic arch and the left main bronchus cross the esophagus, and (3) the diaphragmatic hiatus. Esophageal strictures secondary to gastroesophageal reflux disease and lower esophageal rings are also common anatomic factors that may cause foreign body or food impaction. Achalasia may rarely present with food impaction. Children and mentally impaired adults are more likely to have problems with a foreign body in the esophagus.

Clinical Findings

Younger children and mentally impaired patients may not be able to provide a history of foreign body ingestion. Patients usually complain of difficulties in swallowing, inability to handle oral secretions, and regurgitation. Respiratory symptoms are common in young children because the trachea is easily compressed by an esophageal foreign body. The inability to handle oral secretions is indicative of complete esophageal obstruction and warrants immediate endoscopic intervention to remove the impacted foreign body. Swelling or crepitation in the neck indicates a cervical esophageal perforation. A plain film of the neck, chest, and abdomen should be obtained to rule out complications such as perforation. In addition, the film may better define the location of radiopaque foreign bodies such as bones and coins. A negative radiograph does not rule out the presence of a radiolucent foreign body such as fish bones. Asymptomatic patients with negative plain radiographs need no further treatment. If the patient is symptomatic, upper endoscopy should be obtained. Of note, a barium esophagogram should not be done, as this will interfere with visualization during endoscopy.

Treatment

Treatment is dependent on the type of foreign body and its location upon presentation. Meat impaction at or below the upper esophageal sphincter may compress the airway and can be dislodged in an emergency by the Heimlich maneuver. In managing foreign bodies at the level of the cricopharyngeus, the airway must be maintained at all times, preferably by endotracheal intubation. The foreign body may then be safely extracted by a rigid laryngoscope or flexible endoscope. Patients with a meat impaction in the esophageal body who appear uncomfortable and can manage their oral secretions may be given a trial of intravenous glucagon to promote relaxation of the esophagus. If the bolus does not pass or salivation is evident, endoscopy should be performed to remove the bolus and to determine the cause of obstruction. Most other foreign bodies that remain in the esophagus should be removed by upper endoscopy. Endoscopic removal is not necessary in many cases of foreign bodies in the stomach, since most will pass uneventfully through the gastrointestinal tract. Objects that are more than 5 cm in length; sharp, pointed objects; and razor blades usually should be removed. Disk batteries usually pass readily through the gastrointestinal tract, but if they lodge in the esophagus or remain in the stomach for more than 48 hours, they may cause perforation and should be removed by endoscopy.

ESOPHAGEAL PERFORATION

Esophageal perforation can occur spontaneously **(Boerhaave's syndrome),** from external trauma, or as a result of iatrogenic instrumentation. Spontaneous rupture arises from a combination of elevated intraesophageal pressure and negative intrathoracic pressure associated with vomiting and retching (Figure 20–3). A large meal and alcohol intake are contributory factors. Most cases occur at the distal esophagus within a few centimeters of the diaphragm.

Instrumentation of the esophagus is the most common cause of perforation. The risk of perforation with diagnostic endoscopy is extremely low. Perforations typically occur either in the cervical esophagus (at the cricopharyngeus) or at the site of a benign or malignant stricture. Perforations most commonly occur during therapeutic procedures such as esophageal dilation, sclerotherapy and banding for esophageal varices, palliation of esophageal carcinoma, and foreign body removal (Figure 20–4). Trauma is a rare cause of esophageal rupture.

Clinical Findings

The clinical presentation is dependent on the cause and location of involvement. Most cases of spontaneous perforation are characterized by severe retching and vomiting, followed by the onset of severe

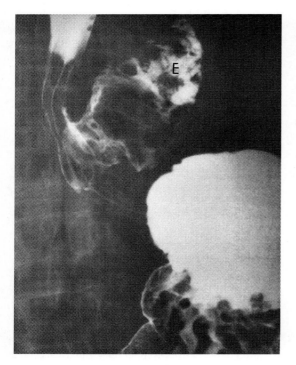

Figure 20–3. Extravasation (E) of contrast material from the lower esophagus from a patient with Boerhaave syndrome.

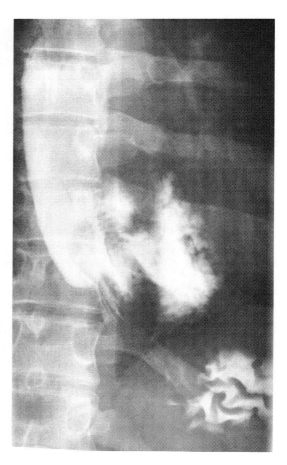

Figure 20–4. Rupture at the lower end of the esophagus following pneumatic dilation for achalasia.

chest and abdominal pain. This may then be followed by the rapid development of fever, tachypnea, and shock. Subcutaneous emphysema is often present but may be absent in the initial 24 hours. With perforation of the thoracic esophagus, chest radiographs are abnormal, revealing pleural effusions, pneumomediastinum, pneumothorax, or subcutaneous emphysema in most cases. The location of the spontaneous laceration is most commonly on the left side of the distal esophagus.

The signs and symptoms of instrumental perforation of the esophagus vary with the site of injury. A contained cervical perforation may result in localized pain, dysphagia, and subcutaneous emphysema (with crepitus in the neck), without signs of significant infection. In contrast, free cervical or thoracic perforations result in clinical signs and symptoms similar to those of spontaneous rupture.

The diagnosis of esophageal perforation should be confirmed by a meglumine diatrizoate water-soluble contrast esophagogram. This will reveal the site and extent of perforation and will be of assistance in designing a therapeutic approach for the patient. If the meglumine diatrizoate study is negative, a barium study should be employed.

Treatment

Esophageal perforation is traditionally treated within 24 hours by surgery, with primary closure and external drainage. In selected patients, conservative medical therapy may suffice. Medical therapy consists of parenteral feeding and intravenous antibiotics, nothing by mouth, and nasogastric suction. Conservative therapy may be indicated in the patient with an iatrogenic perforation who is clinically stable, as evidenced by minimal pain, the absence of shock or clinical sepsis, and only mild to moderate fever or leukocytosis. The perforation must be detected before major mediastinitis occurs and must be well contained within the mediastinum or cervical region with ready drainage into the esophagus on meglumine diatrizoate study.

ESOPHAGEAL DIVERTICULA

An esophageal diverticulum is an outpouching of the esophagus. Most lack a muscular wall and are usually caused by pulsion forces secondary to esophageal motility disorders. Diverticula are classified according to their anatomic location: hypopharyngeal or pharyngoesophageal (Zenker's) diverticula, midesophageal diverticula, epiphrenic diverticula, and intramural pseudodiverticulosis.

1. ZENKER'S DIVERTICULUM

Zenker's (hypopharyngeal or pharyngoesophageal) diverticulum is a protrusion of the mucosa between the oblique fibers of the inferior pharyngeal constrictor and the transverse fibers of the cricopharyngeus muscles. It is the most common form of esophageal diverticulum. Its pathogenesis is uncertain, but speculations center on various forms of oropharyngeal discoordination and dysfunction of the upper esophageal sphincter. The sphincter may be in spasm, fail to relax, have early closure, or have a delay in relaxation. These conditions may result in increased pharyngeal pressure, with herniation of the mucosa in an area where the esophageal wall is the weakest.

Clinical Findings

Many Zenker's diverticula are asymptomatic and are found incidentally on an upper gastrointestinal series (Figure 20–5). Dysphagia and regurgitation are the most common presenting symptoms. Spontaneous regurgitation of food ingested up to several hours previously is characteristic in a patient with a large Zenker's diverticulum. Other symptoms include discomfort in the throat, a palpable mass in the neck area, recurrent pulmonary aspiration, and bad breath.

Barium esophagography is the optimal method for diagnosing Zenker's diverticulum. Endoscopy is not necessary; furthermore, it is selectively contraindicated due to the risk of inadvertent perforation of the diverticulum. If endoscopy is necessary, the instrument must be passed under direct vision through the cricopharyngeus.

Treatment

Surgery is the only treatment for patients with symptomatic Zenker's diverticulum. The operation usually consists of diverticulectomy with or without cricopharyngeal myotomy.

2. MIDESOPHAGEAL & EPIPHRENIC DIVERTICULA

Midesophageal diverticula are outpouchings of the middle third of the esophagus, and epiphrenic diverticula of the distal third (Figures 20–6 and 20–7). Esophageal motility disorders of all types, such as diffuse esophageal spasm, achalasia, and nonspecific esophageal motor disorders, occur in a high percentage of patients with both types of diverticula. It is speculated that abnormal motor activity in the body of the esophagus together with abnormal lower esophageal sphincter function contributes to their formation. "Traction" diverticula may occur in the midesophagus secondary to pathologic changes in the mediastinum.

Clinical Findings

Midesophageal diverticula are usually small and rarely cause symptoms, while epiphrenic diverticula are larger and may be symptomatic. Patients may complain of dysphagia and regurgitation, which may also be caused by the associated esophageal motility disorder.

Diagnosis of diverticula and the associated motor disorder is by barium esophagogram. Endoscopy is useful not only in confirming the diagnosis but also in excluding other structural abnormalities. Esophageal manometry is mandatory in defining the underlying esophageal motility disorder.

Treatment

Almost all patients with midesophageal diverticula and most patients with epiphrenic diverticula are asymptomatic and hence do not require any treatment. Symptomatic epiphrenic diverticula may be treated surgically by diverticulectomy and longitudinal myotomy for the underlying motor disorder.

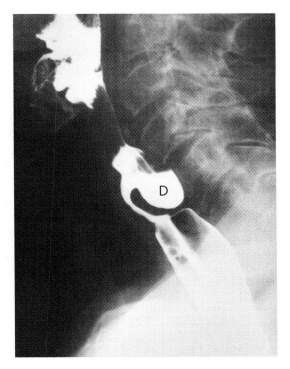

Figure 20–5. Lateral radiograph of the neck showing a Zenker's diverticulum (D).

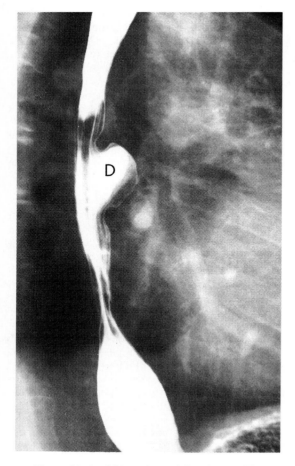

Figure 20–6. Midesophageal diverticulum (D).

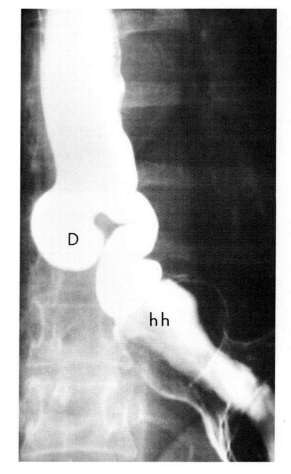

Figure 20–7. Epiphrenic diverticulum (D) of the lower esophagus associated with a hiatal hernia (hh).

RADIATION ESOPHAGITIS

Radiation damage to the esophagus is often seen in patients receiving radiation therapy to the mediastinum for bronchogenic carcinoma, metastatic breast carcinoma, lymphoma, testicular carcinoma, or esophageal carcinoma. Pathologic changes such as inhibition of mitosis, basal cell degeneration, and vascular damage occur early in the course of irradiation. Acutely, sloughing of the mucosa occurs, resulting in erosions and ulcerations. Regeneration of the epithelium occurs after cessation of radiation therapy, with submucosal fibrosis that may result in stricture formation.

Acute radiation esophagitis occurs during or shortly after radiation therapy. Patients usually complain of dysphagia, odynophagia, retrosternal burning, or chest pain. Contrast studies or endoscopy may show esophageal ulceration. Treatment consists of switching the patient temporarily to a liquid diet. If possible, the radiation treatment should be interrupted or modified until symptoms improve.

Chronic radiation esophagitis may occur from 3 months to years after radiation treatment. Patients report progressive dysphagia to both solids and liquids. Chronic radiation changes may result in fibrosis and stricture formation and may also impair esophageal peristalsis. Evaluation with barium esophagography reveals altered esophageal motility, with or without the presence of a fibrotic stricture. Treatment consists of dietary modification and esophageal bougienage, if a stricture is present.

SYSTEMIC DISEASES AFFECTING THE ESOPHAGUS

Many systemic diseases impair esophageal peristalsis. In most cases, the involvement is subclinical and asymptomatic (eg, in diabetes mellitus and hypothyroidism). In other diseases such as progressive systemic sclerosis (scleroderma), esophageal symptoms may be the predominant presentation.

1. PROGRESSIVE SYSTEMIC SCLEROSIS (SCLERODERMA)

Progressive systemic sclerosis can affect the smooth muscle portion of the esophagus. Up to 75% of patients have esophageal involvement consisting of esophageal smooth muscle atrophy and collagen deposition. Patients with concurrent Raynaud's phenomenon are more likely to have esophageal involvement. Esophageal manometry may show low to absent lower esophageal sphincter pressure, with weak or absent peristaltic contractions in the distal esophagus. The upper esophagus is functionally normal. Due to the lack of a functional lower esophageal sphincter barrier and impaired esophageal clearance, patients with scleroderma commonly have severe gastroesophageal reflux disease.

Clinical Findings

Patients with progressive systemic sclerosis tend to have proximal scleroderma, sclerodactyly, digital scars, and pulmonary fibrosis. About 75% have esophageal manometric abnormalities, and two-thirds have esophageal symptoms of gastroesophageal reflux disease (ie, heartburn and regurgitation). Patients may also have dysphagia, which may be due to abnormal esophageal peristalsis, severe esophagitis, or a benign reflux-induced peptic stricture.

An esophagogram may show absent or diminished peristalsis in the distal esophagus and erosive esophagitis with or without the presence of a stricture. Esophageal manometry will reveal low or absent lower esophageal sphincter pressure and weak to absent distal peristalsis.

Treatment

In patients with progressive systemic sclerosis with esophageal symptoms, standard antireflux measures such as elevation of the head of the bed and dietary measures should be instituted. Drug therapy with a histamine-receptor antagonist or proton-pump inhibitor usually is needed. Patients with severe erosive esophagitis should be treated aggressively with omeprazole to prevent the onset of an esophageal stricture. Since the advent of omeprazole, surgery has seldom been necessary.

2. OTHER CONNECTIVE TISSUE DISEASES

Mixed connective diseases commonly have esophageal involvement, but most of these patients are asymptomatic. The manometric abnormalities are similar to those of progressive systemic sclerosis, but the upper esophageal sphincter may also be abnormal. Patients usually present with symptoms of gastroesophageal reflux. As in progressive systemic sclerosis, these symptoms should be treated aggressively to prevent stricture formation.

Esophageal involvement occurs with much less frequency in other types of connective tissue diseases. In rheumatoid arthritis, some patients have diminished peristalsis with decreased lower esophageal sphincter pressure, but most are asymptomatic. Similar changes may be seen in systemic lupus erythematosus. Patients with Sjögren's syndrome may have dysphagia and erosive esophagitis due to diminished esophageal motor function and decreased salivary secretion. In Behçet's syndrome, the characteristic aphthous ulcerations may occur in the esophagus.

Patients with polymyositis and dermatomyositis may have involvement of the skeletal muscle portion of the esophagus, with symptoms of oropharyngeal dysphagia, such as difficulty in initiating a swallow, aspiration, cough, and nasal regurgitation. Involvement of the smooth muscle portion of the esophagus can also occur, with decreased peristalsis and a hypotensive lower esophageal sphincter. Treatment of the underlying disorder results in improvement of esophageal function and symptoms.

3. ENDOCRINE DISEASES

Diabetic patients with evidence of autonomic dysfunction commonly have abnormalities on esophageal motility studies (usually motor abnormalities of the esophageal body and hypotensive lower esophageal sphincter pressure). Most patients are asymptomatic. Diabetic patients are also believed to be prone to esophageal candidiasis, although objective proof of this phenomenon is lacking.

Hypothyroidism may rarely affect the esophagus. Reduction of peristaltic pressure and low esophageal sphincter pressure may be observed.

4. DERMATOLOGIC DISEASES

The autosomal recessive form of epidermolysis bullosa dystrophica is characterized by the formation of blebs, bullas, vesicles, and ulcers of the skin, mucous membrane, and any organ lined with squamous epithelium. Both the mouth and the esophagus may be involved, resulting in severe dysphagia. The lesions in the esophagus may result in scarring and stricture formation. Treatment is symptomatic, and esophageal bougienage should be avoided if possible, since trauma may result in more bulla formation. Esophagectomy and colonic interposition may be necessary in severe cases.

Other dermatologic diseases that may affect the

esophagus include pemphigus vulgaris, bullous pemphigoid, and benign mucous membrane pemphigoid. These are diseases of varying cause in which bullas form in the squamous epithelium, and these may progress to esophageal lesions. Treatment of the underlying disorder is usually adequate.

5. CHRONIC IDIOPATHIC INTESTINAL PSEUDO-OBSTRUCTION

Intestinal pseudo-obstruction is a syndrome in which patients present with recurrent episodes of nausea, vomiting, and intestinal distention without evidence of mechanical obstruction of the small or large intestine. It may be caused by connective tissue disease, endocrine disease, or neuromuscular disease, but in many instances, the cause is unknown. When there is no identifiable cause, the disease is known as chronic idiopathic intestinal pseudo-obstruction.

Esophageal motility is usually abnormal, with absent peristalsis and abnormal lower esophageal sphincter function that may be manometrically indistinguishable from achalasia. Most patients do not have symptoms of esophageal diseases and do not require therapy.

6. INFECTIOUS ESOPHAGITIS

Infectious esophagitis may occur with such pathogens as *Candida,* herpes simplex virus, or cytomegalovirus, usually in an immunocompromised host (see Chapter 2). These infections, particularly candidiasis, may occur occasionally in an immunocompetent host. Disorders that may be associated with these infections are diabetes mellitus, malnutrition, systemic lupus erythematosus, multiple myeloma, and esophageal obstructions such as achalasia and hypoparathyroidism.

REFERENCES

Anderson KD, Rouse TM, Randolph JG: A controlled trial of corticosteroids in children with corrosive injury of the esophagus. N Engl J Med 1990;323:637.

Chowhan NM: Injurious effects of radiation on the esophagus. AmJ Gastroenterol 1990;85:115.

Eckardt VF, Kangler G, Williams D: Single dilation of symptomatic Schatzki rings: A prospective evaluation of its effectiveness. Dig Dis Sci 1992;37:577.

Henderson JAM, Peloquin AJM: Boerhaave revisited: Spontaneous esophageal perforation as a diagnostic masquerader. Am J Med 1989;86:559.

McCord GS, Clouse RE: Pill-induced esophageal strictures: Clinical features and risk factors for development. Am J Med 1990;88:512.

Seeman H, Gates JA, Traube M: Esophageal motor dysfunction years after radiation therapy. Dig Dis Sci 1992;37:303.

Shaffer HA, Valenzuela G, Mittal RK: Esophageal perforation: A reassessment of the criteria for choosing medical or surgical therapy. Arch Intern Med 1992;152:757.

Walton S, Bennett JR: Skin and gullet. Gut 1991;32:694.

Wu WC: Esophageal rings and webs. In: The Esophagus. Castell DO (editor). Little, Brown, 1992.

Section III
Diseases of the Stomach & Small Intestine

Peptic Ulcer Disease

21

Denis M. McCarthy, MD, MSc

From a pathologic perspective, an **ulcer** is a loss of the enteric surface epithelium that extends deeply enough to reach or penetrate the muscularis mucosae. From a clinical perspective, an ulcer is a loss of the mucosal surface, visible by endoscopy or radiography, which, in addition to having depth, must be at least 5 mm in diameter. However, most clinically significant ulcers are 2–5 times this width. Ulcers are distinguished from **erosions,** which are small (< 5 mm) superficial mucosal lesions. Because the superficial mucosa contains only capillaries, erosions may result in clinically mild bleeding (oozing) but are unlikely to give rise to vigorous bleeding, scarring, or perforation through the wall of the affected organ. In contrast, ulcers may give rise to all of these complications.

Peptic ulcer disease refers to the life-long underlying tendency to develop mucosal ulcers at sites that are exposed to peptic juice (acid and pepsin). Most commonly, ulcers have occurred in the duodenum and stomach, but they may also occur in the esophagus, the small intestine, at gastroenteric anastomoses, and, rarely, in areas of ectopic gastric mucosa, eg, in Meckel's diverticula or in the colon.

PATHOPHYSIOLOGY

Etiology

For the past 20 years or so, peptic ulcer disease has been thought to be of multifactorial etiology. Ulcers were believed to arise when one or more of a variety of biological influences noxious to the mucosa overwhelmed the capacity of the mucosa to resist injury, to contain damage, and to heal itself. Until recently, it was regarded as a life-long condition. The notion that a variety of biologic or environmental factors might prove noxious only in subjects who were prone to injury has gradually given way to the recognition that two environmental factors appear to be of overwhelming importance in most persons with ulcer disease: *Helicobacter pylori* infection and the use of aspirin (ASA) or nonsteroidal anti-inflammatory drugs (NSAIDs). Much of the familial aggrega-

tion of ulcer disease that has been observed may reflect intrafamilial infection with *H pylori* rather than genetic susceptibility.

A third important risk factor, interacting with both *H pylori* infections and ASA or NSAID injury, is cigarette smoking. In a minority of cases of peptic ulcer in the United States, other factors—such as hypersecretory states (eg, Zollinger-Ellison syndrome), low-roughage diets, dietary deficiencies in linoleic and other polyunsaturated fatty acids, mucosal infection with viruses, such as herpes simplex, cytomegalovirus, the use of cocaine or "crack," and emotional or psychiatric stress—may play a primary or supplementary etiologic role. Nevertheless, in most cases the prevention or "cure" of ulcer disease will result from eradication of *H pylori* (and the associated chronic active [type B] gastritis) or from the avoidance of ASA or NSAIDs.

Over 90% of all duodenal ulcers and gastric ulcers that occur in subjects who are not using ASA or NSAIDs occur in patients who have chronic active gastritis due to *H pylori* infection. About 5–10% of duodenal ulcer patients and 30% of gastric ulcer patients do not have evidence of *H pylori* infection. These ulcers presumably are due to ASA, NSAIDs, or some other agent of injury. Gastric stasis, pyloroduodenal reflux, ischemia, and age-related diminution in the synthesis of endogenous prostaglandins by gastric mucosa may all have some role in gastric ulcer pathogenesis.

Exactly how *H pylori* infection or ASA/NSAID ingestion leads to ulcer formation is currently unclear. While these are independent risk factors, they may also be synergistic in causing ulcers and, especially, in the development of ulcer complications. Given the high prevalence of asymptomatic peptic ulcers in the general population, many apparently ulcer-free patients who in fact have asymptomatic, occult ulcers may be given ASA or NSAIDs, with resultant adverse effects on ulcer repair and healing.

The risk of complications is accentuated by the analgesic effects of the drugs that may mask the early symptoms of peptic ulcers. These analgesic effects may account for the fact that only 15% of

ASA/NSAID users with endoscopically visible gastroduodenal lesions have dyspeptic symptoms.

PATHOGENESIS

Regardless of the pathogenesis of mucosal injury, the clinical consequences are closely correlated with the amount of acid (pH) and degree of activation of pepsinogen (peptic activity) within the gastric lumen. Suppression of acid secretion with pharmacologic agents results in an increase in the intragastric pH and inactivation of pepsinogen, which in turn results in an amelioration of mucosal damage, a major reduction in bleeding, and a probable reduction in other ulcer complications, although this last has not yet been shown in a randomized prospective study. Until recently, acid-suppressing drugs were the mainstay of anti-ulcer therapy, with antacids, mucosal-protective drugs, and surgery also playing minor roles. That ulcer healing occurred after reducing acidity essentially validated Schwartz's dictum—"No acid-peptic activity, no ulcer." However, there is no evidence that hypersecretion of acid or pepsin is the principal factor in the pathogenesis of most ulcers.

Recent studies in *H pylori*-infected patients have shown that antibiotic therapy alone is as effective as treatment that combines an antibiotic with acid-suppressive therapy, both in promoting ulcer healing and in relieving ulcer symptoms. Thus, most ulcers are a manifestation of an infectious disease, *H pylori* gastritis, but exactly how this chronic infection causes peptic ulcers—especially duodenal ulcers—remains unclear.

Effects of ASA & NSAIDs

ASA particularly and most other NSAIDs interact with peptic ulcer disease in a number of ways. First, small doses of these drugs (eg, 30–80 mg/d of ASA) cause platelet dysfunction that may increase the risk of bleeding from any lesion within the gut, including peptic ulcers. Slightly higher doses may cause acute, usually superficial gastric erosions that result in gastric bleeding, which is generally occult or clinically minor. The mucosa can gradually adapt to this acute injury, minimizing its effects. Much higher doses (eg, 14–21 tablets of ASA/week) taken long-term (longer than 2–4 weeks) are required for ASA to cause focal chronic ulcers. Whether these same or lower ASA/NSAID doses mainly cause complications of *H pylori*-induced peptic ulcers or whether they cause the ulcers which complicate remains unclear.

About two of every three patients on long-term NSAIDs have some gastroduodenal mucosal lesions, most of which are superficial (erosions, hemorrhages, etc). In prevalence studies, about one in four chronic ASA/NSAID users has an ulcer (gastric ulcers= 15%, duodenal ulcers= 10%). Based on infor-

mation from several sources it now seems that only 2% per annum of long-term NSAID users are hospitalized for a severe event (such as hemorrhage, perforation, etc).

Still unknown, however, are: the percentage of minor mucosal lesions that become ulcers; the proportion of ulcers in ASA/NSAID users that are actually caused by the drugs as distinct from those caused by other factors (eg, *H pylori*); the magnitude of the effects of ASA/NSAID therapy on preexisting peptic ulcers (due to *H pylori*, etc); and the percentage of all ulcer complications that arise from peptic ulcer disease exacerbated by ASA/NSAIDs as distinct from those that rise from ulcers actually caused by ASA/NSAIDs. Because much of the underlying peptic ulcer disease can now be cured by eradicating *H pylori* and because most NSAID-associated endoscopic lesions are asymptomatic and of dubious clinical significance, these questions demand attention in planning effective prophylaxis.

In case-control studies of populations in whom the pre-drug prevalence of peptic ulcer disease is unknown, use of ASA/NSAIDs increases the relative risk of suffering the outcomes shown in Table 21–1. The magnitudes of these risks also vary with the type and dose of NSAID and smoking status. Whether they are also affected by age, gender, duration of therapy, blood group, and *H pylori* status remains controversial.

Table 21–1. Relative Risks and Confidence Intervals for ASA/NSAID gastrointestinal outcomes (case-control Studies)[1].

Outcome	Relative Risk	Confidence Interval
Gastric ulcer (ASA)	4.67	3.06–7.14
Gastric ulcer (NSAIDs)	4.03	2.80–5.78
Gastrointestinal bleeding (ASA)	3.30	2.39–4.54
Gastrointestinal bleeding (NSAIDs)	3.09	2.26–4.40
Ulcer perforation (NSAIDs)	5.93	4.0–8.81
Ulcer perforation (ASA)	Similar	Not well studied
Duodenal ulcer (ASA)	1.71	0.69–1.98 (NS)
Duodenal ulcer (NSAIDs)	3.16	1.78–5.61
Death (ASA)[2]	Uncommon	Not well studied
Death (NSAIDs)[2]	7.62	6.17–9.41

[1]Reproduced, with permission, from McCarthy DM: Scand J Gastroenterol 1992;27:9 Data from Hawkey CJ: Br Med J 1990;300:278.
[2]While the association of drug use and death is clear, given the fact that most deaths occur in very old people with multiple diseases, the percentages of deaths truly attributable to NSAID use, to chronic peptic ulcer disease, or to comorbidities remains unclear.

General Considerations

From the turn of the century until 1955, the incidence and prevalence of peptic ulcer disease (PUD) in the USA was rising. However, since then it has been falling steadily in a manner that is not clearly attributable to any medical intervention, such as anti-ulcer drugs or surgery. Factors that may be linked to the recent decline in ulcer disease are an ever-widening use of antibiotics and better sanitation and water supplies, both of which are correlated with a decline in the prevalence of *H pylori* infection. Other factors include less use of salt, higher dietary intake of polyunsaturated fatty acids, and a reduction in cigarette smoking, especially among white-collar males, once the group most prone to develop ulcers.

Despite the decrease in prevalence and incidence, peptic ulcer disease is still a major problem in the population, resulting in direct costs approaching four billion dollars per year in the USA. About half a million new cases and four million recurrences are diagnosed annually. Historical data suggest that the lifetime prevalence of symptomatic ulcers is about 1 in 10 persons. However, based on prospective endoscopic studies which indicate that more than one-half of peptic ulcers are asymptomatic, the true ulcer prevalence could be as high as one in five. Peptic ulcer disease, therefore, is a common ailment, and both the direct costs of diagnosis and treatment and the indirect costs attributable to loss of work and impaired quality of life are of major importance.

Despite the falling incidence and prevalence, the overall mortality rate from ulcer disease has changed little since 1930. Disease-associated deaths, however, are occurring 20–30 years later in life. Duodenal ulcers now appear to be much more common than gastric ulcers (whereas the opposite previously was true). The prevalence ratio of males to females with ulcers has fallen from a previous high of ten to one to almost equal. Peptic ulcer disease now exerts its greatest impact on the elderly, being associated with about 16% of hospitalizations and deaths in persons over age 65. Visits to physicians for ulcer disease increase with age. Hospitalization for gastric ulcers has risen in both sexes, and the proportion of patients over 65 suffering ulcer perforation has climbed steadily, especially in smokers and in those using ASA or other NSAIDs. Deaths from ulcer disease have also risen in the elderly of both genders.

The explanation for the rising incidence of complicated ulcer disease in the elderly remains unclear. Some of the trend may be due to increased longevity in the population, decreased death from other causes, and the increased usage of ASA and NSAIDs in elderly persons. These explanations notwithstanding, some experts are concerned that the anti-ulcer drugs of the past two decades were, ultimately, inadequate. These agents may have suppressed but not cured ulcer disease, and thus may have done little more than delay surgical intervention until patients entered higher-risk age groups. Over age 65, death from ulcer complications, surgery, and postoperative sequelae are greatly increased by the impact of comorbid conditions of the heart, lungs, and other vital organs.

Only recently has medical therapy for ulcer disease been developed that is potentially curative, at least in those patients with *H pylori* infection. Whether this will alter morbidity and mortality of ulcer disease in those using ASA or other NSAIDs has not been determined. The recent developments of several types of newer NSAIDs that appear to be less damaging to the gastrointestinal mucosa may in time lead to major reductions in ulcer disease and associated morbidity and mortality in the population.

CLINICAL FINDINGS

Symptoms & Signs

A. Typical Presentation: The cardinal symptom of peptic ulcer is epigastric pain or dyspepsia, which is often described as "gnawing," "aching," or "like a hunger pain." Classically, the pain of duodenal ulcer is rhythmic, ie, it is regularly relieved by food, milk, or antacids but returns 1 1/2–4 hours after eating. It often awakens the patient from sleep between 1:00 and 3:00 AM, especially if he has taken a snack at bedtime. The pain may radiate into the right hypochondrium, or posteriorly into the back. This latter development, if it becomes persistent, may herald penetration of the ulcer through the posterior wall.

The other major characteristic of ulcer pain is periodicity. That is, ulcer symptoms tend to recur at intervals of weeks or months. During periods of exacerbation, the pain occurs daily for a period of weeks and then remits until the next recurrence. Because the pain is often relieved by food, duodenal ulcer patients like to snack and their body weight tends to be slightly above normal.

The classic pain of gastric ulcer is also periodic and rhythmic, but the pain pattern is different in its rhythmicity. Usually, the pain is least or absent during fasting, but occurs shortly after eating (5–15 minutes) and remains until the stomach empties, either naturally or by vomiting. For this reason, most gastric ulcer patients avoid food, reduce their dietary intake, and lose weight (commonly 8–10 pounds by the time they see the doctor). Gastric ulcer pain may also come on at night, but this occurrence is much less common than in duodenal ulcer patients. The pain may radiate posteriorly and not uncommonly to the left upper quadrant.

With either duodenal ulcer or gastric ulcer, a marked increase in the pain and spread to the whole abdomen may indicate that the ulcer has perforated. This is usually followed rapidly by cessation of bowel sounds and the development of rebound tenderness over a wide area. Similarly, a change from normal rhythmicity to constant pain may herald the development of penetration.

On physical examination, tenderness commonly is detected at or to the left of the midline with gastric ulcer, and 1 inch or more to the right of the midline with duodenal ulcer.

Chronic peptic ulcers in either the stomach or duodenum may cause scarring and impair gastric emptying—a condition known as **gastric outlet obstruction.** This may cause nausea or vomiting, the latter often bringing transient relief of pain or discomfort. The vomiting of gastric outlet obstruction may occur shortly after meals or up to several hours later. Otherwise, nausea and vomiting are very rare in uncomplicated duodenal ulcers and uncommon in gastric ulcers, although some gastric ulcer patients induce vomiting in an effort to relieve their pain. The stool may contain occult blood, and a minority of patients present with anemia because of acute or chronic gastrointestinal blood loss.

Some patients, especially those with duodenal ulcers, may develop **"water-brash,"** a sudden filling of the mouth with clear, colorless, tasteless fluid (ie, saliva), which should not be confused with gastric contents (colored and bitter) resulting from gastroesophageal reflux. Symptoms of acid gastroesophageal reflux, such as heartburn or regurgitation, are not uncommon in ulcer patients, especially in those with some impairment of gastric emptying. However, it is the presence of gastroesophageal reflux and not the presence of peptic ulcer that causes the heartburn.

B. Atypical Presentation: Atypical presentations of ulcer disease are common. In fact, "classic presentations" are the exception rather than the rule. Thus, the history and physical examination alone cannot reliably lead either to the diagnosis of peptic ulcer or to a clear distinction between duodenal and gastric ulcers. In many cases, pain is absent or ill-defined. Patients may be totally asymptomatic or complain only of "indigestion" or other vague dyspeptic symptoms. These symptoms are very nonspecific and in most cases are not due to ulcers.

Fewer than 1% of duodenal bulb ulcers and a higher percentage of postbulbar or jejunal ulcers are associated with the presence of an underlying hypersecretory disorder, such as Zollinger-Ellison syndrome, isolated retained antrum syndrome, systemic mastocytosis, granulocytic leukemia, or hyperparathyroidism, or occur after small bowel resection. The clinical clues to the existence of such an underlying disorder are the presence of diarrhea, weight loss, and a gastric pH value consistently close to 1.0. In the documented presence of such hyperacidity, but not otherwise, fasting serum gastrin and calcium concentrations should be measured. These are rarely indicated in practice and are uninterpretable in the absence of careful studies of gastric acid secretion.

C. Complications:

1. Bleeding–Ulcers may present with a compli-

cation, even in the absence of all antecedent symptoms. Bleeding is the most common complication. Classically, hematemesis is more common in gastric ulcers and melena in duodenal ulcers, though the combination of hematemesis and melena can occur with either ulcer when bleeding is brisk. In the patient with hematochezia, the absence of blood in gastric aspirates is strong evidence against a gastric ulcer. In contrast, a negative gastric aspirate does not reduce the likelihood of bleeding from a duodenal ulcer (which may not reflux through the pylorus) unless it contains bile. Bleeding complications of peptic ulcers often are catastrophic in the elderly and may prove fatal, either in the home or while the patient is being transported to the hospital.

2. Perforation–Much less commonly, patients with sudden perforation of the ulcer often present without antecedent or accompanying symptoms. Perforations most commonly occur in patients using ASA and other NSAIDs, corticosteroids, or cocaine, and in the elderly. In such patients, the history may give little or no indication that a catastrophic event has occurred, and examination may detect only such nonspecific findings as tachycardia, hypotension, altered breathing, or a change in mental status. Patients also may present because the ulcer has penetrated into an adjacent organ, such as the liver, pancreas, aorta, or inferior vena cava. Of these, the most common presentation of gastric or duodenal ulcers is acute pancreatitis. The association of pancreatitis and duodenal ulcer is more common than can be accounted for by the presence of penetration.

Laboratory Findings

Laboratory findings have little or no role in the diagnosis and day-to-day management of peptic ulcer disease per se, but may be involved in defining an underlying disorder or a complication. In uncomplicated disease, laboratory tests are normal.

Investigations

A. Empiric Treatment: Younger patients with classic symptoms of uncomplicated peptic ulcer disease may be treated empirically with H_2-receptor antagonists or proton pump inhibitors and, if they respond within 1 week, no further investigation is necessary. However, if disease symptoms persist or recur, some investigation is warranted. Recommendations as to the nature of these investigations are rapidly changing and controversial.

The role of endoscopy, in particular, is undergoing renewed scrutiny. Academic physicians and clinicians who are concerned with providing the best care to the individual patient may advocate approaches that are very different from those proposed by physicians or health managers who are concerned with the cost-effectiveness of health care delivery to whole populations or groups.

Dyspepsia is an extremely common problem in

general medical practice. Without further testing, it is almost impossible in most cases for the clinician to distinguish patients who have peptic ulcer disease from the much larger group of dyspeptic patients who have nonulcer dyspepsia. One approach might be to perform serologic testing for the presence of *H pylori* antibodies in those dyspeptic patients who obtain pain relief from antacids. Those patients who have positive *H pylori* antibodies could be treated empirically with low-cost triple-drug therapy designed to eradicate *H pylori* (see below). Further investigation with endoscopy would be performed in those *H pylori*-positive patients with persistent symptoms and in *H pylori*-negative patients who fail to respond to reassurance and empiric symptomatic treatment.

At the other extreme, it may be advocated that all patients with dyspepsia should be sent for early endoscopy. In patients with peptic ulcers, antral biopsies should be taken to diagnose *H pylori*-associated chronic active gastritis. Patients with gastric ulcers should undergo biopsy to exclude a malignancy and subsequent endoscopy to document complete ulcer healing. There are some practical and theoretical problems with these and most other intermediate approaches. The unwelcome truth is that the best health care is expensive. The general agreement is that in *H pylori*-infected patients known to have an ulcer, eradication of the infection should be attempted. The role of endoscopy is discussed in the following section.

B. Radiologic Studies: Plain x-ray of the abdomen is of little value in the diagnosis of peptic ulcer disease unless perforation is suspected. In this situation, upright or lateral decubitus x-rays may show the presence of free air. General physicians suspecting the presence of an ulcer will usually obtain a barium meal upper gastrointestinal examination, employing either single-contrast or preferably double-contrast ("air-contrast") techniques. These are widely available, safer and cheaper than endoscopy, and well tolerated by patients, and they provide a permanent record of the findings. Compared to endoscopy, however, the upper gastrointestinal (UGI) series suffers from limited accuracy (20–30% error rate), lack of histologic information, lack of therapeutic potential in bleeding patients, and lack of the capacity to identify most superficial mucosal lesions. However, unlike endoscopy, UGI series are helpful in identifying extrinsic lesions and gastric dysmotility.

If a duodenal ulcer or a scarred duodenal bulb is identified on x-ray, no other endoscopic procedure is necessary before treatment in most cases. This is also true for most radiographically diagnosed gastric ulcers in patients under the age of 40 years. However, if the radiologist is initially uncertain as to the nature of the ulcer or suspects that it may be malignant or lymphomatous, endoscopy should not be delayed.

Repeat x-ray to confirm healing is unnecessary in duodenal ulcer if symptoms resolve and remain absent. In patients with gastric ulcer, either the x-ray should be repeated or endoscopy should be performed after 3 months of therapy to confirm healing, with any residual ulcer referred for endoscopic biopsy. Among ulcers initially called "benign" on a barium study, about 2–6% eventually prove malignant. Patients with chronic symptoms in whom x-rays are reported as normal should also be referred for endoscopy: the false negative rate for gastric ulcer has been up to 40% in some series.

C. Endoscopy: Upper gastrointestinal endoscopy has come to be the "gold standard" in diagnosing peptic ulcers, although it is less than perfect. In most series, upwards of 90% of lesions present are diagnosed at endoscopy. Gastric ulcers or craters may be missed when gastric folds are very prominent, when secretions are copious, when there is food, blood, or clot in the stomach, when ulcers are high in the stomach or in a fundic pouch or hernial sack, when peristalsis or patient movement is excessive, or when the operator is inexperienced. Duodenal ulcers may be missed when the bulb is badly scarred, when ulcers are located in the lateral fornices of the cap, when the ulcer is bleeding, or when peristalsis is active. Practitioners must realize that the procedure is not infallible, and in critical cases, x-ray and endoscopy are complementary and not mutually exclusive diagnostic tests.

Duodenal ulcers are almost always benign and do not require biopsy, except in the setting of Crohn's disease, which rarely may affect the duodenum and mimic peptic ulcer. Duodenal ulcer patients undergoing endoscopy should have antral biopsies to detect active chronic gastritis and *H pylori* organisms. Similar biopsies should be obtained in gastric ulcer patients, regardless of whether or not they are using ASA/NSAIDs. Findings of chemical or type C gastritis in this latter group occasionally lead to identification of unsuspected use of ASA/NSAIDs. However, these histologic appearances are by no means specific.

In gastric ulcer patients over 40 years old, whether or not they are using ASA/NSAIDs, the most important issue is to exclude the possibility of gastric cancer, whose presentation may be similar to that of ulcer. At least six biopsies of the ulcer and surrounding folds should be obtained, supplemented by brushings or irrigation cytology when adequate biopsies are not feasible. Endoscopies without such biopsies do not meet the standard of care. The endoscopic interpretation of benign versus malignant gastric ulcers based solely on visual inspection is subject to considerable error.

In patients with gastric ulcers diagnosed by upper gastrointestinal series in whom the suspicion of a gastric malignancy is deemed low (due to the patient's age or appearance of the ulcer) endoscopy and biopsy can be deferred for 12 weeks to verify complete ulcer healing. On the other hand, when clinical suspicion is high—even when initial endoscopic biopsies are negative or equivocal—endoscopy and biopsy should be repeated in less than 1 month. Patients with gastric ulcers first encountered in the setting of active hemorrhage should probably not undergo ulcer biopsy while bleeding, especially if the they are taking ASA/NSAIDs, heparin, anti-coagulants, or other antiplatelet drugs. The risk of complications in this setting is unclear but most prudent endoscopists defer biopsy for medicolegal and other reasons. Ulcer biopsy in the setting of portal hypertensive gastropathy also is controversial.

Other endoscopic modalities—endoscopic ultrasound, endoscopic Doppler ultrasound, endoscopic reflectance spectrophotometry, and infrared mucosal mapping—are all being investigated for their utility in determining the depth of the ulcer, its blood supply and proximity to major vessels, and its stage of healing. So far, these are not in general clinical use.

D. Determination of *H Pylori* Status: Because eradication of *H pylori* in infected subjects allows ulcers to heal and greatly reduces the chance of ulcer recurrence, determination of the status of infection is of key importance in planning ulcer therapy. Five major types of tests for *H pylori* are available. None are 100% accurate but all have sensitivities and specificities that exceed 90% in untreated patients, with false positive diagnoses being very rare. The sensitivities of these tests in treated patients is much less certain. In clinical trials, it is customary to conclude that eradication has been achieved definitively only when two or three different test modalities are negative, which are obtained at least 1 month after the completion of drug therapy.

1. Serology–After cure of *H pylori* infection, serologic titers for anti-*H pylori* antibodies, as measured in currently available commercial tests, decline gradually over several months to years but do not always become negative. Therefore, the presence of a positive serologic test does not necessarily establish a current infection with viable organisms. Nevertheless, in seropositive patients with a history of proven peptic ulcer, there is a statistically sound reason to conclude that *H pylori* infection is active and playing a causative role. Treatment is therefore warranted. In most situations an empiric course of anti-*H pylori* treatment is much less expensive than the cost of an endoscopy-based diagnosis.

2. Urea breath tests–Breath tests are noninvasive and, unlike serology, a positive test establishes the presence of current infection with *H pylori* with a high degree of sensitivity and specificity. Furthermore, breath tests avoid the sampling error caused by patchy gastritis that may occur with endoscopic biopsies. Hence, these tests seem ideal. Urea breath tests depend on the production by *H pylori* of large amounts of bacterial urease (a nonmammalian en-

zyme). When the patient is administered oral ^{14}C- or ^{13}C-urea, urease from *H pylori* in the stomach breaks down the urea as follows:

$$NH_2 \, {}^*CO \, NH_2 + 3 \, H_2O \rightarrow 2NH_4OH + {}^*CO_2$$

The CO_2 is excreted in exhaled air and collected in a liquid trap. The rate of elimination is calculated from the specific radioactivity of the isotope species. Restrictions on the use of ^{14}C in humans have precluded its widespread clinical use. The isotope ^{13}C, unlike ^{14}C, is nonradioactive but must be measured by mass spectroscopy detectors, which are expensive and not widely available. However, ^{13}C urea breath test kits will soon be available commercially and, if appropriately priced, should prove popular. The test can be performed in most clinical facilities and the liquid sample mailed to a central laboratory for $^*CO_2$ measurement. The result is available to the doctor within a few days. Urea breath tests may be falsely negative in patients in whom the level of *H pylori* infection has been suppressed by recent antibiotic use or treatment with proton pump inhibitors, such as omeprazole or lansoprazoe.

3. Endoscopic biopsy–In patients in whom a peptic ulcer is diagnosed by endoscopy, biopsies should be performed to look for evidence of *H pylori*. At least two gastric biopsies should be performed, one antral and one fundic, and placed in formalin. Even in patients in whom another cause of peptic ulcer is apparent, such as ASA/NSAID use, and in patients with ulcer bleeding, biopsies of antrum and fundus should be obtained.

Another gastric biopsy should be placed into a medium containing urea and phenolphthalein. This is called the **urease or CLO-test** and is very inexpensive. With *H pylori*-urease present, urea is converted to ammonium hydroxide, which turns the indicator from yellow to red. While the test can normally be read rapidly (within 60 minutes), it should not be pronounced negative unless it is devoid of color at 12 hours; reading at 24-hours increase false-positive results. Some clinical centers await the results of the CLO-test before processing the formalin-fixed specimen histologically in order to reduce costs. A positive CLO-test in a patient with ulcer disease is strong evidence of *H pylori* infection. In patients with a negative CLO-test, further histologic assessment is indicated. As with the urea breath test, the CLO-test may be falsely negative in patients in whom *H pylori* infection has been suppressed by antibiotics or the use of proton pump inhibitors.

Routine hematoxylin and eosin staining will often allow recognition of the organism by an experienced pathologist. The finding of polymorphonuclear leukocytes (PMNs) in inflamed gastric tissue is highly suggestive of gastritis due to *H pylori*. Although other causes of gastric injury may be identified in the patient's history, such as the use of ASA,

NSAIDs, or alcohol, none of these lead to significant PMN infiltration. Once PMNs are visualized, the experienced pathologist will search widely for *H pylori* organisms that may be harder to find. Modified Giemsa ("Diffquick"), Warthin-Starry, Genta, and other stains can be used in situations in which *H pylori* is suspected (because of gastritis) but not readily identified. These stains also can help the less experienced pathologist to see the organisms. If all available diagnostic methods fail to reveal *H pylori* organisms but gastritis with PMNs is identified on histology, and the patient is not taking ASA or NSAIDs, a course of therapy aimed at *H pylori* eradication should be recommended provided that the patient has an ulcer.

While the *H pylori* organism can be cultured from gastric biopsies, the process is slow, complicated by the need for special culture media, and rarely used. At the present time, determination of antibiotic sensitivities of *H pylori* in culture is not sufficiently reliable to be of clinical use.

4. Corroboration of *H pylori* eradication– Most patients who successfully complete anti-*H pylori* treatment obtain symptom relief and complete ulcer healing. In current clinical practice, documentation of eradication is seldom necessary in the initial treatment of uncomplicated *H pylori*-associated ulcers unless ulcer symptoms recur. Confirmation of eradication is also suggested in elderly patients with a history of ulcer complications, especially if discontinuation of maintenance antisecretory therapy is contemplated.

DIFFERENTIAL DIAGNOSIS

Other conditions that may give rise to similar upper abdominal pain syndromes include chronic cholecystitis, gastroesophageal reflux disease, chronic pancreatitis, biliary obstruction, cancers of the stomach and pancreas, post-gastrectomy gastritis, and rarely, diseases of the transverse colon. In most cases, other features of these diseases will draw attention to their presence. However, when all such conditions have been excluded, over 50% of all patients with recurrent upper abdominal discomfort or dyspepsia remain, whose symptoms cannot be explained by endoscopic or radiographic tests. These patients are often grouped under the diagnostic heading of "non-ulcer dyspepsia" (see Chapter 22).

When the pain of ulcer becomes severe, the possibility of perforation or penetration should be considered. Severe ulcer pain, while uncommon, also can mimic the pain of myocardial infarction, aortic dissection, biliary or ureteral/colic, acute pancreatitis, cholecystitis or diverticulitis, or mesenteric infarction. The physical findings, including the location of abdominal tenderness, may aid considerably in narrowing the differential diagnosis.

COMPLICATIONS

The complications of ulcer disease are principally hemorrhage, perforation, penetration, and obstruction, in that order, with hemorrhage being the most common and perforation the most lethal. Today, these constitute the main indications for ulcer surgery and account for most deaths from ulcer disease. When emergency surgery is needed, attention is focused on rapid correction of the immediate complication. Until recently, surgery for ulcer complications often included aggressive anti-ulcer operations (vagotomy with partial gastric resection or drainage procedures) that markedly altered normal gastric physiology. The modern trend is towards joint medical and surgical management of the patient, with early performance of the minimum surgical procedure needed for the patient to survive the complication. Specific therapy of the underlying ulcer diathesis can be rendered postoperatively in most patients with anti-*H pylori* eradication therapy, elimination of ASA/NSAID use, or long-term anti-secretory therapy if required.

Hemorrhage

Ulcer hemorrhage may be recognized clinically in five patterns of increasing severity and clinical importance:

1. Occult blood in the stool with or without anemia.
2. Coffee grounds emesis.
3. Hematemesis.
4. Melena.
5. Sudden collapse and shock or focal dysfunction in a vital organ (eg, cerebrovascular accident, coronary ischemia), with or without obvious hemorrhage.

In ulcer patients who are not using ASA/NSAIDs, pain is the most common indication for endoscopy. In contrast, among those with NSAID-induced ulcers, the most common indication for endoscopy is acute blood loss or anemia.

Approximately 90% of clinically significant ulcer bleeds (3, 4, 5 in numbered list, above) stop spontaneously, although blood transfusion may be required. The overall mortality is about 10%, but mortality is much higher in the elderly and in those with serious comorbid conditions. Bleeding ulcers account for about one half of all upper gastrointestinal hemorrhages. Bleeding may be the first sign of an ulcer in 10–15% of clinically recognized cases.

During long-term follow-up, it appears that about 15% of ulcers bleed over 10–15 years of observation, and 25–40% bleed within 15–25 years. These estimates are based on older studies in which ulcer therapy was often sporadic and inadequate. However, more contemporary estimates place the risk at 12%

over 5 years, or 2.7% per year in males and 2.5% per year in females. Of note, this risk is 5% per year in those with a history of bleeding. Ulcer bleeding and re-bleeding rates are greatly reduced in patients taking any kind of maintenance anti-ulcer therapy. Hence, maintenance anti-ulcer therapy (see following discussion) traditionally has been given to almost all patients with a history of a bleeding ulcer. Based on studies involving only a small number of patients, successful *H pylori* eradication also appears to decrease the risk of ulcer re-bleeding dramatically. Because of the high risk of re-bleeding in patients who have had one ulcer-related bleed, if *H pylori* cannot be eradicated, maintenance therapy (discussed below) should continue indefinitely.

Every effort should be made to avoid or minimize surgery in patients who have had a bleeding ulcer that is attributable to ASA/NSAIDs, as the course of their gastric disease may be exacerbated following surgery if drug use is resumed. Long-term prophylaxis with anti-ulcer or cytoprotective drugs may be indicated in such patients. For additional information on the investigation and management of ulcer bleeding, see Chapter 3.

Perforation

Perforation is no longer common in peptic ulcer disease. In most contemporary series, admissions for hemorrhage are between four and six times more common than those for perforation. In older series, estimates suggested that 0.8% of males and 0.3% of females with ulcers suffered perforation each year, with most cases seen in heavy smokers. These perforation rates antedate the impact of the greatly expanded use of ASA/NSAIDs in the elderly, in whom perforation rates are now rising in both sexes. The relative risk of perforations in *H pylori*-infected patients, in *H pylori*-negative ASA/NSAID users, and in persons with both risk factors are currently unknown.

Perforation of an ulcer is usually a dramatic event, the onset of which may be accompanied by severe generalized abdominal pain, loss of bowel sounds, and board-like rigidity of the abdominal wall. The patient experiences a great reluctance to move and a feeling of impending doom. The development of perforation may be the first sign of the presence of an ulcer, particularly in those using ASA or NSAIDs or suffering from Zollinger-Ellison syndrome. The clinical picture may vary greatly. Elderly patients and those using ASA/NSAIDs or steroids may manifest minimal signs until late in the course of their illness, when peritonitis, bacteremia, and shock develop. In others, pain and tenderness may be localized because the perforation has occurred into the lesser sac, leaked contents have tracked into the subhepatic or subphrenic areas, or leaked contents have been limited by the omentum. Other intra-abdominal catastrophic events, eg, dissection or rupture of an aortic aneurysm or mesenteric infarction, may cause simi-larly severe sudden pain but, unlike perforation, these events are usually accompanied by shock from the outset. Acute pancreatitis may closely mimic perforation and may even accompany perforation. However, its onset is not as explosive and it is usually accompanied by a high serum amylase concentration. Aortic and mesenteric vascular injuries, despite severe pain, usually present with a paucity of abdominal findings and rapidly progressing acidosis.

Laboratory tests usually reveal polymorphonuclear leukocytosis. Other findings are unpredictable. A mild rise in serum amylase may be caused by peritoneal absorption of pancreatic enzymes from leaked duodenal secretions. Plain x-ray of the abdomen, in most cases, shows free intraperitoneal air on upright or decubitus views. When x-rays are negative and perforation is suspected, administration of oral soluble radiographic contrast (70% Conray or Gastrografin) may still demonstrate a leak. Barium studies should be avoided when perforation is suspected. Endoscopy should not be performed. In rare cases, urgent laparotomy is required to make the diagnosis.

All patients with suspected perforation should have a nasogastric tube placed in order to evacuate the stomach and minimize further peritoneal soilage. Fluid resuscitation should be aggressively pursued and broad-spectrum antibiotics should be administered. In most circumstances in which perforation is identified early, laparoscopy or laparotomy with closure of the perforation by an omental patch is sufficient, and more definitive anti-ulcer surgery is not required. Mortality is at least 5% but may be as high as 30–50% in elderly subjects with bleeding or other comorbid conditions, particularly when the diagnosis is delayed. For this reason, an initial trial of conservative nonoperative management may occasionally be recommended in the frail patient with serious comorbid illness, especially if no leakage of water-soluble contrast can be demonstrated on an upper gastrointestinal series. Such patients may be followed closely over 12–24 hours for signs of regression of peritonitis, provided that the possibility of other surgical catastrophes can be excluded.

Penetration

Unlike perforation, ulcer penetration into an adjacent viscus, such as liver, pancreas, or the biliary system, is rarely dramatic. Rather, it presents with gradual exacerbation of pain, loss of rhythmicity, increase in local tenderness, increasing requirement for medication, or the development of features of an additional disease process, such as pancreatitis or cholangitis. Its most common manifestation is pancreatitis. The complication of penetration is rarely catastrophic and responds, in most cases, to intensive medical therapy. Only a minority need surgery.

Obstruction

The frequency with which contemporary patients

develop gastric outlet obstruction is unknown, but in older studies 1–3% developed permanent narrowing over 10–20 years of follow-up. Patients may present with gastric outlet obstruction of two types. The first is due to edema and inflammation surrounding an acute ulcer, especially in the antrum or pyloric channel. The second is due to chronic, permanent scarring with fibrosis and outlet narrowing. While intensive medical therapy may reverse the first type, it cannot resolve the second.

Gastric outlet obstruction is the least common complication of peptic (pyloric channel or duodenal) ulcer disease. Other causes besides peptic ulcer disease include carcinomas of the stomach, pancreas, liver, and bile ducts as well as other extrinsic intra-abdominal masses that may compress the stomach or duodenum.

Gastric outlet obstruction must be distinguished from gastroparesis from other causes, in which the stomach fails to empty despite the absence of any obstruction. Patients with gastric outlet obstruction usually complain of postprandial epigastric fullness, early satiety, and vomiting of materials ingested hours to days previously. Vomiting may be worse towards the end of the day. The relationship of vomiting to the ulcer pain is variable. If gastric outlet obstruction is chronic, patients may develop hypochloremic alkalosis, tetany, weight loss, and sometimes aspiration pneumonia.

With chronic obstruction, the stomach may become grossly dilated and contain 200–2000 ml of foul-smelling contents. A succussion splash may be audible on physical examination. The diagnosis may be confirmed using radiographic (barium), endoscopic, or scintigraphic (gastric-emptying) studies. The "saline-load test" is rarely employed, except as a means of following a patient's progress during conservative therapy. In this study, 700 ml of saline is instilled into a nasogastric tube that has been confirmed by radiography to be within the gastric body. After the patient has been kept for 30 minutes in the left lateral decubitus position, the remaining gastric fluid is aspirated, with care taken to roll the patient in several positions to verify complete aspiration. A residual volume of greater than 400 ml is indicative of significant gastric retention.

Most patients with gastric outlet obstruction require suction with a large orogastric tube to fully evacuate the stomach. Thereafter, nasogastric suction with a smaller tube (18 Fr) should be maintained for 4–7 days to allow pyloric edema and spasm to subside and gastric motility to return. Intravenous replacement of fluid and electrolytes is imperative. Intensive antisecretory therapy with intravenous H_2-receptor antagonists should be given to reduce nasogastric fluid losses and to promote ulcer healing. Patients with chronic obstruction and signs of malnutrition should be given parenteral nutrition. A saline load test should be performed after 72 hours of gastric decompression. If this demonstrates significant improvement, a liquid diet may be tried. About one-half to two-thirds of patients fail to improve after 5–7 days of gastric aspiration. Up to 90% of cases of gastric outlet obstruction will come to either surgical or endoscopic dilatation within 1 year.

Where possible, short strictures (< 5 mm long) that are wide enough to allow passage of a pediatric endoscope should be treated with endoscopic balloon dilatation over three or four sessions, combined with intensive acid-suppressive therapy. This drug therapy should be continued indefinitely after symptoms have resolved, especially in high-risk patients. Balloon dilatation therapy has been reported to provide short- and long-term relief of obstructive symptoms in over three quarters of suitable patients without the need for surgery. In patients in whom balloon dilatation therapy is not possible or is unsuccessful, surgical therapy is generally required with either a truncal or parietal vagotomy and a drainage procedure. Surgical treatment is usually necessary when there is extensive scarring, a long stricture, a large ulcer, or a badly deformed bulb. Morbidity following surgery (dumping, diarrhea, stasis, etc.) approaches 10–15%.

TREATMENT

The treatment of peptic ulcer is currently in a state of major change. In the past, therapy consisted of acid-neutralizing or acid–secretory-inhibiting drugs that were useful in the control of symptoms but usually led to only transient healing of the ulcer crater. While the traditional therapies of "acid-peptic" disease remain useful, they are now more relevant to the treatment of peptic esophagitis than to ulcer disease. For peptic ulcer disease, they are playing a secondary role, ie, they are used as supplementary therapy when measures addressing the primary cause of the ulcer are unsuccessful.

Currently, the field is moving rapidly towards a concept of therapy that regards peptic ulcer as an environmental disease for which a permanent cure is possible if the underlying cause can be identified and eliminated. This is not always easy to achieve.

The two major underlying causes of peptic ulcers are chronic active gastritis due to *H pylori* infection and acute or subacute chemical gastritis due to NSAIDs, including ASA. To what extent these independent etiologic factors are also interactive remains unclear. In particular, the issue of whether NSAIDs adversely affect the course of conventional peptic ulcer disease due to *H pylori* is unresolved. There is no doubt that NSAIDs alone can damage the gastroduodenal mucosa, but such damage is very common (67% of cases), is for the most part mild, and is often asymptomatic. In the much smaller percentage of NSAID users who develop severe complications, the proportion of complications arising solely from

NSAID therapy, as distinct from those arising from *H pylori*-associated peptic ulcers that are exacerbated or caused to complicate by NSAID therapy, remains unknown. Such information is crucial to developing effective prophylaxis. Eradication of *H pylori* should be attempted in all *H pylori*-positive cases of ulcer disease, including patients in whom organisms cannot be identified on mucosal biopsy but who have prominent PMNs (highly suggestive of *H pylori*-associated gastritis). Eradication therapy should also be prescribed in *H pylori*-positive patients with NSAID-associated ulcers. Where possible, ASA or NSAID use should be discontinued in all ulcer patients. Nevertheless, there remain numerous patients who need to continue ASA/NSAID therapy.

Treatment of peptic ulcer will be discussed under three major headings; (1) treatment in *H pylori*-positive patients, (2) treatment in *H pylori*-negative, ASA/NSAID users, and (3) treatment in *H pylori*-negative patients who are not using ASA/NSAIDs.

Treatment of *H Pylori* Cases

At the present time, patients who are *H pylori*-positive and have an active ulcer are treated simultaneously with antibacterial therapy to eradicate the *H pylori* and with traditional anti-ulcer drugs, such as antacids, H_2-receptor antagonists, proton pump inhibitors, or sucralfate in order to promote active ulcer healing. Although antimicrobial therapies against *H pylori* may be adequate to induce ulcer healing as well as to eradicate *H pylori,* there is a lack of sufficient studies involving adequate numbers of patients who have been treated solely with antimicrobial drugs. A few such studies suggest that eradicative drugs alone are as effective as combinations of these with anti-ulcer drugs (listed below), both in relieving symptoms and in healing ulcers. Pending further studies, most physicians continue to employ combination therapy with both classes of agents. This approach seems likely to change as better forms of therapy are defined.

A. Antibacterial Therapy: The most widely used, inexpensive, and best validated curative therapy for *H pylori* infection is triple-drug therapy with tetracycline, metronidazole, and bismuth compounds—either tri-potassium dicitratobismuthate, bismuth subsalicylate (Pepto Bismol), bismuth subcitrate, or bismuth subnitrate. Pepto Bismol is the major bismuth compound clinically available in the USA. For patients intolerant of tetracycline, amoxicillin may be substituted, but diarrhea occurs with this drug in about 17% of cases. These and a number of other anti-*H pylori* regimens are outlined in Table 21–2.

Table 21–2. Antimicrobial therapies for treatment of *H pylori* (Hp) infection[1].

Therapy	Hp Drug 1	Hp Drug 2	Hp Drug 3[2]	Notes[2]	Success
Triple	Tetracycline HCl 500 mg qid	Metronidazole 250 mg tid	Bismuth subsalicylate[3] 2 tablets qid	With meals for 14 days plus an antisecretory drug	>90%
Triple	Tetracycline HCl 500 mg qid	Clarithromycin 500 mg tid	Bismuth subsalicylate 2 tablets qid	With meals for 14 days plus an antisecretory drug	>90%
Triple	Amoxicillin 500 mg qid	Clarithromycin 500 mg tid	Bismuth subsalicylate 2 tablets qid	With meals for 14 days plus an antisecretory drug	>90%
Triple	Amoxicillin 500 mg qid	Metronidazole 250 mg tid	Bismuth subsalicylate 2 tablets qid	With meals for 14 days plus an antisecretory drug	>90%
Triple	Clarithromycin 250 mg bid	Metronidazole 500 mg bid	Omeprazole 20 mg bid	For 7–14 days	>90%
Dual	Amoxicillin 750 mg tid	Clarithromycin 500 mg tid		With meals for 14 days plus an antisecretory drug	>90%
Dual	Amoxicillin 750 mg tid	Metronidazole 500 mg tid		With meals for 14 days plus an antisecretory drug	>85%
Dual	Clarithromycin 500 mg tid	Omeprazole 40 mg qam		With meals for 14 days	>70–80%
Dual	Amoxicillin 750 mg tid	Clarithromycin 40 mg tid		With meals for 14 days	>90%
Dual[4]	Amoxicillin 1 mg tid	Omeprazole 20 mg bid		With meals for 14 days	>35–60%

[1]Adapted, with permission, from Graham DY: Peptic Ulcer. In: *Current Practice of Medicine,* Current Medicine (in press).
[2]Generally, one should continue an anti-secretory drug for 6 weeks to ensure ulcer healing.
[3]Bismuth subcitrate can be substituted.
[4]This outcome is based on my impression and estimates based on review of the available data as well as on the results of clinical trials. This particular combination at these or lower dosages is not recommended.

In patients who either have side-effects from metronidazole or a history of exposure to the drug (ie, in whom there is a high probability that *H pylori* will be resistant to the drug, clarithromycin may be substituted for metronidazole.

With any triple-drug regimen, compliance is difficult, especially when side effects develop. The secret of success with these regimens lies in having a physician who is knowledgeable about the effects of the drugs spend sufficient time with patients in advance of therapy. The physician needs to educate the patient about possible side effects, advise the patient when to continue and when to terminate therapy, and be alert to the need to switch to an alternative regimen, if necessary. In the approximately 70% of cases who continue triple therapy for 2 weeks, eradication is accomplished in most (Table 21–2). Nevertheless, compliance is suboptimal in up to one third of patients in practice. Because of problems with compliance, there has been a major search for effective eradication therapy regimens that are simpler and well tolerated. Several studies suggest that 1-week courses of triple therapy are almost as effective as 2-week courses. In addition, numerous two-drug regimens have been evaluated, and efficacies are given in Table 21–2.

The dual drug regimen of omeprazole and amoxicillin initially excited a lot of interest because it combined a single antibiotic with an antisecretory drug. Omeprazole is bactericidal to *H pylori* in vitro; furthermore, by raising the intragastric pH to 5–7, it enhances the antimicrobial efficacy of amoxicillin. However, the results of this dual regimen have been somewhat disappointing in terms of efficacy, with highly variable outcomes in different studies.

Preliminary studies of the dual regimen of omeprazole and clarithromycin suggest that this may have superior efficacy. Since only the doses specified in Table 21–2 can be relied upon, the exact regimens listed should be used. Monotherapy should be avoided. Patients should be encouraged to persist with treatment despite minor side effects, and should be warned that black stools, black tongue, and ammoniacal breath commonly occur during use of bismuth compounds.

Documentation of eradication is not currently warranted in practice. The best evidence of cure is the lack of recurrence of ulcer symptoms. Documentation of continued or recurrent infection should be pursued in patients with ulcer recurrence after an initial attempt at eradicative therapy. Rates of re-infection are estimated at 1–3% per annum in the USA. Vaccination against the organism is currently the focus of much research, and is of major importance to developing areas, eg, Africa, where metronidazole resistance is widespread and the cost of eradication is prohibitive. So far, there has been little success in this area.

B. Traditional Anti-Ulcer Therapies: Because of their excellent efficacy, safety, and relatively low cost, H_2-receptor antagonists are the drugs most widely used to heal peptic ulcers. There are four H_2-receptors clinically available: cimetidine, ranitidine, famotidine, and nizatidine. All inhibit the secretory agonist effect of histamine on the parietal cell, but are less effective in inhibiting cholinergic or gastrin-mediated postprandial secretion. These four drugs are comparable in efficacy and safety.

For the treatment of duodenal ulcers, all are highly efficacious when administered as once-daily nocturnal doses. These agents can also be given twice daily (all agents) or even four times daily (cimetidine). For the treatment of uncomplicated duodenal ulcers, once-daily nocturnal dosing regimens appear equivalent in efficacy to the more frequent dosing regimens, and are therefore recommended. For the treatment of gastric ulcers, once-daily regimens are also efficacious but the more frequent dosing regimens may afford better symptom relief.

Effective daily oral doses are: cimetidine 800 mg at bedtime, 400 mg twice daily, or 300 mg four times daily; ranitidine or nizatidine 300 mg at bedtime or 150 mg twice daily; and famotidine 40 mg at bedtime or 20 mg twice daily. All of the drugs are safe; clinically significant side effects occur in fewer than 3%. Serious side effects are very rare, except at higher doses and with intravenous administration. Duodenal ulcers should be treated for 8 weeks, and gastric ulcers for 12 weeks, unless healing is verified endoscopically or radiographically at an earlier time. At standard doses, ulcer healing rates of greater than 90% can be expected after 8–12 weeks of therapy.

Similar ulcer healing rates may be achieved with sucralfate 4.0 g/d (2 g twice daily or 1 g four times a day), a nonabsorbed, surface-active disaccharide bound to aluminum sulfate whose precise mode of action is unknown. Other "mucosal protective agents," such as bismuth salts, various prostaglandin analogs, carbenoxolone, and numerous other compounds, have not been regarded as comparably safe or effective in the USA and are not approved therapy.

Antacids have enjoyed widespread use for over 100 years in the treatment of peptic ulcers, with efficacy that is similar to other anti-ulcer agents. In the original USA trials, the very high doses of antacids that were employed (7 doses or 1008 mEq of neutralizing capacity per day), were associated with unacceptably high rates of diarrhea. However, in many other countries, studies of low doses of antacids of only 120–240 mEq/d have proven to be as effective as H_2-receptor antagonists, with minimal side effects at a fraction of the cost.

The newest anti-ulcer drugs, and the most effective to date, are the H^+/K^+ ATPase or "proton pump" inhibitors, of which omeprazole is the best known and most widely used. Lansoprazole is now also available in the United States. Other similar drugs, such as pantoprazole are already used in other countries but are not yet available in the United States. These drugs are concentrated in the acidified tubulovesicular membranes of parietal cells where they bind covalently to the enzyme H^+/K^+ ATPase, the final common pathway of acid secretion. Restoration of normal acid secretion is dependent on synthesis of new proton pumps, which have a half-life of approximately 18 hours.

Regardless of the agonist or stimulus, these agents exert profound long-lasting, dose-dependent effects on acid secretion. At the marketed doses, use of the drugs achieves virtually achlorhydric conditions within the gastric lumen, greatly facilitating ulcer healing. Because of the loss of normal acid feedback inhibition of antral gastrin release, fasting and postprandial serum gastrin rise in almost everyone who takes a proton pump inhibitor. In up to 10% of people, the rise in serum gastrin may be dramatic (> 500 pg/ml). So far, this drug-induced hypergastrinemia has not had serious adverse consequences in man.

A single oral dose of omeprazole 20 mg daily achieves greater than 90% ulcer healing within 4 weeks in the case of duodenal ulcers and within 8 weeks in the case of gastric ulcers. Higher doses of omeprazole do not accelerate restoration of the deeper mucosal glandular architecture or benefit the patient clinically. Omeprazole is bactericidal to *H pylori* in vitro. In vivo, it reduces intragastric acidity so much that the organism cannot find enough acid to survive its own endogenous production of NH_4OH from urea. Probably because of this, during omeprazole therapy the organism leaves the antrum and migrates to the pits of gastric fundic glands. Side effects of the drug are clinically negligible. Omeprazole is not available parenterally in the U.S.

For the past fifteen years, the standard practice after an active ulcer has healed has been to continue the patient on a half dose of the anti-ulcer drug indefinitely to reduce the likelihood of an ulcer recurrence. This "maintenance therapy" to prevent endoscopic or symptomatic ulcer recurrence has become largely obsolete, because most of the population who benefitted from it can now be cured of their disease by eradication of *H pylori*. At present, there are insufficient data on the outcome of *H pylori* eradication in high-risk elderly persons—those patients with a previous ulcer hemorrhage or perforation that was not attributable to ASA/NSAIDs—to warrant abandoning maintenance therapy in this group. Therefore, maintenance therapy is still recommended in high-risk patients with a prior ulcer complication, even if *H pylori* has been successfully treated.

H_2-receptor antagonists have been demonstrated to reduce the incidence of recurrent ulcer hemorrhage from almost 40% to less than 10%. The efficacy of half-dose therapy has not been validated in such high-risk cases, and full doses should be given indefinitely. In NSAID users with ulcer disease who must continue to use these ulcerogenic drugs, neither has it been shown that half-dose therapy is of any value in the prevention of recurrent NSAID-associated ulcers. There is some evidence that more powerful drugs, eg, omeprazole, or higher doses of H_2-receptor antagonists (eg, famotidine 40 mg twice daily) are needed for ulcer healing and for maintenance therapy of the NSAID ulcer in the healed state. Thus, classical maintenance (half-dose) therapy is now rarely required. The doses of anti-ulcer drugs are summarized in Table 21–3.

Treatment in *H Pylori*-Negative ASA/NSAIDs Users

The approach to treating ulcers in NSAID users depends on the setting in which the ulcer is encountered. If diagnosed in an elective (nonemergency) setting, treatment is traditional anti-ulcer therapy, except that no eradication therapy is needed. Healing of the ulcer may be achieved with standard doses of an H_2-receptor antagonist, a proton pump inhibitor, or sucralfate. Whenever possible, the drug causing the problem should be stopped and replaced with adequate doses of a non-NSAID compound, such as acetaminophen in doses of up to 1 gm 6-hourly. Doses of 1 or 2 tablets (325 mg) of acetaminophen are usually inadequate in chronic pain syndromes, such as osteoarthritis. Numerous studies have shown that most people using NSAIDs need analgesic rather than anti-inflammatory drugs. In most cases, NSAIDs either can be stopped or their dosage considerably reduced, particularly if supplemented by other analgesics or physical therapy. The availability of the new centrally acting binary analgesic Tramadol, a non-addictive, orally active, non-narcotic agent which is not an NSAID and which is devoid of mucosal erosive properties, promises to be of major use in the management of osteoarthritis.

Table 21–3. Recommended oral doses of drugs used to heal ulcers.[1]

Cimetidine	800 mg hs, 400 mg bid, 300 mg qid
Ranitidine	300 mg hs, 150 mg bid
Famotidine	40 mg hs, 20 mg bid
Nizatidine	300 mg hs, 150 mg bid
Omeprazole	20 mg qd
Lansoprazole	30 mg qd
Sucralfate	1 gm, qid or 2 gm bid

[1]All of these regimens have similar efficacies that have been well validated in prospective, randomized, double-blind, endoscopically-controlled clinical trials. Use and dosages of antacids, bismuth compounds, prostaglandin analogs, or newer proton pump inhibitors are not yet defined with similar level of confidence.

When the patient presents with hemorrhage or perforation, stopping ASA/NSAID therapy appears prudent for both medical and medicolegal reasons. Those who need anti-inflammatory therapy should be treated initially with analgesics and low-to-moderate doses of either corticosteroids or second-line antiarthritic drugs, at least until the ulcer is fully healed. In those taking ASA for prophylaxis against cardiovascular or cerebrovascular thrombosis, the dose of ASA should be reduced. After a loading dose of 150–200 mg of ASA, 30–80 mg daily suffices to inhibit platelets. Use of enteric-coated ASA reduces superficial gastric erosive injury, but unless the dose is lowered, enteric coating does nothing to prevent the systemic prostaglandin inhibitory effects of ASA, which include gastric ulcer. Use of newer and apparently safer NSAIDs, such as nabumetone or etodolac, can also be recommended for managing inflammation, but their analgesic properties may need to be supplemented with acetominophen, codeine, tramadol, or other drugs.

Once ulcers have healed completely, if continued NSAID use is indicated, long-term anti-ulcer prophylactic therapy should be administered. The optimal ulcer prevention regimen in this setting is unclear. Trials of the prostaglandin PGE_1 analog, misoprostol, have systematically excluded all such high-risk ulcer patients from study. Most prospective studies with H_2-receptor antagonists are also flawed.

In less emergent cases of NSAID ulcers, trials have shown that ulcer *healing* is more rapid when NSAID therapy is stopped than when continued. However, when NSAIDs are continued, ulcer healing eventually occurs in most cases treated with antacids, H_2-receptor antagonists, sucralfate, or proton-pump inhibitors. In contrast, effective ulcer *healing* has not been clearly shown during continued use of NSAIDs with the prostaglandin analog misoprostol. With antacids and H_2-receptor antagonists in ordinary dosage, ulcer *healing* is delayed in those patients who continue NSAIDs compared to those who stop using these drugs. No such delay in ulcer healing attends the use of a proton-pump inhibitor while continuing NSAID therapy. However, this observation is based on small numbers of patients. At present, it would appear to be prudent to use omeprazole in patients with active NSAID ulcers who must remain on their NSAID during ulcer therapy.

The prognosis for an NSAID ulcer or its complications appears to be no worse than for a non-NSAID ulcer, in patients matched for age and gender. However, because of the frequency of NSAID use in high doses in the elderly, NSAID use is associated with a higher proportion of poor ulcer outcomes in this age group. Ulcer disease and ASA/NSAID use are both common. Because most complications and deaths from ulcers occur in the elderly, many of whom are using NSAIDs, and because ASA/NSAIDs appear to be independent risk factors for the development of peptic ulcers (especially gastric), there has been much interest in developing prophylactic therapy to prevent adverse outcomes in NSAID users, employing co-therapy with a variety of anti-ulcer drugs, including sucralfate, H_2-receptors antagonists, proton pump inhibitors, and prostaglandins.

The optimal approach to the prevention of NSAID-induced ulcers or ulcer recurrences is highly controversial. From a clinical perspective, it would appear reasonable to assume that any drug that is capable of healing an ulcer in the face of continued NSAID therapy should be capable of maintaining remission and preventing NSAID ulcer recurrence. This explains why H_2-receptor antagonists and omeprazole are widely used in this setting.

The randomized controlled trials done to date on *prophylactic* therapy of NSAID ulcers are seriously flawed in many respects. In most of these trials, patients placed on NSAIDs were given co-therapy with placebo or an active anti-ulcer agent (H_2-receptor antagonist, sucralfate, or misoprostol) and were followed with serial endoscopies over a 2- to 3-month period for the development of endoscopic or symptomatic ulcers. Importantly, the patients at greatest risk from NSAID complications and most likely to benefit from prophylactic therapy—the seriously ill, elderly, and patients with a history of ulcer disease or ulcer complications—have been excluded from most studies. Furthermore, the endpoints of the studies, such as endoscopically visible mucosal lesions 3–5 mm in diameter, have not been shown to be clinically relevant or to predict serious adverse outcomes. Adequate dose-ranging studies for *prophylaxis* have not been performed for sucralfate, H_2-receptor antagonists, or proton pump inhibitors. Serious adverse outcomes, such as hemorrhage, have been routinely attributed to "ulcers" despite much data showing that they can arise from different kinds of lesions throughout the intestinal tract and are frequently attributable to platelet dysfunction rather than to "peptic ulcers." These prophylactic studies often have failed to distinguish between various NSAIDs, despite evidence that some are much more dangerous than others, and the dose of NSAID—which is strongly related to the risk of ulcer development—has been largely ignored.

These major shortcomings notwithstanding, the following may be concluded. Misoprostol 100–200 µg four times daily has been demonstrated to reduce the incidence of endoscopically visible duodenal and gastric lesions of uncertain clinical significance over a 3-month period in patients placed on NSAIDs, but has not affected the development of dyspeptic symptoms. H_2-receptor antagonists in conventional doses have been shown to be comparable to misoprostol in the prevention of duodenal ulcers but inferior in the prevention of gastric ulcers, but famotidine (40 mg twice daily) appears equally effective in reducing the development of gastric ulcers. Until recently no outcome studies had demonstrated a reduction in clinically significant NSAID-associated ulcer complications in patients placed on misoprostol. A major outcome study using misoprostol, which sought as far as possible to exclude patients with preexistent ulcer disease, has ended but is still unpublished in a complete form. Preliminary analysis suggests that one would have to treat 100–200 NSAID users with misoprostol 200 μg four times a day to prevent one major adverse outcome, a yield that does not appear cost-effective. Furthermore, the study did not attempt to identify any high-risk subgroup that might show a worthwhile benefit from prophylactic misoprostol therapy, although the data did show that those with a remote history of ulcer disease or gastrointestinal bleeding benefitted most from co-therapy with misoprostol. Unfortunately, there are no major prospective outcome studies using H_2-receptor antagonists or proton pump inhibitors prophylactically in adequate dosages, although preliminary data suggest that high-dose famotidine 40 mg twice daily and omeprazole 20 mg/d deserve additional evaluation.

For the present, most clinicians use prophylaxis only in elderly patients with a history of clinically significant ulcers or ulcer complications. Long-term full-dose therapy with agents that healed the ulcer in the face of NSAID therapy is most likely to be effective. A minority of physicians employ prophylaxis with omeprazole 20 mg daily, famotidine 40 mg twice a day, or misoprostol 100–200 μg four times a day in high-risk patients for whom a complication, or surgery if a complication developed, would be poorly tolerated. These might include patients with severe medical disease and patients on NSAIDs and co-therapy with corticosteroids or anticoagulants. Routine prophylaxis is not indicated. The use of adequate anti-inflammatory doses of the newer NSAIDs, nabumetone or etodolac, in high-risk NSAID users who need to continue therapy, seems likely to reduce the risks of ulceration and hemorrhage but is costly.

Treatment of Ulcers in *H Pylori*-Negative Subjects Not Using NSAIDs

This category represents a very small proportion of ulcer patients seen in practice. Many who initially appear to belong in this group (based on their volunteered history) on further investigation prove to have been surreptitiously or unconsciously exposed to ASA/NSAIDs. Plasma salicylate or thromboxane B_2 concentrations, platelet function abnormalities, abnormal bleeding time, or gastric biopsies showing marked foveolar hyperplasia in the absence of inflammatory change, may all point the alert clinician towards the possibility of covert or unintentional NSAID use. Asking the patient or a family member to bring in all the medications in the home may also prove revealing.

A minority of ulcer patients, particularly those with complicated duodenal, postbulbar, or jejunal ulcers, may have an underlying ulcer diathesis that is not attributable to *H pylori* or ASA/NSAIDs. Causes of ulcers in such patients may include sporadic Zollinger-Ellison syndrome, multiple endocrine neoplasia type I, primary or secondary hyperparathyroidism, uremia, primary polycythemia, systemic mastocytosis, hyper-histaminemia due to foregut carcinoid syndrome or granulocytic leukemia, hypersecretion following small intestinal resection, or idiopathic gastric hypersecretion. The role of *H pylori* infection has not been examined in most of these conditions, as descriptions of their associations with ulcer disease antedated appreciation of this pathogen's great importance.

A detailed discussion of the diagnosis and management of ulcers in all of these conditions is beyond the scope of this chapter. Briefly, the presence of diarrhea, marked weight loss, poor response to healing, rapid or frequent recurrence, multiple or ectopic ulcers, or the presence of systemic symptoms are all atypical in conventional peptic ulcer disease and should prompt additional investigation. This should start with acid secretory studies, without which serum gastrin concentration is uninterpretable. If hypersecretion is present, fasting serum gastrin, calcium, and blood urea nitrogen (BUN) measurements are indicated, together with a complete blood count. The patient should be referred to a subspecialist who is an expert in ulcer disease. Special investigations, such as provocative tests of gastrin secretion, CT, angiography, MRI, and pancreatic ultrasound, should be undertaken only in centers where there is expertise in their interpretation and in the implementation of related complex management strategies.

Pending this type of comprehensive investigation, the clinical symptoms of ulcer disease in most patients may be treated effectively with omeprazole 20 mg twice daily, or higher doses if diarrhea or pain are not controlled.

PROGNOSIS

In uncomplicated peptic ulcer disease associated solely with *H pylori* gastritis, the prognosis is excellent if the organism is eradicated. However, given the high prevalence of metronidazole-resistant organisms in certain groups (such as females with recurrent urinary tract infections), and the high frequency of side effects of drugs used in therapy, it may take two or three attempts, using different treatment regimens, before eradication is achieved. Reinfection is uncommon in the USA (1–3% per year), except in conditions of poor housing, poor sanitation, over-crowding, etc. Therefore, once eradication is achieved, recurrent ulceration due to reinfection should be uncommon. Treatment of *H pylori*-positive household contacts who do not have symptomatic ulcers currently seems unnecessary, but is still under evaluation.

Whether eradication on its own, in the absence of anti-ulcer drugs, will result in a lowering of the risk of subsequent ulcer complications is unclear. While it seems axiomatic that if there is no ulcer there can be no risk of complication, many physicians believe that the truth of this needs to be established in a large randomized, prospective study in high-risk subjects receiving or not receiving anti-ulcer drug co-therapy.

Similarly, in patients with NSAID-associated ulcers, the prognosis is excellent if ASA or NSAIDs can be stopped. When the therapy cannot be stopped, the prognosis also appears excellent, provided that treatment with an anti-ulcer drug that was shown to heal the ulcer during NSAID therapy is continued indefinitely in the same dosage. Low-dose maintenance therapy, following ulcer healing, has not been shown to be safe in this group.

On the whole, the prognosis is excellent in uncomplicated cases of ulcer disease but is often poor in those with complicated disease, because of advanced age, poor compliance, polypharmacy, and the presence of serious co-morbid conditions. The statistical association of a poor ulcer outcome with death does not establish that the death was truly or solely attributable either to the ulcer or to its underlying cause. Prognosis in ulcer patients with some other underlying condition no longer depends on the ulcer disease, which can be controlled medically in all cases given adequate doses of antisecretory drugs. With overall mortality rates relatively stable over the past 60 years, the prevention of ulcer complications in high-risk elderly patients remains a major challenge. Every effort should be made to avoid "ulcer surgery" in complicated peptic ulcer cases, other then over-sewing perforations or bleeding vessels. Operations such as vagotomy, pyloroplasty, and gastroenterostomy should be avoided in all but the most difficult of ulcer cases.

REFERENCES

Dunn BE: Pathogenetic mechanisms of *Helicobacter Pylori.* Gastroenterol Clin North Am 1993;22:43.

Feldman M, Burton M: Histamine-$_2$-receptor antagonists: Standard therapy for acid peptic disease. N Engl J Med 1990; 323:1672.

Graham DY, Go MF: *Helicobacter Pylori:* Current status. Gastroenterology 1993;105:279.

Hawkey CT: Review: Aspirin and gastrointestinal bleeding. Aliment Pharmacol Ther 1994;8:141.

Kitay W: Peptic ulcer patients with *H pylori* require treatment with antimicrobial agents: Findings of an NIH Consensus Development Conference. Practical Gastroenterology 1994; 18(7):15.

Maton P: Omeprazole. N Engl J Med 1991;324:965.

McCarthy DM: Acid peptic disease in the elderly. Clin Geriatr Med 1991;7:231.

McCarthy DM: Hypergastrinemic peptic ulcer disease. In: *Principles and Practice of Gastroenterology and Hepatology,* 2nd ed. Gitnick G (editor). Appleton & Lange, 1994.

McCarthy DM: Sucralfate. N Engl J Med 1992;325:1017.

Patrono C: Aspirin as an anti-platelet drug. N Engl J Med 1994;330:1287.

Soll AH et al: Nonsteroidal anti-inflammatory drugs and peptic ulcer disease. Ann Int Med 1991;114:307.

Walan A et al: Effects of omeprazole and ranitidine on ulcer healing rates and relapse rates in patients with benign gastric ulcer. N Engl J Med 1989;320:69.

Walt RP: Misoprostol for the treatment of peptic ulcer and anti-inflammatory drugs and peptic ulcer disease. Ann Int Med 1991;114:307.

Walt RP, Langman MJS: Antacids and ulcer healing. Drugs 1991;42:205.

22

Dyspepsia & Nonulcer Dyspepsia

Kenneth R. McQuaid, MD

DYSPEPSIA

Essentials of Diagnosis

- Episodic or persistent pain or discomfort located in the upper abdomen or epigastrium.
- Commonly associated with other symptoms of bloating, early satiety, distention, or nausea.
- Many possible causes; clinical history of limited value.
- Physical examination usually normal. Signs of organic disease warrant further investigation.
- Upper endoscopy is study of first choice.

General Considerations

The word **dyspepsia** is a medical term that refers to a vague constellation of upper abdominal symptoms. Thus, dyspepsia is a symptom, not a disease. Patients more commonly refer to these symptoms as **indigestion,** which is used synonymously. Only about one-fourth of people with dyspepsia report a known history of peptic ulcer disease.

Dyspepsia is an extremely common condition. Based upon surveys of the general population, 15–30% of adults have intermittent dyspepsia lasting for several days. Dyspepsia is the fourth most common medical diagnosis in Sweden and makes up 5–7% of all general medical consultations in Great Britain. The direct and indirect costs of dyspepsia, including diagnostic evaluation, drug therapy, and days lost from work, are staggering.

The lack of a uniform definition of dyspepsia has hampered efforts of clinical investigators to study patients and compare therapeutic efficacy. A consensus conference in Rome, however, has formally defined dyspepsia as episodic or persistent abdominal discomfort that is located in the upper abdomen or epigastrium. Other symptoms, such as bloating, early satiety, distention, and nausea, are commonly present. However, predominant symptoms of substernal burning or regurgitation, or both—which are indicative of gastroesophageal reflux—should not be included in the definition.

Most people with dyspepsia never seek medical attention for their symptoms. The factors that influence patient self-referral have not been well studied. A variety of factors may be important, such as the severity and duration of the pain, the response to over-the-counter medications, and the patient's ethnic or socioeconomic status. In many instances, fear of serious underlying disease may precipitate referral. The physician should attempt to determine why the patient is seeking medical care at a given time in order to fully address the patient's concerns.

In evaluating patients with dyspepsia, the physician must distinguish between a wide spectrum of "organic" causes, such as peptic ulcer disease, and functional or "nonulcer" dyspepsia. In making this distinction, the clinician is confronted with a number of potential diagnostic tests. Deciding on the appropriate level of investigation can be difficult.

Pathophysiology

Dyspepsia may arise from a host of organic disorders intrinsic and extrinsic to the luminal gastrointestinal tract (Table 22–1).

A. Medications: A number of medications can cause gastrointestinal irritation and should not be overlooked. A trial off a potential offending agent may result in symptomatic relief and obviate the need for an expensive evaluation.

B. Dietary Factors: A number of foods are reported by patients to provoke dyspepsia, especially tomatoes, spicy foods, fatty foods, and coffee. The mechanisms by which food might cause dyspepsia include abdominal distention, delayed gastric emptying (cholecystokinin-induced), direct mucosal irritation, and the provocation of gastroesophageal reflux. Lactose intolerance is extremely common, especially in particular racial and ethnic groups, including blacks, Asians, and Hispanics. Patients who are lactose-intolerant often complain only of abdominal discomfort with modest lactose intake. With a larger lactose ingestion, however, flatulence, distention, and diarrhea result.

C. Luminal Gastrointestinal Tract Dysfunction: A number of organic and functional disorders of the upper gastrointestinal tract may cause dyspepsia.

Table 22–1. Causes of dyspepsia and upper abdominal pain.

Luminal GI Tract	Pancreatic disease
Peptic ulcer disease	Chronic pancreatitis
Gastroesophageal reflux	Pancreatic neoplasm
Gastric neoplasms	Systemic conditions
Gastroparesis	Diabetes mellitus
Gastric infiltrative	Thyroid disease
disorders (amyloidosis,	Hyperparathyroidism
Ménétrier's)	Chronic renal insufficiency
Malabsorption syndromes	Pregnancy
Lactose intolerance	Collagen vascular
Parasites (*Giardia lamblia*)	disorders
AIDS	Ischemic heart disease
Chronic intestinal	Intra-abdominal
ischemia	malignancy
Functional gastrointestinal	Miscellaneous causes of
disorders	intermittent abdominal
Nonulcer dyspepsia	pain
Aerophagia	Acute intermittent
Irritable bowel	porphyria
syndrome	Familial Mediterranean
Medications	fever
Nonsteroidal anti-	C_1-esterase deficiency
inflammatory drugs	Diabetic radiculopathy
(NSAIDs)	Nerve entrapment
Theophylline	syndromes
Digitalis	Vertebral nerve
Potassium	compression
Iron	Intussusception or internal
Niacin	hernia
Quinidine	Intermittent small bowel
Antibiotics	obstruction
Alcohol	
Biliary tract disease	
Cholelithiasis with biliary	
colic	
Acute cholecystitis	
Choledocholithiasis	
Sphincter of Oddi dysfunc-	
tion	
Hepatobiliary neoplasms	

1. Peptic ulcer disease–Approximately 20% of patients with dyspepsia have peptic (gastric or duodenal) ulcer disease. That is, the majority of patients with dyspepsia do *not* have ulcer disease. However, recurrent dyspepsia in patients who have a history of peptic ulcer disease is highly suggestive of an ulcer relapse.

2. Gastric neoplasm–Gastric cancer is a rare cause of dyspepsia in patients under age 45. However, it should be considered in the elderly patient with new-onset dyspepsia.

3. Gastroesophageal reflux disease–The symptoms of substernal burning and regurgitation are highly specific for gastroesophageal reflux disease (GERD). When these symptoms dominate the clinical picture, GERD is likely. However, at least one third of patients with GERD experience both epigastric discomfort (dyspepsia) and reflux-like symptoms. Therefore, in patients with dyspepsia who also have some reflux symptoms, a diagnosis of gastroesophageal reflux should be considered.

4. Other intestinal disorders–Less common causes of dyspepsia include malabsorption syndromes, infiltrative disorders, and motility disorders of the stomach or small intestine (see Chapters 23 and 24).

D. Pancreaticobiliary Disorders: Chronic pancreatic diseases (chronic pancreatitis or pancreatic cancer) may cause epigastric or periumbilical pain that can be confused with other causes of dyspepsia. Biliary colic due to symptomatic cholelithiasis may also be confused with other causes of dyspepsia. However, there is no evidence that cholelithiasis causes dyspepsia in the absence of typical biliary colic.

E. Systemic Conditions: Finally, dyspepsia may be present in a number of systemic conditions, including diabetes mellitus, thyroid disease, ischemic heart disease, and collagen vascular disorders. Diabetic patients may have impaired gastric motor activity (**gastroparesis diabeticorum**) which may result in postprandial discomfort, early satiety, nausea, and vomiting. They may also have upper abdominal pain caused by a diabetic radiculopathy of the thoracic nerve roots.

F. Nonulcer Dyspepsia: In approximately one-half of patients with dyspepsia, no apparent cause can be found after evaluation. In these patients, dyspepsia may be a manifestation of a chronic functional gastrointestinal disorder (see Chapter 6). Such patients are labelled as having **nonulcer dyspepsia**. Dyspepsia may also be seen in association with other functional gastrointestinal disorders, such as irritable bowel syndrome.

Clinical Findings

A. Symptoms and Signs: The clinical history is not very useful in distinguishing among the various causes of dyspepsia. The primary usefulness of the history and physical examination is in identifying patients at high risk for organic disease. Previously, it was believed that certain historical features of dyspepsia helped to distinguish between gastric ulcer, duodenal ulcer, nonulcer dyspepsia, and other causes of dyspepsia. Clinicians were taught to ask about the location of abdominal pain, the relationship to meals, the response to antacids, the site of pain radiation, and the pain's rhythmicity and periodicity. With the advent of upper endoscopy, it has become apparent that the low sensitivity and specificity of these features limit their diagnostic value (Table 22–2). Overall, the large overlap of symptoms reduces any diagnosis based on clinical history to an educated guess.

1. Character and location–The epigastrium is the most common site of dyspepsia from all causes. Epigastric pain is the hallmark of peptic ulcer disease, however, only a minority of people with epigastric pain have an ulcer. Furthermore, up to 20% of people with peptic ulcers have pain-free "silent ulcers," which may manifest with bleeding, perfora-

Table 22–2. Symptom comparisons in patients with gastric ulcer, duodenal ulcer, and nonulcer dyspepsia.

Symptom	Gastric Ulcer (%)	Duodenal Ulcer (%)	Nonulcer Dyspepsia (%)
Age	>50 yrs	30–60 yrs	>20 yrs
Features of Pain			
Epigastric	67	61–86	52–73
Frequently severe	68	53	37
Within 30 minutes of food	20	5	32
Relieved by food	2–48	20–63	4–32
Relieved by antacids	36–87	39–86	26–75
Increased by food	24	10–40	45
Occurs at night	32–43	50–88	24–32
Radiation to back	34	20–31	24–28
Clusters (episodic)	16	56	35
Anorexia	46–57	25–36	26–36
Weight loss	24–61	19–45	18–32
Vomiting	38–73	25–57	26–34
Bloating	55	49	52
Belching	48	59	60
Heartburn	19	27–59	28

Modified from Soll A H: Duodenal ulcers and drug therapy. In: *Gastrointestinal Diseases*. Sleisenger M, Fordtran J (editors). WB Saunders Co, 1989, p. 814.

tion, obstruction, or other complications. The pain of uncomplicated peptic ulcers and nonulcer dyspepsia typically is not severe; patients characterize it as "gnawing," "dull," "aching," or "hunger-like." Pain radiation is uncommon in uncomplicated peptic ulcer disease and nonulcer dyspepsia. Pain in the right hypochondrium is unusual in peptic ulcer disease and nonulcer dyspepsia and may suggest biliary tract disease. Severe epigastric pain or pain that radiates to the back should suggest other disease entities, such as a complicated peptic ulcer (with perforation or penetration), biliary tract disease, pancreatitis, or an abdominal aortic aneurysm.

2. Rhythmicity–Most patients with peptic ulcer disease and nonulcer dyspepsia report fluctuating intensity of pain throughout the day and night. Approximately half of ulcer patients report pain relief with antacids or meals and a recurrence of pain 2–4 hours after meals. This is more common in patients with duodenal ulcers than gastric ulcers. However, many ulcer patients deny a relationship between symptoms and meals, and others report worsening with meals. Approximately two thirds of duodenal ulcer patients and one third of gastric ulcer patients experience nocturnal pain that awakens them from sleep. Nonulcer dyspepsia patients are more likely to report an exacerbation of symptoms after meals and seldom have nocturnal pain. Morning nausea or dyspepsia are suggestive of undiagnosed pregnancy or alcoholism.

Biliary colic due to cholelithiasis or choledocholithiasis should be distinguishable in most cases from peptic ulcer disease or nonulcer dyspepsia. The pain usually is severe and felt in the right upper quadrant or epigastrium. It begins abruptly, is steady, and subsides gradually, lasting for up to several hours. In some cases, the pain occurs postprandially, but in many cases there is no relationship to meals. The pain may radiate around the costal margin, to the scapula or to the back. Nausea and vomiting commonly accompany the attack. The frequency of attacks is highly variable, ranging from almost daily to years apart.

The pain of acute pancreatitis should not be confused with dyspepsia. The pain of acute pancreatitis is epigastric, severe, unrelenting and radiates to the back. In contrast, the pain of chronic pancreatitis is epigastric or periumbilical, less severe, and may be interpreted as dyspepsia. It may wax and wane over the course of days. It is often episodic, lasting for days to weeks at a time before resolving for variable periods. Thus, it may be confused with peptic ulcer disease and nonulcer dyspepsia.

3. Associated symptoms–Nausea and anorexia are common in peptic ulcer disease and nonulcer dyspepsia. Weight loss may occur in patients with gastric ulcer but is uncommon in uncomplicated duodenal ulcer or nonulcer dyspepsia. Significant weight loss is worrisome for complicated peptic disease with partial gastric outlet obstruction, for gastric or pancreatic malignancy, or for chronic pancreatitis with malabsorption. Occasional vomiting may be present in peptic ulcer disease or nonulcer dyspepsia. However, repeated vomiting or vomiting of undigested food several hours after meals suggests gastric retention due to structural (gastric outlet obstruction) or functional (gastroparesis) disorders.

4. Physical examination–A complete physical examination is mandatory in every patient with dyspepsia to look for signs of serious underlying disease. However, in most patients the exam is unremarkable. Mild, localized epigastric tenderness to deep palpation commonly is found in most cases of dyspepsia and is neither sensitive nor specific for peptic ulcer disease. Signs of organic disease, such as weight loss, organomegaly, abdominal mass, ascites, hemoccult-positive stool, or jaundice warrant further investigation.

B. Laboratory Findings: Initial laboratory work should include a complete blood count, routine electrolyte measurements, calcium, amylase, and liver chemistry profiles. In the patient with uncomplicated ulcer disease or nonulcer dyspepsia, these usually are normal. Anemia may occur from acute or chronic upper gastrointestinal blood loss and should prompt an endoscopic evaluation. An elevated serum amylase may suggest acute or chronic pancreatitis, a penetrating ulcer, or choledocholithiasis. Elevated liver chemistries may suggest acute hepatitis or biliary tract disease. Other laboratory tests, such as blood alcohol levels, urine pregnancy test, and thyroid function tests, should be obtained as necessary.

C. Upper Endoscopy: In unselected medical populations, fewer than 50% of dyspeptic patients who undergo esophagogastroduodenoscopy (EGD), ie, upper endoscopy, have significant abnormalities: approximately 20% have a gastric or duodenal ulcer, 25% have evidence of reflux esophagitis, and 2% have a gastric malignancy. Over one-half of patients with dyspepsia have either normal exams or nonspecific findings. The majority of these patients are labelled as having nonulcer dyspepsia (see following section). Thus, the primary use of EGD in patients with dyspepsia is to diagnose peptic ulcer disease or atypical reflux esophagitis and to exclude malignancy.

Upper endoscopy has become the study of first choice in the evaluation of most patients with dyspepsia. However, there is great controversy as to how broadly this test should be used. Specifically, there is debate about whether patients first should be given an empiric trial of symptomatic treatment, reserving EGD for patients whose symptoms persist, or whether all patients should undergo early diagnostic endoscopy.

The Public Policy Committee of the American College of Physicians in 1983 issued guidelines for the use of endoscopy in the evaluation of dyspepsia. They recommended that dyspeptics without clinical evidence of underlying disease be given an empiric trial of therapy with an antisecretory agent (H_2-receptor antagonist). Patients who either were unimproved after 7–10 days or had persistent symptoms after 6–8 weeks were recommended for EGD. The principal reason for this approach was that the majority of patients with dyspepsia would have no significant abnormalities at EGD. However, these guidelines had not been subjected to prospective testing, therefore, their impact upon health care utilization and patient satisfaction was unknown. Furthermore, they were based upon assumptions that are no longer valid.

First, they assumed that patients with both peptic ulcer disease and nonulcer dyspepsia were treated optimally with an H_2-receptor antagonist; therefore, there was no pressing need to diagnose uncomplicated ulcer disease. Since that time, it has become clear that more than 90% of duodenal ulcers and 70% of gastric ulcers are caused by infection with *Helicobacter pylori*. For these ulcer patients, optimal therapy now consists of antibiotics to eradicate this organism in order to prevent ulcer recurrence (see Chapter 21). Furthermore, multiple studies suggest that H_2-receptor antagonists have only marginal utility in the symptomatic relief of nonulcer dyspepsia.

Secondly, the committee assumed that it would be less expensive to give patients a trial of empiric therapy prior to recommending endoscopy. Recent studies, however, have shown that prompt endoscopy with specific targeted therapy leads to fewer return visits, less use of medications, lower overall health costs, and greater patient satisfaction with the health care system.

At this time, the optimal, most cost-effective approach to dyspepsia is uncertain. The decision to perform endoscopy in patients with dyspepsia involves a number of different considerations (Figure 22–1). Patients with severe, alarming symptoms, such as pain that radiates to the back, weight loss, dysphagia, or recurrent vomiting, or with organic features, such a palpable abdominal mass, significant tenderness, anemia, or an occult-blood-positive stool should promptly undergo EGD to exclude serious peptic ulcer disease or malignancy.

Patient demographics must also be considered. In patients younger than 45 years of age, the risk of gastric cancer is extremely low. In contrast, the risk of malignancy in older age groups justifies early investigation in an elderly person with new-onset dyspepsia. Dyspepsia in patients from regions with endemic gastric cancer, such as Japan and Chile, also must be evaluated. Endoscopy may also be warranted to allay excessive patient anxiety about serious disease or "cancer phobia." In the remainder of patients who have mild symptoms, discontinuation of offending medications and a judicious trial of dietary and lifestyle modifications or antisecretory therapy may be warranted. However, those patients who either fail to respond completely or relapse after discontinuing medications require EGD.

Future studies will need to refine the endoscopic approach to dyspepsia. For example, it is known that over 99% of peptic ulcers are caused by *H pylori* or nonsteroidal anti-inflammatory drugs (NSAIDs), and most gastric malignancies occur over the age of 50. One study has shown that if endoscopy were restricted to patients with dyspepsia who either had positive *H pylori* serology, were taking NSAIDs, or were over age 50, then almost 40% fewer endoscopies would be performed and no ulcers or malignancies would be missed.

D. Upper Gastrointestinal Series: With the advent of EGD, the upper gastrointestinal (UGI) series has been relegated to a peripheral role for the investigation of the patient with dyspepsia. In general, it should be restricted to health care settings in which

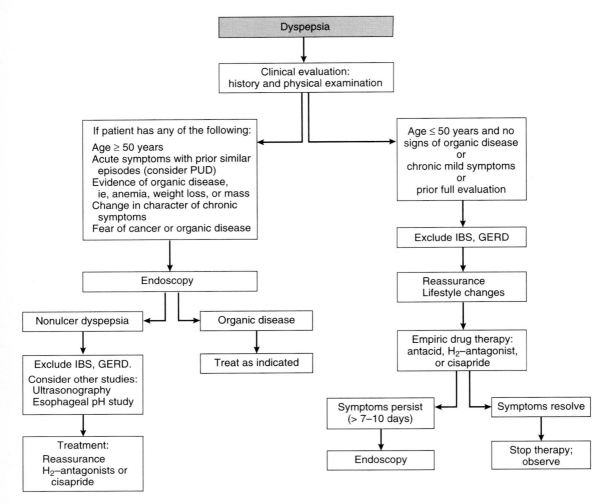

Figure 22–1. Suggested approach to the evaluation of dyspepsia. GERD= gastroesophageal reflux disease; IBS= irritable bowel syndrome; PUD= peptic ulcer disease.

EGD is not readily available. The UGI is less sensitive and specific than EGD for the diagnosis of peptic ulcer disease, early gastric malignancy, and GERD. Properly performed double-contrast UGI studies can detect 80–90% of ulcer craters but may under-diagnose lesions smaller than 5 mm. Factors that confound the diagnostic accuracy include prior ulcer scarring or previous ulcer surgery. The UGI series has limited accuracy in distinguishing benign from malignant gastric ulcers. Therefore, all patients with gastric ulcers identified on UGI series should be fully evaluated by EGD, either immediately or after 8–12 weeks of therapy.

E. Abdominal Imaging: Abdominal ultrasonography is indicated in patients with suspected biliary tract disorders or pancreatic disease. Except in patients with classic biliary colic, one should be extremely hesitant about attributing dyspepsia to

cholelithiasis, which is a common incidental finding. Computed tomography imaging may be obtained in patients with suspected intra-abdominal malignancy or chronic pancreatitis.

Differential Diagnosis

The differential diagnosis of dyspepsia is discussed in the previous sections. Other causes of severe epigastric or periumbilical pain (which should not be confused with typical dyspepsia) include complicated peptic ulcer disease (with perforation or penetration), acute pancreatitis, acute cholecystitis, chronic intestinal ischemia, intermittent or partial small bowel obstruction, aortic dissection, ruptured aortic aneurysm, incarcerated internal or abdominal wall hernia, ureteral colic, and myocardial infarction. Other causes of chronic intermittent abdominal pain (which should not be confused with dyspepsia) include acute intermittent porphyria, familial Mediterranean fever, C_1-esterase deficiency (hereditary angioedema), intermittent intestinal obstruction (intussusception, internal hernia), diabetic radiculopathy, nerve entrapment syndromes, and vertebral root compression.

Treatment

The treatment of dyspepsia is directed at the specific underlying cause, when known. However, in many patients the physician or the patient may decide that diagnostic evaluation is not warranted. In these cases, therapy is empiric. As indicated above, such empiric therapy is best suited for patients under the age of 45 who have no evidence of organic disease or for patients with a longstanding history of mild, intermittent, easily controlled symptoms. Patients who fail to improve with empiric therapy require further diagnostic evaluation. The following are the therapeutic options:

A. Antacids: Antacids are an excellent means of treating the patient with infrequent dyspepsia, especially when related to dietary overindulgence or indiscretion. Antacids are not recommended as primary therapy for patients with daily dyspepsia. Several preparations containing aluminum and magnesium hydroxide are available in liquid and tablet form and may be taken as needed in doses of approximately 60 mEq of acid-neutralizing capacity. Diarrhea and constipation can occur but are infrequent with only one or two doses a day. Treatment more than four to six times daily is not recommended.

Antacids containing calcium carbonate are a satisfactory alternative and offer the added advantage of providing supplemental calcium. Previous concerns that these antacids cause rebound acid hypersecretion are without foundation. One to three tablets containing 500 mg calcium carbonate may be taken as needed for dyspepsia. Doses should not exceed 16 tablets per day. In patients with normal renal function, hypercalcemia or alkalosis do not occur at recommended doses.

B. Bismuth subsalicylate: Bismuth subsalicylate (Pepto Bismol) also may be used on an infrequent basis as needed for intermittent dyspepsia. Doses of 2 tablespoons or tablets (total of 524 mg bismuth) may be taken up to four times daily. Patients should be advised that darkening of the stool is expected. Pepto Bismol contains salicylate, but significant serum levels are not reached in patients with normal renal function. Caution is urged, however, in patients who are also taking aspirin. Because small amounts of bismuth are absorbed, this agent should not be used on a chronic basis.

C. H_2-Receptor Antagonists: H_2-receptor antagonists may be given as an empiric trial for dyspepsia, however, patients who fail to improve significantly after 7–10 days warrant further investigation. Although not generally recommended for intermit-

tent therapy, many patients take them on an "as needed" basis for periodic dyspepsia. Patients should be advised to seek prompt attention if pain is persistent or worsening. These agents are best administered in a twice-daily regimen: cimetidine 400 mg twice a day, ranitidine 150 mg twice a day, nizatidine 150 mg twice a day, or famotidine 20 mg twice a day.

D. Promotility Agents: Metoclopramide 10 mg and cisapride 10 mg taken three to four times daily provide symptomatic relief in patients with gastroesophageal reflux or nonulcer dyspepsia (see section below). Metoclopramide is not recommended on a chronic basis due to its antidopaminergic effects and risk of tardive dyskinesia. In contrast, cisapride is a serotonin $5-HT_4$ agonist that is devoid of antidopaminergic actions. It is an extremely well-tolerated drug with almost no side effects. In patients with clinical features of mild-to- moderate heartburn and dyspepsia, cisapride is an excellent first-line empiric therapeutic agent. Patients with persistent symptoms of reflux or dyspepsia despite cisapride warrant endoscopic evaluation.

NONULCER DYSPEPSIA

Essentials of Diagnosis

- Dyspepsia of at least several weeks duration for which no obvious organic cause can be found.
- No abnormalities on physical examination or laboratory profile that explain symptoms.
- No focal or structural abnormalities at upper endoscopy.

General Considerations

Nonulcer dyspepsia refers to chronic dyspepsia of several weeks duration for which no obvious structural or organic cause is evident on clinical evaluation, laboratory testing, and upper endoscopy. A variety of other terms have been used by clinicians and investigators, more or less synonymously, including nonorganic dyspepsia, essential dyspepsia, functional dyspepsia, and dyspepsia of unknown origin.

Nonulcer dyspepsia is extremely common. Over one-half of patients who undergo endoscopy for dyspepsia have normal or nonspecific findings. Even if one pursues further diagnostic studies in these endoscopy-negative patients to exclude mild (nonerosive) gastroesophageal reflux, irritable bowel syndrome, and pancreaticobiliary disease, at least one fourth of cases of chronic dyspepsia remain unexplained.

The medical costs of evaluating and treating nonulcer dyspepsia have not been well studied but appear to be enormous. It is estimated that the direct costs are $2 billion per year in the United States. The indirect costs also appear to be high. In Sweden, patients with nonulcer dyspepsia take 2.5 times as many sick days per year (or 26 total) for dyspepsia as well as experience a variety of other nonspecific symptoms (headaches, fatigue, etc) compared with other Swedish workers.

From limited studies of the natural history of nonulcer dyspepsia, it appears that 70% of patients continue to experience symptoms after 5 years. Thus, nonulcer dyspepsia is a chronic problem in most cases, which results in tremendous costs to society and the health care system.

Pathophysiology

The causes of nonulcer dyspepsia are poorly understood but appear to be heterogeneous. As with other functional gastrointestinal disorders (see Chapter 6), a number of physiologic and psychological abnormalities have been identified but their relative importance is disputed. These factors are not mutually exclusive, and in many patients a number of factors may be operative.

A. Dietary and Environmental Factors: Patients with nonulcer dyspepsia often cite a number of dietary triggers. Many patients report that tea, alcohol, tomatoes, citrus and other fruits, spicy foods, and rich or fatty foods can exacerbate dyspepsia, although double-blind food challenges dispute their importance. Coffee, however, does appear to provoke dyspepsia, even though total consumption in patients is not greater than in a control population. Patients should be encouraged to eat a balanced diet and to avoid tobacco and excessive alcohol.

B. Gastric Acid Secretion: Basal and peak acid output are normal in patients with nonulcer dyspepsia. There is no evidence of acid hypersecretion. Some studies have suggested an increased sensitivity (heightened visceral nocioception) to intragastric infusions of 0.1 N HCl as well as saline (see section below).

C. Abnormal Gastric Motor Function: Abnormal gastric motor function is present in up to half of patients with nonulcer dyspepsia. Solid phase gastric emptying studies are abnormal in approximately 50% of patients. Similarly, postprandial antroduodenal motility (which can be performed in certain specialty centers) is abnormal in a similar percentage. The cause of this gastroparesis is uncertain. Preliminary studies suggest abnormal gut parasympathetic or sympathetic function in some patients with gastroparesis but also in some dyspeptics with normal emptying. Most patients with gastroparesis do not have abnormalities of esophageal or intestinal motility, ie, there is no evidence of a generalized gastrointestinal myoneuropathy.

Although a significant number of patients with nonulcer dyspepsia appear to have an idiopathic gastroparesis, the clinical importance of this finding and its relationship to symptoms is uncertain. There is a poor correlation between the presence of symptoms and the finding of motor abnormalities. Furthermore, the types of symptoms seen in patients with gastro-

paresis are similar to those in patients with nonulcer dyspepsia. That is, the presence or absence of "dysmotility-like" symptoms of bloating, distention, nausea, or vomiting is not predictive of which patients have abnormal gastric motility. Based upon limited data, it does not appear that patients with gastroparesis have greater symptomatic improvement with promotility agents than other patients with nonulcer dyspepsia. In view thereof, it is not worthwhile in most patients with nonulcer dyspepsia to obtain a gastric emptying study, as it does not influence medical management.

D. Heightened Visceral Nocioception: Many patients with nonulcer dyspepsia appear to have an abnormal or "heightened" perception of physiologic or minor noxious stimuli. As already mentioned, some patients report increased sensitivity to infusions of both saline and acid. Intravenous injection of pentagastrin causes pain in some patients, even when acid secretion is blocked by an H_2-receptor antagonist. This may be similar to the provocation of pain with edrophonium injection in some patients with chest pain of undetermined origin. Several studies report that patients with nonulcer dyspepsia develop pain when balloons are inflated in the proximal stomach. In these patients, pain occurs at significantly lower levels of balloon inflation than in control subjects. These findings are analogous to those found in irritable bowel syndrome, in which there is a lower pain threshold to rectal balloon inflation, and to noncardiac chest pain, in which there is a lower threshold to esophageal balloon inflation.

The basis for this abnormal perception is undetermined. Preliminary evidence suggests that there may be abnormal processing of afferent gut sensation at the spinal or central nervous system level. Abnormal visceral sensation is not related to the presence of gastric motor abnormalities. Of note, somatic pain sensation is normal. Thus, the defect appears to be confined to visceral sensation.

E. Psychosocial Stress: A patient's symptoms may arise from a complex interaction of organic, psychological, and social factors. To understand a patient's illness, one must recognize the interplay of personality traits, life events, social support structure, and coping mechanisms that may be important in the way a patient perceives and reports symptoms.

There is no convincing evidence that for most patients nonulcer dyspepsia is related to psychological abnormalities or chronic stress. The personality profiles are similar to those of patients with other functional gastrointestinal disorders (such as irritable bowel syndrome) or peptic ulcer disease. Patients in all of these groups have higher degrees of neurosis, depression, anxiety, and hypochondriasis on standard inventories. However, these differences are small and unlikely to be of clinical importance, in most cases.

Although patients commonly report a relationship

between dyspepsia and acute or chronic stress, there is no evidence that the mean number of major life stress events is greater for persons with nonulcer dyspepsia than for other people. However, the perceived magnitude of these stresses may be greater. In other words, stress, objectively defined, may not be greater but may subjectively be perceived as being more deleterious to persons with nonulcer dyspepsia.

Psychosocial factors are likely to be important in some patients. Differences in psychosocial factors between those patients with dyspepsia who seek medical attention and those who do not have not been investigated.

F. Aerophagia: Many patients swallow excessive amounts of air, resulting in distention, bloating, flatulence, and frequent belching. Most commonly this occurs subconsciously, often secondary to stress or anxiety. Aerophagia also may occur consciously in patients with severe psychiatric problems. Recognition of this problem is important because it often responds to behavioral modifications.

G. Irritable Bowel Syndrome: There is a large overlap between nonulcer dyspepsia and other functional gastrointestinal disorders (see Chapter 6). Approximately one third of patients with irritable bowel syndrome also report dyspepsia. A similar proportion of patients with nonulcer dyspepsia also have symptoms of irritable bowel syndrome.

H. Gastroesophageal Reflux Disease: Although the symptoms of heartburn and regurgitation are highly specific for gastroesophageal reflux, many patients with GERD do not present such obvious symptoms. Some patients report both heartburn and dyspepsia. Whether these upper abdominal symptoms are due to acid esophageal reflux or concomitant nonulcer dyspepsia of another cause is not clear. In some cases, dyspepsia may dominate the clinical picture or even be the sole symptom.

The actual prevalence of gastroesophageal reflux in patients with chronic dyspepsia is unknown. Approximately one third of patients with chronic dyspepsia also report symptoms of heartburn, suggestive of gastroesophageal reflux. However, the number of patients with dyspepsia who have gastroesophageal reflux has not been well documented.

I. *Helicobacter pylori*-associated Gastritis: *H pylori* is a gram-negative bacterium that commonly colonizes the gastric mucous layer and induces a histologic gastritis. It is the major cause of chronic antral ("Type B") gastritis, a condition that is prevalent in over 35% of asymptomatic adults. It has become quite clear that *H pylori* plays a major contributing role in the pathogenesis of peptic ulcer disease. The organism is present in over 90% of patients with duodenal ulcer and over 70% of those with gastric ulcer.

Successful eradication of the organism with bismuth and antibiotics not only resolves histologic gastritis but decreases ulcer recurrence rates from over 80% to less than 10% per year. Antibiotic treatment is now recommended for all patients with peptic ulcer disease who have documented *H pylori* infection. Of note, only about 15% of people who have *H pylori* gastritis will develop a peptic ulcer over a 25-year period.

The role of *H pylori* in nonulcer dyspepsia is much more controversial. Acute infection with *H pylori* causes transient nausea, abdominal pain, vomiting, and hypochlorhydria. However, it has not been convincingly demonstrated that this organism can cause chronic dyspepsia. *H pylori* is found in approximately 50% of patients with nonulcer dyspepsia, however, this prevalence is not clearly higher than in well-matched asymptomatic controls. A number of trials of therapy directed against *H pylori* in patients with nonulcer dyspepsia have reported a variable effect upon dyspeptic symptoms. Regrettably, these trials have suffered from serious methodologic flaws. Thus, evidence that *H pylori* plays a causative role in nonulcer dyspepsia is unconvincing. While there may be a small number of patients with nonulcer dyspepsia whose symptoms are caused or exacerbated by *H pylori*-associated gastritis, symptoms in the majority of patients are likely caused by the other factors listed above.

Clinical Findings

As discussed previously, nonulcer dyspepsia cannot be reliably distinguished by history and physical examination alone from other causes of dyspepsia. This difficulty may be contrasted with the diagnosis of irritable bowel syndrome, another functional gastrointestinal disorder, which can be made with a high degree of reliability from the clinical findings alone. *The diagnosis of nonulcer dyspepsia is a diagnosis of exclusion: other structural and organic causes must first be excluded by physical examination, laboratory studies, upper endoscopy, and, in some cases, abdominal imaging studies.* A full discussion of the evaluation of dyspepsia is given in the previous section.

A. Symptoms and Signs: Patients complain of vague abdominal discomfort that may be described as gnawing, burning, aching, or a heavy sensation. Many patients complain of bloating, early satiety, nausea, occasional vomiting, belching, heartburn, or exacerbation by meals. Nocturnal symptoms are uncommon. The symptoms tend to wax and wane over time, with periods of minimal symptomatology often alternating with symptomatic periods that range from days to weeks.

Some investigators have attempted to classify patients with nonulcer dyspepsia into symptom subgroups. **Ulcer-like** dyspepsia is pain that is well-localized to the epigastrium, is relieved by food or antacids, occurs between meals, and may awaken the patient from sleep. **Reflux-like** dyspepsia is upper abdominal discomfort that is accompanied by heartburn or regurgitation. **Dysmotility-like** pain consists of upper abdominal discomfort that is aggravated by meals and is associated with bloating, nausea, early satiety, and postprandial fullness.

With the exception of "reflux-like" dyspepsia, this classification system is of little clinical utility. Many patients do not fall into any category; many others fall into more than one subgroup. Furthermore, these clinical categories do not correlate with pathophysiologic disturbances or clinical response. For example, patients with "dysmotility-like" symptoms do not have a higher prevalence of gastroparesis than other subgroups and do not necessarily have a better response to promotility agents. Patients with "reflux-like" symptoms do appear to have a higher prevalence of gastroesophageal reflux and a better response to anti-reflux therapies.

The physical examination in nonulcer dyspepsia should be normal. Mild epigastric tenderness is common. Signs of organic disease such as serious pain, weight loss, a palpable abdominal mass, or an occult-blood-positive stool cannot be attributed to nonulcer dyspepsia and mandate further investigation.

B. Laboratory Studies: Laboratory studies (as described in the section on dyspepsia) should be normal.

C. Endoscopy: The indications for endoscopy are discussed in the section on dyspepsia. All patients with either chronic unexplained dyspepsia or dyspeptic symptoms that do not respond to empiric medical therapy warrant an upper endoscopy examination. Careful attention should be given to the gastroesophageal junction to look for evidence of mild gastroesophageal reflux. By definition, all patients with nonulcer dyspepsia have either normal or nonspecific findings on endoscopy.

D. Abdominal Imaging: Abdominal ultrasonography is commonly ordered in patients with chronic dyspepsia who have normal endoscopic findings to screen for pancreatic or biliary tract disorders or for intra-abdominal malignancy. The yield of this study in patients with a normal physical examination, normal laboratory data, and nonspecific dyspepsia is extremely low. Further imaging with computed tomography or magnetic resonance imaging should be obtained only when there is a strong suspicion of intra-abdominal disease.

E. Other Studies: Nuclear solid-phase gastric emptying studies and gastroduodenal manometry are not very useful clinically and should not be generally obtained in patients with nonulcer dyspepsia. Although they are abnormal in up to half of patients, they do not help establish the diagnosis or guide medical therapy.

Neither the clinical history nor endoscopy reliably excludes gastroesophageal reflux in patients with chronic dyspepsia. Ambulatory esophageal pH monitoring is a valuable tool to diagnose gastroesophageal reflux in patients with atypical symptoms. In most cases, however, it is more practical simply to treat patients with suspected GERD with an anti-reflux regimen, reserving pH monitoring for selected cases.

Differential Diagnosis

The differential diagnosis of dyspepsia and intermittent upper abdominal pain is discussed under the section on dyspepsia, above. Patients with nonulcer dyspepsia should be distinguished from those with idiopathic chronic intractable abdominal pain (CIAP). More than 70% of patients with CIAP are women, many of whom have a history of physical or psychological abuse. These patients typically report a long history of abdominal pain (more than 6 months) that is diffuse and is described in vague or bizarre terms that do not conform to normal physiology. They commonly report a number of other somatic symptoms outside the abdomen. Most have undergone extensive diagnostic tests and procedures with negative findings.

The majority of patients with CIAP have severe underlying psychological problems, including depression, anxiety, and somatoform disorders. Unfortunately, these patients usually have little insight into their psychological condition. They can be extremely difficult to manage, often insisting that they have a serious condition and demanding further testing. In most cases, referral to a multidisciplinary pain clinic is appropriate, in which a combination of psychological, behavioral, and pharmacologic therapies can be rendered in a consistent fashion.

Treatment

A. General Management: The approach to the patients with functional gastrointestinal disorders is discussed in detail in Chapter 6. In general, the most important aspect of therapy is the development of a solid therapeutic relationship between the physician and patient. The physician should foster the trust and confidence of the patient by taking a careful history and performing a thorough physical examination. An attempt should be made to determine the reason that the patient with chronic symptoms has presented at a given time. The patient's fears (ie, cancer phobia) should be addressed and allayed. Life stresses should be explored; those related to the patient's family, workplace, personal relationships, or living situation may cause a decompensation in a patient who was previously coping adequately with chronic symptoms. Recent changes in diet or medications should be reviewed. The physician should be aware of the patient's psychological state, as gastrointestinal symptoms may be a somatic manifestation of serious psychiatric disease, such as depression, anxiety, or psychosis.

After the initial evaluation, the differential diagnosis should be discussed with the patient, including the possibility of nonulcer dyspepsia. A reasonable, cost-effective diagnostic workup should be proposed that addresses the patient's concerns as well as the physician's needs. Although in most cases this will include upper endoscopy, an empiric therapeutic trial may be appropriate in many younger patients. After the diagnostic evaluation, the patient should be told that the diagnosis is nonulcer dyspepsia and that this is a recognized clinical entity. The tendency to "over-investigate" must be resisted. The emphasis must shift from finding the cause of the pain to helping the patient cope with symptoms.

Reassurance and education are extremely important. What is known about the pathogenesis of nonulcer dyspepsia and functional gastrointestinal disorders should be explained. Patients should be told that there are a large number of nerves and hormones in the gut that respond to a variety of poorly understood factors. Symptoms may arise from either an increased sensitivity to minor pain or distention, or from an increased reactivity to environmental or psychological factors that result in abnormal motility. It should be emphasized that the vast majority of people with functional disorders do not have psychological or functional impairment, lest the patient infer that the physician is implying he or she is "crazy" or that "it's all in my head." Fear that the symptoms will progress or degenerate into other illness should also be allayed.

It is important, early on, for the physician to set reasonable goals and expectations for the patient. The symptoms tend to be chronic and characterized by periods of exacerbation and remission. It will be necessary to learn to cope with these symptoms through lifestyle changes. While the physician can assist, he or she cannot "cure" the illness. On the other hand, the physician should reassure the patient that he or she will continue to follow and work with the patient, as necessary. The majority of patients will be reassured by the above approach and require little or no ongoing care. A follow-up visit should be scheduled initially to determine the patient's course and response to treatment. A subset of patients will require ongoing care, either intermittently during periods of symptom exacerbation or on a regular basis. The importance of this ongoing relationship cannot be overemphasized. In multiple clinical trials, the symptomatic response to placebo therapy has been over 50%. Although most primary care practitioners are not psychotherapists, patients clearly derive great benefit from a stable relationship with a concerned physician. Over the course of time, life events that trigger symptoms may become more apparent. Similarly, psychological difficulties that were not evident initially may become so with time. In some cases, referral to a trained psychologist, family counselor, or social worker may be indicated. If a trusting physician-patient relationship has been established, most patients will acquiesce to such a referral.

B. Lifestyle Changes: The patient's diet and medications should be reviewed for possible factors that may exacerbate symptoms. Although the role of foods in chronic dyspepsia is unclear, many patients report symptomatic improvement with dietary alterations. Coffee and excessive alcohol should be eliminated.

In some cases, a food diary may be helpful. In the diary, the patient should record foods ingested, level of symptoms, and daily activities. These chronicles may suggest foods or life stresses that may be precipitating symptoms but were previously not apparent to the patient.

Life stresses are present in virtually everyone's life, but modifying these factors may be impossible. Patients should be counseled on stress reduction measures, such as exercise and good eating and sleeping habits. Classes in stress reduction or meditation may be suitable for some people.

C. Medications: Drugs have been extremely disappointing in the management of nonulcer dyspepsia, and no agent is approved by the FDA for this indication. A large number of therapeutic trials have produced a hodgepodge of conflicting results. It should be borne in mind that most studies have shown a placebo response of 30–60%, which makes it difficult for active agents to demonstrate clear superiority. Furthermore, dyspeptic patients who respond well to standard therapies may be less inclined to enter clinical trials. Thus, these studies may select for a more unresponsive group of patients.

While symptoms may "improve" with pharmacologic therapy, complete symptom resolution is unusual. Moreover, it should be kept in mind that improvement may relate to the natural waxing and waning of the symptom course or to the placebo benefit, rather than to direct salutary effects of the drug. The focus of therapy should be upon lifestyle alterations and positive coping strategies rather than a search for a pharmacologic panacea. Short courses of drug therapy may be helpful for periods of symptom exacerbation, but attempts should be made to stop these agents. Chronic therapy should be continued only when there is a demonstrated benefit.

The following are the pharmacologic options for these patients.

1. Antacids–Many patients with intermittent dyspepsia report symptomatic benefit from antacids. Nevertheless, antacids have failed to demonstrate obvious benefit in controlled clinical trials. Given their safety and ease of use, it is reasonable to try these agents in patients with occasional dyspepsia.

2. Antisecretory agents–H_2-receptor antagonists have been tested in a number of clinical studies; approximately half of these studies have shown a therapeutic benefit over placebo and half have not. A meta-analysis of these studies suggests a therapeutic gain of about 20% for H_2-receptor antagonists over placebo. The greatest benefit is derived in patients with reflux-like dyspepsia. In contrast, patients with ulcer-like dyspepsia do not respond any better than other patients with dyspepsia. Given their excellent safety profile, a trial of H_2-antagonists is warranted in patients with chronic symptoms, particularly when atypical GERD is suspected. Proton pump inhibitors have not undergone testing in nonulcer dyspepsia.

3. Prokinetic drugs–Metoclopramide is a dopaminergic receptor antagonist that increases lower esophageal sphincter pressure and enhances gastric emptying. Cisapride is a serotonin 5-HT_4 agonist that has similar actions but also increases colonic motility. Due to its central antidopaminergic effects, metoclopramide causes significant central nervous system side effects in 10–20%, including lethargy, anxiety, and extrapyramidal effects. To avoid the risk of tardive dyskinesia it should not be used on a long-term basis. Cisapride is devoid of these actions and is extremely well tolerated.

These agents have demonstrated superiority to placebo in multiple European clinical trials but have not been sufficiently tested in the United States.

Overall, these studies report symptomatic improvement in 65–90% of patients. The mechanism of symptom improvement in unclear. Symptomatic benefit is not confined to the subset of patients with idiopathic gastroparesis or to patients with dysmotility-like symptoms. Similarly, there is an inconsistent correlation between symptom improvement and enhancement of gastric emptying. In patients with refractory symptoms, a trial of cisapride 10 mg three to four times a day, or metoclopramide 5–10 mg three times a day, is warranted.

4. Anti-*H pylori* treatment–As discussed above, there is no convincing evidence that *H pylori* plays a role in nonulcer dyspepsia. Many clinicians may choose to administer a trial of anti-*H pylori* therapy in patients with nonulcer dyspepsia who are known to harbor the organism. However, such therapy is not recommended outside of controlled clinical trials.

REFERENCES

Bytzer P et al: Empirical H_2-blocker therapy or prompt endoscopy in the management of dyspepsia. Lancet 1994;343:811.

Jones R: When is endoscopy appropriate in dyspepsia? Am J Gastroenterol 1993;88:981.

Malagelada JR: When and how to investigate the dyspeptic patient. Scand J Gastroenterol 1991;26(suppl 182):70.

Mayer E, Gebhart G: Basic and clinical aspects of visceral hyperalgesia. Gastroenterology 1994;107:271.

Richter JE: Dyspepsia: Organic causes and differential characteristics from functional dyspepsia. Scand J Gastroenterol 19991;26(Suppl 182):11.

Sobala G et al: Screening dyspepsia by serology to *Helicobacter pylori*. Lancet 1991;338:94.

Talley NJ: A critique of therapeutic trials in *Helicobacter pylori*-positive functional dyspepsia. Gastroenterology 1994;106:1174.

Talley NJ: Drug treatment of functional dyspepsia. Scand J Gastroenterol 1991;26(Suppl 182):47.

Talley NJ: Nonulcer dyspepsia: Current approaches to diagnosis and management. Am Fam Physician 1993;47:1407.

Talley NJ: Non-ulcer dyspepsia: Myths and realities. Aliment Pharmacol Ther 1991;5(Suppl 1):145.

Talley NJ et al: Lack of discriminant value of dyspepsia subgroups in patients referred for upper endoscopy. Gastroenterology 1993;105:1378.

Motility Disorders of the Stomach & Small Intestine

23

Michael Camilleri, MD, & Michael D. O'Brien, MD

Motility disorders of the stomach (**gastroparesis**) and small intestine (**chronic intestinal pseudo-obstruction**) are being increasingly recognized in clinical practice. They are typically characterized by acute, recurrent, or chronic symptoms of stasis in the stomach or small intestine in the absence of any obstruction within the lumen of the gut. These disorders result from impaired control of the gut by the nervous and muscular systems. They are sometimes associated with a generalized disease process that influences the extrinsic autonomic nervous system supply to the gut. This process may not only affect the stomach and small bowel but also other regions of the gastrointestinal tract and even extraintestinal organs, particularly the urinary bladder. Other motility disorders are characterized by accelerated transit of material through the stomach and small bowel.

Gastric & Small Bowel Motility

The motor functions of gastric and small bowel motility are characterized by distinct patterns of activity in the fasting and postprandial periods. The fasting period is characterized by the occurrence of a cyclic motor phenomenon called the **interdigestive migrating motor complex.** In healthy individuals, one cycle of this complex is completed every 60–90 minutes. This cycle has three phases: a period of quiescence (phase 1), a period of intermittent pressure activity (phase 2), and an activity front (phase 3), during which the stomach and small intestine contract at the highest frequency typical of each site (three frequencies per minute in the stomach and 11 or 12 per minute in the small intestine). The interdigestive activity front migrates for a variable distance down the small intestine; the frequency of contractions may be as high as 12 per minute in the duodenum and as low as 5 per minute in the ileum. Another characteristic motor pattern is seen in the distal small intestine; this is a propagated prolonged contraction, or power contraction, which serves to empty residue from the ileum to the colon in bolus transfers.

In the postprandial period, the cyclic activity previously described is replaced by a more irregular, but more consistent, pressure response, which is observed in all stomach and small bowel regions that are in contact with food. The maximum frequency of contractions is lower than that noted during phase 3 of the interdigestive migrating motor complex. Segments of the small intestine that are not in contact with digestive material may still be subject to the interdigestive process, so that interdigestive activity may be occurring in the distal small bowel at the same time that irregular postprandial contractile activity is occurring in the proximal small bowel, which is in contact with digestive material.

The contractile patterns previously described are associated with aboral movement of chyme in the stomach and small intestine. Liquids empty from the stomach in an exponential manner (eg, for nonnutrient liquids, the half-emptying time of the stomach in a healthy person is approximately 20 minutes or less). Solids are initially selectively retained within the stomach until particles have been triturated to a size of less than 2 mm diameter, at which point they can be emptied in a linear fashion from the stomach. Thus, the gastric emptying of solids is characterized by an initial lag period, followed by a more linear postlag gastric emptying phase. The small intestine transports solids and liquids at approximately the same rate, but because of the two phases of transport for solids in the stomach, liquids may arrive in the colon before the first portion of the solid material.

Control of Gastrointestinal Motor Function

Motor function of the gut is dependent on the contraction of smooth muscle cells and their integration and modulation by enteric and extrinsic nerves (Figure 23–1). The contractile state of the smooth muscle cells results from fluctuation of ions, which alter the electrical potential of the cell membrane. The enteric nervous system, a vast population of cells organized in ganglionated plexuses (with submucosal and myenteric plexuses predominant), consists of approximately 100 million neurons and is organized in intricate excitatory and inhibitory programmed circuits that have essential controlling function over such processes as peristalsis and the migrating motor

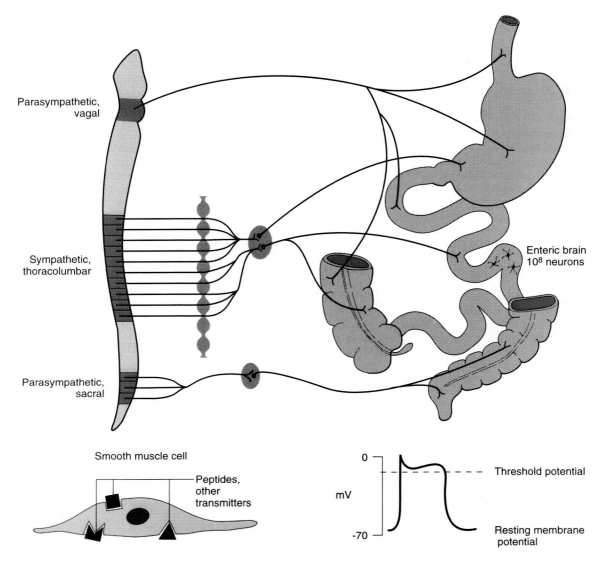

Figure 23–1. Control of gut motility. Interactions between extrinsic neural pathways and the intrinsic nervous system ("enteric brain") modulate contractions of gastrointestinal smooth muscle. Peptide-receptor interactions alter muscle membrane potentials by stimulating bidirectional ion fluxes. In turn, membrane characteristics dictate whether or not the muscle cell contracts. (Reproduced, by permission of Mayo Foundation, from Camilleri M, Phillips SF: Disorders of small intestinal motility. Gastroenterol Clin North Am 1989;18:405.)

complex. Enteric nerves are also important in visceral afferent function. The gastrointestinal tract has myelinated A δ fibers, which respond to phasically encoded stimuli, and polymodal unmyelinated C fibers, which tend to respond to more tonic stimuli; this is similar to somatic afferent function. These fibers may be important in producing pain and also the autonomic and emotional responses seen in patients with functional gastrointestinal disease. The extrinsic neural control is subdivided into the cranial and sacral parasympathetic outflow and the thoracolumbar sympathetic supply. The cranial outflow is predominantly through the vagus nerve, which supplies the region from the stomach down to the right side of the colon, and the sacral parasympathetic outflow, which supplies the left colon. The supply of sympathetic fibers to the stomach and small bowel arises from approximately levels T-5 to T-10 of the intermediolateral column of the spinal cord. The prevertebral sympathetic ganglia play an important role in the integration of afferent impulses from the gut with the central nervous system. Derangement of any of these intrinsic or extrinsic control mechanisms may lead to altered gut motor function.

Structural Diseases & Their Effect on Small Bowel Motility

Disturbances of proximal small bowel motility are frequently observed in symptomatic patients following gastric surgery. Uncoordinated phasic pressure waves occur in the Roux limb after Roux-en-Y gastrectomy. Dysfunction in the vagotomized gastric remnant may also play a role in producing symptoms, because tonic contractile activity of the gastric remnant is deranged after vagotomy and partial gastric resection, and, in practice, further resection of the gastric remnant relieves the symptoms of upper gut stasis in about two-thirds of patients.

Subacute mechanical obstruction is often associated with one of two contractile patterns of small bowel motility. Rhythmic, clustered contractions are a feature of partial obstruction; these occur postprandially, with each cluster lasting approximately 1 minute and each separated from the next by an interval of 1–2 minutes. These are nonspecific patterns, however. In other patients with distal mechanical obstruction, manometric studies of the proximal small bowel have revealed simultaneous prolonged contractions separated by periods of quiescence (Figure 23–2). This pattern was subsequently shown to have a positive predictive value of 80%. If such contractile patterns are present, mechanical obstruction must be excluded by careful enteroclysis, laparoscopy, or even laparotomy.

Small bowel fistulas, diverticula, and postsurgical blind loops are all associated with bacterial overgrowth, but the pathogenic sequence is not always clear. Experimentally, bacterial toxins induce migrating action potential complexes in the rabbit ileum, abnormal motility, rapid transit through the small bowel, diarrhea, and steatorrhea. It has also been suggested that multiple jejunal diverticulosis may result from abnormal neuromuscular function.

GASTROPARESIS & CHRONIC INTESTINAL PSEUDO-OBSTRUCTION

Pathogenesis

Although several factors are involved in the development of gastric or small bowel motility disturbances (Table 23–1), they can generally be characterized as neuropathic processes involving enteric and extrinsic nerves, and myopathic processes involving smooth muscle.

A. Neuropathic Processes:

1. Extrinsic nerves–Processes involving the extrinsic nervous system include diabetic autonomic neuropathy, amyloidosis, and a paraneoplastic syndrome usually associated with small cell carcinoma of the lung. Surgical vagotomy also disrupts these nerves. Use of certain medications, such as α_2-adrenergic agonists, calcium channel blockers, anticholinergic drugs, or opiate agents, may lead to motility disorders (eg, tricyclic antidepressants,

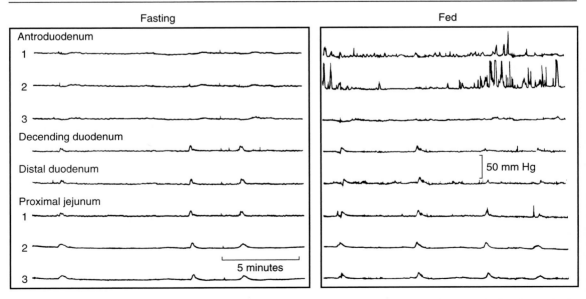

Figure 23–2. Gastroduodenal manometric recording of a 54-year-old female patient with systemic sclerosis and mechanical bowel obstruction. Note simultaneous prolonged contractions of low amplitude during fasting and following meals. (Reproduced, with permission, from Frank JW, Sarr MG, Camilleri M: Use of gastroduodenal manometry to differentiate mechanical and functional intestinal obstruction: An analysis of clinical outcome. Am J Gastroenterol 1994;89:339.)

Table 23–1. Classification of gastroparesis and chronic intestinal pseudo-obstruction.

Type	Myopathic	Neuropathic	Comments
Familial	Familial visceral myopathies (autosomal dominant or recessive)	Familial visceral neuropathies, von Recklinghausen's disease	Rare, often present in neonatal period or childhood; neurofibromas may also cause mechanical obstruction
Sporadic			
Infiltrative	Progressive systemic sclerosis Amyloidosis	Early progressive systemic sclerosis Amyloidosis	Manometry essential to differentiate pathophysiology
General neurologic disease	Myotonic and other dystrophies	Diabetes, porphyria, spinal cord transection, dysautonomias, multiple sclerosis, brain stem tumor	For review, see Camilleri M, 1990
Infectious		Chagas' disease, Norwalk virus, cytomegalovirus, Epstein-Barr virus	Nonspecific "postviral" causes appear to be common
Drug-induced		Tricyclic antidepressants, narcotics, anticholinergics, antihypertensives, vincristine, laxative abuse	Exclusion of drug side effects essential in all patients
Neoplastic		Paraneoplastic (small cell lung, carcinoid lung)	May require chest CT scan to exclude bronchial tumor if chest x-ray is negative
Idiopathic	Sporadic hollow visceral myopathy	Chronic idiopathic intestinal pseudo-obstruction	Variable manifestations and severity

nifedipine, narcotic analgesics, and antihypertensives such as clonidine).

2. Enteric nerves–Disorders of the enteric nervous system are usually the result of a degenerative, immune, or inflammatory process (Figure 23–3). Schuffler and co-workers have defined the morphologic characteristics of familial and sporadic abnormalities of enteric nerves by means of silver staining techniques. Although the cause can only rarely be ascertained, there clearly are examples of gastroparesis or pseudo-obstruction induced by Norwalk virus, cytomegalovirus, and Epstein-Barr virus. Degenerative disorders associated with infiltration of the myenteric plexus with inflammatory cells, including eosinophils, have also been identified. Idiopathic gastroparesis and chronic intestinal pseudo-obstruction are thought to occur in patients in whom there is no disturbance of extrinsic neural control and no underlying cause for the enteric neural abnormality.

B. Myopathic Processes: Disturbances of smooth muscle, including progressive systemic sclerosis and amyloidosis, may result in significant disorders of gastric emptying or small bowel transit. Rarely, dermatomyositis, dystrophia myotonica, and metabolic muscle disorders such as mitochondrial myopathy may be causes. There may be a positive family history with these disorders. A condition known as **hollow visceral myopathy** may occur either sporadically or in families. Rarely, motility disturbances may be the result of metabolic disorders such as hypothyroidism or hyperparathyroidism, but these more commonly manifest with constipation.

Clinical Findings

A. Symptoms and Signs:

1. Motility disorders in adults–The clinical features of gastroparesis and chronic intestinal pseudo-obstruction are quite similar. They typically include nausea, vomiting, early satiety, abdominal discomfort, distention, bloating, and anorexia. If stasis and vomiting are significant problems, there may be considerable weight loss, and disturbances of mineral and vitamin stores may result. The severity of the motility problem often manifests itself most clearly in the degree of nutritional and electrolyte depletion. The presence of abdominal distention and disturbances of bowel movements such as diarrhea or constipation indicate that the motility disorder is more extensive than gastroparesis. Significant vomiting may be complicated by the development of Mallory-Weiss tears, with gastrointestinal hemorrhage, and, on rare occasions, aspiration pneumonitis. As stated above, a more generalized motility disorder may have symptoms referable to abnormalities in esophageal clearance or colonic transit.

A careful family and medication history is crucial in defining underlying causes. A thorough review of all organ systems will help to identify patients with an underlying collagen vascular disease (such as scleroderma) or disturbances of extrinsic neural control that may be affecting the abdominal viscera. Symptoms include orthostatic dizziness; difficulties with erection or ejaculation; recurrent urinary tract infections; dry mouth, eyes, or vagina; difficulties with visual accommodation in bright lights; or absence of sweating.

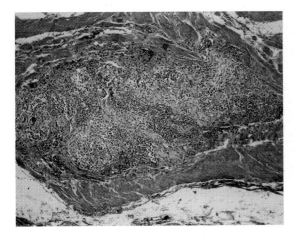

A

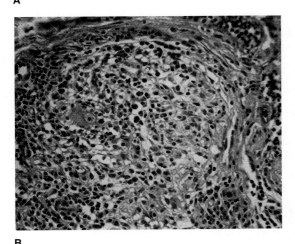

B

Figure 23–3. Mononuclear infiltration in the gastric enteric plexus from a patient with small cell lung cancer and paraneoplastic gastroparesis. **A:** The portion of the plexus rich in ganglion cells was expanded, but no necrosis was observed. Intact nerve fiber bundles can be seen. (Hematoxylin-eosin stain, original magnification × 100.) **B:** High-power view of the same field shows mature small lymphocytes and abundant plasma cells. Although neurons were decreased in number, a normal-appearing ganglion cell can be seen just above the center. (Hematoxylin-eosin stain, original magnification × 400.) (Reproduced, with permission, from Lennon VA et al: Enteric neuronal autoantibodies in pseudo-obstruction with small-cell lung carcinoma. Gastroenterology 1991;100:137.)

On physical examination, the presence of a succussion splash is usually indicative of a region of stasis within the gastrointestinal tract. The hands and mouth may show signs of Raynaud's phenomenon or scleroderma. Pupillary responses should be noted, the blood pressure should be taken in the supine and standing positions, and general features of peripheral neuropathy should be sought and external ocular

movements tested, to identify a possible neurologic disturbance or oculogastrointestinal dystrophy.

2. Pseudo-obstruction in children—In a survey of the North American Society of Pediatric Gastroenterology and Nutrition, 87 pediatric patients were identified, 19 of whom had symptoms at birth and 37 (43%) within the first month of life. This survey excluded Hirschsprung's disease, which should always be considered in the differential diagnosis of abnormal colonic motility or distention in children. Sixty-four percent of children with pseudo-obstruction were diagnosed by the first year of life. The predominant clinical features were distention (80%), vomiting and constipation (both 57%), diarrhea and failure to thrive (23%), and urinary tract abnormalities and failure to void (12%). Diagnosis was established by clinical features, radiologic studies, and laparotomy. Esophageal manometric findings were abnormal in all 14 patients in whom the procedure was performed. Anorectal manometric findings were usually unhelpful, being abnormal in only 1 of 16 patients studied. Full-thickness biopsies of the intestine were abnormal in 12 cases reported in this series (eight plexus disorders, four disorders of muscle degeneration), whereas 22 other miscellaneous gut biopsies were noncontributory. Among the group with adequate follow-up, 31.4% died; almost half the deaths were attributed to complications of central parenteral nutrition within the first 6 months of starting treatment. Other reports showed that antroduodenal pressure profiles and histopathologic features revealed abnormalities similar to those reported in adults.

3. Localized forms of pseudo-obstruction—There are numerous reports of localized forms of chronic pseudo-obstruction, usually affecting the entire colon or the duodenal loop in "superior mesenteric artery syndrome." Surgical treatment is sometimes justifiable and efficacious in these disorders, particularly when the colon is affected.

B. Diagnostic Steps: Four questions should be considered in the diagnosis of each patient:

(1) Is the presentation an acute or chronic problem?
(2) Is the disease due to a neuropathy or a myopathy?
(3) What is the status of hydration and nutrition?
(4) Which regions of the digestive tract are affected?

These questions can be answered by the thorough physiologic assessment described below. These steps are essential for planning therapy for each patient.

1. Suspect and exclude mechanical obstruction—The presence of a motility disorder of the stomach or small bowel should be suspected whenever a large volume of material is aspirated from the stomach, particularly after overnight fasting. Another sign is nondigestible solid food or large volumes of liquids observed during esophagogastroduodenoscopy. Barium studies may fortuitously suggest the presence of a motor disorder, particularly if there is gross dilatation or dilution of barium, or retained solid food within the stomach. These studies rarely identify the causative factor, except in the case of small bowel systemic sclerosis, which is characterized by megaduodenum and the presence of packed valvulae conniventes in the small intestine. Diagnosis of a motility disorder, therefore, depends on careful history taking and confirmation by functional tests. The standard approach is to exclude mechanical obstruction by means of endoscopy and a small bowel x-ray.

2. Assess gastric and small bowel motor activity—Once mechanical obstruction or an alternative diagnosis such as Crohn's disease has been excluded, a transit profile of the stomach or small bowel, or both, is indicated (Figure 23–4). In the authors' experience, efficiency in the emptying of solids is the best indicator of normal or abnormal activity (Figure 23–5). These tests can now be performed relatively simply and at fairly low cost, and are especially helpful when scanning is done immediately after ingestion of a radiolabeled meal and then 2, 4, and 6 hours later (Figure 23–6). Once functional impairment of motor activity has been documented, history taking should focus on an obvious causative factor such as a medication or other disease

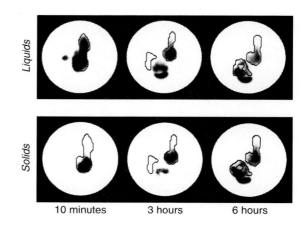

Figure 23–5. Transit of radiolabeled solids and liquids in a patient with chronic (neuropathic) intestinal pseudo-obstruction. Note the prolonged retention of both phases of the meal in the stomach and small bowel. The upper outline depicts the stomach, and the lower outline depicts the right side of the colon on 3- and 6-hour scans. (Reproduced, with permission, from Camilleri et al: Impaired transit of chyme in chronic intestinal pseudo-obstruction: correction by cisopride. Gastroenterology 1986;91:619.)

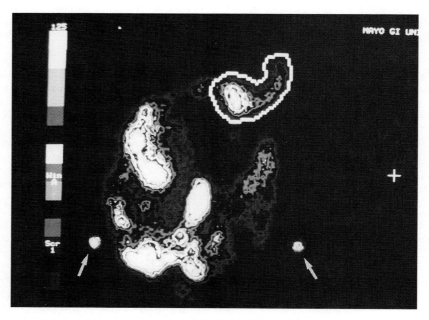

Figure 23–4. Radioscintigraphic image from a gastrointestinal transit study performed in the same patient. Arrows indicate reference markers placed on the iliac crests; the gastric area has been outlined, and the dilated duodenum and pooling of radiolabeled material in the distal ileum is again apparent. (Reproduced, with permission, from Greydanus MP et al: Ileocolonic transfer of solid chyme in small intestinal neuropathies and myopathies. Gastroenterology 1990;99:158.)

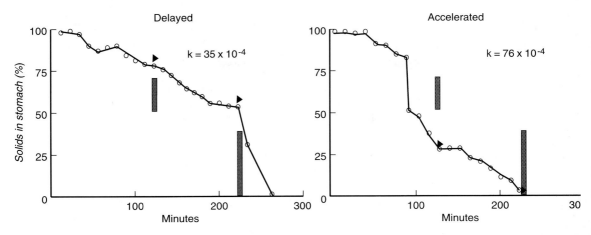

Figure 23–6. Simplified measurement of gastric emptying. The bar shows normal gastric retention at 2 and 4 hours. The graph on the right shows a gastric emptying curve in a patient with rapid transit (k as shown). The simplified analysis at 2 hours correctly detects rapid transit, as compared with data from a healthy person. The graph on the left shows a gastric emptying curve in a patient with slow transit (k as shown). The simplified analyses *(solid triangle)* at 2 and 4 hours correctly detect slow gastric emptying, as compared with data from a healthy person. k = emptying rate constant by power exponential analysis ($N = 41 - 66 \times 10^{-4}$). (Reproduced, with permission, from Thomforde GM et al: Prospective evaluation of an inexpensive screening scintigraphic test of gastric emptying. J Nucl Med 1995;36:93–96.)

such as diabetes mellitus that might account for the impairment.

If the cause is obvious, it is usually unnecessary to pursue any further investigations. If the cause is unclear, upper gastrointestinal manometry, using a multilumen tube with sensors strategically placed in the distal stomach and proximal small intestine (Figure 23–7), will differentiate between a neuropathic and myopathic process (Figure 23–8). Neuropathic conditions are characterized by normal contraction amplitude but uncoordinated contractile activity at the level of the stomach and small intestine. The neuro-pathic pressure profile shows a reduction in frequency of contractions, with normal contraction amplitude at the level of the stomach (antral hypomotility) or abnormalities in the propagation or coordination of fasting migrating motor complexes or postprandial motor patterns. Myopathic conditions are characterized by markedly reduced contraction amplitude but well-coordinated contractile activity.

The role of other noninvasive tests such as electrogastrography, impedance tomography, and ultrasound is controversial, because it is still unclear whether they provide clinically useful information.

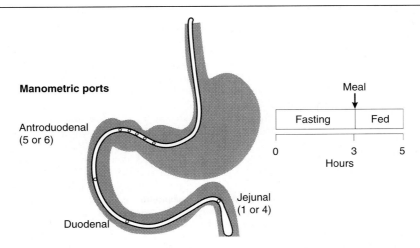

Figure 23–7. Experimental protocol for measuring upper gastrointestinal motility. The patient has taken no medications for 48 hours and eats a 535-kcal meal during the study.

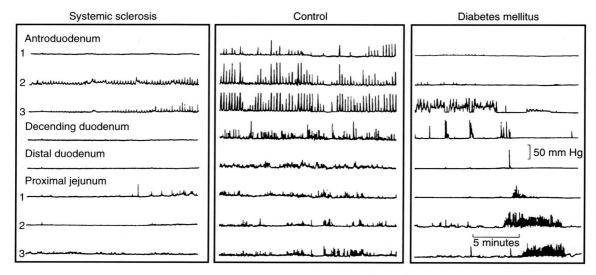

Figure 23–8. Postprandial manometric profile in small bowel dysmotility due to myopathy (systemic sclerosis) and neuropathy (diabetes mellitus). (Reproduced, with permission, from Camilleri M et al: Medical treatment of chronic intestinal pseudo-obstruction. Practical Gastroenterol 1991;15:10.)

The chief benefits of manometry are differentiation of neuropathic and myopathic dysmotility and assessment of both stomach and small bowel. The information obtained facilitates diagnosis and treatment.

3. Identify the pathogenesis—In the presence of a neuropathic pattern of motor activity in the small intestine, it is necessary to pursue further investigations, such as autonomic function tests, search for an antineuronal enteric antibody (a feature of paraneoplastic motility disorders), MRI of the brain, and, on rare occasions, a laparoscopically obtained full-thickness biopsy of the small intestine. Autonomic testing identifies the presence of sympathetic adrenergic, sympathetic cholinergic, or vagal neuropathies. These abnormalities are revealed by orthostatic hypotension, changes in plasma norepinephrine levels when the patient is in the supine and standing positions, abnormal quantitative sudomotor axon reflex tests, and abnormal tests for vagal function (eg, the heart interval change during deep breathing and the plasma pancreatic polypeptide response to modified sham feeding). These investigations will identify an underlying cause of the neuropathic process.

Current researchers are attempting to characterize the neuronal transmitters in enteric plexuses. Several conditions in which there is absence of relaxation of a gut segment have been shown to be associated with deficiencies of the inhibitory transmitters, vasoactive intestinal polypeptide, somatostatin, and nitric oxide (eg, achalasia, congenital esophageal stenosis, congenital hypertrophic pyloric stenosis, and Hirschsprung's disease). It is hypothesized that altered neurotransmitter populations result in some of the "idiopathic" syndromes causing gastroparesis or pseudo-obstruction.

Myopathic disorders are characterized by low amplitude but well-coordinated pressure profiles in the stomach or small intestine; such a pattern should lead to a search for amyloidosis (immunoglobulin electrophoresis, fat aspirate, or rectal biopsy), systemic sclerosis (SCL-70), or a family history of hollow visceral myopathy. Special staining techniques of a full-thickness biopsy specimen may be needed to identify metabolic muscle disorders such as mitochondrial myopathy.

4. Identify complications—It is important to look for complications of the motor disorder, including nutritional deficiencies, inadequacies in essential elements and vitamins, and bacterial overgrowth in patients presenting with diarrhea. Bacterial overgrowth is relatively uncommon in neuropathic disorders but more common in myopathic conditions, presumably because the amplitude of contractions is insufficient to clear residue from the small intestine.

Differential Diagnosis

The major conditions to be differentiated are mechanical obstruction, such as may occur because of peptic stricture or Crohn's disease in the small intestine, and the eating disorders, particularly anorexia nervosa. There is impairment of gastric emptying in anorexia nervosa, but to a minor degree compared with that of the more obvious motor disturbances such as diabetic gastroparesis or postvagotomy gastric stasis.

Treatment

A thorough physiologic assessment must be done for each patient, as described in the preceding section, "Diagnostic Steps," before a therapeutic plan can be designed. The principle methods of management are correction of hydration and nutritional deficiencies, use of prokinetic and antiemetic medications, suppression of bacterial overgrowth, decompression, and surgical treatment.

A. Correction of Hydration and Nutritional Deficiencies: Correction of dehydration and electrolyte and nutritional depletion is particularly important during acute exacerbations of gastroparesis or chronic intestinal pseudo-obstruction syndromes. Nutritional support should be tailored to the severity of the deficiencies of trace elements and dietary constituents in each individual patient. Initial dietary measures include use of low-fiber supplements with addition of iron folate, calcium, and vitamins D, K, and B_{12}. In patients with more worrisome symptoms, such as severe diabetic gastroparesis or myopathic pseudo-obstruction, enteral or parenteral supplementation of nutrition may be necessary. If it is anticipated that enteral supplementation may be required for more than 3 months, it is usually best to provide feedings through a jejunostomy tube, which can now be placed with laparoscopic techniques in most patients. Gastrotomy tubes should not be used, because of gastroparesis. In more severely affected patients, parenteral nutrition may be necessary, although experience suggests that many patients continue to tolerate some oral feeding.

B. Prokinetics and Medications: Medications are being increasingly used for the treatment of neuromuscular motility disorders. Regrettably, there is little evidence that they are effective in myopathic disturbances, except for the rare case of dystrophia myotonica affecting the stomach and for small bowel scleroderma.

1. Erythromycin—Erythromycin, a macrolide antibiotic that stimulates motilin receptors, possibly by a cholinergic mechanism, results in the dumping of solids from the stomach. This drug markedly facilitates the emptying of nondigestible solid residue from the stomach (eg, bezoars in patients with diabetic gastroparesis). The effect of oral erythromycin appears to be restricted by tolerance. Although initial studies demonstrated effectiveness in patients with diabetic gastroparesis treated for 2 weeks, there is little evidence that continued therapy results in improvement of emptying problems and associated symptoms in these patients. Many patients develop gastrointestinal upset, which precludes use of erythromycin for longer than 1 month. Erythromycin is most effective when it is used intravenously during acute exacerbations, particularly while the patient is hospitalized for dehydration and electrolyte depletion. The usual dose of erythromycin lactobionate is 3 mg/kg by an infusion every 8 hours.

2. Cisapride—Cisapride is a substituted benzamide that acts as a serotonin 5-HT$_4$ agonist, but it has none of the central antidopaminergic or hormonal side effects associated with the other substituted benzamide, metoclopramide. Cisapride is probably the most effective prokinetic drug available at the present time, and there is evidence that it stimulates clearance from the esophagus, emptying from the stomach, transit in the small bowel, and, possibly, transit through the colon. Cisapride has been effective in correcting objective parameters of altered motility, such as impaired gastric emptying in patients with both gastroparesis and chronic intestinal pseudo-obstruction. In long-term trials, it has been associated with weight gain and has facilitated oral supplementation of nutrition. It may be given in doses of 5–20 mg orally, 3 or 4 times daily.

3. Octreotide—Octreotide, a cyclized analog of somatostatin, has been shown to induce activity fronts in the small intestine that mimic the interdigestive migrating motor complex. There was hope initially that this drug would improve small intestinal motor function in patients with small bowel scleroderma, since patients given the drug in an open trial for up to 15 days appeared to improve. More recent experience suggests that the small bowel motility induced is not well coordinated and is characterized by a simultaneous or very rapidly propagated activity front through the small intestine. In healthy individuals, relatively low dosages of octreotide (50 μg three times a day) result in marked impairment of small bowel transit. Its therapeutic efficacy in patients with intestinal dysmotility needs to be further assessed in clinical trials.

4. Antiemetics—There is an important role for standard antiemetics such as diphenhydramine, trifluoperazine, or metoclopramide in relieving symptoms of nausea and vomiting. The more expensive serotonin 5-HT$_3$ antagonists (eg, ondansetron) have not proved to be of greater benefit than these less expensive medications.

5. Antibiotics—In patients with symptomatic bacterial overgrowth, antibiotic therapy is indicated. Although no trials have actually been performed, it is common practice to use a different antibiotic for 7–10 days each month, in an attempt to avoid development of resistance. Typical antibiotics used are doxycycline, 100 mg twice daily; metronidazole, 500 mg three times daily; ciprofloxacin, 500 mg twice daily; or double-strength trimethaprim-sulfamethoxazole, two tablets twice daily. These measures usually result in significant symptomatic relief in patients with diarrhea and fat malabsorption.

C. Decompression: Decompression is rarely necessary in patients with chronic pseudo-obstruction. Venting enterostomy (jejunostomy) is effective in relieving abdominal distention and bloating, and has been shown to significantly reduce the frequency of nasogastric intubations or hospitalizations required for acute exacerbations in patients with severe intestinal pseudo-obstruction requiring central parenteral nutrition. Access to the small intestine by enterostomy also provides a way to deliver nutrients by the enteral route. This may even be possible in patients with chronic intestinal pseudo-obstruction, where the motility disorder is often intermittent and not persistent. Currently available enteral tubes allow for aspiration and feeding by a single apparatus.

D. Surgical Treatment: Surgical treatment should be considered whenever the motility disorder is localized to a portion of the gut that can be resected. In clinical practice, the three instances that most commonly lend themselves to this approach are: colectomy and ileoproctostomy for intractable constipation associated with chronic colonic pseudo-obstruction; duodenojejunostomy, or duodenoplasty for patients with megaduodenum or duodenal atresia in children; and completion gastrectomy for patients with postgastric surgical stasis syndrome.

E. Pseudo-obstruction in Children: Neonatal pseudo-obstruction rarely occurs as a single disorder; it is more often found in association with other anomalies requiring surgical correction, including gastroschisis, duodenal atresia, or megalocystis. Prokinetic medications are usually ineffective, and many patients require parenteral nutrition and bowel decompression, including gastrostomy or enterostomy.

Prognosis

The prognosis depends on the severity of the individual case. Patients with suspected postviral gastroparesis appear to have an overall positive prognosis, with restoration of nutrition and reduction of symptoms over the first 2 years. Patients with myopathic, dilated bowel have persistent symptoms, are more prone to develop bacterial overgrowth, and usually require long-term parenteral nutrition, with its inherent complications. Between these two ends of the spectrum are patients with mild to moderately severe motility disorders, who have recurrent or chronic symptoms. They can usually be managed on an outpatient basis with maintenance of nutrition, if certain dietary supplementations and measures are instituted to provide symptomatic relief, including medications and decompression. There is no formal analysis of the natural history of motility disorders, and current impressions are based on anecdotal reports or data from open 1-year trials of medications for these disorders.

DUMPING SYNDROME & ACCELERATED GASTRIC EMPTYING

Typically, these conditions follow truncal vagotomy and gastric drainage procedures. Now that vagotomy is being used more selectively in the surgical treatment of peptic ulcer disease, the prevalence of these problems seems to be decreasing.

The pathophysiology of rapid gastric emptying is thought to be related to an impaired accommodation response of the stomach upon ingestion of food. Intragastric pressure is relatively high and results in active propulsion of liquid foods from the stomach. A high caloric (usually carbohydrate) content of the liquid phase of the meal evokes a rapid insulin response, with secondary hypoglycemia. These patients may also have impaired antral contractility and gastric stasis of solids, which may paradoxically result in a clinical picture of both gastroparesis (for solids) and dumping (for liquids).

The most useful investigation is a dual-phase radioisotopic gastric emptying test (Figure 23–9).

Management of dumping includes patient education regarding dietary maneuvers (avoidance of high-nutrient liquid drinks and, possibly, addition of guar gum or pectin to retard emptying) and, rarely, pharmacologic treatment with a drug such as octreotide, 50–100 µg given subcutaneously before meals.

Accelerated gastric emptying of liquids occurs in patients with non-insulin-dependent diabetes mellitus who do not have autonomic dysfunction. Recent data refute an earlier hypothesis that this was an important mechanism of postprandial hyperglycemia in these patients. The mechanism and significance of accelerated liquid emptying in this disorder is the subject of ongoing investigation.

RAPID TRANSIT DYSMOTILITY OF THE SMALL BOWEL

Rapid transit of material through the small bowel may be a minor component of an illness (eg, irritable bowel syndrome) or a major component that results in significant loss of fluid and osmotically active solutes, so that colonic capacitance and reabsorptive capacity are overwhelmed and severe diarrhea results. Examples include postvagotomy diarrhea, short bowel syndrome, diabetic diarrhea, and carcinoid diarrhea.

Clinical Findings

These disturbances may be confirmed by scintigraphic studies or by the lactulose-hydrogen breath test. Manometric studies of the small bowel may reveal prolonged duration, high amplitude, and rapid propagation of contractions, and rapidly propagated spike bursts may be seen on intraluminal electromyographic studies. These studies are not widely available in most clinical settings, however. Similar myoelectric activity has been noted in a series of bacterial or toxic diarrheas induced in experimental animals.

Idiopathic bile acid catharsis may represent an inability of the distal ileum to reabsorb bile acids because of rapid transit and reduced contact time with ileal mucosa. It may then induce cholerrheic enteropathy with colonic secretion.

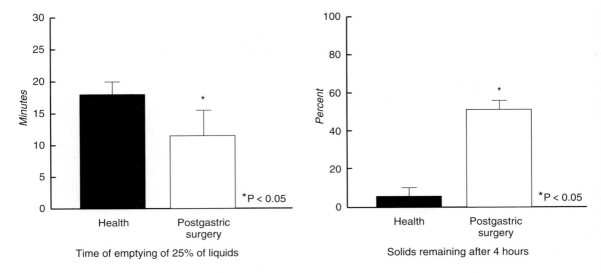

Figure 23–9. Gastric emptying of liquids and solids in healthy controls (black bars; n = 17) and postgastric surgery patients (white bars; n = 16). The time necessary for 25% of the liquids to empty is shorter in the postsurgical group; the proportion of solid radiolabeled material remaining in the stomach after 4 hours is larger in the postsurgical group. Data are means plus or minus standard error of the mean. (Reproduced, with permission, from Fich A et al: Stasis syndromes following gastric surgery: Clinical and motility features of 60 symptomatic patients. J Clin Gastroenterol 1990;12:505.)

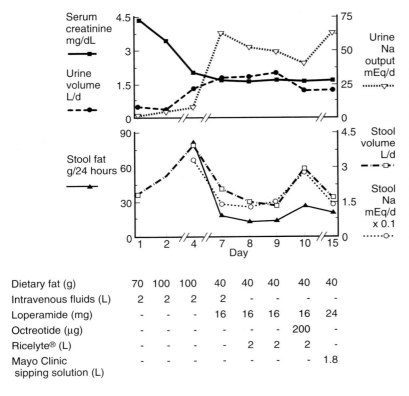

Figure 23–10. *Top:* Renal function during therapeutic trials and balance studies in a 54-year-old woman with short-gut syndrome. Note the improvement in renal function and steady increase in output of urinary sodium; a slight impairment occurred after administration of octreotide. *Bottom:* Stool output in the same woman. Note the dramatic decrease in stool fat, sodium, and volume after institution of a 40-g fat diet; a temporary increase occurred during treatment with octreotide. Note also the close parallelism between output of fat, volume, and sodium; this finding suggests an important role for malabsorbed products of digestion of fat in high stomal output. (Reproduced, with permission, from Camilleri M et al: Balance studies and polymeric glucose solution to optimize therapy after massive intestinal resection. Mayo Clin Proc 1992;67:755.)

Dietary fat (g)	70	100	100	40	40	40	40	40
Intravenous fluids (L)	2	2	2	2	-	-	-	-
Loperamide (mg)	-	-	-	16	16	16	16	24
Octreotide (μg)	-	-	-	-	-	-	200	-
Ricelyte® (L)	-	-	-	-	2	2	2	-
Mayo Clinic sipping solution (L)	-	-	-	-	-	-	-	1.8

Treatment

The objectives of treatment are restoration of hydration and nutrition and retardation of small bowel transit.

A. Nutritional Therapy: Dietary interventions include the avoidance of hyperosmolar drinks (eg, virtually all soft drinks), and the use of isosmolar or hyposmolar rehydration solutions. The fat content in the diet should be reduced to approximately 50 g, to avoid delivery of unabsorbed fat to the colon, where the metabolites are cathartic. All nutritional deficiencies (commonly, deficiencies of calcium, magnesium, potassium, and water- and fat-soluble vitamins) should be corrected (Figure 23–10).

B. Drug Therapy: An approach that has been shown to be effective is an opioid agent given at a high dosage (eg, loperamide, 4 mg three times daily) 30 minutes before each meal and at bedtime to suppress the gastrocolonic response, then verapamil, 40 mg twice daily, or clonidine, 0.1 mg twice daily, is added. If these are ineffective or produce unacceptable side effects, octreotide is used, starting at 50 µg given subcutaneously three times daily.

In patients with less than 1 meter of residual small bowel, it may be impossible to maintain fluid and electrolyte homeostasis without parenteral support, but in patients with a longer residual segment, oral nutrition, pharmacotherapy, and supplements are almost always effective for this purpose.

SUMMARY

Disorders of gastric and small bowel motility may result in either stasis or accelerated transit; understanding the mechanisms that control motility and pathophysiology in an individual patient is the key to optimal management. Simple, quantitative measures of transit and an algorithmic approach to identifying the underlying cause may lead to correction of abnormal function. Alternatively, correction of dehydration and nutritional depletion and symptomatic relief constitute important steps to manage these chronic, often debilitating conditions. Patient education is essential to avoid aggravation of symptoms because of dietary indiscretions.

REFERENCES

Camilleri M: Appraisal of medium- and long-term treatment of gastroparesis and chronic intestinal dysmotility. Am J Gastroenterol 1993;169.

Camilleri M: Disorders of gastrointestinal motility in neurologic diseases. Mayo Clin Proc 1990;65:825.

Camilleri M, Ford MJ: Functional gastrointestinal disease and the autonomic nervous system: A way ahead? (Editorial.) Gastroenterology 1994;106:1114.

Camilleri M et al: Balance studies and polymeric glucose solution to optimize therapy after massive intestinal resection. Mayo Clin Proc 1992;67:755.

Camilleri M et al: Effect of six weeks of treatment with cisapride in gastroparesis and intestinal pseudo-obstruction. Gastroenterology 1989;96:704.

Camilleri M et al: Towards a less costly but accurate test of gastric emptying and small bowel transit. Dig Dis Sci 1991;36:609.

Colemont L, Camilleri M: Chronic intestinal pseudo-obstruction: Diagnosis and treatment. Mayo Clin Proc 1989;64:60.

Farthing MJ: Octreotide in dumping and short bowel syndromes. Digestion 1993;54:47.

Frank JW, Sarr MG, Camilleri M: Use of gastroduodenal manometry to differentiate mechanical and functional intestinal obstruction: An analysis of clinical outcome. Am J Gastroenterology 1994;89:339.

Greydanus MP et al: Ileocolonic transfer of solid chyme in small intestinal neuropathies and myopathies. Gastroenterology 1990;99:158.

Haruma K, Wiste JA, Camilleri M: Effect of octreotide on gastrointestinal pressure profiles in health, functional and organic gastrointestinal disorders. Gut 1994;35:1064.

Krishnamurthy S, Schuffler MD: Pathology of neuromuscular disorders of the small intestine and colon. Gastroenterology 1987;93:610.

Pitt HA et al: Chronic intestinal pseudo-obstruction: Management with total parenteral nutrition and a venting enterostomy. Arch Surg 1985;120:614.

Soudah HC, Hasler WL, Owyang C: Effect of octreotide on intestinal motility and bacterial overgrowth in scleroderma. N Engl J Med 1991;325:1461.

Vantrappen G et al: The interdigestive motor complex of normal subjects and patients with bacterial overgrowth of the small intestine. J Clin Invest 1977;59:1158.

Vargas JH, Sachs P, Ament ME: Chronic intestinal pseudo-obstruction syndrome in pediatrics: Results of a national survey by members of the North American Society of Pediatric Gastroenterology and Nutrition. J Pediatr Gastroenterol Nutr 1988;7:323.

von der Ohe M et al: Motor dysfunction of the small bowel and colon in patients with the carcinoid syndrome and diarrhea. N Engl J Med 1993;329:1073.

von der Ohe MR, Thomforde GM, Camilleri M: Differential regional effects of octreotide on human gastrointestinal motor function. Gut 1995;36:743–748.

Malabsorption Disorders

24

Lawrence R. Schiller, MD

Each day the average person consumes 2000–3000 kcal of food. Most of this caloric load is in the form of polymers or other complex compounds that must be broken down into smaller molecules, to be transported across the small intestinal mucosa. Thus, proteins are cleaved into dipeptides and amino acids, starches are split into monosaccharides, and fats are broken down into fatty acids and monoglycerides. The processes of digestion and absorption are complex and often go awry. Nearly 200 conditions are associated with defects in this process and can produce substantial disability.

General Considerations

Strictly speaking, **maldigestion** refers to impaired hydrolysis of luminal contents, and **malabsorption** refers to impaired transport across the mucosa. In clinical practice, malabsorption is used to describe the end result of either defect.

Malabsorption may involve a broad range of nutrients (**panmalabsorption**) or only an individual nutrient or class of nutrients (specific malabsorption). This distinction can be helpful in the differential diagnosis of malabsorption.

The many causes of malabsorption can be sorted pathophysiologically into conditions that are associated with: (1) impaired luminal hydrolysis, (2) impaired mucosal function (mucosal hydrolysis, uptake, and packaging), and (3) impaired removal of nutrients from the mucosa (Table 24–1).

Essentials of Diagnosis

- Steatorrhea (foul-smelling, greasy stools with increased fat excretion) or chronic watery diarrhea
- Increased flatus
- Weight loss, signs of vitamin and mineral deficiencies (anemia, easy bruising, tetany, osteoporosis)

Clinical Findings

A. Symptoms and Signs (Table 24–2): Most patients with malabsorption have changes in their stools. Classically, steatorrhea (excess fat) is present. Typical characteristics of steatorrhea include a pale color, bulkiness, greasiness, and tendency to float (because of incorporated gas). Less commonly, patients with malabsorption present with watery stools resulting from the osmotic effects of unabsorbed carbohydrates and short-chain fatty acids.

Abdominal distention and gaseousness are common and most often a result of fermentation of unabsorbed carbohydrates by colonic bacteria. The presence of excess flatus may be the only finding in patients with some specific malabsorptive problems, such as lactase deficiency.

Weight loss is common in patients with severe panmalabsorption, but may not be seen in patients with more limited forms of malabsorption. It usually is substantial early in the course of the illness, but usually levels off with time as body weight and calorie absorption again come into balance. This is contrast to the progressive weight loss seen with tuberculosis or cancer. If weight loss is progressive with malabsorption, conditions such as inflammatory bowel disease or lymphoma should be considered.

Vitamin and mineral deficiencies can lead to several problems. Anemia is common, but not universal. Iron deficiency anemia may be the only finding in some patients with celiac disease, for instance. More typically anemia is part of a spectrum of findings. Microcytic anemia may also be seen in Whipple's disease (in which occult blood loss is frequent) and in lymphomas presenting with malabsorption. Macrocytic anemias complicate malabsorption when folate or B_{12} deficiency is present.

Deficiencies of the fat soluble vitamins, D, K, and A, sometimes produce symptoms. Since substantial stores of these vitamins are maintained in the body, deficiency indicates longstanding malabsorption or inadequate intake. Vitamin D deficiency can produce osteomalacia, bone pain, cramps, and tetany resulting from hypocalcemia. Vitamin K deficiency can cause easy bruising and ecchymosis. Vitamin A deficiency sometimes produces night blindness.

Deficiencies of water soluble vitamins (other than folate and B_{12} seldom produce identifiable clinical manifestations by the time patients seek medical attention. Glossitis and cheilosis are probably the most common manifestations; findings of overt beriberi,

Table 24–1. Causes of malabsorption or maldigestion.

Impaired luminal hydrolysis or solubilization
  Pancreatic exocrine insufficiency
  Bile acid deficiency
  Zollinger-Ellison syndrome
  Post-gastrectomy malabsorption
  Rapid intestinal transit
  Small bowel bacterial overgrowth
Impaired mucosal hydrolysis, uptake or packaging
  Brush border or metabolic disorders
    Lactase deficiency
    Sucrase-isomaltase deficiency
    Glucose-galactose malabsorption
    Abetalipoproteinemia
  Mucosal diseases
    Celiac sprue
    Collagenous sprue
    Nongranulomatous ulcerative jejunoileitis
    Eosinophilic gastroenteritis
    Systemic mastocytosis
    Immunoproliferative small intestinal disease (IPSID)
    Lymphoma
    Crohn's disease
    Radiation enteritis
    Amyloidosis
  Infectious diseases
    Tropical sprue
    Whipple's disease
    Parasitic diseases
    Mcyobacterium avium-intracellulare
    AIDS enteropathy
  After intestinal resection
Impaired removal of nutrients
  Lymphangiectasia
  Chronic mesenteric ischemia

pellagra, scurvy and other classic vitamin-deficiency syndromes are rarely seen unless a substantial period of malnutrition has been present.

Constitutional symptoms of chronic fatigue and weakness are often present. Appetite is typically well-maintained until vitamin and other deficiencies

Table 24–2. Symptoms and signs of malabsorption.

Changes in stools
  Pale, bulky, greasy stools
  Watery diarrhea
  Floating stools
Increased colonic gas production
  Abdominal distention
  Borborygmi
Weight loss, muscle wasting
Vitamin and mineral deficiencies
  Anemia
  Cheilosis
  Glossitis
  Dermatitis
  Neuropathy
  Night blindness
  Osteomalacia
  Paresthesia
  Tetany
  Ecchymosis
Fatigue, weakness
Edema

develop. Edema is uncommon until late in the course, unless there is coexisting protein-losing enteropathy.

Abdominal pain is not usually present with malabsorption syndrome. Usually it involves only modest cramping associated with diarrhea. If pain is more severe, the physician should consider the possibilities of chronic pancreatitis, Zollinger-Ellison syndrome, lymphoma, Crohn's disease, or intestinal ischemia.

Signs and symptoms elsewhere in the body may also be related to malabsorption or to the disorder causing malabsorption. Aphthous ulcers in the mouth may be associated with celiac disease, Behçet's syndrome or Crohn's disease. Iritis may be seen with Crohn's disease and conjunctivitis with Behçet's syndrome. Skin abnormalities may be seen in some conditions. Whipple's disease is associated with hyperpigmentation, and dermatitis herpetiformis (which produces a pruritic, blistering skin eruption) is associated with celiac disease. Tightening of the skin, digital ulceration, nail changes and Raynaud's phenomenon suggest scleroderma. A history of chronic sinusitis, bronchitis, and pneumonia should raise the question of cystic fibrosis in a child or young adult.

Several systemic diseases can produce malabsorption (Table 24–3). Symptoms and signs suggesting these conditions may be present.

B. Laboratory Tests (Table 24–4):

1. Routine blood tests—Patients with established panmalabsorption typically have several laboratory abnormalities. Conversely, patients with isolated malabsorption may have no laboratory abnormalities.

The complete blood cell count may show a microcytic or macrocytic anemia depending on the specific condition causing malabsorption. The white blood cell count and platelet counts are usually normal. Lymphopenia may be present in patients with AIDS or lymphangiectasia. High platelet counts can be seen with iron deficiency.

Biochemical screening tests often will show one or more abnormalities. Hypokalemia, chloride depletion and acid-base abnormalities may be present, due to a combination of poor intake and excessive loss in

Table 24–3. Systemic diseases associated with malabsorption.

Endocrine diseases
  Diabetes mellitus
  Hyperthyroidism
  Hypothyroidism
  Addison's disease
  Hypoparathyroidism
Collagen-vascular diseases
  Scleroderma
  Vasculitis (systemic lupus erythematosus, polyarteritis nodosa)
Amyloidosis
AIDS

Table 24–4. Laboratory tests in malabsorption.

Routine blood tests	
Complete blood count	
Microcytic anemia	Blood loss, iron malabsorption
Macrocytic anemia	Vitamin B_{12} or folate deficiency
Lymphopenia	AIDS, lymphangiectasia
Thrombocytosis	Iron deficiency
Biochemical screening tests	
Hypokalemia	Poor patassium intake, excessive stool losses
Low blood urea nitrogen	Poor protein intake
Low serum creatinine	Muscle wasting
Low serum calcium	Calcium malabsorption, vitamin D deficiency, fat malabsorption, hypomagnesemia
Low serum albumin	Protein losing enteropathy, concurrent acute disease
Prothrombin time	
Extended	Poor vitamin K intake, chronic steatorrhea, colectomy
Blood levels of potentially malabsorbed substances	
Serum iron, vitamin B_{12}, folate, 25-OH vitamin D, carotene	Reduced in malabsorption or prolonged inadequate intake
Tests of fat absorption	
Qualitative fecal fat	May be normal with mild or moderate steatorrhea
Quantitative fecal fat	Useful for follow-up, affected by stool weight
Tests of protein absorption	
Fecal nitrogen excretion	Adds little to assessment
α-antitrypsin clearance	Useful to identify protein-losing enteropathy
Tests of carbohydrate absorption	
Quantitative excretion (anthrone)	Does not account for colonic salvage
Stool pH <5.5	Characteristic for carbohydrate malabsorption
Osmotic gap in stool water	Not specific
Stool reducing substances	May be positive with reducing substances other than carbohydrates
D-xylose absorption test	Measure urine and blood concentrations, low results suggest proximal intestinal dysfunction
Oral glucose, sucrose, lactose tolerance tests	May be misleading in patients with diabetes mellitus, bacterial overgrowth
Breath hydrogen tests	Simple and inexpensive test for malabsorption of a specific substrate
Schilling test with intrinsic factor	
Low urinary recovery	Suggests ileal dysfunction, may be abnormal with pancreatic exocrine insufficiency or bacterial overgrowth
Dual-labeled study	Corrects for pancreatic exocrine insufficiency
Tests of bile acid malabsorption	
Fecal bile acid excretion	"Gold standard," but difficult assay
Radiolabeled bile acid excretion	Correlates with fecal bile acid excretion
[75]SeHCAT retention	Sensitive indicator of ileal bile acid malabsorption
[14]C-glycocholic acid breath test	Abnormal with small bowel bacterial overgrowth or bile acid malabsorption
Tests for small bowel bacterial overgrowth	
[14]C-glycocholic acid breath test	Sensitivity may be low
[14]C-xylose breath test	Sensitivity may be low
Glucose breath hydrogen test	Inexpensive, some false-negatives
Quantitative culture of jejunal aspirate ($>10^5$/ml)	"Gold standard" for this diagnosis
Tests for exocrine pancreatic insufficiency	
Stool chymotrypsin concentration	Low concentration in presence of steatorrhea highly suggestive of pancreatic insufficiency
Dual-labeled Schilling test	Complex test
Bentiromide test	May be abnormal if mucosal disease present
Secretin/CCK tests	Involve intubation, complex analysis

stool. Renal function is well-maintained in most conditions causing malabsorption; blood urea nitrogen may be low due to poor protein intake or absorption and serum creatinine concentration may be low due to reduction in muscle mass. Serum calcium concentration may be low as a result of malabsorption, vitamin D deficiency, or intraluminal complexing of calcium by fatty acids. In addition, concurrent hypomagnesemia may produce hypocalcemia that is resistent to intravenous repletion. Serum phosphorus, cholesterol, and triglyceride concentrations may be low because of poor intake or malabsorption. Liver tests (AST, ALT, and bilirubin) remain normal in most individuals; refeeding (either enterally or parenterally) may be complicated by fatty infiltration and mild to moderate liver test abnormalities. Serum total protein and albumin levels are well-maintained in most patients with malabsorption. Albumin levels may be depressed, if protein-losing enteropathy or a concurrent acute illness is present.

Prothrombin time and partial thromboplastin time are usually normal unless vitamin K malabsorption due to prolonged poor intake, chronic steatorrhea, antibiotic therapy, or colectomy has been present.

2. Blood levels of potentially malabsorbed substances–Additional circumstantial evidence of malabsorption can be obtained by measuring blood levels of several substances that may be reduced when malabsorption is present, including serum iron, vitamin B_{12}, folate, 25-OH vitamin D and carotene. The rationale is that generalized malabsorption will reduce serum concentrations of one or more of these substances. One problem with this concept, however, is that several of these substances have substantial body stores and thus depletion may take a long time. Another problem is that prolonged inadequate intake may also cause reduced serum levels. Thus, the sensitivity and specificity of low serum concentrations of these substances for malabsorption is poor. To make a firm diagnosis of malabsorption, more direct evidence of malabsorption should be obtained.

3. Tests of fat absorption–The simplest approach to detect the presence of fat malabsorption is a qualititative examination of stool. A spot specimen is smeared on a microscope slide and is gently heated with a drop of glacial acetic acid for a few seconds to allow fat droplets to form. A fat-soluble stain such as Sudan III is then applied and the slide is examined under the microscope. Stained fat droplets are sought and the number of droplets is assessed semiquantitatively.

This test is regularly positive (more than 5 droplets per high power field) when substantial steatorrhea is present, but may be equivocal if not done properly or with lesser degrees of steatorrhea. It has the additional advantage of being relatively simple and inexpensive. Light microscopy cannot be used to evaluate treatment (unless steatorrhea is completely eliminated) and is subject to false positive results with some drugs (eg, mineral oil).

A more comprehensive evaluation of fat malabsorption can be obtained by chemical measurement of fat excretion. This test is best done as a 48-hour or 72-hour metabolic balance. Fat intake should be assessed by a dietician based on diet diaries to adjust for potentially large differences in fat intake. This works better than prescribing a 100 g fat diet or assuming that the patient is eating 100 g of fat each day. Stools need to be collected quantitatively; kits (consisting of a collection pan, preweighed containers and coolant) can be made which simplify this task for outpatients. Once completed, the collected stools should be homogenized, weighed, and analyzed. Direct measurement of fat content by the VanderKamer (titrimetric) method or by gravimetric methods is preferable to indirect methods, such as near infrared spectroscopy.

Daily fecal fat output needs to be evaluated against stool weight. As stool weight increases, more fat is excreted even without any mucosal pathology. While normal fat excretion on an intake of 100 g/d is less than 7 g/d fat, outputs of up to 15 g/d may result solely from large stool weights. The stool fat concentration (gram fat per 100 g stool) may also be helpful. Pancreatic exocrine insufficiency is associated with high stool fat concentrations (> 10 g per 100 g stool), since, unlike hydrolyzed fat, unhydrolyzed fat does not stimulate colonic water and electrolyte secretion that would dilute stool fat. Results can be affected by intake of mineral oil or other poorly absorbed lipids.

Measuring stool fat excretion is moderately difficult and somewhat expensive, but provides a reliable benchmark for the sequential assessment of therapy. It remains the gold standard for assessing of generalized malabsorption. Attempts to replace it with "cleaner" tests, such as the ^{14}C-triolein breath test, have not been successful.

4. Tests of protein absorption–Measuring fecal nitrogen excretion is not widely used to test for malabsorption. While in theory, the test can be conducted simultaneously with a quantitative stool fat collection, in practice it does not add much to the assessment of the patient.

When protein-losing enteropathy is suspected because of hypoalbuminemia, α_1-antitrypsin clearance can be measured. In this technique α_1-antitrypsin is used as a marker for serum protein loss into the intestine. It is about the same size as albumin, but is relatively resistant to hydrolysis by luminal enzymes. α_1-antitrypsin is thought to leak into the intestine at the same rate as albumin, but passes into the stool with relatively little loss. By measuring α_1-antitrypsin concentration in serum and in a timed stool collection, clearance can be calculated by dividing stool output (concentration × volume) by serum concentration. This gives a result that can be interpreted as milliliters of serum leaked into the intestine each day. Values of more than 25 ml/d are associated with hypoalbuminemia.

5. Tests of carbohydrate absorption–Carbohydrate losses into the stool can be gauged by measuring total carbohydrate excretion in a quantitative stool collection by means of the anthrone method, but this does not measure small bowel malabsorption accurately because of fermentation of carbohydrate to short chain fatty acids by colonic bacteria. The short chain fatty acids can be absorbed by the colon, reducing the calorie loss and osmotic diarrhea that would otherwise occur with small intestinal carbohydrate malabsorption. This colonic salvage decreases the loss of carbohydrate calories, but the capacity for colonic short chain fatty acid absorption is limited to about 80 g/d. Loss of unabsorbed short-chain fatty acids can be accounted for by measuring their output in stool. This measurement can be converted back to carbohydrate fermented to short chain fatty acids by applying an empiric fermentation formula. This calculated carbohydrate loss can be added to directly measured carbohydrate loss to give a better picture of overall carbohydrate malabsorption. Because of its complexity such careful quantification is not done often for clinical purposes. Research studies on patients with chronic diarrhea have shown a wide range for carbohydrate malabsorption in various disorders.

More readily available, but indirect, tests for carbohydrate malabsorption are available on routine stool chemical analysis. Because of carbohydrate fermentation in the colon, stool pH tends to be low when carbohydrate is malabsorbed. Stool pH less than 5.5 is characteristic, but may not always be present because other factors may alter stool pH. If a large amount of unfermented carbohydrate is present in stool water, an osmotic gap may be noted. The osmotic gap is an estimate of the amount of substances other than sodium, potassium, and their accompanying anions in stool water. The osmotic gap should be calculated by doubling the sum of the stool sodium and potassium concentrations (in mmol/L) and subtracting this from 290 mosm, the osmolality of colonic contents within the body. Gaps greater than 50 mosm, suggest the presence of a substantial amount of some unmeasured solute, such as a simple sugar. Measured osmolalities in stool water should not be used for this calculation; they are often quite high due to fermentation of carbohydrate in the collection can in vitro. Another simple test on stool water is to measure reducing substances with a semi-quantitative test, like Glucotest tablets. If a substantial amount of unfermented reducing sugar is present, the test will be positive.

Another approach to evaluating carbohydrate malabsorption is an oral tolerance test in which a test sugar, such as glucose, sucrose, or lactose, is administered and blood glucose concentrations are measured over time. If no rise in blood sugar is seen, malabsorption is implied. A variant of this is the d-xylose test. In this test, d-xylose is given orally, usually in a dose of 25 g. Blood xylose concentration is measured after 2 hours and urinary excretion is measured for 5 hours after ingestion. Failure of blood xylose levels to rise about 30 mg/dL or urinary output to exceed 5 g/5 h suggests malabsorption. For any of these oral tolerance tests a finding of malabsorption suggests mucosal dysfunction because none of these sugars depends on pancreatic enzymes or bile acids for absorption. These tests can be misleading if diabetes mellitus is present, if body fluid compartments are abnormal (ie, because of dehydration or ascites), or if renal function is impaired. They also can be abnormal in the presence of bacterial overgrowth in the upper intestine (or urinary tract infection for d-xylose) in which substrate may be destroyed.

Breath hydrogen tests are another approach to evaluating carbohydrate malabsorption. Substrates such as lactose or sucrose can be ingested orally. If these are not absorbed in the small intestine, they pass into the colon, where in most individuals, the colonic bacteria can ferment the carbohydrate, producing hydrogen as a byproduct. This hydrogen is transported through the circulation to the lungs and exhaled, raising the hydrogen concentration in expired air. This can be measured with a simple gas chromatograph. Rises of more than 10–20 ppm after ingestion are consistent with malabsorption of the ingested substrate. This test is simple and inexpensive and is ideal for investigating patients in whom malabsorption of a specific carbohydrate is suspected (eg, due to disaccharidase deficiency). False-positives can be a result of small bowel bacterial overgrowth. (This produces an increase in breath hydrogen, but usually soon after ingestion.) False-negative results can be seen in individuals in whom the colonic flora does not produce hydrogen and in patients on antibiotic therapy.

6. Measurement of vitamin B_{12} absorption– In the context of evaluating malabsorption, vitamin B_{12} absorption is measured as an index of ileal function. Hence, part I of Schilling's test (measurement of B_{12} absorption in the absence of intrinsic factor) is not necessary, and part II (measurement of B_{12} absorption with intrinsic factor) can be done as the first step. In this test, radiolabeled B_{12} and exogenous intrinsic factor are given simultaneously by mouth, unlabeled B_{12} is given by injection to saturate internal B_{12} binding sites, and 24-hour urinary recovery of the radiolabel is measured. Recovery of less than 9% of the administered dose is abnormal and suggests ileal dysfunction. The test can be falsely positive for ileal dysfunction if pancreatic exocrine insufficiency is present (because endogenous R-protein may not be cleaved from R-protein-B_{12} complexes), if bacterial overgrowth is present, or if renal failure is present.

A dual-labeled Schilling Test has been developed to investigate the possibility of exocrine pancreatic insufficiency as a cause for B_{12} malabsorption. In this study two isotopes of cobalt are used to study the relative absorption of B_{12} coupled to R-protein and B_{12} coupled to intrinsic factor. Both complexes are labeled separately and given orally simultaneously. Urinary recovery of each isotope is measured. If pancreatic insufficiency is present, the B_{12} coupled with R-protein is malabsorbed and the ratio of isotopes in urine changes from the ratio that was administered. If bacterial overgrowth or ileal dysfunction is present, both B_{12} coupled to R-protein and B_{12} coupled to intrinsic factor are malabsorbed equally and the ratio of the two isotopes is unchanged. Though not regularly performed because of its complexity, this test is becoming more available in large centers.

7. Evaluation of bile acid malabsorption– Selective malabsorption of bile acids by the ileum has been proposed as a common cause of chronic watery diarrhea and malabsorption of bile acid has been considered to be one factor contributing to chronic diarrhea in patients with ileal disease. Several tests have been developed to evaluate bile acid absorption.

The gold standard is to measure fecal bile acid concentration and output. This is difficult because of the complexity of the chemical analysis of bile acids, and therefore has been used mainly in research studies. Another test that has not been used widely is to feed radiolabeled bile and to measure recovery of the isotope in stool over several days. Results only correlate with total fecal bile acid output, but the test is technically easier to perform.

More extensively used is the SeHCAT (75-selenium-labeled taurohomocholic acid) test. The radioactive taurocholic acid analog is administered orally and total body retention is measured over several days by repeated gamma scintigraphy. Retention of less than 50% after 3 days is abnormal and suggests bile acid malabsorption. Studies have suggested that this is a sensitive measure of bile acid malabsorption. Indeed, it may be too sensitive, producing a positive result when bile acid malabsorption may be too slight to produce diarrhea.

The ^{14}C-glycocholic acid breath test has also been tested as a method of identifying bile acid malabsorption. This test was originally designed to evaluate small bowel bacterial overgrowth. ^{14}C is used to label the glycine residue of this conjugated bile acid and is liberated when the bile acid is deconjugated and glycine is metabolized by bacteria. Radioactive CO_2 is expired and measured. The test is positive when there is small bowel bacterial overgrowth or if glycocholic acid is malabsorbed by the ileum and enters the colon. The specificity and sensitivity of this test for ileal dysfunction has not been identified.

8. Tests for small bowel bacterial overgrowth–In addition to the ^{14}C-glycocholic acid breath test mentioned above, several other indirect tests have been developed. Each of these work on the principle that bacterial metabolism of a substrate will release some substance that is measurable in exhaled air. ^{14}C-xylose is one of these substrates. In healthy individuals, xylose is absorbed from the small intestine and undergoes relatively slow metabolism in the body. If bacteria are present in the upper gastrointestinal tract or jejunum, xylose can be fermented and radioactive CO_2 will be exhaled in the breath. Recent studies indicate that the sensitivity of this test may be as low as 65%, making it of limited value.

A similar rationale is behind the glucose-breath hydrogen test. A bolus of glucose is ingested and breath hydrogen concentrations are measured sequentially. If no bacteria are present in the upper gastrointestinal tract or jejunum, the glucose is absorbed by the intestine and no hydrogen is generated since human metabolic pathways do not produce hydrogen gas as a byproduct. If bacteria are present, the glucose can be fermented before it can be absorbed and the hydrogen produced can be exhaled. This test also has sensitivity problems in some series, but is inexpensive and avoids exposure to radionuclides. Because of this, it is probably the indirect screening test of choice.

The gold standard for demonstrating bacterial overgrowth is quantitative culture of jejunal aspirate. A tube or long endoscope is inserted into the jejunum under radiographic or direct visual guidance and a sample of jejunal contents is aspirated and cultured quantitatively. Colony counts of more than 10^5/ml are abnormal. Care must be taken to avoid contamination of the specimen with oral flora or with antibacterials or bacteriostats that may have been used to clean the equipment.

9. Tests for exocrine pancreatic insufficiency–Whenever steatorrhea is present, exocrine pancreatic insufficiency needs to be considered. This insufficiency may result from pancreatic disease (eg, chronic pancreatitis) or lack of effective pancreatic stimulation (eg, because of mucosal atrophy in celiac disease, or as a sequela to gastric surgery that bypasses the duodenum). One of the simpler screening tests for exocrine pancreatic insufficiency is measurement of stool chymotrypsin concentration. In patients with steatorrhea, a low stool chymotrypsin concentration suggests the likelihood of exocrine pancreatic insufficiency, but does not prove it. Coupled with other information (eg, history of pancreatic disease, pancreatic calcification by x-ray), it may offer sufficient evidence to proceed with a therapeutic trial of high-dose pancreatic enzyme replacement. A low stool chymotrypsin concentration in the absence of steatorrhea does not have the same significance; most often this reflects dilution in a large stool volume.

Two other tubeless, indirect tests of pancreatic exocrine function are available. The dual-labeled Schilling test has already been discussed. The other test is the bentiromide test. In this technique, patients are fed an artificial substrate that can be hydrolyzed by chymotrypsin, N-benzoyl-L-tyrsyl-para-amino benzoic acid (bentiromide). If adequate chymotrypsin activity is present, this substrate is hydrolyzed and the free para-aminobenzoic acid (PABA) is absorbed and excreted in the urine. Measurement of the amount of PABA recovered provides an idea of the activity of chymotrypsin in the intestine. More than 50% reduction in enzymatic activity is necessary for PABA excretion to be reduced. The test can be "falsely" abnormal if mucosal disease, liver disease, or kidney disease alters the absorption, metabolism, distribution or excretion of PABA. Attempts have been made to correct for some of this by simultaneously giving a tracer dose of ^{14}C-PABA or the closely related nonradioactive compound, para-aminosalicylate (PAS). Several drugs can interfere with analysis of PABA and these should be discontinued before the test.

The gold standard tests for exocrine pancreatic insufficiency involve duodenal intubation and stimulation of the pancreas with either secretin, secretin and cholecystokinin, or a test meal (Lundh meal). Duodenal contents are aspirated and volume, bicarbonate secretion and enzyme secretion can be measured.

Steatorrhea usually does not occur until less than 10–20% of pancreatic secretory capacity remains.

These tests are infrequently performed because of their complexity; therapeutic trials of exogenous enzyme therapy are used instead. If a therapeutic trial is undertaken, several precautions should be used to prevent misinterpretation: (1) give a large dose of an active enzyme preparation, (2) make sure that the patient knows exactly how to take the enzyme supplement, and (3) measure the response of stool fat to the trial. If these steps are not done, an equivocal trial may result.

C. Imaging: Visualization of the absorptive surface of the small intestine by means of a small bowel follow-through study or by enteroclysis is an important step toward defining the cause of malabsorption. Table 24–5 details some of the many findings that have been associated with various conditions producing malabsorption. It is important to realize that differences in technique and contrast materials may accentuate or minimize some of these findings and therefore the reliability of some of the softer findings is questionable. It is also important to realize that severe malabsorption may be present despite no radiologic findings. Radiography cannot be used as a sub-

stitute for functional testing. Neither can the radiologist make a diagnosis of a malabsorptive disease with certainty. For example, the same findings could represent mucosal edema, lymphoma, or an acute viral syndrome. The radiologist can exclude some conditions and suggest others, but the definite diagnosis of these disorders depends on a clinical aggregation of history, laboratory findings, and pathology.

Use of CT scans is patients with malabsorption disorders is frequently helpful. The CT scan allows visualization of the pancreas, lymph nodes, and mesentery in addition to the small intestine. This often permits additional conditions to be considered or eliminated from consideration.

Some mucosal diseases produce gross changes that can be visualized by upper gastrointestinal endoscopy or enteroscopy. In general, it is not worthwhile doing endoscopic examination solely for the purpose of inspecting the intestine. However, endoscopy can be used to aspirate jejunal contents or to obtain mucosal biopsies.

D. Pathology: Most patients with panmalabsorption will require a small bowel biopsy to identify or exclude diffuse mucosal disease as a cause for their problem. Table 24–6 indicates conditions in

Table 24–5. Small bowel radiographic findings in malabsorption.

	Luminal Caliber	Luminal Fluid	Folds	Gut Wall	Extra-luminal Mass	Other
Celiac disease	Dilated	Increased	Thin, effaced ("moulage")	—	—	Segmentation of barium column, painless intussusceptions
Whipple's disease	Normal	—	Thick, wild pattern	—	—	Patchy micronodularity
Scleroderma	Dilated, especially the duodenum	—	—	—	—	Delayed peristalsis, hypomotility
Lymphoma	Variable	—	Coarse	Infiltrated, stiff	Often	—
Amyloidosis	Normal	—	Symmetric thickening, no edema	Stiff	—	Micronodularity
Lymphangiectasia	—	Increased	Thick, edematous	—	—	Micronodularity
Crohn's disease	Stenotic	—	Deformed	Rigidity, ulceration, thickening	Sometimes	—
Dysgammaglobulinemia	—	—	Thick	—	—	Nodular lymphoid hyperplasia
Giardiasis	—	Increased	Thick in duodenum & jejunum	—	—	Spasm, rapid transit
Zollinger-Ellison syndrome	Dilated duodenum	Increased	Thick in duodenum	—	—	Peptic ulcers, reticulated small bowel pattern
Cystic fibrosis	Dilated duodenum	—	Thick in duodenum	—	—	Nodularity in duodenum
Abetalipoproteinemia	—	—	Thick	—	—	Fine mucosal graininess
Mastocytosis	—	—	—	Thick	—	Mucosal nodularity, "bull's eye" lesions

which small bowel biopsy is useful and offers diagnostic considerations for various findings.

For the pathologist to interpret the histology correctly, the gastroenterologist must provide enough tissue. In most cases, endoscopic biopsies from the distal duodenum can be interpreted, but it is important that multiple biopsies be obtained. Capsule biopsies provide larger samples of tissue and can be obtained more distally in the bowel, features that are important in some situations. When possible, biopsies should be oriented so that sections can be made perpendicular to the surface, since tangential sections are difficult to evaluate. When possible, the gastroenterologist should review the biopsy slides with the pathologist to ascertain both the confidence of the pathologist in the diagnosis and the adequacy of the tissue provided.

Differential Diagnosis & Descriptions of Specific Entities

The differential diagnosis of malabsorption is quite broad (see Table 24–1). For clinical purposes, it is useful to divide these into five categories:

1. Mucosal disorders causing generalized malabsorption.
2. Infectious diseases causing generalized malabsorption.
3. Luminal problems causing malabsorption.
4. Postoperative malabsorption.
5. Disorders that cause malabsorption of specific nutrients.

A. Mucosal disorders causing generalized malabsorption:

1. Celiac sprue—Celiac disease is characterized by malabsorption usually of a variety of nutrients, villous atrophy of the small intestine, and clinical improvement following withdrawal of dietary gluten, a protein component of several grains.

The malabsorption is due to damage to the absorptive mucosa of the small intestine. Surface area is reduced substantially because of the villous atrophy, and the remaining absorptive cells are damaged, often lacking membrane-bound disaccharidases and peptidases, which are essential for mucosal hydrolysis. In contrast, the crypts undergo substantial hyperplasia and lengthen. The extent of malabsorption depends on the length of intestine affected. Patients with duodenal involvement only may have isolated iron deficiency, whereas those with more extensive involvement have panmalabsorption. Involvement is typically more severe proximally in the intestine and diminishes distally. In a few patients with celiac disease, the loss of the absorptive surface is so extensive that a secretory diarrhea is present even when the patient is fasting.

The current thinking about the cause of celiac disease is that it represents an abnormal immune response to gluten (specifically gliadin), a component of wheat, barley, rye, and some varieties of oats. Rice and corn do not contain gluten. The immune response is both humoral and cellular and can produce damage to the mucosa within hours of exposure to gluten. Genetic factors are important as in many immunologically mediated disorders. HLA-B8 and HLA DR3 are present in most European and North American patients with celiac disease. Environmental factors, such as prior exposure to type 12 adenovirus, the coat of which shares some homology to gluten, may also be important.

The clinical course of celiac disease is variable. Symptoms frequently develop in childhood and malabsorption may be severe enough to stunt growth. Children may be pale, thin, and spindly; often their symptoms subside in adolescence, only to reappear in middle age. Other patients first develop symptoms in adulthood.

The diagnosis of celiac sprue depends on the demonstration of malabsorption, typical histologic features on small intestinal biopsies, and response to a gluten-free diet. Additional tests such as antigliadin antibodies have not had sufficient specificity to preclude biopsy.

Table 24–6. Interpretation of pathologic findings on small bowel biopsy in malabsorption.

Brush border abnormalities	
Sickle-shaped organisms	Giardiasis
Basophilic dots	Cryptosporidium
Inclusions	Microvillous inclusion disease
Abnormal enterocytes	
Intracytoplasmic organisms	Isosporiasis
Foamy vacuolation	Abetalipoproteinemia
Abnormal basement membrane	
Collagenous band	Collagenous sprue
Villous atrophy	
Total or partial	Celiac disease, tropical sprue, bacterial overgrowth, dysgammaglobulinemia, dermatitis herpetiformis, radiation enteritis, IPSID[1], acute viral infection, ischemia, nongranulomatous ulcerative jejunoileitis, microsporidiosis
Lamina propria abnormalities	
Noncaseating granulomas	Crohn's disease
Infiltrating eosinophils	Eosinophilic gastroenteritis
Infiltrating malignant lymphocytes	Lymphoma, IPSID
Infiltrating mast cells	Mastocytosis
PAS-positive macrophages	Whipple's disease (bacilli on EM), *Mycobacterium avium-intracellulare* (acid-fast bacilli)
Dilated lymphatics	Lymphangiectasia

[1]IPSID = Immunoproliferative small intestinal disease

Treatment of celiac disease consists of strict exclusion of gluten from the diet. This is more difficult than it seems, because gluten is present in a number of prepared foods that have no obvious connection to grains containing gluten. Initially, lactose intake should be restricted as well, because of the likelihood of secondary lactase deficiency. Patients need rigorous instruction by a dietician to assure compliance with this diet. Symptoms should respond to gluten withdrawal within a few weeks. If they do not, adherence to the diet needs to be reevaluated. Failure to respond to a strict diet excludes celiac diseases; other diagnoses then need to be considered.

Because adherence to the gluten-free diet is difficult and must be continued for a lifetime, objective evidence of improvement should be obtained. Ideally, the patient should undergo another small bowel biopsy to document a return to normal. If this is impossible, repeating the quantitative stool fat or some other test of absorption should be considered.

The prognosis of patients with celiac disease is generally excellent with treatment. Absorptive defects resolve promptly and most deficiencies can be repaired with refeeding. Serious complications occur in a minority of patients. These include malignant neoplasms, progression to refractory sprue and ulceration. Malignant disease may complicate the course of celiac sprue in up to one-eighth of patients. Most tumors are T-cell lymphomas; there is also an excess incidence of small intestinal adenocarcinoma. Refractory sprue is an unusual pattern of disease in which a patient responds to treatment, but then symptoms return despite continued adherence to a gluten-free diet. The cause for this is not clear. Some of these patients respond to corticosteroid therapy; others need to be maintained with parenteral nutrition. Ulceration occurs in very few patients and can be complicated by perforation or stricture formation.

2. Collagenous sprue–This rare condition of unknown cause presents with symptoms and signs of malabsorption, not unlike celiac sprue. Biopsy of the small intestine shows a flat mucosa with collagen deposition in the lamina propria and few crypts. It does not improve with a gluten-free diet or other therapy. Without parenteral nutrition, it is invariably fatal.

3. Nongranulomatous ulcerative jejuno-ileitis–Patients with this disorder present with severe malabsorption and diarrhea related to extensive ulceration of the small intestine. The absorptive surface between ulcers is often abnormal with variable degrees of villous atrophy. The relationship to celiac disease is not clear, but some patients respond to gluten withdrawal or to corticosteroids. The disease is progressive and fatal. Enterectomy has been performed in a few patients with mixed results.

4. Eosinophilic gastroenteritis–Eosinophilic gastroenteritis is another rare condition that is associated with malabsorption. In this disorder, the wall of the intestine is infiltrated with eosinophils, which can disrupt absorptive function. It is most often a component of systemic eosinophilia, but 20% of cases may have no abnormality in the peripheral blood.

The cause of eosinophilic gastroenteritis is unknown. Food allergies have been implicated in one-half of cases and insensitivity to drugs or toxins in others. Eosinophils infiltrate the mucosa and submucosa and villous atrophy can be present. This is the form of the disease that is associated with malabsorption. Involvement of the muscular layers or serosa typically produces intestinal obstruction or ascites, respectively.

Laboratory tests may show peripheral blood eosinophilia (in 80% of patients), iron deficiency anemia (due to blood loss) and hypoalbuminemia (due to protein-losing enteropathy). In some patients, Charcot-Leyden crystals can be detected in stools, but the specificity of this for the diagnosis of eosinophilic gastroenteritis is unknown.

Intestinal biopsy is essential for diagnosis. The finding of increased eosinophils in the mucosa should prompt consideration of a diagnosis of eosinophilic gastroenteritis, but other conditions need to be considered as well. These include parasitic diseases, connective tissue diseases, vasculitis, systemic mastocytosis, inflammatory bowel disease, celiac disease, specific food allergies, (eg, cow's milk, milk protein sensitivity) and hypereosinophil syndrome. Local infiltration with eosinophils can be seen in some benign polyps (eosinophilic granuloma).

Treatment consists of an elimination diet (sequential elimination of individual sources of protein, such as milk, beef, or eggs) and corticosteroids. Experience with other immunosuppressive agents is quite limited. The prognosis for this disease is generally good with treatment.

5. Systemic mastocytosis–Some patients with mastocytosis have malabsorption in addition to other symptoms, such as nausea, vomiting, diarrhea, and flushing. In this disorder, mast cells infiltrate the intestinal wall and other organs and release mediators, such as histamine, eosinophil chemotactic factor, platelet-activating factor and other cytokines. Release can be triggered by several different agents, such as exogenous and endogenous antigens.

Diagnosis of mastocytosis may be difficult because of the protean manifestations of this disease. If typical cutaneous involvement (urticaria pigmentosa), flushing and gastrointestinal symptoms are present, only confirmatory tests may be necessary; measurement of plasma and urine histamine concentrations can provide indirect evidence for the presence of mastocytosis. Otherwise, intestinal biopsy can be useful. Mast cells are not well demonstrated by standard histochemical stains, such as hematoxylin and eosin, and impressive numbers may be overlooked with routine biopsy processing. Special stains, such as toluidine blue, may be necessary.

Treatment depends on the severity of the disease.

For mild cases without much in the way of lymph node or splenic infiltration, therapy with oral sodium chromoglycate, H_1, and H_2-antagonists and low-dose aspirin may be sufficient. For extensive disease, therapy with interferon may cause a marked reduction in mast cell burden. The outlook for patients with mastocytosis is generally good, if symptoms can be controlled and organ infiltration is not extensive.

6. Immunoproliferative small intestinal disease (IPSID)–This disorder, once called alpha chain disease, is thought to be related to proliferation of the cells of the intestinal immune system in response to chronic antigenic stimulation, probably by bacteria. Signs include dense infiltration of the mucosa and submucosa of the entire small intestine with lymphocytes and plasma cells in association with flattening of the villi. The infiltrate may be benign-appearing or have features consistent with a low-grade or intermediate-grade malignant lymphoma. Patients suffer from severe malabsorption and weight loss because of disruption of the absorptive surface of the small intestine.

The disease mainly affects adolescents and young adults in the Middle East, North Africa, and South Africa. Clinical manifestations include severe diarrhea, crampy abdominal pain, anorexia, and marked, progressive weight loss. Fever may be prominent in some patients. Organomegaly and abdominal mass are not seen early in the course, but may develop later.

Diagnosis depends on demonstration of diffuse intestinal involvement by radiography, the characteristic histological findings by small bowel biopsy, and typical changes in serum proteins. Serum protein electrophoresis may show a broad band in the α_2 or β regions. This paraprotein is the Fc portion of IgA. No light chains are present in the serum, and Bence Jones proteins are absent from the urine.

Treatment is empiric. For early stage disease, prolonged antibiotic therapy (tetracycline 250 mg four times a day or ampicillin plus metronidazole) may induce a remission within 6–12 months. Once malignant changes have occurred, combination cytotoxic chemotherapy can be tried; results have been variable. Surgery for cure is not feasible because of the extent of involvement.

7. Lymphoma–Several types of lymphoma involve the small intestine. T-cell lymphomas complicate the course of celiac disease. Tumors of the mucosa-associated lymphoid tissue (MALToma) affect the B-lymphocytes associated with Peyer's patches. Multiple lymphoid polyposis is a multicentric polypoid mucosal tumor of B-cells. The most common types are diffuse large cell lymphoma and small non-cleaved lymphoma, in which involvement is initially segmental.

Malabsorption syndrome occurs with more extensive lymphomas, especially T-cell lymphomas. Localized B-cell lymphomas are more likely to produce pain, obstruction and abdominal mass, unless bacterial overgrowth or terminal ileal involvement predisposes to malabsorption.

8. Lymphangiectasia–Protein-losing enteropathy can complicate the course of several malabsorptive diseases, particularly when accompanied by mucosal ulceration or lymphatic obstruction (Table 24–7). It can also occur as an isolated phenomenon without generalized malabsorption. In such cases the only clinical finding may be hypoalbuminemia and lymphopenia.

Intestinal lymphangiectasia is a disease of children and young adults characterized by the formation of dilated lymphatic channels in the small bowel mucosa. These dilated channels are patchy and several biopsies may be necessary to make a diagnosis. The dilated lymphatics rupture easily and leak lymph containing a variety of plasma proteins, lymphocytes, and chylomicrons. If the lesions are proximal, the processes of luminal digestion and mucosal absorption distally may remove most of the leaked protein and fat from the lumen so that measured stool protein or fat losses may be very low. When steatorrhea is present, it is typically mild (< 10 g excretion per day). Diarrhea is usually not severe. Edema is the major sign at presentation.

Diagnosis depends on recognizing the possibility of protein-losing enteropathy and excluding other malabsorptive disorders associated with it (Table 24–7). Measurement of α_1-antitrypsin clearance with a timed stool collection can confirm protein-losing enteropathy. Mucosal biopsy can show dilated lymphatic channels, but does not necessarily show the cause of the condition. Small bowel x-rays, abdominal CT scan, and cardiac catheterization may be needed to exclude primary causes.

Treatment of lymphangiectasia consists of dietary manipulation and supportive measures. Intestinal lymph flow varies with meal composition; a low-fat diet can reduce protein loss. Breakdown products of medium chain triglycerides (MCT) are transported in portal blood and therefore do not increase lymph flow. MCT oil can be used to improve caloric intake without worsening enteric protein loss. Supportive

Table 24–7. Malabsorptive disorders associated with protein-losing enteropathy.

Mucosal diseases
  Celiac disease
  Tropical sprue
  Whipple's disease
  Eosinophilic gastroenteritis
  Small bowel bacterial overgrowth
  Ulcerative jejunoileitis
Lymphatic obstruction
  Congenital lymphangiectasia
  Lymphoma
  Crohn's disease
  Constrictive pericarditis

measures include appropriate (limited) use of diuretics and elastic support hose to control edema. With these measures the prognosis for patients with intestinal lymphangiectasia is good.

9. Crohn's disease—Crohn's disease can produce malabsorption in four ways:

1. Extensive direct mucosal involvement.
2. Stricture formation and bacterial overgrowth.
3. Fistula formation leading to bacterial overgrowth.
4. Surgical resection of small intestine.

Crohn's disease is discussed further in Chapter 7.

10. Radiation enteritis—Radiation therapy directed to the abdomen or pelvis routinely produces gastrointestinal dysfunction and often, symptoms as well. These abnormalities can develop acutely or after many years. Whereas diarrhea may present acutely or chronically, and absorption tests may be abnormal acutely, clinically important malabsorption typically occurs only late after irradiation.

The pathogenesis of malabsorption involves several mechanisms. Acutely, subclinical malabsorption is due to mucosal damage, but this usually resolves as the mucosa regenerates. Chronic malabsorption can occur years after irradiation and may be due to: (1) ileal dysfunction causing bile acid malabsorption and deletion, (2) bacterial overgrowth due to intestinal strictures, and (3) enteroenteral or enterocolic fistulas. Other contributing factors can be lymphatic obstruction, ischemia, and radiation-induced motility disorders.

Diagnosis depends on a careful history and typical radiographic findings. Because several mechanisms can contribute to diarrhea and malabsorption, it may be useful to define the mechanism of malabsorption so that the correct treatment can be selected. This may involve tests for bile acid malabsorption or bacterial overgrowth (see previous section, "Tests for small bowel bacterial overgrowth").

Therapy is aimed at correcting malnutrition, maximizing absorption of nutrients, and correcting remediable processes, such as small bowel bacterial overgrowth. Parenteral nutrition and bowel rest may be needed to control symptoms and to allow time to institute other therapeutic measures. Maximizing absorption involves dietary manipulation (elemental diet if hydrolysis is impaired, medium-chain triglyceride if bile acid deficiency is present, frequent feedings to maximize exposure of the mucosa to nutrients), and antiperistaltic agents (opioids or anticholinergics) to slow transit and increase the contact time of luminal contents with the absorptive surface. Surgery should be limited to correction of obstruction or fistulous disease.

With adequate therapy the prognosis of malabsorption in radiation enteritis is good. Patients rarely need long-term parenteral nutrition.

11. Chronic mesenteric ischemia—Patients with chronic mesenteric ischemia often develop weight loss and evidence of malabsorption in addition to the cardinal feature of postprandial abdominal pain. Weight loss is frequently due to sitophobia, but many of these patients have mild to moderate steatorrhea, too.

This syndrome can occur when blood flow through two of the three mesenteric vessels is compromised. Audible bruits are heard in some of these patients, but diagnosis is prompted by history rather than physical or laboratory findings. Angiography shows vascular occlusion and collateral formation. In the presence of typical symptoms, such findings should prompt surgery. Revascularization can be accomplished by several methods and can produce a good long-term result with reversal of malabsorption and weight gain.

B. Infectious diseases causing generalized malabsorption:

1. Small bowel bacterial overgrowth—The upper gastrointestinal tract ordinarily supports the growth of a very sparse bacterial flora ($<10^4$/ml). This is somewhat surprising in view of the large amount of nutrients and warm, dark environment that should be conducive to bacterial growth. This paradox is due to a series of defenses that limit bacterial proliferation, including gastric acidity, and immunologic, secretory, and motility mechanisms (migrating motor complex) that tend to clear the upper tract of luminal contents and prevent stasis.

When disease or therapy interferes with these protective mechanisms, bacteria can proliferate in the lumen and can produce malabsorption. Fat malabsorption results from bacterial deconjugation of bile acid. This allows the free bile acid to be reabsorbed, lowering luminal bile acid concentration and limiting micelle formation. In addition, patchy mucosal damage (villous blunting and increased lamina propria cellularity) due to bacterial toxins or the toxic effects of free bile acids may also contribute to fat malabsorption. Carbohydrate and protein malabsorption can also be related to mucosal damage or to intraluminal bacterial metabolism of these nutrients. To some extent bacteria can also compete for nutrients. For example, vitamin B_{12} is absorbed by gram-negative, anaerobic bacteria and is sequestered from ileal absorption sites. (Intrinsic factor protects vitamin B_{12} from uptake by aerobic bacteria.) In contrast, luminal bacteria release folate into the intestine, and deficiency of this vitamin is unlikely with bacterial overgrowth.

Conditions that predispose to bacterial overgrowth include achlorhydria or hypochlorhydria (due to atrophic gastritis or antisecretory drug therapy), motility disorders of the upper gut (diabetes mellitus, scleroderma, chronic intestinal pseudo-obstruction), and anatomic problems, such as blind loops, diverticulosis, intestinal obstruction, afferent loop syndrome, and gastrocolic or enterocolic fistula. Although many of these predisposing conditions are "permanent," the severity of malabsorption and diarrhea may wax and wane as the bacterial population rises and falls.

The clinical features of bacterial overgrowth are those typical for malabsorption: steatorrhea or watery diarrhea, weight loss, and anemia. When present, anemia is macrocytic and is due to vitamin B_{12} malabsorption.

Diagnosis is made by showing both evidence of malabsorption and direct or indirect evidence of bacterial overgrowth. A quantitative culture of luminal contents is the gold standard, but breath hydrogen testing and other indirect tests (see previous section, "Tests for small bowel bacterial overgrowth") may be sufficient if the clinical findings are very suggestive. Small bowel x-ray studies should be done in all of these patients to look for anatomical problems. Small bowel biopsies done in the course of evaluation of steatorrhea may show villous blunting and increased cellularity of the lamina propria, but these changes are not specific.

Treatment consists of antibiotic therapy, if no correctable anatomic problems are discovered. Tetracycline is no longer universally effective in these patients. Amoxicillin with clavulinic acid, cephalosporins, chloramphenicol, ciprofloxacin, and metronidazole have been recommended in its place. Therapy should be given for 1–2 weeks and then discontinued. Patients should be retreated when symptoms recur. If symptoms recur quickly, intermittent expectant courses of antibiotic should be tried. Very few patients with this syndrome need to be on continuous antibiotic therapy. If anatomic problems are present, surgical correction should be considered. This may not be practical for some lesions (eg, duodenal diverticulum), but may be useful in others (eg, fistula).

2. Tropical sprue—Tropical sprue is a progressive, chronic malabsorptive disease occurring in people living in certain tropical countries. It is characterized by abnormalities in intestinal structure and function, symptoms related to malabsorption, and responsiveness to treatment with folic acid, tetracycline, or both. It must be differentiated from subclinical malabsorption, an endemic condition in tropical countries that may produce similar structural changes, but which does not produce symptoms. Subclinical malabsorption is quite common in indigenous populations in the Caribbean, Central America, northern South America, Equatorial and South Africa, the Indian subcontinent, and Southeast Asia. Tropical sprue occurs both in the indigenous population and in foreigners who reside in tropical places for extended periods.

It is unclear whether the incidence of tropical sprue is declining or not. Americans who fought in Vietnam and Peace Corps volunteers working in endemic areas did not have as much trouble with tropical sprue as expected. Whether improved nutrition, better sanitation, or prompt treatment of acute diarrhea with antibiotics is responsible for this is not known.

The leading hypothesis about the cause of tropical sprue is that it represents a form of small bowel bacterial overgrowth. Most individuals with tropical sprue have evidence of aerobic gram negative bacterial overgrowth and at least some of these strains appear to secrete enterotoxins. What distinguishes individuals with tropical sprue from other patients with bacterial overgrowth (other than the obvious epidemiology) is not clear.

Tropical sprue typically begins as an acute diarrheal disorder which then develops into a chronic persistent diarrhea. Over the course of several months, evidence of more substantial malabsorption develops, associated with progressive weight loss. Megaloblastic anemia (due to folate or combined folate and B_{12} deficiency) then becomes prominent along with variable evidence of other deficiency states. Untreated tropical sprue can be fatal.

The basis for malabsorption is dysfunction of the mucosa. Histologically, the villi are shortened and thickened (partial villous atrophy); the flat mucosa of celiac sprue is not usually observed. The enterocytes themselves are abnormal with disruption of microvilli and reduced brush border enzyme levels. A chronic inflammatory infiltrate is present in the submucosa. Megaloblastic changes may be seen in the crypt epithelium.

Diagnosis of tropical sprue depends upon recognition of malabsorption in an individual complaining of diarrhea who was a resident of one of the endemic countries. The finding of B_{12} or folate deficiency and typical biopsy changes should suggest the diagnosis. It is important to exclude other infectious problems, such as giardiasis or cryptosporidiosis (see following section, "Parasitic diseases").

Treatment of tropical sprue includes pharmacological doses of folic acid (5 mg daily), injection of B_{12} (if deficient), and antibiotic therapy. Tetracycline (250 mg four times a day) or sulfonamide is the treatment of choice; newer antibiotics have not been extensively tested. Antibiotic therapy should be continued for 1–6 months. Optimal therapy includes both folate and an antibiotic; therapy with folic acid alone does not allow resolution of all of the structural changes in the intestine and therapy with antibiotic alone delays correction of the vitamin deficiencies until structural integrity is restored. Improvement should be seen with optimal therapy over the course of a few weeks.

The prognosis with treatment is excellent, but recurrences can occur, particularly in patients indigenous to endemic areas. There does not seem to be an excess risk for lymphoma or other cancers in patients with tropical sprue. Subclinical malabsorption may be associated with the development of low-grade lymphoma of the small intestine (MALToma) in some populations.

3. Whipple's disease—Whipple's disease is an uncommon chronic bacterial infection with multisystem involvement. The small bowel is usually involved and gastrointestinal symptoms are prominent. Typically, the intestinal mucosa is heavily infiltrated by foamy macrophages containing periodic acid-Schiff (PAS) positive material, distorting the villi. Under electron-microscopy or high-resolution light microscopy, bacteria can be visualized in the lamina propria. PAS-positive macrophages and bacteria have been demonstrated outside the intestine in lymph nodes, spleen, liver, central nervous system, heart, and synovium.

The bacterium responsible for Whipple's disease has not been cultured. Genetic analysis shows that it is related to actinobacter and tentatively it has been named *Tropheryma whippleii*. It does not appear to be very contagious; no cases of direct person-to-person transmission have been published. Presumably, differences in host resistance or reaction to the organism allow proliferation without clearance of the bacteria.

Whipple's disease occurs mainly in older white men, but women and all races are susceptible. Most patients have diarrhea or other gastrointestinal symptoms of malabsorption, but some present with only joint or neurologic symptoms. Extraintestinal symptoms, including arthritis, fever, cough, dementia, headache, and muscle weakness are common and can predate gastrointestinal symptoms. Unlike most other malabsorptive disorders, gastrointestinal bleeding, either gross or occult, can occur. Protein-losing enteropathy (and resultant hypoalbuminemia and edema) may occur due to blockage of lymphatic drainage by infiltrated lymph nodes.

When gastrointestinal symptoms predominate, diagnosis depends upon recognition of the clinical syndrome, proof of malabsorption and small-intestine biopsy. Diagnosis can be difficult if the patient presents with arthritis, fever, or neurologic symptoms and no intestinal symptoms.

Care must be taken to differentiate biopsies in Whipple's disease from those in infection with *Mycobacterium avium intracellulare* (MAI) in patients with AIDS. Both disorders have infiltration of the lamina propria with PAS-positive macrophages. MAI, however, is an acid-fast organism, whereas the Whipple's bacterium is not. Electron microscopy can also be used to differentiate the two conditions.

Antibiotic therapy produces an excellent response in most patients within days to weeks, but must be continued for months to years. Several different regimens have been recommended, including penicillin, erythromycin, ampicillin, tetracycline, chloramphenicol, or trimethoprim-sulfamethoxazole. Relapses are common with any of these regimens. If central nervous system involvement is present, chloramphenicol should be administered, and antibiotic therapy should be continued for a long time (if not permanently). The role of rebiopsy to confirm clearance of the organisms from the intestine is uncertain, but makes sense before discontinuing antibiotic therapy. PAS-positive macrophages may persist for years after bacteria disappear.

4. Parasitic diseases—Although many organisms parasitize humans on a regular basis, only a few produce malabsorption with any regularity (Table 24–8). Potential mechanisms producing malabsorption include competition for luminal nutrients, mechanical occlusion of the absorptive surface and epithelial damage. It is also possible that immune responses to the organisms or their products alter intestinal motility or stimulate secretion.

Giardia lamblia is a cosmopolitan parasite that can be acquired from contaminated water in the United States. The organism can also be spread person-to-person by fecal-oral transmission, especially in day care centers for infants and in facilities for the mentally retarded. *Giardia* is found encysted and as trophozoites. The cysts are relatively resistent to environmental stresses, but can be killed by boiling or chemical disinfectants. Patients with dysgammaglobulinemia (decreased IgA and IgM levels) are particularly likely to be infected.

Patients with giardiasis complain of diarrhea, bloating, dyspepsia, fatigue, and weight loss. Symptoms can become chronic, but may be intermittent. Secondary disaccharidase deficiency can lead to flatulence and other symptoms of lactase deficiency.

Diagnosis depends on finding the *Giardia* organism or its antigens in stool, or by small bowel biopsy. Standard ova and parasite examination of stool is only positive in 50% of infected patients. Concentration and staining techniques can improve the yield somewhat, but the organism may never be seen in stool in up to 25% of patients. Immunologic studies (immunoelectrophoresis or ELISA) for *Giardia* antigens in stool are alternative methods of detecting giardiasis and may gain wider use for diagnosis because of a sensitivity of greater than 90%. Small bowel biopsy is another way to find the organism. Most patients with giardiasis have structurally normal small bowel mucosa and the organisms can be

Table 24–8. Parasites associated with malabsorption.

Protozoa
  Giardia lamblia
  Coccidia
    Isospora belli
    Cryptosporidium
  Microsporidia (Enterocytozoon bieneusi)
Tapeworms
  Taenia saginata (Beef tapeworm)
  Hymenolepis nana (Dwarf tapeworm)
  Diphyllobothrium latum (fish tapeworm)

missed on casual inspection. Microscopic examination of duodenal contents or "touch preps" (in which a biopsy is pressed against a glass slide, leaving a layer of mucus that is then stained with Giemsa stain) may have a higher yield for the organisms than routine biopsies. Biopsies from patients with dysgammaglobulinemia may have changes resembling celiac disease and these patients may have more severe malabsorption.

Therapy consists of quinacrine 100 mg or metronidazole 250 mg three times a day for a week. Patients with immunodeficiency require longer courses of therapy (from 6 weeks to 6 months) to clear their infection. When clearance does occur, combination therapy with quinacrine and high-dose metronidazole (750 mg three times a day) can be used. Furazolidone (100 mg four times a day) is an alternative.

Coccidia are protozoa that invade the epithelium, producing functional disruption. *Isospora belli* enters the enterocytes and reproduces within the cytoplasm. This can produce disruption of the cells, villous abnormalities, or even necrotizing enterocolitis. The onset is usually acute with diarrhea, weight loss, abdominal pain, and fever. Oocysts can be found on concentrated stool specimens and are pink with acid-fast stains. The parasites can also be seen on appropriately stained mucosal biopsies, but many sections may need to be examined. The disease is usually self-limited and runs its course over 1 week to 6 months. Treatment with trimethoprim-sulfamethoxazole or furazolidone may shorten the course.

Cryptosporidia are also classified as *Coccidia*. Unlike *Isospora*, *Cryptosporidia* do not enter cells, but instead attach to the brush border, destroying microvilli. This reduces absorptive capacity and produces a watery diarrhea associated with evidence of malabsorption of various nutrients. Acid-fast smears of stool or concentrated stool specimens can identify the organism. Mucosal biopsy with detection of basophilic bodies in the brush border is diagnostic. Normal subjects have a self-limited course lasting about 2 weeks. Patients with AIDS have a prolonged course that sometimes subsides with paromomycin 500 mg four times a day.

Microsporidia are intracellular protozoa that have been associated with diarrhea and malabsorption in patients with AIDS and other immunodeficiency diseases. They produce partial villous atrophy and may be difficult to see with light microscopy. Electron microscopy shows typical changes, however. Examination of stool with special trichrome stains has sometimes been helpful in finding the organism. No treatment has been shown to clear the organism reliably in AIDS patients. Metronidazole has been tried and may help some with symptoms.

Tapeworms compete with their hosts for nutrients in the lumen. In most cases substantial malabsorption does not occur. *Diphyllobothrium latum,* the fish tapeworm, can produce vitamin B_{12} deficiency. *Tae-*

nia solium, the pork tapeworm, produces cysticercosis (from ingestion of eggs) more often than it produces tapeworms (from ingestion of larva in infected meat). *Taenia saginata* (beef tapeworm) is more commonly found in the United States and may produce weight loss. *Hymenolepis nana* (dwarf tapeworm) is the most common tapeworm in the United States. There is no intermediate host and infection results from ingestion of human feces containing embryonated eggs; autoinfection is possible. Diagnosis of any tapeworm infection depends on careful examination of stool for eggs and proglottids. Treatment of *Diphyllobothrium latum, Taenia solium,* or *Taenia saginata* is niclosamide 2 g in a single dose. Praziquantel 25 mg/kg or paromomycin 4 g can also be used. For the treatment of *Hymenolepis nana,* a single dose of praziquantel is preferred to niclosamide, which must be given for 7 days to prevent autoinfection. Paromomycin 45 mg/kg can also be given for seven days.

5. *Mycobacterium avium-intracellulare*–Diarrhea and weight loss are common manifestations of AIDS. These symptoms may be due to any of a variety of infections, impaired oral intake, difficulty swallowing, or malabsorption. When malabsorption occurs in this setting, infection with *Mycobacterium avium-intracellulare* needs to be considered. Mucosal biopsy is diagnostic, but the changes can be confused with Whipple's disease (see previous discussion). Antibiotic therapy can reduce the intensity of infection in these patients, but rarely eradicates the organism.

C. Luminal problems causing malabsorption:

1. Pancreatic exocrine insufficiency–When pancreatic enzyme secretion is reduced by 90% or more, maldigestion and malabsorption will occur. There can be important clinical differences between the malabsorption of pancreatic exocrine insufficiency and that due to mucosal disease, like celiac sprue. When fat is not digested, it is transported through the gastrointestinal tract as triglyceride. When fat is digested, but not absorbed, it enters the colon as fatty acids and monoglyceride. This difference in chemical composition has several ramifications: (1) oil is seen in stool in pancreatic exocrine insufficiency, but not in celiac disease; (2) stool volumes are greater for equal fat outputs in celiac disease than in pancreatic exocrine insufficiency because of inhibition of colonic fluid absorption by fatty acids; (3) fecal fat concentration is accordingly higher with pancreatic exocrine insufficiency than with mucosal disease; and (4) hypocalcemia due to formation of complexes containing calcium and fatty acids (soap formation) is seen in celiac disease, but not pancreatic exocrine insufficiency. In addition, patients with pancreatic exocrine insufficiency tend to have fewer problems with vitamin deficiencies than those with celiac disease.

Carbohydrate malabsorption and protein malabsorption can be quite significant in pancreatic exocrine insufficiency. Symptoms related to carbohydrate malabsorption, such as bloating, flatulence, and watery diarrhea, may be prominent. Although protein malabsorption may be substantial, hypoproteinemia is usually not present until late in the course of the disease.

Tests to document pancreatic exocrine insufficiency have been discussed earlier in this chapter. The diagnosis and differential diagnosis of chronic pancreatitis are discussed in Chapter 32.

Treatment of pancreatic exocrine insufficiency involves replacing the missing enzymes with exogenous pancreatic enzymes. Adequate amounts of potent enzyme supplements (particularly enteric coated preparations that release the enzymes only when luminal pH is > 5.5) are needed to reduce steatorrhea. The effectiveness of therapy should be judged by comparing fecal fat excretion before and after therapy.

2. Bile acid deficiency—Adequate concentrations of bile acids are necessary for micelle formation and fat digestion. If this critical concentration is not present, fat maldigestion ensues. Lack of micelle formation also impairs absorption of fat-soluble vitamins. Other nutrients continue to be absorbed normally.

Bile acid deficiency can develop in the course of chronic cholestatic liver disease, such as primary biliary cirrhosis, in patients with complete extrahepatic biliary obstruction or diversion, in patients after extensive terminal ileal resection, and in some patients with ileal dysfunction. As with pancreatic exocrine insufficiency, stools tend to have high fat concentration when bile acid deficiency is due to hepatic or biliary disease. With ileal resection or dysfunction, bile acid loss into the colon leads to a secretory diarrhea and dilution of fat by increased stool water.

Diagnosis of bile acid deficiency is made by measuring postprandial bile acid concentration in the duodenum. Feeding exogenous bile acid with meals can reduce fat malabsorption, but may worsen diarrhea if ileal bile acid malabsorption leads to sufficiently high colonic bile acid concentrations. This can be reduced to some extent by the concurrent use of opiate antidiarrheal drugs.

3. Zollinger-Ellison syndrome—The high rates of gastric acid secretion in Zollinger-Ellison syndrome produce malabsorption by several mechanisms. First, persistently low pH in the duodenum precipitates bile acid and can secondarily affect fat absorption. Second, low intraduodenal pH may inactivate pancreatic enzymes. Third, the excess acid and pepsin may damage the mucosal absorptive cells directly. Removal of acid by aspiration or by inhibitory drugs can promptly reduce the secretory diarrhea seen in some of these patients. Steatorrhea may take several days to weeks to respond to acid inhibition.

D. Postoperative Malabsorption:

1. After gastric surgery—Many patients operated upon for peptic ulcer disease lose weight after surgery. In most cases this results from reduced food intake due to early satiety and to the development of food-related symptoms (pain, nausea, vomiting, and diarrhea). In some patients malabsorption is responsible for weight loss.

Malabsorption after gastric surgery is multifactorial. Most operations for ulcer are designed to reduce gastric acidity. This also reduces pepsin secretion and may allow bacterial overgrowth in the stomach and small intestine. Truncal vagotomy or gastric resection impairs the grinding of solid food into small particles, reducing the surface area that can be attacked by digestive enzymes. Gastric emptying of liquid is somewhat more rapid after most traditional ulcer surgeries. This results in dilution of pancreatic enzymes and bile acid in the duodenum (when chyme has access to the duodenum) and mismatching of chyme delivery and absorptive capacity. Rapid transit through the intestine may reduce contact time with the absorptive surface, reducing absorptive capacity. In some patients gastrectomy brings out latent celiac sprue or lactase deficiency as independent causes of malabsorption. Malabsorption of specific nutrients, such as iron, calcium, or vitamin B_{12} may also occur after gastric surgery.

Although there are many potential mechanisms of malabsorption after surgery, malabsorption is usually only mild to moderate unless complicating features like small bowel bacterial overgrowth occur. Steatorrhea is typically less than 15–20 g daily.

Treatment depends on the specific findings of an evaluation for the mechanism of malabsorption. Bacterial overgrowth should be assessed, since it is readily treatable with antibiotics. Trials of antiperistaltic agents, such as anticholinergics or opiates, may reduce rapid gastric emptying and intestinal transit and redress some of the pathophysiology leading to malabsorption. In some patients exogenous pancreatic enzymes administered with food may improve intraluminal digestion and reduce steatorrhea. Reoperation is indicated in patients with anatomical problems causing malabsorption, such as blind loop syndrome, afferent loop obstruction, or gastrocolic fistula.

2. After intestinal resection—Short intestinal resections are usually well tolerated without symptoms. Extensive small bowel resections produce diarrhea and malabsorption of variable severity, commonly known as short bowel syndrome. The extent of resection necessary to produce malabsorption varies and depends upon the portion of the intestine removed, since functional capacity differs from segment to segment. Nutrient absorptive needs can generally be met if at least 100 cm of jejunum is preserved. However, fluid absorptive needs may not be met by this length of residual bowel. Moreover, the specific transport abilities of the ileum (eg, absorbing vitamin B_{12} or bile acid) will be lost if that segment of the intestine is removed. The issue of the extent of resection necessary to produce symptoms is further complicated by intestinal adaption. Absorptive capacity for some nutrients can increase with time; thus, initially inadequate absorption may become adequate over weeks to months. The factors leading to hyperplasia and hypertrophy of the remaining intestine are not understood completely.

Malabsorption in short bowel syndrome is not due solely to loss of absorptive surface. Other factors contributing include: (1) gastric acid hypersecretion; (2) bile acid deficiency; (3) loss of the "ileal brake," a neurohumoral mechanism slowing gastric emptying and intestinal transit when nutrients enter the ileum; and (4) bacterial overgrowth, particularly when the ileocecal valve has been compromised. It is claimed that small ileal resections (< 100 cm) produce diarrhea due to bile acid malabsorption and that larger resections produce steatorrhea due to loss of absorptive surface.

Treatment of short bowel syndrome consists of maximizing absorptive capacity by slowing intestinal transit with antiperistaltic agents, ingestion of a diet designed to take advantage of remaining absorptive capacity, and correction of specific vitamin, mineral, and electrolyte abnormalities. Patients may need parenteral nutrition if they cannot be maintained with enteral intake (either orally or via continuous tube feeding). Small bowel transplantation is now under investigation as a long-term solution for selected patients with short bowel syndrome.

Complications of short bowel syndrome include cholesterol gallstones, oxalate kidney stones, and lactic acidosis. Prognosis depends on the ability to maintain nutritional status, to prevent fluid and electrolyte depletion, and to avoid complications of therapy, such as sepsis or loss of venous access.

E. Disorders Which Cause Malabsorption of Specific Nutrients:

1. Disaccharidase (carbohydrase) deficiency—Ingested disaccharides, such as lactose or sucrose, and starch breakdown products, such as maltotriose and alpha-limit dextrins, are hydrolyzed by brush border enzymes into monosaccharides that can be transported across the apical membrane of the enterocyte. These enzymes include lactase, maltase, sucrase-isomaltase, and trehalase and are glycoproteins inserted into the brush border membrane of villous cells after intracellular processing. If these hydrolytic enzymes are not active because of defective synthesis or processing, or if the luminal surface of the villous cell is damaged, carbohydrate malabsorption results. Gaseousness occurs regularly and osmotic diarrhea can occur, if the load of carbohydrate entering the colon exceeds the capacity for colonic bacterial fermentation and short-chain fatty acid absorption.

Congenital deficiencies of these enzymes occur, but are rare diseases. For example, congenital lactase deficiency is an autosomal recessive trait (as are all of these genetic deficiencies) that has been described in fewer than 50 individuals. Symptoms begin as soon as milk is given to the newborn and disappear when milk is removed from the diet. Similar rare syndromes have been described for sucrase-isomaltase and trehalase, but symptoms do not begin until later in life when their substrates are introduced into the diet. (Trehalase, a disaccharide in mushrooms and insects, may never be consumed in large enough amounts to produce symptoms, even if trehalase activity is deficient.)

In contrast, secondary deficiency of lactase is quite common. In most human populations (as in most mammals) intestinal lactase activity declines to low levels after weaning. By early adulthood, most people have <10% of normal lactase activity and many develop symptoms with ingestion of milk or other lactose-containing foods. The one exception to this is the western European population, in which lactase activity is well-maintained into adulthood. Thus, acquired lactase deficiency can be looked on as the rule and persistent lactase activity as the exception. Nevertheless, unrecognized hypolactasia may be the cause of symptoms when it develops in a person who previously could tolerate milk and must be considered when patients present with gaseousness or intermittent diarrhea. Secondary deficiencies of other disaccharidases also occur but are much less common unless there has been extensive compromise of the brush border membrane.

Symptoms of disaccharidase deficiency are diet-dependent. They therefore vary widely from day to day, depending upon dietary intake of the malabsorbed substrate. Gaseousness, bloating, flatulence, and variable stool consistency are typical symptoms. Stools are usually acid and, when diarrhea is profuse, an osmotic gap may be present in stool water. Diagnosis can be suggested by breath hydrogen testing after ingestion of the malabsorbed substrate and can be proven by assay for enzyme activity in mucosal biopsy specimens. Dietary management by elimination of substrate should be completely successful in abolishing symptoms, but dietary indiscretion is common, since many processed foods have fillers, such as non-fat dried milk, added to them. Pretreatment of food with exogenous lactase before ingestion may reduce symptoms, but is usually ineffective, incompletely relieving them.

2. Transport defects at the brush border— Glucose-galactose malabsorption is a rare congenital disease that presents like congenital lactase deficiency soon after birth. In this condition hydrolysis of lactose is intact, but the hexose transporter is defective, preventing entry of glucose and galactose into the cell. Transport of fructose is normal. Hexose transport in the renal tubule is often abnormal also, producing glycosuria. Recognition of the disorder soon after birth is essential, since diarrhea is quite severe and dehydration occurs quickly. Feeding fructose and eliminating glucose and galactose from the diet prevents symptoms and allows normal development.

There are several other congenital transport defects producing malabsorption of specific nutrients, including Hartnup disease (neutral aminoacid transport) and cystinuria. These do not produce prominent gastrointestinal symptoms.

3. Abetalipoproteinemia–This rare autosomal recessive disease is due to failure to produce apolipoprotein B and the lipoproteins containing apolipoprotein B (chylomicrons, very low density lipoproteins and low density lipoproteins). Since long chain triglyceride transport by enterocytes is linked to formation of chylomicrons, triglyceride "backs up" in the mucosal cells producing a foamy appearance under the microscope. Mild steatorrhea beginning in childhood, fat-soluble vitamin deficiencies, failure to gain weight, anemia with acanthocytosis, retinitis pigmentosa, and progressive peripheral neuropathy are the usual clinical manifestations. Several similar syndromes have been described, including normotriglyceridemic abetalipoproteinemia and chylomicron retention disease, which occur in patients with defects in apolipoprotein B-48 metabolism. A low fat diet supplemented by medium chain triglyceride (not requiring chylomicron formation for malabsorption) and fat-soluble vitamin replacement can reduce symptoms in all of these conditions.

Malabsorption in Specific Settings

A. Malabsorption in Childhood: Malabsorption developing in infancy and childhood should bring to mind a distinct differential diagnosis (Table 24–9). For example, congenital enzyme deficiency states may become manifest as nutrients are added to the infant's diet. Other conditions may be more or less likely to occur in young individuals. Two conditions should be considered in particular, celiac disease and cystic fibrosis. Celiac disease can develop any time after wheat and other gluten-containing foods are added to the diet. Cystic fibrosis produces malabsorption when pancreatic insufficiency manifests itself. The diagnosis of cystic fibrosis should be considered when respiratory disease is accompanied by evidence of malabsorption.

The presentation of malabsorption may also be different than that in adults. Children may be less likely to complain of changes in stool consistency after toilet training is completed. Growth retardation may be more prominent than weight loss. Patients whose growth is slowed should be screened for malabsorption. Growth failure can be reversed if caught in time and adequate nutrition is provided.

B. Malabsorption in the Elderly: Almost any cause of malabsorption can present in old age. Several should be considered more prominently. These include small bowel bacterial overgrowth (due to

Table 24–9. Differential diagnosis of malabsorption in childhood.

Problem	Mechanism
Congenital	
[1]Intestinal malrotation	Blind loop syndrome
Intestinal duplication	Blind loop syndrome
[1]Short small bowel	Lack of absorptive surface
Lymphangiectasia	Lymphatic obstruction
[1]Primary lactase deficiency	Enzyme deficiency
Sucrase-isomaltase deficiency	Enzyme deficiency
Glucose-galactose malabsorption	Transport protein dysfunction
Cystinuria	Transport protein dysfunction
Hartnup disease	Transport protein dysfunction
Abetalipoproteinemia	Metabolic disorder
Familial dysautonomia	Abnormal transit time
[1]Cystic fibrosis	Pancreatic exocrine insufficiency
Familial pancreatitis	Pancreatic exocrine insufficiency
[1]Biliary atresia	Bile acid deficiency
Immune deficiency syndromes	Small bowel bacterial overgrowth
Acquired	
Short bowel syndrome	Lack of absorptive surface
[1]Giardiasis	Parasitosis
[1]Necrotizing enterocolitis	Mucosal damage
[1]Milk allergy	Mucosal damage
Eosinophilic gastroenteritis	Mucosal damage
[1]Celiac disease	Mucosal damage
Tropical sprue	Mucosal damage
Dermatitis herpetiformis	Mucosal damage
[1]Adrenal insufficiency	Mucosal damage
Chronic pancreatitis	Pancreatic exocrine insufficiency
Neoplasm (ganglioneuroma, carcinoid, lymphoma)	Abnormal transit time, others
[1]Crohn's disease	Multiple

[1]More common diagnoses in North America.

hypochlorhydria, motility disorders, and jejunal diverticula), pancreatic exocrine insufficiency, and diabetes mellitus.

C. Systemic Diseases Causing Malabsorption:

1. Diabetes mellitus and other endocrine disease–Gastrointestinal symptoms occur regularly in patients with diabetes mellitus and are usually attributed to the effects of autonomic neuropathy. These include nausea and vomiting, constipation, diarrhea, and fecal incontinence. In some diabetics, steatorrhea is prominent (usually with chronic diarrhea). The mechanism of diabetic steatorrhea is not always understood. Three conditions should be excluded: (1) small bowel bacterial overgrowth, (2) celiac disease, and (3) pancreatic exocrine insufficiency. These conditions occur with increased frequency in diabetics. Steatorrhea occurring in the absence of these conditions can sometimes be attributed to rapid intestinal transit. The mechanism of steatorrhea in diabetes is important to work out since it is likely to be a recurrent problem. Treatment depends on the cause of the malabsorption.

Both hyperthyroidism and hypothyroidism can be associated with malabsorption. In hyperthyroidism, rapid intestinal transit, hyperphagia, and altered intestinal secretion have all been implicated. Correction of hyperthyroidism with drugs, radioiodine, or surgery corrects steatorrhea. In hypothyroidism, celiac disease or partial villous atrophy may occur. This seems to respond to gluten withdrawal.

Some patients with Addison's disease develop malabsorption that can be reversed by treatment with corticosteroids. Autoimmune adrenal insufficiency is associated with celiac disease; this responds to gluten withdrawal.

Hypoparathyroidism has been associated with malabsorption that may be due to villous atrophy, motility disorders, and lymphangiectasia.

2. Collagen-vascular diseases—Advanced scleroderma is often associated with small intestine problems. Replacement of the smooth muscle with fibrous tissue and the presence of small bowel diverticula predispose to bacterial overgrowth. This can produce steatorrhea of varying severity. Antibiotic therapy is quite helpful, but recurrence is the rule and episodic therapy may be necessary.

Vasculitis is sometimes associated with severe weight loss that has been attributed to small bowel ischemia.

3. Amyloidosis—Amyloidosis can produce malabsorption by several mechanisms. Infiltration of the mucosa can affect enterocyte function, but ischemia (from vascular compromise), pancreatic exocrine insufficiency, bacterial overgrowth and dysmotility (from muscle infiltration) probably contribute as well. The diagnosis can be suggested by small bowel x-ray and confirmed by biopsy, but most experts advise avoiding intestinal biopsy, if possible, for fear of inducing bleeding. Biopsy of abdominal fat is easy, safe, and frequently positive.

4. AIDS—Chronic wasting is a common presentation of AIDS in Africa and is seen elsewhere, as well. Diarrhea and malabsorption in AIDS is usually due to any of several opportunistic infections. Careful search for potential pathogens can result in improvement with therapy. The role of HIV-1 in causing enterocyte dysfunction by itself is controversial. Pancreatic exocrine insufficiency can also occur in the course of this illness and may be readily treated. Lymphoma can produce malabsorption during the course of AIDS and is not amenable to treatment. *Mycobacterium avium intracellulare* infection is frequent in patients with AIDS and probably accounts for many cases of malabsorption in this patient group (see previous section, *"Mycobacterium-avium intracellulare"*).

REFERENCES

Anonymous. Choosing and using a pancreatic enzyme supplement. Drug & Therapeutic Bulletin 1992;30:37.

Beebe DK, Walley E: Diabetic diarrhea. An underdiagnosed complication? Postgrad Med 1992;91:179.

Casellas F, Chicharro L, Malagelada JR: Potential usefulness of hydrogen breath test with D-xylose in clinical management of intestinal malabsorption. Dig Dis Sci 1993;38:321.

Cosnes J et al: Adaptive hyperphagia in patients with postsurgical malabsorption. Gastroenterology 1990;99:1814.

Donald IP et al: The diagnosis of small bowel bacterial overgrowth in elderly patients. J Am Geriat Soc 1992;40:692.

Edes TE: Clinical management of short-bowel syndrome. Enhancing the patient's quality of life. Postgrad Med 1990;88:91.

Ehrenpreis ED et al: D-xylose malabsorption: characteristic finding in patients with the AIDS wasting syndrome and chronic diarrhea. J Acquired Immune Defic Synd 1992;5:1047.

Ehrenpreis ED et al: Histopathologic findings of duodenal biopsy specimens in HIV-infected patients with and without diarrhea and malabsorption. Am J Clin Path 1992;97:21.

Eusufzai S: Bile acid malabsorption in patients with chronic diarrhoea. Scand J Gastroenterol 1993;28:865.

Fernandez-Banares F et al: Sugar malabsorption in functional bowel disease: clinical implications. Am J Gastro 1993;88:2044.

Ford GA et al: Use of the SeHCAT test in the investigation of the diarrhoea. Postgrad Med J 1992;68:272.

Gillanders L et al: Dietary management of the patient with massive enterectomy. New Zealand Med J 1990;103:322.

Grunfeld C, Kotler DP: Wasting in the acquired immunodeficiency syndrome. Semin Liver Dis 1992;12:175.

Gudmand-Hoyer E: The clinical significance of disaccharide maldigestion. Am J Clin Nutri 1994;59(Suppl):735S.

Gueant JL et al: Malabsorption of vitamin B_{12} in pancreatic insufficiency of the adult and of the child. Pancreas 1990;5:559.

Haboubi NY, Montgomery RD: Small-bowel bacterial overgrowth in elderly people: clinical significance and response to treatment. Age & Ageing 1992;21:13.

Hammer HF et al: Carbohydrate malabsorption. Its measurement and its contribution to diarrhea. J Clin Invest 1990;86:1936.

Hjelt K, Paerregaard A, Krasilnikof PA: Giardiasis causing chronic diarrhoea in suburban Copenhagen: Incidence, physical growth, clinical symptoms and small intestinal abnormality. Acta Paediatr 1992;81:881.

Holt PR: Diarrhea and malabsorption in the elderly. Gastro Clin of North Amer 1990;19:345.

Kapembwa MS et al: Ileal and jejunal absorptive function in patients with AIDS and enterococcidial infection. J of Infection 1990;21:43.

Ladas SD et al: Effect of forceps size and mode of orientation on endoscopic small bowel biopsy evaluation. Gastrointest Endo 1994;40:51.

Nightingale JM et al: Jejunal efflux in short bowel syndrome. Lancet 1990;336:765.

Peled Y et al: D-xylose absorption test. Urine or blood? Dig Dis Sci 1991;36:188.

Perman JA: Clinical application of breath hydrogen measurements. Canad J Physiol & Pharmacol 1991;69:11.

Riby JE, Fujisawa T, Kretchmer N: Fructose absorption. Am J Clin Nutri 1993;58(Suppl):748S.

Riley SA, Turnberg LA: Maldigestion and Malabsorption. In: *Gastrointestinal Disease: Pathophysiology, Diagnosis, Management,* 5/e. Sleisenger MH, Fordtran JS (editors). Saunders, 1993.

Robinson PJ, Smith AL, Sly PD: Duodenal pH in cystic fibrosis and its relationship to fat malabsorption. Dig Dis Sci 1990;35:1299.

Rubesin SE, Rubin RA, Herlinger H: Small bowel malabsorption: Clinical and radiologic perspectives. How we see it. Radiology 1992;184:297.

Saverymuttu SH et al: Impact of endoscopic duodenal biopsy on the detection of small intestinal villous atrophy. Postgrad Med J 1991;67:47.

Spickett GP, Misbah SA, Chapel HM: Primary antibody deficiency in adults. Lancet 1991;337:281.

Strocchi A et al: Detection of malabsorption of low doses of carbohydrate: Accuracy of various breath H_2 criteria. Gastroenterology 1993;105:1404.

Suhr O, Danielsson A, Steen L: Bile acid malabsorption caused by gastrointestinal motility dysfunction? An investigation of gastrointestinal disturbances in familial amyloidosis with polyneuropathy. Scand J Gastroenterol 1992;27:201.

Toskes PP: Bacterial overgrowth of the gastrointestinal tract. Advances in Intern Med 1993;38:387.

Turk E et al: Glucose/galactose malabsorption caused by a defect in the Na^+/glucose cotransporter. Nature 1991;350:354.

Williams AJ, Merrick MV, Eastwood MA: Idiopathic bile acid malabsorption—a review of clinical presentation, diagnosis, and response to treatment. Gut 1991;32:1004.

25

Tumors of the Stomach & Small Intestine

Samuel B. Ho, MD

Pathophysiology

Gastrointestinal neoplasms arise by the accumulation of genetic mutations. Predisposing conditions are associated with increased proliferation of mucosal epithelial cells. Increased cell proliferation increases the likelihood of genetic mutation, amplification, deletion, or rearrangement resulting in the loss of tumor suppressor gene function or activation of proto-oncogenes.

Several case control studies have suggested an association between *Helicobacter pylori* infection and gastric cancer, including gastric lymphomas and both intestinal and diffuse types of adenocarcinoma. However, only a small proportion of individuals infected with *H pylori* subsequently develop cancer, indicating that other carcinogenic factors are necessary for disease to develop. *H pylori* infection is associated with chronic atrophic gastritis (type B, predominantly involving the antrum), intestinal metaplasia, and impaired gastric acid secretion. Investigators have speculated that this latter condition may lead to bacterial overgrowth and increased bacterial production of N-nitroso compounds from nitrates in the diet. Chronic gastritis is associated with increased cell proliferation, which increases epithelial susceptibility to genetic alterations. In addition, altered mucous production associated with gastritis and metaplasia may increase mucosal susceptibility to luminal factors or carcinogens.

Intestinal metaplasia is defined as the replacement of normal gastric epithelium with columnar epithelium similar to the small intestine or colon. Three types of intestinal metaplasia have been described, based on morphologic criteria and mucin histochemistry. Type I intestinal metaplasia is characterized by straight crypts with well-developed goblet and absorptive cells. Goblet cells contain sialomucins and absorptive cells are nonsecretory. Type II intestinal metaplasia contains less well-differentiated small intestinal epithelium. Type III intestinal metaplasia has tortuous crypts with immature columnar cells and goblet cells containing sulphomucins. Several studies have shown that type III intestinal metaplasia is most commonly associated with gastric cancer, usually of the intestinal type. A recent cohort study from Filipe and coworkers determined that the relative risk for gastric cancer was 2.14 for type II and 4.58 for type III, compared with type I intestinal metaplasia. Type III intestinal metaplasia may be a possible predictive factor for the development of gastric cancer. Molecular features associated with different types of intestinal metaplasia remain to be determined.

Numerous epidemiologic studies have identified other potential contributing factors to gastric cancer, including diets with low fat and protein intake, low vitamin A and C intake, high intake of salted meat and fish, and high intake of nitrates. Low socioeconomic status is associated with increased cancer risk, which may be explained by poor food preparation, poor nutrition, lack of refrigeration and increased *H pylori* infection rates. Whereas smoking increases the risk of gastric cancer, alcohol intake does not.

Other conditions associated with chronic gastritis have also been associated with increased risk of gastrointestinal cancer. Chronic gastritis due to pernicious anemia is categorized as type A (autoimmune) and typically involves the body and fundus rather than the antrum. The increased risk attributable to pernicious anemia is small. In a recent large retrospective study of patients with pernicious anemia, the ratio of observed to expected gastric cancers was 3:2. Increased risk of stomach cancer is also found in patients who have undergone partial gastrectomy with a Billroth II anastomosis, and also in patients who have had a Billroth I anastomosis or a vagotomy and pyloroplasty. The increased risk following gastric surgery occurs after a period of 15–20 years. In addition to atrophic gastritis, contributing factors for the development of gastric cancer include: achlorhydria, a vagotomy, and duodenogastric reflux. Patients with congenital or acquired immunodeficiency states, including AIDS, are at increased risk for gastrointestinal lymphomas. Celiac sprue is a risk factor for intestinal lymphomas, which usually occur in the jejunum; these lymphomas also may be multifocal. Inflammatory bowel disease is a risk factor for adenocarcinoma and possibly lymphoma. The increased cancer risk in these patients described above is not considered to be high enough to warrant routine endoscopic screening.

Gastric cancer can be divided into two histologic

subtypes, with differing biologic characteristics which may reflect differing etiologic factors (see Table 25–2). The first type, "intestinal," is characterized by gland formation, and often appears similar to colon carcinoma. The second type, "diffuse," is characterized by poorly differentiated cells that cluster in sheets or nodules; this type is devoid of gland-like structure. The intestinal-type is the predominant form found in areas with epidemic gastric cancer and is associated with atrophic gastritis and intestinal metaplasia. This type is more common in males and the elderly. The diffuse-type is more common in endemic areas and is not typically associated with precursor lesions in the stomach. This type is more common in women and in younger patients.

Aneuploidy is defined as an abnormal amount of DNA per cell and can be detected by flow cytometry in fresh or formalin-fixed specimens. A number of studies have determined that aneuploidy is present in 40–70% of gastric adenocarcinomas. The presence of aneuploidy correlates with increased pathologic stage and worse survival.

A number of specific genetic abnormalities have been described in gastric adenocarcinomas, which appear similar regardless of the country of origin. Chromosomal alterations include frequent deletions of portions of chromosomes 5q, 17p, and 18q—the sites of tumor suppressor genes APC, p53, and DCC, respectively. These sites are frequently altered in other cancers, also such as adenocarcinoma of the colon. In general, more advanced cancers are associated with more numerous chromosomal abnormalities. The p53 gene product is a DNA-binding phosphoprotein that plays a role in proliferation, apoptosis, and DNA repair, and is the most common genetic abnormality found in cancers. Altered p53 is found more frequently in advanced gastric cancers and is associated with a worse prognosis.

Several alterations of dominantly-acting oncogenes have been described in gastric adenocarcinomas. Oncogenes related to fibroblast growth factor (*hst-1/int-2*) and fibroblast growth factor receptors (K-*sam*) are frequently amplified or overexpressed. Amplification or overexpression of *HER2/NEU* (also known as *erb*B-2, a receptor related to the epidermal growth factor receptor) is associated with lymph node metastases and a worse prognosis, and, in multivariant analysis, is an independent predictor of survival. In contrast with colon adenocarcinomas, mutations or overexpression of the *ras* family of oncogenes occurs rarely in gastric adenocarcinomas. Precursor lesions such as superficial gastritis or gastric dysplasia may also demonstrate genetic alterations, such as altered expression of tyrosine kinase growth factor receptor *met, ras* oncogenes, and p53. However, the relationship of specific genetic abnormalities and progressive stages of gastric carcinogenesis has not been completely defined.

Prior *H pylori* infection has been associated with primary gastric lymphomas, but not with lymphomas of other sites. *H pylori*-induced gastritis is characterized by infiltration of the mucosa with lymphocytes. This is thought to give rise to low grade gastric lymphomas that resemble mucosa-associated lymphoid tissue (MALT) rather than lymphomas associated with lymph nodes. Low grade MALT lymphomas and high grade B-cell lymphomas may be found together in patients with gastric lymphoma, and it is thought that low grade MALT lymphomas may be a precursor to high grade gastric lymphomas.

Chromosomal abnormalities play an important role in the pathogenesis of lymphocytic lymphomas of the gastrointestinal tract. More than 90% of lymphocytic lymphomas display cytogenetic abnormalities, and greater numbers of these abnormalities are associated with higher grade tumors. The molecular genetics of lymphoma is characterized by translocation of DNA from one chromosome to another. Clinically important translocations appear to bring oncogene regions in proximity to immunoglobulin genes. The t(8;14) and t(8;22) translocations bring the *myc* oncogene on chromosome 8 close to immunoglobulin heavy chain or light chain loci, respectively. This results in upregulation of *myc* gene expression, which is a DNA-binding protein involved in control of proliferation. The t(14;18) translocation juxtaposes the B-cell leukemia lymphoma-2 gene (*BCL2*) and the immunoglobulin heavy chain joining region on chromosome 14. These lead to increased *BCL2* protein expression, which is an inner mitochondrial membrane protein that contributes to tumor proliferation by blocking programmed cell death (apoptosis). Other genes that are implicated in translocations in lymphomas include *BCL1, PRAD1* (a cell-cycle regulatory protein or cyclin), and T-cell receptor genes (*TCRα, TCRδ, TCRβ TCRγ*). Interestingly, low grade MALT-type lymphomas of the stomach characteristically do not demonstrate rearrangement of the *BCL2* gene. The differences in molecular alterations in gastrointestinal and nongastrointestinal lymphomas, and the relationship of molecular changes in precursor and early stage lymphomas with late stage lymphomas have not been well characterized.

Essentials of Diagnosis

- Common gastric and small intestinal malignancies include adenocarcinoma, lymphoma, metastatic carcinoma, leiomyoma, and carcinoid. These must be differentiated from benign ulcerative lesions and polyps by endoscopic or surgical biopsy.
- Symptoms and signs include abdominal pain, weight loss, obstructive symptoms, and evidence of intestinal blood loss or iron deficiency anemia.
- Diagnosis of early stage gastric cancer requires a high index of suspicion for patients who are at increased risk, eg, new symptoms in patients aged 40–45 or older, history of prior gastric surgery, prior history of pernicious anemia, celiac sprue,

immunodeficiency or gastric polyps. Diagnosis requires referral for endoscopy or barium radiologic examinations.

- Diagnosis of small bowel tumors often requires a barium enteroclysis examination performed by an experienced radiologist or endoscopy using small bowel enteroscopes.

General Considerations

The stomach, and less frequently the small intestine, give rise to a variety of benign and malignant tumors (Table 25–1). In 5000 endoscopic examinations of the stomach conducted over a 7-year period at the University of Chicago, approximately 119 gastric malignant growths (2.4%) and 125 benign gastric polyps (2.5%) were diagnosed. The most frequent gastric malignant growth is adenocarcinoma, followed by primary gastric lymphoma, metastatic carcinoma, and less frequently leiomyosarcoma, carcinoid, and Kaposi's sarcoma. These present as ulcerated or polypoid lesions which must be differentiated from benign tumors by endoscopic or operative biopsies.

Gastric adenocarcinoma is the second most common malignant growth world wide. Gastric cancer is particularly common, or epidemic, in Japan, Eastern Europe, and South America. In Japan, the gastric cancer incidence is 100 per 100,000 persons and is the leading cause of cancer deaths. In the United States, the overall annual incidence of gastric cancer has declined from 33 cases per 100,000 population in 1935 to less than 6 cases per 100,000 in the 1990s, and is currently the seventh leading cause of death due to malignant tumor among males and eleventh among females. However, the incidence of adenocarcinoma of the gastric cardia and gastroesophageal junction has been increasing in both the United States and Europe over the last 15 years.

Lymphoma is the second-most common malignancy encountered in the stomach. Primary gastric lymphomas account for 3–5% of gastric neoplasms. The large majority of these lymphomas are B-cell non-Hodgkin's lymphomas of the diffuse, large cell type. Gastric lymphoma is the most common extranodal lymphoma, accounting for 20–24% of primary extranodal lymphomas. Less frequent primary gastric malignancies include carcinoid tumors and leiomyosarcomas. The occurrence of carcinoids in the stomach is rare; approximately 95% of all carcinoid tumors occur in the rectum, appendix, and small intestine. Leiomyosarcomas can occur in all segments of the intestine. Leiomyomas can be distinguished from leiomyosarcomas by the number of cells in mitosis per high power field and the cellularity of the tumor.

Tumors of the small intestine are much less com-

Table 25–1. Tumors of the stomach and small intestine.

	Tumors	Percentage of total	Benign polyps	Percentage of total
		Endoscopic series		Endoscopic series
Gastric	Adenocarcinoma	86	Hyperplastic	71
	Lymphoma	8	Adenomatous	11
	Metastatic carcinoma	4	Leiomyoma	6
	Leiomyosarcoma	<2	Pancreatic rest	<2
	Carcinoid	<2	Myoepithelial hamartoma	<2
	Kaposi's sarcoma		Peutz-Jeghers hamartoma, eosinophilic granuloma, no histologic diagnosis, neurogenic tumors, lipoma	5
		Surgical series		Surgical series
Small intestine	Adenocarcinoma	29–40	Adenomas (polypoid, Brunner gland, islet cell)	25–38
	Carcinoid	29–49	Leiomyoma	35
	Leiomyosarcoma	15–22	Lipoma	4–20
	Lymphoma	4–11	Hamartomas, fibromas, neurogenic	
	Metastatic carcinoma		Angiomas, myxomas, other rare types	
	Kaposi's sarcoma		Pseudotumors, lymphoid hyperplasia, hyperplastic inflammatory, pancreatic rests, Brunner gland hyperplasia, Amyloidosis, Endometrioma	

mon than gastric tumors, and account for only 1–2% of all gastrointestinal malignant growths. During a 20-year period at Case Western Reserve University, 64 patients underwent surgical resection for primary small bowel tumors; of these, 38 (59%) were malignant and 26 (41%) were benign. The relative frequencies of different histologic types of small bowel tumors are listed in Table 25–1. The majority of small bowel adenocarcinomas and leiomyosarcomas occur in the duodenum and jejunum. In contrast, the majority of small bowel carcinoids and lymphomas occur in the ileum.

Clinical Findings

A. Symptoms and Signs: Symptoms associated with early gastrointestinal tumors are often minimal or nonspecific. The initial symptoms attributable to a tumor depend on its location. Obstructing lesions of the lower esophagus and gastric cardia often cause dysphagia to solid foods. Because of this location, tumors of the lower esophagus and gastric cardia may be diagnosed at an earlier stage compared with tumors of the body or antrum. Early tumors in the body or antrum are asymptomatic or cause vague abdominal discomfort or "fullness," dyspepsia-like symptoms, nausea, or diminished appetite. Patients often will alter their diet in an attempt to ameliorate these symptoms. Symptoms of gastric outlet obstruction, early satiety, and weight loss indicate a large or advanced-stage tumor. Early satiety results from infiltration of the gastric wall and loss of distensibility. Gastric tumors may also cause occult gastrointestinal blood loss and the development of symptoms associated with iron deficiency anemia.

Since the symptoms of early stage gastric tumors are minimal or mimic those of acid-peptic disease, the diagnosis is often delayed. Consequently, the proportion of patients diagnosed with advanced stage tumors is high. Diagnosis of operable gastric cancers requires a high index of suspicion and early referral for endoscopy or radiologic studies. If dyspeptic symptoms are accompanied by weight loss, vomiting, dysphagia, or evidence of gastrointestinal blood loss, then endoscopy should be performed first before any therapeutic trials are initiated. Of particular concern are new "dyspeptic" symptoms that develop in patients over 40–45 years of age. Predisposing factors such as prior gastric resection, pernicious anemia, or prior gastric adenomas should also be taken into consideration when considering early diagnostic studies.

The indications for endoscopy in patients presenting with dyspepsia and no other symptoms are evolving. Currently, many physicians elect to treat dyspeptic symptoms with a course of H_2 blocker therapy, and proceed to endoscopy only for persistent symptoms following a 1- to 2-month course of therapy. Others will attempt to diagnose *H pylori* infection and associated ulcers prior to initiating treatment.

Tumors of the small intestine usually present with pain, obstructive symptoms, or bleeding. The pain is cramping and intermittent and results from partial lumenal obstruction. Other symptoms include nausea, vomiting, anorexia, altered bowel habits, and weight loss. Gastrointestinal bleeding is usually self-limited or occult. Patients presenting with melena or iron deficiency anemia should have a dedicated radiologic examination of the small intestine or enteroscopy if endoscopic studies of the gastroduodenum and colon do not reveal a cause. Similarly, occult fecal blood loss associated with anemia or symptoms should be evaluated in a similar fashion.

Less frequently, gastric and small intestinal tumors may present with a gastrointestinal emergency, such as massive hemorrhage, acute obstruction, intussusception, or perforation. Adenocarcinomas, lymphomas, and leiomyosarcomas may present with acute gastrointestinal hemorrhage and require blood transfusion and management in an intensive care unit. Diagnosis is initially attempted using endoscopic procedures. Injection or thermal endoscopic therapies which have been shown to be effective for bleeding peptic ulcers are often not successful if the bleeding is caused by a malignant growth. Continued bleeding should be treated by urgent laparotomy or angiographic vessel occlusion. Leiomyosarcomas may present with acute bleeding into the peritoneal cavity with little intraluminal blood loss.

Patients with acute obstruction present with persistent nausea, vomiting, and abdominal pain. Flat and upright films of the abdomen may demonstrate dilated small intestine and air fluid levels above the site of obstruction. Perforation should be considered if the pain is severe, constant, and associated with rebound tenderness, fever, or leukocytosis. The primary diagnostic and therapeutic procedures for patients with acute obstruction or perforation are surgical; therefore, early consultation with the surgical service is mandatory for patients with these symptoms. Perforation is a sign of an advanced tumor, and is associated with a worse prognosis.

Symptoms do not distinguish carcinoid from other tumors of the intestine, unless the carcinoid is advanced and produces the carcinoid syndrome. Carcinoid syndrome results from a large tumor mass that drains into the caval circulation. This is found with hepatic metastases, with carcinoids developing in large teratomas of the ovaries or testes, or with large tumors that invade retroperitoneal vessels. Symptoms are thought to result from serotonin or other vasoactive substances synthesized by the tumor. The majority of patients complain of diarrhea and facial flushing. Asthma and pellagra may occur in up to 10% of patients. Diagnosis of carcinoid syndrome is made by the demonstration of elevated urinary 5-HIAA levels.

Physical examination often is unhelpful in patients with early gastrointestinal tumors. Guaiac tests of stool obtained on rectal examination should be performed. Pallor and cachexia often indicate an advanced stage of gastric cancer. Palpation of the abdomen occasionally reveals an epigastric mass; this, however, is also only evident with advanced disease. Gastrointestinal lymphomas and leiomyomas may present with a palpable mass in 20–50% of cases. Advanced gastric adenocarcinomas may be associated with physical signs of distant metastases. These include hepatomegaly, ascites (due to peritoneal involvement or secondary to portal hypertension from extensive liver metastases), left supraclavicular lymph adenopathy (Virchow's node), left anterior axillary adenopathy (Irish's node), umbilical nodules (Sister Mary Joseph's node), a rigid rectal prominence above the prostate (Blumer's shelf), and ovarian metastases (Krukenberg tumor). Rare skin abnormalities associated with gastric cancer include acanthosis nigricans, dermatomyositis, metastatic nodules, or warty keratosis and pruritus (sign of Leser-Trelat).

B. Laboratory Findings: Evidence of iron deficiency anemia should always prompt an evaluation of the gastrointestinal tract, including upper and lower gastrointestinal endoscopic procedures. If these procedures are negative, a small bowel barium examination should be performed. Abnormalities of liver function tests may suggest hepatic metastases. Asymptomatic patients without anemia who are found to have a positive stool guaiac on routine screening should have a colonoscopic or barium examination of their colon only, since the finding of gastric or small intestinal malignant growths under these conditions (in North American patients) is exceedingly small.

C. Endoscopy: Upper gastrointestinal endoscopy provides a sensitive and specific method to diagnose gastric tumors. The size and location of abnormalities should be carefully documented during endoscopy. All abnormal mucosal lesions such as ulcers, polyps, strictures, and thickened gastric folds should be biopsied. One study has shown that accurate histologic diagnosis of gastric adenocarcinoma is possible in 95% of cases when four biopsies are taken from a specific lesion. Diagnostic accuracy increases to 98% when 7 biopsies are taken, and if 7–8 biopsies and cytologic brushings or aspirates are taken, diagnostic accuracy approaches 100%. Biopsies should be taken from both the margin and base of ulcer-like lesions. Since visual endoscopic discernment of malignant growths is often inaccurate, it is recommended that at least 4–7 biopsies with or without cytology be obtained from all gastric ulcers and suspicions lesions.

Several endoscopic features of gastric ulcers are more commonly associated with malignancies, however, differentiation of benign and malignant gastric ulcers by endoscopic appearance alone is not reliable. The size of an ulcer is an important risk factor for malignancy, since up to 20% of ulcers over 3 cm in diameter are malignant. Other endoscopic features more frequently associated with malignancy include an irregular base, an irregular ulcer margin (which can be interrupted by tumor nodules), and disruption or abruptly cut-off folds adjacent to the ulcer. All gastric ulcers (with the possible exception of superficial ulceration associated with aspirin and nonsteroidal anti-inflammatory drugs, or NSAIDs), should be followed with repeat endoscopy and biopsy until healed.

Gastric adenocarcinomas have been classified according to their gross appearance. The original classification system was proposed by Borrmann in 1926, and contrasted protruding types with flat or depressed types of cancers; the protruding type was considered to have a better prognosis (Table 25–2). This classification was modified by the Japanese Research Society for Gastric Cancer in 1981. The relationship of tumor contour and prognosis has not been consistent. The most common endoscopic appearance of gastric lymphoma is the presence of large folds in the body or antrum with diffuse ulceration. This is similar to the Bormann IV appearance of advanced gastric adenocarcinoma.

The majority of gastric polyps are benign, and again there are no reliable endoscopic features to differentiate benign from malignant. Polyp size larger than 1 cm is a risk factor for the presence of neoplasia (adenoma) or a malignant growth (Figure 25–1). Biopsy of small polyps (<1 cm) is sufficient for diagnosis. Although larger polyps should be biopsied to determine whether they are neoplastic, this may miss neoplastic foci within the polyp. Before removal of large polyps by endoscopic polypectomy or other surgery, the physician must consider the histology obtained on biopsy, clinical symptoms attributable to the polyp, and the patient's age and medical status, to determine if polyp removal warrants the risk of the procedure. Endoscopic removal of large gastric polyps may be associated with a 4% risk of postpolypectomy bleeding, which may require surgery.

Submucosal polyps are less common than epithelial polyps (see Table 25–1). For submucosal polyps, especially in suspicious areas such as central ulcerations, large forceps biopsies and double biopsies (biopsies within previous biopsy sites) should be performed. Infiltrating adenocarcinoma and lymphomas may also occur in the submucosa. Infiltrating adenocarcinoma (linitis plastica) may be difficult to recognize endoscopically. Subtle changes in gastric folds and areas with poor distensibility should be biopsied. Again, large biopsies and biopsies within biopsies may be required to make a diagnosis. If clinical or endoscopic findings suggest malignancy and biopsies and brushings are negative, large-particle snare biopsy or needle aspiration cytology should be performed. Laparotomy may be required to obtain a histologic diagnosis.

Small bowel enteroscopes may be used to examine the small intestine, and have primarily been used in

Table 25–2. Morphologic and histopathologic classification systems for gastric adenocarcinoma.

Classification	Characteristics	Associations	Prognosis (Compared with average survival)
Lauren			
Intestinal	Gland-like structures	Epidemic prevalence, associated with precursor lesions, men and older patients	Better
Diffuse	Poorly differentiated, unorganized sheets of cells	Endemic prevalence, younger patients and women	Worse
Broder's			
I	Well differentiated, tubular-like arrangement of cells		Better
II	Moderately differentiated, irregular tubules		
III	Poorly-differentiated, irregular sheets of cells		
IV	Anaplastic		Worse
Ming			
Expansive	Discrete tumor nodules growing by expansion	Associated with intestinal metaplasia, M:F = 2:1, 6% under age 50	Better
Infiltrating	Tumor cells individually invade surrounding tissue	M:F = 1:1, 14% under age 50	Worse
Borrmann			
I	Polypoid or fungating		Better
II	Ulcerated with elevated borders		
III	Ulcerated and infiltrating gastric wall		
IV	Diffusely infiltrating		Worse
V	Unclassifiable		

patients with gastrointestinal bleeding and no identifiable source on standard upper and lower gastrointestinal endoscopies. "Push" enteroscopy entails the use of colonsocopes 135–160 cm in length or special 167 cm-long enteroscopes that are inserted through the mouth and into the proximal small intestine under direct visualization. Examination of 50–60 cm beyond the ligament of Treitz can be accomplished with this method. "Sonde-type" enteroscopes are more effective for examination of the distal small intestine. These contain a balloon at the tip which allows for peristalsis to propel the enteroscope into the

Size (mm)	Lesion configuration				Total
	I	II	III	IV	
≤ 4	○2	○8			10
5–9	○2	○13 ◐2	○24	○12	53
10–19	○7	◐2	○8 ◐4	○31	52
20–29	○1	○2	◐1 ●1	○4 ◐2	11
≥ 30	○1	◐5 ●1	◐8 ●9	◐1 ●1	26
Total	13	33	55	51	152

○ Benign
◐ Early gastric cancer
● Advanced gastric cancer

Figure 25–1. The relationship of lesion size, shape or configuration, and histology for 217 elevated lesions of the stomach diagnosed with double contrast radiography. Malignancy occurs more frequently in lesions over 1 cm in diameter. (Reproduced, with permission, from Yamada T, Ichikawa H: X-ray diagnosis of elevated lesions of the stomach. Radiology 1974;110:79–83.)

ileum. Using "sonde-type" enteroscopy, small intestinal lesions have been identified in one-quarter to one-third of patients examined for unexplained gastrointestinal blood loss. Small intestinal tumors have been found in 5% of patients examined by small bowel enteroscopy under these conditions. Diagnosis of small bowel tumors by small bowel enteroscopy has been reported in cases when other imaging modalities, including enteroclysis and angiography, have been negative. The "sonde" technique is limited by the length of time required for passage of the enteroscope (mean 4–8 hours) and lack of tip deflection and biopsy capabilities. Intraoperative endoscopy of the small bowel can also be performed. This involves passage of a colonoscope through the mouth or anus by the endoscopist. The surgeon then manually telescopes loops of bowel over the endoscope.

D. Imaging: Computed tomography (CT) scans of the chest and abdomen are the primary imaging modalities for preoperative staging of stomach and small intestine tumors. In stomachs that are well-distended with contrast, wall thickness of greater than 2 cm may indicate transmural extension of the tumor (Figure 25–2). Evidence of direct invasion of perigastric fat, diaphragm, pancreas, transverse colon, and left lobe of the liver should be sought. Metastases to the liver, lung, and other organs can also be documented. For gastric adenocarcinoma, overall accuracy of preoperative CT scans ranges from 61–72%. CT scans are particularly unreliable in assessing regional lymph nodes and invasion of adjacent organs, resulting in understaging of the disease. CT scans may also overstage gastric adenocarcinoma, resulting in labeling the cancer as unresectable when in fact the tumor may be resectable. One study comparing preoperative CT scanning with surgical staging found that 31% of patients were understaged and 16% were overstaged by CT. Careful review of preoperative CT scans by the gastroenterologist, surgeon, and radiologist is necessary before making a decision regarding resectability.

Endoscopic ultrasound is able to increase the accuracy of preoperative staging by determining the depth of invasion and possibly the involvement of regional lymph nodes. Several studies have compared endoscopic ultrasound, CT scans, and subsequent operative staging. Endoscopic ultrasound demonstrated 83–88% accuracy for determining depth of invasion compared with 35% accuracy for CT. For determining nodal involvement, endoscopic ultrasound is 66–72% accurate compared with 45% accuracy for CT.

Although radiologic examination of the stomach can identify advanced gastric cancers, it is less accurate than endoscopy for identification of early gastric cancer. All ulcers identified by x-ray examination should be referred for endoscopic biopsy. Radiologic criteria that suggest a benign ulcer include radiating folds and a normal-appearing mucosal surface around the crater. Linitus plastica is suggested by ra-

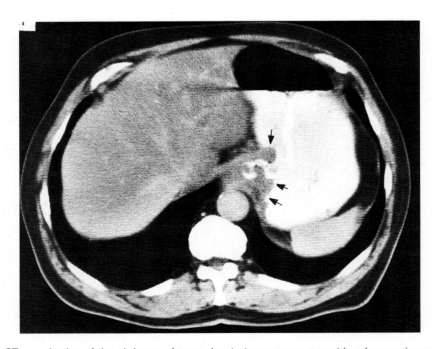

Figure 25–2. CT examination of the abdomen. Arrows denote tumor mass, a gastric adenocarcinoma of the cardia. (Courtesy of Howard Ansel, MD.)

diologic studies that demonstrate a nondistensible stomach.

Radiologic examination of the small bowel remains the most widely used method for diagnosis of small intestinal tumors (Figure 25–3). It is essential to communicate with the radiologist that a small bowel tumor is suspected, so that a dedicated small bowel examination can be performed. The "small bowel follow-though" that accompanies an upper gastrointestinal x-ray is often inadequate for diagnosis of small bowel tumors. Enteroclysis, performed following placement of a naso-duodenal tube, is the most sensitive test for diagnosis of intestinal tumors, particularly if they occur in the jejunum. If an ileal lesion is suspected, a small bowel follow-through with air insufflated in the colon should be performed, which provides a clear air-contrast examination of the ileum. Patients actively bleeding from a suspected small bowel source should undergo a nuclear medicine tagged-RBC examination followed by angiography if the bleeding is continuous. Patients with gastrointestinal blood loss who are not actively bleeding and in whom a small bowel lesion is suspected should undergo a nuclear medicine Meckel's scan before barium studies. In addition to identification of Meckel's diverticula, this scan will occasionally identify leiomyomas or leiomyosarcomas, and can be followed by angiography or laparotomy to confirm the diagnosis.

Differential Diagnosis

Ulcerative and polypoid lesions of the stomach and intestine must be differentiated into benign and malignant categories. All ulcers found in the stomach require endoscopic biopsies and brushings at the time of initial diagnosis. A history of aspirin or NSAID use should be sought. Ulcers should also be followed with repeat endoscopy after a course of therapy, to determine if they have healed, and repeat biopsies taken if healing is not demonstrated. Occasionally, malignant ulcers may appear to heal or partially heal following antacid therapy, and therefore repeated biopsies and brushings are important.

Most polyps found in the stomach are hyperplastic, and usually occur in response to inflammation (see Table 25–1). Adenomatous polyps are the second most frequent type of gastric polyp and are considered precancerous. Adenomas should be removed by endoscopic polypectomy or by surgical means. The risk of malignancy increases in polypoid lesions greater than 1 cm in diameter, and surgical resection should be considered if a definitive diagnosis cannot be made by endoscopic biopsy. Less frequently, benign gastric polyps may represent carcinoid, leiomyoma, lipoma, and pancreatic rests. The latter represent ectopic pancreatic tissue, usually located in the submucosa of the antrum. Pancreatic rests may have a central umbilication or ulceration, and may present with bleeding, obstruction, or rarely, clinical pancreatitis.

Gastric polyps frequently occur in patients with familial polyposis coli. Typically, hyperplastic polyps are found in the fundus and adenomatous polyps in the distal stomach and duodenum. Duodenal and peri-ampullary adenocarcinoma can occur in 1 of 21 patients with familial polyposis coli over a lifetime. Screening endoscopy with careful attention to the duodenal ampulla and removal of all polyps has been recommended for these patients every 4 years. Peutz-Jeghers syndrome is an autosomal dominant condition characterized by intestinal polyps and pigmenta-

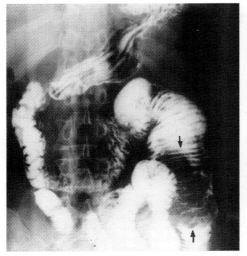

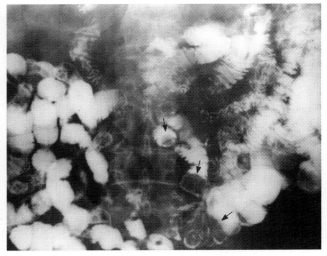

A

B

Figure 25–3. *A:* Primary jejunal adenocarcinoma *(arrows)* diagnosed with a small bowel follow-through barium examination. Bowel proximal to the tumor is dilated. *B:* Metastatic adenocarcinoma of the small bowel *(arrows)* diagnosed with a small bowel follow-through examination. (Courtesy of Howard Ansel, MD.)

tion of the lips, buccal mucosa, hands, feet, or eyelids. Gastric hamartomas occur in 25% of patients with Peutz-Jeghers syndrome. Large folds (> 1 cm in height) in the stomach that may resemble infiltrative malignancy may occur with hypertrophic gastritis and Menetrier's disease. The latter is a very rare condition characterized by mucosal hyperplasia and cystic dilation of gastric glands. Gastric folds in the fundus, body, and occasionally, antrum, appear enlarged, erythematous, and convoluted. Patients present with abdominal pain and hypoproteinemia.

Metastatic cancers may occur in the stomach and should be considered in any patient with gastrointestinal symptoms and history of a prior nongastric malignant growth. The most common metastatic cancers to the stomach or small intestine include lung, breast, and melanoma (Figure 25–3B). These may appear as polypoid lesions with or without erosions or ulceration. Metastatic melanoma characteristically may appear as target or "bull's eye" lesions on a barium x-ray of the stomach, and at endoscopy often appear as small, discrete brown tumor nodules. Larger melanomas may appear as plaques with peripheral pigmentation, submucosal tumors with central ulceration, or as large amelanotic masses. Metastatic breast carcinoma may present with a linitus plastica-type appearance. Other cancers that may metastasize to the stomach include cancer of the ovary, testes, liver, colon, and parotid gland.

Kaposi's sarcoma, a common tumor in patients with AIDS, may be found in the gastrointestinal tract in up to 50% of patients with AIDS-related Kaposi's sarcoma. The endoscopic appearance may consist of erythematous nodules ranging in size from 1 to 5 mm or larger, with or without central erosions. The appearance may also resemble gastric lymphoma with polypoid-type lesions.

Pseudotumors are lesions that simulate common tumors in the intestine. These include inflammatory pseudotumors or fibroid polyps (accumulation of fibroblasts), invasion of the gut wall by nematodes (helminthic pseudotumor), intestinal endometrioma, and amyloidosis.

Staging

A. Gastric Adenocarcinoma: Initial staging of gastric adenocarcinoma includes determination of operative resectability. This requires a complete history and physical examination to evaluate for concomitant medical problems and ability to undergo abdominal surgery. Local staging of the actual tumor includes determination of the size and location of the tumor by endoscopy. Biopsies should be taken of apparently normal mucosa distal and proximal to the lesion to rule out infiltrative or submucosal spread. CT scans of the abdomen and chest are required to determine extent of disease into adjacent organs, possible lymph node involvement, and distant metastases. Careful questioning for new skeletal symptoms may

direct x-ray or bone scan evaluations for osseous metastases. Patients with gastric tumors are generally considered operative candidates if they have no serious concurrent medical problems and when there is no evidence of distant metastases to liver, lung, or other organs.

The most commonly used staging system in the United States is the American Joint Committee on Cancer Staging System (Table 25–3). This system incorporates depth of invasion (T), location of nodal metastases (N), and distant metastases (M). This staging system is similar to the Union Internationale Contre le Cancer (UICC) TNM system used in Europe. Japanese surgeons have developed a rigorous staging system that requires extensive nodal dissection at the time of surgery. This staging system also

Table 25–3. American Joint Committee on Cancer staging of gastric cancer.

Stage	Classification			5-year survival rate
0	Tis	N0	M0	>90%
IA	T1	N0	M0	70–80%
IB	T1	N1	M0	55–70%
	T2	N0	M0	
II	T1	N2	M0	40–50%
	T2	N1	M0	
	T3	N0	M0	
IIIA	T2	N2	M0	10–20%
	T3	N1	M0	
	T4	N0	M0	
IIIB	T3	N2	M0	
	T4	N1	M0	
IV	T4	N2	M0	<1%
	Any T	Any N	M1	

Primary Tumor (T)

TX	Primary tumor cannot be assessed
T0	No evidence of primary tumor
Tis	Carcinoma-in-situ
T1	Tumor invades lamina propria or submucosa
T2	Tumor invades muscularis propria
T3	Tumor invades adventitia
T4	Tumor invades adjacent structures

Regional Lymph Nodes (N)

NX	Regional nodes cannot be assessed
N0	No regional lymph node metastases
N1	Metastasis in perigastric lymph nodes within 3 cm of edge of primary tumor
N2	Metastasis in perigastric lymph nodes more than 3 cm from edge of primary tumor, or in lymph nodes along left gastric, common hepatic, splenic, or celiac arteries

Distant Metastasis (M)

MX	Presence of distant metastasis cannot be assessed
M0	No distant metastasis
M1	Distant metastasis present

incorporates gross (Bormann's classification) and microscopic (Lauren's classification) pathologic characteristics of the cancers. As a consequence, comparison of cancers by stage from Japan and other countries is not often accurate.

"Early" gastric cancers are characterized by their location in the mucosa and submucosa (T1), and may or may not have nodal metastases. By definition, early gastric cancers include stage IA (T1N0), stage IB (T1N1), and stage II (T1N2) tumors. Not surprisingly, early gastric cancers are associated with excellent survival from surgical resection. Early gastric cancers account for only 15% of the cases in the United States. In contrast, they comprise 40% or more of cancers reported in Japan, most likely because of extensive endoscopic surveillance programs.

B. Lymphoma: Primary gastrointestinal lymphoma staging is adapted from the Ann Arbor staging system for lymphoma (Table 25–4). This staging system, however, does not take into account several other criteria that have been shown to be associated with an adverse prognosis. These include size of tumor at presentation larger than 7 cm, B-type symptoms (fever, sweats, weight loss), elevated serum lactate dehydrogenase and beta-2 microglobulin, advanced depth of invasion and level of lymph node involvement, abdominal perforation, increased number of sites, non-resectability, advanced age of the patient, and the presence of comorbid disease. In addition to a physical examination, staging can be accomplished by intestinal barium studies, CT scans of the chest, abdomen, and pelvis, indirect laryngoscopy, and bilateral bone marrow biopsy and aspirates. Gallium scanning, bipedal lymphangiography and a laparoscopic liver biopsy may also be used to complete the workup. One-third of patients are diagnosed with stage IE lymphoma, one-third to one-half with Stage IIE, and less than one-quarter with stage IV disease.

Treatment & Prognosis

A. Gastric Adenocarcinoma: The overall 5-year survival for gastric adenocarcinoma has

Table 25–4. Modified Ann Arbor staging system for primary gastrointestinal lymphoma.

Stage	Extent of involvement
IE	Limited to one area of the GI tract with no other site.
IIE	Localized involvement of an extranodal GI site and its lymph node chain.
II₁E	Limited to the GI site and immediately draining lymph nodes.
II₂E	A primary GI extranodal site and involvement of immediate and noncontinuous subdiaphragmatic lymph node groups.
IIIE	Involvement of lymph nodes on both sides of the diaphragm and localized involvement of a dominant extranodal GI site.
IV	Diffuse or dissemenated involvement.

changed little in the last several decades in the United States, and currently remains at 10–15%. Early gastric cancer is curable with surgical resection, however, this type only comprises 5–16% of patients undergoing resection for gastric cancer. In the United States, approximately 60% of patients with gastric cancer will have unresectable disease at the time of diagnosis. Of the remaining 40% who have a "curative" resection, only 25% will survive 5 years (Figure 25–4).

Gastric adenocarcinomas are optimally resected using wide margins and with extensive lymph node dissections. Total gastrectomy is not routinely performed because of the increased morbidity associated with this procedure, however, it is occasionally required if the tumor is extensive or multifocal. The Japanese Research Society for Gastric Cancer groups gastric lymph nodes (N1–N4) according to their proximity to the stomach. Curative resection requires resection of tumor-free lymph nodes in at least one group distant to involved lymph nodes. Curative resections also often include removal of the omentum and spleen. Extended or radical lymph node dissections have long been performed in Japan and may contribute to the extended survival found in Japanese patients with early stage cancer. The use of extended lymphadenectomies in Western countries is controversial, and several studies have not demonstrated a survival advantage with this procedure (probably because of inadequate control of the quality of the lymph node dissections). Whereas extended lymphadenectomies may benefit patients with serosal invasion or limited regional node disease, it most likely is not beneficial for patients with N3 node involvement, linitus plastica, and extensive invasion of adjacent organs. Surgical resection should be considered even if CT scans suggest locally advanced disease. Occasionally a curative resection can be performed by en-bloc resection of the tumor and adjacent involved organs. If the lesion is extensive and complete removal does not appear possible, a palliative resection can be planned. Survival and symptoms are improved if a palliative resection is performed instead of a simpler bypass procedure. Bypassing obstructing lesions with a gastrojejunal anastomosis may be the only surgical option for maintenance of fluid intake in some cases of advanced gastric cancer.

Both combination chemotherapy and radiation have been used as adjuvant therapy for patients with gastric cancer following surgery. Although several large multicenter trials have investigated mitomycin and fluorouracil and the combination of mitomycin, doxorubicin, and fluorouracil, no regime has demonstrated a clinically relevant and reproducible survival benefit compared with surgery alone. Similarly, adjuvant radiotherapy has not been shown to alter survival or the incidence of local recurrence. Currently, adjuvant therapy for gastric adenocarcinoma cannot be recommended outside a clinical trial.

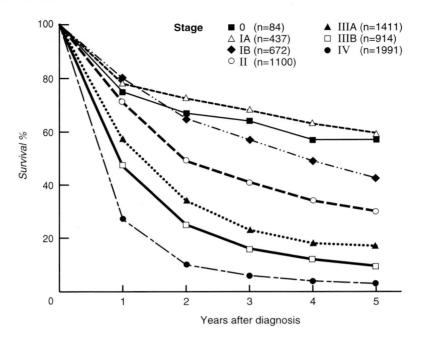

Figure 25–4. Survival by TNM classification and staging of 6609 patients with gastric adenocarcinoma. IA vs IB p<0.01, II vs IB, IIIA, or IIIB p<0.01. (Reproduced, with permission, from Thompson GB, van Heerden JA, Sarr MG: Adenocarcinoma of the stomach: Are we making progress? Lancet 1993;342:713.)

Patients with unresectable disease demonstrated by preoperative staging or following a laparotomy may be offered chemotherapy. Palliation of obstructive symptoms can be accomplished with chemotherapy if the cancer responds to therapy. A positive tumor response is defined as a 50% or greater reduction in the size of a measurable tumor. Single chemotherapeutic agents with response rates of 20–25% include 5-fluorouracil (5-FU), mitomycin C, doxorubicin, nitrosoureas, and cisplatin. Combination chemotherapy with 5-fluorouracil, doxorubicin (Adriamycin), and mitomycin (FAM) or etoposide, Adriamycin, and cisplatin (EAP) have a response rate of 22–50%. Several combinations have been described that demonstrate response rates of up to 50% in a limited number of trials. These include 5-FU, Adriamycin, and cisplatin (FAP); etoposide, leucovorin, and 5-FU (ELF); and 5-FU, Adriamycin, and methotrexate (FAMTx). Significant toxicities may occur with these regimes. Studies to date have not shown any advantage for the addition of radiation to chemotherapy regimes for advanced disease.

Palliation of obstructive or bleeding complications due to disseminated or recurrent gastric cancer represents a difficult management problem. For obstruction of the distal esophagus, endoscopic laser therapy or prosthetic wire mesh stents have been used successfully. For obstruction of the distal stomach, a simple gastrojejunostomy or partial gastrectomy can be performed. Although palliative resection may pro-

vide superior results compared with palliative bypass, this comes at the expense of increased morbidity. Palliation of obstructing cancer at the gastric outlet may also be managed by wire mesh stents placed by endoscopy. Laser or thermal cautery therapy may be used for persistently bleeding lesions. Occasionally, an obstructing tumor may respond to localized radiation therapy. The dose of radiation, however, is often limited by the low tolerance of surrounding tissues.

B. Lymphomas: Recommendations for therapy of gastrointestinal lymphoma have been made on the basis of the experience of small, retrospective series of patients which used varying staging criteria. The type of primary therapy used for the treatment of gastrointestinal non-Hodgkin's lymphomas is controversial. Many oncologists prefer to use combination chemotherapy as primary therapy for both localized or advanced disease, beginning as soon as possible after the lymphoma is diagnosed. In this situation surgical therapy is reserved for the management of complications related to bleeding or perforation. Conversely, in many centers patients with apparent stage IE or IIE disease undergo an initial attempt at surgical excision of the tumor and lymph nodes. Total gastrectomies are avoided. Patients with extensive stage IE lesions or stage IIE lesions are often treated with adjuvant combination chemotherapy. Radiation therapy is sometimes added to help prevent local recurrence at sites of bulk disease. Patients with stage

III or IV disease generally undergo combination chemotherapy as the primary treatment modality. Although proponents of surgical therapy state that surgical debulking of stage III or stage IV disease may enhance survival and prevent the infrequent complications of perforation or bleeding during chemotherapy, there is no study that demonstrates an advantage for elective surgery before definitive systemic treatment.

The prognosis of gastrointestinal lymphoma, like nodal lymphomas, is strongly influenced by the histologic subtype, number of extranodal sites at presentation, tumor bulk, and patient performance status. Patients with diffuse, large cell lymphoma treated with combination chemotherapy can be grouped into risk categories based on these factors. Patients treated with combinations of surgery, radiation, and combination chemotherapy experience a long term survival of 70–80% with stage IE disease and 50–67% with stage IIE disease. Most relapses will occur in the first 2 years. Long term survival in patients with advanced stage disease treated with combination chemotherapy may also occur.

The optimal treatment strategies for recently recognized subtypes of lymphoma (MALT lymphoma, mantle zone lymphoma) remain to be defined. For example, recent reports indicate that low grade (MALT) lymphomas may regress after antibiotic therapy for *H pylori*.

C. Carcinoid: Carcinoid tumors are characterized by a slow rate of invasion and metastases. Carcinoid localized to the intestine will be cured by surgical resection in over 90%. Patients with carcinoid tumors with nodal metastases at the time of surgery will have an 80% recurrence-free rate at 5 years; however, after 25 years, only 23% of patients will be recurrence-free. Patients with unresectable abdominal tumors and patients with unresectable hepatic metastases will have a 50% and 30% survival rate at 5 years, respectively (Figure 25–5). Current therapies for treating hepatic metastases may extend these survivals, and include a multispecialty approach using surgical debulking, cryoablation, hepatic artery embolization, octreotide, and possibly, combination chemotherapy. For example, promising results have been obtained in treating unresectable hepatic carcinoid by hepatic artery occlusion with or without adjuvant chemotherapy. Patients with advanced carcinoid and the carcinoid syndrome can be palliated by

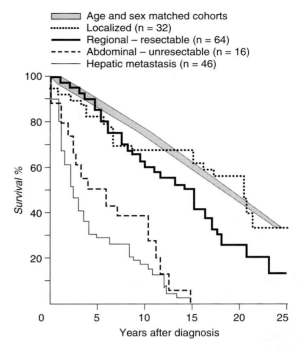

Figure 25–5. Carcinoid tumors of the small bowel. Survival according to stage at initial surgical diagnosis (Reproduced, with permission, from Moertel CG: An odyssey in the land of small tumors. J Clin Oncology 1987;5:1503.)

treatment with octreotide, a somatostatin analog. Chemotherapy is generally ineffective, and is often not recommended except on an experimental basis. Active agents include 5-fluorouracil, doxorubicin, dacarbazine, cyclophosphamide, or streptozotocin. The response rate to these drugs is poor (approximately 20%) and the median duration of tumor regression has been reported to be 4 months.

D. Leiomyosarcoma: Preoperative staging is necessary to identify disseminated disease. Approximately 67% of patients with leiomyosarcoma will have extragastric extension at laparotomy, and surgical resection with curative intent is successful in up to one-half of patients. Radiotherapy for residual or recurrent tumor may be considered. Overall, the 5-year survival for leiomyosarcoma is between 25 and 30%.

REFERENCES

Alexander HR, Kelsen DP, Tepper JE: Cancer of the stomach. In: *Cancer: Principles and Practice of Oncology,* 4/e. DeVita VT, Hellman S, Rosenberg SA, (editors). Lippincott, 1993.

Blackstone, MO: *Endoscopic interpretation. Normal and pathologic appearances of the gastrointestinal tract.* Raven Press, 1984.

Davis, GR. Neoplasms of the stomach. In: *Gastrointestinal Disease. Pathophysiology, Diagnosis and Management,* 5/e. Sleisenger MH, Fordtran JS (editors). Saunders, 1993.

Filipe MI et al: Intestinal metaplasia types and the risk of gastric cancer: A cohort study in Slovenia. Int J Cancer 1994;57:324.

Frazee RC, Roberts J: Gastric lymphoma treatment: medical versus surgical. Surg Clin No Amer 1992;72:423.

Freedman AS, Nadler LM: Non-Hodgkin's lymphomas. In: *Cancer Medicine,* 3/e. Holland JF et al (editors). Lea & Febiger, 1993.

Moertel CG: Gastrointestinal carcinoid tumors and the malignant carcinoid syndrome. In: *Gastrointestinal Disease. Pathophysiology, Diagnosis and Management,* 5/e. Sleisenger MH, Fordtran JS (editors). Saunders, 1993.

Thompson GB, van Heerden JA, Sarr, MG: Adenocarcinoma of the stomach: Are we making progress? Lancet 1993;342:713.

Wright PA, Williams GT: Molecular biology and gastric carcinoma. Gut 1993;34:145.

Zollinger RM, Sternfeld WC, Schreiber HS: Primary neoplasms of the small intestine. Am J Surgery 1986;151:654.

Miscellaneous Disorders of the Stomach & Small Intestine

26

James H. Grendell, MD

A variety of "miscellaneous" disorders can involve the stomach and small intestine. Although these diseases are not as common as most of those described in other chapters, it is important that clinicians have some basic familiarity with their presentation.

STOMACH

Gastric Volvulus

Gastric volvulus is the twisting of the stomach. Most commonly, the stomach rotates on its longitudinal axis, a condition associated with paraesophageal hernia, although other patterns of rotation can occur.

Acute gastric volvulus presents with sudden, severe pain of the upper abdomen or chest, persistent retching producing only a little vomitus, epigastric distention, and the inability to pass a nasogastric tube. Upper gastrointestinal series demonstrates an abrupt obstruction at the site of the volvulus. Acute gastric volvulus requires emergency surgical evaluation because of the substantial risk of mortality related to gastric ischemia or perforation.

Chronic gastric volvulus may be asymptomatic or present with nonspecific symptoms of dyspepsia, heartburn, or postprandial bleeding. Diagnosis is made by performing an upper gastrointestinal series, and treatment consists of gastropexy and repair of any associated paraesophageal hernia.

Gastric Diverticula

Gastric diverticula are uncommon and typically asymptomatic, although the clinician may have difficulty in differentiating them from gastric ulcers on upper gastrointestinal series. Usually, no treatment is required, although diverticulectomy rarely may be necessitated owing to inflammation or hemorrhage.

Gastric Rupture

Gastric rupture may occur following blunt trauma, gastroscopy, vomiting, and overdistention of the stomach by massive overeating or ingestion of large doses of sodium bicarbonate. Patients usually present with abdominal pain and distention, and on examination usually have tympany and may have subcuta-

neous emphysema. Chest x-ray or upright or lateral abdominal x-rays typically demonstrate free intraperitoneal air. Emergency surgical repair is mandatory, and morbidity (eg, fistula, intra-abdominal abscess) and mortality rates are high.

Bezoars

Bezoars are persisting accumulations of foreign material in the stomach. Although they can occur as a result of unusual eating habits (eg, trichobezoars from ingesting hair or persimmon bezoars), most bezoars in adults consist mainly of plant material in patients who have undergone surgery affecting gastric motor function (eg, vagotomy, particularly when associated with antrectomy or partial gastrectomy).

Patients typically present with abdominal pain, nausea, vomiting, and early satiety. Less commonly bezoars may result in mucosal ulceration, which may lead to acute or chronic gastrointestinal blood loss or perforation. The diagnosis may be made by upper gastrointestinal series or endoscopy.

Most gastric bezoars can be mechanically disrupted and can either be removed or will pass spontaneously from the stomach. This is accomplished using endoscopic tools or lavage either through the endoscope or through a large-bore gastric tube. Bezoars that cannot be removed in these ways or that result in serious complications may require surgery.

Following successful treatment of a bezoar, patients should be advised to avoid raw citrus fruits and persimmon. Prokinetic agents such as metoclopramide or cisapride may also help prevent recurrence. Habitual ingestion of hair or other foreign indigestible material requires psychiatric evaluation and therapy.

Eosinophilic Gastroenteritis

This rare disease results from eosinophilic infiltration of the gut wall that can occur anywhere in the gastrointestinal tract, but it most commonly involves the stomach and small intestine. The cause of this disorder in most patients is unknown, however, allergies (eg, to foods) or drug or toxin exposures are thought to play a role in some cases.

There are three main patterns of involvement:

1. Mucosal and submucosal disease: These patients typically have cramping or colicky abdominal pain, nausea, vomiting, weight loss, and diarrhea.
2. Muscle layer disease: These patients have symptoms and signs of pyloric or intestinal obstruction.
3. Serosal layer disease: These patients usually present with eosinophilic ascites.

Peripheral blood eosinophilia is found in about 75–80% of patients and ranges from about 1000/μL in patients with muscle layer disease to 8000/μL in patients with serosal disease.

Upper gastrointestinal series or abdominal computed tomography may show thickened folds in the stomach or small intestine with or without nodules. These findings, however, are nonspecific. Endoscopy usually demonstrates prominent mucosal folds, nodularity, erythema, and, in some cases, ulcerations. However, endoscopic abnormalities may be subtle. Endoscopic biopsy of involved areas is the best way of making the diagnosis. In patients with disease that primarily involves the muscle layer or serosa, endoscopic biopsies may be negative, and the diagnosis is made on the basis of clinical, laboratory and radiologic findings, or on full-thickness operative biopsy.

Patients with disease involving the mucosa may respond to dietary manipulation if they have a history suggestive of a specific food allergy or intolerance. Patients with mucosal disease failing to respond to elimination diets and those with muscle layer or serosal disease usually respond to treatment with corticosteroids. In some patients requiring high doses of steroids to keep them symptom-free, azathioprine can be added in an attempt to reduce the maintenance corticosteroid dose. Because obstructive symptoms usually respond to medical therapy, surgery is generally not necessary and should be avoided unless it is required to confirm the diagnosis and exclude cancer.

SMALL INTESTINE

Small Bowel Obstruction

Mechanical obstruction of the small intestine is a common problem that usually is due to adhesions resulting from previous abdominal surgery. However, a variety of other causes can be found (Table 26–1).

The presentation depends on the level of the obstruction in the small intestine. High or proximal small bowel obstruction results in variable upper abdominal pain and profuse vomiting. Mid- or distal small bowel obstruction presents with cramping or colicky periumbilical or diffuse abdominal pain, abdominal distension, and episodic vomiting frequently associated with crescendos of pain. The more distal the obstruction, the greater the abdominal distension and the more feculent the vomitus or nasogastric drainage. When small bowel obstruction is complete, obstipation results.

Table 26–1. Causes of mechanical small bowel obstruction.

Postoperative adhesions
Congenital adhesive bands
External or internal hernias
Tumors
Strictures (eg, from Crohn's disease, ischemia, radiation injury)
Intussusception
Volvulus
Gallstones
Foreign bodies
Hematomas (eg, from trauma or spontaneously in patients on anticoagulants)

Physical examination may demonstrate postural or resting changes in pulse and blood pressure owing to hypovolemia and dehydration. On abdominal examination, mild diffuse tenderness often is present and high-pitched "tinkling" bowel sounds and peristaltic "rushes" may be noted on auscultation of the abdomen. The patient should be evaluated carefully for incarcerated external hernias.

Depending on the duration of obstruction and degree of hypovolemia, patients may demonstrate leukocytosis, hemoconcentration, and varying degrees of electrolyte abnormalities. Supine and upright (or lateral) abdominal x-rays strongly suggest the diagnosis with a paucity of air in the colon and a ladderlike arrangement of small bowel loops with air-fluid levels (Figure 26–1). A radiologic examination of the small intestine with contrast or abdominal computed tomography may provide additional information concerning the level and cause of obstruction.

The differential diagnosis includes colonic obstruction, intestinal ileus, and intestinal pseudo-obstruction. In colonic obstruction, abdominal x-rays demonstrate dilated colon proximal to the site of obstruction. Intestinal ileus may occur as a result of an intra-abdominal inflammatory process (eg, acute pancreatitis, acute appendicitis), following abdominal surgery or as a multifactorial process in the hospitalized patient related to immobility, electrolyte abnormalities, and the administration of drugs (eg, narcotics and anticholinergics). Both symptoms and abdominal findings in intestinal ileus tend to be milder than in small bowel obstruction, and abdominal x-rays typically show gas mainly in the colon without a pattern of numerous air-fluid levels. Patients with intestinal pseudo-obstruction due to neuromuscular disease of the gastrointestinal tract have chronic or recurring symptoms that may involve one or more of the hollow digestive organs. In cases where the differential diagnosis is in doubt, contrast radiographic studies of the small intestine, colon, or both need to be performed to determine if mechanical obstruction is present.

The initial treatment of small bowel obstruction is fluid and electrolyte resuscitation and nasogastric decompression. Partial small bowel obstruction will

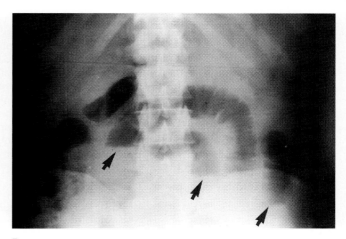

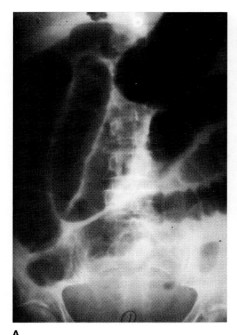

Figure 26–1. ***A:*** Dilated loops of intestine on a supine abdominal x-ray of a patient with small bowel obstruction. ***B:*** Air-fluid ***(arrows)*** on an upright abdominal x-ray of a patient with small bowel obstruction.

usually resolve spontaneously within a few days. Operative therapy is required for cases of partial obstruction that fail to resolve with expectant management and for most cases of complete obstruction.

Diverticular Disease of the Small Intestine

Diverticula may occur throughout the small intestine but are most commonly found in the duodenum or jejunum. In the duodenum about 3/4 of the diverticula are within 2 cm of the ampulla of Vater and are termed **juxtapapillary.** These duodenal diverticula are usually asymptomatic and require no treatment, but can occasionally bleed or perforate. Furthermore, juxtapapillary diverticula have been suggested to contribute to gallstone disease or acute pancreatitis in some patients.

Jejunal diverticula (other than Meckel's diverticulum) are acquired and are associated with disorders of impaired intestinal motility such as progressive systemic sclerosis and intestinal pseudo-obstruction. Symptoms are usually related to the underlying motility disorder although bacterial overgrowth leading to malabsorption, bleeding, and perforation have been reported.

Enteropathy from Radiation and from Nonsteroidal Anti-inflammatory Drugs

Radiation therapy to the abdomen frequently produces acute intestinal mucosal injury characterized by self-limited abdominal pain, nausea, vomiting, and diarrhea (at times, bloody). In addition, radiation can injure blood vessels in the intestinal wall, causing a chronic fibroproliferative response leading to obliteration of the vessels and chronic intestinal ischemia. This process may result in symptomatic disease presenting anytime from several months to many years after completion of the course of radiation therapy with bleeding, stricture formation with obstruction, and occasionally, perforation with abscess or fistula formation. Depending on the presentation and the patient's overall condition, the treatment is usually operative resection or bypass of the involved segment of intestine.

Long-standing use of nonsteroidal anti-inflammatory drugs (NSAIDs) can produce mucosal injury to the small intestine leading to chronic gastrointestinal blood loss. In a small number of patients, overt intestinal ulcerations or transmural injury occurs and this can result in diaphragm-like intestinal strictures. Withdrawal of NSAIDs will result in eventual resolution of intestinal mucosal inflammation, although strictured areas may require resection.

Pneumatosis Cystoides Intestinalis

Pneumatoses cystoides intestinalis is an uncommon condition in which gas-filled cysts are found in the small intestine, colon, and occasionally in the stomach or mesentery. Cysts are subserosal and range from a few millimeters to several centimeters and can be single or in clusters. About 15% of cases are considered to be primary (idiopathic) and usually involve only the left colon. The remaining 85% of cases termed **secondary pneumatosis** are associated with a variety of gastrointestinal diseases, endoscopic and operative procedures, and pulmonary disease.

Patients with pneumatosis intestinalis are usually asymptomatic, with the diagnosis being an unexpected finding on a radiologic study. When present, symptoms are more likely related to the gastrointestinal process presumably producing the pneumatosis. Patients with gas in the bowel wall in other settings such as intestinal ischemia or a severe infectious process (eg, *Clostridium difficile* colitis) typically have obvious manifestations of sepsis.

Most patients with pneumatosis only require treatment of any associated disease process. Patients with symptomatic disease (usually colonic) can be treated with oxygen therapy by mask or in a hyperbaric chamber. Avoidance of nonabsorbable carbohydrates (eg, sorbitol, lactulose) and correction of any carbohydrate malabsorption (eg, lactase deficiency) may also be helpful.

REFERENCES

Chiu KW, Changchien CS, Chuah SK: Small-bowel diverticulum: Is it a risk for small-bowel volvulus. J Clin Gastroenterol 1994;19:176.

Cho KC, Baker SR: Extraluminal air. Diagnosis and significance. Radiol Clin North Am 1994;32:829.

Hughes W, Pierce WS: Surgical implications of gastric diverticula. Surg Gynecol Obstet 1970;131:99.

Milne LW et al: Gastric volvulus: Two cases and a review of the literature. J Emerg Med 1994;12:299.

Palder SB, Frey CB: Jejunal diverticulosis. Arch Surg 1988;123:889.

Robles R et al: Gastrointestinal bezoars. Br J Surg 1994;81:1000.

Talley NJ et al: Eosinophilic gastroenteritis: A clinicopathological study of patients with disease of the mucosae, muscle layer, and subserosal tissue. Gut 1990;31:54.

Welch JP: *Bowel obstruction. Differential diagnosis and clinical management.* Saunders, 1990.

Section IV
Diseases of the Colon & Rectum

Malignant & Premalignant Lesions of the Colon

27

Robert S. Bresalier, MD

ESSENTIALS OF DIAGNOSIS

- Ninety percent of colorectal cancers occur in patients over 50 years of age.
- Adenomas precede carcinomas.
- Early cancers are asymptomatic.
- Fecal occult blood testing can detect preneoplastic lesions and early cancers.
- Microcytic anemia in the elderly suggests the presence of colorectal cancer.
- Hematochezia may be a sign of colorectal cancer (especially of the distal colon and rectum).
- Weight loss and obstructive symptoms are late findings.

GENERAL CONSIDERATIONS

Cancers of the colon and rectum (colorectal cancers) are a major cause of illness and death in patients living in the United States and other Western countries. There will be an estimated 138,000 new cases of colorectal cancer in the USA in 1995, accounting for 55,000 cancer-related deaths (second only to lung cancer). Because these cancers arise over a long period of time as the result of interactions between genetic predisposition and environmental influences, it is possible to identify preneoplastic and early neoplastic lesions and improve survival rates. Rapidly evolving knowledge of the pathogenesis of colorectal cancer, especially in high-risk groups, is leading to the development of new tools for identifying people who will most benefit from cancer surveillance and adjuvant therapy following potentially curative surgery.

A rapid proliferation of knowledge about the molecular biologic characteristics of colorectal cancer has provided useful insights into the pathogenesis of not only colonic neoplasia but of cancer in general. The importance of the DNA mismatch repair genes associated with hereditary nonpolyposis colorectal cancer, for example, is emphasized in one recent article entitled "Molecule of the Year." "Molecular diagnosis" of at-risk individuals is now clinically possible in families with familial adenomatous polyposis and may soon be possible for hereditary nonpolyposis colorectal cancer patients. A panel of molecular markers may in the future allow for identification of those in the general population at risk for sporadic cancer, as well.

Screening for colorectal cancer has been advocated for some time because of the high prevalence of the disease in the USA and the potential for cure if preneoplastic or early neoplastic lesions are removed endoscopically or surgically. Although screening has been advocated by many, others have been resistant because the many false-positive fecal occult blood tests have made it an expensive procedure and because it has been difficult to demonstrate definite improvements in survival rates following screening. Recent prospective and case-control studies do indeed suggest improved rates in those screened with fecal occult blood testing and sigmoidoscopy; these observations will no doubt increase the acceptance of screening of persons in the general population who are over 50 years of age, but more specific, cost-effective methods are clearly needed.

Removal of preneoplastic adenomatous polyps and early colorectal cancers improves survival rates, and screening methods to date have focused on eliminating preexisting lesions. The ideal goal, however, would be to prevent the development of cancer in the general population (primary prevention). Ongoing clinical trials are concentrating on dietary manipulation (eg, decreased amount or altered composition of fat, increased fiber), use of antioxidants, dietary calcium supplementation, and use of aspirin and nonsteroidal anti-inflammatory agents (NSAIDs), which affect prostaglandin synthesis (based on studies of familial adenomatous polyposis). The efficacy of any such manipulation remains unproved, however, for prevention of cancer in the general population.

PATHOPHYSIOLOGY

Colorectal cancers arise through complex interactions between genetic and environmental influences. The relative contribution of each varies. Genetic factors predominate in defined hereditary syndromes such as familial adenomatous polyposis and hereditary nonpolyposis colorectal cancer. Sporadic colon cancers develop over longer periods of time as environmental influences produce genotoxic events eventually leading to cancer. In both types, tumors do not develop all at once but rather evolve from progressive identifiable changes in the colonic mucosa (eg, dysplasia, adenoma).

Environmental Influences

Several pieces of evidence suggest that the environment plays a role in the development of colorectal cancers. The frequency of colorectal cancer varies remarkably worldwide, with the highest rates in North America, Australia, and Europe, and much lower rates in regions of Asia, South America, and sub-Saharan Africa. The risk of cancer rises rapidly in populations migrating from low-risk to high-risk areas, again suggesting that environmental factors, especially dietary differences, are important in its development. Environmental influences that may potentially influence carcinogenesis in the colon are listed in Table 27–1.

Descriptive epidemiologic studies and studies of experimental carcinogenesis both suggest that diets containing high amounts of fat predispose to colorectal cancers, especially those arising in the descending and sigmoid colon. Total dietary fat accounts for 40–45% of total caloric intake in countries with high incidence rates of colorectal cancer, whereas in low-risk populations, it accounts for only 10–15%. Several case-control studies confirm a relationship between dietary fat intake and the incidence and mortality rates of colorectal cancer. Experimental animals fed diets high in polyunsaturated and saturated fats also develop greater numbers of carcinogen-induced colonic adenocarcinomas than those on low-fat diets. Dietary fat enhances cholesterol and bile acid synthesis by the liver. These substances are converted by colonic bacteria to secondary bile acids, cholesterol metabolites, and other potentially toxic compounds that may damage the colonic mucosa, leading to increased cellular proliferation (Figure 27–1). Actively proliferating cells are most susceptible to the effects of carcinogens and other genotoxic influences. Such carcinogens may result from the processing or cooking of foods or from the action of colonic bacteria on dietary components.

While dietary fat may promote carcinogenesis in the colon, dietary fiber appears to have the opposite effect. Dietary fiber consists of plant material resistant to digestion, which includes a heterogeneous mix of carbohydrate and noncarbohydrate components. Cereals such as bran cereals may increase stool bulk, thereby diluting carcinogens and tumor promoters, decreasing their contact with the mucosa, and enhancing their elimination. Cellulose and hemicellulose decrease the level of bacterial enzymes, and may diminish the activation of carcinogens and co-carcinogens.

Dietary calcium may also have a protective role in preventing colonic carcinogenesis. Epidemiologic studies indicate that men consuming the least amount of calcium and vitamin D have twice the cancer risk of those who consume high amounts of these compounds. Calcium increases the fecal excretion of bile acids and decreases the ratio of dihydroxy to trihydroxy bile acids in duodenal bile. Supplemental calcium also decreases proliferation of the colonic mucosa, both in humans and experimental animals, by mechanisms that appear to be independent of its effects on bile acids.

While high dietary intake of yellow-green cruciferous vegetables, micronutrients such as selenium salts, and vitamins A, C, and E (antioxidants) has been linked to a reduction in colon cancer development, the influence of these foods in preventing colonic carcinogenesis remains controversial.

Genetic Influences

Although it is convenient to categorize colorectal cancers as hereditary (familial) and nonhereditary (sporadic), it is more appropriate to consider all colorectal cancers as having genetic components that are inherited or acquired to varying degrees. Individuals with familial adenomatous polyposis, hereditary nonpolyposis colorectal cancer, and other familial syndromes are born with genetic alterations that make them susceptible to the development of colonic neoplasia. Environmental factors then contribute additional "hits," leading to malignant transformation. In the case of "sporadic" cancers, multiple somatic mutations are contributed by the environment.

Table 27–1. Environmental factors that may influence colorectal carcinogenesis.

Probably related
  High dietary fat consumption
  Low dietary fiber consumption
Possibly related
  Environmental carcinogens and mutagens
    Heterocyclic amines (from charbroiled or fried foods)
    Products of bacterial metabolism
  Beer and ale consumption (rectal cancer)
  Low dietary selenium
Probably protective
  Dietary fiber consumption (wheat bran, cellulose, lignin)
  Dietary calcium
Possibly protective
  Yellow-green cruciferous vegetables
  Foods rich in carotene (vitamin A)
  Vitamins C and E
  Selenium
  Folic acid

Risk factors: diets high in fats, cholesterol, and fried foods and foods low in fiber

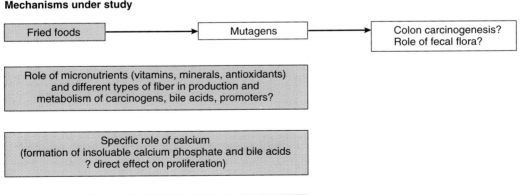

Figure 27–1. Scheme of current concepts of the environmental causation of colon cancer, based on epidemiologic considerations and experimental models of carcinogenesis. Many of the relationships depicted remain speculative. (Reproduced, with permission, from Bresalier RS, Kim YS: Malignant neoplasms of the large intestine. In: *Gastrointestinal Disease,* 5/e. Sleisenger MH, Fordtran JS (editors). Saunders, 1993.)

Genetic changes that may lead to the development of colorectal cancer can be organized into three major classes: alterations in proto-oncogenes, loss of tumor-suppressor gene activity, and abnormalities in genes involved in DNA repair. While much of what is known about the molecular genetics of colorectal cancer has come from the study of familial syndromes, similar changes are associated with the development of sporadic cancers (Table 27–2).

Cellular proto-oncogenes are human genes containing a DNA sequence homologous to that of acute transforming retroviruses. Many of these genes play a role in the normal regulation of cell growth, and their altered expression contributes to abnormal proliferation and eventual carcinogenesis. Mutations of the K-ras gene, for example, can be found in approximately 60% of sporadic colon cancers.

Allelic losses in chromosomes 5q, 18q, and 17p are commonly found in colorectal cancers (Table 27–2). Originally described in association with familial adenomatous polyposis, alterations of the APC gene on chromosome 5 can be found in 60% of sporadic adenomas, suggesting that this is an early event in colonic carcinogenesis. APC abnormalities may lead to disruption of normal cell-to-cell adhesion through altered association with molecules called catenins and the cellular adhesion molecule E-cadherin. The DCC (deleted in colon cancer) gene is deleted in 70% of colon cancers. This gene, found on chromosome 18q, may also be involved in normal cell-to-cell adhesive interactions. Patients whose tumors have deletions of the DCC gene have a worse prognosis than those in whom the gene is intact. Deletions of chromosome 17p, present in approximately 75% of colorectal cancers, involve the p53 gene, which normally prevents cells with damaged DNA from progressing beyond the G1-S boundary in the cell cycle. This is a late, important event in colonic carcinogenesis.

Genes designated hMSH2 and hMLH1 play a role in repairing base pair mismatches occurring during DNA replication. Alterations in these genes (and in two related genes, hPMS1 and hPMS2) lead to DNA replication errors (RER+ phenotype) and increased mutation. These genes appear to play a major role in hereditary nonpolyposis colorectal cancers, but similar alterations may be found in approximately 15% of sporadic cancers.

Colorectal cancers thus arise as the result of complex interactions between hereditary and environmental factors. A proposed sequence of genetic events is outlined in Figure 27–2. Cancers develop from an accumulation of events in a multistep process.

Progression of Dysplasia to Carcinoma

Colorectal cancers do not arise de novo, but the colonic mucosa progresses through a sequence of morphologic events that eventually culminate in invasive carcinoma. **Dysplasia** refers to abnormalities in crypt architecture (ie, reduced number, irregular branching, crowding resulting in a "back-to-back" appearance) and cytologic detail (ie, enlarged, hyperchromatic nuclei with multiple mitoses and pseudostratification) (Figure 27–3). In nearly all cases, dysplasia is manifested in macroscopic adenomatous polyps. Sometimes, as in ulcerative colitis, dysplasia may occur as a microscopic lesion in the mucosa (see discussion following).

Risk Factors for Development of Colorectal Cancer

A. Age: Colorectal cancer is predominantly a disease of older age-groups. Ninety percent of cancers occur in persons over 50 years of age, with the peak incidence in the seventh decade (Figure 27–4). A person who is 50 years of age has an approximately 5% chance of developing colorectal cancer by age 80 years, and a 2.5% risk of dying from the disease. While the risk of developing colorectal cancer rises sharply after age 50 years in the general population, these cancers also occur in younger individuals, especially those with a family history of the disease (see discussion following).

B. Adenomatous Polyps: The vast majority of colorectal cancers in the general population arise in adenomatous polyps. These are macroscopic le-

Table 27–2. Genes altered in colon cancer.

Gene	Chromosome	Sporadic Tumors With Alterations	Class	Function
K-ras	12	60%	Proto-oncogene	Signal transduction
APC	5	60%	Tumor supressor	?Cell adhesion
DCC	18	70%	Tumor supressor	?Cell adhesion
p53	17	75%	Tumor supressor	Cell cycle control
hMSH2	2		DNA mismatch repair	Maintains DNA replication
hMLH1	3		DNA mismatch repair	Maintains DNA replication

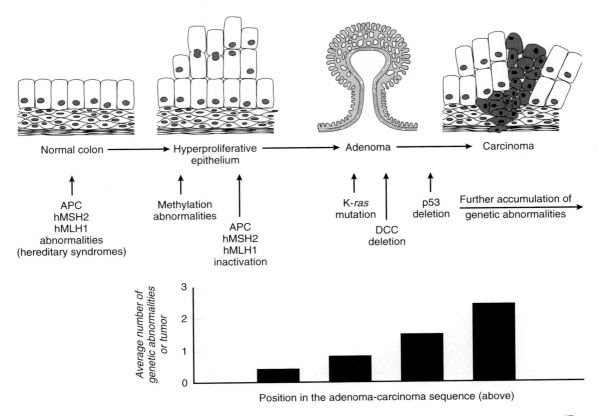

Figure 27–2. Proposed sequence of molecular genetic events occurring during the evolution of colorectal cancer. (Reproduced and modified, with permission, from Bresalier RS, Toribara NW: Familial colon cancer. In: *Premalignant Conditions of the Gastrointestinal Tract.* Eastwood GL (editor). Elsevier, 1990.)

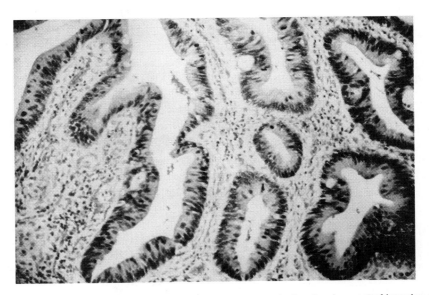

Figure 27–3. Dysplastic changes in the colonic mucosa are precursors to the development of invasive cancer. Glands are branched, irregular, and crowded together. Nuclei are hyperchromatic and do not line up on the basement membrane but are arranged in pseudopalisades (pseudostratification). Adenomatous polyps by definition contain dysplastic changes.

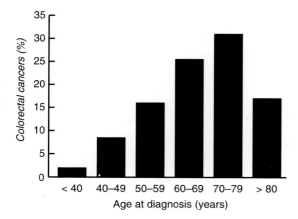

Figure 27–4. Colorectal cancer incidence by age at diagnosis, based on the United States population.

sions made up of dysplastic epithelium. They may be peduncluated, attached to the colonic wall through a fibrovascular stalk (Figure 27–5), or sessile with a broad base attachment. Tubular adenomas are characterized by a complex network of branching adenomatous glands (Figure 27–6A). Villous adenomas have glands extending straight down from the surface toward the base of the polyp (Figure 27–6B). Many polyps are tubulovillous adenomas, having characteristics of both types (Figure 27–6C). All adenomas by definition contain dysplastic epithelium. These are benign neoplasms that have the potential for malignant degeneration. The risk of evolution from adenoma to carcinoma is related to polyp size and histologic characteristics (Figure 27–7). Large polyps and

those with a higher proportion of villous architecture are more likely to contain carcinoma. Likewise, polyps containing higher degrees of architectural distortion and cellular atypia (moderate to severe dysplasia) will more often contain coincident cancer. These features are interdependent. Large polyps often have higher degrees of villous architecture and dysplasia.

Adenomatous polyps are associated with abnormal cellular proliferation. In the normal colon, DNA synthesis and cellular proliferation occur only in the lower and middle regions of the crypt. Cells that have migrated to the upper crypt become terminally differentiated and can no longer divide. Disordered proliferative activity is characteristic of adenomas and a hallmark of neoplasia. Abnormal proliferation can be detected even in the normal-appearing mucosa of some individuals at especially high risk for cancer development (eg, members of kindreds with familial adenomatous polyposis, Gardner's syndrome, and nonpolyposis hereditary colorectal cancer). These abnormalities may be associated with alterations in biochemical markers of cellular proliferation such as ornithine decarboxylase and protein kinase C activity, and molecular markers such as APC gene inactivation and K-ras proto-oncogene mutations. Clinical studies suggest that the evolution of colon cancer may take as long as a decade, and as much as 5 years for progression from recognizable adenoma to invasive carcinoma. This has implications for screening, as will be discussed in later sections.

Several pieces of evidence support the view that colonic adenomas are the precursors to carcinoma. The epidemiologic description of colonic adenomas parallels that of carcinomas. Adenomatous polyps are

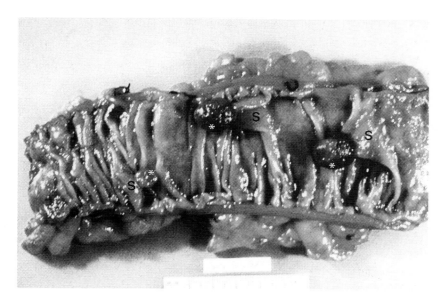

Figure 27–5. Colectomy specimen containing multiple pedunculated polyps *(asterisks)*. S, polyp stalk.

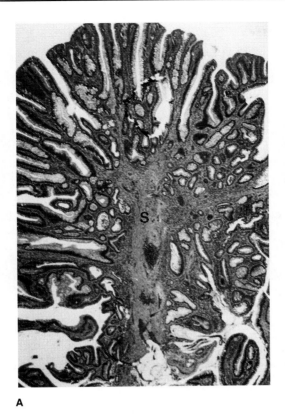

A

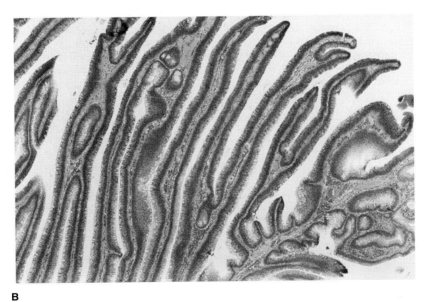

B

Figure 27–6. Adenomatous polyps contain various degrees of tubular and villous components. **A:** Tubular adenomas are characterized by a complex network of branching glands. **B:** Villous adenomas contain adenomatous glands that extend straight down from the surface to the center of the polyp.

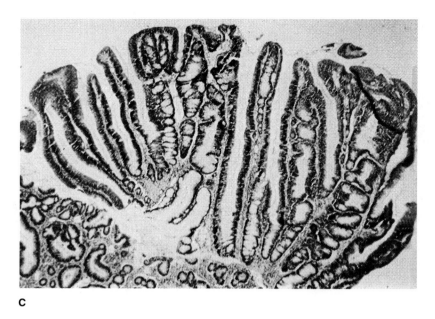

C

Figure 27–6. *C:* Many adenomas are mixed villotubular adenomas.

rare in geographic regions with low colon cancer prevalence, and the distribution of adenomas in different segments of the colon mimics that of carcinomas. Adenomas often occur in anatomic proximity to colon cancers (**sentinel polyps),** and cancer risk is proportional to the number of adenomas present synchronously (at the same time) or metachronously (at different times) in the colon. Cancer is often present in polyps removed endoscopically or surgically, and the risk of cancer is proportional to the degree of dysplasia in the polyp. Most importantly, several

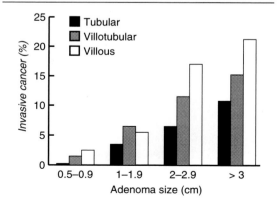

Figure 27–7. The risk that an adenoma will evolve into carcinoma is related to polyp size and histologic characteristics. Shown here is the percentage of adenomas containing invasive cancer by size and histologic findings, based on an analysis of 7000 endoscopically removed polyps.

clinical studies now suggest that removal of adenomatous polyps in the context of surveillance proctosigmoidoscopy decreases the risk of death from colon cancer.

C. Family History:

1. Sporadic cancer–It has become increasingly clear that there exists an inherited susceptibility to the development of colon cancer. This is not only true of well-defined hereditary syndromes such as familial adenomatous polyposis and hereditary nonpolyposis colorectal cancer, but also of so-called sporadic, or common, colorectal cancers. Cancer incidence and mortality studies suggest that the incidence of colon cancer in first-degree relatives of those with the disease is two to three times higher than that of the general population. This is echoed by more recent case-control and prospective family analyses, which demonstrated a risk 1.8 times higher for those with one affected relative, and 2.75–5.7 times higher for those with two affected relatives. The risk is greater if an affected relative has cancer diagnosed before age 45 years. Similar trends have been demonstrated for adenomatous polyps.

2. Familial adenomatous polyposis and Gardner's syndrome–Familial adenomatous polyposis and its variant, Gardner's syndrome, are inherited in an autosomal dominant fashion, with inactivation of the APC gene located on chromosome 5q. These syndromes have served as models for the study of the sequence of events in which adenoma develops into carcinoma in the large bowel. Hundreds to thousands of adenomatous polyps progressively develop in the colon and rectum of affected individuals (Figure 27–8). Polyps often begin to appear

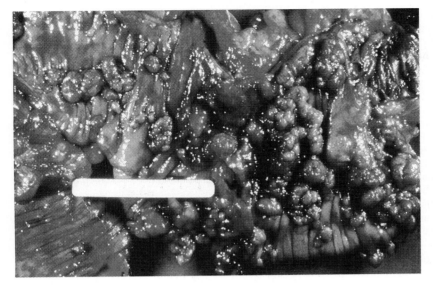

A

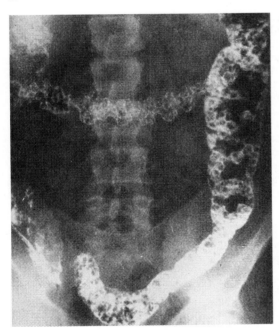

B

Figure 27–8. **A:** Colectomy specimen from a patient with familial adenomatous polyposis. Hundreds of polyps of varying size can be seen arising from the colonic mucosa. **B:** Barium enema study in a patient with familial adenomatous polyposis. Numerous filling defects represent polyps throughout the colon.

by 15–20 years of age. If the colon is not removed, cancer development is inevitable, usually within a decade of the appearance of adenomas. Histologic examination reveals numerous microadenomas, which may not yet be evident on gross examination. Hyperproliferation of the colonic mucosa can be detected by labeling with tritiated thymidine and as an increase in the polyamine biosynthetic enzyme ornithine decarboxylase. Abnormalities can be detected on in vitro studies of skin fibroblasts, including ab-

normal responses to tumor promoters. Importantly, it is now possible to detect at-risk individuals in kindreds of familial adenomatous polyposis patients by means of practical, sensitive assays, which detect truncated APC gene products in patients who will manifest the disease (ie, molecular diagnosis). Once at-risk individuals develop adenomas, colectomy should be performed. Subtotal colectomy with ileorectal anastomosis, combined with frequent endoscopic surveillance plus medical management with

NSAIDs, has been advocated by some, but the possibility of rectal cancer exists (see following section, "Treatment").

Gardner's syndrome is a variant of familial adenomatous polyposis in which extracolonic manifestations occur in conjunction with polyposis. Like familial adenomatous polyposis, Gardner's syndrome is an autosomal dominant disease linked to the APC gene, and both share similar features. In both cases, the small intestine as well as the colon is at risk for neoplastic growth. Duodenal adenomas occur, and the periampullary region is especially susceptible to neoplastic degeneration. Extracolonic manifestations of Gardner's syndrome include osteomas of the mandible, skull, and long bones (Figure 27–9), epidermoid cysts, fibromas, lipomas, mesenteric fibromatosis, and desmoid tumors. Fundic gland hyperplasia of the stomach is common. Congenital hypertrophy of the retinal pigmented epithelium occurs in over 90% of patients with Gardner's syndrome.

3. Hereditary nonpolyposis colorectal cancer–Hereditary nonpolyposis colorectal cancer **(Lynch syndrome)** is a disease of autosomal dominant inheritance in which colon cancers arise in discrete adenomas, but polyposis (ie, hundreds of polyps) does not occur. Table 27–3 lists the criteria for this disease, as defined by the International Collaborative Group on Hereditary Nonpolyposis Colorectal Cancer. Families must have at least three relatives with colorectal cancer, one of which is a first-degree relative of the other two. Colorectal cancer must involve at least two generations, and at least one case must occur before age 50 years. Clinical features of cancers arising in hereditary nonpolyposis

Table 27–3. Hereditary nonpolyposis colorectal cancer.

≥ 3 relatives with colorectal cancer (one must be first-degree relative of other two)
Colorectal cancer involving at least 2 generations
One or more colorectal cancer cases before age 50 years

colorectal cancer are compared with those of sporadic cancer in Table 27–4. Cancers arising in hereditary nonpolyposis colorectal cancer occur at an earlier age (age 40–50 years), are often proximal in location and multiple, and are more commonly mucinous or poorly differentiated. Patients with hereditary nonpolyposis colorectal cancer type b **(Lynch syndrome II; cancer family syndrome)** are prone to develop cancers of the female genital tract (eg, ovary, endometrium) and other sites in addition to the colon. Colon cancers sometimes arise in flat, slightly raised lesions in the proximal colon, with foci of adenomatous change confined to the upper crypt ("flat" adenomas). The exact frequency of hereditary nonpolyposis colorectal cancer in the population is yet to be determined, but it appears to account for at least 4–6% of colorectal cancers. Genes that play a role in DNA repair are altered in this type of cancer. Loss of the hMSH2 and hMLH1 genes (two additional genes, hPMS1 and hPMS2, may also be involved) leads to increased susceptibility to mutation from failure to repair base pair mismatches. This is manifested in DNA replication errors (the so-called RER+ phenotype), whose detection may eventually be important in clinical screening.

4. Other hereditary syndromes–
a. Peutz-Jeghers syndrome and familial ju-

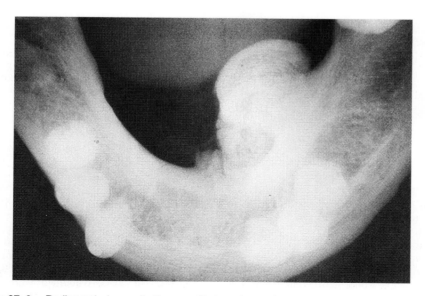

Figure 27–9. Radiograph demonstrating mandibular osteoma in a patient with Gardner's syndrome.

Table 27–4. Clinical features of hereditary nonpolyposis colorectal cancer and sporadic colon cancer.

	Hereditary Nonpolyposis Colorectal Cancer	Sporadic Cancer
Mean age at diagnosis	44.6 years	67 years
Multiple colon cancers Synchronous Metachronous	34.5% 18.1% 24.3%	4–11% 3–6% 1–5%
Proximal location	72.3%	35%
Excess malignant tumors at other sites	Yes	No
Mucinous and poorly differentiated cancers	Common	Infrequent
RER+ phenotype	79%	17%

venile polyposis–Peutz-Jeghers syndrome (mucocutaneous pigmentation and hamartomas of the gastrointestinal tract) and the familial form of juvenile polyposis have been associated with a slightly increased risk of large and small bowel cancer, because of the coexistence of scattered adenomas in conjunction with nonneoplastic hamartomas.

b. Cronkhite-Canada syndrome–Adenomas may also occur in Cronkhite-Canada syndrome (gastrointestinal hamartomas, cutaneous hyperpigmentation, dystrophic nails, alopecia, intestinal malabsorption), conferring an increased risk of carcinoma.

c. Torres's syndrome (Muir's syndrome)–Torres's syndrome is a variant of hereditary nonpolyposis colorectal cancer in which adenomas of the colon occur in conjunction with multiple skin lesions (eg, sebaceous adenomas and carcinomas, basal cell and squamous cell carcinomas, keratoacanthomas).

D. Inflammatory Bowel Disease:

1. Ulcerative colitis–Patients with inflammatory bowel disease are at increased risk for developing colorectal carcinoma; this is best documented in idiopathic ulcerative colitis. The risk of cancer correlates most closely with the duration of the colitis; the risk is lowest in patients who have had the disease for less than 7–10 years and rises 0.5–1% for each additional year of disease. Cancer risk is greatest in those who have pancolitis involving the entire bowel, but those with left-sided colitis (distal to the splenic flexure) are also at risk. Cancer develops in dysplastic epithelium. Unlike in the general population, where dysplasia occurs in adenomatous polyps, dysplasia associated with ulcerative colitis often occurs in flat mucosa. The risk of cancer is highest where dysplasia arises in visible plaques or masses (dysplasia-associated mass lesion). Dysplasia in ulcerative colitis is divided into low-grade and high-grade categories. The presence of high-grade dysplasia is asso-

ciated with a significant risk of synchronous cancer or subsequent cancer development. Colonoscopic screening programs are therefore aimed at identifying dysplasia through multiple biopsies of the colonic mucosa. If high-grade dysplasia is detected or dysplasia occurs in a macroscopic lesion (ie, dysplasia-associated mass lesion), total colectomy is advised. While the significance of low-grade dysplasia is less clear, its presence mandates frequent surveillance.

2. Crohn's disease–Some studies have reported an increased risk for development of dysplasia and colorectal cancer in the setting of Crohn's disease, but a recent population-based cohort study failed to confirm the association. The exact risk of cancer in Crohn's disease patients therefore remains unclear.

Pathologic Findings

A. Gross Features: Colorectal cancers most often present as mass lesions. Carcinomas of the cecum and ascending colon are often polypoid and may become large and bulky prior to presentation because of the larger circumference of the right colon. Bulky mass lesions occur elsewhere in the colon as well. In the distal colon and rectum, where the bowel circumference is smaller, tumors may involve the entire circumference of the bowel to produce an annular constricting ("napkin ring") lesion, which may obstruct the lumen (Figure 27–10). Cancers occasionally have a flatter appearance, spreading intramurally. This feature is more common in the setting of inflammatory bowel disease. As tumors expand, they outgrow their blood supply, undergo necrosis, and ulcerate. This is a common feature of larger cancers.

B. Microscopic Features: Carcinomas of the colon and rectum are adenocarcinomas that form glandular structures of varying degrees of differentiation. Most are moderately well to well differentiated in appearance (Figure 27–11) and secrete variable amounts of mucin. In poorly differentiated tumors, gland formation is less prominent or absent. Mucinous or colloid cancers contain scattered collections of tumor cells floating in "lakes" of mucin, while signet-ring cell carcinomas contain cells in which large vacuoles of mucin displace the nuclei. Poorly differentiated, colloid, and signet-ring cell carcinomas tend to have a poorer prognosis than well-differentiated cancers. While it is convenient to categorize tumors in this fashion, most cancers are actually heterogeneous in their microscopic appearance, and may contain multiple populations of cells (Figure 27–12). Other pathologic features such as venous, lymphatic, or neural invasion may also affect the prognosis (see discussion following).

Tumors that are not adenocarcinomas represent less than 5% of malignant tumors in the large intestine. Primary lymphomas and carcinoid tumors together make up less than 0.1% of colorectal neoplasms. Other rare tumors include squamous cell,

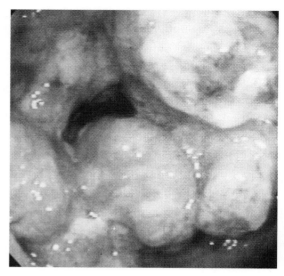

A

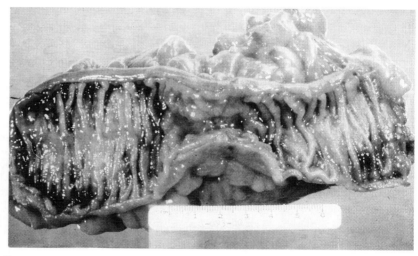

Figure 27–10. Obstructing carcinomas of the sigmoid colon. **A:** Endoscopic view showing bulky tumor mass nearly obstructing the lumen. **B:** Resected surgical specimen showing circumferential constricting lesion.

B

cloacogenic, and transitional cell carcinomas and melanocarcinomas at the anorectal junction.

Tumor Progression, Natural History, & Staging

Colorectal cancers evolve over long periods of time, beginning as intraepithelial lesions arising in dysplastic or adenomatous tissue. Microscopic analyses of biopsy or surgical specimens have demonstrated adenomatous change in even single glands. In most cases, the growth of adenomatous epithelium gives rise to macroscopic polyps. Further evolution is associated with increasing degrees of cellular atypia and glandular disorganization, eventuating in intraepithelial carcinoma (carcinoma in situ). Further growth leads to invasion of the muscularis mucosa

and eventual penetration of the bowel wall. Invasion of lymphatic and vascular structures gives rise to regional lymph node and distant metastases. This process occurs over a period of years. Approximations based on clinical observations indicate that it may take as long as a decade for the initial molecular changes to become invasive carcinoma, and half that time for adenoma to become carcinoma. Patterns of spread of the tumor depend to some extent on its location. Rectal cancers tend to spread locally to involve lymph nodes and adjacent structures, while colon cancer spreads to regional lymph nodes and more distant sites (eg, liver, lung). Metastasis is a complex multistep process involving numerous biologic events (Figure 27–13). The long natural history of cancer evolution in the colon and rectum has sig-

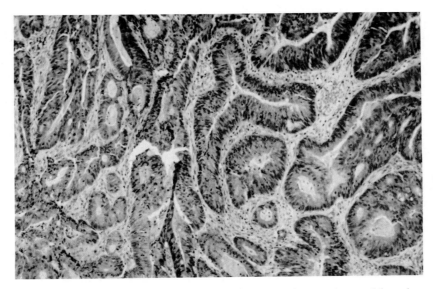

Figure 27–11. Photomicrograph of a well-differentiated adenocarcinoma of the colon.

nificant implications for screening and diagnosis, and affects the ability to improve survival rates and achieve cure (see discussion of diagnosis following).

Staging systems for colorectal cancer are based on the assumption that invasion and metastasis of colorectal neoplasms occur as an orderly progression. Clinical and pathologic correlations confirm that the prognosis depends on the depth of bowel wall invasion at the time of diagnosis. Lymph node involvement is associated with further decreased survival rates, while distant metastases are associated with the worst prognosis of all (see following discussion,

"Prognosis"). The two major staging systems used are modifications of the Dukes' classification (Table 27–5) and the TNM classification of the American Joint Committee on Cancer Staging for Colorectal Cancer (Table 27–6).

CLINICAL FINDINGS

Symptoms & Signs

Adenocarcinomas of the colon and rectum grow slowly and remain asymptomatic for long periods of

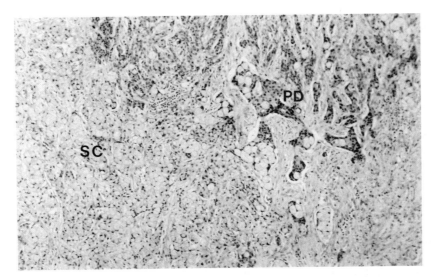

Figure 27–12. Photomicrograph of colonic carcinoma demonstrating heterogeneity in histologic morphologic study. This tumor contains areas of signet-ring cell *(SC)* as well as poorly differentiated *(PD)* carcinoma.

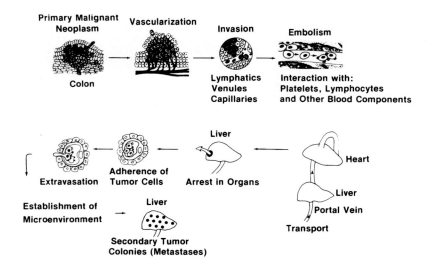

Figure 27–13. Metastasis is a multistep process involving numerous biologic events.

time. When symptoms do occur, they depend to some degree on the location of the tumor in the large intestine. Cancers of the proximal colon and cecum usually attain a large size before becoming symptomatic because of the diameter of the bowel in this region. It is common for such right-sided cancers to present with microcytic anemia secondary to chronic blood loss.

Constitutional symptoms resulting from anemia may be the first indication of a problem when elderly patients present with fatigue, shortness of breath, or even angina. Occasionally, more acute bleeding results in the presentation of dark red blood admixed with stool. Vague abdominal discomfort or even a palpable mass may be late findings. Cancers of the descending and sigmoid colon often involve the bowel circumferentially. As they grow into the lumen, patients present with obstructive symptoms such as cramping, abdominal pain, or a change in bowel habits. Constipation may alternate with postobstructive diarrhea as stool moves beyond the obstructing lesion. Rectal cancers often present with hematochezia (red blood per rectum) or obstruction. These tumors may invade locally to involve surrounding structures such as the bladder or female genital tract. Pain due to involvement of the sacral plexus is a late occurrence.

Diagnostic Studies

A. Diagnostic Procedure in Symptomatic Patients: When the presence of colorectal cancer is suggested by clinical signs and symptoms such as microcytic anemia, hematochezia, abdominal pain, weight loss, or change in bowel habits (see preceding discussion "Symptoms & Signs"), prompt diagnostic evaluation should be undertaken endoscopically or radiographically (Figure 27–14). The finding of oc-

cult blood in the stool heightens the suspicion that neoplasia may be present, but its absence does not rule out a significant lesion and should not deter evaluation when cancer is suspected.

1. Colonoscopy–Colonoscopy is the most accurate means of evaluating the colonic mucosa, and allows biopsy of suspicious lesions. Colonoscopes have flexible shafts that accommodate the curves of the colon, high-resolution optics with 20- to 30-fold magnification at close range, and instrument and suction channels that allow washing, mucosal biopsy, and electrocauterization. Video imaging and instant printing make a permanent record available. Complete examination of the colon to the cecum can be accomplished in over 90% of patients (most colonoscopes are 165 cm in length). The potential discomfort of the procedure is somewhat dependent on the operator, but in most cases, the procedure can be comfortably performed with modest intravenous conscious sedation. While the risk of colonic perforation or bleeding exists, complication rates for diagnostic procedures are less than 0.5%. The combined diagnostic accuracy is 90–95% for detecting polypoid lesions. Small polyps located behind folds, intramucosal lesions in the setting of ulcerative colitis, and abnormalities present in areas of extensive diverticulosis, stricture, or spasm account for missed lesions. Colonoscopy is approximately 12% more accurate than air contrast barium enema, especially in detecting small lesions such as adenomas (studies claim both lower and higher rates). The cost of the examination is an important issue, especially in reference to the value of screening examinations (see discussion following). Colonoscopy is most accurate and highly cost effective in the evaluation of symptomatic patients, however.

2. Barium enema examination–Air contrast

Table 27–5. Dukes classification for carcinoma of the rectum and its modifications for colorectal carcinoma.

Stage	Dukes, 1932 (Rectum)	Gabriel, Dukes, Bussey, 1935 (Rectum)	Kirklin et al, 1949 (Rectum and Sigmoid)	Astler-Coller, 1954 (Rectum and Colon)	Turnbull et al, 1967 (Colon)	Modified Astler-Coller (Gunderson & Sosin, 1974) (Rectum and Colon)	GITSG, 1975 (Rectum and Colon)
A	Limited to bowel wall	Limited to bowel wall	Limited to mucosa	Limited to mucosa	Limited to mucosa	Limited to mucosa	Limited to mucosa
B	Through bowel wall	Through bowel wall	—	—	Tumor extension into pericolic fat	—	—
B1	—	—	Into muscularis propria	Into muscularis propria	—	Into muscularis propria	Into muscularis propria
B2	—	—	Through muscularis propria	Through muscularis propria (and serosa)	—	Through serosa (m = microscopic, m + g = gross)	Through serosa
B3	—	—	—	—	—	Adherent to or invading adjacent structures	—
C	Regional nodal metastases	—	Regional nodal metastases	—	Regional nodal metastases	—	—
C1	—	Regional nodal metastases near primary lesion	—	Same as B1 plus regional nodal metastases	—	Same as B1 plus regional nodal metastases	1–4 regional nodes positive
C2	—	Proximal node involved at point of ligation	—	Same as B2 plus regional nodal metastases	—	Same as B2 plus regional nodal metastases	> 4 regional nodes positive
C3	—	—	—	—	—	Same as B3 plus regional nodal metastases	—
D	—	—	—	—	Distant metastases (liver, lung, bone) or due to parietal or adjacent organ invasion	—	—

Reproduced, with permission, from Bresalier RS, Kim YS: Malignant neoplasms of the large intestine. In: *Gastrointestinal Disease,* 5/e. Sleisenger MH, Fordtran JS (editors). Saunders, 1993.

barium enema is an alternative to colonoscopy, but may miss small lesions. Nonetheless, if colonoscopy is unavailable, technically difficult, or refused by the patient, this examination is still highly accurate in detecting carcinomas and larger adenomas. Barium enema may also be effective in visualizing areas beyond strictures not accessible to the colonoscope. Full column barium enemas detect most large mass lesions, but are less accurate than air contrast examinations for detecting smaller lesions. Distal lesions, especially those in the rectum, are sometimes diffi-

cult to detect radiographically, and flexible fiberoptic sigmoidoscopy with retroflexion should complement the barium enema.

B. Screening Procedures in Asymptomatic Patients: Because colorectal cancer is curable if detected at an early stage, screening for preneoplastic adenomas and early cancers has received a great deal of attention. Screening pertains to detection in large asymptomatic populations. Screening in the general population has concentrated on fecal occult blood testing and proctosigmoidoscopy. It has been known

Table 27–6. Staging of colorectal cancer by the American Joint Committee on Cancer (TNM classification.)[1]

Stage 0	Carcinoma in situ	Tis	N0	M0
Stage I	Tumor invades submucosa	T1	N0	M0
Stage II	Tumor invades through muscularis propria into subserosa, or into nonperitonealized pericolic or perirectal tissues	T3	N0	M0
	Tumor perforates the visceral peritoneum or directly invades other organs or structures	T4	N0	M0
Stage III	Any degree of bowel wall perforation with regional lymph node metastasis			
	N1	1–3 pericolic or perirectal lymph nodes involved		
	N2	4 or more pericolic or perirectal lymph nodes involved		
	N3	Metastasis in any lymph node along a named vascular trunk		
	Any T	N1	M0	
	Any T	N2, N3	M0	
Stage IV	Any invasion of bowel wall with or without lymph node metastasis, but with evidence of distant metastasis			
	Any T	Any N	M1	

[1]Based on American Joint Committee on Cancer Staging for Colorectal Cancer (3rd ed.) Lippincott, 1988. Dukes B (corresponds to stage II) is a composite of better (T3, N0, M0) and worse (T4, N0, M0) prognostic groups, as is Dukes C (corresponds to stage III) (any T, N1, M0) and (any T, N2, N3, M0).

for some time that colorectal cancer screening with these modalities can detect early cancers. Importantly, recent studies now suggest improved survival rates in patients in colorectal cancer screening programs.

1. Fecal occult blood testing–Annual fecal occult blood testing in persons over 40–50 years of age has been recommended for several years by the American Cancer Society (in conjunction with sigmoidoscopy every 3–5 years), American College of Physicians, and National Cancer Institute. Standardized slide tests, such as Hemoccult II, employ guaiac-impregnated paper (Figure 27–15). In the presence of the pseudoperoxidase activity of hemoglobin (blood) and hydrogen peroxide (supplied in the developing solution), the colorless phenolic guaiac is converted to a blue-pigmented quinone that is visually apparent. Adequate performance of the examination (Table 27–7) requires that the patient avoid red meat and peroxidase-rich foods for 3 days before the test, in order to prevent false-positive results, and that two samples from each of three consecutive stools be supplied. Slides should be developed within 4–6 days, since low levels of peroxidase activity may be degraded by fecal bacteria. Although adding a drop of water to the slide (rehydration) increases sensitivity, this is usually not recommended, because of the excess cost of evaluating false-positive tests. Immunologic tests for fecal occult blood that are more specific for human hemoglobin have recently become available, and have demonstrated a high degree

of sensitivity and specificity for detecting colonic lesions in preliminary trials.

Five major controlled trials have examined the potential benefit of fecal occult blood testing in screening asymptomatic individuals for colorectal neoplasms (Table 27–8). Compliance in these studies ranged from 50% in a clinical practice setting to 75% at a tertiary care center. Positive tests were obtained in approximately 2% of individuals. This was remarkably similar in all studies. The predictive value of a positive test for adenomas ranged from 26 to 41%, while the predictive value for carcinomas was much lower, ranging from 5 to 17% (about 10% in most studies). In all five trials, cancers at an earlier stage of development (Dukes' A and B cancers) were found in the screened group compared with those in the control group. One study demonstrated that annual fecal occult blood testing decreased the 13-year cumulative mortality rate from colorectal cancer by 33%. It should be noted, however, that this study used rehydrated test samples, yielding a high number of false-positive tests.

2. Sigmoidoscopy–Routine proctosigmoidoscopy and removal of adenomatous polyps detected by this method can reduce the incidence and mortality rates due to colorectal cancers found within reach of the sigmoidoscope by as much as 70%. The 60-cm flexible sigmoidoscope has supplanted the rigid scope, because it causes less discomfort to the patient, visualizes at least 2.5 times more surface area, and detects two to three times more adenomas. Flexible sigmoidoscopy can be learned by paramedical personnel, and has been successfully used in screening programs employing nurse-practitioners. Current recommendations suggest that screening flexible sigmoidoscopy be performed every 3–5 years in asymptomatic individuals over 50 years of age. This should be combined with yearly fecal occult blood testing, since only half of carcinomas will be found within reach of the flexible sigmoidoscope (Figure 27–16).

3. Other screening methods–Instillation of water into the colon followed by extracorporeal ultrasound examination (hydrocolonic sonography) has been suggested as a means of detecting carcinomas and large adenomas, but recent evidence has demonstrated a low sensitivity for this method. Detection of shed cancer cells by cytometry, biochemical and immunologic detection of fecal cancer-associated antigens, and detection of mutated proto-oncogenes such as K-ras in stool may be possible, but the feasibility of such methods for screening programs remains unproved.

C. Laboratory Findings: Laboratory findings are most often absent until colorectal cancers are advanced. Microcytic anemia and iron deficiency with low transferrin saturation results from chronic blood loss. Abnormalities in liver function tests are rare accompaniments to extensive metastatic disease. Ele-

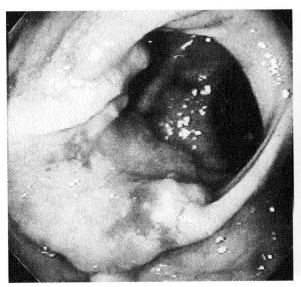

A

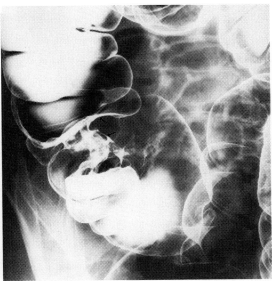

B

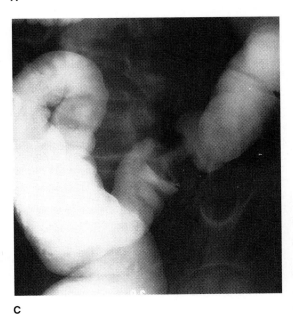

C

Figure 27–14. Modalities for detecting colorectal cancer include colonoscopy and radiography. ***A:*** Colonoscopic view of cancer of the ascending colon. Cancer is seen infiltrating a colonic fold and growing semicircumferentially and into the lumen. ***B:*** Air contrast barium enema demonstrating cancer similar to that seen in ***A (arrows)***. ***C:*** Constricting "apple core" lesion of the left colon seen on full column barium enema.

vated serum levels of tumor-associated glycoprotein antigens such as carcinoembryonic antigen also occur late in the course of disease and have negative prognostic implications. Because mutations in the APC gene are germline mutations in patients with familial adenomatous polyposis, these may be detected in at-risk individuals in kindreds through examination of peripheral blood leukocytes (see discussion following). This is not possible, however, in sporadic colon cancer, where epithelial cell mutations are somatic (acquired). The expression of certain glycoprotein antigens in resected tumors or deletions in tumor

suppressor genes such as DCC and p53 have prognostic implications that will be further discussed (see following discussion, "Prognosis").

D. Diagnostic and Imaging Studies: The general roles of colonoscopy, flexible sigmoidoscopy, and radiology in diagnosing colorectal cancer in symptomatic patients and in screening asymptomatic individuals has been discussed earlier. The specific roles of these modalities in screening patients who are at average or high risk will now be discussed.

1. Individuals with average risk—Because

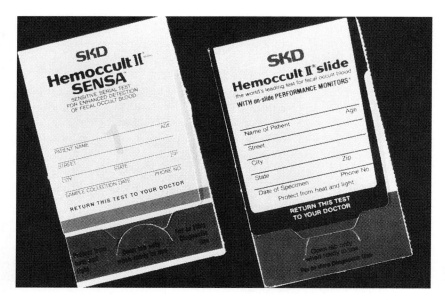

Figure 27–15. Standardized slide tests for performance of fecal occult blood testing. Proper performance is necessary to avoid false-positive and false-negative tests (see text). (Reproduced, with permission, from SmithKline Diagnostics.)

colorectal cancer occurs in an older age-group in the general population, individuals over age 40 or 50 years should be targeted for screening. This should at present include annual digital rectal examination and fecal occult blood testing in individuals over 40 years of age, and flexible sigmoidoscopy every 3–5 years after age 50 years (in keeping with the recommendations of the American Cancer Society and other groups). The presence of fecal occult blood in this age-group dictates a diagnostic evaluation. Colonoscopy or air contrast barium enema combined with flexible sigmoidoscopy should be performed in those with positive fecal occult blood tests to rule out colonic lesions. Screening programs should include educational components to heighten the awareness of both patients and physicians as to the frequency and curability of colorectal cancer. Given the high cost of

Table 27–7. Performance of the slide guaiac test for fecal occult blood.

1. For three days prior to and during testing, patients should avoid
   a. Rare red meat
   b. Peroxidase-containing vegetables and fruits (eg, broccoli, turnips, cantaloupe, cauliflower, radishes)
   c. The following medications:
      Vitamin C (antioxidant)
      Aspirin
      NSAIDs
2. Two samples of each of three consecutive stools should be tested (it is proper to sample areas of obvious blood)
3. Slides should be developed within 4–6 days
4. Slides should not be rehydrated prior to developing (for average-risk screening)

colorectal cancer screening in the general population and the long natural history of the disease, some have advocated the performance of a single barium enema or even colonoscopy at age 50 years, with no further evaluation in asymptomatic individuals with negative examinations. The appropriateness of such an approach has not, however, gained wide acceptance.

2. Patients with a family history of colorectal cancer–The familial pattern of colorectal cancer has already been discussed. Obtaining an accurate family history is an important component of evaluating patients at risk for this disease. Screening procedures are controversial for someone with only one first-degree relative who has had colon cancer. Many experts do not believe that the increased risk (two to three times that of the general population) warrants the added cost of screening modalities beyond those recommended for those with no family history. Others, however, feel that a single screening colonoscopy at age 50 years is warranted in this group, especially if the index case had colon cancer before age 50 years. When two first-degree relatives have had colon cancer, colonoscopic examination at periodic intervals (eg, every 5 years) has been suggested (beginning at an age 5 years younger than that of the youngest affected relative). The effectiveness of such a program remains to be determined. If three or more relatives have had colorectal cancer, a familial syndrome should be suspected.

a. Hereditary nonpolyposis colorectal cancer–Hereditary nonpolyposis colorectal cancer is defined by three relatives with colon cancer (one of whom is a first-degree relative of the other two), co-

Table 27–8. Controlled trials of fecal occult blood testing in screening asymptomatic persons for colorectal cancer.[1]

Site	Cohort	Screening Interval	Rehydrated	Percentage of Dukes Stage A or B Screened	Percentage of Dukes Stage A or B Control
New York	21,961	—	No	66	33
Minnesota	46,961	1 and 2 years	Yes	61[2]	58
England	142,690	2 years	No	76	46
Sweden	51,325	14–22 months	Yes	64	35
Denmark	61,938	2 years	No	81	46

[1]Reproduced and adapted, with permission, from Bresalier RS, Kim YS: Malignant neoplasms of the large intestine. In: Gastrointestinal Disease, 5th ed. Sleisinger MH, Fordtran JS (editors). Saunders, 1993.
[2]A 33% decrease in cumulative mortality rates over 13 years was demonstrated due to a significant decrease in Dukes D tumors.

lorectal cancer involving at least two generations, and one case of cancer occurring before age 50 years. At present, members of such families should be screened by colonoscopy every 3 years, beginning at age 20 years or at an age 10 years younger than that of the index case. The ability to detect defects in DNA mismatch repair genes or DNA replication errors (RER+ phenotype) may make it possible to identify at-risk individuals in a given family in the future.

b. Familial adenomatous polyposis–Family members of kindreds with familial adenomatous polyposis should be screened for colonic polyposis by colonoscopy beginning at age 15–20 years. The recent availability of sensitive methods for detecting APC gene product abnormalities in at-risk individuals may supplant the need for routine colonoscopy in all family members in the future. Molecular diagnosis should be performed in all family members of kindreds to help determine who is at risk and facilitate genetic counseling.

3. Patients with a history of adenoma–The vast majority of colorectal cancers arise in adenomatous polyps. Substantial clinical evidence indicates that patients who have one adenoma are not only likely to have additional adenomas elsewhere in the colon, but to develop subsequent adenomas in the future (32% at 3 years after initial polypectomy in one study, and 42% in a second study). It is therefore suggested that patients with a history of adenomatous polyps undergo routine surveillance colonoscopy. It has become clear, however, that due to the slow growth of adenomas and their progression to carcinoma, repeat colonoscopy need not be performed at intervals less than every 3 years in patients whose index polyp demonstrates no evidence of high-grade dysplasia or carcinoma. Patients with multiple adenomas, large adenomas, and adenomas occurring before 60 years of age are more likely to develop recurrent adenomas. Multiplicity, however, seems to be the major risk factor for development of recurrent adenomas with advanced pathologic features (ie, large adenomas and those with high-grade dysplasia or invasive cancer). It should be borne in mind that although most cancers arise in adenomatous polyps, only a small percentage of adenomas will eventually demonstrate malignant degeneration. A case in point is "diminutive polyps" less than 5 mm in size. The chance of these polyps containing cancer and the long-term risk of development of cancer after excision of such polyps is low. Some have therefore advocated that persons whose index polyp is a single tubular adenoma under 1 cm in size with only mild to moderate dysplasia need not be routinely screened for polyp recurrence; this has not yet gained general acceptance, however.

4. Patients with a history of colorectal cancer–Patients who have had resection of colon cancer for cure require surveillance for two reasons: to detect cancer recurrence and to screen for new metachronous cancers, which occur in 1–5% of patients. Such patients should have colonoscopy 6

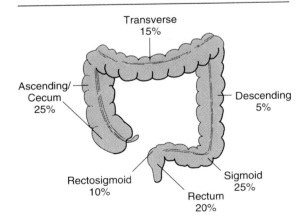

Figure 27–16. Distribution of colorectal cancers within the large intestine. Only half of the cancers are found within reach of the flexible sigmoidoscope.

months after surgery and twice at yearly intervals to rule out local recurrence. Screening colonoscopy should then be performed every 3 years.

Elevated serum carcinoembryonic antigen levels may signal recurrence and should be measured at regular intervals following surgery. The ideal frequency of such testing is unclear, but one reasonable approach is 2-month intervals for 2 years and then 4-month intervals for an additional 3 years. If levels of carcinoembryonic antigen are elevated, "second-look" operations may improve survival rates in selected persons, and may help identify isolated hepatic metastases that are amenable to surgical resection.

The use of CT scanning of the pelvis to detect local recurrence of rectal cancer and of the abdomen to detect distant liver metastasis has been suggested by some, but the cost effectiveness of such an approach compared with that of physical examination plus serial carcinoembryonic antigen determinations is unproved.

5. Patients with inflammatory bowel disease–

a. Ulcerative colitis–Patients with long-standing ulcerative colitis (> 7 years' duration) should undergo routine surveillance colonoscopy with serial biopsies of the colonic mucosa, since dysplasia in this setting may occur in flat, normal-appearing mucosa. Biopsy specimens should be taken throughout the colon at 10-cm intervals. Any macroscopic lesion should be biopsied, since dysplasia occurring in polypoid masses or plaques suggests a high likelihood of coincident cancer. Common recommendations as to the interval between examinations vary from yearly to every 3 years. Given that the mucosa in ulcerative colitis must still undergo transition from dysplasia to carcinoma, colonoscopy every 3 years seems reasonable in such patients.

b. Crohn's disease–The need for routine surveillance in Crohn's disease is less clear. Patients undergoing colonoscopy for other reasons should of course have any suspicious lesions and all strictures biopsied.

DIFFERENTIAL DIAGNOSIS

Symptomatic patients with colorectal cancer are often initially misdiagnosed. Abdominal pain, bleeding, or a change in stool caliber may be wrongly diagnosed as diverticular disease, and rectal bleeding is often attributed to hemorrhoids. A high index of suspicion is necessary, especially in those over 50 years of age. Anyone in this age-group presenting with microcytic anemia, hematochezia, or new onset of cramping abdominal pain should be properly evaluated for the presence of colorectal cancer. Table 27–9 lists some clinical situations that may be confused with colorectal cancer.

Table 27–9. Differential diagnosis of colorectal cancer.[1]

Mass lesions
  Benign tumors (mucosal and submucosal)
  Diverticulosis
  Inflammatory masses
    Diverticulitis
    Inflammatory bowel disease
    Ischemia
    Infections (tuberculosis, amebiasis, fungal infection)
  Fatty infiltration of the ileocecal valve
  Endometriosis
Strictures
  Inflammatory bowel disease (Crohn's colitis)
  Ischemia
  Radiation (late sequelae)
Rectal bleeding
  Diverticulosis
  Ulcerative colitis
  Infectious colitis
  Ischemic colitis
  Solitary rectal ulcer
  Hemorrhoidal bleeding
Abdominal pain
  Ischemia
  Diverticulitis
  Inflammatory bowel disease
  Irritable bowel syndrome
Change in bowel habits
  Inflammatory bowel disease
  Infectious diarrhea
  Medications (constipation or diarrhea)
  Irritable bowel syndrome

[1]This list includes common clinical situations that may be initially confused with signs or symptoms of colorectal cancer, but it is not meant to be inclusive.

COMPLICATIONS

Complications of colon cancer include chronic and acute blood loss, bowel obstruction, bowel perforation, and the illness (ie, cachexia) and death associated with metastatic disease. Rectal cancers may invade locally to involve adjacent structures, creating rectovesical or rectovaginal fistula, ureteral obstruction, or neurologic symptoms referable to invasion at the sacral plexus.

TREATMENT

Polypectomy

Endoscopic polypectomy (Figure 27–17) is adequate treatment for an adenomatous polyp that contains carcinoma if it can be demonstrated to be confined to the mucosa in the head of the polyp (carcinoma in situ; Figure 27–18). The adequacy of simple polypectomy remains controversial in cases where malignant cells have invaded the polyp stalk, but most studies indicate that this is adequate treatment, provided that a margin of more than 2 mm is present, there is no vascular or lymphatic invasion, and the cancer is not poorly differentiated. These cri-

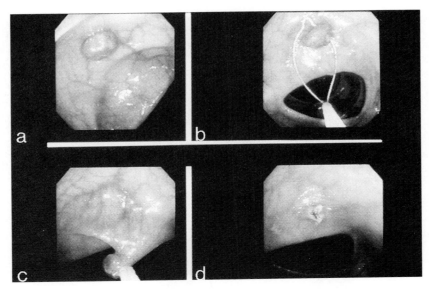

Figure 27–17. Endoscopic polypectomy prevents eventual malignant degeneration to carcinoma, and is adequate treatment when carcinoma is confined to the mucosa of the polyp (carcinoma in situ). **A:** Pedunculated polyp. **B:** The polypectomy snare is placed around the neck of the polyp. **C:** The polyp is brought into the lumen. **D:** The polypectomy site after removal of the polyp.

teria are more difficult to assess in sessile than pedunculated polyps. If an adequate margin cannot be demonstrated or negative histologic indicators are present, surgery is recommended to rule out regional metastases.

Surgical Resection

A. Primary Tumor Resection: Surgical resec-

tion of primary colorectal cancer with curative intent is the treatment of choice in most patients. This involves wide resection of the involved bowel segment and removal of its lymphatic drainage (Figure 27–19). The extent of colonic resection is determined in part by the vascular supply of the large bowel and the distribution of regional lymph nodes. A minimum surgical margin of 5 cm on either side of the tumor is

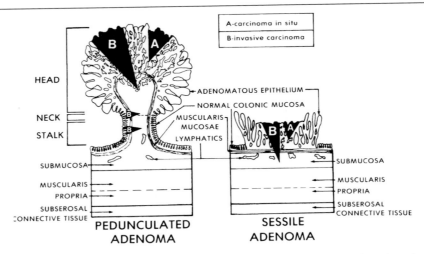

Figure 27–18. Diagrammatic representation of carcinoma within a polyp. Endoscopic polypectomy is adequate treatment for carcinoma in situ **(A).** If submucosal invasion occurs in a pedunculated polyp **(B),** polypectomy may be adequate if a sufficient margin (> 2 mm) can be demonstrated and histologic features are favorable (see text). The depth of invasion in sessile polyps is often difficult to determine, and surgery may be required to rule out lymph node metastases. (Reproduced and adapted, with permission, from Haggitt et al: Prognostic factors in colorectal carcinomas arising in adenomas: Implications for lesions removed by endoscopic polypectomy. Gastroenterology 1985;89:328.)

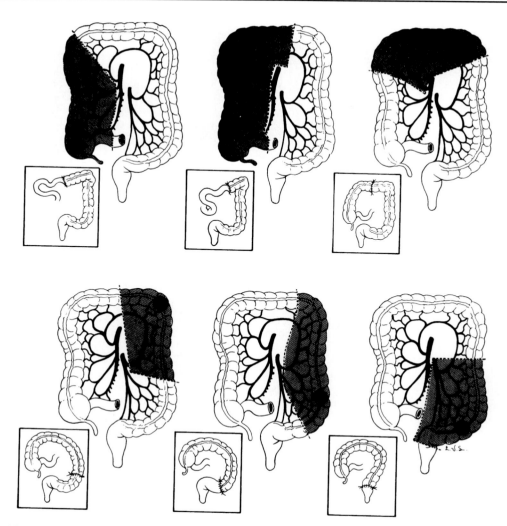

Figure 27–19. Surgical resection of colorectal cancer based on location of the primary tumor, blood supply, and lymphatic drainage. (Reproduced, with permission, from Schrock T: Large intestine. In: *Current Surgical Diagnosis and Treatment,* 10/e Way LW (editor). Lange, 1994.)

required, although segmental resection is not always possible, due to compromise of the vascular supply to portions of the colon. Rectosigmoid and many rectal lesions can be removed with a low anterior resection through an abdominal incision, combined with primary anastomosis of the remaining bowel. Primary anastomoses can now be performed even for low rectal lesions using end-to-end stapling devices and sphincter-saving operations. If an adequate uninvolved distal margin (usually at least 2 cm) cannot be obtained, the tumor is large and bulky, or the pelvis is involved by extensive local tumor spread, an abdominoperineal resection with ileostomy may be necessary for cancer of the distal rectum.

B. Resection of Liver Metastases: Synchronous metastases to the liver are grossly evident at the time of initial surgery in 10–25% of patients with colorectal cancer. If adequate surgical margins have been obtained at resection of the primary tumor and there is no evidence of extrahepatic disease, resection of isolated hepatic lesions with curative intent is possible. Resection is usually confined to those with no more than four hepatic lesions, although even those with bilobar metastases may be resected for cure. Five-year survival rates exceed 25% in selected patients, with a low operative mortality rate of less than 2% in experienced hands. Seventy to eighty percent of hepatic metastases appear within 2 years following primary resection. Hepatic resection of isolated lesions subsequent to initial surgery follows the same principles as those for resection of synchronous lesions, and repeat hepatic resection can result in long-term survival times in selected individuals. Those with extrahepatic disease at presentation or bilobar metastases are at increased risk for recurrence after hepatic resection. Patients with underlying liver disease are poor candidates for hepatic resection because of limited functional hepatic reserve.

Adjuvant Chemotherapy

Chemotherapy of colon cancer can be divided into adjuvant chemotherapy and chemotherapy of advanced disease. Adjuvant therapy is aimed at eradicating microscopic metastases in patients who have undergone resection with curative intent but are at high risk for recurrence due to the presence of lymph node metastases or poor prognostic features. Recent data indicate that adjuvant chemotherapy with fluorouracil (a fluoropyrimidine) plus levamisole (an agent with possible immunomodulatory activity) decreases cancer recurrence by 42% and mortality rates by 33% after surgery in patients with Dukes C (stage III) tumors. Data for Dukes B2 (stage II) disease are equivocal, but if the primary tumors are poorly differentiated; demonstrate lymphatic, vascular, or perineural invasion; or demonstrate invasion into adjacent structures, patients should receive adjuvant therapy as well. A great deal of ongoing research is aimed at defining prognostic variables that will help determine who will most benefit from adjuvant chemotherapy (see following discussion, "Prognosis").

While cancers of the colon tend to recur at distant sites, rectal cancers often recur both locally and distantly. Patients with rectal cancer who are treated with postoperative irradiation have a decreased incidence of local tumor recurrence, but die from metastatic disease. Recent trials demonstrate that combined adjuvant therapy with postoperative irradiation plus fluorouracil chemotherapy reduces cancer-related deaths in stage II and III rectal cancers (Dukes B2 and C disease) by 36% compared with tumors treated by surgery alone. The effect of combined treatment as postoperative adjuvant therapy in patients with high-risk rectal cancer is enhanced by administering fluorouracil as a protracted infusion during pelvic irradiation rather than as an intermittent bolus. The addition of the chemotherapeutic agent semustine to the regimens does not further improve survival rates but increases toxicity.

Chemotherapy for Advanced Disease

Chemotherapy of advanced colorectal cancer is usually associated with short-lived responses and lack of improvement in survival rates. The fluoropyrimidines (fluorouracil and fluorodeoxyuridine) inhibit DNA synthesis by interacting with thymidylate synthase and inhibiting the methylation of deoxyuridylic to thymidylic acid. These agents may be administered by bolus or continuous intravenous in-

fusion, with response rates as single agents of approximately 20%. Combinations of fluorouracil plus high-dosage intravenous leucovorin (tetrahydrofolate) are superior to fluorouracil alone, with response rates of up to 50%, but prolongation of survival rates has not been convincingly demonstrated. Addition of recombinant α_2-interferon increases response rates but not survival rates, and also increases toxicity. Selective infusion of chemotherapeutic agents such as fluorodeoxyuridine into the hepatic arterial system achieves objective response rates of 50–80% for liver metastases, but, again, the impact on survival rates is unclear. Selective infusion of fluoropyrimidines combined with hepatic arterial occlusion has also been advocated as treatment of hepatic metastases, with promising preliminary results. Others have attempted to deliver chemotherapeutic agents through liposomes linked to monoclonal antibodies that recognize tumor-associated antigens (immunotargeted therapy). While conceptually appealing, this approach must be considered experimental.

Postoperative irradiation decreases local recurrence in patients with high-risk rectal cancers. The incidence of local recurrence in stage II or III disease is 40–50%, and these patients should receive postoperative irradiation. As previously noted, postoperative irradiation combined with chemotherapy improves survival rates when used in an adjuvant setting. Irradiation may also be used preoperatively in an attempt to convert large bulky tumors or those with fixation to pelvic organs to resectable lesions.

Endoscopic therapy using the neodymium yttrium aluminum garnet (ND:YAG) laser can be used for palliation of patients with obstructing rectal cancer or persistent bleeding who are poor surgical candidates. Photodynamic therapy, in which a hematoporphyrin derivative is used to sensitize tumor cells to phototherapy with a tunable dye laser, has also been used as experimental therapy in patients who are poor surgical risks.

PROGNOSIS

The prognosis of patients with colorectal cancer is most closely related to tumor stage at the time of diagnosis (see earlier discussion, "Pathophysiology"). Tumor stage, in turn, is related to the degree of bowel wall penetration and presence or absence of involved lymph nodes or distant metastases. Thus, patients whose tumors are confined to the mucosa or submucosa (Dukes A, or T1 N0 M0, disease) or extend beyond the submucosa but are confined to the bowel wall (Dukes B1, or T2 N0 M0, disease) have excellent survival rates (Figure 27–20). Survival rates decrease with bowel wall penetration (Dukes B2, or stage II, disease) and lymph node involvement (Dukes C, or stage III, disease). The number of involved lymph nodes also has an impact on prognosis;

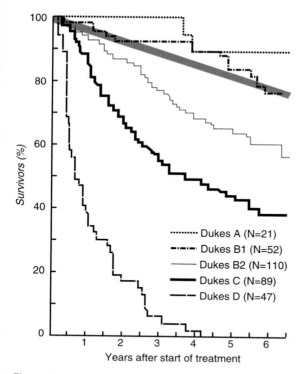

Figure 27–20. Survival rates after surgical resection, according to modified Dukes' staging system for colorectal cancer. Expected survival times of age- and sex-matched individuals in the general population are indicated by the shaded area. (Reproduced, with permission, from Moertel CG et al: The preoperative carcinoembryonic antigen test in the diagnosis, staging, and prognosis of colorectal cancer. Cancer 1986;58:603.)

Figure legend:
- ········ Dukes A (N=21)
- —·—·— Dukes B1 (N=52)
- —— Dukes B2 (N=110)
- **——** Dukes C (N=89)
- — — Dukes D (N=47)

patients having one to three involved nodes have better survival rates than those with four or more involved nodes. Distant metastatic disease (Dukes D, or stage IV, disease) is associated with a poor prognosis, with 5-year survival rates of only 5–10%.

Other histologic and clinical features may have an impact on the prognosis but are less important than the surgical and pathologic stage (Tables 27–10 and 27–11). Patients with poorly differentiated, colloid, or signet-ring cell cancers tend to have a poorer prognosis than those with moderately well or well-differentiated tumors. Tumor size (independent of penetration) seems to have less impact on prognosis. Venous, lymphatic, and perineural invasion indicate a diminished prognosis, while evidence of local inflammation and immunologic reaction (peritumoral lymphocytes) seems to indicate a better prognosis. Certain clinical features such as bowel obstruction or perforation, young age at diagnosis (in those without familial syndromes), and high preoperative serum carcinoembryonic antigen levels are associated with a poor prognosis.

Table 27–10. Pathologic features that may affect prognosis in patients with colorectal cancer.

Pathologic Features	Effect on Prognosis

Surgical or pathologic stage
  Depth of bowel wall penetration
  Number of regional lymph nodes involved by tumor
	Increased penetration diminishes prognosis; 1–4 nodes better than > 4 nodes

Histologic findings Degree of differentiation	Well-differentiated better than poorly differentiated
Mucinous (colloid) or signet-ring cell histologic findings	Diminished prognosis
Scirrhous histologic findings	Diminished prognosis
Venous invasion	Diminished prognosis
Lymphatic invasion	Diminished prognosis
Perineural invasion	Diminished prognosis
Local inflammation and immunologic reaction	Improved prognosis
Tumor size	No effect in most studies
Tumor morphologic findings	Polypoid or exophytic better than ulcerating or infiltrating
Tumor DNA content	Increased DNA content (aneuploidy) diminishes prognosis

Table 27–11. Clinical features that may affect prognosis in patients with colorectal cancer.

Clinical Features	Effect on Prognosis
Diagnosis in asymptomatic patients	?Improved prognosis
Duration of symptoms	No demonstrated effect
Rectal bleeding as presenting symptom	Improved prognosis
Bowel obstruction	Diminished prognosis
Bowel perforation	Diminished prognosis
Tumor location	?Colon better than rectum ?Left colon better than right colon
Age less than 30 years	Diminished prognosis
Preoperative serum carcinoembryonic antigen	Diminished prognosis with high level of carcinoembryonic antigen
Deletions in chromosome 18q (DCC gene)	Diminished prognosis
Deletions in chromosome 17p (p53)	Diminished prognosis
Distant metastases	Markedly diminished prognosis

In a search to better understand the natural history of tumor progression and identify patients who will most benefit from potentially toxic adjuvant therapies, molecular analysis of colorectal cancers has been recently employed. Patients whose tumors have abnormal chromosome numbers and, specifically, deletions of chromosomes 17p (p53) and 18q (DCC) have been demonstrated to have a worse prognosis than those whose tumors do not contain such allelic deletions. The status of chromosome 18q can be determined clinically after microdissection of even formalin-fixed, paraffin-embedded tumors using the polymerase chain reaction to amplify polymorphic microsatellite markers. Such studies reveal that the survival rate of patients with stage II disease whose tumors have chromosome 18q allelic loss is similar to that of patients with stage III disease, whereas patients whose tumors retain both alleles of chromosome 18q have a significantly better outcome. These assays can be readily adapted for clinical use and may be used in the future to help determine who should receive adjuvant therapy after surgical resection.

REFERENCES

Atkin WS, Morson BC, Cuzick J: Long-term risk of colorectal cancer after excision of rectosigmoid adenomas. N Engl J Med 1992;326:658.

Fuchs CG et al: A prospective study of family history and the risk of colorectal cancer. N Engl J Med 1994;331:1669.

Jen J et al: Allelic loss of chromosome 18q and prognosis in colorectal cancer. N Engl J Med 1994;331:213.

Lynch HT et al: Genetics, natural history, tumor spectrum, and pathology of hereditary nonpolyposis colorectal cancer: An updated review. Gastroenterology 1993;104:1535.

Mandel JS et al: Reducing mortality from colorectal cancer by screening for fecal occult blood. N Engl J Med 1993;328:1365.

Moertel CG et al: Levamisole and fluorouracil for adjuvant therapy of resected colon carcinoma. N Engl J Med 1990;322:352.

Neugut AI et al: Dietary risk factors for incidence and recurrence of colorectal adenomatous polyps: A case control study. Ann Intern Med 1993;118:91.

O'Connell MJ et al: Improving adjuvant therapy for rectal cancer by combining protracted-infusion fluorouracil with radiation therapy after curative surgery. N Engl J Med 1994;331:502.

Powel SM et al: Molecular diagnosis of familial adenomatous polyposis. N Engl J Med 1993;329:1982.

St. John DBJ et al: Cancer risk in relatives of patients with common colorectal cancer. Ann Intern Med 1993;118:785.

Selby JV et al: A case-control study of screening sigmoidoscopy and mortality from colorectal cancer. N Engl J Med 1993;326:653.

Willet WC et al: Relation of meat, fat, and fiber to the risk of colon cancer in a prospective study among women. N Engl J Med 1990;323:1664.

Winawer SJ et al: Prevention of colorectal cancer by colonoscopic polypectomy. N Engl J Med 1993;329:1977.

Winawer SJ et al: Randomized comparison of surveillance intervals after colonoscopic removal of newly diagnosed adenomatous polyps. N Engl J Med 1993;328:901.

28 Diverticular Disease of the Colon

Bruce E. Stabile, MD

Diverticula occur more often in the colon than in any other segment of the gastrointestinal tract. A true diverticulum contains all layers of the intestinal wall while a false, or pseudodiverticulum, represents a herniation of the mucosa and submucosa through a defect in the muscular layer of the intestine. True colonic diverticula are rare, occur almost exclusively in the cecum or ascending colon, are typically single, and are occasionally quite large. In contrast, pseudo-diverticula are very common, affect the left hemi-colon more often than the right, are almost always multiple, and are usually small. In common usage, the term **diverticulosis** refers to the presence of pseudodiverticula of the colon. Approximately 95% of diverticulosis cases involve the sigmoid colon, and approximately two-thirds of cases involve the sigmoid exclusively. The cecum alone is involved in only approximately 5% of cases.

Diverticulosis coli is among the most common diseases of Western civilization. In the United States, approximately one-third of the population develops diverticulosis by age 50 years and approximately two-thirds by the age of 80. While the exact pathogenesis is unknown, development of colonic diverticula is clearly related to advanced age, decreased dietary fiber intake, and elevation of colonic intraluminal pressure. In recent years the condition appears to be affecting greater numbers of adults younger than 40 years of age. There is no significant difference in incidence between the genders.

Pathophysiology

Increasing longevity and a highly refined, low fiber diet appear to contribute to a segmental abnormality of the colonic wall musculature that is believed to be central to the pathogenesis of **diverticulosis.** A low food fiber content results in decreased stool volume, which requires a high intraluminal pressure for fecal propulsion. Work hypertrophy is manifest by the colonic wall muscle layers in two ways: as thickening, and by the longitudinal fore-shortening known as myochosis coli. These wall muscle abnormalities are associated with exaggerated mucosal infoldings that create segmented high pressure cells within the bowel lumen. Manometric recordings have identified high colonic pressures in response to meals and pharmacologic stimuli as well as increased nonpropulsive segmental contractions that are most prominent in the sigmoid. By the law of Laplace, the small radius and high pressure within the sigmoid lumen make this the most vulnerable segment to mucosal herniation at sites of weakness in the muscularis propria. Thus, pulsion pseudodiverticula occur at sites where the penetrating nutrient blood vessels (vasa recta) traverse the circular smooth muscle layer between the serosa and submucosa (Figure 28–1). Since the blood vessels penetrate the colonic wall between the taenia coli, the vast majority of diverticula are found in these areas of weakness. Colonic diverticula are frequently obscured by the pericolic fat of the mesocolon and the appendices epiploicae. This explains the greater sensitivities of barium enema and colonoscopy in identifying diverticula compared with direct visual inspection of the serosal surface of the bowel.

The derangements of colonic muscular anatomy and motility observed in diverticulosis are similar to those present in the irritable bowel syndrome. To a degree, the two conditions may be viewed as different parts of a spectrum of colonic dysmotility; at one end of the spectrum are intense muscular contractions causing very high intraluminal pressures and severe pain; at the other end of the spectrum, extreme weakness of the bowel wall with mucosal herniation at relatively modest pressures and without symptoms. Only about one-quarter of patients with colonic diverticula experience symptoms. There is poor correlation between symptoms and location, size, or number of diverticula. While diverticular disease of the colon is most often asymptomatic, approximately 10–20% of patients develop acute diverticular infection or hemorrhage.

Diverticulitis describes the complication of acute infection that is far more common in the sigmoid colon than in other areas. In the vast majority of cases, diverticulitis is confined exclusively to the sigmoid with involvement of the descending colon, transverse colon, or ascending colon being distinctly

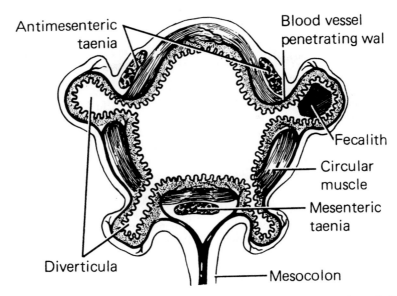

Figure 28–1. Cross section of the colon illustrating pseudodiverticula formation at sites of penetration of nutrient blood vessels through the circular muscle layer between the taenia coli. The presence of a fecalith within the lumen of a diverticulum may predispose to development of diverticulitis.

rare. Infection of a solitary cecal diverticulum is an infrequent though well-recognized entity that is clinically indistinguishable from acute appendicitis. The pathogenic mechanisms responsible for acute diverticulitis may be twofold. A fecalith inhabiting a diverticulum may slowly erode the attenuated wall of the diverticulum, leading to perforation and microscopic or macroscopic leakage of colonic contents. Alternatively, an empty diverticulum may simply burst as a result of unusually high intraluminal pressure. In either circumstance, an infectious process ensues that may involve only the colonic wall and adjacent paracolic fat, or may widely contaminate the free peritoneal cavity. Thus, diverticulitis always implies perforation of one or more diverticula that manifests as a phlegmonous inflammatory mass and localized peritonitis, a pericolic or pelvic abscess, or a generalized purulent or feculent peritonitis. By direct extension of the infectious process, sigmoid diverticulitis may cause fistulization to the urinary bladder, vagina, or less frequently, to adjacent small intestine or through the abdominal wall to the skin. Acute colonic obstruction related to severe edema or compression by an adjacent abscess occasionally accompanies acute diverticulitis. With repeated episodes of acute diverticulitis, a cicatricial scar slowly develops that causes a progressive fibrotic colonic stricture.

Acute lower gastrointestinal hemorrhage develops in approximately 5–10% of patients with colonic diverticulosis. The bleeding is thought to result from the close anatomic relationship between diverticula and the penetrating arterioles of the vasa recta. While the exact mechanism precipitating hemorrhage is unknown, the evidence suggests that a slow development of chemical or mechanical damage to the vessel wall results in rupture into the associated diverticulum. The diverticular bleeding that follows is typically massive but self-limited and may recur. Chronic occult blood loss is atypical of diverticular bleeding.

DIVERTICULOSIS

Essentials of Diagnosis
- Characteristic radiologic or endoscopic signs
- Intermittent left lower quadrant pain
- Constipation or diarrhea
- No fever or leukocytosis

General Considerations
Diverticulosis uncomplicated by acute inflammation or bleeding is often asymptomatic and diagnosed incidentally on barium enema or colonoscopy obtained for some other indication or for cancer screening purposes. When symptomatic, diverticulosis typically presents with abdominal pain and altered bowel habits typical of the irritable bowel syndrome. Symptoms are probably related to the dysmotility disorder accompanying diverticulosis rather than to the diverticula themselves. In the absence of perforation or hemorrhage, diverticula are probably incapable of causing symptoms. Thus, the major clinical importance of diverticulosis lies in the propensity for diverticula to perforate and bleed.

Clinical Findings

A. Symptoms and Signs: The pain of symptomatic diverticulosis typically is located in the left lower quadrant and is intermittent and cramping in nature. The pain may be associated with constipation, diarrhea, or both. Pain episodes are correlated with spastic contractions of the colonic musculature. Examination of the abdomen may elicit mild to moderate left lower quadrant tenderness but involuntary guarding and rebound tenderness are absent. In thin individuals, a palpable left lower quadrant mass may be present as a result of intense spastic contraction of the sigmoid colon. Because of the absence of diverticular perforation and inflammation, no fever is present.

B. Laboratory Findings: In the absence of bleeding and inflammation, the hematocrit, hemoglobin level, and white blood cell count are normal. The stool test for occult blood is negative.

C. Imaging: Plain film x-rays of the abdomen are unremarkable, but the barium enema study reveals multiple diverticula, typically involving the sigmoid colon with or without involvement of other colonic segments (Figure 28–2). Segmental spasm with a narrowed luminal diameter resulting in the typical sawtooth pattern may also be present. Any evidence of contrast extravasation, fistulization, or sinus tract formation indicates diverticulitis rather than simple uncomplicated diverticulosis. Abdominal computerized tomography (CT) in uncomplicated diverticulosis may reveal localized wall thickening and luminal narrowing of the involved colonic segment but no inflammatory changes of the pericolic fat.

D. Endoscopy: Endoscopic evaluation by means of rigid proctosigmoidoscopy, flexible fiberoptic sigmoidoscopy, or colonoscopy reveals the orifices of the diverticular sacs, but these may be obscured by mucosal folds. Luminal narrowing as a result of segmental colonic spasm may also be evident.

Differential Diagnosis

Symptomatic diverticulosis with intermittent bouts of pain and bowel irregularity may be difficult to differentiate from the irritable bowel syndrome and from mild acute diverticulitis. The presence of diverticula on barium enema establish the diagnosis of diverticular disease, but the absence of fever and leukocytosis do not exclude acute diverticulitis. If fever and leukocytosis are present and the diagnosis of diverticulitis is being entertained, the barium enema examination should be delayed until after resolution of the acute illness. In many instances where the systemic signs of inflammation are absent, the distinction between symptomatic diverticulosis and mild acute diverticulitis can only be made by observation of the clinical course of the episode.

When less than severe, a number of inflammatory conditions of the lower abdomen and pelvis such as appendicitis, Crohn s disease, endometriosis, pelvic inflammatory disease, as well as ruptured or torsed ovarian cyst, ischemic colitis, and colorectal carcinoma can present with pain patterns that may be confused with symptomatic diverticulosis. It is the irritable bowel syndrome, however, that is particularly indistinguishable when based solely on the clinical presentation; demonstration of diverticula on barium enema or endoscopy is required to make the diagnosis of diverticulosis.

Complications

Indolent perforation or acute rupture of a diverticulum results in diverticulitis. Erosion or rupture of the penetrating nutrient arteriole associated with a diverticulum causes acute lower gastrointestinal hemorrhage. Unlike simple diverticulosis, both of these complications are potentially life-threatening.

Treatment

A. Medical: The need for any specific treatment of patients with asymptomatic diverticulosis is controversial. Although a diet low in vegetable fiber is thought to be a causative factor, there is no convincing evidence that high fiber diets can prevent the development of additional diverticula or protect against the complications of diverticulosis. However, because high fiber diets and fiber supplements such as bran, psyllium seed products, or methylcellulose

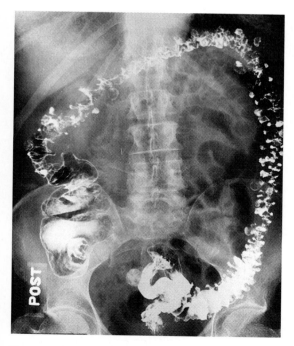

Figure 28–2. Barium enema demonstrating extensive diverticulosis of the left hemicolon. (Reproduced, with permission, from Stabile BE: Therapeutic options in acute diverticulitis. Comp Ther 1991;17:26.)

have theoretical value in minimizing the progression of the disease, they are frequently prescribed.

For patients with pain or bowel dysfunction attributable to otherwise uncomplicated diverticular disease, the efficacy of high fiber diets has been demonstrated. In animal models, progressive decreases in intracolic pressures with increasing dietary fiber has been shown. Similar diets have eliminated or greatly diminished the gastrointestinal symptoms associated with diverticulosis in numerous clinical trials. It appears that increasing stool bulk and water content has a salutary effect on the ease and regularity of bowel movements and decreases painful spasms. Thus, the benefits of such a diet appear to derive from its effects on colonic dysmotility rather than on the diverticula per se. Once present, there is no evidence that diverticula regress under the influence of any medical therapy. Rather, medical treatment is aimed at ameliorating symptoms and possibly halting progression of the disease.

In general, the least expensive and most widely recommended dietary source of added vegetable fiber is unprocessed wheat bran. The relative effectiveness of various brans is thought to be related to their particle size and hydrophilia. Increasing the bran content of the diet typically gives rise to abdominal distention and increased flatus production. It is therefore recommend that the dosage be increased slowly over a period of 1–2 months to 10–25 grams per day in divided portions with meals. Palatable sources of wheat fiber include whole grain bread and breakfast cereals. Alternative sources of vegetable fiber probably have similar therapeutic benefits, but less is known about their physiochemical properties. A number of hydrophilic colloids refined from vegetable sources, as well as bran tablets, are commercially available but relatively expensive.

Other than stool bulking agents, additional specific therapy is rarely required for patients with uncomplicated but symptomatic diverticular disease. Anticholinergic and other motility altering agents have no proven efficacy. Likewise, sedative-hypnotic agents, tranquilizers, antidepressants, and antibiotics are of no value. For patients requiring potent analgesia, pentazocine has been demonstrated to reduce the motility of the sigmoid colon in patients with diverticular disease while providing adequate pain relief. Morphine and related narcotics are relatively contraindicated, because they can significantly increase the intraluminal pressure of the sigmoid colon.

B. Surgical: Several operations that divide the thickened muscle layer of the colon have been proposed for the treatment of symptomatic diverticulosis. Longitudinal myotomy of the circular fibers of the muscularis propria throughout the length of the sigmoid and rectosigmoid colon has been associated with a high postoperative complication rate (including rectal perforation) and only marginal results on long-term follow-up. Multiple transverse myotomies of the antimesenteric taenia coli designed to counteract the colonic foreshortening associated with myochosis have also had minimal if any beneficial results. Prophylactic resection of the colon for diverticulosis has been proposed but is not indicated for uncomplicated disease.

Prognosis

Despite its high prevalence, diverticulosis is most often unattended by complications. Nevertheless, an occasional patient with severe pain and colonic dysmotility may be nearly disabled. Such symptoms, however, are not predictive of life-threatening complications. For the 10–20% of patients who develop either diverticulitis or lower gastrointestinal hemorrhage, the prognosis is much more worrisome. Three-quarters of patients who develop life-threatening complications do so in the absence of any prior colonic symptoms. Thus, acute diverticulitis or hemorrhage are often the presenting manifestations of diverticular disease. Fortunately, most episodes of acute diverticulitis and diverticular hemorrhage are self-limited or can be managed medically, but outcomes are age-related with considerable morbidity and mortality among the very elderly.

DIVERTICULITIS

Essentials of Diagnosis

- Acute abdominal pain
- Constipation or bowel irregularity
- Left lower quadrant tenderness and mass
- Fever and leukocytosis
- Characteristic radiographic signs

General Considerations

Acute diverticulitis results from perforation of a diverticulum with infection and inflammation extending into the colon wall, epiploic appendages, mesentery, and adjacent organs. As such, diverticulitis is more accurately termed peridiverticulitis, as the inflammatory response extends immediately or far beyond the diverticulum itself. In most instances diverticulitis follows indolent microperforation of the diverticular mucosa by a contained fecalith. The infectious process typically results in phlegmonous swelling of the bowel wall in which microabscesses, sinus tracts, and intramural fistulae can be found, but there is no macroabscess or free perforation into the peritoneal cavity. This represents the most common variant of acute diverticulitis, or stage I disease (Table 28–1). If the infectious process penetrates the serosa of the bowel wall, but is confined locally by adjacent abdominal wall, omentum, small intestine, urinary bladder, or female reproductive organs, a pericolic or pelvic macroabscess results. This represents stage II disease. Alternatively, if there is no containment of the spreading infection or if a con-

Table 28–1. Clinical stages of acute diverticulitis.

Stage	Description
I	Peridiverticular phlegmon with microabscesses
II	Pericolic or pelvic macroabscess
III	Generalized purulent peritonitis
IV	Generalized feculent peritonitis

tained abscess ruptures, diffuse purulent peritonitis or stage III disease results. On rare occasion a colonic diverticulum suddenly ruptures with diffuse fecal contamination of the peritoneal cavity. The ensuing feculent peritonitis is rapid in development and particularly lethal. This represents stage IV disease.

Fistulization of diverticulitis to adjacent organs or through the abdominal wall occurs by direct extension of microscopic or macroscopic peridiverticular abscesses that decompress into the adjacent organ lumen or through the skin. The clinical manifestations of fistulization depend on the organ involved, the size of the fistula, and the degree of abscess decompression through the fistula. In most instances the acute systemic sepsis is alleviated by decompression of the abscess through the fistula.

Colonic obstruction due to diverticulitis is usually transient and subsides with resolution of acute swelling in conjunction with treatment. Unrelenting obstruction is the result of segmental fibrosis of the bowel wall, usually as a sequela of repeated episodes of acute inflammation and healing. Such instances of obstruction sometime occur in the absence of a recent acute attack and inevitably require surgical intervention.

Clinical Findings

A. Symptoms and Signs: In concert with the gradual development of the inflammatory process, patients with acute diverticulitis generally present with left lower quadrant abdominal pain of gradual onset and progression. The pain is constant, unrelenting and may be accompanied by intermittent exacerbations associated with colonic spasms that are followed by loose bowel movements. In contrast to symptomatic diverticulosis uncomplicated by infection, the pain of acute diverticulitis does not subside within minutes or hours, but persists for days to weeks if untreated.

In patients with stage I disease the infectious process is largely confined to the bowel itself, although the omentum or other adjacent structures may become inflamed because of their proximity. Such patients generally have abdominal pain confined to the left lower quadrant, but in some instances it may extend to the mid lower abdomen or right lower quadrant if the sigmoid loop is long and redundant. Patients with pericolic or pelvic abscesses, or stage II disease, have pain that is indistinguishable from that of patients with phlegmonous inflammation only, al-

though it may be more constant and severe. Associated anorexia, nausea, and emesis are relatively frequent, particularly among those with significant localized peritonitis or large abscesses. Fever may be low grade or high, depending on the severity and extent of the septic process.

In patients with diffuse purulent peritonitis, or stage III disease, the abdominal pain is severe and generalized and inhibits movement. There is associated ileus with constipation or obstipation, bloating, nausea, and emesis. Patients with feculent peritonitis, or stage IV disease, present with a precipitous illness characterized by acute onset of severe generalized abdominal pain and high fever. Patients rapidly progress to a septic state that is often accompanied by prostration and cardiovascular collapse.

The findings on physical examination reflect the severity and localization of the septic process and the associated systemic response. Patients with localized peritonitis from phlegmonous inflammation or abscess present with lower abdominal tenderness with guarding and rebound tenderness, whether or not a mass is palpable. In cases of diffuse peritonitis, generalized severe abdominal tenderness and rigidity are typical, and bowel sounds are usually absent. Marked abdominal distention suggests bowel obstruction in cases of localized disease and diffuse paralytic ileus in patients with generalized peritonitis. High fever or hypothermia, diaphoresis, and tachycardia reflect systemic sepsis and possible impending cardiovascular decompensation. Mental obtundation, anuria, and hypotension indicate advanced septic shock.

Nonspecific urinary symptoms such as urgency and frequency suggest proximity of the inflammatory process to the urinary bladder. The presence of pneumaturia or fecaluria are pathognomonic for the presence of a colovesical fistula. Localized tenderness, swelling, and erythema of the lower abdominal wall suggest the presence of an underlying pericolic abscess and impending colocutaneous fistulization.

B. Laboratory Findings: The diagnosis of acute diverticulitis is largely a clinical exercise; laboratory investigations are not particularly useful in refining the diagnosis. Leukocytosis is commonly present, although one-half of patients with mild diverticulitis have normal white blood cell counts. Marked leukocytosis is usually present only with macroabscess or diffuse peritonitis. When the urinary bladder is involved in the inflammatory process, mild pyuria, hematuria, or both may be present. Gross pyuria bacteriuria or fecaluria indicate the presence of a colovesical fistula.

C. Imaging: The findings on plain abdominal films depend on the stage of the disease. With phlegmonous inflammation or localized abscess, radiologic signs may be minimal or absent. A localized ileus pattern or mass effect may be present and partial colonic obstruction may be reflected by proximal dilatation of the bowel. On upright abdominal x-rays, an air-fluid level may be seen in a large pericolic abscess having communication with the bowel lumen, or because of the presence of gas-forming organisms. Likewise, an air-fluid level in the urinary bladder indicates colovesical fistula. In cases of diffuse peritonitis, a generalized ileus pattern is typical and a pneumoperitoneum may be present. A massive amount of intraperitoneal air often accompanies feculent peritonitis.

If the diagnosis of acute diverticulitis can be confidently made based on the clinical findings and the plain films of the abdomen, no additional imaging studies need be pursued. Barium enema has in the past been used to confirm the diagnosis but has been replaced almost entirely by abdominal CT. CT is generally reserved for patients with suspected abscesses, perforations, and those who fail to respond to medical therapy or in whom the diagnosis is in doubt. It is also particularly useful in the elderly and in patients immunocompromised as a result of corticosteroid or other immunosuppressive medication use. In such patients the abdominal examination may be deceptively unremarkable, and thus there is a greater reliance on imaging studies to secure the diagnosis.

Numerous studies have shown the superiority of abdominal CT over contrast enema in the diagnosis of acute diverticulitis. CT also has the advantage of better definition of the extraluminal complications of diverticulitis such as abscess and fistula, as well as identification of alternative diagnoses such as appendiceal abscess, tubo-ovarian abscess, ischemic colitis, pancreatitis, and various intra-abdominal tumors.

The typical findings of phlegmonous diverticulitis include wall thickening of the involved colonic segment with associated inflammatory edema of the pericolic fat. Pelvic and pericolic macroabscesses are readily defined by CT (Figure 28–3). In some instances fistulization to adjacent organs is demonstrable. The ability of the CT scan to identify small volumes of free intraperitoneal air make the study extremely sensitive in the diagnosis of perforated diverticulitis.

Ultrasonography has also been shown to be a useful investigation in acute diverticulitis, particularly in identifying the presence of pericolic abscess. The test is highly examiner-dependent, however, and the presence of large bowel obstruction or significant paralytic ileus renders the examination relatively useless because of the presence of large amounts of intraluminal gas. Under optimal conditions, however, ultrasonography has the ability to identify focal colonic wall thickening, inflamed diverticula, inflammatory changes in the pericolic fat, as well as abscesses and fistulae.

Although no longer frequently used, contrast enema x-ray examination of the colon and rectum can provide highly specific diagnostic information in acute diverticulitis. Because of the danger of precipitating or exacerbating bowel perforation, contrast radiography is reserved for patients in whom the diagnosis is in doubt. Only water soluble contrast material should be used because spillage of barium into the peritoneal cavity may be associated with a particularly lethal peritonitis. Water soluble contrast agents are readily absorbed by the peritoneum and

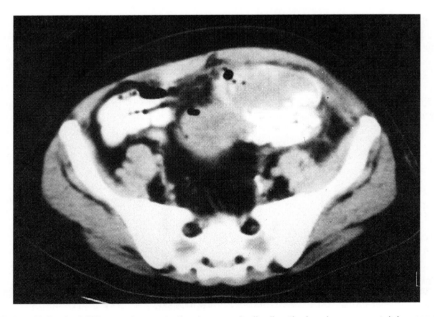

Figure 28–3. Abdominal CT scan demonstrating large pericolic diverticular abscess containing gas bubbles.

obviate the risks associated with particulate materials such as barium sulfate. No preparation of the bowel should precede a water soluble contrast enema. Communication with the radiologist is essential for two reasons: (1) to limit the study to the colonic segment in question, and (2) to ensure that excessive installation pressures are avoided. The mere presence of colonic diverticula on contrast enema examination is insufficient to make the diagnosis of diverticulitis, because other specific indicators of an infectious component must also be observed (Table 28–2). Included among these are the presence of an intramural fistula, sinus tract (Figure 28–4), extrinsic bowel compression by a pericolic mass, or demonstration of an extraluminal collection of contrast medium (Figure 28–5). The presence of luminal narrowing and a sawtooth appearance of the mucosa in the presence of colonic diverticula may be secondary to muscular spasm alone and are insufficient criteria to make the diagnosis of diverticulitis.

D. Endoscopy: Endoscopic evaluation including rigid proctosigmoidoscopy, flexible sigmoidoscopy, and colonoscopy are generally contraindicated in suspected acute diverticulitis. Insufflation of air is required, and this predisposes to acute perforation with fecal contamination of the peritoneal cavity. As with barium enema examination, a period of 6–8 weeks is allowed to pass after resolution of an acute attack before endoscopy is performed. Early endoscopy may be employed, however, if the diagnosis is in real doubt, and particularly when high grade obstruction is present and colorectal carcinoma must be ruled out. Because of the necessity of bowel preparation for adequate flexible fiberoptic endoscopy, rigid proctosigmoidoscopy is the prudent choice when early endoscopic examination is required. Indicators of acute diverticulitis include edema, spasm, and erythema, with the occasional definitive finding of purulent discharge from a diverticular orifice.

In cases of suspected colovesical fistula, diagnostic cystoscopy is a useful adjunct. Although the fistula is rarely visualized, erythema and bullous edema of the bladder mucosa are virtually diagnostic of fistula presence.

Table 28–2. Radiographic signs of diverticulitis seen on contrast enema examination.

Sinus tract
Fistula
Abscess
Deformed diverticula
Stricture
Spasm
Obstruction
Segmental narrowing
Extraluminal mass effect
Pneumoperitoneum
Colonic wall thickening

Differential Diagnosis

The differential diagnosis of acute diverticulitis encompasses a wide range of inflammatory, mechanical, vascular, and neoplastic processes with the pertinent inclusions being dictated by the stage of acute diverticulitis under consideration. Thus, patients with very mild diverticulitis associated with only minimal abdominal findings and no radiographic abnormalities, fever, or leukocytosis, might be misinterpreted as having irritable bowel syndrome or uncomplicated symptomatic diverticulosis. In general, the duration of acute symptoms, the degree of abdominal tenderness and the ultimate development of fever and leukocytosis make the diagnosis of diverticulitis apparent. In more severe cases of phlegmonous diverticulitis, the differential diagnosis includes acute appendicitis, inflammatory bowel disease, pelvic inflammatory disease, ischemic colitis, and colorectal carcinoma with or without contained perforation. In the uncommon circumstance of cecal diverticulitis, the clinical differentiation from acute appendicitis is virtually impossible. Similar confusion arises in instances of sigmoid diverticulitis when the inflammatory focus is in the apex of an elongated sigmoid loop that resides in the right lower quadrant.

In cases of diverticular pericolic or pelvic abscess, the differential list may include a variety of other causes of hollow viscus perforation such as appendiceal abscess, tubo-ovarian abscess, and abscesses related to inflammatory bowel disease, colorectal and other intra-abdominal cancers, foreign body and iatrogenic perforations, as well as perinephric and pancreatic abscesses. The symptoms and clinical course prior to appearance of the abscess, together with imaging studies and endoscopy, clarify the cause of the abscess. Occasionally only contrast enema x-ray examination can settle the issue of diverticular disease versus colonic Crohn's disease or carcinoma, by clear demonstration of a diverticulum as the source of the abscess.

For patients presenting with diffuse peritonitis, the differential diagnosis again includes all variety of gastrointestinal perforations including peptic ulcer disease, Crohn's disease, appendicitis, and gastrointestinal malignant growths. In addition, pelvic inflammatory disease, ischemic bowel, severe pancreatitis, and spontaneous bacterial peritonitis in patients with ascites require consideration. When a large volume pneumoperitoneum is evident, the source is almost invariably colonic or gastroduodenal. In patients with AIDS, perforation of the small or large intestine as a result of cytomegalovirus infection also warrants serious consideration.

Among patients with colovesical, colovaginal, coloenteric, or colocutaneous fistulae, Crohn's disease and malignant growths arising from the fistulized organs must also be included in the differential diagnosis. Endoscopic biopsy of the fistulous tract is often diagnostic.

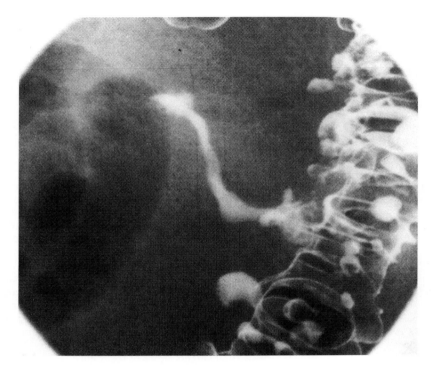

Figure 28–4. Barium enema illustrating extraluminal contrast in a sinus tract due to diverticular perforation into the sigmoid mesocolon. This radiographic sign is diagnostic of diverticulitis.

In cases of large bowel obstruction, the differential diagnosis includes all potentially obstructing lesions, but most prominently, colorectal carcinoma. Crohn's disease, ischemic strictures, colonic endometriosis, colonic tuberculosis, and ameboma, as well as atypical presentation of sigmoid volvulus occasionally require serious consideration. CT, endoscopy, and contrast enema radiography generally clarify the issue.

Complications

The important complications of acute diverticulitis include pericolic and pelvic macro-abscesses, diffuse purulent or feculent peritonitis, fistulization to adjacent organs, and colonic obstruction. All of the complications represent a virulent extension of the disease beyond the colonic wall. Abscesses may rupture to cause purulent peritonitis; they may involve adjacent organs and lead to fistula formation or hollow viscus obstruction; or they may slowly lead to systemic sepsis. Diffuse peritonitis almost inevitably progresses to septic shock and death if untreated. Among survivors it is often the source of recurrent small bowel obstructions due to adhesions. Fistulae to the urinary bladder are often complicated by severe urinary tract infections and urosepsis, while those involving the small intestine can lead to bacterial overgrowth with associated malabsorption and diarrhea. Fistulae involving the vagina or the abdominal wall are less dangerous but may be responsible

for fluid losses and significant local irritation of the perineum or abdominal skin. Colonic obstruction due to diverticular disease is typically partial but may precipitate acute colonic dilatation and cecal perforation.

Treatment

A. Medical Therapy: Most patients with acute diverticulitis require hospitalization. Patients with minimal evidence of inflammation, no paralytic ileus, and good functional status can be given a trial of outpatient therapy consisting of a liquid diet and an oral broad spectrum antibiotic. Failure to improve after 48 hours should dictate immediate hospitalization. For those presenting with more severe disease, inpatient treatment with intravenous hydration, antibiotics, bowel rest, and nasogastric tube decompression are required. The antibiotic regimen should be designed to cover both aerobic and anaerobic colonic flora. Since diverticulitis is by definition infection extending beyond the colonic mucosa, nonabsorbable intraluminal antibiotics are ineffective. Because of its propensity to increase colonic intraluminal pressure, morphine sulfate is relatively contraindicated as an analgesic, and pentazocine or meperidine hydrochloride are preferred. Anticholinergic agents, glucagon, and other smooth muscle relaxing agents have not been found to be effective in acute attacks.

In most cases, aggressive medical therapy results

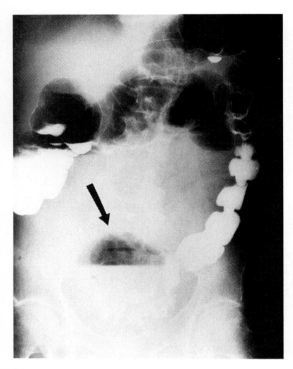

Figure 28–5. Barium enema demonstrating a large diverticular pelvic abscess **(arrow)** containing an air-fluid level. (Reproduced, with permission, from Stabile BE: Therapeutic options in acute diverticulitis. Comp Ther 1991;17:26.)

Table 28–3. Indications for operation in diverticulitis.

Diffuse peritonitis
Pneumoperitoneum
Obstruction
Abscess
Persistent mass
Fistula
Stricture
Failure to improve on medical therapy
Clinical progression on medical therapy
Recurrent attacks
Younger than 40 years old
Inability to exclude carcinoma
Immunosuppressed patient

in rapid and dramatic clinical improvement with resolution of pain, fever, and ileus within 48–72 hours. Broad spectrum antibiotics should be continued for 7–10 days. Oral feedings are gradually reintroduced as ileus and any partial colonic obstruction resolve. Approximately 1 month after successful medical treatment of an acute attack, the patient should be prescribed a high fiber diet supplemented by psyllium grains or hydrophilic colloids. This may protect against the development of additional acute attacks. Longitudinal studies of patients following resolution of the initial episode of acute diverticulitis suggests that approximately two-thirds to three-fourths of patients have no further problems. About 10–20% of patients suffer repeated serious attacks and require surgical intervention.

B. Surgical Therapy: Operation for diverticulitis and its complications may be required as either an elective or emergency procedure (Table 28–3). Indications for elective operation include: (1) two or more acute attacks of diverticulitis successfully treated medically; (2) one attack with evidence of perforation, colonic obstruction, or inflammatory involvement of the urinary tract; and (3) inability to rule out colonic carcinoma. Because the occurrence of a second acute episode of diverticulitis portends a

clinical course of additional recurrent attacks, elective operation is advised unless the patient's overall ill health precludes safe elective operation. Since the natural history of diverticular disease appears to be more fulminant in young patients, an initial attack requiring hospitalization in a patient younger than 40 years of age should be considered an indication for colon resection. Regardless of age, the development of perforation, colonic obstruction, or urinary tract involvement signifies aggressive disease that is highly prone to recurrence with abscess, fistulization, or generalized peritonitis. Any patient with persisting colonic stricture after an attack of presumed diverticulitis should undergo elective colon resection because of the possibility of carcinoma.

Because the overwhelming majority of patients with acute diverticulitis have sigmoid involvement, resections of other portions of the colon are infrequent. Patients deemed to be candidates for elective operation following successful medical treatment of an acute attack usually undergo sigmoid colectomy with primary anastomosis as a single stage procedure (Figure 28–6). On occasion the descending colon will be severely involved with myochosis coli and a left hemicolectomy will be required. The distal anastomosis should be made at the level of the proximal rectum, because anastomosis to the distal sigmoid colon is associated with a higher incidence of recurrent diverticulitis. Isolated cecal or ascending colon diverticulitis is relatively rare and usually prompts emergency operation for presumed acute appendicitis. Once the true diagnosis is appreciated, a right hemicolectomy is performed.

Elective operation for diverticular disease is always preceded by a thorough mechanical and oral nonabsorbable antibiotic bowel preparation. Mortality rates for elective resection and primary anastomosis range from 0–2% compared to rates of 5–20% for emergency operations. While it is essential that resections for diverticulitis encompass all inflamed and thickened bowel, it is unnecessary to resect all diverticula present, as recurrent diverticulitis proximal to the resection is distinctly uncommon. If an unexpected abscess or severe active inflammation is en-

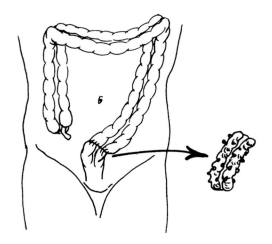

Figure 28–6. Single stage sigmoid colectomy with primary anastomosis. (Reproduced, with permission, from Stabile BE: Therapeutic options in acute diverticulitis. Comp Ther 1991;17:26.)

countered at elective operation, an end descending colostomy and distal mucous fistula or Hartmann closure of the rectal stump may be required. Colostomy closure is then electively performed 2–4 months later. Recently, all phases of elective surgery for diverticular disease have been performed by using laparoscopic techniques.

Patients who present with diffuse peritonitis or pneumoperitoneum require prompt fluid resuscitation, intravenous antibiotics, and emergency surgical exploration. Resection of the perforated colonic seg-

ment (almost always the sigmoid) with descending end colostomy should be performed (Figure 28–7). Since the morbidity and mortality attending these cases derive from inadequately controlled sepsis, removal of the perforated colonic segment clearly has distinct advantages over the older approach of proximal diverting colostomy and drainage of the area of perforation. Numerous studies have documented substantial improvements in patient survival, complication rates, and lengths of hospitalization and disability with the two-stage approach of primary resection and colostomy followed by colostomy closure, as compared with the older three-stage approach of: (1) proximal colostomy and drainage, (2) resection, and (3) colostomy closure (Figure 28–8). The three-stage approach has lost favor because of an appreciation that leaving a column of stool above a colonic perforation does not consistently allow control of the septic process. Since there is no evidence that the initial dissection associated with primary colonic resection contributes to spread of infection, it is considered most prudent to remove the diseased colonic segment whenever technically possible. In most instances, sigmoid colectomy and descending end colostomy with Hartmann closure of the rectal stump is employed. If the distal rectosigmoid segment is of sufficient length to reach the abdominal wall, a mucous fistula may be created in lieu of the Hartmann pouch. This approach requires subsequent additional resection of the rectosigmoid segment at the time of colostomy takedown.

Patients who deteriorate or fail to improve after 48–72 hours of maximal medical therapy for severe diverticulitis should undergo prompt CT scanning of the abdomen. If inflammation without an abscess is

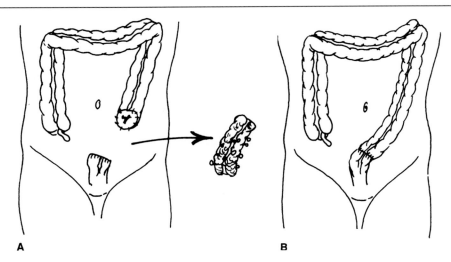

A   **B**

Figure 28–7. **A:** Sigmoid colectomy, descending end colostomy and Hartmann closure of the rectal stump. **B:** Colostomy takedown and anastomosis as a second procedure. (Reproduced, with permission, from Stabile BE: Therapeutic options in acute diverticulitis. Comp Ther 1991;17:26.)

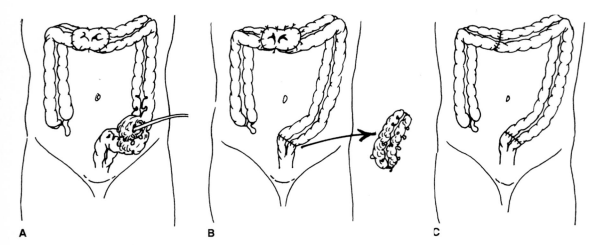

Figure 28–8. *A:* Transverse loop colostomy with catheter drainage. *B:* Sigmoid colectomy and anastomosis as a second procedure. *C:* Closure of transverse colostomy as a third procedure. (Reproduced, with permission, from Stabile BE: Therapeutic options in acute diverticulitis. Comp Ther 1991;17:26.)

found, immediate laparotomy and colon resection is performed. Small (1–4 cm) intramural or intermesenteric abscesses are commonly present in such cases and can usually be resected en bloc with the colon. Traditionally, a colostomy has been required in most such instances because of the severity of the acute inflammation and the unprepared condition of the bowel. More recently the technique of on-table lavage and resection with primary anastomosis is becoming more widely used. The technique involves the introduction of physiologic saline through a temporary tube appendicostomy, cecostomy, or ileostomy with copious irrigation of the colonic lumen and emptying of the bowel by means of a large tube introduced into the distal colon at the level of proximal resection.

For patients failing medical therapy who are found on CT scanning to have a large (5 cm or greater) pericolic or pelvic abscess, two therapeutic options are available. The standard approach is immediate surgical exploration with drainage of the abscess, resection of the perforated colonic segment, and end colostomy. This approach is time-tested, widely accepted, and has a mortality rate of about 5%. This approach has recently been modified by the introduction of the on-table lavage and primary anastomosis technique. The reported experience with abscess drainage combined with colon resection and immediate primary anastomosis is limited and concerns regarding its safety remain. The second therapeutic option in patients with large diverticular abscesses is initial nonoperative percutaneous catheter drainage under CT guidance (Figure 28–9) followed by elective colon resection and primary anastomosis. This approach is designed to first control sepsis and then definitively treat the diseased bowel segment while

avoiding both the inconvenience of initial colostomy and the risks of initial primary anastomosis. The experience to date suggests that 80% of patients with large abscesses can be treated successfully by initial percutaneous drainage without increased morbidity or mortality, compared with standard multiple stage surgical treatment. However, the percutaneous catheter drainage technique has been found to poorly control the septic process in the few patients who evidence grossly feculent abscess drainage. Urgent colon resection is required in these cases. Despite the presence of radiographically demonstrable small fistulas in one-half of patients with abscesses, sepsis can be promptly and reliably controlled, provided good catheter function is maintained. Patient satisfaction with the technique is great, because temporary colostomy is avoided.

Patients whose acute diverticulitis is complicated by colovesical, colovaginal, or other fistulae rarely require emergent operative intervention. Development of a fistula represents spontaneous decompression of the associated abscess and subsidence of the acute inflammation routinely follows. Patients with fistulae are best treated medically at first, and then subsequently with elective colon resection and primary anastomosis. In most instances of colovesical fistula, the bladder defect is small and can be managed without bladder resection. If acute severe inflammatory changes or an abscess is encountered at the time of fistula takedown, colon resection with end colostomy and Hartmann closure of the rectum is utilized.

The vast majority of patients with colonic obstruction from diverticular disease present with partial obstruction and can be initially managed with bowel rest, nasogastric tube decompression, and intra-

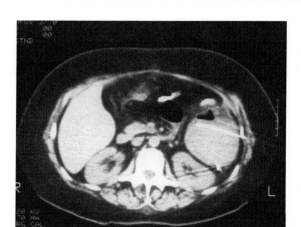

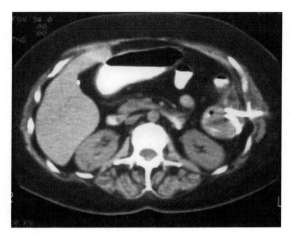

Figure 28–9. *A:* Abdominal CT scan showing aspirating needle in a large left pericolic diverticular abscess. *B:* Repeat CT scan showing coiled percutaneous drainage catheter in collapsed abscess cavity. (Reproduced, with permission, from Stabile BE et al: Preoperative percutaneous drainage of diverticular abscesses. Am J Surg 1990;159:99.)

venous fluids. Endoscopic examination of the colon should subsequently be performed with biopsy of the stricture to rule out a malignant growth. As the obstruction is usually incomplete, a gentle mechanical and antibiotic bowel preparation is usually possible. Colon resection with primary anastomosis can then be performed. In the uncommon instance where complete or high grade partial obstruction precludes bowel preparation, a colostomy with or without colon resection is required. If proximal colonic distention is not severe, the on-table lavage with resection and primary anastomosis technique can be employed.

Prognosis

Approximately 15–20% of patients presenting with an initial attack of acute diverticulitis require surgical intervention for peritonitis, abscess, or fistula. Among patients whose initial attack is successfully treated medically, only 10–20% return with repeat attacks, but the need for surgical intervention in this group is very high. The mortality for elective colon resection and primary anastomosis following resolution of acute diverticulitis is approximately 1%, while emergency operations carry a 5–20% mortality, depending on the age of the patient and the severity of the sepsis. Following successful resection and colonic anastomosis, the rate of recurrent acute diverticulitis is well below 5%, but is higher if the resection has not encompassed all inflamed or thickened bowel.

DIVERTICULAR HEMORRHAGE

Essentials of Diagnosis

- Elderly patient
- Hematochezia or melena
- Gastric aspirate negative for blood
- Transfusion often required
- Characteristic angiographic or endoscopic findings

General Considerations

It is estimated that 5–15% of patients with known diverticulosis develop the complication of acute hemorrhage. Progressive enlargement of a colonic diverticulum leads to stretching and splaying of the small associated arteriole over the dome of the lesion. Hemorrhage results from weakening and finally rupture of the vessel with decompression into the bowel lumen. Histopathologic observations have confirmed changes in the intima and media of the arteriole, suggesting that the primary lesion resides within the vessel wall rather than the mucosa of the diverticulum. Thus, the hemorrhage associated with diverticulosis tends to be rather massive, owing to its arterial origin. Right-sided colonic diverticula, while much less common than left-sided or sigmoid diverticula, are considered to be responsible for a disproportionately higher incidence of diverticular hemorrhage. This finding has not been well confirmed, however, because there is often difficulty differentiating between diverticula and arteriovenous malformations in the absence of detailed angiographic or endoscopic evidence. While the overall high prevalence of diverticulosis in the population suffering lower gastrointestinal bleeding makes the exact cause of many bleeding episodes problematic, it appears that the condition is responsible for greater than 50% of cases. In some instances, diverticular hemorrhage is associated with the use of anticoagulants such as warfarin or antiplatelet agents such as aspirin.

Clinical Findings

A. Symptoms and Signs: The presentation of diverticular bleeding is dark to bright red blood per rectum in moderate to large amounts. The more distal the source in the colon, the more likely the hematochezia is to be bright red and contain clots. Occasionally, slow right colonic diverticular bleeding produces melena, thus mimicking an upper gastrointestinal bleeding source. Because of the cathartic effect of blood in the colon, some abdominal cramping may be present, but otherwise the bleeding is painless. In approximately 80–90% of patients, the bleeding stops spontaneously, and this often has occurred by the time the patient presents. In the 10–20% of patients whose bleeding is massive and unrelenting, pallor, tachycardia, and orthostatic hypotension or frank shock may be present. The abdominal examination may reveal slight distention and active bowel sounds but there is no tenderness or mass palpable. The rectal examination demonstrates gross blood ranging from bright red to melena. Passage of a nasogastric tube reveals no blood in the stomach aspirate.

B. Laboratory Findings: It is important to note that a normal hematocrit or hemoglobin level does not negate the diagnosis of acute diverticular hemorrhage; this is because anemia develops only when sufficient time elapses for hemodilution to occur. Intravenous fluid resuscitation hastens the hemodilution. A low initial hematocrit or hemoglobin level suggests bleeding ongoing for a number of hours or days, or the presence of chronic anemia from chronic slow blood loss or some unrelated cause. A hypochromic microcytic anemia suggest chronic blood loss. Abnormalities of platelet count, prothrombin time, partial thromboplastin time, liver function tests or bleeding time suggest specific associated medical conditions or drug therapy that may contribute to the severity of bleeding.

C. Imaging: Plain abdominal x-rays reveal no diagnostic clues. Nuclear scintigraphy bleeding scans incorporating technetium sulfur colloid or ^{99m}-technetium labeled red blood cells utilize external gamma counters to detect intraluminal extravasation of blood. The sulfur colloid scans are very sensitive in detecting active bleeding and can be completed in less than 1 hour. The labeled red blood cell scans allow repeated scanning for up to 24 hours and are able to detect intermittent bleeding. They also provide better bleeding site localization by demonstration of anatomic contours within the gastrointestinal tract.

Because of the intermittent nature of lower gastrointestinal bleeding, angiographic examination should only be performed on actively bleeding, hemodynamically stable patients. Selective injection of the superior and inferior mesenteric arteries identifies the sight of active bleeding in 60–80% of patients. The technique allows detection of bleeding rates as low as 0.5 ml per minute. A positive arteriogram demonstrates accumulation of contrast material at the sight of the bleeding diverticulum. In some instances the diverticular sac is defined by the extravasated contrast (Figure 28–10).

Although once considered the diagnostic standard in acute lower gastrointestinal bleeding, barium enema no longer has a major role in the care of patients with active hemorrhage. Because of retention of barium within the lumen of the lower gastrointestinal tract, the examination obscures the findings of other more specific tests such as angiography and endoscopy. After cessation of bleeding, however, barium enema may be useful to make the diagnosis of diverticulosis following nondiagnostic angiography and endoscopy. Unfortunately, the detection of diverticula does not imply causality of the bleeding episode nor localization of the bleeding site.

D. Endoscopy: Whenever the nasogastric aspirate is negative for blood and the clinical presentation suggests a lower gastrointestinal source, the first specific diagnostic maneuver should be rigid proctosigmoidoscopy. Although most lower gastrointestinal hemorrhages are found to be emanating from more than 25 cm above the anal verge, proctosigmoidoscopy allows accurate evaluation for the presence of bleeding internal hemorrhoids, rectal tumors, or polyps, or diffuse hemorrhagic mucosal disorders. These sources must be ruled out prior to pursuit of more proximal colonic bleeding with more invasive procedures.

The utility of fiberoptic colonoscopy in patients with massive lower gastrointestinal bleeding remains

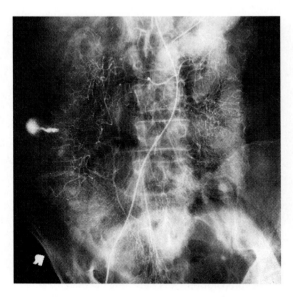

Figure 28–10. Superior mesenteric arteriogram demonstrating extravasated contrast material in a bleeding diverticulum of the ascending colon. This angiographic sign is diagnostic of diverticular hemorrhage.

somewhat controversial. Direct visualization of actual bleeding is relatively uncommon, and indirect indicators such as adherent blood clots and mucosal lesions must often be relied upon. If active bleeding from the orifice of a diverticulum is seen, the diagnosis is secure, but this is an uncommon event. Tattooing of the bleeding sight with submucosal injection of methylene blue or India ink should be performed, because this allows intraoperative localization of the site should the patient require emergency surgery. This permits segmental resection or hemicolectomy rather than a more extensive operation.

Differential Diagnosis

In the majority of cases, massive lower gastrointestinal hemorrhage derives from one of two lesions: colonic diverticula or arteriovenous malformations. It is debatable which of these lesions is more common, but both are prevalent in the aged population. Arteriovenous malformations are also referred to as angiodysplasia and have been reported with dramatically increased frequency since the introduction of diagnostic visceral angiography and fiberoptic colonoscopy. As is the case with colonic diverticula, a disproportionate number of bleeding episodes attributable to arteriovenous malformations seem to derive from the cecum and ascending colon. Also like diverticula, the pattern of bleeding from arteriovenous malformations is typically one of recurrent episodes. The intermittent nature of the bleeding frequently foils attempts at definitive diagnosis if they are not performed emergently during the bleeding episode. The lesions can be identified colonoscopically between bleeding episodes, but active hemorrhage tends to obscure their true identity. Visceral angiographic criteria that identify arteriovenous malformation include: (1) early and prolonged filling of the draining vein, (2) clusters of small arteries, and (3) visualization of a vascular tuft. Extravasation of contrast material may be seen if active bleeding is present at a rate of 0.5–1.0 ml per minute or greater.

Ulcerative colitis, ischemic colitis, and, to a lesser degree Crohn's colitis, occasionally present with massive lower gastrointestinal hemorrhage. Although other colitides may present with bleeding, it is usually less than massive. Although massive hemorrhage as the presenting symptom is unusual, rigid proctosigmoidoscopy or colonoscopy demonstrates the mucosal lesion in virtually all cases.

Colorectal neoplasms account for less than 10% of major lower gastrointestinal bleeding episodes. The majority of symptomatic bleeds are due to malignant tumors of the colon and rectum while major bleeding from benign polyps is quite rare.

Colonic and anorectal varices associated with portal hypertension are capable of precipitating massive hemorrhage but hemorrhoids in the absence of portal hypertension rarely bleed massively. Meckel's diverticulum, a congenital true diverticulum of the distal ileum, occasionally contains gastric mucosa that is responsible for peptic ulceration of the adjacent normal ileal mucosa. These ulcers occasionally precipitate major lower gastrointestinal hemorrhage, but such episodes are most commonly seen in children and young adults, rather than in middle aged or elderly patients.

Because exact diagnosis of the lesion responsible for massive lower gastrointestinal hemorrhage is often impossible without pathologic examination of the bleeding tissue, the clinical approach is directed more at localizing the site of the bleeding lesion rather than its exact identity. As lower gastrointestinal bleeding from all sources tends to be intermittent and self-limited, most patients can be thoroughly evaluated with endoscopy and barium contrast radiography following cessation of the bleeding episode. When neoplasms are found, excision is required. Treatment of non-neoplastic lesions is individualized, based on the nonoperative therapies available as well as the risk-benefit ratio associated with operative resection.

Complications

The complications associated with diverticular hemorrhage include all of those associated with acute massive blood loss. Myocardial ischemia, cerebral vascular accidents, and acute oliguric renal failure are the principal organ injuries that account for the major morbidity and mortality in the elderly population disposed to diverticular hemorrhage.

Treatment

A. Medical Therapy: The medical therapy for acute diverticular hemorrhage is largely supportive and consists of intravenous fluid administration, red blood cell transfusion and specific support of coagulation, if needed, through the provision of vitamin K, fresh frozen plasma, cryoprecipitate, and platelet transfusions. Anticoagulants, aspirin, and nonsteroidal anti-inflammatory drugs (NSAIDs) are discontinued. Hemodynamically unstable patients are resuscitated, monitored, evaluated, and treated in intensive care units. Only stable patients are allowed to be transported to endoscopy, angiography, or nuclear medicine suites for diagnostic evaluation.

In the event of endoscopic localization of a bleeding diverticulum, a variety of transendoscopic therapeutic modalities are of potential benefit. These include bicap electrocautery, heater probe coagulation, injection sclerotherapy, and laser photocoagulation. Because the bleeding site is typically located at or near the apex of the diverticulum, electrocautery or coagulation of the vessel is often difficult or impossible and carries a high risk of perforation. For these reasons injection therapy with epinephrine solution or a sclerosant is the preferred endoscopic approach.

Upon successful angiographic visualization of a bleeding colonic diverticulum, the catheter is advanced superselectively into the feeding vessel for intra-arterial infusion of vasopressin. This agent causes arterial and venous vascular constriction as well as contraction of bowel wall smooth muscle. These combined effects markedly reduce local blood flow and promote thrombosis at the bleeding site. Confirmation of control of bleeding is obtained by repeat angiography and, if effective, the infusion is continued for 24–48 hours and then slowly tapered. Following initial control of bleeding, rebleeding occurs in as many as 50% of patients with most failures occurring within 12 hours of discontinuation of vasopressin infusion. If transcatheter intra-arterial vasopressin fails to control the bleeding, the patient is prepared for emergency surgery. Patients who are at prohibitive risk for an operation may be considered for transcatheter embolization using gelfoam, wire coils, or autologous blood clot. Unfortunately, a significant incidence of postembolic infarction of the colon limits application of these techniques.

B. Surgical Therapy: Despite optimal medical therapy, including angiographic and endoscopic maneuvers to control diverticular hemorrhage, a small subset of patients requires emergent operative intervention. In general, patients who have had preoperative localization of the bleeding site are candidates for segmental colectomy that includes the bleeding diverticulum. For patients with bleeding cecal or ascending colon diverticula, a right hemicolectomy is performed with anastomosis of the terminal ileum to the midtransverse colon. For bleeding diverticula of the sigmoid or descending colon, a left hemicolectomy is performed with anastomosis of the transverse colon to the proximal rectum. Primary anastomosis is usually possible because solid stool has been removed by the cathartic effect of passage of large volumes of blood. If the colon is not adequately emptied of fecal material the proximal bowel end can be ex-

ternalized as a stoma and the distal bowel end as a mucous fistula. The alternative to stoma creation is on-table colonic lavage to prepare the colon for primary anastomosis. Segmental resection of the colon is highly curative for preoperatively localized bleeding diverticular disease and is attended by an operative mortality of about 5%.

Without the benefit of accurate preoperative localization of the bleeding site, blind segmental colectomies have no place in the treatment of diverticular hemorrhage. Segmental colectomy may be an option if on-table colonic lavage and intraoperative colonoscopy successfully localizes the bleeding site. In the absence of preoperative or intraoperative localization of the bleeding source, subtotal colectomy is the accepted standard of treatment. A primary ileorectal anastomosis can be safely performed in most cases. The procedure has an acceptable operative mortality rate of less than 10%, a rebleeding rate of less than 10%, and acceptable postoperative bowel function for virtually all patients with adequate anorectal sphincter control. In contrast, blind segmental colectomies are attended by rebleeding rates of 20–50% and a mortality somewhat higher than that for subtotal colectomy.

Prognosis

Approximately 80–90% of patients with acute diverticular hemorrhage experience spontaneous cessation of bleeding. The risk of rebleeding following a self-limited hemorrhage is approximately 25% but increases to 50% among patients who have suffered two prior episodes of diverticular bleeding. Among the minority of patients who require surgical intervention to control exsanguinating or persistent hemorrhage, the operative mortality rate is 5–10% and far less than those of other treatment modalities in this subset of patients.

REFERENCES

Ambrosetti P et al: Acute left colonic diverticulitis: A prospective analysis of 226 consecutive cases. Surgery 1994;155:546.

Deckmann RC, Cheskin LJ: Diverticular disease in the elderly. J Am Geriatr Soc 1993;41:986.

Elfrink RJ, Meidema BW: Colonic diverticula. When complications require surgery and when they don't. Postgrad Med 1992;92:97.

Freeman SR, McNally PR: Diverticulitis. Med Clin N Am 1993;77:1149.

Rege RV, Narhrwold DL: Diverticular disease. Curr Probl Surg 1989;26:135.

Reinus JF, Brandt LJ: Vascular ectasias and diverticulosis.

Common causes of lower gastrointestinal bleeding. Gastroenterol Clin N Am 1994;23:1

Roberts PL, Veidenheimer MC: Current management of diverticulitis. Adv Surg 1994;27:189.

Rothenberger DA, Wiltz O: Surgery for complicated diverticulitis. Surg Clin N Am 1993;73:975.

Stabile BE: Therapeutic options in acute diverticulitis. Comp Ther 1991;17:26.

Stabile BE et al: Preoperative percutaneous drainage of diverticular abscesses. Am J Surg 1990;159:99.

Ure T, Vernava AM, Longo WE: Diverticular bleeding. Sem Col Rect Surg 1994;5:32.

Anorectal Diseases

29

Mark Lane Welton, MD

GENERAL ANATOMIC CONSIDERATIONS

The rectum, endodermal in origin, is the dorsal component of the cloaca, which is partitioned by the anorectal septum. The anal canal is an invagination of ectodermal tissue. The anorectum develops from the fusion of the rectum and the anal canal, which occurs at 8 weeks when the anal membrane ruptures. The dentate line marks the point of fusion and the transition from endodermal to ectodermal tissue. These anatomic considerations are important when one considers the epithelium, innervation, vascular supply, and venous and lymphatic drainage of the anorectum.

The rectum is approximately 12–15 cm long. It extends from the rectosigmoid junction, marked by the fusion of the tenia, to the anal canal, marked by the passage into the pelvic floor musculature (Figure 29–1). The rectum lies in the sacrum and forms three distinct curves, creating folds that, when visualized endoscopically, are known as the **valves of Houston.** The proximal and distal curves are convex to the left, and the middle curve is convex to the right. The middle curve roughly marks the anterior peritoneal reflection, which is generally 6–8 cm above the anus. The rectum gradually transitions from intraperitoneal to extraperitoneal beginning posteriorly at 12–15 cm from the anus and becoming completely extraperitoneal at 6–8 cm from the anus. The rectum is "fixed" posteriorly, laterally, and anteriorly by the presacral or Waldeyer's fascia, the lateral ligaments, and Denonvilliers fascia, respectively.

The anatomic anal canal starts at the dentate line and ends at the anal verge. However, for practical purposes the surgical anal canal extends from the muscular diaphragm of the pelvic floor to the anal verge. The **anal canal** is a 3- to 4-cm-long collapsed anteroposterior slit. The **anal verge** is the junction of the highly specialized anoderm of the anal canal and the surrounding perianal skin. The anal canal is "supported" by the surrounding **anal sphincter mechanism,** composed of the internal and external sphincters. The **internal sphincter** is a specialized continuation of the circular muscle of the rectum. It is an involuntary muscle that is normally contracted at rest. The **external sphincter** is a group of three U-shaped muscular loops acting as a single functional unit. It is composed of voluntary striated muscle that appears to act as a continuation of the puborectalis. The **intersphincteric plane,** created by the fibrous continuation of the longitudinal muscle of the rectum, separates the internal and external sphincters.

Familiarity with the histology of the rectum and anal canal is critical for understanding the pathophysiology of disease processes of these two organs. The rectum is composed of an innermost layer of mucosa, over which lies the submucosa, two continuous sheaths of muscle, the circular and longitudinal muscles, and in the upper rectum, serosa. The mucosa is subdivided into three layers: (1) epithelial cells, (2) lamina propria, and (3) muscularis mucosa. The **muscularis mucosa** is a fine sheet of muscle containing a network of lymphatics. Lymphatics are not present above this level, making the muscularis mucosa critical in defining metastatic potential of malignancies.

As the rectum enters the narrow musculature of the pelvic floor and becomes the anal canal, the tissue is thrown into folds known as the **columns of Morgagni.** At the lower end of the columns lie small pockets called **crypts,** some of which communicate with anal glands lying in the intersphincteric plane. The epithelium of the anal canal is composed of three types: columnar epithelium in the upper anal canal, transitional epithelium just above the dentate line, and anoderm, a specialized squamous epithelium below the dentate line. The anoderm is rich in nerve fibers but lacking in secondary appendages (hair follicles, sebaceous glands, or sweat glands). The dentate line marks the true mucocutaneous junction.

The innervation of the rectum is via the sympathetic and parasympathetic nervous systems. The

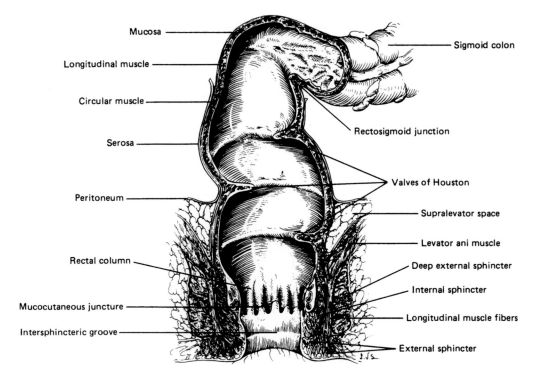

Figure 29–1. Anatomy of the anorectum. (Reproduced, with permission, from Russell TR: Anorectum. In: *Current Surgical Diagnosis & Treatment,* 10/e. Way LW (editor). Appleton & Lange, 1994.)

sympathetic nerves originate from the lumbar segments L_{1-3}, form the inferior mesenteric plexus, travel through the superior hypogastric plexus, and descend as the hypogastric nerves to the pelvic plexus.

The parasympathetic nerves arise from the second, third, and fourth sacral roots and join the hypogastric nerves anterior and lateral to the rectum to form the pelvic plexus, from which fibers pass to form the periprostatic plexus. Sympathetic and parasympathetic fibers pass from the pelvic and periprostatic plexi to the rectum and internal anal sphincter as well as the prostate, bladder, and penis. Injury to these nerves or plexi can lead to impotence, bladder dysfunction, and loss of normal defecatory mechanisms.

The internal anal sphincter is innervated with sympathetic and parasympathetic fibers. Both are inhibitory and keep the sphincter in a constant state of contraction. Stool entering the rectal vault distends the rectum and leads to reflex relaxation of the internal anal sphincter. This is the **rectoanal inhibitory reflex.** It allows the rectal contents to descend into the anal canal and be sampled by the exquisitely sensitive anal epithelium. Continued distention of the rectum leads to relaxation of the external anal sphincter. This sphincter is also under voluntary con-

trol and can be maximally contracted for approximately 1 minute before fatiguing.

Above the dentate line, noxious stimuli are experienced as ill-defined dull sensations conducted through afferent fibers of the parasympathetic nerves. Below the dentate line, the epithelium is exquisitely sensitive. Cutaneous sensations of heat, cold, pain, and touch are conveyed through the inferior rectal and perineal branches of the pudendal nerve.

The arterial supply of the anorectum is via the superior, middle, and inferior rectal arteries. The superior rectal artery is the terminal branch of the inferior mesenteric artery and descends in the mesorectum. It supplies the upper and middle rectum. The middle rectal arteries arise from the internal iliac arteries and enter the rectum anterolaterally at the level of the pelvic floor musculature. They supply the lower two thirds of the rectum. Collaterals exist between the middle and superior rectal arteries. The inferior rectal arteries, branches of the internal pudendal arteries, enter posterolaterally, do not anastomose with the blood supply to the middle rectum, and provide blood supply to the anal sphincters and epithelium.

The venous drainage of the anorectum is via the superior, middle, and inferior rectal veins draining into the portal and systemic systems. The superior rectal veins drains the upper and middle third of the rectum. They empty into the portal system via the inferior mesenteric vein. The middle rectal veins drain the lower rectum and upper anal canal into the systemic system via the internal iliac veins. The inferior rectal veins drain the lower anal canal, communicating with the pudendal veins and draining into the internal iliac veins. There is communication between the venous systems. This allows low rectal cancers to spread via the portal and systemic systems.

Lymphatic drainage of the upper and middle rectum is into the inferior mesenteric nodes. Lymph from the lower rectum may also drain into the inferior mesenteric system or into the systems along the middle and inferior rectal arteries, posteriorly along the middle sacral artery, and anteriorly through channels in the retrovesical or rectovaginal septum. These drain to the iliac nodes and ultimately to the periaortic nodes. Lymphatics from the anal canal above the dentate line drain via the superior rectal lymphatics to the inferior mesenteric lymph nodes and laterally to the internal iliac nodes. Below the dentate line, drainage occurs primarily to the inguinal nodes but can occur to the inferior or superior rectal lymph nodes.

Gordon PH: Surgical Anatomy. In: *Principles and Practice of Surgery for the Colon, Rectum, and Anus.* Gordon PH, Nivatvongs S (editors). Quality Medical Publishing, 1991.
Kodner IJ et al: Colon, Rectum, and Anus. In: *Principles of Surgery,* 6/e. Schwartz SI (editor). McGraw-Hill, 1994.
Levi AC, Borghi F, Garavaglia M: Development of the anal canal muscles. Dis Colon Rectum 1991;34:262.
Shafik A: A concept of the anatomy of the anal sphincter mechanism and the physiology of defecation. Dis Colon Rectum 1987;30:970.

NORMAL FUNCTION OF THE ANORECTUM

The normal function of the anorectum is storage and appropriate release of intestinal waste products. The rectum functions mainly as a storage capacitance vessel. The normal rectum holds 650–1200 ml of liquid. Resting rectal pressure is approximately 10 mm Hg. Changes in intrarectal pressure are primarily a reflection of intra-abdominal pressure changes, as the rectum itself has little peristaltic function. The anal sphincters function mainly as the regulator of appropriate release of intestinal waste. Resting anal pressure is generated by the internal sphincter (80–85%) and external sphincter (15–20%), while the external sphincter generates 100% of the maximum squeeze pressures.

Integration of the functions of the rectum and the anus provide for normal defecation and continence. These actions are complex, poorly understood, coordinated functions that can be disrupted at many levels, leading to alterations in continence. Altered rectal capacity or compliance may decrease the capacitance of the rectum, resulting in urgency and incontinence, even in the face of normal sphincters.

Normal defecation can be divided into four components: (1) movement of feces into the rectum, (2) rectoanal inhibitory reflex or "sampling reflex," (3) voluntary relaxation of the pelvic floor and external sphincter mechanism, and (4) voluntary increase in intra-abdominal pressure. Stool enters the rectum two to three times a day associated with mass movement of the more proximal colon. When this occurs the rectum distends, eliciting the rectoanal inhibitory reflex. The relaxation is asymmetrical in that the proximal sphincter relaxes more than the distal sphincter. This allows the "sampling" of the rectal contents at the transitional zone. If it is a socially acceptable time to pass flatus or stool, steps three and four occur. However, if it is not, then the external sphincters are actively contracted and continence is maintained. In the act of defecation, the pelvic floor and external sphincters are relaxed and intra-abdominal pressure is increased. The act of passing flatus is more complex and requires the selective relaxation of some but not all of the external sphincter.

Bielefeldt K, Enck P, Erckenbrecht JF: Sensory and motor function in the maintenance of anal continence. Dis Colon Rectum 1990;33:674.
Burleigh DE: Pharmacology of the internal anal sphincter. In: *Coloproctology and the Pelvic Floor,* 2/e. Henry M, Swash M (editors). Oxford, Butterworth-Heinemann, 1992.
Rune Sjödahl, Olof Hallböök: Incontinence and normal sphincter function. In: *Colorectal Physiology: Fecal Incontinence.* Kuijpers HC (editor) CRC Press, 1994.

DYSFUNCTION OF THE ANORECTUM

INCONTINENCE

Essentials of Diagnosis
- Inability to control elimination of rectal contents.
- Characterization of rectal contents that are uncontrolled.
- Characterization of timing of incontinence.

General Considerations
Incontinence results from mechanical or neurogenic defects. Obstetrical trauma during delivery is the major cause of mechanical injury and a cause of

partially reversible neurogenic injury. There is an increased incidence of disruption of the external sphincter, resulting in incontinence after fourth degree perineal tears, multiple vaginal deliveries with midline episiotomies, and infection of an episiotomy repair. The injury after prolonged labor may be twofold, with mechanical disruption of the sphincter and stretch of the pudendal nerve.

Incontinence may result from the treatment of cryptogenic abscess/fistula disease, or perianal Crohn's disease, where the external sphincter may be divided during a fistulotomy. In women, the external sphincter is a thin band of muscle anteriorly, and therefore especially susceptible to complete transection in this location. If it is surgically disrupted, or destroyed by chronic inflammation, continence is lost.

Neurogenic causes of incontinence include pudendal nerve stretch secondary to prolonged labor at childbirth or chronic history of straining to defecate. In the latter instance, the pudendal nerve is stretched over the ischial spine as the perineum descends, leading to "idiopathic" fecal incontinence in elderly patients.

Other causes of incontinence include systemic diseases effecting either the muscular or neurologic systems (eg, scleroderma, multiple sclerosis, dermatomyositis, and diabetes), and causes unrelated to the function of the sphincter itself (severe diarrhea, fecal impaction with overflow incontinence, radiation proctitis with fibrosis, and tumors of the distal colon and rectum).

Clinical Findings

A. Symptoms and Signs: Complete incontinence is lack of control of gas, liquid, and stool. Inability to control liquid and gas or gas alone is **partial incontinence.** Urgency, seepage, and soiling may occur regularly or intermittently, depending on the nature of the stool presenting to the rectum. Elicitation of these symptoms is important in localizing the deficit. Patients who complain of soiling with urgency may have a poorly distensible rectum and normal sphincters, whereas those patients complaining of inability to sense stool until it has passed, may have a neurologic injury. The signs of incontinence may include a patulous anus, a focal loss of corrugation of the anal verge, maceration of the perianal skin, decreased sphincter tone, and loss of anal sensation.

B. Laboratory and Imaging Studies: Evaluation with anorectal manometry, transrectal ultrasound, pudendal nerve latency studies, electromyography (EMG), and defecography may all be part of the evaluation of the incontinent patient.

Anorectal manometry defines the limits of the injury by measuring the maximum resting pressure, maximum squeeze pressure, sphincter length and symmetry, minimum sensory volume, presence or absence of the rectoanal inhibitory reflex, and ability to relax the puborectalis muscle. Normal maximal resting pressures generally range from 40–80 mm Hg while maximal squeeze pressures range from 80–160. The internal sphincter gives rise to 80–85% of the resting maximal pressure while the external sphincter provides 15–20% of the resting pressure and 100% of the maximal squeeze pressures. The sphincter is typically 3 cm in length, asymmetrical (longer in back), and the whole complex is shorter in women. The minimum sensory volume is usually approximately 10 ml. The rectoanal inhibitory reflex is seen as a decrease in resting anal pressure when an air-filled balloon distends the rectum. Finally, the patient is asked to pass a fully inflated 60 ml latex balloon at the completion of the procedure. This task requires normal relaxation of the puborectalis.

Transrectal ultrasound is useful in the evaluation of sphincteric defects. Although EMG has been used for mapping sphincter defects, transrectal ultrasound has largely replaced the more painful and poorly tolerated EMG procedure. Excellent resolution is possible. The exact location and extent of the sphincter defect can be mapped.

Pudendal nerve latency studies further define the nature of the injury in incontinent patients. The study is performed by placing a gloved finger with a stimulating electrode on the finger tip in the rectum and stimulating the pudendal nerve as it traverses the ischial spine. An electrode at the base of the examining finger records the delay between stimulation and contraction of the external sphincter. A "normal" delay is 2.0 seconds. This may be prolonged with age, after childbirth, in individuals with a history of excessive straining to defecate and perineal descent, and in certain systemic disease states, such as diabetes and multiple sclerosis.

As noted above, electromyography has generally been replaced by transrectal ultrasound. However, in some individuals' hands it is still quite useful in identifying certain systemic diseases (eg, dermatomyositis) based on their characteristic EMG patterns.

Defecography is useful in patients with both constipation and incontinence, as some patients with incontinence may be straining to defecate and intussuscept the rectum into itself, causing obstruction and apparent constipation, which is followed by uncontrolled release of liquid stool after the straining is stopped.

Differential Diagnosis

Obstructed defecation secondary to tumor or intussusception may lead to incontinence. Obstetrical injury, either from excessive straining and pudendal nerve injury or disruption of the sphincter mechanism, may cause varying degrees of incontinence. Incontinence may present immediately or after many years as the patient ages, sphincter tone decreases, and an occult injury is uncovered. Chronic straining at defecation stretches the pudendal nerve over the ischial spine, leading to "idiopathic fecal incontinence" in the elderly. An extreme example of this is seen in rectal prolapse, where 30% of patients may be incontinent after repair because of stretch injury from chronic prolapse. Consideration of systemic diseases, such as multiple sclerosis, dermatomyositis, and diabetes mellitus, is also necessary. Finally, incontinence may be unrelated to dysfunction of the anal sphincter mechanism, but may be secondary to other diseases that overwhelm a normally functioning sphincter, such as severe diarrhea, fecal impaction with overflow, inflammatory bowel disease of the rectum, radiation proctitis, and fibrosis.

Treatment

The algorithm for the diagnosis and treatment of incontinence is summarized in Figure 29–2. If a muscular defect is limited and there is no neurologic injury, surgical correction with an overlapping sphincter reconstruction restores continence by reestablishing a complete ring of muscle. However, if there is extensive loss of sphincter muscle or severe neurologic injury, simple overlapping repair is not as successful, and consideration must be given to muscle flap or encirclement procedures. Gracilis or gluteal muscle flap procedures have been reserved for those patients with complete neurologic injury or extensive muscle loss who wish to avoid a colostomy. Currently, a pacemaker for retraining the gracilis is under investigation, but true continence with any of these procedures is questioned.

Incomplete neurologic injuries may respond to retraining with biofeedback. Decreased sensation and muscle weakness may also be improved with this technique.

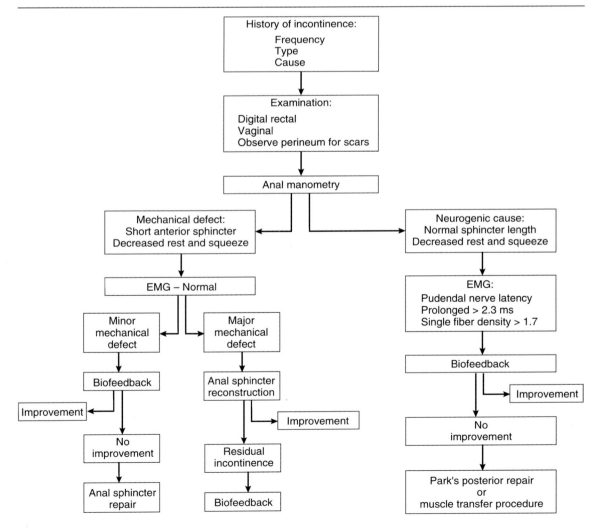

Figure 29–2. Algorithm for workup and treatment of fecal incontinence.

Anal encirclement procedures with foreign material (wire, mesh, or silicon) have been reserved for the critically ill or patients with a short life expectancy. Patients are given daily enemas to evacuate the rectum, providing a form of continence with artificial obstruction and stimulated evacuation. However, the foreign material is prone to infection and erosion into the rectum, which often necessitates removal.

The incontinence associated with prolapse is fixed during the repair of the prolapse if there has not been significant nerve injury. The prolapsing segment often stimulates the rectoanal inhibitory reflex, decreasing internal sphincter pressure and leading to incontinence.

Bielefeldt K et al: Anorectal manometry and defecography in the diagnosis of fecal incontinence. J Clin Gastroenterol 1991;13:661.

Burleigh DE: Pharmacology of the internal anal sphincter. In: *Coloproctology and the Pelvic Floor,* 2/e. Henry M, Swash M (editors). Oxford, Butterworth-Heinemann, 1992.

Burnett SJD et al: Confirmation of endosonographic detection of external anal sphincter defects by simultaneous electromyographic mapping. Br J Surg 1991;78:448.

Fleshman JW et al: Anal sphincter reconstruction. Anterior overlapping muscle repair. Dis Colon Rectum 1991;34:739.

Law PJ, Kamm MA, Bartram CI: Anal endosonography in the investigation of faecal incontinence. Br J Surg 1991;78:312.

Shorvon PJ et al: Defaecography in normal volunteers: Results and implications. Gut 1989;30:1737.

OBSTRUCTED DEFECATION

Essentials of Diagnosis

- Inability to voluntarily evacuate rectal contents.
- Normal colonic transit time.

General Considerations

Obstructed defecation results from anal stenosis, non-relaxing puborectalis syndrome, or internal intussusception.

The most common cause of anal stenosis is scarring after anal surgery. In particular, inexpertly performed hemorrhoidectomies or the circumferential "Whitehead" hemorrhoidectomy lead to stenosis. Other causes include anal tumors, Crohn's disease, radiation injury, recurrent anal ulcers, infection, and trauma.

Nonrelaxing puborectalis syndrome is a component of the disease syndrome of pelvic floor dysfunction, which includes internal intussusception, solitary rectal ulcer, and true prolapse. Nonrelaxation of the puborectalis is a functional disorder in that the muscle is normal but control is dysfunctional. The puborectalis is normally contracted "at rest," pulling the rectum forward and maintaining an acute anorectal angle. During defecation the muscle relaxes and evacuation occurs. In nonrelaxing puborectalis syndrome the muscle does not relax and maintains the anorectal angle. The patient therefore performs a Valsalva maneuver against an obstructed outlet, and elimination does not occur or is significantly obstructed.

Internal intussusception causes outlet obstruction because of laxity of attachments of the rectum to the sacrum that allows the upper rectum to move away from the sacrum and telescope into the more distal rectum, leading to obstruction (see following section, "Abnormal rectal fixation").

Clinical Findings

A. Symptoms and Signs: Anal stenosis presents with increasing difficulty and straining at defecation, thin and sometimes painful bowel movements, and bloating. Patients with nonrelaxing puborectalis syndrome similarly complain of straining and anal or pelvic pain, but also complain of constipation, incomplete evacuation, and a need to perform digital maneuvers to evacuate rectal contents. As with nonrelaxing puborectalis syndrome, patients with internal intussusception complain of constipation, sensations of rectal fullness, or incomplete evacuation, but in contrast to the above causes of obstructed defecation, they also note mucous discharge, rectal bleeding, and tenesmus.

Examination of the patient with anal stenosis will reveal postsurgical changes and a stenotic anal canal. Digital examination may be quite painful or impossible. Digital examination of the patient with nonrelaxing puborectalis syndrome may reveal a tender pelvic muscular diaphragm but it is otherwise unremarkable. Sigmoidoscopic examination of the patient with internal intussusception may reveal an anterior solitary rectal ulcer. The ulcer, which develops anteriorly 4–12 cm from the anal verge, is the lead point of the internal intussusception.

B. Laboratory and Imaging Studies: No additional studies of the patient with anal stenosis are required, but patients with nonrelaxing puborectalis syndrome and internal intussusception should have defecography, colonic transit studies, anorectal manometry with the balloon expulsion test, and barium enema or colonoscopy.

The patient with nonrelaxing puborectalis syndrome will have a normal colon on barium enema or colonoscopy and normal colonic transit to the rectosigmoid, but will demonstrate persistent anterior displacement of the rectum on the lateral view of a cinedefecogram and be unable to expel the balloon at the completion of anorectal manometric evaluation.

In the patient with internal intussusception, colonic transit time will be normal to the rectosigmoid, and barium enema or colonoscopy will document a normal colon. Defecography will document the intussusception. Patients with intussusception secondary to nonrelaxing puborectalis will be unable to expel the latex balloon.

Differential Diagnosis

Causes of anal pain include fissure, external hemorrhoids, perirectal abscess, malignancy, foreign body, and proctalgia fugax. Proctalgia fugax (levator syndrome), a diagnosis of exclusion, is suggested when a patient complains of pain that awakens him or her from sleep. The pain is generally left-sided, short-lived, and relieved by heat, dilation, or muscle relaxants. The patient often has a history of migraines and may report the occurrence of pain in relation to stressful events.

Complaints suggestive of obstructed defecation arise in patients with fecal impaction, rectal or anal cancer, descending perineum syndrome, rectocele, internal intussusception, and nonrelaxing puborectalis syndrome. The workup of these complex patients is diagrammed in Figure 29–3.

Fecal impaction may occur as a result of nonrelaxing puborectalis syndrome, and therapy is therefore directed towards that disorder.

Treatment

A. Medical: Mild anal stenosis may be treated successfully with gentle dilation and bulk agents. Nonrelaxing puborectalis syndrome is best treated with biofeedback. The puborectalis is retrained to relax during the act of defecation, which allows the act to proceed without obstruction. Mild-to- moderate intussusception is treated with bulk agents.

B. Surgical: Severe anal stenosis is treated surgically if there is no evidence of active disease (Crohn's) and healthy tissue is available to perform the anoplasty. Nonrelaxing puborectalis should not be treated surgically. Treatment of severe intussusception is discussed later.

Prognosis

The prognosis for anal stenosis is excellent if there is no evidence of active disease. Patients with nonrelaxing puborectalis have excellent results with biofeedback, but may require retraining episodes. Most patients with mild-to-moderate intussusception do quite well, once they are reassured that an abnormality exists and it is not malignant.

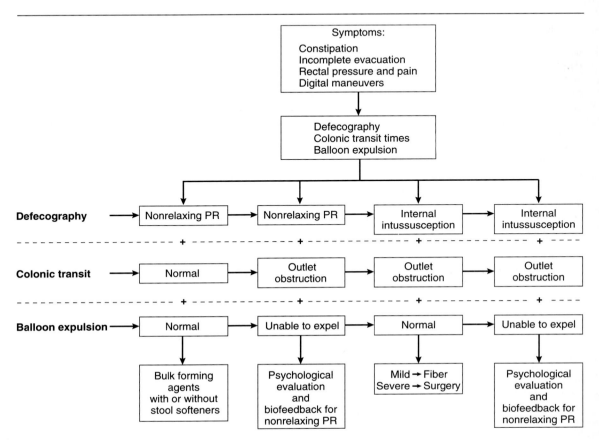

Figure 29–3. Algorithm for workup and treatment of obstructed defecation.
PR = puborectoris

Caplin DA, Kodner IJ: Repair of anal stricture and mucosal ectropin by simple flap procedures. Dis Colon Rectum 1986;29:92.

Kodner IJ et al: Rectal prolapse and other pelvic floor abnormalities: Current state of the art as related to physiologic studies and surgical alternatives. In: *Surgery Annual.* Appleton & Lange, 1992.

Levine DS: Solitary rectal ulcer syndrome. Are "solitary" rectal ulcer syndrome and "localized" colitis cystica profunda analogous syndromes caused by rectal prolapse? Gastroenterology 1987;92:243.

ABNORMAL RECTAL FIXATION

Essentials of Diagnosis

- Increased mobility of the rectum.
- Altered defecation (constipation, incontinence, or both).
- Digital maneuvers to defecate.

General Considerations

Abnormal rectal fixation is a group of diseases in which the attachment of the rectum to the sacrum has lengthened, allowing the rectum to block the act of defecation, to protrude into the vagina, or to prolapse through the anus. The reason for the increased mobility appears to be related to chronic straining. This may be secondary to colonic dysmotility or nonrelaxing puborectalis syndrome.

Clinical Findings

A. Symptoms and Signs: Internal intussusception leads to complaints of rectal fullness, urge to defecate, and if associated with solitary rectal ulcer syndrome, complaints of rectal bleeding, mucous discharge, or tenesmus. Patients with rectal prolapse complain of mucous discharge, progressive incontinence, pain, and bleeding, and upon direct questioning, they may report their rectum "falls out."

Digital examination of the patient with internal intussusception may reveal a mass. This is the lead point of the intussusceptum and may be mistaken for a malignancy. It may be a solitary rectal ulcer or may have progressed to colitis cystica profunda, which develops as the healing solitary rectal ulcer entraps glands in the rectal submucosa. Biopsy reveals diffuse submucosal cysts that must be differentiated from rectal adenocarcinoma. Colitis cystica profunda may also be associated with radiation injury, postoperative changes, adenomatous polyps, malignancy, or inflammatory bowel disease.

Physical examination of the patient who presents with an acute episode of rectal prolapse is not difficult. A large mass of prolapsed tissue with concentric mucosal rings will be apparent. However, the patient with a history of prolapse but without active prolapse may be more difficult. It may be necessary to give the patient an enema, allow him to evacuate, and then examine the perineum. This often induces prolapse, allowing confirmation of the diagnosis in the office. An alternative is to demonstrate the prolapse on defecography. Digital examination may reveal decreased or absent sphincter tone.

B. Laboratory and Imaging Studies: Patients with internal intussusception and rectal prolapse need anorectal manometry, electromyography, pudendal nerve latency studies, defecography, and barium enema or colonoscopy. Defecography will document the intussusception or prolapse and may reveal the cause. Evaluation of the entire colon with either barium enema or colonoscopy is necessary to rule out a malignancy. The surgical approach may be chosen based on the pudendal nerve latency studies and EMG.

Differential Diagnosis

Internal intussusception must be differentiated from adenocarcinoma. The patient presentation, physical appearance, and histologic characteristics of the ulcer may be confused with malignancy.

Rectal prolapse should be distinguished from hemorrhoidal disease. Rectal prolapse is seen as uninterrupted circumferential rings of mucosa, while hemorrhoidal prolapse will be seen as prolapsing tissue with deep grooves between areas of prolapsing edematous tissue.

Complications

The complications of intussusception and prolapse include progression of intussusception to prolapse; nerve injury from prolapse or chronic straining; descending perineum syndrome; bleeding; and incontinence. Severe cases of rectal prolapse may become too edematous to allow reduction and may progress to necrosis of the prolapse.

Treatment

A. Medical: As noted earlier, mild-to-moderate intussusception is treated with bulk agents and reassurance, producing excellent results.

B. Surgical: Severe intussusception with impending pudendal nerve damage is treated surgically. The abdominal procedures for patients with severe intussusception or rectal prolapse with normal sphincter function are low anterior resection or rectopexy. Rectopexy corrects the mobility of the rectum but does not correct the underlying disorder. Therefore, symptoms often persist or recur. Low anterior resection removes the intussusception and the mobile portion of colon. In the constipated patient or the patient with a redundant sigmoid colon, resection is preferable. In either operation, rectopexy or resection, complete mobilization of the entire rectum is required to avoid distal intussusception.

Of those patients with rectal prolapse and incontinence, 60–70% will have return of sphincter function. However, reliable means of preoperatively identifying these patients do not exist. Those that do not have return of sphincter function will not tolerate low anterior resection. Therefore, transabdominal rectopexy with a synthetic sling or perineal proctectomy and posterior sphincter enhancement are recommended in these patients. The posterior reconstruction may alter the angle of the rectum or obstruct the outlet sufficiently to allow for continence.

Finally, in those patients with prolapse who either have prohibitively high operative risk or who are elderly with limited life expectancy, an anal encirclement procedure may be performed. Thiersch originally described the use of a silver wire to encircle the external sphincter in the ischiorectal fat, but currently synthetic mesh, silicone tubes, or muscle flaps are preferred. With any of the above, an outlet obstruction is created and laxatives or enemas are required for rectal evacuation. The encirclement procedures are complicated by erosion of the foreign material into the rectum and infection. This procedure is utilized less frequently as the perineal approach with the patient under spinal or epidural anesthesia gains favor.

Prognosis

The prognosis for patients with mild-to-moderate intussusception who are treated with bulk agents is excellent. Those individuals with severe intussusception and those who have rectal prolapse without sphincter dysfunction should do well. Those with sphincter dysfunction have a 60–70% chance of regaining function. The long-term follow-up of patients repaired by the perineal approach is not available, but this approach appears promising, especially in the high-risk patients in whom an abdominal operation is undesirable.

Ballantyne GH: The historical evolution of anatomic concepts of rectal prolapse. Semin Colon Rectal Surg 1991;2:170.

Corman ML: Rectal prolapse. Surgical techniques. Surg Clin North Am 1988;68:1255.

Kodner IJ et al: Rectal prolapse and other pelvic floor abnormalities: Current state of the art as related to the physiologic studies and surgical alternatives. In: *Surgery Annual.* Appleton & Lange, 1992.

Levine DS: Solitary rectal ulcer syndrome. Are "solitary" rectal ulcer syndrome and "localized" colitis cystica profunda analogous syndromes caused by rectal prolapse? Gastroenterology 1987;92:243.

Mackle EJ, Parks TG: Solitary rectal ulcer syndrome. Aetiology, investigation, and management. Dig Dis 1990;8:294.

Madden MV et al: Abdominal rectopexy for complete prolapse: Prospective study evaluating changes in symptoms and anorectal function. Dis Colon Rectum 1992;35:48.

Madoff RD et al: Long-term functional results of colon resection and rectopexy for overt rectal prolapse. Am J Gastroenterol 1992;87:101.

McKee RF et al: A prospective randomized study of abdominal rectopexy with and without sigmoidoscopy in rectal prolapse. Surg Gynecol Obstet 1992;174:145.

Prasad ML et al: Perineal proctectomy, posterior rectopexy, and postanal levator repair for the treatment of rectal prolapse. Dis Colon Rectum 1986;29:547.

Sun WM et al: A common pathophysiology for full-thickness rectal prolapse, anterior mucosal prolapse and solitary rectal ulcer. Br J Surg 1989;76:290.

HEMORRHOIDS

Essentials of Diagnosis: Internal Hemorrhoids

- Bright red blood per rectum.
- Mucous discharge.
- Rectal fullness or discomfort.

Essentials of Diagnosis: External Hemorrhoids

- Sudden, severe perianal pain.
- Perianal mass.

General Considerations

Hemorrhoidal tissues are part of the normal anatomy of the distal rectum and anal canal (Figure 29–2). **Internal hemorrhoids** are vascular and connective tissue cushions that originate above the dentate line and are lined with rectal or transitional mucosa. **External hemorrhoids** are vascular complexes underlying the richly innervated anoderm. Hemorrhoids function as protective pillows that engorge with blood during the act of defecation, protecting the anal canal from direct trauma due to passage of stool. Hemorrhoidal tissues engorge when intra-abdominal pressure is increased. This occurs with obesity, pregnancy, lifting, and defecation.

The disease state of "hemorrhoids" may involve the internal complex, external complex, or both. Internal hemorrhoids become symptomatic when the internal complex becomes chronically engorged or the tissue prolapses into the anal canal due to laxity of the surrounding connective tissue and dilation of the veins. The external hemorrhoids become symptomatic with thrombosis, which leads to acute onset of severe perianal pain. When the thrombosis resolves, the overlying skin may remain enlarged, creating a skin tag.

Pathophysiology of abnormal hemorrhoidal tissue development is related to chronic straining that leads to engorgement, vascular dilatation, and stretching of the supporting connective tissue. The most common cause of prolonged straining is the act of defecation.

Internal hemorrhoids are traditionally classified by the following scheme: first-degree hemorrhoids bleed; second-degree hemorrhoids bleed and prolapse, but reduce spontaneously; third-degree hemorrhoids bleed, prolapse, and require manual reduction; fourth-degree hemorrhoids bleed, incarcerate, and cannot be reduced.

Clinical Findings

A. Symptoms and Signs: Internal hemorrhoids typically do *not* cause pain but rather bright red bleeding per rectum, mucous discharge, and a sense of rectal fullness or discomfort. Infrequently, however, internal hemorrhoids will prolapse into the anal canal, incarcerate, thrombose, and necrose. In this instance, patients may complain of pain. Visual inspection of the perineum may reveal a normal-appearing perineum, edema near the involved hemorrhoid, a prolapsed hemorrhoid or an edematous, gangrenous, incarcerated hemorrhoid. The perineum may be macerated from chronic mucous discharge, the resulting moisture, and local irritation. Anoscopy may reveal tissue with evidence of chronic venous dilatation, friability, mobility, and squamous metaplasia.

External hemorrhoids may present acutely with a clot in an external vein. This is extremely painful. The clot may occasionally erode through the anoderm, causing bleeding. Repeated episodes of dilatation and thrombosis may lead to enlargement of the overlying skin, which is seen as a skin tag on physical examination. The acutely thrombosed external hemorrhoid is seen as a purplish, edematous, tense subcutaneous perianal mass that is quite tender.

B. Laboratory and Imaging Studies: Chronic bleeding from internal hemorrhoids may cause anemia. However, until all other sources of blood loss have been ruled out, anemia must not be attributed to hemorrhoids, regardless of a patient's age. Barium enema or colonoscopy are necessary to rule out malignancy and inflammatory bowel disease. Defecography is helpful in the patient in which obstructed defecation and rectal prolapse is suspected.

Differential Diagnosis

Patients with perianal pathology often present, or are referred, with a chief complaint of "hemorrhoids." A thorough history frequently suggests the diagnosis. Those individuals with painless bleeding due to hemorrhoids must be distinguished from those with rectal bleeding from colorectal malignancy, inflammatory bowel disease, diverticular disease, and adenomatous polyps. Painful bleeding associated with a bowel movement is often due to an ulcer or fissure. Straining at stool may be attributed to hemorrhoids but is likely secondary to obstructed defecation. Similarly, rectal prolapse must be distinguished from hemorrhoids because it is safe to band a hemorrhoid but not a prolapsed rectum. Moisture or maceration may be secondary to hemorrhoids or condylomata acuminata.

Complications

The complications of internal or external hemorrhoids are the indications for medical or surgical intervention. They are bleeding, pain, necrosis, mucous discharge, moisture, and, rarely, perianal sepsis.

Treatment

A. Medical: Initial medical management for all but the most advanced cases is recommended. Dietary alterations, including elimination of constipating foods (eg, cheeses), addition of bulking agents, stool softeners, and increased intake of liquids, are advised. Changing daily routines by adding exercise and decreasing time spent on the commode is often beneficial.

B. Surgical: First- and second-degree hemorrhoids generally respond to medical management. Hemorrhoids that fail to respond to medical management may be treated with elastic band ligation, sclerosis, photocoagulation, cryosurgery, excisional hemorrhoidectomy, and many other local techniques that induce scarring and fixation of the hemorrhoids to the underlying tissues. The three most common techniques—elastic band ligation, sclerosis, and excisional hemorrhoidectomy—will be discussed.

Elastic band ligation is used most frequently in patients with second- and third-degree hemorrhoids. Hemorrhoidal tissue 1–2 cm above the dentate line is grasped and pulled into the barrel of an elastic band applier, and a band is placed at the base of the hemorrhoidal complex. After 7–10 days, the hemorrhoid sloughs, leaving a scar that inhibits further prolapse and bleeding. Patients must avoid nonsteroidal anti-inflammatory agents and aspirin for 10 days after ligation, as significant bleeding may otherwise occur when the hemorrhoid sloughs.

If the band is placed in the transitional zone or below, patients may experience sudden severe pain, as this mucosa and skin is highly innervated. The band should be immediately removed. Immune-compromised patients or those with rectal prolapse have developed severe sepsis after banding. This complication is heralded by inordinate pain, fever, and urinary retention. Treatment requires intravenous antibiotics, band removal, and observation.

Injection sclerotherapy is often tried for first-degree and second-degree hemorrhoids that continue to bleed despite medical measures. Sclerosant, 1–2 ml, is injected into the loose submucosal connective tissue above the hemorrhoidal complex, causing inflammation and scarring. This inhibits prolapse and bleeding of the remaining hemorrhoidal tissue. The depth of injection is critical. If the injection is too superficial, mucosal sloughing may occur, and if it is too deep full-thickness injury, necrosis, and life-threatening infection may occur.

Excisional hemorrhoidectomy is reserved for the larger third- and fourth-degree hemorrhoids, mixed internal and external hemorrhoids not amenable to banding of the internal component, and incarcerated internal hemorrhoids requiring urgent intervention. The base of the hemorrhoid is visualized with an anoscope. The vascular pedicle is suture-ligated. The hemorrhoidal tissue is excised using the "knife" (scalpel, scissors, cautery, laser) preferred by the surgeon. Care must be taken to avoid the underlying internal sphincters while dissecting the vascular cushion and overlying mucosa afree. The mucosal and skin defect is then closed with the suture used for control of the vascular pedicle.

Urinary retention is the most common acute complication of excisional hemorrhoidectomy. Anal stenosis is a long-term complication that may be avoided by leaving adequate anoderm between excised hemorrhoidal complexes.

The acutely thrombosed external hemorrhoid may be treated with excision of the hemorrhoid or clot evacuation if the patient presents less than 48 hours after onset of symptoms. Excision removes the clot and hemorrhoidal tissues, thereby decreasing the incidence of recurrence significantly. However, many surgeons simply evacuate the thrombus, relieving the pressure and pain. If the patient presents over 48 hours after onset of symptoms, the thrombus has begun to organize and evacuation will not be successful. Conservative management with warm sitz baths, high-fiber diet, stool softeners and reassurance is advised.

Prognosis

The prognosis for recurrence of hemorrhoidal disease is most related to success in changing the patient's bowel habits. Increasing dietary fiber, decreasing constipating foods, introducing exercise, and decreasing time spent on the toilet all decrease the amount of time spent straining in the squatting position. These behavioral modifications are the most important steps in preventing recurrence.

American Society of Colon and Rectal Surgeons, Standards Task Force. Practice parameters for the treatment of hemorrhoids. Dis Colon Rectum 1991;34:992.

Johanson JF, Sonnenberg A: Temporal changes in the occurrence of hemorrhoids in the United States and England. Dis Colon Rectum 1991;34:585.

Johanson JF, Sonnenberg A: The prevalence of hemorrhoids and chronic constipation: An epidemiologic study. Gastroenterology 1990;98:380.

Leff EI: Hemorrhoidectomy: Laser vs. nonlaser. Outpatient surgical experience. Dis Colon Rectum 1992;35:743.

Mazier WP: Hemorrhoids. In: *Surgery of the Colon, Rectum, and Anus.* Mazier WP et al (editors). Saunders, 1995.

Senagore A et al: The treatment of advanced hemorrhoidal disease: A prospective randomized comparison of cold scapel vs. contact Nd:YAG laser. Dis Colon Rectum 1993;6:1042.

Wolkomir AF, Luchtefeld MA: Surgery for symptomatic hemorrhoids and anal fissures in Crohn's disease. Dis Colon Rectum 1993;36:545.

ANAL FISSURE & ULCER

Essentials of Diagnosis

- Tearing pain upon defecation.
- Blood on tissue or stool.
- Persistent perianal pain or spasm following defecation.
- Sphincter spasm.
- Disruption of anoderm.

General Considerations

An **anal fissure** is a split in the anoderm. An **anal ulcer** is a chronic fissure. When mature, an ulcer is associated with a skin tag (**sentinel pile**), and an hypertrophied anal papilla. Fissures occur in the midline just distal to the dentate line. About 90% are posterior, 10% are anterior, and fewer than 1% occur simultaneously in the anterior and posterior positions.

Fissures result from forceful dilation of the anal canal, most commonly during defecation. The anoderm is disrupted, exposing the underlying internal sphincter muscle. The muscle spasms in response to exposure and fails to relax with the next dilations. This leads to further tearing, deepening of the fissure, and increased muscle irritation. Typically, the initial insult is believed to be a firm bowel movement. The pain associated with the initial bowel movement is great, and the patient therefore ignores the urge to defecate for fear of experiencing the pain again. This allows a harder stool to form, which tears the anoderm more as it passes, because of its size and the poor relaxation of the sphincter.

Clinical Findings

A. Symptoms and Signs: Fissures cause pain and bleeding with defecation. The pain is often tearing or burning, worst during defecation, and subsides over a few hours. Blood is noted on tissue and on the stool but is not mixed in the stool or toilet water. Constipation develops secondarily due to fear of recurrent pain.

Physical examination by simple gentle traction on the buttocks will evert the anus sufficiently to reveal a disruption of the anoderm in the midline at the mucocutaneous junction. In the acute fissure this may be all that is present. In the chronic fissure, a sentinel pile may be visualized at the inferior margin of the ulcer. Gentle, limited, digital examination will confirm internal sphincter spasm. Anoscopy and proctosigmoidoscopy should be deferred until healing occurs or the procedure can be performed under anesthesia.

B. Laboratory and Imaging Studies: Anal manometry is unhelpful. Studies have shown increased pressures in patients with ulcers, but patients with high pressures have not been found to be at increased risk for fissure/ulcer disease.

Differential Diagnosis

Fissure/ulcer disease occurs in the anterior or posterior midline and involves the mucocutaneous junction. Ulcers occurring off the midline, or away from the mucocutaneous junction, are suspect. Crohn's disease, anal tuberculosis (TB), anal malignancy, abscess/fistula disease, cytomegalovirus, herpes, chlamydia, syphilis, acquired immunodeficiency syndrome, and some blood dyscrasias may all mimic certain aspects of fissure/ulcer disease. Initial manifestations of Crohn's disease are limited to the anal canal in 10% of patients. Anal TB will be associated with a prior or concomitant history of pulmonary TB. Anal cancer may present as a painless ulcer. Patients with nonhealing ulcers must undergo biopsy to rule out malignancy.

Complications

The complications are related to persistence of the disease and its associated pain, bleeding, and alteration in bowel habits. The ulcers do not become malignant.

Treatment

A. Medical: Stool softeners, bulk agents, and sitz baths are successful in healing 90% of anal fissures. A second episode has a 60–80% chance of healing with this regimen. Sitz baths after painful bowel movements soothe the muscle spasm. Patients are instructed to contract the sphincters to identify the muscle in spasm and then focus on relaxing that muscle. The effect is twofold: it decreases the pain associated with the spasm and improves blood flow to the fissure, allowing for improved healing. Stool softeners and bulk agents make the stool more malleable, decreasing the trauma of each successive bowel movement. Chronic (1-month history) or chronic recurrent ulcers should be considered for surgery.

B. Surgical: Lateral internal anal sphincterotomy is the procedure of choice for most surgeons. This may be performed "open," where an incision is made in the skin and the hypertrophied distal one third of the internal sphincter is divided under direct vision, or "closed," where a scalpel is passed in the intersphincteric plane and swept medially, dividing the internal sphincter blindly. Both techniques are associated with similar results. It is possible to disrupt the internal sphincter with a four-finger stretch but this is an uncontrolled disruption of the internal sphincter and is associated with a higher rate of recurrence and incontinence.

Prognosis

Lateral internal anal sphincterotomy is 90–95% successful in the treatment of chronic anal fissure/ulcer disease. Fewer than 10% of patients so treated are incontinent to mucous and gas. Recurrence is less than 10%.

Case JB: Chronic anal fissure. Dis Colon Rectum 191;34:198.

Khubchandani IT, Reed JR: Sequelae of internal sphincterotomy for chronic fissure in ano. Br J Surg 1989;76:431.

Laucks SS II: Anal fissures. In:*Surgery of the Colon, Rectum, and Anus.* Mazier WP et al (editors). Saunders, 1995.

Lewis TH et al: Long-term results of open and closed sphincterotomy for anal fissure. Dis Colon Rectum 1988;31:368.

Lin JK: Anal manometric studies in hemorrhoids and anal fissures. Dis Colon Rectum 1989;32:839.

Rosen L et al: Practice parameters for the management of anal fissure. Dis Colon Rectum 1992;35:206.

INFECTIONS OF THE ANORECTUM

ANORECTAL ABSCESS & FISTULA

Essentials of Diagnosis

- Severe anal pain.
- A palpable mass is usually present on perineal or digital rectal examination.
- Systemic evidence of sepsis.

General Considerations

Perirectal abscess fistulous disease is most commonly cryptoglandular in origin. The anal canal has 6–14 glands that lie in the intersphincteric plane between the internal and external sphincters. Projections from the glands pass through the internal sphincter and drain into the crypts at the dentate line. Glands may become infected when a crypt is occluded, trapping stool and bacteria within the gland. If the crypt does not decompress into the anal canal, an abscess may develop in the intersphincteric plane. The abscess may track within or across the intersphincteric plane. Abscesses are classified by the space they invade. Regardless of abscess location, the extent of disease is difficult to determine without examination under anesthesia.

Antibiotics given while allowing the abscess to "mature" are not helpful. Early surgical consultation and operative drainage are the best measures to avoid the disastrous complications associated with undrained perineal sepsis. When the abscesses are drained, either surgically or spontaneously, 50% will have persistent communication with the crypt, creating a fistula from the anus to the perianal skin or fistula in ano. A fistula in ano is not a surgical emergency.

Clinical Findings

A. Symptoms and Signs: An abscess creates severe anal pain, which may worsen with ambulation and straining. Occasionally, patients present with fever, urinary retention, and life-threatening sepsis. This is especially true in diabetics and the immunocompromised host. A patient with fistula in ano may report a history of severe pain, bloody purulent drainage associated with resolution of the pain, and subsequent chronic mucopurulent discharge.

Physical examination of the patient with an abscess reveals a tender perianal or rectal mass. The size is often difficult to assess until the patient is provided adequate anesthesia. An apparently small abscess may extend high into the ischiorectal or supralevator space. A fistula is present when internal and external openings are identified. A firm connecting tract is often palpable.

B. Laboratory and Imaging Studies: Transrectal ultrasound is used in the complex fistula in ano patients where extent of sphincter involvement may be unclear yet critical to determining operative approach. Computed tomography (CT) scan may be helpful in finding the undiagnosed supralevator abscess.

Differential Diagnosis

Abscess fistula disease of cryptoglandular origin must be differentiated from complications of Crohn's disease, pilonidal disease, hidradenitis suppurativa, TB, actinomycosis, trauma, fissures, carcinoma, radiation, chlamydia, local dermal processes, retrorectal tumors, diverticulitis, and ureteral injuries.

About 10% of patients with Crohn's disease will present with anorectal abscess fistulous disease with no antecedent history of inflammatory bowel disease. TB may cause indolent, pale, granulomatous perianal disease but is usually associated with a known history of TB. Hidradenitis suppurativa is considered in the patient with multiple chronic, draining fistulas, as might be seen with undiagnosed horseshoe abscess fistula disease. Pilonidal disease may extend towards the perineum but may be distinguished from cryptoglandular disease by the presence of inspissated hairs, direction of the tract, and presence of other openings in the sacrococcygeal area. A colonic source may be suspected in a patient with known inflammatory bowel disease or diverticular disease. Other less common causes include tumors, radiation, infections, and urologic injuries.

Complications

The complications of an undrained anorectal abscess may be severe. If the abscess is not drained surgically or spontaneously, the infection may spread rapidly, which may result in extensive tissue loss, sphincter injury, and even death. In contrast, a fistula in ano, which may develop when the abscess is drained, is not a surgical emergency. A chronic fistula may be associated with recurring perianal abscesses and, rarely, with cancer of the fistulous tract.

Treatment

Abscesses need to be drained surgically. Most patients require drainage in the operating room where anesthesia allows for adequate evaluation of the extent of the disease. Abscesses that are thought to be superficial in the office examination may extend above the levators. Intersphincteric abscesses are treated by internal sphincterotomy, which drains the abscess and destroys the crypt. Perirectal and ischiorectal abscesses should be drained by a catheter or with adequate excision of skin to prevent premature closure and reaccumulation of the abscess. If the internal opening of the fistula is identified and significant external sphincter is not involved, a fistulotomy may be performed when the abscess is drained. However, the internal opening is often hard to find due to the inflammation, and drainage is all that can be achieved. In this instance, catheter drainage is preferred over skin excision, as the catheter: (1) establishes drainage with a minimal disruption of normal perianal skin, (2) facilitates identification of the internal opening at subsequent evaluation, and (3) facilitates patient compliance by eliminating the need for packing or "wicking" the wound open.

Patients with chronic or recurring abscesses after apparent adequate surgical drainage often have undrained deep postanal space abscesses that communicate with the ischiorectal fossa via a "horseshoe fistula." Treatment involves opening the deep postanal space and counter-draining the tract through the ischiorectal external opening. Once the postanal space heals, the counter drain may be removed.

Immunocompromised patients are a particular challenge. In the moderately compromised host, such as the diabetic patient, urgent drainage in the operating room is required, as they are more prone to necrotizing anorectal infections. In the severely compromised host, such as patients receiving chemotherapy, an infection may be present without an "abscess" due to neutropenia. In these patients it is important to attempt to localize the process, establish "drainage," localize the internal opening, and obtain a biopsy for tissue examination and culture (to rule out leukemia and to select antibiotics).

The treatment of fistulas is dictated by the course of the fistula. Goodsall's rule is of assistance in identifying the direction of the tract (Figure 29–4). If the tract passes superficially and does not involve sphincter muscle, then a simple incision of the tract with ablation of the gland and "saucerization" of the skin at the external opening is all that is necessary. A fistula that involves a small amount of sphincter may be treated similarly but a tract that passes deep, or that involves an undetermined amount of muscle, is best treated with a mucosal advancement flap (described in the section on rectovaginal fistulas), because immediate or delayed (as with a seton) muscle division is associated with a high rate of incontinence.

Prognosis

The prognosis for cryptoglandular abscess fistula disease is excellent, once the source of infection is

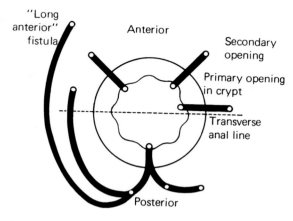

Figure 29–4. Goodsall's Rule. (Reproduced, with permission, from Russell TR: Anorectum. In: *Current Surgical Diagnosis & Treatment,* 10/e. Way LW (editor). Appleton & Lange, 1994.)

identified. Fistulas persist when the source has not been identified or adequately drained, when the diagnosis is incorrect, or when postoperative care is insufficient.

Corman ML: Anal rectal abscess and anal fistula. In: *Colon and Rectal Surgery,* 3/e. Corman ML (editor). Lippincott, 1993.

MacKeigan JM: Anal rectal abscess and fistula in ano. In: *Surgery of the Colon, Rectum, and Anus.* Mazier WP et al (editors). Saunders, 1995.

Schouten WR, van Vroonhoven TJ: Treatment of anorectal abscess with or without primary fistulectomy: Results of a prospective randomized trial. Dis Colon Rectum 1991;34:60.

Ustynoski K, Rosen L, Riether R: Horseshoe abscess fistula: Seton treatment. Dis Colon Rectum 1990;33:602.

RECTOVAGINAL FISTULA

Essentials of Diagnosis

- Passing stool and flatus via vagina.
- Altered continence.
- Tract generally visible or palpable.

General Considerations

Rectovaginal fistulas occur as a result of obstetrical injuries, Crohn's disease, diverticulitis, radiation, undrained cryptoglandular disease, foreign body trauma, surgical extirpation of anterior rectal tumors, and malignancies of the rectum, cervix, or vagina. The fistulas are classified as low, middle, or high. The location and cause of the fistula determine the operative approach.

Clinical Findings

A. Symptoms and Signs: Passing stool and flatus through the vagina is characteristic of recto-

vaginal fistulas. Patients will also note varying degrees of incontinence. An opening in the vagina or rectum may be visualized or palpated on physical examination.

B. Laboratory and Imaging Studies: A vaginogram or barium enema may identify the fistula. If the fistula is not demonstrated on radiographic or physical examination, a dilute methylene blue enema may be administered with a tampon in the vagina. If a fistula is present, it should be confirmed by the methylene blue staining of the tampon.

Differential Diagnosis

The signs and symptoms of a rectovaginal fistula are fairly unmistakable. The important differential is the cause of the fistula, as this impacts on the management, which is discussed below.

Complications

The major complication of a rectovaginal fistula is impaired hygiene and incontinence.

Treatment

Treatment of rectovaginal fistulas is determined by cause and location of the fistula. Involvement of surrounding tissue by the disease process that leads to the fistula may limit the surgical options. For example, in patients with active Crohn's disease or radiation injury in the surrounding tissue, the fistula cannot be repaired with local procedures; the Crohn's disease must go into remission prior to local repair of fistulas. Radiation injuries require that normal healthy tissues be brought from outside the irradiated field.

Low rectovaginal fistulas (rectal opening near the dentate line and vaginal opening just above the fourchette) commonly result from obstetrical injuries, trauma from foreign bodies, cryptoglandular disease, or Crohn's disease. Obstetrical injuries often heal within the first 3 months. Waiting 3 months allows inflammation to resolve, which facilitates repair and allows for closure of those fistulas that will spontaneously heal. Similarly, traumatic fistulas may be repaired most easily after inflammation resolves. Fistulas secondary to cryptoglandular disease may close spontaneously once the primary process is drained.

Fistulas secondary to Crohn's disease rarely heal spontaneously. Aggressive medical therapy and surgical control of perianal sepsis are necessary to conserve the sphincters. Once the disease is in remission, local advancement flap procedures may be performed. The principal is to bring fresh, uninvolved tissue down over the fistulous tract and excise the old rectal opening. This often delays proctectomy and preserves the rectal sphincter and rectum. Patients with severe disease that does not respond to local measures may require a temporary diverting colostomy. After diversion, a single focus of disease is often found and an advancement procedure may be performed while the fecal stream is diverted. Extensive destruction of the rectum or sphincters may mandate immediate proctectomy without attempts at local preservation. This situation may be postponed by early surgical intervention and conservative drainage or diversion.

Midrectal fistulas from cryptoglandular disease, Crohn's disease, or obstetrical injury should be treated as outlined above. Those that occur secondary to radiation are not amenable to local procedures, as the surrounding tissue is similarly effected. Transabdominal resection and coloanal anastomosis is preferred. These are particularly challenging patients. Other surgical options are beyond the scope of this chapter.

High rectal fistulas result from Crohn's disease, diverticular disease, operative injury, malignancy, and radiation. High rectovaginal fistulas are best treated via a transabdominal approach. This allows for resection of the diseased bowel that created the fistula.

Prognosis

The prognosis is determined by the cause of the fistula.

Corman ML: Anal rectal abscess and anal fistula. In: *Colon and Rectal Surgery*, 3/e. Corman ML (editor). Lippincott, 1993.

Fry RD et al: Techniques and results in the management of anal and perianal Crohn's disease. Surg Gynecol 1989;168:42.

Jacobs PP et al: Obstetric fecal incontinence: Role of pelvic floor denervation and results of delayed sphincter repair. Dis Colon Rectum 1990;33:494.

Scott NA, Nair A, Hughes LE: Anovaginal and rectovaginal fistula in patients with Crohn's disease. Br J Surg 1992;79:1379.

Senagore A: Treatment of acquired anovaginal and rectovaginal fistulas. Semin Colon Rectal Surg 1990;1:219.

Shemesh EI et al: Endorectal sliding flap repair of complicated anterior anoperineal fistulas. Dis Colon Rectum 1988;31:22.

Wise WE et al: Surgical treatment of low rectovaginal fistulas. Dis Colon Rectum 1991;34:271.

PRURITUS ANI

Essentials of Diagnosis

- Severe perianal itching, often at night.
- When chronic, skin is white, leathery, thickened.

General Considerations

Pruritus ani is usually idiopathic. Most patients have tried many over-the-counter preparations without relief. Preparations may exacerbate the problem by keeping the perineum moist, causing further irritation, or by creating a contact dermatitis (especially local anesthetics). Poor cleaning of the perineum may lead to irritation of the exquisitely sensitive anoderm and subsequent pruritus. In contrast, frequent washing with soaps and detergents dries the skin, also leading to pruritus. Pinworms (*Enterobius vermicularis*) are the most common cause of perianal itching in children.

Clinical Findings

A. Symptoms and Signs: The patient experiences severe perianal itching, often worse at night. Skin is thickened, white, and leathery in the chronic state but may be normal-to-weeping in the acute stage. In children with pinworms, perianal itching is most severe at night when the pinworm deposits its eggs on the perianal skin.

B. Laboratory and Imaging Studies: The diagnosis of pinworms is made by applying cellophane tape to the perianal skin, which collects the eggs and allows them to be viewed under a microscope. Scrapings of the perianal skin viewed microscopically may reveal fungi or parasites. Biopsy and histologic evaluation may be necessary in refractory cases to rule out underlying malignancy.

Differential Diagnosis

Pruritus may be associated with other perianal lesions that distort normal anal anatomy, such as hemorrhoids, fistulas, fissures, tumors of the anorectum, previous surgery, and radiation therapy. As noted above, it may be secondary to excessive cleaning or application of ointments in the perianal region. Presence of yeast, pinworms, or parasites should be identified. Other causes include contact dermatitis from local anesthetic creams and various soaps, primary dermatologic problems such as psoriasis, recent oral antibiotic usage, and rare perianal neoplasms, such as Bowen's or Paget's disease. Careful history and physical examination will generally reveal these causes, and any remaining patients fall under the category of idiopathic pruritus ani.

Complications

Complications include severe excoriation, ulceration, and secondary infection of the perineum.

Treatment

Identifiable causes of pruritus ani such as hemorrhoids, yeast infection, or parasites, should be treated. Patients should be educated about proper perineal care. Use of soaps and topical ointments should be discouraged. The perineum should be kept dry. Use of a blow dryer on the perineum after bathing may be helpful. Alteration in dietary habits may be necessary. Coffee, tea, cola, beer, chocolate, and tomatoes cause perianal itching and should be removed from the diet for a minimum of 2 weeks. Symptoms should resolve with alterations in dietary and cleaning habits. After resolution of symptoms, each food group may be added sequentially to identify the causative agent.

Prognosis

Relapse is common and re-education effective. In

refractory cases, dermatologic and psychiatric consultation may be necessary.

Corman ML: Cutaneous conditions. In: *Colon and Rectal Surgery,* 3/e. Corman ML (editor). Lippincott, 1993.

Graham BD: Pruritis ani. In: *Surgery of the Colon, Rectum, and Anus.* Mazier WP et al (editors). Saunders, 1995.

PROCTITIS & ANUSITIS

General Considerations

Proctitis and anusitis are general, nonspecific terms that indicate varying degrees of inflammation due to infectious or inflammatory diseases. The causative agent or event determines the symptoms, signs, and appropriate management. In considering these diseases, particular attention should be paid to sexual practices and sexually transmitted diseases. The differential diagnoses for the following diseases are the diseases discussed in this section.

1. HERPES PROCTITIS

Essentials of Diagnosis

• Painful perianal vesicles and ulcers.

Clinical Findings

A. Symptoms and Signs: Lesions appear as vesicles, which rupture to form ulcers that may become secondarily infected. Patients may present early with anal pain and vesicles or later with ulcerations, discharge, rectal bleeding, tenesmus, and even fear of defecation secondary to severe pain. Fever and generalized malaise are often noted. No history of anoreceptive intercourse is required, as the disease may spread by extension from the vagina.

B. Laboratory and Imaging Studies: The diagnosis is made by viral culture of the vesicle or biopsy of the ulcer. Herpes simplex type II is most common.

Treatment & Prognosis

Oral acyclovir is the treatment of choice but is not curative. It decreases the duration of outbreaks and viral shedding, and increases the interval between attacks. The first episode is associated with the most pain and longest duration of ulceration. Subsequent episodes are generally shorter and not as painful.

2. ANORECTAL SYPHILIS

Essentials of Diagnosis

• Asymptomatic perianal or anal ulcers (chancre).

Clinical Findings

A. Symptoms and Signs: The **chancre** is an indurated, nontender perianal ulcer at the site of inoculation. Proctitis, pseudotumors, and condylomata lata may also be present. **Condylomata lata** are contagious hypertrophic papules associated with secondary syphilis.

B. Laboratory and Imaging Studies: Dark-field microscopy of exudate and serologic testing are the preferred methods of diagnosis. Serologic tests may initially be negative and should be repeated several months later.

Treatment & Prognosis

Penicillin is the treatment of choice. Prognosis is good. Contacts must be sought and treated.

3. GONOCOCCAL PROCTITIS

Essentials of Diagnosis

• Cultures of anus, vagina, urethra, and pharynx.

Clinical Findings

A. Symptoms and Signs: Symptoms range from asymptomatic to painful defecation. Rectal bleeding and discharge, perianal excoriation, and fistulas may develop. The mucosa may appear friable and edematous.

B. Laboratory and Imaging Studies: Cultures of anus, vagina, urethra, and pharynx should be obtained and plated on a Thayer-Martin medium. The gram-negative diplococcus *Neisseria gonorrhoeae* is the causative agent.

Treatment & Prognosis

Intramuscular procaine penicillin G and oral probenecid is the treatment of choice. Follow-up examination and cultures should be performed to confirm adequate therapy. The prognosis is excellent. Resistant strains should be treated with spectinomycin.

4. CHLAMYDIA PROCTITIS & LYMPHOGRANULOMA VENEREUM

Essentials of Diagnosis

• Inguinal adenopathy.
• Small, shallow ulcer.

Clinical Findings

A. Symptoms and Signs: As in gonococcal proctitis, symptoms of chlamydia proctitis range from none to rectal pain, bleeding, and discharge. The small shallow ulcer of lymphogranuloma venereum (LGV) may be unnoticed but the inguinal adenopathy may become quite marked. Late findings include hemorrhagic proctitis and rectal stricture.

B. Laboratory and Imaging Studies: The causative agent, *Chlamydia trachomatis*, is an intracellular parasite that is spread by anal intercourse or direct extension through the lymphatics of the rectovaginal septum. The diagnosis is made with the LGV complement fixation test. Tissue cultures are also used.

Treatment & Prognosis

Treatment with 21 days of tetracycline is recommended, but erythromycin is an acceptable alternative. Early strictures may be dilated. Although uncommon, strictures may cause bowel obstruction and require colostomy.

5. CONDYLOMATA ACUMINATA

Essentials of Diagnosis

• Characteristic perianal cauliflower-appearing warts.

Clinical Findings

A. Symptoms and Signs: The most frequent complaint is that of a perianal growth. Pruritus, discharge, bleeding, odor, and anal pain are present to a lesser degree. Physical examination reveals the classic cauliflower-like lesion, which may be isolated, clustered, or coalescent. The lesions may be surprisingly large at the time of presentation.

B. Laboratory and Imaging Studies: Anoscopy and proctosigmoidoscopy are essential because the disease may extend into the anal canal. Cultures and serologic tests for other venereal diseases may be performed.

Differential Diagnosis

These lesions must be distinguished from condylomata lata, which are the lesions of secondary syphilis. The syphilitic lesions are flatter, paler, and smoother.

Complications

Squamous cell carcinoma of the anal canal (discussed below) is the major complication.

Treatment & Prognosis

The treatment is determined by the extent of the disease. Minimal disease is treated in the office with topical agents, such as bichloracetic acid or 25% podophyllin in tincture of benzoin. The former is preferred because the latter must be washed off within 4–6 hours to limit pain. Patients should be seen again at regular intervals until the treatment is complete. More extensive disease may require initial treatment under anesthesia, where random lesions may be excised for pathologic evaluation to rule out dysplasia and the remainder may be coagulated. Electrocautery coagulates the lesions. Care is taken to spare the surrounding skin. Follow-up evaluation may reveal residual disease, but this is often easily treated with topical agents in the office. Refractory disease may respond to intralesional interferon or autogenous vaccine created from excisional biopsies of the lesions. The recurrence rate is approximately 65%.

Human papilloma viruses 16 and 18 appear to be associated with squamous cell carcinoma of the anal canal. The association of anal condylomata with squamous cell carcinoma of the anus has led to new screening techniques to evaluate high-risk patients for early, not grossly visible, disease. These techniques include Pap smears and acetic-acid-assisted "colposcopy" of the anus. These techniques aid in identifying otherwise occult disease. Excisional biopsies of grossly apparent condylomata may reveal dysplasia, low-grade or high-grade intraepithelial neoplasia, or squamous cell carcinoma of the anal canal. Treatment of anal carcinoma will be discussed later.

Buschke-Löwenstein tumors are giant condylomata acuminata that are locally aggressive and exhibit malignant behavior. Radical excision is the only therapeutic option for either palliation or cure.

6. CHANCROID

Essentials of Diagnosis

• Multiple soft, painful lesions that bleed easily.

Clinical Findings

A. Symptoms and Signs: *Haemophilus ducreyi* causes a soft perianal ulcer that is painful, often multiple, and bleeds easily. Autoinoculation is common. Inguinal lymph nodes become fluctuant, rupture, and drain.

B. Laboratory and Imaging Studies: Cultures are diagnostic.

Treatment & Prognosis

Sulfonamides are the treatment of choice.

7. INFLAMMATORY PROCTITIS

General Considerations

Inflammatory proctitis is a mild form of ulcerative colitis that involves only the rectum. About 90% of the patients never develop colonic manifestations of ulcerative colitis.

Clinical Findings

A. Symptoms and Signs: Rectal bleeding, discharge, diarrhea, and tenesmus are common. The rectal mucosa is inflamed and friable but the remainder of the colon appears normal on examination.

B. Laboratory and Imaging Studies: Biopsies are taken at endoscopy to rule out infectious processes and Crohn's disease.

Differential Diagnosis

An infectious process must be ruled out before initiating steroid therapy. Distinguishing between Crohn's disease and inflammatory proctitis may be difficult. Lack of response to appropriate therapy is an indication to reassess the patient. The patient may have Crohn's disease or ulcerative colitis.

Treatment & Prognosis

Steroid retention enemas are given for 2 weeks. If patients do not respond, a short course of oral steroids may be given. In addition, 5-aminosalicylic acid (5-ASA) may be given either orally or rectally in an enema or suppository. Patients should avoid milk and milk products, fruit, and fiber. A bulk-forming agent should be added. The disease usually responds to these measures and resolves quite rapidly.

8. RADIATION PROCTITIS

Essentials of Diagnosis

• History of pelvic radiation.

Clinical Findings

A. Symptoms and Signs: Early symptoms include diarrhea, rectal bleeding, discharge, tenesmus, pain, and incontinence. Late disease may develop months to years after the injury. Symptoms of late disease are secondary to strictures, fistulas, and telangiectasias and include bleeding, changes in bowel habits, urinary tract infections, and vaginal discharge.

B. Laboratory and Imaging Studies: Endoscopy may reveal friable edematous mucosa, telangiectasias, or strictures, and may document internal openings of fistulas.

Complications

The complications are those of late disease—strictures, fistulas, and telangiectasias. These may present as recurrent urinary tract infections, vaginal discharge, fecal incontinence, rectal bleeding, changes in stool caliber, and constipation.

Treatment & Prognosis

Initial therapy includes bulk-forming agents, antidiarrheals, and antispasmodics. Topical steroids or 5-ASA preparations may be useful in early disease. Dilatation of strictures and laser coagulation of telangiectasias are the treatments of choice of late disease. Fistulas to the bladder and vagina can be particularly challenging. The key to surgical success is interposition or transposition of healthy non-irradiated tissue into the field. Only infrequently is the rectum so badly irradiated that it must be removed. Prognosis, therefore, is good.

Corman ML: Infectious and noninfectious colitides. In: *Colon and Rectal Surgery,* 3/e. Corman ML (editor). Lippincott, 1993.

Gottesman L: Anal rectal sexually transmitted diseases and anal rectal disease in AIDS. In: *Surgery of the Colon, Rectum, and Anus.* Mazier WP et al (editors). Saunders, 1995.

Palefsky JM: Human papillomavirus-associated anogenital neoplasia and other solid tumors in human immunodeficiency virus-infected individuals. Curr Opin Oncol 1991;3:881.

Palefsky JM: Human papillomavirus infection among HIV-infected individuals. Implications for development of malignant tumors. Hematol Oncol Clin North Am 1991;5:357.

Palefsky JM et al: Anal intraepithelial neoplasia and anal papillomavirus infection among homosexual males with group IV HIV disease. JAMA 1990;263:2911.

Smith LE: Sexually transmitted diseases. In: *Principals and Practices for the Colon, Rectum, and Anus.* Gordon PH, Nivatvongs S (editors). Quality Medical Publishing, 1991.

Sonnex C et al: Anal human papillomavirus infection: A comparative study of cytology, colposcopy, and DNA hybridization as methods of detection. Genitourin Med 1991;67:21.

Wexner SD: Sexually transmitted diseases of the colon, rectum, and anus: The challenge of the nineties. Dis Colon Rectum 1990;33:1048.

ANAL NEOPLASMS

TUMORS OF THE ANAL MARGIN

Prediction of the biology and planning for treatment of tumors of the perianal region is dependent on precise localization of the tumor with respect to anal landmarks, such as the dentate line, the anal verge, and the anal sphincters. Two classes of perianal neoplasms are identified by these landmarks–tumors of the anal margin and tumors of the anal canal.

The Histologic Typing of Intestinal Tumors (adopted by the World Health Organization) arbitrarily defines the **anal canal** as the area above the anal verge and the **anal margin** as the area outside the anal verge. Squamous cell tumors of the anal margin are well-differentiated, keratinizing tumors that behave similarly to squamous cell tumors of the skin elsewhere. Tumors of the anal canal are aggressive, high-grade tumors with significant risk for metastasis.

1. SQUAMOUS CELL CARCINOMA

Essentials of Diagnosis

• Rolled, everted edges, central ulceration.
• Arises in perianal skin.

Clinical Findings

A. Symptoms and Signs: Patients frequently

complain of bleeding, itching, pain, or tenesmus (complaints common to most lesions of this region). The lesions occur more commonly in men. They are centrally ulcerated with rolled, everted edges.

Treatment & Prognosis

Biopsies should be done on all chronic or nonhealing ulcers of the perineum to rule out squamous cell carcinoma. Small lesions are treated by wide local excision with a 2-cm margin. Deep lesions that involve the sphincters require an abdominoperineal resection of the rectum. Chemotherapy and radiation therapy have been used in larger lesions. Spread is to the inguinal lymph nodes and may occur in 8–40%. Inguinal dissection is reserved for palpable disease. Disease recurring in the skin may be treated with excision alone. Patients with lesions less than 5 cm have a 60–80% 5-year survival.

2. BASAL CELL CARCINOMA

Clinical Findings

A. Symptoms and Signs: Bleeding, itching, and pain are presenting symptoms. The lesions appear with raised edges and central ulceration. They are more frequent in men.

Treatment & Prognosis

As with squamous cell carcinoma of the margin, treatment is wide local excision, when possible. Deeply invasive lesions may require abdominal perineal resection. Metastasis is rare, but local recurrence rates are 30%. Local recurrences are treated with re-excision.

3. BOWEN'S DISEASE

Essentials of Diagnosis

- Intraepidermal squamous cell carcinoma.
- Associated with condylomata in young patients.

Clinical Findings

A. Symptoms and Signs: As with the lesions above, patients often complain of perianal burning, itching, or pain. Lesions are often found on routine histologic evaluation of specimens acquired at unrelated procedures. When grossly apparent, the lesions appear scaly, discrete, and erythematous.

B. Laboratory and Imaging Studies: In high-risk HIV-positive patients a Pap smear is a useful screening technique to detect evidence of intraepithelial neoplasia. If the Pap smear is positive, anal colposcopy and acetic acid "painting" may reveal "occult" condylomata with intraepithelial neoplasia.

Treatment & Prognosis

Wide local excision is the treatment of choice.

Four quadrant biopsies are necessary to establish that no residual disease persists. Skin grafts may be necessary for larger lesions. Fewer than 10% of patients develop invasive squamous cell carcinoma of the anus. Presence of an ulcer suggests invasive cancer has developed. Fewer than 3–5% of Bowen's disease patients have lymph node metastasis.

4. PAGET'S DISEASE

Essentials of Diagnosis

- Intraepithelial adenocarcinoma.
- Often associated with underlying gastrointestinal malignancy.

Clinical Findings

A. Symptoms and Signs: In contrast to the above three diseases, this disease occurs predominantly in women. Patients are usually in their seventh or eighth decade. Severe intractable pruritus is characteristic. On physical examination an erythematous, eczematoid rash is apparent. As above, biopsies of any nonhealing lesion should be taken to rule out this diagnosis.

Treatment & Prognosis

Wide local excision with multiple perianal biopsies is the treatment of choice. An abdominal perineal resection may be indicated for advanced disease. Lymph node dissection should only be done for palpable adenopathy. If metastatic disease or an underlying neoplasm exists, patients do poorly; otherwise, the prognosis is good.

TUMORS OF THE ANAL CANAL

1. EPIDERMOID (SQUAMOUS, BASOLOID, MUCOEPIDERMOID) CARCINOMA

Clinical Findings

A. Symptoms and Signs: Generally, there is a long history of minor perianal complaints, such as bleeding, itching, or perianal discomfort. A mass may or may not be associated with the above symptoms. These cancers are more common in women. Digital rectal examination and anoscopy are useful in determining depth of invasion, size, presence of perirectal nodes, and proximal extent of disease. Biopsy of the mass is done under anesthesia to confirm the diagnosis. Both groins should be palpated for gross disease.

B. Laboratory and Imaging Studies: An abdominal CT and chest radiograph are used to visualize the liver and chest for distant disease. Endorectal ultrasound can determine the depth of invasion and may identify perirectal nodes.

Treatment

Early lesions that are small, confined to the submucosa, and well differentiated may be treated with local excision, but recurrence rates are high with local excision alone. Radiation therapy or combined radiation and chemotherapy are the preferred treatment options for larger lesions of the anal canal. Nigro introduced combined therapy, which is generally preferred, but some centers use radiation therapy alone. Randomized prospective trials comparing the two are ongoing. The combined regimen varies but is based on Nigro's protocol of 30 Gy to the primary tumor, pelvic, and inguinal nodes with mitomycin C ($15mg/m^2$ intravenous bolus) on day 1 of radiation therapy and 5-fluorouracil (4-day infusion) on days 1 and 28. Failures are treated with salvage chemoradiation protocols or abdominoperineal resection.

Prognosis

About 30–40% of the patients have metastatic disease at the time of presentation. Metastatic disease is more likely with increasing depth of invasion, size, and worsening histologic grade. Distant disease is uncommon at the time of diagnosis but usually involves the liver when present. The overall survival rate is 83%. The presence of lymph nodes at the time of presentation is a bad prognostic sign.

Beahrs OH et al (editors): *Manual for Staging of Cancer,* 4/e. Lippincott, 1992.

Beck DE, Wexner SD (editors): Anal neoplasms. In: *Fundamentals of Anorectal Surgery.* McGraw-Hill, 1992.

Fenger C: Anal neoplasia and its precursors: Facts and controversies. Semin Diagn Pathol 1991;8:190.

Gordon PH: Current status—perianal and anal canal neoplasms. Dis Colon Rectum 1990;33:799.

Jass JR, Sobin LH: *Histologic Typing of Intestinal Tumors,* 2/e. Springer-Verlag, 1989.

Lopez MJ et al: Squamous cell carcinoma of the anal canal. Am J Surg 1991;162:580.

Lorenz HP et al: Squamous cell carcinoma of the anus and HIV infection. Dis Colon Rectum 1991;34:336.

Nigro ND: The force of change in the management of squamous-cell cancer of the anal canal. Dis Colon Rectum 1991;34:482.

Papillon J, Chassard JL: Respective roles of radiotherapy and surgery in the management of epidermoid carcinoma of the anal margin. Series of 57 patients. Dis Colon Rectum 1992;35:422.

Schutze WP, Gleysteen JJ: Perianal Paget's disease. Classification and review of management: Review of two cases. Dis Colon Rectum 1990;33:502.

Surawicz CM et al: Anal dysplasia in homosexual men: Role of anoscopy and biopsy. Gastroenterology 1993;105:658.

Miscellaneous Diseases of the Colon

Bret A. Lashner, MD, MPH

COLLAGENOUS & LYMPHOCYTIC COLITIS

Patients with chronic, voluminous watery diarrhea that does not improve with fasting, does not exhibit fecal leukocytes, and does not have an inordinate osmolar gap have a **secretory diarrhea.**

The most common causes of chronic secretory diarrhea are enterotoxin-mediated from *Vibrio cholerae, Escherichia coli,* or *Clostridium perfringens.* Other causes include hormone-mediated diarrhea (VIPoma, carcinoid syndrome, and medullary carcinoma of the thyroid), laxative abuse, hyperthyroidism, intestinal ischemia, amyloidosis, irritable bowel syndrome, secreting villous adenoma, and bile salt malabsorption. Collagenous and lymphocytic colitis account for up to 5% of patients with this diagnosis.

Pathophysiology

Since the clinical features, treatment, and prognosis of collagenous and lymphocytic colitis are identical, many suggest that they are different manifestations of the same disease. In fact, lymphocytic submucosal infiltration may precede collagen deposition. Still others suggest that collagenous and lymphocytic colitis patients have "malabsorption" of water and electrolytes, which represents a colonic immune response to a dietary toxin. Indeed, many of the histologic features of celiac sprue of the small bowel are shared with collagenous and lymphocytic colitis, with the inflammatory change occurring principally in the lamina propria and sparing the crypts. Submucosal collagen is deposited in one-third of sprue patients, and lymphocytic infiltration in the lamina propria is characteristic. Furthermore, collagenous colitis may develop in celiac sprue patients after successful treatment with a gluten-free diet.

Essentials of Diagnosis
- More common in females.
- Chronic watery diarrhea.
- Mucus discharge with mild steatorrhea.
- Eosinophilic bands of type III collagen and fibronectin.

General Considerations

The mean age at presentation is in the sixth decade but ranges between the third and ninth decades. Females outnumber males 10:1 in some published series. Collagenous colitis has been associated with many diseases, including rheumatoid arthritis, scleroderma, atrophic gastritis, chronic active hepatitis, primary biliary cirrhosis, hypothyroidism, hyperthyroidism, Hodgkin's disease, and non-Hodgkin's lymphoma.

Clinical Findings

A. Symptoms and Signs: The typical clinical presentation of patients with collagenous colitis is chronic watery diarrhea, usually greater than 1/2 L/d. There is acute onset of the diarrhea, but symptoms are chronic and may be intermittent. There may be mucus discharge with mild steatorrhea. Nausea, vomiting, abdominal pain, abdominal distention, flatulence, incontinence, and weight loss also are presenting features of the disease.

B. Histologic Findings: The diagnosis can be confirmed by eliminating some of the above causes of chronic secretory diarrhea, finding normal-appearing colonic mucosa at endoscopy, and finding characteristic histologic patterns. Specimens from collagenous colitis patients have a band of eosinophilic deposits under the surface epithelium that can measure 7–100 μ in thickness. This eosinophilic band is composed mostly of type III collagen and fibronectin, the usual submucosal deposits following injury or inflammation in the intestine. In contrast, normal basement membrane is less than 4 μ thick and composed mostly of type IV collagen. Patients with lymphocytic colitis, a related disorder with secretory diarrhea and a normal endoscopic appearance to the colon, have no excess eosinophilic deposits but have an excess of lymphocytes as well as plasma cells, eosinophils, and mast cells in the lamina propria. Histologic abnormalities may be limited to the proximal colon, sparing the rectum, and may be discontinuous. There are usually no crypt abscesses, granulomas, alterations of goblet cells or crypt architecture, or immune complex deposits. The intact epithelium causes no increase in intestinal permeability to dietary toxins.

Treatment & Prognosis

Collagenous and lymphocytic colitis are usually short-lived. Diarrhea may resolve, even without resolution of collagen deposition. Histologic regression of the collagen bands and improvement of diarrhea have been reported with prednisone or sulfasalazine use. Metronidazole and loperamide also can control symptoms, but histologic improvement has not been documented with these agents. There is no malignant potential and no risk of development of inflammatory bowel disease.

PNEUMATOSIS CYSTOIDES INTESTINALIS

Pneumatosis cystoides intestinalis (PCI) is characterized by the pathologic finding of air-filled cysts in the submucosa of the large or small bowel. Cysts also may be found in the stomach, mesentery, or omentum. Two clinical syndromes have been described—a fulminant process and an asymptomatic process—that have pathogenetic and therapeutic distinctions.

Essentials of Diagnosis

- Cysts may produce cramping, bleeding, and popping sound when punctured.
- On abdominal examination, tympany over abdomen, no dullness over liver.
- Common form often an incidental finding.
- Rare fulminant form associated with other diseases, especially inflammatory or ischemic bowel disease.

General Considerations

The rare fulminant form of PCI usually is associated with inflammatory or ischemic bowel disease in adults or necrotizing enterocolitis in children. Other associated diseases include graft-versus-host disease, complications from liver or kidney transplantation, cytomegalovirus colitis, and ulcerations from cancer chemotherapy. Cyst formation may occur from luminal gas entering through a disrupted mucosa or from the migration of gas-forming organisms to the subepithelial layers.

The more common form of PCI is chronic and often an incidental finding in the evaluation of unrelated complaints. Predisposing conditions for PCI include obstructive lung disease, scleroderma, nitrous oxide anesthesia, lactulose, steroids, or recent intestinal surgery. Cysts in these patients are sterile; rupture and pneumoperitoneum does not cause peritonitis. The gas in the cysts have a marginally increased concentration of hydrogen and methane and have nitrogen: oxygen ratios similar to atmospheric air. The epithe-lial-lined cysts may vary in size, be single or multiple, and do not communicate with the luminal surface.

Clinical Findings

When symptomatic, larger cysts may produce cramping abdominal pain, rectal bleeding, mucus discharge, tenesmus, change in bowel habits, or even obstruction from volvulus, cyst impaction, or intussusception.

Clues to the diagnosis include tympany throughout the abdomen, no dullness over the liver, and a popping sound when the cysts are punctured with a needle during endoscopy.

Treatment

Usually, no therapy is necessary for the common form of PCI other than treatment of the predisposing condition. Indeed, cysts may resolve spontaneously. When therapy is necessary, increasing the partial pressure of oxygen in inspired air to 200–250 mm Hg for 1–2 weeks will diffuse nitrogen in the cysts to the bloodstream, thereby reducing the size of the cysts.

COLITIS CYSTICA PROFUNDA

The presence of benign mucus-filled cysts in layers deeper than the muscularis mucosae defines **colitis cystica profunda (CCP)**. The similar entity known as **colitis cystica superficialis** has asymptomatic cystic structures superficial to the muscularis mucosae; it is a rare condition usually associated with pellagra or celiac sprue, and resolves with treatment of the underlying disease.

Essentials of Diagnosis

- Hematochezia, mucus discharge, diarrhea, pain.
- Movable mass in anterior of rectum.

General Considerations

Colitis cystica profunda (CCP) most likely represents an unusual complication from colonic mucosal inflammation or trauma. Associated conditions include solitary rectal ulcers, rectal prolapse, and chronic ulcerative colitis. Epithelial-lined cysts often are large, are few in number, and can penetrate the muscularis propria. Overlying mucosa may be ulcerated or intact. There is a proliferation of muscular elements in the lamina propria, similar to those found in the solitary rectal ulcer syndrome.

Clinical Findings

A. Symptoms and Signs: CCP typically affects men and women in their third or fourth decade. Presenting symptoms most often include hematochezia, mucus discharge, diarrhea, tenesmus, and abdominal and rectal pain. Digital examination may reveal a smooth, rubbery, movable mass in the anterior aspect of the rectum.

B. Endoscopy: Lesions appear as sessile adenomatous polyps requiring biopsy or polypectomy for confirmation of diagnosis. Polypoid lesions of the colon detected by barium enema require colonic polypectomy to differentiate CCP from an adenomatous polyp.

Differential Diagnosis

Lesions in the differential diagnosis include juvenile polyps, adenomatous polyps, adenocarcinoma, intestinal lymphoma, lipoma, leiomyoma, pseudopolyps from inflammatory bowel disease, and cysts from pneumatosis cystoides intestinalis or endometriosis.

Treatment

Colonoscopic polypectomy usually is insufficient to control symptoms. The bulky symptomatic lesions will require surgical resection. Rectal prolapse, a predisposing condition, may require surgical repair.

SOLITARY ULCERS OF THE COLON & RECTUM

Patients who present with abdominal pain and hematochezia, especially in the setting of chronic constipation, straining at stool, and rectal prolapse, may be suffering from the solitary rectal ulcer syndrome (SRUS) or, more generally, solitary ulcers of the colon and rectum. In fact, rectal ulcers account for only 5% of this clinical entity, with the remainder accounted for by ulcers in the cecum (45%), ascending colon (20%), and sigmoid (16%). SRUS affects more women than men, and the peak age range is 20–35 years old.

Pathophysiology

In the SRUS there is often evidence of colitis cystica profunda, with glands buried in the adjacent mucosa, implying a common pathogenetic mechanism for these two disorders. Both entities are believed to be caused by a reaction to chronic constipation and prolonged straining at stool, with high intrarectal pressures.

Prolapse, seen in up to 95% of SRUS patients, and self-induced trauma from manual disimpaction may lead to ulceration of the mucosa. In the SRUS, the response to ulceration is the deposition of excessive amounts of collagen and muscular fibers in the lamina propria that extend to the deeper layers past the muscularis mucosae. More proximal ulcers are most likely caused by localized trauma from prolapse of the ileocecal valve, or even a short-lived intussusception.

Essentials of Diagnosis

- Abdominal cramps or hematochezia.
- Digital rectal examination may suggest carcinoma.
- Rectal prolapse, constipation common.

Clinical Findings

The location of the ulcer determines the clinical syndrome, with more proximal ulcers causing cramping abdominal pain and more distal ulcers causing hematochezia. The ulcers are frequently multiple, between 5 mm and 5 cm, and concentrated in the anterior wall of the rectum 6–12 cm above the anal verge. Findings by digital examination of the firm tissue surrounding the ulceration can resemble carcinoma.

The diagnosis of solitary ulcers of the colon and rectum depends on endoscopic and pathologic correlation in the proper clinical setting. The pathologic findings are crucial in confirming the diagnosis. Endoscopy and defecagraphy will suggest, but not confirm, the diagnosis.

Differential Diagnosis

The differential diagnosis includes colonic ischemia, adenocarcinoma, Crohn's colitis, infectious colitis, colitis from nonsteroidal anti-inflammatory drug (NSAID) use, and stercoral ulceration.

Treatment

Treatment options for solitary ulcers of the colon and rectum are not wholly satisfactory. The use of bulking agents and stool softeners as well as counseling to avoid straining and digital manipulation are the only medical options available. Sulfasalazine, 5-aminosalicylic acid agents, corticosteroids, and sucralfate enemas are largely unsuccessful. Defecagraphy may show internal sigmoid or rectal prolapse or incomplete relaxation of the puborectalis muscle that may be amenable to surgical repair. Severely symptomatic ulcers proximal to the rectum that do not respond to bulking agents will require surgical resection.

FECAL IMPACTION & STERCORAL ULCERS

Fecal impaction is defined as a large, firm, immovable fecal mass in the rectum or colon. Fecal impactions are usually rock-hard and may be calcified and, consequently, radiopaque. Most are in the rectum, but impactions may occur in the colon when the lumen is narrowed from a malignancy or fibrous stricture.

Pathophysiology

Predisposing conditions include chronic debility, pseudo-obstruction, spinal cord injuries, diabetes, chronic renal failure, cystic fibrosis, immobility, painful anal disease (such as hemorrhoids, fissures, stricture, and cancer), chronic dehydration, and altered mental status, especially in institutionalized patients. Narcotics, anticholinergics, antihypertensives, aluminum-containing compounds such as sucralfate and antacids, and bulk-forming laxatives without sufficient hydration also may predispose to impaction.

Barium examination without adequate evacuation may cause barium concretions and impaction.

Essentials of Diagnosis

- Firm fecal mass that is palpable.
- Vague abdominal pain.
- Numerous predisposing conditions.

Clinical Findings

Clinically, patients may complain of vague abdominal pain, rectal fullness, tenesmus, anorexia, incontinence, and small amounts of watery stool, the so-called "diarrhea around a fecal impaction."

Complications

Unless promptly treated, fecal impactions eventually may lead to obstruction and possibly perforation, ureteral obstruction from local compression, sigmoid volvulus, rectal prolapse, and perirectal fistulae.

Fecal impactions are also involved in the pathogenesis of **stercoral ulceration,** which are rectal ulcers from pressure necrosis. These ulcers have been dubbed the "decubitus ulcers" of the rectum and usually are irregular in appearance, conforming to the shape of the fecal mass. There is minimal inflammation surrounding this ulceration, but ischemic injury to the deeper layers makes localized perforation relatively common. Patients with stercoral ulceration often present with hematochezia, fever, and localized tenderness. Free peritoneal air from perforation is rare. In the proper clinical setting, the diagnosis is confirmed by a digital examination.

Treatment

Fecal impaction and stercoral ulceration can be prevented by recognizing the predisposing conditions and intervening in high-risk patients. Preventive intervention includes adequate hydration, bulk-forming agents, periodic enemas, judicious laxative use, and frequent rectal examinations. Once formed, fecal impactions usually require manual fracture of the mass with tap water enemas to assist expulsion. Oral laxatives or mineral oil may be helpful once manual disimpaction has been performed. A local anesthetic may be required to assist with anal relaxation during the disimpaction process.

DIVERSION COLITIS

Diversion colitis—also known as bypass colitis, exclusion colitis, and disuse colitis—is characterized by the occurrence of inflammation in a segment of colon surgically diverted from the fecal stream that completely resolves with re-anastomosis. With the possible exception of Crohn's colitis, there is no evidence of inflammation in the affected distal segment prior to surgery.

Pathophysiology

The pathogenesis of diversion colitis has been purported to include stasis of enteric secretions, colonization from pathogenic bacteria, and loss of luminal nutrients. Recent work has documented loss of luminal nutrients as the most important factor. Because saline enemas are ineffective treatment for diversion colitis, stasis of toxic material is an unlikely cause. Colonization of bacteria also appears unlikely. The anaerobic bacteria count in the diverted colon drops by a factor of 100 after surgery. Even antibiotic treatment designed to restore presurgical proportions of bacterial species do not improve findings. However, replacement of luminal nutrients markedly improves symptoms and findings, making this the most likely cause.

Colonocytes are nourished from the bloodstream as well as from luminal contents. Nonabsorbed carbohydrates are metabolized by colonic flora to synthesize, among other compounds, short-chain fatty acids (SCFAs). In vitro studies indicate that these SCFAs are preferred over glucose or ketone bodies as a metabolic substrate. The most favored nutrient source for colonocytes is butyrate, but propionate and acetate also are used efficiently. Blood concentrations of SCFAs are negligible. From a normal diet in an intact colon, 100–200 mM/L of SCFAs are delivered into the colon; a diverted segment has less than 5 mM/L. The preference of colonocytes for SCFAs increases aborally, making privations worse in diverted distal colonic segments. In laboratory animals, metabolic inhibition of the utilization of SCFAs induces a colitis similar to diversion colitis in humans.

Essentials of Diagnosis

- A complication of bowel bypass surgery.
- Blood and mucus discharge from 1 month to 3 years later.
- Pain and fever, or asymptomatic.

Clinical Findings

A. Symptoms and Signs: Affected persons develop a blood and mucus discharge from the rectum or mucus fistula as early as 1 month after surgery but symptoms may develop up to 3 years after diversion. There also may be pelvic pain, fever, and anal irritation, although asymptomatic disease is not rare.

B. Endoscopy and Histology: Even though clinical symptoms are not universal, pathologic or endoscopic evidence of colitis usually is present. Changes are more evident in the most distal segments. Histologic findings include mucin depletion, mucosal edema, decreased number and depth of crypts, superficial ulcerations, expansion of cellular elements of the lamina propria, granulocyte infiltration, and fibrosis of the lamina propria. The endoscopic appearance of a diverted segment may show narrowing, erythema, ulceration, friability, exudate, or a distorted mucosal vascular pattern.

Treatment

Palliation is best achieved with twice-daily 60-ml SCFA enemas delivered into the diverted segment; this procedure completely resolves symptoms and evidence of endoscopic or histologic inflammation. Such a dramatic response is not typical with corticosteroid or 5-aminosalicylic acid enemas. SCFA enemas can be manufactured by a local pharmacy or laboratory. One formulation that works well is a combination of 60 mM acetate, 30 mM propionate, and 40 mM butyrate with sufficient sodium chloride and sodium hydroxide to bring the osmolality to 280 mosm and the pH to 7.0. Success also has been achieved with 100 mM butyrate enemas at the same osmolality and pH.

The best curative therapy for diversion colitis is re-anastomosis. Even in the face of mucosal inflammation in a patient with Crohn's colitis, surgery should proceed if indicated. In a symptomatic patient who cannot be re-anastomosed, twice-daily SCFA enemas should provide adequate treatment within 6 weeks, usually by 3 weeks. Enemas given daily or even every other day can be used to maintain remission until re-anastomosis becomes a feasible option.

DRUG-INDUCED COLITIS

Mucosal inflammation of the colon is a rare adverse effect of some commonly used medications. Oral contraceptives and NSAIDs, especially, may simulate inflammatory bowel disease symptoms and endoscopic appearance. Even if the incidence of colitis is exceedingly low, the widespread use of these medications makes drug-induced colitis potentially a more important problem than inflammatory bowel disease.

Pathophysiology

The pathogenesis of colitis from oral contraceptives is unknown but is believed to be a result of an occlusive vascular phenomenon. The leading theory regarding the development of NSAID-induced colitis involves cyclo-oxygenase inhibition and the loss of cytoprotective prostaglandins.

Other medications that may cause a drug-induced colitis include methyldopa, penicillamine, potassium supplements, 5-fluorouracil, oral gold, and isoretinoin.

Essentials of Diagnosis

- With oral contraception use, mimics Crohn's colitis: chronic diarrhea, aphthoid ulcers.
- With NSAID use, mimics ulcerative colitis: bleeding, diarrhea, and superficial ulcers.
- Symptoms resolve when drugs discontinued.

General Considerations

The distinction between drug-induced colitis and idiopathic inflammatory bowel disease is important, because drug-induced colitis is usually treated with withdrawal of the medication whereas inflammatory bowel disease often requires the institution of potentially toxic medications.

Clinical Findings

The colitis from oral contraceptives can be indistinguishable from Crohn's colitis. Patients present with chronic diarrhea and aphthoid ulcers scattered throughout the colon. Symptoms and signs of oral contraceptive colitis completely resolve without sequelae upon discontinuation of the agents. The colitis from oral NSAID use mimics ulcerative colitis. The inflammation is diffuse with superficial ulcers, and patients most often present with bleeding and diarrhea. The distinction between inflammatory bowel disease and NSAID-induced colitis is further complicated by the fact that arthritis, a condition usually treated with NSAIDs, is common to both diseases. An older patient with arthritis who develops symptoms and signs suggestive of ulcerative colitis certainly should have drug-induced colitis ruled out before being diagnosed as having inflammatory bowel disease; this is done by observing symptoms after NSAIDs are discontinued. NSAID-induced colitis should completely resolve. NSAIDs also may induce a flare of ulcerative colitis in remission.

Diagnosis

Observing resolution of symptoms with the withdrawal of medications and ruling out inflammatory bowel disease from the differential diagnosis are the key diagnostic elements.

Complications

Besides bleeding and diarrhea, severe complications include stricture from submucosal fibrosis and perforation from deep ulceration. Diaphragmatic-like narrowing from fibrosis has been reported in the small bowel but similar lesions have not been reported in the colon.

Treatment

Withdrawal of the offending agent is the only effective therapy.

RADIATION COLITIS

It is estimated that one-half of patients diagnosed with cancer will receive radiation therapy. In previous years, the dose-limiting organ was the skin. Now, with newer concentrating techniques, toxicity to the gastrointestinal tract limits the dose. Radiation colitis occurs in approximately 5–10% of patients receiving therapy. The malignancies most likely to result in radiation colitis are transitional cell carcinoma of the bladder, squamous cell carcinoma of the cervix, endometrial cancer, and adenocarcinoma of the prostate or rectum.

Pathophysiology

Radiation colitis is dependent on the port, total dose, dose rate (fractionation), and type of energy (photon, neutron, or alpha particle). Cell death is exponentially related to the total dose, and rapid delivery is more lethal than slower delivery in fractions. Radiation causes molecules in the path of the beam to ionize and thereby damage living cells. Nuclear DNA is the prime target, resulting in either immediate cell death or loss of reproduction/division capacity. Most damage is done in the mitotic phase or late second rest phase (M or G2 phase) of the cell cycle. Cell function may be altered by damage to cell membrane proteins.

Early toxicity from radiation therapy is caused by injury to the crypt cells of the epithelium, whereas late injury is caused by damage to the vascular endothelium and connective tissue. The presence of early symptoms does not correlate with the development of late symptoms. Delivery of 6,000 rads to the region of the colon or 8,000 rads to the region of the rectum will induce early or late radiation colitis, or both, in approximately 50% of patients. There is a narrow margin of safety, since these doses are close to what is required for treatment of the tumor.

Essentials of Diagnosis

- Early disease: diarrhea, hematochezia occurring within first month after radiation therapy.
- Late disease: abdominal pain, diarrhea usually within 5 years of treatment but still possible years later.

EARLY RADIATION COLITIS

Clinical Findings

A.   Symptoms and Signs: Early radiation colitis usually occurs within the first month of therapy. Because the epithelium is disrupted, the most common symptoms are diarrhea and hematochezia. Tenesmus and mucus discharge also are common complaints.

B.   Endoscopy: Endoscopically, the mucosa will appear edematous with a loss of mucosal vascular pattern. There will be friability and superficial ulcerations, similar findings to ulcerative colitis. Involvement will be limited to the radiation port and will not necessarily be continuous, as it is in ulcerative colitis patients.

C.   Laboratory Findings: Histologic findings include a decrease in the height of the epithelial cells, mucin depletion, ulceration, and crypt abscesses. Anterior rectal ulcerations, luminal narrowing, radio-

logic "thumbprinting," and loss of haustrations are further radiologic signs of early toxicity.

Treatment

Successful symptomatic treatment of early toxicity includes antispasmodics, antidiarrheals, bulking agents, and topical anesthetics. Steroid enemas are of moderate benefit but 5-aminosalicylic acid agents are of no help.

Attempts to prevent or to minimize the risk of developing early radiation injury include surgical fixation of bowel away from the anticipated port and administration of free radical scavengers, such as diallyl sulfide (garlic), or cyclo-oxygenase inhibitors, such as aspirin.

LATE RADIATION COLITIS

Clinical Findings

A.   Symptoms and Signs: Late injury from radiation therapy usually occurs within 5 years but may be first manifest several decades after therapy. Symptoms are insidious and progressive and are related to changes in the submucosal layers. The most common presenting complaints are abdominal pain and diarrhea referable to the development of fibrous strictures and partial obstruction. Fistulas, perforation, and impaired motility also may occur. Patients also may present with proctitis, tenesmus, mucous discharge, change in stool caliber, and hematochezia.

B.   Endoscopy: Telangiectasias, granularity, friability, discrete ulcers in the anterior rectum, and strictures are commonly found on endoscopy.

C.   Laboratory Findings: In late radiation injury, histologic findings resembles ischemia, with submucosal fibrosis, telangiectasias of small vessels, hyalinized endothelium of larger blood vessel walls, fistulas, and fissures.

Treatment

Treatment of late complications of radiation therapy is not satisfactory. Steroid enemas or other forms of medical therapy are of marginal benefit. Nd:YAG laser or bipolar electrocoagulation of bleeding telangiectasias may help. Sometimes strictures can be dilated manually or with endoscopically-placed balloon dilators. Because of the brittle nature of radiated bowel, perforation is a frequent complication of bowel dilation. Surgery for obstruction, bleeding, fistulas, or perforation should be considered high-risk, since there often is delayed healing of the wound and surgical anastomosis.

FOREIGN BODIES OF THE RECTUM & COLON

Foreign bodies in the rectum and colon may occur from a variety of circumstances, ranging from the accidental to criminal assault. Oral ingestion of smaller objects able to traverse the ileocecal valve, anal eroticism, and voluntary rectal insertion are other methods of entry of foreign bodies into the large bowel. Because of both a narrower pelvis that more easily leads to impaction and male homosexual eroticism, men more commonly present with foreign bodies than do women.

Clinical Findings

There are no specific signs or symptoms. Findings are directly related to the size and type of the foreign body.

Diagnosis & Treatment

With a history, physical examination, and biplane x-ray, the clinician usually can identify the foreign body and assess the advisability of removal in the outpatient setting. Low-lying objects are palpable and usually are situated in the ampulla. Their extraction is more difficult than was their insertion because of the presence of spasm, blood, or edema either from the object or from previous efforts at removal. The object usually can be removed with sedation and a local anesthetic through an anoscope with snare, forceps, or uterine tenaculum. Enemas should be avoided, since objects may be pushed out of reach, and blind removal should not be attempted. Anal dilation under general anesthesia with transanal removal usually is required for larger objects.

High-lying objects are not palpable on digital examination. Most will descend within 24 hours with sedation. Bimanual manipulation under general anesthesia may be required. If laparotomy is necessary, the surgeon often may manipulate the object to the rectum and remove it transanally, thereby avoiding a colotomy on the unprepared colon. High-lying objects in the colon that have been swallowed are thin enough to traverse proximal areas of physiologic narrowing, and will usually pass within 48 hours on a high-fiber diet. Sharp objects may become impacted and perforate or bleed, making laparotomy necessary.

REFERENCES

Bjarnason I et al: Nonsteroidal anti-inflammatory drug-induced intestinal inflammation in humans. Gastroenterology 1987;93:480.

Davila M, McQuaid K: Management of rectal foreign bodies. In: *Consultations in Gastroenterology.* Snape W (editor). Saunders, 1994 (in press).

Ernest DL, Trier JS: Radiation enteritis and colitis. In: *Gastrointestinal Disease,* 5/e. Sleisenger MH, Fordtran JS (editors). Saunders, 1993.

Galandiuk S, Fazio V: Pneumatosis cystoides intestinalis: A review of the literature. Dis Colon Rectum 1986;29:358.

Guest CB, Reznick RK: Colitis cystica profunda: Review of the literature. Dis Colon Rectum 1989;32:983.

Harig JM et al: Treatment of diversion colitis with short-chain fatty acid irrigation. N Engl J Med 1989;320:23.

Stampfl DA, Friedman LS: Collagenous colitis: Pathophysiologic considerations. Dig Dis Sci 1991;36:705.

Womack NR et al: Pressure and prolapse—the cause of solitary rectal ulceration. Gut 1987;28:1228.

Wrenn J: Fecal impaction. N Engl J Med 1989;321:658.

Section V
Diseases of the Pancreas

Acute Pancreatitis

31

James H. Grendell, MD

Acute pancreatitis is an acute inflammatory process of the pancreas, with variable involvement of peripancreatic tissue or remote organ systems. It ranges in severity from a mild self-limited disease to a catastrophic one with multiple severe complications and the risk of death.

GENERAL CONSIDERATIONS

Gallstone disease and excessive alcohol use account for 70–80% of cases of acute pancreatitis in industrialized countries. Other important but less common causes include genetic hyperlipidemia (serum triglyceride levels typically > 1000 mg/dL at the time of hospital admission for symptoms of pancreatitis), chronic hypercalcemia, surgery, abdominal trauma (blunt or penetrating), endoscopic retrograde cholangiopancreatography (ERCP), infection (eg, ascariasis, clonorchiasis, mumps, cytomegalovirus infection), and a variety of drugs (eg, azathioprine, mercaptopurine, didanosine, pentamidine, sulfonamides, 5-aminosalicylates). Pancreatic cancers and ampullary tumors can infrequently present as acute pancreatitis. Table 31–1 lists some of the causes of acute pancreatitis.

Patients with acquired immunodeficiency syndrome (AIDS) have an increased incidence of acute pancreatitis. In part, this is due to infections involving pancreatic tissue (eg, cryptosporidiosis, cryptococcosis, or infection with cytomegalovirus, *Mycobacterium tuberculosis*, or *Mycobacterium avium* complex) and in part to use of medications (eg, didanosine, pentamidine, trimethoprim-sulfamethoxazole). In these patients, serum amylase concentrations are also frequently elevated in the absence of evidence of pancreatitis; this may be due to abnormalities in renal tubular function and increases in the salivary isoamylase fraction of total serum amylase.

Although most series classify 10–30% of patients as having idiopathic acute pancreatitis, recent reports suggest that occult gallstones (biliary microlithiasis

or gallbladder sludge) can be demonstrated in 50–75% of these patients by microscopic examination of the bile or duodenal juice or by repeated abdominal ultrasound examinations. Treatments directed at gallstone disease (eg, cholecystectomy, endoscopic sphincterotomy, ursodeoxycholic acid therapy) appear to reduce the likelihood of recurrent pancreatitis in these patients.

Gallstone disease results in acute pancreatitis when a stone (usually only a few millimeters in diameter) migrates from the gallbladder into the common bile duct and reaches the duodenal papilla. This may lead to a sudden increase in pressure in the pancreatic duct, resulting in a "secretory block" of digestive enzymes at the level of the acinar (enzyme-secreting) cell, or may lead to reflux of bile or duodenal juice into the pancreatic duct.

The mechanism by which acute pancreatitis is induced by causative factors other than gallstone disease and direct trauma remains unknown. Experimental studies and some clinical observations suggest that development of a secretory block may be a common feature of acute pancreatitis, whatever the cause.

Identification of Occult Causes of Acute Pancreatitis

In most patients, the cause of acute pancreatitis will be identified by an initial evaluation consisting of history taking (looking for excessive alcohol use, medications, previous episodes of gallstone disease), physical examination, determination on admission of serum triglyceride and calcium concentrations, and abdominal ultrasound (or, previously, oral cholecystography). In most series, however, 10–30% of patients have been considered to have "idiopathic" acute pancreatitis.

Several recent reports suggest that about one-half of these patients have occult gallstone disease (eg, microlithiasis, biliary sludge), which is best identified by examination of bile for cholesterol and calcium bilirubinate crystals or by repeated abdominal

Table 31–1. Major causes of acute pancreatitis.

Gallstone disease
Chronic excessive alcohol use
Drugs (eg, azathioprine, mercaptopurine, didanosine,
    pentamidine, sulfonamides, salicylates, valproic acid,
    furosemide, methyldopa)
Infections (eg, ascariasis, clonorchiasis, mumps,
    coxsackievirus, cytomegalovirus, tuberculosis, *M avium*
    complex)
Blunt or penetrating abdominal trauma
Surgery
ERCP
Genetic hypertriglyceridemia
Chronic hypercalcemia
Pancreatic or ampullary tumors
Sphincter of Oddi dysfunction
Duodenal disease (eg, peptic ulcer, Crohn's disease,
    periampullary diverticula)
Toxins (eg, organophosphate insecticides, scorpion venom)
Pancreas divisum
Vasculitis (eg, polyarteritis nodosum, systemic lupus
    erythematosus, thrombotic thrombocytopenic purpura)
Cystic fibrosis
Hereditary disease
Idiopathic disease

ultrasound examinations. Additionally, genetic hyperlipidemia is frequently missed because serum triglycerides are not measured until after the patient has been fasting for several days, by which time triglyceride levels may have fallen substantially.

The more common identifiable causes of "idiopathic" acute pancreatitis and the means of diagnosing them are given in Table 31–2.

PATHOPHYSIOLOGY

Acute pancreatitis is believed to begin as an autodigestive process within the gland as a result of premature activation of zymogens (digestive enzyme precursors) within the pancreatic secretory (acinar) cells, duct system, or interstitial space. This results in acinar cell damage and necrosis, edema, and inflammation. In addition to digestive enzyme activation, oxidative stress and impaired microcirculation of blood in the pancreas may also be important contributors to pancreatic injury.

Extension of this inflammatory process beyond the pancreas frequently leads to localized complications (Table 31–3) and can result in a variety of systemic complications (Table 31–4).

In about 75% of patients, the inflammatory process is self-limited, involving only the pancreas and immediate peripancreatic tissue and resolving spontaneously in a few days to a week. In the other 25%, a severe course ensues, with multiple localized and systemic complications, prolonged hospitalization, and risk of death. The overall mortality rate for hospitalized patients with acute pancreatitis is 5–10%.

CLINICAL FINDINGS

Symptoms & Signs

Abdominal pain is the cardinal manifestation of acute pancreatitis, present in about 95% of patients. Pain is epigastric and radiates to the back in one-half to two-thirds of patients. Nausea, vomiting, and abdominal distention are also frequent symptoms.

On examination, abdominal tenderness is usually present, along with guarding and rebound tenderness in more severe cases. Depending on the severity of the disease, patients may also exhibit fever, tachycardia, tachypnea, and hypotension.

Laboratory Findings

Because the history and physical findings are nonspecific, confirmation by laboratory tests or abdominal imaging is necessary. The serum amylase concentration is increased in 80–85% of patients with

Table 31–2. Possible occult causes of acute pancreatitis.

Cause	Useful Diagnostic Tests
Occult gallstone disease (negative abdominal sonogram)	Biliary drainage for crystal analysis Repeated abdominal sonograms ERCP
Undiagnosed hypertriglyceridemia	Previous serum triglyceride concentration, if available Serum triglyceride determination *after* patient is placed on regular diet and medications
Abnormalities of bile and pancreatic ducts	ERCP
Sphincter of Oddi dysfunction	ERCP Sphincter of Oddi manometry
Pancreatic cancer, ampullary and other tumors	CT scanning and fine-needle aspiration biopsy of suspicious areas ERCP Serial determination of CA 19-9 levels
Cystic fibrosis	Measurement of sweat chloride Genetic testing

Table 31–3. Local complications of acute pancreatitis.

Pancreatic complications
  Phlegmon (inflammatory mass)
  Peripancreatic effusions
  Infected necrosis or pancreatic abscess
Nonpancreatic complications
  Gastrointestinal ileus
  Pancreatic ascites and pleural effusions
  Bile duct obstruction

acute pancreatitis but in only 65–70% with pancreatitis resulting from alcohol use. Amylase levels may also be elevated in a variety of conditions that can mimic acute pancreatitis (eg, cholangitis, gastrointestinal perforation or ischemia, ruptured ectopic pregnancy), as well as in salivary gland disease and acute or chronic renal failure. Serum lipase determination, at least by some methods, is as sensitive as amylase determinations but has greater specificity, and lipase levels may remain elevated longer than amylase levels. Measurement in serum or urine of other pancreatic enzymes (eg, trypsin, elastase) or amylase isoenzymes has not proved useful.

Because serum amylase levels tend to be lower in alcoholic acute pancreatitis than in other forms (particularly gallstone-induced disease), whereas lipase levels are about the same in all forms, an elevated lipase to amylase ratio has been proposed as an indicator of alcohol-induced disease. The optimal discriminant value for the ratio differs in various studies, however, and substantial overlapping diminishes the usefulness of this ratio. A threefold or greater increase in measurements of alanine aminotransferase (ALT) is suggestive of gallstones as the cause for acute pancreatitis.

Table 31–4. Systemic complications of acute pancreatitis.

Cardiovascular complications
  Hypovolemia
  Hypotension or shock
Renal complications
  Oliguria
  Azotemia or renal failure
Hematologic complications
  Vascular thrombosis
  Disseminated intravascular coagulation
Pulmonary complications
  Hypoxemia
  Atelectasis or pleural effusion
  ARDS or respiratory failure
Metabolic complications
  Hypocalcemia
  Hyperglycemia
  Hypertriglyceridemia
  Metabolic acidosis
Gastrointestinal bleeding
  Stress gastritis
  Pseudoaneurysm
  Gastric varices
Other complications
  Peripheral fat necrosis
  Encephalopathy

Imaging Studies

Abdominal imaging, particularly CT scanning, has made the greatest contribution to the accurate diagnosis of acute pancreatitis and many of its complications. Abdominal ultrasound is useful in determining whether gallstone disease may be the cause of an episode of acute pancreatitis; however, the sensitivity of this modality in diagnosing acute pancreatitis is relatively low, and examinations are frequently technically inadequate in patients with significant ileus. CT scans may be normal in 15–30% of patients with mild acute pancreatitis but are virtually always abnormal in moderate to severe attacks (Figure 31–1). Thus, CT scanning is the most useful means of differentiating severe acute pancreatitis from other intra-abdominal catastrophic processes that may mimic pancreatitis.

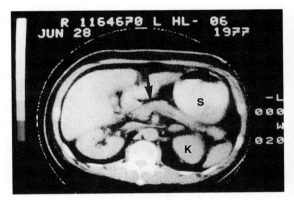

A

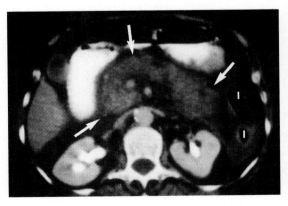

B

Figure 31–1. **A:** The normal pancreas on computed tomography. The gland **(arrows)** is homogeneous in appearance and, like the adjacent stomach **(S)** and left kidney **(K)**, sharply demarcated. **B:** The pancreas on computed tomography in acute pancreatitis **(arrows)** is enlarged and inhomogeneous because of edema and inflammation. In addition, inflammatory changes have increased the density of the tissue surrounding loops of intestine **(I)** near the tail of the pancreas.

So far, magnetic resonance imaging (MRI) has not improved upon CT scanning as a diagnostic technique for pancreatic inflammatory disease, but it may be useful in evaluating patients unable to receive intravenous contrast medium for CT scanning.

Criteria for Assessing the Severity of Acute Pancreatitis

Extensive efforts have been devoted to establishing a method for predicting the severity of acute pancreatitis, so that the approximately 75% of patients who will have a relatively mild course can be differentiated from those destined for serious illness and death (Table 31–5).

Ranson's criteria have been the prognostic indicator most commonly used in the United States (Table 31–6). Patients with two or fewer risk factors have a low probability of serious illness or death; with three or more risk factors, both of these probabilities increase, and they continue to increase as the number of risk factors increases.

The modified Glasgow (Imrie) criteria are similar to Ranson's criteria and have been used extensively in the United Kingdom. Neither the Ranson nor the Glasgow score can be computed until the patient has been hospitalized for 48 hours, and neither can be used to follow the patient's course after that point. The Acute Physiologic and Chronic Health Evaluation (APACHE) II system is a complex scoring system that can be calculated prior to 48 hours of hospitalization and then recalculated throughout the course of hospitalization to measure progress. The Ranson and Glasgow criteria and APACHE II scoring system are similar in their abilities to predict the severity of disease at 48 hours of hospitalization. CT scanning is just as accurate but is costly (if done only to estimate prognosis) and associated with the risk of renal toxicity from intravenous contrast medium. The other predictors listed in Table 31–5 have not been as extensively validated as these three scoring methods or CT scanning.

Table 31–5. Predictors of severity in acute pancreatitis.

Multiple clinical criteria
  Ranson's criteria
  Glasgow (Imrie) criteria
  APACHE II
  Multiple-organ failure score
CT scanning criteria
  Anatomic findings
  Bolus contrast (dynamic pancreatography)
MRI
Abdominal paracentesis
Individual laboratory tests
  Methemalbumin
  Phospholipase A_2
  C-reactive protein
  Granulocyte elastase
  Interleukin-6
  Trypsinogen activation peptide

Table 31–6. Ranson's criteria of severity.

Gallstone pancreatitis
  On admission to hospital:
    Age > 70 years
    WBC > 18,000/μL
    Glucose > 220 mg/dL
    Lactate dehydrogenase > 400 U/L
    AST > 250 U/L
  Within 48 hours of hospital admission:
    Decrease in hematocrit > 10 points
    Increase in blood urea nitrogen > 2 mg/dL
    Serum calcium < 8 mg/dL
    Base deficit > 5 mmol/L
    Fluid deficit > 4 L
Pancreatitis due to causes other than gallstones
  On admission to hospital:
    Age > 55 years
    WBC > 16,000/μL
    Glucose > 200 mg/dL
    Lactate dehydrogenase > 350 U/L
    AST > 250 U/L
  Within 48 hours of hospital admission:
    Decrease in hematocrit > 10 points
    Increase in blood urea nitrogen > 5 mg/dL
    Calcium < 8 mg/dL
    PaO_2 < 60 mm Hg
    Base deficit > 4 mmol/L
    Fluid deficit > 6 L

Although several of these predictors function reasonably well (particularly APACHE II) in defining or stratifying patient populations for clinical research, none so far is clearly superior to close observation and careful clinical judgment as a basis for making therapeutic decisions for an individual patient.

TREATMENT

The goals of therapy of acute pancreatitis are to provide supportive care; decrease pancreatic inflammation and its results; and prevent, identify, and treat complications.

Mild Acute Pancreatitis

Most patients will have a mild, self-limited course requiring only bed rest, no oral intake, intravenous hydration and electrolytes, and analgesia. Traditionally, meperidine has been the analgesic of choice because of reports that it is less likely than other opiates to raise the sphincter of Oddi pressure. The clinical importance of this is uncertain, however, and other narcotics can be substituted if needed. Nasogastric suction does not shorten the course of the disease but is useful in relieving symptoms of nausea, vomiting, or abdominal distention. Patients may be cautiously fed once abdominal pain has mostly abated, nausea (if present) has resolved, and serum amylase or lipase values have begun to return to normal.

Severe Acute Pancreatitis

A. Early Management: Care of the patient with severe pancreatitis poses a much greater challenge. In the earliest stages, vigorous resuscitation with intravenous hydration and electrolytes is critical. Volume requirements may be staggeringly large, and these patients will frequently require an intensive care unit setting, with careful attention to monitoring of hemodynamics, urine output, and renal and respiratory function. Acute renal failure may require dialysis, and respiratory failure (due to adult respiratory distress syndrome) may necessitate mechanical ventilation. The presence of renal or respiratory failure markedly increases mortality rates; however, both complications are reversible if the underlying pancreatic inflammation abates and other complications (eg, sepsis) do not supervene. Large amounts of intravenous analgesics are frequently needed for pain and nasogastric suction for severe ileus, nausea, and vomiting.

A number of pharmacologic agents have been tried to inactivate proteases (eg, aprotinin, gabexate), decrease pancreatic secretion (eg, atropine, somatostatin), or reduce inflammation (eg, indomethacin). None of these has been shown to be beneficial in good controlled studies, however. Additionally, the efficacy of peritoneal lavage and early operative approaches (eg, "necrosectomy," débridement and drainage) in the absence of documented infection remains to be demonstrated.

B. Management of Gallstones: Several recent randomized controlled studies have examined the value of ERCP with sphincterectomy and stone extraction, if indicated, in diminishing the severity of presumed gallstone pancreatitis. Gallstones should be suspected as the cause of acute pancreatitis in high-incidence areas (eg, Hong Kong) and in patients who abstain from alcohol or use it moderately, are of female gender, are over 60 years of age, have a greater than threefold elevation in ALT levels, or have a history of gallstones or a dilated common bile duct visualized on abdominal ultrasound or CT scanning. Patients with moderate to severe presumed gallstone pancreatitis should undergo ERCP if they have not improved following 24–36 hours of vigorous supportive care or if cholangitis is suspected on the basis of right upper quadrant pain or fever (> 39.5 °C) or a white blood cell count (> 20,000/μL) that is unusually high for pancreatitis alone. In Western societies, cholangitis complicates acute gallstone pancreatitis in less than 10% of cases.

C. Management of Infected Necrosis or Abscess: Patients with moderate to severe acute pancreatitis are at risk for lethal septic complications resulting from infected necrosis or abscess, usually presenting a week or more after admission to the hospital as clinical deterioration (eg, worsening pain or nausea and vomiting), fever (especially if > 39.5 °C), or leukocytosis (especially if > 20,000/μL). Early studies of attempts to prevent infected necrosis or abscess by prophylactic administration of antibiotics failed to show a benefit; however, the patients studied were on the milder end of the spectrum of severity, and the antibiotics used were later shown not to penetrate inflamed pancreatic tissue well. In two recent small studies of imipenem and of ofloxacin and metronidazole, all of which may reach significant blood levels in pancreatic tissue, there were some beneficial effects but no clear improvement in survival rates. The results of further studies will be required to determine whether prophylactic antibiotics should be used.

Although the value of prophylactic antibiotics is currently uncertain, over the past 20 years the earlier diagnosis and aggressive treatment of pancreatic infected necrosis and abscess has resulted in a reduction in mortality rates for this complication, from 70–80% to 10–20%. This has resulted from the widespread use of CT scanning in the early evaluation of patients with suspected infected necrosis or abscess. Suspicious (low-density) areas in the pancreas or fluid collections adjacent to it should be aspirated and material sent for culture and, most importantly, immediate preparation of gram-stained smears. The presence of both bacterial organisms and polymorphonuclear white blood cells (PMNs) on gram-stained smear is strongly indicative of infected necrosis or abscess, and patients with this finding should undergo emergency operation, with extensive débridement and drainage. Because of the viscous nature of the infected material and the frequent presence of loculations, percutaneous catheter drainage is usually inadequate for treatment of infected necrosis.

Needle aspiration in the evaluation of suspected infected necrosis or abscess is safe and highly reliable if adequate sampling has been achieved. The presence in aspirates of PMNs without bacterial organisms indicates a sterile necrotizing process. Operative débridement and drainage are sometimes performed in patients with sterile necrosis because of failure to improve (eg, persisting multiple-organ failure); however, the benefits of these procedures are unclear.

D. Nutritional Management: Care should be taken not to resume feeding by mouth too early in patients with severe acute pancreatitis or major complications (eg, organ failure, sepsis), as this may lead to further exacerbation of the disease. Such patients should receive either total parenteral nutrition or enteral tube feedings (preferably of an elemental diet delivered to the distal jejunum to diminish pancreatic stimulation) until any complications have been effectively treated and the patient is free of pain and nausea and has normal serum amylase and lipase concentrations. At the time of operative débridement and drainage of infected necrosis or abscess, surgical placement of a tube jejunostomy greatly facilitates subsequent nutritional management.

Management of Pseudocysts & Hemorrhage

As many as two-thirds to three-fourths of patients with acute pancreatitis will have fluid collections (peripancreatic effusions) demonstrated early in their illness by abdominal ultrasound or CT scanning. Most of these will resolve spontaneously. Only about 15% of patients with acute pancreatitis develop an encapsulated collection of inflammatory fluid and pancreatic juice (**pseudocyst**). If asymptomatic or mildly symptomatic (eg, mild pain), pseudocysts should be followed by ultrasound studies or CT scanning for at least 6 weeks to see if they will resolve or decrease in size without treatment. Asymptomatic pseudocysts less than 5–6 cm in diameter can be watched without treatment indefinitely.

Pseudocysts larger than 6 cm in diameter and persisting for more than 6 weeks after an episode of acute pancreatitis should be considered for therapy. The standard definitive treatment has been open internal surgical drainage of the cyst into the stomach, duodenum, or a Roux loop of jejunum. Other techniques currently being evaluated include minimally invasive (laparoscopic) surgical techniques, percutaneous catheter drainage, and endoscopic internal drainage. The efficacy and risks of these newer approaches compared with standard operative open internal drainage remain to be determined, except in the case of clinically infected pseudocysts (patients who typically have fever, leukocytosis, and pseudo-cyst aspirates demonstrating both PMNs and bacterial organisms on gram-stained smear). Percutaneous catheter drainage of infected pseudocysts is as effective as the previous operative approach (open external drainage), with a lower rate of pseudocyst recurrence and fistula formation.

Significant hemorrhage (requiring transfusion) is only rarely seen as a complication of acute pancreatitis. Potential causes include stress gastritis, development of pseudoaneurysm in the peripancreatic arterial circulation, bleeding from small vessels in the wall of a pseudocyst into the cyst contents, or gastric varices due to splenic vein thrombosis. Stress gastritis and gastric varices usually present with hematemesis, melena, and a falling blood hemoglobin and are best diagnosed by upper gastrointestinal endoscopy. Bleeding from a pseudoaneurysm or into a pseudocyst may not communicate with the intestinal tract (best diagnosed by abdominal CT scanning) or may result in bleeding via the pancreatic duct (hemosuccus pancreaticus) with melena and blood or clots in the region of the duodenal papilla at endoscopy without the finding of any luminal lesion that could account for it.

Angiography is of great value in identifying the site of bleeding from a pseudoaneurysm. Some pseudoaneurysms can be definitively treated by angiographic embolization, whereas others require direct operative control.

REFERENCES

Adler JA, Barkin JS: Management of pseudocysts, inflammatory masses, and pancreatic ascites. Gastroenterol Clin North Am 1990;19:863.

Fan S-T et al: Early treatment of acute biliary pancreatitis by endoscopic papillotomy. N Engl J Med 1993;328:228.

Fernandez-del Castillo C, Rattner DW, Warshaw AL: Acute pancreatitis. Lancet 1993;342:475.

Forsmark CE, Grendell JH: Complications of pancreatitis. Semin Gastrointest Dis 1991;2:165.

Gerzof SG et al: Early diagnosis of pancreatic infection by computed tomography-guided aspiration. Gastroenterology 1987;93:315.

Grendell JH: Idiopathic acute pancreatitis. Gastroenterol Clin North Am 1990;19:1120.

Lee SP, Nichols JF, Park HZ: Biliary sludge as a cause of acute pancreatitis. N Engl J Med 1992;326:589.

Mulvihill SJ, Debas HT: Surgical treatment of pancreatitis and its complications. Semin Gastrointest Dis 1991;2:194.

Neoptolemos JP et al: Controlled trial of ERCP-sphincterotomy vs conservative treatment for acute pancreatitis due to gallstones. Lancet 1988;2:979.

Pederzoli P et al: A randomized multicenter clinical trial of antibiotic prophylaxis of septic complications in acute necrotizing pancreatitis with imipenem. Surg Gynecol Obstet 1993;176:480.

Peynaert MS, Dugernier TH, Kestens PV: Current therapeutic strategies in severe acute pancreatitis. Intensive Care Med 1990;16:352.

Ros E et al: Occult microlithiasis in "idiopathic" acute pancreatitis: Prevention of relapse by cholecystectomy or ursodeoxycholic acid therapy. Gastroenterology 1991;101:1701.

Steinberg W, Tenner S: Acute pancreatitis. N Engl J Med 1994;330:1198.

Steinberg WM: Predictors of severity of acute pancreatitis. Gastroenterol Clin North Am 1990;19:849.

Chronic Pancreatitis & Pancreatic Insufficiency

32

Chris E. Forsmark, MD

Patients with chronic pancreatitis seek medical attention primarily because of chronic abdominal pain, consequences of maldigestion (eg, steatorrhea, weight loss, or malnutrition), or recurrent attacks of clinically evident acute pancreatitis. Although most patients develop pain, approximately 15% will develop steatorrhea in the absence of pain, and a substantial number will suffer from pain alone and never develop pancreatic exocrine insufficiency. This variability of symptoms, coupled with the inability to obtain histologic confirmation of disease in most cases, has made classification of chronic pancreatitis difficult. A series of international panels have attempted to draw up categories and definitions. In the most recent effort (the Marseilles-Rome classification), three types of disease were defined: chronic calcifying pancreatitis, chronic obstructive pancreatitis, and chronic inflammatory pancreatitis. **Chronic calcifying pancreatitis,** characterized by diffuse calcification of the gland on radiographic imaging and the development of calcified pancreatic duct stones, is the most common and is usually associated with alcohol abuse. **Chronic obstructive pancreatitis** is believed to occur as a consequence of "downstream" obstruction of the pancreatic duct, with subsequent damage, atrophy, and fibrosis of "upstream" acini (eg, inflammatory or traumatic stricture of the pancreatic duct). In both of these forms, damage to the main pancreatic duct is usually substantial, and ductal abnormalities are often easy to appreciate on radiographic imaging with either CT scanning or endoscopic retrograde pancreatography (ERP) ("big-duct" disease). **Chronic inflammatory pancreatitis** is more difficult to define, but is perhaps best described as a process affecting only the acinar tissue and small ductules, with sparing of the main pancreatic duct until late in the clinical course. This form is clearly underdiagnosed and underappreciated by many clinicians, primarily because of the difficulty in establishing the presence of chronic pancreatitis in the absence of obvious abnormalities in the main pancreatic duct ("small-duct" disease). Chronic damage to the pancreas occurs in all three forms of chronic pancreatitis, and these changes are usually ir-

reversible, making cure improbable. Despite this, medical and surgical therapy can often produce substantial improvement in the major complaints of abdominal pain and maldigestion.

DEMOGRAPHIC FINDINGS

The true incidence and prevalence of chronic pancreatitis is unknown. The fact that estimates of incidence and prevalence vary widely should not be surprising, given the various presentations, definitions, causative factors, and diagnostic tests used in the disease. Autopsy studies suggest a prevalence of 0.04–5%. Retrospective clinical studies also vary widely, ranging from less than 1 to more than 10 new cases per 100,000 population. The only prospective study (Copenhagen Pancreatitis Study) found a prevalence of 27.4 cases per 100,000 population and an incidence of 8.2 new cases per 100,000 population. All data are based on populations primarily having alcohol-induced chronic pancreatitis and therefore vary with the overall magnitude of alcohol abuse in that population. None of these studies reflect the incidence or prevalence of other forms of chronic pancreatitis, in particular, forms where obvious damage to the main pancreatic duct is not apparent (small-duct disease). Recent clinical studies have clearly demonstrated histologic findings of chronic pancreatitis in patients with severe chronic pain in the absence of abnormalities of the main pancreatic duct, as defined by CT scanning or ERP. If these patients with small-duct disease were included, the true incidence and prevalence of chronic pancreatitis would be higher than the figures suggested by the available epidemiologic studies.

PATHOPHYSIOLOGY & ETIOLOGY

The exact pathophysiologic mechanism producing pancreatic injury and chronic pancreatitis is unknown for all of the common underlying conditions. It is probable that different causes have different mechanisms of injury. Regardless of the cause, the ultimate effect is damage to the pancreatic acini, ducts, nerves, and islet-cells. This damage is responsible for the cardinal manifestations of abdominal pain, maldigestion, and diabetes mellitus. The specific causes of chronic pancreatitis and their presumed pathophysiology are discussed below and presented in Table 32–1.

Alcohol Consumption

Alcohol consumption is the major cause of chronic pancreatitis in Western societies. The incidence of chronic pancreatitis at autopsy is 50 times higher in alcoholics than in nondrinkers, and there appears to be a direct relationship between daily alcohol consumption and the risk of chronic pancreatitis. Prolonged alcohol intake is usually required before chronic pancreatitis will develop (eg, four pints of beer or 800 mL of wine per day for 6–12 years). Only 15% of alcoholics with this level of intake ultimately develop chronic pancreatitis, and this suggests that other factors such as diet (particularly one high in fat) or genetic predisposition are also important. In Western societies, 70% of cases of chronic pancreatitis are due to alcohol consumption, with the remaining 30% due to other causes or idiopathic disease. The mechanism by which alcohol produces pancreatic injury and chronic pancreatitis is unknown. Alcohol appears to interfere with intracellular transport and secretion of digestive enzymes and augments the pancreatic response to cholecystokinin. In addition, alcohol promotes the formation of protein precipitates in the pancreatic duct. Whether these changes explain the development of chronic pancreatitis remains to be elucidated.

Malnutrition (Tropical Pancreatitis)

Chronic pancreatitis is commonly seen as a consequence of malnutrition in certain areas of Indonesia, India, and Africa. Although rare in people born in the United States, this disease can be seen in immigrants to the USA. Patients typically present with abdominal pain beginning in childhood, diabetes, malnutrition, and diffuse pancreatic calcifications. Most people ultimately die from complications of the disease. While malnutrition is important in the development

Table 32–1. Causes of chronic pancreatitis.

Alcohol abuse
Obstruction
Trauma to pancreatic duct
Ductal stricture or stone
Long-standing pancreatic duct stent
Pancreas divisum, with associated accessory papillary stenosis
Hyperlipidemia
Cystic fibrosis
Familial pancreatitis
Malnutrition (tropical pancreatitis)
Idiopathic pancreatitis

of chronic pancreatitis, toxic products contained in the diet (eg, cassava or sorghum) or the environment may also play a role in pancreatic injury.

Pancreatic Duct Obstruction

Obstruction of the main pancreatic duct by tumors, strictures, or scarring; stents; or anatomic variants can lead to chronic pancreatitis. The pathologic hallmarks are acinar atrophy and fibrosis and dilatation of the pancreatic duct "upstream" of the obstruction. Longstanding obstruction can lead to irreversible chronic pancreatitis, but both functional and structural improvement can be seen if the obstruction is discovered and relieved. Obstruction may be due to posttraumatic strictures, ampullary stenosis or neoplasms, pancreatic tumors or pseudocysts, endoscopically placed pancreatic duct stents, or, rarely, inflammatory strictures resulting from a severe episode of acute pancreatitis.

Pancreas divisum, or failure of fusion of the dorsal and ventral pancreatic ducts, may also lead to obstruction to flow and chronic pancreatitis. In this condition, the small ventral pancreas drains through the major papilla, while the larger dorsal pancreas drains through the accessory papilla. Pancreas divisum may occur in up to 10% of the population, and the vast majority of patients with this congenital abnormality have no symptoms. In fact, two large studies of several thousand patients did not find pancreas divisum to be associated with either acute or chronic pancreatitis. There is a subset of patients with both divisum and obstruction to flow at the accessory papilla, however, in whom clinical pancreatic disease does occur. The clinical challenge arises in attempting to determine which patients have obstruction at the accessory papilla. Significant structural abnormalities limited to the dorsal pancreatic duct (eg, dilatation) is the most specific finding and usually confirms that pancreas divisum is responsible for the clinical pancreatic disease. The finding of a normal dorsal duct does not exclude the possibility that pancreas divisum is responsible for chronic pain or chronic pancreatitis, but additional confirmatory evidence is required. This issue is discussed in more detail in the section on diagnostic studies following.

Hyperlipidemia

Hypertriglyceridemia may precipitate episodes of acute pancreatitis. Triglyceride levels above 1000 mg/dL are usually required to initiate acute pancreatitis, commonly as a result of familial hyperlipidemias (types IV and V) exacerbated by estrogen use or poorly controlled diabetes. What is not appreciated is that recurrent attacks of hyperlipidemic pancreatitis may ultimately produce chronic pancreatitis. While rare, this cause of both acute and chronic pancreatitis should not be forgotten, as effective therapy is available. The incidence of hyperlipidemic pancreatitis may be increasing because of the use of estrogens for prevention of postmenopausal osteoporosis.

Familial Pancreatitis

A number of kindreds have been described with the clinical features of recurrent acute pancreatitis beginning at an early age, which ultimately culminates in a markedly dilated pancreatic duct, diffuse calcifications, steatorrhea, and diabetes mellitus. Symptoms typically begin in childhood. The pattern of inheritance appears to be autosomal dominant with incomplete penetrance.

Cystic Fibrosis

Cystic fibrosis is the most common cause of pancreatitis in children but can also be seen in young adults as improved overall medical care leads to more prolonged survival times in these patients. A defect in the chloride channel causes reduced flow of pancreatic secretions, the development of supersaturated pancreatic juice, and the precipitation of protein plugs within the duct.

Idiopathic Pancreatitis

Despite careful evaluation, 10–30% of patients may not have a definable cause of chronic pancreatitis. Idiopathic chronic pancreatitis is the second most common cause of chronic pancreatitis in adults, behind alcohol abuse. Some of these patients abuse alcohol surreptitiously, but a substantial number are not imbibers. Many of these patients do not have easily identifiable abnormalities of the pancreatic duct and are commonly misdiagnosed. There do appear to be demographic differences between these patients and those with the more common alcoholic chronic pancreatitis (Table 32–2).

CLINICAL FINDINGS

Symptoms & Signs

A. Pain: For most patients with chronic pancreatitis, abdominal pain is the predominant symptom and the one that most affects life-style. There are no characteristic features, and the pain varies tremendously in severity, pattern, quality, and frequency. An episode of acute pancreatitis superimposed on an already irreversibly damaged gland may produce the more abrupt abdominal pain associated with acute pancreatitis. In up to one-third of patients, these acute exacerbations are absent, and a more gradual onset of chronic pain is noted. The most commonly noted type of chronic pain is dull, constant, located in the epigastrium with associated back pain, and often made worse by eating. Food may be avoided, leading to weight loss and malnutrition. Episodes of pain usually last from days to weeks, although some patients develop continuous pain. The pain may be quite mild or severe, requiring narcotics for relief in up to 20% of patients. Pain never develops in up to 15% of patients with alcoholic chronic pancreatitis and up to 25% or more with idiopathic chronic pancreatitis.

The cause of pain in chronic pancreatitis is not well understood and is certainly multifactorial. Factors that may contribute include inflammation within the gland or affecting neural pain fibers supplying the pancreas through the celiac plexus; elevated pressures within the pancreatic ductal system or the parenchyma of the gland; associated extrapancreatic complications such as bile duct or duodenal obstruction; associated pancreatic pseudocysts; and hyperstimulation of the pancreas due to interruption of the normal negative-feedback control of the pancreas. The specific contribution of these (or other mechanisms) to pain in an individual patient is often impossible to determine.

In many patients, the pain may "burn out" after many years of chronic pancreatitis. Substantial relief may also occur if a patient with alcoholic chronic pancreatitis stops drinking, particularly if the disease is less advanced.

B. Malabsorption: Steatorrhea due to pancreatic exocrine insufficiency does not occur until the secretory capacity of the pancreas is reduced to less

Table 32–2. Differences between idiopathic and alcoholic chronic pancreatitis.

	Alcoholic Pancreatitis	Idiopathic Pancreatitis
Sex	Male predominance	Female > male
Calcification	Common	Less common
Steatorrhea	More common	Less common
Painless disease	Rare (5%)	Not uncommon (25%)
Progression to steatorrhea	Earlier	Later or not at all
Big-duct disease[1]	Common	Rare
Response to enzymes[2]	Uncommon	Common

[1]See text for definitions.
[2]Pain relief with use of high-dosage, non–enteric-coated pancreatic enzymes (see text for further discussion).

than 10% of normal. This degree of damage is not usually present until late in the clinical course of disease, so that steatorrhea is most often a marker of far advanced chronic pancreatitis. The ability of the pancreas to secrete proteases tends to be preserved longer than the ability to secrete lipase, so that protein malabsorption occurs later than fat malabsorption. In addition, carbohydrate malabsorption may rarely occur. Malabsorption is not only due to diminished secretion of pancreatic enzymes; reduced secretion of bicarbonate from the pancreatic ductal system also lowers the duodenal pH and further interferes with digestion. Weight loss occurs as a consequence of malabsorption, but may be worsened by avoidance of food due to pain or by inadequate dietary intake due to chronic alcoholism. Signs and symptoms of specific vitamin deficiencies are rare, although folate deficiency may be seen as a consequence of dietary deficiency in chronic alcoholics.

C. Diabetes Mellitus: The pancreatic islet-cells appear to be more resistant to damage than the acinar and ductal cells, so that diabetes occurs less frequently than steatorrhea. Diabetes mellitus ultimately develops in up to 30% of patients with chronic pancreatitis and as many as 70% when diffuse pancreatic calcifications (a marker of far advanced disease) are present. This secondary diabetes is characterized by frequent treatment-associated episodes of hypoglycemia (due to inadequate glucagon reserve) and infrequent findings of ketosis. Complications such as diabetic retinopathy or neuropathy occur as frequently as in other diabetics, if corrected for the duration of diabetes.

Diagnostic Studies

The diagnosis of chronic pancreatitis is usually suggested by clinical features such as abdominal pain or steatorrhea. A wide range of diagnostic tests for evaluation of pancreatic function and structure is available. Chronic pancreatitis is a slowly progressive disease, with severe exocrine insufficiency sometimes developing over a period of 20 years or more. As the disease progresses, easily recognizable radiographic abnormalities may be seen, and this makes the diagnosis straightforward. In less advanced disease, however, the diagnosis can be quite challenging, particularly in idiopathic chronic pancreatitis, in which characteristic radiographic features develop less frequently. When evaluating these patients, it is important for the physician to know the value of the various tests and to have a plan for using them. The true "gold standard" for diagnosis is pancreatic biopsy, which demonstrates pancreatic inflammation, fibrosis, destruction of acinar tissue, and intraductal concretions and plugs. Pancreatic tissue is rarely available, however, so another test usually must be substituted. Diagnostic tests used for chronic pancreatitis are listed in Table 32–3.

A. Diagnostic Strategy: The ideal diagnostic

Table 32–3. Diagnostic tests and studies for chronic pancreatitis, listed in order of decreasing sensitivity.

Function	Structure
Secretin and secretin-cholecystokinin test	Endoscopic retrograde pancreatography
Bentiromide test	CT scanning
Pancreolauryl test	Endoscopic ultrasound[1]
Serum trypsin	Magnetic resonance imaging[1]
Fecal chymotrypsin	Ultrasonography
Dual-label Schilling test	Plain abdominal radiograph
Fecal fat	
Blood glucose	

[1]The exact sensitivity of endoscopic ultrasound and MRI is unknown, but appears to be close to that of CT scanning.

test, which is highly accurate in both early and advanced disease and is also inexpensive, safe, and widely available, does not yet exist. The strategy for evaluating patients should therefore initially focus on tests that are safe, simple, and inexpensive. More invasive, risky, or costly tests should be reserved for cases where diagnostic uncertainty remains or where therapeutic rather than diagnostic information is required. Simple tests that identify more advanced disease are used first (ie, usually a plain abdominal radiograph or serum trypsin measurement, or both). Second-echelon tests include hormonal stimulation tests, ultrasound, CT scanning, or a bentiromide test. Invasive or risky tests such as ERP are used last and only in a subset of patients where diagnostic uncertainty exists. A general diagnostic algorithm is outlined in Figure 32–1.

B. Imaging Studies:

1. X-ray studies—Plain abdominal radiographs are inexpensive, simple, and noninvasive. The finding of diffuse pancreatic calcification is specific for chronic pancreatitis but is seen only in far advanced disease. Focal pancreatic calcification is not specific for chronic pancreatitis and may be due to trauma, islet-cell tumors, or hypercalcemia. The test is insensitive in less advanced disease; in addition, these calcifications may disappear as the disease progresses.

2. Abdominal ultrasonography—Abdominal ultrasonography may also demonstrate calcifications or a markedly dilated pancreatic duct in advanced disease. The sensitivity of ultrasonography is also low, and the procedure has a limited ability to visualize the pancreas because bowel gas may obstruct the view.

3. CT scanning—CT scanning is more accurate and more sensitive in detecting chronic pancreatitis than plain abdominal radiography or ultrasonography. CT findings that suggest chronic pancreatitis include atrophy of the gland, irregular contour of the

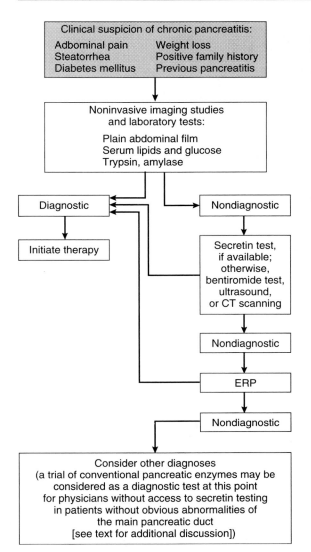

Figure 32–1. Diagnostic strategy for chronic pancreatitis.

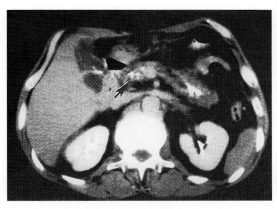

Figure 32–2. A CT scan demonstrating a dilated pancreatic duct and multiple pancreatic calcifications *(arrow)*.

pancreas, dilatation or irregularity of the pancreatic duct, and calcified pancreatic calculi (Figure 32-2). CT scanning is the most sensitive method for detecting pancreatic calcification and is also useful in screening for complications of chronic pancreatitis (eg, pancreatic pseudocyst). CT scanning is an accurate diagnostic test in advanced chronic pancreatitis, with reported sensitivities of 74–90%, but is substantially less sensitive in less advanced disease. The use of "spiral" CT scanning technology has not been extensively evaluated, but this technique can more readily reveal small structures such as the pancreatic duct; in the author's experience, it has a sensitivity approaching that of ERP.

4.   MRI–Magnetic resonance imaging (MRI) has also not been extensively evaluated, but the use of new contrast agents and "turboflash" technology has markedly improved image quality.

5.   Endoscopic ultrasonography–Early work with endoscopic ultrasound suggests it may be even more sensitive than CT scanning or MRI, but further evaluation is required to confirm this.

6.   Endoscopic retrograde pancreatography–ERP is a commonly used imaging technique in the evaluation of patients with chronic pancreatitis or symptoms suggestive of that disease. ERP remains the most sensitive method for viewing pancreatic duct structure but is associated with substantial cost and risk. Diagnosis of chronic pancreatitis by ERP is based on changes in both the main pancreatic duct and the side branches. The most widely used criteria include duct dilatation, narrowing or stricture formation, irregular contour, associated filling of cavities or pseudocysts, and filling defects (ie, pancreatic ductal calculi) (Figure 32–3). At its most advanced stage, the "chain-of-lakes" appearance is quite characteristic of chronic pancreatitis. The reported sensitivity of ERP is 67–90%, and the specificity 89–100%. The test is quite accurate in advanced disease but, like all tests of pancreatic structure, is insensitive in less severe disease. It has not usually been appreciated that many patients with clear-cut chronic pancreatitis may have normal or only minimally abnormal ERP findings. ERP is also limited by a number of complicating factors, including the following: (1) in up to 30% of patients the pancreatogram is of inadequate quality to allow a definitive conclusion; (2) a variety of clinical conditions such as pancreatic carcinoma, acute pancreatitis, pancreatic duct stenting, and even normal aging may produce changes in the pancreatic duct that are indistinguishable from those of chronic pancreatitis; (3) the procedure requires substantial experience and skill to perform; (4) complications occur in up to 10% of patients undergoing ERP; and (5) it is extremely expen-

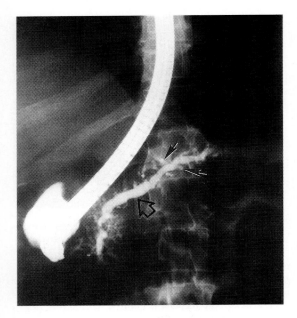

Figure 32–3. An ERP demonstrating moderate changes of chronic pancreatitis, with a dilated main pancreatic duct *(big arrow)* and dilated, clubbed side branches *(small arrows).*

sive. These factors make ERP a late step in the evaluation of patients with suspected chronic pancreatitis.

In addition to providing diagnostic information, ERP can be used to develop a therapeutic plan. Surgical decompression of the main pancreatic duct (Peustow procedure) can only be accomplished if the duct is sufficiently dilated (> 7–8 mm), and this is best confirmed by ERP.

C. Pancreatic Function Tests:

1. Laboratory tests—The measurement of serum glucose levels as a marker of diabetes mellitus is too insensitive to be of any clinical use in chronic pancreatitis, and serum amylase or lipase levels are often normal and also not of diagnostic importance. Serum trypsin levels appear to be a more accurate marker of chronic pancreatitis, particularly when steatorrhea is also present; levels below 20 mg/dL appear to be quite specific for chronic pancreatitis.

Measurement of fecal chymotrypsin as a marker of intraluminal concentration of pancreatic enzymes and, hence, pancreatic function has also been evaluated. Overall, the sensitivity approaches 85% in advanced disease but is less than 50% in less advanced disease. Measurement of 72-hour fecal fat concentrations can document steatorrhea, but this is an overly cumbersome, insensitive test. With the exception of serum trypsin values, these simple laboratory evaluations are not helpful.

2. Indirect tests of pancreatic function—Indirect tests of pancreatic function are based on documentation of exocrine insufficiency. Since this does

not occur until 90% of exocrine function has been lost, these tests will be accurate in advanced or end-stage disease but inaccurate in earlier disease.

a. Bentiromide test—The bentiromide, or nitroblue tetrazolium-*p*-aminobenzoic acid test (NBT-PABA test), is the most widely used test. It requires the cleavage of a synthetic peptide by pancreatic chymotrypsin. The *p*-aminobenzoic acid that is released is absorbed and then removed from the circulation by renal excretion. Recovery of a metabolite of *p*-aminobenzoic acid in the urine or blood reflects the relative amount of intraluminal chymotrypsin. The test is accurate in advanced disease (overall sensitivity of approximately 70%) but much less sensitive and probably useless in mild or early chronic pancreatitis (overall sensitivity of approximately 45%). A similar test, the pancreolauryl test, is not available in the USA. Both tests may have false-positive results in the presence of hepatic disease, biliary disease, kidney disease, or small bowel disease, and in patients who have undergone a Billroth II gastrectomy.

b. Dual-label Schilling test—Absorption of vitamin B_{12} is impaired in advanced chronic pancreatitis due to inability of the pancreas to degrade R protein. This is the basis of the dual-label Schilling test for diagnosing chronic pancreatitis. The sensitivity of this test is too inadequate to be helpful in general clinical use.

3. Direct tests of pancreatic function—The only tests that can detect chronic pancreatitis in its less severe form are direct tests of pancreatic secretory capacity. The secretin and secretin-cholecystokinin tests both require the collection of pancreatic secretions with a tube placed in the duodenum after stimulation of the pancreas with one or both of these hormonal secretagogues. These tests depend on the adequate collection of pancreatic secretions and on the technical ability to measure bicarbonate or proteases in the collected fluid. The sensitivity of these tests, like all diagnostic tests, depends on the severity of the disease (sensitivities are 74–90%, and specificities 80–90%). A number of studies have compared these tests of pancreatic function with other diagnostic tests, especially ERP documentation of changes in the pancreatic duct. All of these studies have reached similar conclusions: that these hormonal stimulation tests are more sensitive, more accurate, and more able to diagnose chronic pancreatitis in its less severe stages, compared with other tests. All of these studies have also documented patients who have normal pancreatic appearance on radiographic imaging (CT scanning or ERP) but abnormal results of hormonal stimulation tests. In the absence of pancreatic histologic studies documenting chronic pancreatitis, it was not clear if these patients actually had the disease. Two recent studies have been able to document histologic findings of chronic pancreatitis in patients with normal pancreatic duct anatomy, confirming the suspicion that small-duct disease, or "minimal-change" disease, exists in some patients.

Direct hormonal stimulation tests therefore appear to diagnose chronic pancreatitis at an earlier stage than any other available test. Substantial expertise is required for these tests to be performed reliably, and they are used at only a few referral centers and are unavailable to many clinicians.

DIFFERENTIAL DIAGNOSIS

The abdominal pain associated with chronic pancreatitis is not specific, and a variety of other abdominal conditions may mimic it. These usually include acid peptic disease, biliary tract disease, acute pancreatitis, mesenteric ischemia or infarction, aortic dissection, and a variety of others. Some of these conditions may also be associated with elevations in amylase or lipase levels, and they are more often confused with acute pancreatitis than chronic pancreatitis. They should be kept in mind, however, when a patient with chronic pancreatitis develops a more acute flare-up of pain.

Acute pancreatitis may be confused with chronic pancreatitis, and several clinical issues should be kept in mind: Patients with chronic pancreatitis may initially present with acute pancreatitis as the first manifestation or may develop flare-ups of disease during their course; acute pancreatitis may induce changes in the pancreatic duct which mimic chronic pancreatitis but which will eventually resolve; and acute pancreatitis will temporarily interfere with pancreatic function, so that a hormonal stimulation test will remain abnormal for weeks after an acute attack. The major diagnostic dilemma is, however, none of these conditions, but rather the differentiation of chronic pancreatitis from pancreatic cancer.

Pancreatic carcinoma may closely mimic the symptoms, signs, and radiographic appearance of chronic pancreatitis. The use of CT scanning, ERP, pancreatic duct cytologic studies, percutaneous biopsy, tumor markers such as CA 19-9, and, possibly, endoscopic ultrasound allow pancreatic carcinoma to be distinguished from chronic pancreatitis in most patients. In a subset of patients, laparotomy is required to establish the diagnosis. This is discussed more fully in Chapter 33.

TREATMENT

Treatment of Direct Manifestations of Chronic Pancreatitis

A. Steatorrhea: Steatorrhea occurs primarily as a consequence of inadequate delivery of pancreatic digestive enzymes to the gut lumen, and only when 90% of pancreatic output has been lost. Deficient delivery of bicarbonate may also contribute to steatorrhea, because gastric acid may be inadequately neutralized, and this may cause inactivation of digestive enzymes and precipitation of bile salts. Therapy for steatorrhea is directed at delivering adequate amounts of exogenous pancreatic enzymes to the gut lumen. Appropriate use of these enzymes leads to resolution of diarrhea and weight loss, despite the fact that steatorrhea cannot usually be totally corrected.

The lipase content of pancreatic enzyme preparations is the critical determinant of efficacy in treating steatorrhea. Most of the commercially available preparations are of low potency, although newer, more concentrated preparations have been developed. The enzymes are either packaged in a conventional form, which begins to dissolve in the stomach, or are contained in enteric-coated microspheres, which do not release their contents until the pH rises above 5.5. These preparations are listed in Table 32–4.

Effective treatment of steatorrhea usually requires the delivery of at least 28,000 IU of lipase to the duodenum during a 4-hour postprandial period. Patients using the lower-potency preparations must therefore take three to eight pills with each meal. Fewer pills must be taken with the newer, more concentrated forms, which contain more than 25,000 IU of lipase per pill, but these forms have been recalled by the manufacturers after colonic strictures were noted in young patients with cystic fibrosis taking high dosages of these preparations. No such complications have been reported in adults or patients with other forms of chronic pancreatitis. The most common reason for failure of pancreatic enzymes to correct steatorrhea is the patient's unwillingness to take the number of pills required. The second most common reason is inactivation of lipase by gastric acid; to prevent this, the gastric pH must be kept above 4.0 by using sodium bicarbonate, H_2-receptor antagonists, or omeprazole. Alternatively, one of the enteric-coated preparations of lipase may be used, although the enteric-coated microspheres contained in these preparations are often too large to empty easily from the stomach and dissolve too slowly.

Dietary manipulations may also be helpful in the management of malabsorption and malnutrition. The diet should usually contain a moderate amount of fat (30%), high amount of protein (24%), and low amount of carbohydrates (40%). Decreasing the amount of long-chain triglycerides in the diet or adding medium-chain triglyceride supplements, or both, may improve steatorrhea in selected patients.

B. Pain:

1. Medical treatment–The management of pain is often unsatisfactory, in large part because there are many causes of pain, so that one treatment will not be effective in all patients, and also because there is no effective treatment for many causes. Ab-

Table 32–4. Pancreatic enzymes for the treatment of steatorrhea[1] or pain.[2]

Conventional Enzyme Preparations

Brand Name	Units of Lipase Per Pill
Viokase	8000
Cotazym	8000
Ku-Zyme HP	8000

Enteric-Coated Enzyme Preparations

Brand Name	Units of Lipase Per Pill
Cotazym-S	5000
Pancrease MT 4, MT 10, MT 16	4000, 10,000, 16,000, respectively
Creon	10,000
Ultrase MT 6, MT 12, MT 18, MT 20	6000, 12,000, 18,000, 20,000, respectively

[1]For the treatment of steatorrhea, both conventional and enteric-coated preparations can be used. The dosage depends on the lipase content. Low-potency formulations (5000–8000 units of lipase per pill) require five to eight pills with each meal. Higher-potency formulations require three to five pills with each meal. Unlike with the treatment of pain, it is often useful to spread these out during the course of the meal. The highest-potency formulations containing more than 20,000 units of lipase per pill (Pancrease MT 25, Pancrease MT 32, Ultrase MT 24, Ultrase MT 30, and Creon 25) have been withdrawn by the manufacturers because of the development of colonic strictures in patients with chronic pancreatitis due to cystic fibrosis.

[2]For the treatment of pain, conventional enzyme preparations are used, eight pills before meals and at night. An adjuvant agent to reduce gastric acid is usually required, either H_2-receptor antagonists or omeprazole.

stinence from alcohol should be strongly encouraged, as this often produces pain relief. Analgesics are often required, and nonnarcotic analgesics should be used first. Narcotic agents are required in a subset of patients, and the least potent formulation should be tried first (eg, Darvocet-N 100). Narcotic addiction occurs less frequently than is commonly thought but is a risk in patients requiring these agents.

Complications of chronic pancreatitis such as pseudocyst, bile duct obstruction, or duodenal obstruction may produce pain and are usually amenable to therapy. In any patient with chronic pancreatitis and refractory or severe pain, these complications should be sought.

Several controlled trials have demonstrated that conventional (nonenteric-coated) pancreatic enzymes can provide pain relief in some patients with chronic pancreatitis. These preparations are felt to reestablish normal negative feedback of pancreatic secretion, reducing hyperstimulation of the gland by cholecystokinin and thereby reducing pain. This feedback loop is operative only in the duodenum, so enteric-coated preparations that do not release enzymes until they reach the jejunum are ineffective. Patients who respond best to the use of conventional enzymes are those with mild to moderate chronic pancreatitis (without steatorrhea) and minimal abnormalities on ERP (ie, small-duct disease). In some studies, up to 75% of these patients responded to the use of these enzymes. Conversely, patients with steatorrhea or marked abnormalities of the pancreatic duct (big-duct disease) are unlikely to respond. Eight tablets or capsules of a potent non–enteric-coated preparation (eg, Viokase, Ku-Zyme HP) should be given at meals and at bedtime, along with an adjuvant agent to reduce gastric acid.

2. Celiac plexus block and other blocks– Ablation of the celiac plexus by radiographically guided injection of alcohol can be effective for the pain of pancreatic cancer but is usually ineffective or provides short-lived relief in patients with chronic pancreatitis. This technique has generally been abandoned. Use of percutaneous splanchnic nerve blocks or thoracoscopic splanchnicectomy has also been recorded, but their efficacy remains to be established in chronic pancreatitis.

3. Surgical treatment–Surgical therapy can be considered for complications of chronic pancreatitis (pseudocyst, bile duct obstruction, duodenal obstruction) or big-duct disease with refractory pain. Performance of a lateral pancreaticojejunostomy (Peustow procedure), with or without partial pancreatic resection, leads to immediate pain relief in 70–80% of patients. Long-term pain control is achieved in 50% after 1–3 years of follow-up. The pancreatic duct must usually be dilated to 7–8 mm or more for the technical performance of a Peustow procedure. This is usually defined by ERP preoperatively. The procedure carries acceptable rates of complications (5%) and mortality (2%). Surgical pancreatic duct decompression may also slow the progression of chronic pancreatitis. Subtotal or total pancreatic resections are rarely needed for pain control and are associated with more significant rates of complications and death than a Peustow procedure. For selected patients with an inflammatory mass involving the head of the pancreas, pancreaticoduodenectomy (eg, modified Whipple procedure) or duodenum-sparing resection of the pancreatic head may be beneficial.

Prospective Treatments

A. Endoscopic Therapy of Chronic Pancreatitis: The endoscopic therapies of chronic pancreatitis include pancreatic duct stenting and pancreatic duct sphincterotomy of both the major and minor papilla, dilation of strictures, removal of pancreatic calculi, and treatment of complications such as pseudocyst or biliary obstruction. Endoscopic stenting of the bile duct for biliary decompression, particularly in the setting of cholangitis, is effective but is not usually an acceptable long-term solution due to the need for repeated stent changes. The use of metal biliary prostheses has also been reported, although obstruction of these prostheses will eventually occur. Endoscopic biliary stents should usually be considered a temporizing measure or a "bridge" to surgical biliary bypass.

No randomized trials have been performed for any of these endoscopic techniques in patients with chronic pancreatitis. In many series, the response rate to endoscopic therapy is no greater than that due to placebo (approximately 35%). Complications are not infrequent from endoscopic treatment of the pancreatic duct, including pancreatitis, bleeding, perforation, and sepsis. In addition, pancreatic stents can in and of themselves induce ductal changes resembling those of chronic pancreatitis in up to half of patients treated, and these changes may not resolve. Endoscopic therapy should still be considered unproved, and randomized trials are sorely needed.

B. Octreotide: Use of the somatostatin analog octreotide has also begun to be evaluated. This agent appears to be able to reduce pancreatic secretion, perhaps by interfering with the feedback control of secretion by cholecystokinin. Anecdotal reports suggested that pain relief might be achieved in some patients. A multicenter trial in the United States designed to evaluate the optimal dosage demonstrated pain relief in 65% of patients given 200 μg subcutaneously three times a day (compared with 35% in placebo-treated patients). This study is still only reported in abstract form. Further studies are required before the efficacy of this agent can be established.

C. Cholecystokinin Antagonists: Like octreotide, antagonists of cholecystokinin might reduce pancreatic secretion and pain by interfering with feedback control of secretion and reducing the "hyperstimulation" of the pancreas. Early studies have demonstrated that these agents reduce pancreatic secretion. Whether this is accompanied by pain relief remains to be studied.

Treatment of Complications of Chronic Pancreatitis

A. Episodes of Acute Pancreatitis: Patients with chronic pancreatitis may experience flare-ups of disease or episodes of acute pancreatitis superimposed on an already irreversibly damaged gland. These flare-ups tend to be mild and decrease in severity with evolution of the disease. A subset of patients will experience a more severe attack and may develop all of the complications associated with severe acute pancreatitis, such as renal failure or adult respiratory distress syndrome. These complications and their management are discussed fully in Chapter 31.

B. Pancreatic Pseudocyst: Collections of pancreatic fluid in and around the pancreas may occur as a consequence of acute or chronic pancreatitis. Pseudocysts occurring in the setting of acute pancreatitis are usually due to ductal disruption and necrosis, with the escape of pancreatic juice containing activated enzymes. Pseudocysts complicating chronic pancreatitis are more often due to downstream obstruction of the pancreatic duct, causing a "retention cyst" filled with inactive enzymes. These different pathophysiologic mechanisms are reflected in somewhat different clinical presentations and natural histories. Pseudocysts occurring in the setting of acute pancreatitis are more likely to produce complications than pseudocysts associated with chronic pancreatitis but are also paradoxically more likely to resolve.

Patients with a pseudocyst complicating acute pancreatitis may remain asymptomatic or may present with complications such as pseudocyst rupture or infection. While patients with pseudocysts complicating chronic pancreatitis may present in a similar fashion, they are also likely to notice worsening chronic pain, develop a wasting syndrome, or remain asymptomatic.

The diagnosis of pseudocyst is best made by CT scanning. Pseudocysts are characterized as rounded collections of fluid surrounded by a visible capsule (Figure 32–4). Other fluid collections that have not matured into this form are better termed acute pancreatic fluid collections. It appears to take at least 6 weeks for an acute pancreatic fluid collection to mature into a pseudocyst, although many will resolve without developing into pseudocysts.

The natural history of pseudocysts is variable. Initial studies suggested that complications developed in up to 40% of patients and that only 20% of pseudocysts spontaneously resolved. Resolution of pseudocysts usually happened within the first 6 weeks, and many of the complications occurred after this period. Six weeks was also approximately the amount of time it took for an acute pancreatic fluid collection to develop into a mature pseudocyst, and

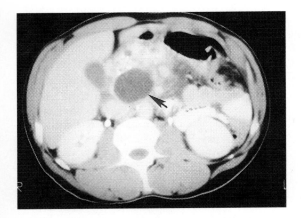

Figure 32–4. A CT scan demonstrating a pseudocyst *(arrow)* in the head of the gland, with areas of associated calcification.

was considered the most appropriate time for surgical intervention. These early studies appear to have overestimated the severity of the natural history of pseudocysts. Several recent studies using CT scanning have noted resolution rates as high as 64%, with complications occurring in less than 10%. In addition, the long-term risk of pseudocysts less than 6 cm in diameter producing complications appears to be extremely small. The risk of complications has probably been overestimated and the chance of spontaneous resolution underestimated. In practice, relatively small (< 6 cm) pseudocysts that are asymptomatic can be safely followed without therapy, especially if the patient can stop drinking alcohol.

Symptomatic pseudocysts that have not caused significant complications can be treated with both surgical techniques and percutaneous drainage. Surgical therapies include decompression into an adjacent hollow viscus (eg, cystjejunostomy, cystgastrostomy) or resection of the pseudocyst along with a portion of the pancreas (typically for pseudocysts in the tail of the pancreas). Percutaneous aspiration of pseudocysts with catheter drainage can also be tried and is the treatment of choice for clinically infected pseudocysts. This therapy is often effective in the short term (90% success rate), but the long-term results are unknown. In many patients, these pseudocysts recur when the catheter is removed, although this may take months and the recurrent pseudocyst often remains asymptomatic. In addition, catheter drainage does not allow differentiation of pseudocysts from cystic neoplasms of the pancreas. Despite these drawbacks, percutaneous drainage is used widely due to its technical simplicity and low rate of complications. The use of inhibitors of pancreatic secretion, particularly octreotide, may improve the success rate of percutaneous catheter drainage.

1. Hemorrhage due to pseudocyst—Only

2–7% of patients with pancreatic pseudocysts bleed, but the development of bleeding is associated with a substantial rate of mortality (up to 35%). Bleeding from a pseudocyst can originate in small vessels in the pseudocyst capsule or in larger visceral arteries that are damaged and disrupted by the pseudocyst or associated pancreatitis, producing a pseudoaneurysm. Pseudoaneurysms most commonly form in the splenic artery, followed by the gastroduodenal and pancreaticoduodenal arteries. Blood may remain in the pseudocyst, enter the gut via the pancreatic duct (hemosuccus pancreaticus) (its passage may also transiently obstruct the bile duct at the ampulla), or rupture into an adjacent hollow viscus. Rarely, the pseudocyst or pseudoaneurysm may rupture into the peritoneal cavity.

Pseudocyst-associated bleeding should be suspected when gastrointestinal bleeding develops in a patient with a known or suspected pseudocyst, when sudden abdominal pain develops in association with an enlarging abdominal mass, when a patient with a pseudocyst develops sudden unexplained blood loss, or when evidence of bile duct obstruction and gastrointestinal bleeding is seen at the same time in a patient with pancreatic disease. Upper endoscopy is usually performed first, after fluid resuscitation, to search for other potential sources of bleeding. If no obvious abnormality is documented, radiographic evaluation is required. An initial ultrasound study may reveal the pseudocyst and even occasionally a pulsatile pseudoaneurysm, but CT scanning is usually more accurate and associated with fewer inadequate examinations. The finding of high-density fluid (blood) within a pseudocyst or blood in the pancreatic duct should prompt further investigation, primarily angiography. Angiography can be used to document the presence of a pseudoaneurysm and also allows therapeutic embolization for stabilization or definitive therapy. Definitive therapy may require surgical ligation of the pseudoaneurysm and cystenterostomy or resection.

2. Infected pseudocyst—Pseudocysts may become infected in up to 15% of patients. Gram-negative enteric organisms are most commonly involved, but streptococci and anaerobes also may be causative organisms. In up to 40% of patients, more than one organism is responsible. Pseudocyst infection presents clinically with abdominal pain, fever, and leukocytosis. The presence of gas in a pseudocyst demonstrated by ultrasonography or CT scanning is strongly suggestive of pseudocyst infection but is insensitive. Most infected pseudocysts will not have gas present. The diagnosis can usually be established by puncture of the pseudocyst, with gram-stained smear and culture of the fluid.

Treatment requires the initiation of broad-spectrum antibiotics and drainage. Both percutaneous catheter drainage and surgical drainage are usually effective. Percutaneous drainage is preferred, if pos-

effective. Percutaneous drainage is preferred, if possible, but should not be used if the infected material cannot be adequately removed through a small-bore tube, as is the case with infected pancreatic necrosis and fluid collections containing solid necrotic tissue or multiple septations.

3. Obstruction of surrounding organs by pseudocyst–Pseudocysts in the head of the pancreas may obstruct the common bile duct as it passes through the head of the pancreas. Bile duct obstruction due solely to pseudocyst is rare; usually, the bile duct is primarily obstructed from fibrosis due to chronic pancreatitis. Although common duct obstruction is common, clinically important obstruction is less common. Radiographic evidence of bile duct narrowing, seen on ERP, in and of itself is not an indication for therapy. Conservative management is usually appropriate, unless clinical evidence (eg, cholangitis) or biochemical evidence (eg, markedly elevated alkaline phosphatase levels) of biliary obstruction develops; this is an indication for surgical biliary bypass along with cyst decompression (if present). Duodenal obstruction may also occur as a result of an inflammatory mass in the head of the pancreas or large pseudocyst (1–7% of patients with pancreatic pseudocysts). Persistent symptomatic obstruction is an indication for gastrojejunostomy. Obstruction of the portal vein, ureters, and colon has also been rarely observed.

4. Rupture of pseudocyst–Pseudocyst rupture occurs in less than 10% of patients and is associated with a mortality rate of 14–40%. The rate is highest with abrupt rupture into the peritoneal cavity or rupture associated with bleeding. Rupture into a surrounding hollow viscus is often well tolerated, creating a spontaneous cystenterostomy, which obviates the need for further therapy. Rupture into the peritoneal cavity often produces a severe chemical peritonitis and usually requires surgical therapy, with external cyst drainage the treatment of choice.

C. Pancreatic Fistula: Disruption of the pancreatic duct or rupture of a pseudocyst may lead to a controlled leak of pancreatic secretions. This fluid may enter a number of spaces, including the peritoneal cavity and pleural spaces. The fluid may become walled off as a pseudocyst or remain connected to the pancreatic duct (internal pancreatic fistula) due to persistent leakage. Pancreatic ascites is usually associated with persistent leakage and a fistula on the anterior surface of the pancreas. Posterior fistulas usually reach the pleural space or mediastinum, producing pancreatic pleural effusions from a pancreaticopleural fistula. These persistent fistulas occur almost exclusively in patients with chronic pancreatitis. Surprisingly, signs and symptoms of pancreatitis are often absent, and patients may instead complain of abdominal distention or dyspnea. Abdominal pain is absent in up to one-fifth of these patients, and only one-half have a history compatible with previous attacks of pancreatitis. These fistulas should be suspected when an exudative pleural effusion or ascites with an elevated amylase level is found. The amylase value in the fluid is usually markedly elevated (median > 18,000 IU/L). Radiographic studies, including CT scanning and ERP, can often document chronic pancreatitis and localize the fistulous tract and any associated pseudocyst.

Medical therapy may be effective in up to 40% of patients and includes allowing nothing by mouth, using hyperalimentation, repeatedly draining fluid that has collected, and giving octreotide to reduce pancreatic secretion. Surgical therapy is effective for patients who fail medical therapy and usually includes repair of the duct leak and drainage of any associated pseudocyst.

D. Gastrointestinal Bleeding: In addition to the bleeding associated with pseudocysts, bleeding may occur in acute and chronic pancreatitis due to thrombosis of the splenic vein. This typically results in segmental portal hypertension. The endoscopic correlates of this left-sided portal hypertension are isolated gastric varices or large gastric varices with minor or trivial esophageal varices. The diagnosis of splenic vein thrombosis can usually be documented by Doppler ultrasound, CT scanning, or angiography. The treatment of this condition is splenectomy, which is usually curative.

E. Pancreatic Carcinoma: Several recent large case control studies have suggested that chronic pancreatitis is a risk factor for the development of pancreatic carcinoma. These studies are provocative but do not provide clear-cut information on the nature and magnitude of the risk or the potential value of screening.

REFERENCES

Amann RW et al: Course and outcome of chronic pancreatitis: Longitudinal study of a mixed medical-surgical series of 245 patients. Gastroenterology 1984;86:820.

Bockman DE et al: Analysis of nerves in chronic pancreatitis. Gastroenterology 1988;94:1459.

Buchler MW, Binder M, Friess H: Role of somatostatin and its analogues in the treatment of acute and chronic pancreatitis. Gut 1994;Suppl 3:S15.

Burtin P et al: Pancreas divisum and pancreatitis: A coincidental association? Endoscopy 1991;23:55.

DiMagno EP, Go VLW, Summerskill WHJ: Relations between pancreatic enzyme outputs and malabsorption in severe pancreatic insufficiency. N Engl J Med 1973; 288:813.

Forsmark CE, Grendell JH: Complications of pancreatitis. Semin Gastrointest Dis 1991;2:165.

Forsmark CE, Toskes PP: What does an abnormal pancreatogram mean? Gastrointest Endosc Clin North Am 1995;5:105.

Gulliver DJ et al: Stent placement for benign pancreatic disease: Correlations between ERCP findings and clinical response. AJR 1992;159:751.

Hayakawa T et al: Relationship between pancreatic function and histologic changes in chronic pancreatitis. Am J Gastroenterol 1992;87:1170.

Jacobson DG et al: Trypsin-like immunoreactivity as a test for pancreatic insufficiency. N Engl J Med 1984; 310:1307.

Kalthoff L et al: The course of alcoholic and nonalcoholic chronic pancreatitis. Dig Dis Sci 1984;29:953.

Lowenfels AB et al: Pancreatitis and the risk of pancreatic cancer. N Engl J Med 1993;328:1433.

Lumsden A, Bradley EL: Secondary pancreatic infections. Surg Gynecol Obstet 1990;170:459.

Mulvihill SJ, Debas HT: Surgical treatment of pancreatitis and its complications. Semin Gastrointest Dis 1991;2:194.

Nealon WH, Thompson JC: Progressive loss of pancreatic function in chronic pancreatitis is delayed by main pancreatic duct decompression: A longitudinal prospective analysis of the modified Peustow procedure. Ann Surg 1993;217:458.

Neiderau C, Grendell JH: Diagnosis of chronic pancreatitis. Gastroenterology 1985;88:1973.

Sarles H et al: The pancreatitis classification of Marseilles-Rome 1988. Scand J Gastroenterol 1989;24:641.

Singh M: Pathophysiology of alcohol-related pancreatitis. Semin Gastrointest Dis 1991;3:140.

Stabile BE, Wilson SE, Debas HT: Reduced mortality from bleeding pseudocysts and pseudoaneurysms caused by pancreatitis. Arch Surg 1983;118:45.

Steinberg W: The clinical utility of the CA 19-9 tumor-associated antigen. Am J Gastroenterol 1990;85:350.

Toskes PP: Hyperlipidemic pancreatitis. Gastroenterol Clin North Am 1990;19:783.

Toskes PP: Medical therapy of chronic pancreatitis. Semin Gastrointest Dis 1991;2:188.

Twersky Y, Bank S: Nutritional deficiencies in chronic pancreatitis. Gastroenterol Clin North Am 1989;18:543.

van Sonnenberg E et al: Imaging and interventional radiology for pancreatitis and its complications. Radiol Clin North Am 1989;27:65.

Vitas GJ, Sarr MG: Selected management of pancreatic pseudocysts: Operative versus expectant management. Surgery 1992;111:123.

Walsh TN et al: Minimal change chronic pancreatitis. Gut 1992;33:1566.

Yeo CJ et al: The natural history of pancreatic pseudocysts documented by computed tomography. Surg Gynecol Obstet 1990;170:411.

Tumors of the Pancreas

33

John P. Cello, MD

The vast majority of pancreatic neoplasms are adenocarcinomas of ductal epithelial origin. A relatively small percentage of pancreatic tumors consist of islet-cell tumors, cystadenomas, adenoacanthomas, or pancreatic lymphomas. The clinician caring for patients with pancreatic neoplasms needs to be aware that most of these tumors grow rapidly and are fatal.

Incidence & Risk Factors

About 30,000 patients with pancreatic neoplasms are diagnosed annually in the United States, and there are 25,000 cancer-related deaths. The estimated annual incidence in the USA is nearly 10 per 100,000 persons over the age of 75, making carcinoma of the pancreas the fourth most common cause of cancer death in men, and the fifth in women. The disease is somewhat more common in men than in women, and risk increases with age to a mean age of onset within the seventh and eighth decades of life. Certain ethnic and racial groups are noted to have an increased incidence: blacks, Polynesians, and native New Zealanders.

Additional risk factors include cigarette smoking (male smokers have four times the risk of nonsmokers), alcohol consumption, gallbladder stones, diabetes mellitus, chronic pancreatitis, and high intake of animal fat. Other dietary factors that may well be associated with an increased risk of pancreatic cancer include high protein consumption and the use of highly refined flour. Coffee consumption was once identified as a risk factor but now appears not to be associated with pancreatic cancer. Certain environmental agents are statistically associated with pancreatic cancer, including prolonged contact with petroleum products and wood pulp.

Pathophysiology

The clinical manifestations, laboratory features, and abdominal imaging characteristics can be explained by the pathology of most pancreatic neoplasms. Adenocarcinoma of the pancreas, the histologic type of over 90% of neoplastic processes of the gland, is characterized by a dense, fibrotic reaction surrounding a compact mass of hard pancreatic tissue. Because the pancreas lacks a mesentery and is adjacent to the bile duct, duodenum, stomach, and colon, the most common clinical presentations are those related to duct invasion or compression of these adjacent structures. Neoplasms such as islet-cell tumors, lymphomas, and cystadenomas tend to be less fibrotic and softer, thus distortion rather than compression or encasement is more common with these neoplasms of the pancreas.

Essentials of Diagnosis

- Vague, dull midepigastric abdominal discomfort
- Weight loss
- Anorexia
- Dysguesia
- Diarrhea, weakness, and vomiting
- Jaundice

ADENOCARCINOMA

Clinical Findings

A. Symptoms and Signs: There are few characteristic signs or symptoms early in the clinical course of pancreatic neoplasms that suggest the diagnosis. The most common pain presentation is vague, dull midepigastric abdominal discomfort, occasionally radiating through to the back. Weight loss, anorexia, dysgeusia, diarrhea, weakness, and vomiting are also commonly seen in patients with pancreatic neoplasms, particularly adenocarcinoma. Jaundice is noted in over 50% of patients with pancreatic neoplasms, particularly those involving the head of the gland. Most of these tumors are quite large and bulky, encasing the distal portion of the common bile duct. On occasion, however, a very small focal pancreatic mass involving only the periampullary area obstructs the common bile duct and produces jaundice at a very early stage of the disease, at which time the neoplasm is only 1–2 cm in diameter. Unfortunately, for those 30–40% of patients who develop the pancreatic malignant neoplasm in the body or tail of the gland, jaundice is a very late manifestation of the disease, commonly associated with a large retroperitoneal mass or with extensive hepatic metastases.

On occasion, obstruction of the distal common bile duct by a pancreatic neoplasm will be accompanied by a palpably distended nontender gallbladder, called **Courvoisier's sign**. This same feature may be noted in patients with bile duct obstruction from carcinoma of the ampulla of Vater, duodenal carcinoma, or even cholangiocarcinoma. Even rarer manifestations of pancreatic neoplasms include severe back pain, thrombophlebitis, pruritus, acute pancreatitis, psychiatric disturbances, or diabetes. Infrequently, patients may present with signs and symptoms of upper gastrointestinal tract bleeding because of erosion of the pancreatic neoplasm into the duodenal lumen. From the above it should be evident that most pancreatic neoplasms present very late in the course of the disease, at which time diagnosis confirms a nonresectable neoplasm.

B. Laboratory Findings:

1. Abnormalities—The most common clinical laboratory abnormalities include anemia, elevation of the erythrocyte sedimentation rate (ESR), and elevation of the serum alkaline phosphatase, bilirubin, and transaminases. Because most patients with pancreatic neoplasms have adenocarcinoma, and the most common site of pancreatic cancer is the head of the gland, high-grade common bile duct obstruction is frequently encountered. Malignant obstruction of the distal common bile duct characteristically elevates the serum alkaline phosphatase over four to five times the upper limits of normal. Furthermore, serum alkaline phosphatase levels increase out of proportion to bilirubin until late in the course of the disease, when alkaline phosphatase levels greater than 1000 IU/L and serum bilirubin values greater than 20 mg/dl are noted. Cholangitis with right upper quadrant pain, fever, leukocytosis, and modest elevations of the serum aminotransferases is distinctly uncommon. Elevations of serum amylase may occasionally be seen, and, rarely, patients will present with acute pancreatitis related to pancreatic duct obstruction.

2. Early markers—The search for "early" tumor markers has generated tremendous enthusiasm (Table 33–1). An elevated carcinoembryonic antigen (CEA) has been noted in over 70% of patients with confirmed pancreatic neoplasm. Other tumor markers such as alpha-fetoprotein, RNase, galactosyltransferase II (GT-II), and oncofetal antigen are elevated in small numbers of patients with pancreatic neoplasms. Other peptides have been investigated but largely dismissed as markers of patients with early pancreatic cancer.

Most recently, a carbohydrate antigen, CA19-9, has been identified as a promising new marker for well-differentiated pancreatic adenocarcinoma. The CA19-9 antigen is detected by monoclonal antibody and seems to correlate with the degree of differentiation of the tumor and with advancing stages of the disease. When a laboratory cutoff value of greater than or equal to 37 U/ml is used, approximately 80% of patients with pancreatic cancer have an elevated CA19-9 level. Unfortunately, only a very small percentage of patients with pancreatic cancer confined

Table 33–1. Percentage of positive findings suggesive of pancreatic cancer.[1]

Diagnostic Tests	Pancreatic Cancer (n = 61)	Other Gastrointestinal Cancer/Unknown Primary (n = 28)	Nongastrointestinal Cancer (n = 14)	Benign Disease (n = 167)
Ultrasonography (n = 236)	64	19	0	1
Computed tomography (n = 74)	79	0	25	4
ERCP[2] (n = 79)	93	0	0	0
Angiography (n = 12)	100	—	—	0
Alpha-Fetoprotein (n = 270)	3	6	7	1
Ferritin (n = 270)	50	45	64	22
RNase (n = 270)	30	39	8	14
CEA[3] >4 ng/dl (n = 270)	34	38	7	2
GT II[4] (n = 270)	67	71	21	2

Adapted from Podolsky DK et al. N Engl J Med 1981; 304:1313.
[1]In 270 patients evaluated by different means.
[2]ERCP = Endoscopic retrograde cholangiopancreatography.
[3]CEA = carcinoembryonic antigen.
[4]GT-II = galactosyltransferase isoenzyme II.

entirely to the pancreatic bed have elevated serum levels of CA19-9. Furthermore, CA19-9 can be elevated in patients with acute pancreatitis, chronic pancreatitis, chronic liver disease, and biliary tract disease.

Elevations of serum trypsin levels and trypsin-creatinine clearance have also been demonstrated in patients with pancreatic cancer. These and other biochemical and serologic markers for pancreatic cancer will need extensive evaluation in larger prospective trials.

C. Diagnostic Studies:

1. Noninvasive imaging–Noninvasive abdominal imaging is commonly done in patients with suspected pancreatic neoplasms; this often includes an upper gastrointestinal tract series and upper endoscopy. On occasion, the upper gastrointestinal series will show widening of the duodenal loop or even a mass indentation along the second portion of the duodenum. Endoscopy might likewise reveal gastric outlet obstruction or even invading mass within the descending duodenum. Neither of these techniques, however, is sensitive or specific for pancreatic cancer.

Other noninvasive imaging modalities include ultrasound, computed tomography (CT) (Figure 33–1), and magnetic resonance imaging (MRI). By these modalities, a pancreatic neoplasm presents as a heterogeneous asymmetric mass in the pancreas, or, rarely, a uniform enlargement of the pancreas. In addition, there may be loss of tissue fat planes between the pancreas and the retroperitoneum. Because most pancreatic adenocarcinoma arises in the head of the gland and will obstruct both the pancreatic duct and the common bile duct, dilation of these ducts is commonly noted by noninvasive imaging modalities.

The reported sensitivity and specificity of both ultrasound and CT in pancreatic carcinoma easily exceeds 90%. The main problem with these noninvasive imaging modalities is that their lower limits of resolution are generally in the range of 1–2 cm, therefore, small foci of the pancreatic cancer may be missed. In patients with a very strong index of suspicion for pancreatic carcinoma, however, CT should be the initial noninvasive diagnostic procedure. A CT "pancreatic protocol" is most appropriate in imaging these patients, with 5-mm transverse sections following intravenous contrast enhancement. Oral contrast is also important in order to outline the adjacent stomach and small bowel. It is important to realize that in patients strongly suspected of having pancreatic cancer, even in the face of a negative ultrasound, CT, or MRI, an endoscopic retrograde cholangiopancreatogram (ERCP) may be warranted (Figure 33–2).

2. Endoscopic retrograde cholangiopancreatography–ERCP provides the only means for directly viewing the entire pancreatic duct. Though on occasion transhepatic cholangiography and direct surgical pancreatography may be helpful, they cannot be a substitute for ERCP, given its widespread availability and high sensitivity (over 90% in most series). Because the vast majority of pancreatic neoplasms are ductal adenocarcinomas, even small mass lesions obstruct the pancreatic duct, leading to its dilation (Figure 33–3). The most common features of pancreatic neoplasms on ERCP include a solitary irregular pancreatic duct narrowing or an abrupt cutoff of the main pancreatic duct with a dilated bile duct (Figures 33–3 and 33–4). While these changes are usually quite different from those seen in chronic pancreatitis, in some instances, there may be overlap.

The best ERCP criterion for diagnosis of carcinoma of the pancreas appears to be a single, irregular, abrupt focal stricture of the pancreatic duct with the absence of other changes seen in chronic pancreatitis. In addition to contrast imaging of the pancreatic duct, pure pancreatic juice or directed brushings of the pancreatic duct have been used in some centers to confirm the diagnosis of a malignant neoplasm.

It is important to recognize that noninvasive abdominal imaging studies such as CT, MRI, and ultrasound are not competitive with ERCP in the diagnosis of pancreatic malignancy. In most studies the combined accuracy of ERCP and CT in patients with pancreatic neoplasms approaches 100%. Thus, a definite abnormality on either CT or ERCP can justify proceeding with the other technique in an attempt to detect mass lesions that are resectable for cure.

3. Cytology–Despite a low clinical threshold for ordering invasive and noninvasive imaging, the majority of patients with pancreatic neoplasm are diagnosed by direct needle aspiration cytology (see Figure 33–2). Most patients present late in the course of the disease and are found to have large mass lesions on CT, ultrasound, or both. These patients should undergo cytologic studies as a part of initial

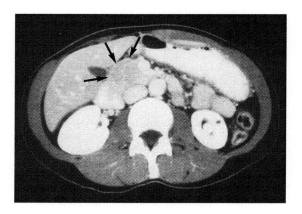

Figure 33–1. Computed tomography of the abdomen in a patient with carcinoma of the head of the pancreas. An irregular, low-density mass is noted in the head of the pancreas **(arrows)**. Pancreatic carcinoma was subsequently confirmed by fine-needle aspiration cytology.

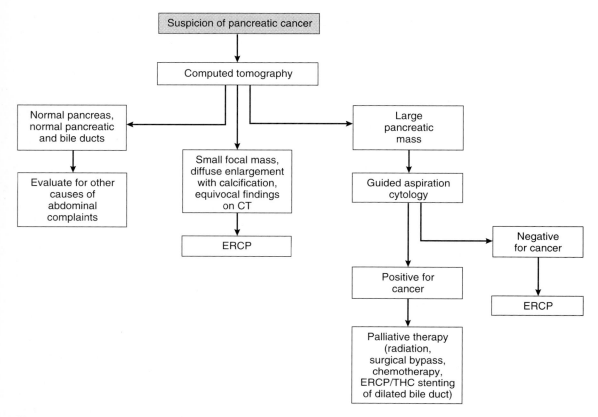

Figure 33-2. Scheme for the diagnosis of pancreatic cancer. CT = computed tomography; ERCP = endoscopic retrograde cholangiopancreatography; THC = transhepatic cholangiography.

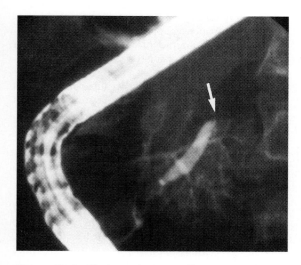

Figure 33-3. Endoscopic retrograde pancreatogram in patient with carcinoma of the head of the pancreas. An abrupt cutoff of the pancreatic duct is noted, with filling of secondary pancreatic ductules in the head and uncinate process. Such an abrupt cutoff (arrow) is invariably due to pancreatic adenocarcinoma arising in the main pancreatic duct.

noninvasive imaging, either by CT or ultrasound guidance.

Cytology is now the principal means for establishing the diagnosis of pancreatic cancer. In most series, cytology has demonstrated 80–90% sensitivity and 100% specificity with virtually no false-positive biopsy results in patients with chronic inflammatory disease of the pancreas. The absence of malignant cells in a single aspirated cytologic sample does not, however, definitively exclude pancreatic neoplasm. Multiple attempts should be made to secure an adequate number of cells for cytologic examination. The safety, sensitivity, and specificity of this technique have made cytologic examination the principal means of firmly establishing the diagnosis of pancreatic neoplasms.

Differential Diagnosis

Because most pancreatic neoplasms present as solid masses in the pancreas, the primary differential diagnosis is chronic pancreatitis. Rare cystic neoplasms must be differentiated from pancreatic pseudocysts.

Patients with focal or generalized enlargement of

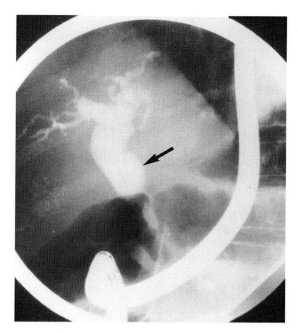

Figure 33–4. Endoscopic retrograde cholangiogram in a patient with pancreatic carcinoma. The common bile duct is markedly dilated to greater than 2 cm (normal is less than 8 mm) *(arrow)*. Dilation is also noted of the intrahepatic bile ducts.

the pancreas should have cytologic examination of the gland by fine- needle aspiration cytology, which usually confirms the histologic diagnosis of pancreatic neoplasm (see Figure 33–2). For those patients with negative or equivocal results on cytologic studies, an ERCP will likely differentiate between chronic pancreatitis and pancreatic neoplasms.

Carcinoma of the ampulla of Vater must also be differentiated from pancreatic cancer in patients who have jaundice. Patients with ampullary cancer are usually identified on CT or ultrasonography by dilation of the extrahepatic bile ducts and the pancreatic duct without detectable distal bile duct mass lesion.

Endoscopic examination of the medial wall of the duodenum is essential prior to surgery for patients with likely ampullary carcinoma. The duodenal papilla must be adequately viewed, and biopsy and pancreatography must be confirmatory.

Treatment

A. Surgery: The minority of patients with pancreatic neoplasms undergo curative surgical resection, primarily because only 10% present early enough with potentially curable disease. For example, over 300 patients with pancreatic carcinoma were referred to UCLA Medical Center over a 15-year period, but only 15% underwent pancreatic resection while 50% underwent nonresective operative

procedures to relieve biliary or gastric outlet obstruction. Fully one-third of the patients had neither resection nor surgical bypass because of obvious widespread disease, advanced age, or debility.

For patients with confirmed carcinoma of the head of the pancreas, the Whipple resection is the procedure of choice. Candidates for this resective procedure should have adequate preoperative staging by CT, ERCP, and endoscopic ultrasonography. There is now an acceptable operative mortality rate of less than or equal to 5% for resected patients. For patients with pancreatic carcinoma overall, however, there remains only a 4–5% survival at 5 years following Whipple resection.

The main source of morbidity and mortality from the Whipple procedure is the pancreaticojejunostomy, through which anastomotic leaks and hemorrhage have occurred. Despite overall poor operative results, Whipple resection is the only real hope of cure for patients with carcinoma of the head of the pancreas and in the best of surgical hands may provide superior palliation, particularly among good-risk patients who have small periampullary neoplasms.

On-block resection of the entire pancreas, duodenum, spleen, and greater omentum with subtotal gastrectomy has been suggested by some investigators to have definite advantages over the Whipple procedure for patients with carcinoma of the head of the pancreas. Total pancreatectomy obviates the need for the difficult and problematic pancreaticojejunal anastomosis. Furthermore, for many patients who have carcinoma in the pancreas, the body and tail of the pancreas may be quite fibrotic and unlikely to function normally postoperatively. Some studies have also shown that even among patients whose carcinoma seems confined to the head of the pancreas, microscopic or macroscopic tumor foci can often be found far from the margin of pancreatic resection. One recent study from the Mayo Clinic failed to demonstrate a significant difference in 5-year survival between patients undergoing Whipple procedure versus those having total pancreatectomy. Clearly, surgical resection provides the only real chance for cure among patients with malignant neoplasms of the pancreas. Patients who have obvious nonresectable disease should be carefully excluded before pancreatic resection.

As previously mentioned, pancreatic neoplasm at the time of presentation is usually large and bulky, with either metastases, retroperitoneal extension, high-grade common bile duct obstruction, or all these findings. For those patients with the accompanying symptoms of pruritus, fever, or jaundice, strong consideration must be given to palliative decompression of the bile duct. Unfortunately, the mean survival following surgical bypass is only about 6 months, however, this procedure should be considered in otherwise good-risk patients, particularly those who have coexistent obstruction of the pylorus or the second portion of the duodenum. Surgical biliary and gastric bypass can be performed rapidly and safely and is usually effective. Percutaneous transhepatic stenting has been employed by experienced hands to palliatively decompress the dilated bile duct and relieve the symptoms of obstructive jaundice. Endoscopic biliary stenting, however, remains the preferred initial therapeutic palliative procedure for obstruction of the distal common bile duct (Figure 33–5). The procedure is usually performed at the time of the diagnostic ERCP. It is, however, advantageous for the endoscopist to have already established a malignant diagnosis so that large metal stents, such as the Wallstent, may be placed immediately over guidewires selectively passed into the common bile duct. Problems may be encountered at ERCP with very distal high-grade common bile duct obstructions, since there may be virtually no lumen available for cannulation. Problems may also occur in the patient whose tumor has eroded into the duodenum since no normal papilla is visible. In patients in whom endoscopic stent placement is not feasible, backup interventional radiologic support is necessary to decompress bile ducts. Close cooperation and consultation among the primary care physician, surgeon, gastroenterologist, and interventional radiologist ensure that palliation is individualized to patient need and anatomy.

B. Chemotherapy: Single-agent chemotherapy does not provide substantive palliation and improvement in survival for patients with non-resectable pancreatic cancer (Table 33–2). The mean survival time after the administration of 5-fluorouracil (5-FU) is less than 20 weeks, with a response rate of only 10–15%. Mitomycin, streptozotocin, ifosfamide, and doxorubicin likewise provide only a 10–25% response rate without improvement in long-term survival. Current chemotherapeutic regimens employ combinations of 5-FU and other agents. The FAM regimen (fluorouracil, doxorubicin [Adriamycin], and mitomycin) in preliminary studies produced response rates only in the range of 9–40%. Other studies have noted that mean survival time, mean interval to progression of tumor, and objective response rates are not significantly better for combination chemotherapy than fluorouracil alone. Promising new chemotherapeutic modalities, however, are becoming available, including cisplatin, epirubicin, and ifosfamide. Most recent studies, however, have not provided strong and compelling evidence that combination chemotherapy is helpful in either prolonging survival or enhancing the quality of life among patients who clearly have advanced pancreatic cancer. Clearly, extensive controlled clinical trials are needed before chemotherapy can be routinely recommended.

C. Radiation Therapy: When used alone, orthovoltage radiation therapy gives very disappointing results, with median survivals of only 6–12 months. Moreover, radiation can produce substantial injury to adjacent organs, such as the spinal cord, liver, and duodenum. Several techniques appear promising, however, improvements in survival or quality of life have not been documented. These include combination external beam radiation therapy and chemotherapy, surgically- or endoscopically-implanted iodine-125 seeds, or the intraoperative delivery of massive doses of radiation. A few studies have described the use of high linear energy transfer particle radiation therapy. This is an extremely demanding technique, requiring CT assistance. Neutron beam radiation can be delivered accurately to the tumor alone, with only limited injury to adjacent organs. Future studies of this technique are necessary, however, before it can be recommended over standard radiation therapy.

D. Celiac Plexus Block: For many patients, extensive retroperitoneal infiltration produces disabling, intractable pain. While narcotics and radiation therapy may be helpful, percutaneous neurolytic celiac plexus block can help patients who do not respond to standard narcotics or radiation therapy. An experienced anesthesiologist should perform this technique, usually guided by plain radiography, fluoroscopy, or CT. While no prospective randomized trials have examined this therapy, complications are few and adequate palliation can be achieved with very low risk. For those patients who do not obtain adequate pain relief from a celiac plexus block, percutaneous splanchnic nerve blocks or thoracoscopic splanchnicectomy can be tried.

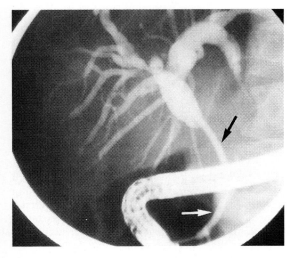

Figure 33–5. Endoscopic retrograde stenting of the common bile duct. A long polyethylene stent has been placed **(arrows)** with the proximal margin of the stent draining the dilated ductal system. The distal portion of the stent is left within the duodenum.

Table 33–2. Combination chemotherapy in advanced pancreatic cancer.

Regimen	Number of Patients	Responders	Response Rates	Median Survival
SMF	23	10	43%	6 months
SMF	22	7	32%	6 months
FAM	27	10	37%	6 months
FAM	15	6	40%	6 months
FAMS	25	12	48%	7 months
FAP	15	3	20%	NS
FAP	29	6	21%	4 months
FAP	19	9	47%	14 months
HEXA-FAM	30	5	17%	4 months
HEXA-FM	21	2	10%	10 months
EF	44	6	14%	4 months
EIFOS	26	3	12%	5 months
	n = 296	n = 79	27%	5–6 months

Adapted from: Wils JA. AntiCancer Research 9:1027, 1989.
A = Adriamycin
E = Epirubicin
F = 5-Flourouracil
HEXA = Hexamethylmelamine
IFOS = Ifosamide
M = Mitomycin
P = Cisplatin
S = Streptozotocin
NS = not stated

PANCREATIC ISLET-CELL TUMORS

Pancreatic islet-cell tumors constitute about 2% of all pancreatic neoplasms. Most patients with pancreatic islet-cell tumors present very early in the course of their disease, with clinical manifestations related to the secretion of hormonally-active substances. While tumors expressing amine precursor uptake and decarboxylation (APUD-cell tumors) will not be discussed extensively in this chapter, several points need to be emphasized.

Clinical Findings

The vast majority of patients with pancreatic islet-cell tumors present with signs and symptoms of excess hormone secretion. The most common tumor of islet-cell origin, namely the insulinoma, usually is manifested by profound hypoglycemia with diaphoresis, confusion, and syncope. Occasionally, hormonally inactive islet-cell tumors of the pancreatic head present with jaundice, pruritis, or abdominal pain.

Diagnostic Studies

In most patients, an elevated hormone level or other serologic test documents the presence of a syndrome likely to include a pancreatic islet-cell tumor. Transhepatic portal venous sampling for APUD-cell hormones along the splenic vein generated initial enthusiasm several years ago, but currently enjoys only limited clinical use. Clearly, the initial diagnostic procedure for localizing the tumor should be contrast-enhanced dynamic CT of the pancreas, employing 5-mm sections. In most instances, pancreatic islet-cell tumors are hypervascular; the use of the "pancreatic protocol" CT imaging technique can pick up small lesions, even those under a centimeter. Additional techniques for locating small APUD-cell tumors not seen by CT include preoperative endoscopic ultrasonography, intraoperative surgical inspection of the gland, and intraoperative ultrasonography. Endoscopic ultrasonography is especially helpful in localizing small islet-cell tumors and demonstrating resectability by showing normal tissue planes between the pancreas and adjacent great vessels.

Treatment

The vast majority of pancreatic islet-cell neoplasms can be treated by segmental resection of the gland or enucleation of the tumor. Although there may be some advantage to preoperative angiography, results have generally been quite disappointing.

CYSTIC NEOPLASMS

Pancreatic carcinomas other than adenocarcinoma of pancreatic ductal origin and islet-cell tumors are uncommon, representing only 5% of pancreatic cancers. A special mention needs to be made of cystadenomas and cystadenocarcinomas because they are often mistaken for benign pancreatic pseudcysts.

Clinical Findings

A. Symptoms and Signs: Most commonly, cystadenomas and cystadenocarcinomas present with abdominal pain, a palpable mass, weight loss, nausea, and vomiting. Jaundice, pruritis, cholangitis, and upper gastrointestinal tract bleeding are less common presentations.

B. Diagnostic Studies: Usually, because of vague abdominal complaints, a CT or sonogram (including endoscopic ultrasonography) demonstrates a large cystic mass within the pancreas. It may be difficult, however, to differentiate cystic pancreatic neoplasms from non-neoplastic pancreatic pseudocysts. The absence of trauma, alcoholism, clinically acute pancreatitis, or biliary tract disease makes cystic neoplasm of the pancreas more likely in patients who are found to have an isolated cystic lesion of the gland. In most instances, however, diagnosis is confirmed by laparotomy with resection. It is important to carefully exclude cystic neoplasms of the pancreas in patients who present with isolated cystic lesions without risk factors for pancreatic pseudocysts.

Treatment

These patients should be strongly considered for surgical resection, even if the cystic neoplasm appears to be large and bulky. Long-term survival following resection of pancreatic cystic neoplasms is excellent.

PANCREATIC LYMPHOMAS

Pancreatic lymphomas are infrequent, probably representing 1–3% of all pancreatic neoplasms. An increase in pancreatic lymphomas is now being described among patients with AIDS. These latter patients have B-cell non-Hodgkin's lymphomas arising primarily in the pancreas, wall of the duodenum, or even common bile duct.

Clinical Findings

The differentiation of pancreatic lymphoma from pancreatic adenocarcinoma is important preoperatively because the primary form of therapy for lymphoma is chemotherapy rather than surgical resection. In general, patients with pancreatic lymphoma present with signs and symptoms identical to those with adenocarcinoma. However, patients with pancreatic lymphoma have lower levels of serum bilirubin and alkaline phosphatase than patients with comparably bulky pancreatic adenocarcinoma. Percutaneous transabdominal aspiration cytology usually establishes the diagnosis of lymphoma. However, an uncertain preoperative diagnosis may necessitate surgery.

Treatment

Surgery may also be warranted when there is clear-cut high-grade biliary or gastric outlet obstruction, or both. When patients with pancreatic lymphoma are diagnosed preoperatively, chemotherapy can be initiated with cyclophosphamide, prednisone, and doxorubicin.

REFERENCES

INCIDENCE & RISK FACTORS, PATHOPHYSIOLOGY

Gold EB et al: Diet and other risk factors for cancer of the pancreas. Cancer 1985;55:460.

Haddock G, Carter DC: Aetiology of pancreatic cancer. Br J Surg 1990;77:1159.

Olsen GW et al: A case-control study of pancreatic cancer and cigarettes, alcohol, coffee and diet. Am J Public Health 1989;79:1016.

DIAGNOSTIC STUDIES

Moss AA et al: The combined use of computed tomography and endoscopic retrograde cholangiopancreatography in the assessment of suspected pancreatic neoplasm: A blind clinical evaluation. Radiology 1980;134:159.

Schmiegel W: Tumor markers in pancreatic cancer—current concepts. Hepatogastroenterology 1989;36:446.

Snady H, Cooperman A, Siegel J: Endoscopic ultrasonography compared with computed tomography with ERCP in patients with obstructive jaundice or small peripancreatic mass. Gastrointest Endosc 1992; 38:27.

Van Dyke JA, Stanley RJ, Berland LL: Pancreatic imaging. Ann Intern Med 1985;102:212.

TREATMENT

Fietkau R, Sauer R: Future prospects of radiotherapy in pancreatic cancer. Eur J Surg Oncol 1991;17:201.

McGrath PC et al: Management of biliary obstruction in patients with unresectable carcinoma of the pancreas. Ann Surg 1989;209:284.

Sharfman WH, Walsh TD: Has the analgesic efficacy of neurolytic celiac plexus block been demonstrated in pancreatic cancer pain? Pain 1990;41:267.

Singh SM, Longmire WP, Reber HA: Surgical palliation for pancreatic cancer. Ann Surg 1990;212:132.

Topham C et al: Randomised trial of epirubicin alone versus 5-fluorouracil, epirubicin and mitomycin C in locally advanced and metastatic carcinoma of the pancreas. Br J Cancer 1991;64:179.

Wils JA: Current status of chemotherapy of metastatic pancreatic cancer. Anticancer Res 1989;9:1027.

Section VI
Diseases of the Liver & Biliary System

Approach to the Patient With Suspected Liver Disease

34

Kurt O. Bodily, MD, & J. Gregory Fitz, MD

The clinical manifestations of liver injury are diverse, ranging from isolated and clinically silent laboratory abnormalities to dramatic and rapidly progressive liver failure. This spectrum relates in part to the broad range of pathophysiologic processes that can damage the liver, and in part to the reserve capacity of the organ, which is large and can mask significant injury. It is estimated that approximately 40% of patients with cirrhosis are asymptomatic. Once symptoms develop, however, the prognosis is poor and the human and economic costs of liver disease are high. Cirrhosis accounts for around 26,000 deaths each year in the United States, and more than 228,145 years of potential life lost. The average patient with alcoholic liver disease loses 12 years of productive life, a much larger loss than that for heart disease (2 years) and cancer (4 years). The poor outcome and high cost of treatment of advanced liver disease reinforce the need for early diagnosis and intervention.

This chapter provides general guidelines for evaluating suspected liver disease. Clinical categories that reflect common patterns of liver injury are emphasized and include: isolated aminotransferase elevation in the absence of symptoms; jaundice and cholestasis; and chronic liver disease. There is obvious overlapping between these categories, but recognition of the dominant pattern of injury provides an important framework for subsequent diagnosis of the underlying causes of liver injury. Indeed, this accounts for much of the challenge of clinical practice in liver disorders. Specific disease processes are described in more detail in subsequent chapters.

CLINICAL EVALUATION OF SUSPECTED LIVER DISEASE

Liver disease is identified in most patients by suggestive laboratory abnormalities or signs or symptoms that result from hepatocyte necrosis or from fibrosis. These abnormalities are often nonspecific, initiating a more focused evaluation to establish the extent of liver damage, identify the underlying causes, and guide therapy. Points of the history, physical, and laboratory examinations that merit special emphasis are summarized here.

Clinical History: Risk Factors for Liver Disease

Evaluation of suspected liver disease begins first with a detailed assessment of risk factors. Initially, basic demographic factors (ie, age, gender, and race) are used to establish a hierarchy of possibilities. Usually, males and nonwhites represent high-risk groups for liver disease, as evidenced by an increased number of hospital admissions. Men under 20 years of age are at risk for acute viral hepatitis, but with increasing age, overuse of alcohol, biliary disease, and chronic hepatitis are more commonly identified. Men over 55 years of age are at increased risk for cirrhosis, biliary disease, and hepatobiliary malignancies. Women are subject to the same general processes, but in addition are much more likely to develop autoimmune hepatitis in young and middle-aged cohorts, or primary biliary cirrhosis in those above age 40 years. Primary biliary cirrhosis is about nine times more common in women as compared with men.

Attention to the family history can also identify patients at risk. Classic genetic diseases such as hemochromatosis, α_1-antitrypsin deficiency, or Wilson's disease are the best defined. Hemochromatosis involves men more than women, and is associated with coexisting diabetes, heart disease, and pigmentation in many patients. Deficiency of α_1-antitrypsin is associated with pulmonary disease and younger age of onset. Wilson's disease is suggested by coincidence of neurologic abnormalities and an earlier age of onset. These familial disorders are relatively uncommon, however, and together account for less than 5% of visits to most hepatology practices. Instead, a positive family history of liver disease usually indicates either shared risks (eg, exposure to viral hepatitis) or more common inherited traits that have a much more complex genetic basis. Alcoholism, hyperlipidemia, and diabetes represent important risk factors that have unequivocal but poorly understood genetic links. These disorders are more common and likely to be associated with a family history of liver disease, and therefore may require the appropriate use of other diagnostic tests.

Personal habits and exposures also represent important risk factors (Table 34–1). As a rule, focused questions about high-risk behavior are required because of the temporal delay between the actions and the onset of clinical symptoms. Among these risk factors, alcohol abuse deserves special emphasis because of its prevalence. Alcohol-related liver disease accounts for 30% or more of hepatologic consultations. The precise mechanisms responsible for alcohol-related liver damage remain uncertain; there is evidence both for direct damage to liver cells by alcohol and its metabolites, and for indirect damage because of nutritional depletion (see Chapter 40). Most individuals have a history of substantial exposure. In men, it is estimated that consumption of 60–80 g of alcohol daily (approximately four beers, glasses of wine, or mixed drinks) establishes a clear risk for subsequent cirrhosis. In women, only 40–60 g/d establishes the same risk. Alcohol use must usually be continued for 10 years or more before cirrhosis develops. There is a broad range of susceptibility, however, and lower levels of consumption can be

toxic in some individuals. In addition, binge drinking, with exposure to higher alcohol levels, can cause alcoholic hepatitis and fatty liver. While these usually resolve with cessation of drinking, a history of alcoholic hepatitis identifies individuals at high risk for subsequent cirrhosis.

Attention to past medical events represents a final focus of the initial history. Male homosexuality, prior episodes of hepatitis, jaundice, or blood transfusions indicate increased risk for acute or chronic viral hepatitis, and a history of alcohol-related pancreatitis or hepatitis identifies a cohort with sufficient consumption to be at risk for cirrhosis. Prior cholecystectomy or biliary surgery represents a major risk for development of biliary strictures. Finally, many general medical conditions are accompanied by hepatic manifestations (Table 34–1).

Physical Examination

Physical manifestations of liver disease can result from loss of hepatocyte mass, bile duct obstruction, or development of portal hypertension. Chronic hepatitis and cirrhosis are clinically silent in a significant portion of patients because of the large reserve capacity of the liver. Consequently, the absence of physical findings provides no guarantee that liver disease can be ruled out, thus emphasizing the importance of a systematic evaluation.

A. Jaundice: Jaundice results from an increase in serum bilirubin concentration (see following discussion) and is detected as a yellow-green coloration of skin, mucous membranes, and sclerae. The onset usually coincides with a rise in serum bilirubin to over 3.5 mg/dL, and is of sufficient concern to most patients that they seek medical attention quickly. Unfortunately, not all patients are careful observers, and the multiple potential causes of jaundice limit the specificity of this finding. Instead, the clinical interpretation depends on the duration of the hyperbilirubinemia as well as laboratory and radiographic testing to assess whether there is intra- or extrahepatic cholestasis.

Jaundice accompanying acute liver necrosis that results from acetaminophen overdose, viral hepatitis, or hypotension is due to the loss of hepatocellular mass and impaired bilirubin secretion. In the early stages, detection of right upper quadrant tenderness and an increase in liver size (span > 12 cm) support active hepatocellular necrosis and inflammation. Appearance of asterixis, confusion, or coma mark further deterioration, and the onset of bleeding may indicate profound synthetic defects and coagulopathy. Liver size may decrease in the later stages, and decorticate or decerebrate posturing and neurogenic hyperventilation accompany irreversible damage.

The abrupt onset of jaundice accompanied by abdominal pain, fever, and right upper quadrant tenderness suggests acute cholangitis with or without cholecystitis. The liver is not usually enlarged, and a

Table 34–1. Risk factors for liver disease.

Risk Factors	Associated Liver Diseases
Family history	Hemochromatosis, Wilson's disease, α-1-antitrypsin deficiency, cystic fibrosis, thalassemia
Alcohol consumption (usually $\geq$ 50 g/d)	Alcoholic fatty liver, alcoholic hepatitis, cirrhosis
Hyperlipidemia, diabetes, obesity	Fatty liver
Previous blood transfusion	Hepatitis B, C, non-A, non-B
Autoimmune diseases	Autoimmune hepatitis, primary biliary cirrhosis
Medications	Drug-induced liver injury
Parenteral exposures, (IV drug use, health care workers)	Hepatitis B and C
Male homosexuality	Hepatitis B
Foreign travel	Hepatitis A and B
Ulcerative colitis	Primary sclerosing cholangitis
History of jaundice or hepatitis	Chronic viral hepatitis, autoimmune hepatitis, cirrhosis
Hepatobiliary surgery	Postoperative stricture of bile ducts, recurrent gallstones

history of previous gallbladder stones or surgery is suggestive. A more indolent onset of jaundice in the absence of tenderness may indicate underlying transport abnormalities, cirrhosis, or duct obstruction.

B. Manifestations Resulting from Loss of Hepatocellular Mass and Portal Hypertension: Other physical manifestations of chronic liver disease result from sustained loss of hepatocellular mass and development of portal hypertension (see Chapter 43). A small liver (< 8 cm) or a liver with a nodular contour suggests the presence of established cirrhosis, although interobserver variability limits the reproducibility of this finding. As the metabolic capacity of the liver deteriorates, the estrogen precursor androstenedione can accumulate and lead to gynecomastia, testicular atrophy, and palmar erythema. In addition, spider angiomas are common and most frequently involve the face, shoulders, and trunk. These may result from increased circulating levels of angiogenic factors.

Anatomic distortion of the liver caused by fibrosis and regeneration leads to distortion and loss of sinusoidal area and an increase in portal vein pressures. Portal hypertension may remain clinically silent but more commonly leads to predictable clinical sequelae, including renal Na^+ retention, which results in ascites and edema; hypersplenism with thrombocytopenia; portal-systemic shunting, resulting in hemorrhoids and distended superficial and periumbilical (caput medusa) abdominal veins; and esophageal varices. In chronic cirrhosis, hepatic encephalopathy correlates more closely with the degree of portal hypertension and shunting of blood away from the liver than with the loss of hepatocyte mass. While any one of these features may predominate in an individual patient, they often coexist and may change over time.

C. Manifestations More Common to Specific Disorders: Some physical findings have more specificity in that they occur with greater frequency according to the underlying cause of cirrhosis. Chronic alcohol use is associated with fibrosis of the palmar fascia, leading to Dupuytren's contractures involving the fourth and fifth fingers, atrophy of proximal muscles, and peripheral neuropathy. Hemochromatosis is accompanied by a characteristic metallic-gray pigmentation related to melanin deposition on sun-exposed areas of the body; pigmentation can also be seen in the genital regions and in areas of scarring. Hemochromatosis is also accompanied by a characteristic arthropathy involving the small joints of the hands, particularly the second and third metacarpophalangeal joints. Wilson's disease can cause acute liver failure with hemolytic anemia, or chronic liver failure with associated neurologic findings due to involvement of basal ganglia; findings include movement disorders, tremors, spasticity, rigidity, chorea, and dysarthria. Kayser-Fleischer rings due to deposition of copper in Descemet's membrane are highly suggestive of Wilson's disease.

Laboratory Findings

Because many of the clinical features of liver injury are nonspecific, the history and physical examination are routinely supplemented by "liver function" tests, which are so widely available that they have become a standard and essential component of the evaluation. In this section, a brief overview of standard laboratory tests is provided to serve as a basis for later definition of specific clinical syndromes.

A. Hepatocellular Injury: Aminotransferases: Aspartate aminotransferase (AST) and alanine aminotransferase (ALT) are found in high concentrations inside hepatocytes, where they catalyze transfer of α-amino groups from their respective amino acids to ketoglutaric acid, resulting in the formation of oxaloacetic acid and pyruvate plus glutamate. The aminotransferases are detectable in serum in concentrations of less than 60 IU/L, as a result of normal cell turnover and regeneration. Any insult that leads to liver cell injury or necrosis releases intracellular enzymes and results in increases in serum AST and ALT concentrations. Consequently, the aminotransferases provide a sensitive but relatively nonspecific measure of liver inflammation. Aminotransferase levels may be elevated to the same degree in patients with benign conditions such as fatty liver, or more serious conditions, including chronic viral hepatitis and cancer. Thus, detection of elevated aminotransferases mandates more specific evaluation to identify the underlying cause.

Recognizing that there are exceptions to every rule, some useful generalizations regarding interpretation of aminotransferase elevations appear consistently and have enhanced their utility in the clinical setting. First, an AST to ALT ratio greater than 2 with AST levels of less than 300 IU/L is suggestive of alcohol-related liver disease. In contrast, viral hepatitis, ischemia, and other causes of injury result in more equivalent increases in AST and ALT and can produce higher serum concentrations. Second, increases in AST are not always related to liver injury, since this enzyme is also found in heart, muscle, kidney, brain, and pancreatic tissue and in erythrocytes. Because there are no tissue-specific isoenzymes of AST, it is important to suspect extrahepatic origins and confirm hepatic inflammation by measurement of ALT, which is found almost exclusively in the liver. Third, acute elevations of aminotransferases to values of more than 1000 IU/L usually reflect severe necrosis and necessitate rapid evaluation, with the aim of implementing specific therapy as soon as possible. Viral hepatitis, toxin-induced hepatitis (acetaminophen overdose, *Amanita phylloides* ingestion), and hepatic ischemia represent important causes of markedly elevated aminotransferases and should be considered according to the clinical presentation.

B. Alternative Markers for Hepatocellular Injury: Other hepatic enzymes have been used to supplement measurements of aminotransferase activity, with the aim of improving sensitivity or permitting early detection of alcohol-related injury. These include glutamate dehydrogenase, alcohol dehydrogenase, and lactate dehydrogenase. Their clinical utility has been limited by a lack of specificity, however, and they provide little information beyond that provided by AST and ALT.

C. Ductular Injury and Cholestasis: Alkaline Phosphatase and 5′-nucleotidase: The alkaline phosphatases represent a family of enzymes that hydrolyze organic phosphate esters in an alkaline environment. In the liver, they are localized to the canalicular region of hepatocytes and to bile duct cells. Ductular obstruction and cholestasis lead to increased production of alkaline phosphatase and to release of alkaline phosphatase from damaged cells. Consequently, elevation of serum alkaline phosphatase levels provides an important marker for duct cell injury, duct cell proliferation, and cholestasis.

Increases in alkaline phosphatase to levels four times normal or more are highly suggestive of ductular injury; representative causes include intrahepatic cholestasis, infiltrative processes, extrahepatic biliary obstruction, primary sclerosing cholangitis, primary biliary cirrhosis, malignant liver disease, and organ rejection after liver transplantation (Table 34–2). Lesser increases in alkaline phosphatase can accompany a broader range of injuries, including viral hepatitis, cirrhosis, and congestive hepatopathy.

Elevations of alkaline phosphatase also accompany diseases affecting bone, adrenal cortex, placenta, intestine, kidney, and lung. These diverse sources mandate that the hepatic origin of elevated alkaline phosphatase levels be confirmed by detection of associated evidence of liver disease and by evaluation for nonhepatic sources. Traditionally, this was done by fractionation of the alkaline phos-

phatase, since the hepatic and nonhepatic isoenzymes can be separated on the basis of different electrophoretic mobilities and susceptibility to urease and heat. This has largely been replaced by measurement of 5′-nucleotidase, which is a reliable and relatively specific marker of cholestasis and ductular injury. 5′-nucleotidase activity is also abundant in the canalicular region, and usually increases in parallel with hepatic alkaline phosphatase levels.

Elevations of γ-glutamyl transpeptidase (GGT) also accompany the rise in alkaline phosphatase and 5′-nucleotidase levels. GGT is frequently elevated in patients ingesting alcohol, dilantin, barbiturates, and other drugs, and this has led to its use as a possible marker for occult alcohol use or liver disease. Isolated elevations of GGT in the absence of other findings are nonspecific, however, and most cases are not associated with clinically significant liver disease. This represents an obvious limitation for the use of GGT as a screening test.

D. Cholestasis: Bilirubin: Under normal conditions, serum bilirubin levels are maintained at less than 1.2 mg/dL, despite a continuous bilirubin load related to catabolism of heme molecules from senescent red blood cells. Maintenance of low serum levels requires three basic steps, which are illustrated in Figure 34–1. These steps include: (1) hepatic uptake of bilirubin from the circulation, an efficient process mediated by specific carrier proteins in the basolateral membrane; (2) intracellular conjugation of bilirubin to glucuronic acid to improve water solubility; and (3) canalicular secretion of bilirubin into the canalicular space between cells. From there, bilirubin conjugates are directed through the intrahepatic network of bile ducts and ultimately into the duodenum. Bilirubin is deconjugated in the intestinal lumen by bacteria. This secretory cycle can be interrupted at many levels, resulting in accumulation of bilirubin in the serum and clinical jaundice.

The subtleties of bilirubin metabolism and the susceptibility of the metabolic pathways to nonspecific injury complicate the interpretation of individual tests. Canalicular secretion is usually the rate-limiting step in the bilirubin cycle, however. Consequently, most jaundice encountered in adults is caused by conjugated hyperbilirubinemia resulting from defective canalicular transport and regurgitation of conjugated bilirubin out of the hepatocyte and back into the circulation. Unconjugated hyperbilirubinemia is encountered less commonly, and relevant causes include Gilbert syndrome and hemolysis. Bilirubin elevations in the hospitalized patient with other medical or surgical problems are most often multifactorial, with contributions from increased bilirubin production and impaired secretion. Systemic bacteremia, for example, causes a selective defect in secretion of conjugated bilirubin. In the absence of specific diagnostic tests, this syndrome is suggested by elevations of bilirubin out of proportion

Table 34–2. Common clinical findings in hepatic disease.

Test	Hepatocellular Injury	Cholestatic Disorders
Aminotransferases	> 8 times normal	< 3 times normal
Alkaline phosphatase	< 3 times normal	> 4 times normal
Bilirubin	Variably elevated	Elevated
5′-nucleotidase	Variably elevated	Elevated
Prothrombin	Prolonged, poorly responsive to vitamin K	Prolonged, responsive to vitamin K
Abdominal pain	Uncommon	Common in extrahepatic obstruction
Fever, leukocytosis	Uncommon	Common in extrahepatic obstruction

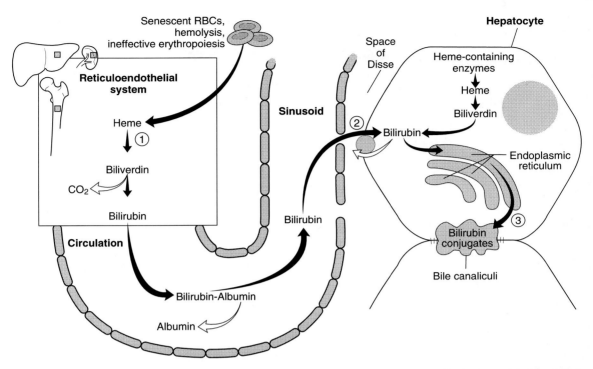

Figure 34–1. Bilirubin metabolism. Senescent red blood cells are removed from the circulation by reticuloendothelial cells in the liver, spleen, and bone marrow. Heme oxygenase (1) catalyzes cleavage of the tetrapyrrole ring to the linear tetrapyrrole biliverdin. Biliverdin is subsequently reduced to bilirubin. After production in the reticuloendothelial system, bilirubin is released into the circulation, where it is bound primarily to albumin. Fenestrations in the endothelial cells lining the hepatic sinusoids allow proteins access to Disse's space, where free bilirubin is transported into the hepatocyte (2). Bilirubin is poorly soluble in water and requires conjugation with glucuronide for excretion into the bile canaliculi (3). Conjugated bilirubin is actively transported into the bile canaliculi, where it is carried to the biliary tree and ultimately the duodenum.

to alkaline phosphatase levels, without evidence of biliary obstruction.

Most clinical laboratories use the van den Bergh reaction to measure serum bilirubin levels. This colorimetric approach detects conjugated bilirubin as a "direct" fraction, and unconjugated bilirubin as an "indirect" fraction. Conjugation of bilirubin to glucuronide greatly increases its water solubility. Because conjugated bilirubin is then freely excreted by the kidneys, it has a short half-life in the circulation. The van den Bergh approach tends to overestimate the direct fraction as compared with high-resolution chromatography methods, which indicate that almost all circulating bilirubin in normal individuals is unconjugated. With intra- or extrahepatic cholestasis, there are increases in both the conjugated and unconjugated forms, but conjugated bilirubin usually predominates, since uptake and conjugation continue despite limited canalicular secretion. Over time, a third form of bilirubin appears that is covalently bound to albumin. This is often referred to as a delta fraction, which increases with the degree and duration of the

bilirubin elevation. Protein-bound bilirubin is detected as part of the "direct" fraction by colorimetric assays, but protein-bound bilirubin is not secreted by the kidneys and has a much longer half-life in the circulation. Consequently, hyperbilirubinemia may persist for weeks after resolution of cholestasis if there is an appreciable amount of protein-bound (delta) bilirubin present.

E. Synthetic Functions of the Liver: Loss of hepatocyte mass results in impairment of the biosynthetic functions of the liver and is reflected in common symptoms, including fatigue and loss of muscle mass. Measurement of the serum albumin concentration and the prothrombin time provides a more quantitative assessment of functional impairment. Decreases in serum albumin result primarily from decreased production, and sustained values of less than 3 mg/dL indicate substantial impairment. Because albumin has a half-life in the circulation of approximately 28 days, several weeks or months of impaired synthesis are required before there are detectable decreases in serum concentrations. Nonhepatic causes of hypoalbuminemia include protein-losing enteropathies, nephrosis, and malnutrition.

Prolongation of the prothrombin time is a more reliable indicator of defective synthetic function. Maintenance of normal values requires synthesis of multiple vitamin K–dependent factors in the coagulation cascade. With loss of hepatocyte mass, the decrease in factor levels leads to incremental defects in coagulation. A decrease in factor VII levels to less than 30% of normal or an increase in the prothrombin time of more than 3 seconds correlates with marked impairment. Since cholestasis, malabsorption, and nutritional deprivation can all contribute to vitamin K deficiency, it is important to replete vitamin K stores to ensure that the prothrombin time accurately reflects synthetic capacity rather than vitamin K depletion.

Clinical Assessment & Prognosis

Although individual laboratory findings lack specificity, the use of a panel of laboratory and clinical findings has been shown to provide important insights into the severity of the underlying disease and the long-term prognosis. This approach helps to quantitate functional reserve and is becoming increasingly important with the advent of newer therapies. The appropriate timing of transplantation, for example, is critical to successful and cost-effective outcomes (see Chapter 54). Transplantation too early in the clinical course would improve surgical outcomes at the expense of some unnecessary operations, while transplantation late in the clinical course at a time when hepatic reserve is exhausted predicts poorer outcomes and increased costs.

Several methods for evaluating functional hepatic reserve have been developed. One of the best validated and easiest to use is the **Child-Pugh score,** which is based on the original observations of Child and Turcotte. This approach uses a graded system to assign a numerical risk on the basis of serum albumin and serum bilirubin measurements, the presence of ascites and encephalopathy, and nutritional status, as shown in Table 34–3. The sum of these clinical and laboratory parameters, on a scale of 0–15, provides an important overall assessment of the severity of cirrhosis. A total score of less than 6 is considered

grade A (well-compensated) disease; 7–9 grade B (significant functional compromise) disease; and 10–15 grade C (decompensated) disease, which has the highest risk for subsequent complications. The ease and prognostic utility of this scoring system provides important advantages for routine assessment of most patients with cirrhosis. Separate disease-specific measures may be more reliable in primary biliary cirrhosis, where alkaline phosphatase and bilirubin are specifically influenced by the illness.

CLINICAL PRESENTATIONS OF LIVER INJURY

The following sections delineate several of the more common clinical presentations that account for most consultations to liver specialists. Since the hepatic response to diverse injuries may be similar, emphasis is placed on pattern recognition and categorization into basic pathophysiologic syndromes. It is important to emphasize that this is not an end unto itself but is useful as a guide to management and provides a framework for the efficient evaluation of the underlying cause of liver damage. Specific etiologic diagnoses, as described in subsequent chapters, are always preferred, since they allow better definition of the natural history and potential complications.

Isolated Aminotransferase Elevation in the Asymptomatic Patient

A. Clinical Presentation: Most patients with liver disease are asymptomatic during much of the course of the disease due to the large reserve capacity of the organ. They come to medical attention only when abnormal blood tests suggest underlying liver damage, usually in the form of modest AST or ALT elevations (or both). Unfortunately, lack of symptoms is no assurance of a benign cause, since chronic active hepatitis, cirrhosis, and other threatening processes are not distinguished from transient and clinically insignificant processes without further assessment. A systematic evaluation such as the one shown in Figure 34–2 is warranted, to identify patients with significant disease and initiate treatment to prevent progression to cirrhosis.

B. Pathophysiologic Findings: AST and ALT are widely used as screening tests because they provide a sensitive index of active liver inflammation. In the absence of symptoms, values are usually less than 400 IU/L; higher values more often reflect an acute process such as viral or ischemic hepatitis with accompanying clinical manifestations. The increase in aminotransferases alone provides little insight into the underlying cause; and the degree of transaminase elevation has only a weak correlation with the degree of inflammation as assessed histologically. Consequently, even modest transaminase ele-

Table 34–3. Modified Child-Pugh classification of the severity of liver disease.[1]

Parameter	Points Assigned		
	1	**2**	**3**
Ascites	Absent	Slight	Moderate
Bilirubin (mg/dL)	≤ 2	2–3	> 3
Albumin (g/dL)	> 3.5	2.8–3.5	< 2.8
Prothrombin time (seconds over control)	1–3	4–6	> 6
Encephalopathy	None	Grade 1–2	Grade 3–4

[1]Total score of 1–6, grade A; 7–9, grade B; 10–15, grade C.

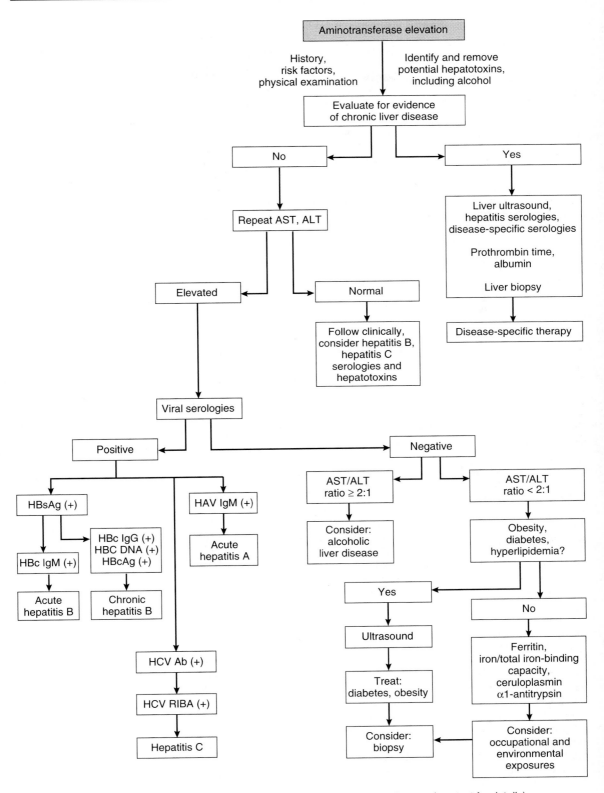

Figure 34–2. An approach to the patient with elevated aminotransferases (see text for details).

vations should not be dismissed without further consideration.

It is helpful to consider some of the more common causes of increased aminotransferase elevation in asymptomatic populations as a guide to designing an appropriate evaluation. Alcohol overuse, fatty liver, chronic viral and autoimmune hepatitis, and drug toxicity account for two-thirds of cases. Unsuspected cirrhosis, liver tumors, and genetic diseases such as hemochromatosis are less common.

C. Diagnostic Evaluation: Evaluation of increased aminotransferase values is challenging for both the patient and the physician. While many of the causes are benign and self-limited, the recognition that a potentially serious disease could be present necessitates a systematic approach in order to identify the underlying cause and establish the severity. The approach summarized in Figure 34–2 is predicated upon the lack of symptoms and no evidence for cholestasis; coexisting increases in alkaline phosphatase and bilirubin levels mandate concomitant evaluation for ductular diseases (eg, primary biliary cirrhosis), cirrhosis, and bile duct obstruction.

1. Initial evaluation—The initial evaluation of these patients begins with a careful history to identify risk factors and a physical examination to identify features of unrecognized chronic liver disease. Use of alcohol or potential hepatotoxic medications should be prohibited, and in the absence of symptoms, there is usually a window of opportunity for observation to determine whether test abnormalities will improve without further intervention. More commonly, persistent or intermittent elevations require more focused testing. Initially, this should include testing for viral hepatitis, with emphasis on hepatitis B surface antigen and hepatitis C viral antibodies to identify those at risk for chronic viral disease (see Chapter 37). Positive tests for autoimmune markers, including antinuclear antibodies, might suggest an autoimmune basis for the disease; autoimmune disease is less common in men. The evaluation of persistent aminotransferase elevations in the setting of positive viral or autoimmune markers usually requires a liver biopsy for confirmation of the diagnosis, assessment of disease activity, and guidance of therapy.

2. Fatty liver—If viral and autoimmune markers are unrevealing, the possibility of fatty liver, which is found in up to 20–60% of these patients, should be considered. Obesity, hyperlipidemia, and glucose intolerance represent important risk factors for fatty liver, which is characterized histologically by accumulation of lipids inside hepatocytes. The clinical course of fatty liver is usually benign. Since the abnormalities reflect a systemic metabolic abnormality, treatment is aimed at correction of the underlying risk factors. Even when fatty liver is suspected on clinical grounds, an ultrasound examination is warranted in most patients to address the possibility of

an unsuspected mass lesion. In more severe cases, ultrasound may reveal a diffuse increase in echogenicity because of increased fat accumulation. A more worrisome entity referred to as nonalcoholic steatohepatitis occurs with greater frequency in overweight women and can mimic simple fatty liver or autoimmune liver disease (see Chapter 45). Unlike fatty liver, nonalcoholic steatohepatitis can progress to hepatic fibrosis and cirrhosis. Consequently, if there is uncertainty about the diagnosis, or if the test abnormalities do not respond to treatment of the underlying risk factors, a liver biopsy is warranted.

3. Drug-induced liver disease—A common clinical quandary is that many of the drugs used to treat hyperlipidemia or hyperglycemia can themselves cause elevation of aminotransferases. While this is limited to less than 5% of patients, drug-induced liver disease can have serious sequelae. As a general rule, the benefits of these medications in controlling the risk factors outweigh their potential for liver toxicity. Careful surveillance for an increase in AST or ALT is warranted however. Control of risk factors through diet and exercise is important but not always successful.

4. Other diseases—In patients without a clear working diagnosis, or in whom a conservative course of observation and risk factor reduction fails, additional studies should be performed. These include ultrasound examination of the liver to minimize the possibility of an unsuspected anatomic abnormality or mass lesion, and screening for genetic diseases, including hemochromatosis, Wilson's disease, and α_1-antitrypsin deficiency. Suspicion of these disorders usually requires liver biopsy for definitive diagnosis.

Jaundice & Cholestasis

A. Clinical Presentation: Cholestasis is detected clinically by the onset of jaundice and an increase in serum bilirubin concentrations. Due to the central role of the liver in bilirubin metabolism, the onset of jaundice localizes the abnormality to the hepatobiliary system in most patients. An efficient diagnostic approach helps to minimize unnecessary tests in those with benign causes, focuses the workup in those with extrahepatic causes, and provides a clear therapeutic rationale for those with significant underlying pathologic changes.

When cholestasis develops acutely, impaired bile flow is often associated with jaundice, pruritis, and anorexia. Nausea and vomiting are nonspecific but frequently present. With sustained cholestasis, the decrease in bile flow has more far-reaching metabolic effects. Weight loss and fat malabsorption are related to impaired intestinal micelle formation; coagulopathy and bleeding to impaired absorption of dietary vitamin K; and osteomalacia to malabsorption and impaired metabolism of vitamin D.

A central focus of the diagnostic evaluation is to determine whether jaundice results from "medical" causes, including increased bilirubin load and intrahepatic cholestasis, or from "surgical" causes, such as obstruction of the bile ducts. Clinical judgment based on a careful history, physical examination, and routine laboratory studies is a powerful tool in differentiating between intrahepatic and extrahepatic jaundice. Clinical judgment is more sensitive but less specific than duct visualization by ultrasonography. Clinical features that suggest extrahepatic obstruction include fever, leukocytosis, right upper quadrant pain, elevated alkaline phosphatase values, or previous biliary surgery; features that suggest intrahepatic cholestasis include a history of chronic hepatitis, cirrhosis, portal hypertension, or exposure to hepatocellular toxins.

B. Pathophysiologic Findings: Cholestasis in the strictest sense refers to impaired bile formation. While this is usually associated with a rise in bilirubin, it is important to emphasize that the formation of bile does not depend upon bilirubin but is driven by the transport of other organic and inorganic solutes, including bile salts, glutathione, and HCO_3^-. The increase in bilirubin itself is not harmful, but in the presence of cholestasis, it is a marker for underlying changes in bile flow. Indeed, parallel increases in the serum concentrations of bile salts and other solutes may contribute more importantly to the clinical symptoms of cholestasis.

Figure 34–1 shows an outline of bilirubin production, metabolism, and secretion. A working knowledge of these pathways provides an important framework for clinical evaluation, since disorders at any of these steps can lead to an increase in bilirubin concentrations. Unconjugated (indirect) hyperbilirubinemia suggests increased bilirubin production or defective conjugation, while conjugated (direct) hyperbilirubinemia suggests impaired secretion or obstruction. Since secretion of conjugated bilirubin across the canalicular membrane is rate limiting, most patients with hepatitis or cirrhosis have an increase in conjugated bilirubin levels.

C. Diagnostic Evaluation: Evaluation of jaundice or hyperbilirubinemia begins with a careful history to determine whether risk factors of liver disease are present, a review of routine liver function tests, and a physical examination focusing on liver size, tenderness, and evidence of chronic liver disease. In addition, conjugated and unconjugated bilirubin fractions should be measured. One algorithm for evaluation of jaundice is shown in Figure 34–3.

1. Intravascular Hemolysis and Gilbert Syndrome—In the absence of other liver function test abnormalities, the differential diagnosis of unconjugated hyperbilirubinemia centers either on increased bilirubin production resulting from intravascular hemolysis or impaired conjugation as in Gilbert syndrome. A large number of other possibilities exist but are rarely encountered clinically. As a general rule, hemolysis sufficient to elevate serum bilirubin levels is not subtle and is readily detected by routine studies. Note that AST but not ALT can be released from damaged red blood cells, and that a large hematoma can have similar effects on bilirubin production. In the absence of hemolysis, Gilbert syndrome is suggested when peak bilirubin values are less than 3–5 mg/dL, an appreciable portion is unconjugated, and other liver function tests are normal. Gilbert syndrome is not a disease but a genetic variant characterized by diminished bilirubin UDP-glucuronyl transferase, the enzyme that catalyzes the conjugation of bilirubin to glucuronide. This benign variant is important to keep in mind because it is common, occurring in 4–7% of the population, and does not have known clinical sequelae. Consequently, recognition of Gilbert syndrome may limit unnecessary testing and concern in the future. Typically, episodes of jaundice are mild and occur intermittently. An increase in serum bilirubin levels is brought out by fasting, exercise, or stress. Values usually return to normal with resumption of normal activities. If the diagnosis is in doubt, patients should be subjected to supervised fasting for 1–2 days to determine if there is an increase in unconjugated bilirubin concentrations. Assurance and counseling about the benign course and familial basis for the disease are the only treatments needed.

2. Conjugated hyperbilirubinemia—Conjugated hyperbilirubinemia with otherwise normal liver tests is relatively uncommon. Attention to medication exposure, including antibiotics, sulfa derivatives, and azathioprine, may suggest drug-induced cholestasis. Potential offending agents should be discontinued and tests followed over time to ensure resolution. Occasionally, conjugated hyperbilirubinemia is the only manifestation of well-compensated cirrhosis; the normal aminotransferase and alkaline phosphatase values indicate the lack of clinically active hepatocellular necrosis and duct obstruction, respectively. Sustained hyperbilirubinemia following acute hepatitis or other events may persist for many weeks due to the persistence of protein-bound bilirubin, which forms slowly over time in the setting of prolonged cholestasis. Genetic disorders such as Rotor's disease and Dubin-Johnson syndrome result in conjugated hyperbilirubinemia but are distinctly uncommon.

3. Bile duct obstruction or proliferation—Concomitant elevations of alkaline phosphatase, 5′-nucleotidase, or GGT mandate a careful evaluation of the bile ducts to rule out obstruction or duct proliferation. Chronic cholestasis with elevated alkaline phosphatase values presents indolently with pruritis and malabsorption. Acute presentations with associated pain, fever, and leukocytosis increase the index of suspicion for cholangitis. Common duct stones with or without cholecystitis are encountered frequently. Increases in bilirubin levels above 5 mg/dL are uncommon in uncomplicated stone disease, and suggest a more complete obstruction resulting from duct strictures or cancer. Again, direct visualization

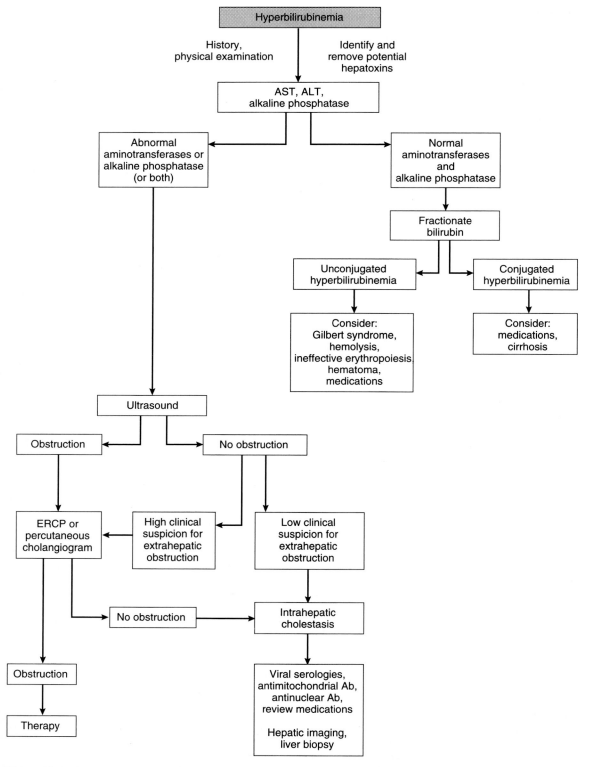

Figure 34–3. An approach to the patient with hyperbilirubinemia. ERCP = endoscopic retrograde cholangiopancreatography.

of the ducts is required, along with consideration of chronic duct-oriented diseases such as primary biliary cirrhosis and sclerosing cholangitis.

Ultrasonography is the preferred initial screening test for duct obstruction, and offers the advantages of relatively low cost, high sensitivity for gallstones and duct dilatation, and wide availability. False-negative studies can occur in patients with cirrhosis and previous biliary tract surgery. Consequently, if the index of suspicion for an obstructive lesion is high, it is reasonable to proceed with endoscopic retrograde cholangiopancreatography or percutaneous cholangiography for definitive diagnosis. Similarly, direct duct visualization is required for the diagnosis of primary biliary cirrhosis, sclerosing cholangitis, duct strictures, and most duct tumors.

4. Intrahepatic disorders—If jaundice is accompanied by significant elevation of aminotransferases out of proportion to alkaline phosphatase concentrations, the origin is more likely to be intrahepatic. Evaluation focusing on acute or chronic hepatitis, cirrhosis, and primary hepatocellular disorders as described below is indicated. There is obviously overlapping between these presentations. When in doubt, visualize the biliary tree. If there is no obstruction, consider a liver biopsy for definitive diagnosis of the underlying disease process.

Chronic Hepatocellular Injury & Cirrhosis

A. Clinical Presentation: Chronic hepatocellular injury is suspected when there are clinical or laboratory findings suggesting poorly compensated liver function. These may be subtle, such as sustained fatigue or decreased albumin concentrations, or life threatening, such as variceal hemorrhage or prolongation of the prothrombin time. Evidence of decompensation imparts a sense of urgency because of the potential benefits of treatment and the poor prognosis of established cirrhosis. Consequently, efforts to treat the manifestations of liver injury and establish the diagnosis should proceed in parallel (eg, treatment of ascites should not await an etiologic diagnosis). This is particularly true since no definitive cause can be ascertained in more than 30% of cirrhotic patients.

Clinical symptoms related to loss of hepatocyte mass are nonspecific outside of the setting of fulminant liver failure (see Chapter 43). Fatigue, weight loss, poor memory, and inability to concentrate are common. Menstrual irregularities or a decrease in libido also develop relatively early; direct questioning may be required to elicit the history. Hepatic origin of the symptoms is suspected when there are suggestive physical features such as jaundice, gynecomastia, or cutaneous angiomas or associated liver test abnormalities.

Development of portal hypertension contributes importantly to the clinical manifestations of chronic hepatocellular injury (see Chapter 43). The increase in portal pressure leads directly to engorged varices or hemorrhoids, and the probability of bleeding increases with the degree of pressure elevation. Accompanying abnormalities of renal function lead to Na^+ and water retention and, if uncorrected, to ascites and edema. While the pathophysiologic basis is complex, defective Na^+ secretion is thought to initiate the cascade leading to fluid retention. The hepatorenal syndrome marks the most extreme manifestation and is characterized by severe Na^+ retention (urine Na^+ concentrations < 10 meq/L), oliguria, and a decrease in creatinine clearance. This is reversible with correction of liver function, but untreated disease can result in uremia.

Hepatic encephalopathy deserves special emphasis as a clinical manifestation of chronic liver injury because it is often unrecognized in the early stages, when it responds best to therapy. Indeed, most patients with cirrhosis will have subtle impairment of fine motor skills and memory that can be improved with moderate protein restriction, lactulose intake, and a decrease in portal pressures. Attention to subtle symptoms, measurement of serum ammonia levels, and cognitive testing are helpful when the diagnosis is suspected. More often, a therapeutic trial will be instrumental in establishing the diagnosis. Usually, overt encephalopathy with asterixis, mental confusion, and disturbed sleep patterns is readily detectable.

B. Pathophysiologic Findings: The pathophysiologic processes that result in the clinical manifestations of chronic liver injury are directly related to loss of liver cell mass or development of portal hypertension (or both), as described above. Clinically, it is important to establish a time course or rate of change of symptoms as an aid to understanding the pathophysiologic changes. Chronic liver injury due to viral hepatitis, autoimmune diseases, and sometimes alcohol abuse is most often indolent, with a clinical course developing over many months or years. More acute presentations suggest either acute injury (ie, toxic, infectious, or vascular cause) or decompensation of previously unrecognized chronic disease. The latter is surprisingly common.

Chronic liver injury also predisposes patients to predictable complications that can cause rapid clinical deterioration. Portal vein thrombosis deserves special mention as an important but underrecognized complication of chronic liver disease. Liver function depends upon portal flow for maintaining the cellular supply of nutrients and oxygen, so even small decreases in portal flow can result in significant functional deterioration, particularly when there is preexisting hepatocellular disease. Portal vein thrombosis can occur in the absence of preexisting liver disease (eg, as a manifestation of hypercoagulability or portal bacteremia), but it is more often observed as a complication of chronic liver disease and cirrhosis.

Doppler sonography is a reliable screening test that allows visualization of portal flow to assess patients at risk. The relative risk for hepatocellular carcinoma is markedly increased in the setting of preexisting cirrhosis, particularly if cirrhosis is related to chronic hepatitis B or C infection or hemochromatosis. Again, an ultrasound study of the liver is a reasonable screening test for identification of a liver mass. The utility of α-fetoprotein for screening and early diagnosis in high-risk patients has not been firmly established, but its use is widespread (see Chapter 46). Finally, an increased rate of infection is associated with cirrhosis and portal hypertension. This is due in part to increased seeding of the portal vein with enteric pathogens, and in part to defective clearance of circulating microorganisms by the reticuloendothelial system. Attention to these complications of chronic liver disease may account for unexplained deterioration in liver function or worsening of ascites and encephalopathy.

C. Diagnostic Evaluation: When chronic liver disease or cirrhosis is suspected on clinical grounds, the first goals are to establish the degree of functional impairment and look for reversible causes of deterioration. The history focuses on assessment of risk factors (see Table 34–1) and the physical examination on detection of portal hypertension, encephalopathy, liver size, and cutaneous manifestations of cirrhosis. The clinical findings are used in association with laboratory studies to calculate a Child-Pugh score, which should be followed routinely to assess changes in functional hepatic reserve (see Table 34–3).

Laboratory studies also provide some insight into the causes of liver damage by suggesting whether the underlying pathologic basis is primarily obstructive ductular disease or hepatocellular damage (Figure 34–4). Patients with alkaline phosphatase or bilirubin levels elevated out of proportion to aminotransferase levels are more likely to have duct-centered pathologic causes such as sclerosing cholangitis, primary biliary cirrhosis, infiltrative liver diseases, or biliary obstruction. Accordingly, an evaluation focusing on imaging of the biliary system and screening for antimitochondrial antibodies is appropriate. Patients with sustained aminotransferase elevation usually have ongoing cell necrosis such as that caused by toxic injury (due to alcohol, medications, or occupational exposures), chronic viral hepatitis, or autoimmune hepatitis. An evaluation focusing on viral and autoimmune markers, alcoholism, and medications is appropriate. In each case, the laboratory findings are rarely definitive, so liver biopsy is required for staging and diagnosis.

While such an approach is orderly and logical, most findings are nonspecific. Consequently, the authors' impression is that every patient with chronic or poorly compensated liver disease suspected of having underlying cirrhosis should undergo a detailed evaluation, which includes abdominal ultrasound examination with Doppler flow studies, screening tests for chronic hepatitis, and definitive assessment of ductular anatomy. This approach is based on the premise that early investigation offers the best chance of definitive diagnosis and correction, but it may or may not be cost effective.

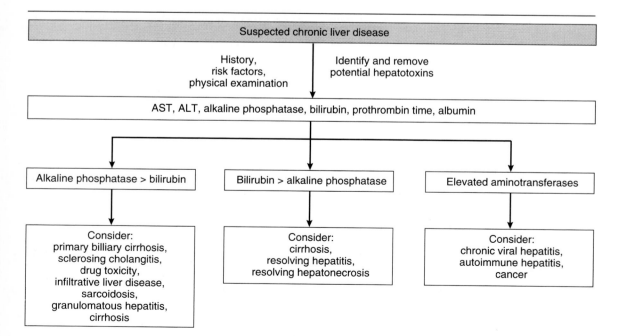

Figure 34–4. An approach to the patient with chronic hepatocellular injury or suspected cirrhosis.

Ultrasound study is readily justified, since it is noninvasive, widely available, and provides information about the liver parenchyma, biliary tree, and vasculature. Findings suggestive of cirrhosis, including a diffuse increase in echogenicity and a nodular contour, provide presumptive evidence of chronic disease with established fibrosis. More importantly, findings of duct dilatation, gallstones, mass lesions, or portal vein thrombosis rapidly alter the diagnostic and therapeutic approaches.

Screening for unsuspected hepatitis B and C is also justified because of the prevalence of these viruses and the potential for treatment with α-interferon. Since serologic testing for hepatitis B surface antigen and hepatitis C antibodies is relatively inexpensive, even patients with alternative diagnoses such as alcoholic liver disease or primary biliary cirrhosis should be tested. Moreover, identification of unsuspected viral hepatitis has important long-term ramifications, including a risk for viral transmission and effects of immunosuppressive drugs if liver transplantation is considered.

Guidelines for appropriate screening for genetic diseases in patients with established liver disease are not clear. Liver disease related to Wilson's disease and α_1-antitrypsin deficiency has an earlier age of onset, while that related to hemochromatosis typically appears later and affects men more than women. The authors' approach is a pragmatic one.

Since patients at this stage of evaluation already have active liver disease, they represent a high-risk group. In the absence of another clear cause, ferritin, ceruloplasmin, and α_1-antitrypsin levels are obtained, since these tests are relatively inexpensive and positive results have clear implications for treatment and family counseling. Among these, serum ferritin levels are particularly important due to the higher prevalence of hemochromatosis and the beneficial effects of phlebotomy. Suggestive or equivocal results are evaluated by liver biopsy for definitive diagnosis.

Two final caveats in the evaluation of chronic hepatocellular injury merit emphasis. First, always have a high index of suspicion for biliary obstruction, since it may lead to cirrhosis, and endoscopic or percutaneous cholangiography allows definitive diagnosis and treatment in many situations. If the sonogram is unrevealing but other features suggest obstruction, proceed to direct visualization of ductular anatomy with a cholangiogram. Second, rapid advances in liver transplantation have made this the treatment of choice for many patients with decompensated cirrhosis (see Chapter 54). Operating on patients with minimal functional reserve and multiple medical complications leads to higher costs and poorer outcomes, however. Because the timing of transplantation is so important, early referral to a transplant center is warranted for appropriate candidates.

REFERENCES

EPIDEMIOLOGY

Dufour MC: Chronic liver disease and cirrhosis. In: *Digestive Diseases in the United States: Epidemiology and Impact.* Everhart JE (editor). US Department of Health and Human Services, Public Health Service, National Institutes of Health, National Institute of Diabetes and Digestive and Kidney Diseases, Washington, DC. US Government Printing Office, 1994. NIH Publication no. 94-1447.

PHYSICAL EXAMINATION

Naylor CD: Physical examination of the liver. JAMA 1994;271:1859.

HEPATOCELLULAR INJURY

Cohen JA, Kaplan MM: The SGOT/SGPT ratio: An indicator of alcoholic liver disease. Dig Dis Sci 1979;24:835.

Goddard CJR, Warnes TW: Raised liver enzymes in asymptomatic patients: Investigation and outcome. Dig Dis Sci 1992;10:218.

Katkov WN et al: Elevated serum alanine aminotransferase levels in blood donors: The contribution of hepatitis C virus. Ann Intern Med 1991;115:882.

Reichling JJ, Kaplan MM: Clinical use of serum enzymes in liver disease. Dig Dis Sci 1988;33:1601.

Sherman KE: Alanine aminotransferase in clinical practice. Arch Intern Med 1991;151:260.

Simko V: Alkaline phosphatase in biology and medicine. Dig Dis Sci 1991;9:189.

HYPERBILIRUBINEMIA & JAUNDICE

Anciaux ML et al: Prospective study of clinical and biochemical features of symptomatic choledocholithiasis. Dig Dis Sci 1986;31:449.

Borsch G et al: Clinical evaluation, ultrasound, cholescintigraphy, and endoscopic retrograde cholangiography in cholestasis: A prospective comparative clinical study. J Clin Gastroenterol 1988;10:185.

Frank BB: Clinical evaluation of jaundice: A guideline of the patient care committee of the American Gastroenterological Association. JAMA 1989;262:3031.

Matzen P et al: Ultrasonography, computed tomography, and cholescintigraphy in suspected obstructive jaundice: A prospective comparative study. Gastroenterology 1983;64:1492.

Richter JM, Silverstein MD, Schapiro R: Suspected obstructive jaundice: A decision analysis of diagnostic strategies. Ann Intern Med 1983;99:46.

Sherlock S, Scheuer PJ: The presentation and diagnosis

of 100 patients with primary biliary cirrhosis. N Engl J Med 1973;289:674.

CHRONIC LIVER DISEASE

Child CG, Turcotte JG: Surgery in portal hypertension. In: Major Problems in Clinical Surgery: The Liver and Portal Hypertension. Child CG (editor). Saunders, 1964.

Pugh RNH et al: Transection of the oesophagus for bleeding oesophageal varices. Br J Surg 1973;60: 646.

Saunders JB et al: A 20-year prospective study of cirrhosis. Br Med J 1981;282:263.

Van Ness MM, Diehl A: Is liver biopsy useful in the evaluation of patients with chronically elevated liver enzymes? Ann Intern Med 1989;111:473.

Acute Liver Failure

35

Emmet B. Keeffe, MD

Essentials of Diagnosis

- An acute liver disease which evolves rapidly and is complicated by coagulopathy and hepatic encephalopathy.
- Most common underlying causes include acute viral hepatitis and drug-induced liver injury.
- Nonspecific symptoms are followed rapidly by jaundice and altered mental status, with or without coma.
- Laboratory findings include markedly elevated serum aminotransferases, hyperbilirubinemia, hypoprothrombinemia, and, in advanced cases, hypoglycemia and metabolic acidosis.

General Considerations

Acute liver failure is a relatively rare but catastrophic illness resulting from sudden marked impairment of liver cell function. In most cases, acute liver failure evolves from a severe, rapidly progressive course of an acute liver disease such as viral or drug-induced hepatitis. In a few cases, acute liver failure is the first manifestation of an underlying chronic liver disease that has been asymptomatic (eg, Wilson's disease). By convention, however, reactivation of chronic viral hepatitis that results in liver failure, such as chronic hepatitis B, is usually not categorized as acute liver failure. Multiorgan failure often accompanies acute liver failure, and the mortality rate with supportive care only ranges from 50 to 90%.

Acute liver failure is a term reserved for the presence of acute liver disease associated with significant coagulopathy, which has been arbitrarily defined by a prothrombin time or factor V level of less than 50% of normal (Table 35–1). The term **fulminant hepatic failure** was introduced by Trey and Davidson in 1970 to designate acute liver failure associated with hepatic encephalopathy developing within 8 weeks of the onset of illness. The term is now widely used, although changes in the time interval between the onset of symptoms and encephalopathy have been proposed. In addition, some investigators use the time interval between the onset of jaundice, rather than symptoms, and the development of hepatic en-

cephalopathy to define acute liver failure. Finally, alternative terminology has been introduced to characterize a group of patients with a more delayed onset of encephalopathy.

Bernuau and colleagues at the Hôpital Beaujon base their classification of acute liver failure on the interval between the first detection of jaundice and the appearance of encephalopathy (Table 35–1). They define fulminant hepatic failure as the development of hepatic encephalopathy within 2 weeks of the onset of jaundice. The term **subfulminant hepatic failure** is used to designate another subgroup of acute liver failure disorders characterized by the development of encephalopathy 2 weeks to 3 months after the appearance of jaundice. By contrast, Gimson and colleagues at King's College Hospital in London define fulminant hepatic failure as originally proposed by Trey and Davidson. They use the term late-onset hepatic failure as synonymous with subfulminant hepatic failure, but the interval between the onset of illness and encephalopathy is defined as 8 weeks to 6 months. To further confuse the terminology issue, the same investigators at King's College Hospital have more recently proposed new terminology based on the interval between the onset of jaundice and encephalopathy:

1. Hyperacute liver failure, with an interval of less than 7 days
2. Acute liver failure, with an interval of between 8 and 28 days
3. Subacute liver failure, with an interval of between 5 and 12 weeks.

This latter terminology has only recently been proposed and is not accepted, and thus will not be used in this chapter.

The distinction between fulminant and subfulminant hepatic failure is important clinically, because patients with the shortest interval between jaundice and the onset of encephalopathy have the best prognosis. Moreover, the causes of acute liver failure are usually different in patients experiencing fulminant and subfulminant hepatic failure. The management of

Table 35–1. Definitions of acute liver failure.

Acute liver failure	Acute liver disease, with prothrombin time or factor V less than 50% of normal
Fulminant hepatic failure	Acute liver failure with hepatic encephalopathy, developing less than 2 weeks[1] (or 8 weeks[2]) after onset of jaundice[1] (or illness[2])
Subfulminant hepatic failure[3]	Acute liver failure with hepatic encephalopathy, developing from 2 weeks[1] (or 8 weeks[2]) to 3 months[1] (or 6 months[2]) after onset of jaundice[1] (or illness[2])

[1]Criteria from Bernuau J, Rueff B, Benhamou J-P: Fulminant and subfulminant liver failure: Definitions and causes. Semin Liv Dis 1986;6:97.
[2]Criteria from Trey C, Davidson LS: The management of fulminant hepatic failure. In: Progress in Liver Diseases. Vol 3. Popper H, Schaffner F (editors). Grune & Stratton, 1970; and Gimson AES et al: Clinical and prognostic differences in fulminant hepatitis type A, B, and non-A, non-B. Gut 1983;24:1194.
[3]Also called late-onset hepatic failure.

Table 35–2. Known causes of acute liver failure.

Viral hepatitis
  Hepatitis A, B, C, D, and E viruses
Hepatitis due to other viruses
  Herpesviruses 1, 2, and 6
  Adenovirus
  Epstein-Barr virus
  Cytomegalovirus
Drug-induced liver injury
  Acetaminophen overdose
  Idiosyncratic drug reaction
Toxins
  Amanita phalloides
  Organic solvents
  Phosphorus
Metabolic disorders
  Acute fatty liver of pregnancy
  Reye's syndrome
Vascular events
  Acute circulatory failure
  Budd-Chiari syndrome
  Veno-occlusive disease
  Heat stroke
Miscellaneous disorders
  Wilson's disease
  Autoimmune hepatitis
  Massive infiltration with tumor
  Liver transplantation with primary graft nonfunction

patients with acute liver failure must be individualized according to the pace and tempo of the illness, which can often be predicted by the cause of liver failure. The overall goal of treatment is to provide supportive care and buy time to allow hepatic regeneration, while at the same time assessing for prognostic indices that suggest a poor outcome and the need to proceed rapidly to orthotopic liver transplantation.

As noted above, a small subset of patients with acute liver failure will, in reality, have a previously unrecognized chronic liver disease. For example, Wilson's disease may initially present with the symptoms and signs of acute hepatitis or, if severe, acute liver failure, usually subfulminant hepatic failure. Wilson's disease, however, more commonly presents as a chronic illness with a clinical picture of chronic hepatitis or cirrhosis. Another example of a chronic liver disease that may present acutely is autoimmune hepatitis, which occasionally is first recognized in a rapidly progressive form that meets the criteria of acute liver failure.

The true incidence of acute liver failure is unknown. Because it is an uncommon condition, patients tend to be referred to tertiary centers that are able to provide aggressive supportive intensive care and orthotopic liver transplantation. Thus, referral bias certainly influences the published information regarding the causes and outcome of acute liver failure.

The causes of acute liver failure are diverse, but viral hepatitis and drug-induced liver injury account for 80–85% of all cases for which a cause can be determined (Table 35–2). Toxins, metabolic diseases, vascular events, and a few miscellaneous conditions explain the remaining causes. The distribution of causes may vary in different geographic regions. For example, in the United Kingdom, acetaminophen

overdose is the most common cause. In an impressive series from King's College Hospital, 431 of 763 patients (56%) had acetaminophen overdose as the cause of fulminant hepatic failure. There also is emerging evidence that the use of excessive therapeutic doses of acetaminophen by heavy drinkers of alcohol accounts for an increasing percentage of acute liver failure in the United States, with one center reporting that two-thirds of cases could be explained by this combination of events.

Acute viral hepatitis is overall the most common cause of acute liver failure. In the large referral experience with this disorder at Hôpital Beaujon, 72% of 330 cases in adults could be attributed to viral hepatitis. All five hepatotropic viruses have been implicated as a cause of acute liver failure, although the contribution of hepatitis C virus remains uncertain. According to previous compilations of the causes of acute liver failure at referral centers, non-A, non-B hepatitis, a designation based on the exclusion of hepatitis A, hepatitis B, and other causes of acute liver failure and presumed to represent an unidentified specific viral agent, was typically second in prevalence to hepatitis B as the cause of acute liver failure. The currently preferred terminology for a patient with an unknown cause of acute liver failure is "indeterminate" or "sporadic." Acute liver failure caused by one of the hepatotropic viruses usually follows a course compatible with fulminant rather than subfulminant hepatic failure. Finally, one must keep in mind that viral hepatitis is complicated by the development of acute liver failure in less than 1% of cases.

Hepatitis A virus is only rarely complicated by the

development of fulminant hepatic failure (0.1–0.5% of cases). In addition, patients who experience fulminant hepatitis A have a relatively good prognosis, with a survival rate of 50–60% and a less frequent need for orthotopic liver transplantation. Fulminant hepatitis A may be more common in intravenous drug users, older patients, and individuals with pre-existing chronic liver disease.

Hepatitis B virus is the single most common cause of fulminant hepatic failure, being responsible for 30–60% of all cases. Most patients who experience fulminant hepatitis B are young adults. Immunosuppressed patients who are acutely infected with hepatitis B virus are less likely to experience fulminant hepatic failure. Massive hepatic necrosis with fulminant hepatic failure has also been reported in asymptomatic chronic hepatitis B surface antigen (HBsAg) carriers after withdrawal of immunosuppressive drugs. Patients with acute liver failure secondary to acute hepatitis B may have rapid clearance of hepatitis B virus in one-third to one-half of cases, most likely related to a major immunologic attack on infected hepatocytes; these individuals will not have detectable HBsAg several days after the onset of illness. For this reason, occult hepatitis B virus infection may explain some cases of fulminant hepatic failure classified in the past as non-A, non-B hepatitis. This hypothesis is supported by the finding of serum or hepatic (or both) hepatitis B virus DNA in some patients undergoing orthotopic liver transplantation for fulminant non-A, non-B hepatitis (indeterminate fulminant hepatic failure, by current terminology). Mutants of hepatitis B virus, as well as the more common wild type of this virus, have been shown to cause fulminant hepatic failure. The most common hepatitis B virus mutant has a stop codon inserted in the precore region of the C gene, such that hepatitis B e antigen is not released from hepatocytes.

Hepatitis D virus is also associated with the development of acute liver failure, particularly in intravenous drug users, who are often infected with this virus. Between 30 and 50% of HBsAg-positive patients with fulminant hepatic failure also test positive for antibody to hepatitis D virus and have concomitant hepatitis D (or delta hepatitis). Patients with fulminant hepatic failure may be acutely coinfected with hepatitis B and hepatitis D viruses; alternatively, patients with chronic hepatitis B may develop fulminant hepatic failure secondary to superinfection with hepatitis D virus. Some data suggest that the risk of fulminant hepatic failure is higher in patients coinfected with hepatitis B and hepatitis D viruses than in patients having acute hepatitis B alone.

The recently identified enteric hepatitis E virus often causes infection in the setting of epidemics and is characterized by an unusually high incidence of fulminant hepatic failure in pregnant women, who experience a case fatality rate approaching 40%. Overall, however, fulminant hepatic failure appears to be an infrequent complication of hepatitis E, and hepatitis E virus infection is not commonly found in patients with acute liver failure of indeterminate cause. To date, hepatitis E has only rarely been identified in the United States.

As noted above, the designation non-A, non-B hepatitis had in the past been applied to patients with fulminant hepatic failure and no viral markers or other recognized cause of acute liver failure. This terminology had implied that hepatitis C virus, or some other viral agent, was the likely causative factor. In fact, hepatitis C virus RNA or antibody (or both) to hepatitis C virus have been inconsistently, and in most series rarely, identified in patients designated as having non-A, non-B or indeterminate fulminant hepatic failure. It thus seems unlikely that hepatitis C virus plays an important role in the development of acute liver failure. On the other hand, there are studies from Asian countries suggesting that multiple viral infections (hepatitis B and D viruses, as well as hepatitis B and C viruses) are common in patients with acute liver failure. In cases of fulminant hepatic failure of indeterminate cause, there may be one or more novel viral agents causing this syndrome. In some studies, viruslike particles have been identified in the cytoplasm of infected liver cells in patients with fulminant hepatic failure of uncertain cause (ie, a candidate hepatitis F virus). Other cases of indeterminate fulminant hepatic failure may be explained by cryptic hepatitis B virus or hepatitis C virus infection, including mutant forms of hepatitis B or different genotypes of hepatitis C.

Acute liver failure has rarely been attributed to hepatitis caused by other viruses, including herpes viruses 1, 2, and 6, adenovirus, Epstein-Barr virus, and cytomegalovirus.

Drug-induced liver injury is the second major cause of acute liver failure, accounting for 15–20% of all cases. Acute liver failure complicates drug-induced hepatitis ($\leq$ 20% of cases) relatively more frequently than acute viral hepatitis (< 1% of cases). Drug-induced liver injury occurs most often in individuals older than 40 years of age. It has classically been divided into two categories: predictable and idiosyncratic. Predictable hepatotoxicity occurs in a dose-dependent fashion, while idiosyncratic liver injury occurs in less than 1% of users of an individual drug; the latter is therefore unpredictable, and is unrelated to the administered dose (see Chapter 44).

Acetaminophen hepatotoxicity is an example of dose-dependent, predictable liver injury, but its effect can be exaggerated by drugs, including alcohol, which induce its cytochrome P-450 isoenzyme, or by starvation, which depletes glutathione. Neither acetaminophen nor its major sulfate or glucuronide metabolites are toxic. A small percentage of acetaminophen, however, is metabolized via its P-450 isoenzyme to a reactive metabolite that is conjugated to a nontoxic product by glutathione. Acetaminophen hepatotoxicity with acute liver failure may occur as the result of a suicidal overdose following the ingestion of more than 10 g of a drug or by high or excessive therapeutic doses used by alcoholics who have induced cytochrome P-450 enzymes. From either the ingestion of a large dose of acetaminophen that overwhelms available glutathione, or from the excessive therapeutic use of acetaminophen by alcoholic patients with induced P-450 isoenzymes or reduced glutathione stores, or both, the toxic intermediate of acetaminophen accumulates, binds to liver cytoplasmic proteins, and causes liver cell necrosis. While the fatality rate for acetaminophen overdose approximates 50%, excessive ingestion of acetaminophen by the alcoholic is associated with as much as a 20% fatality rate. Markedly elevated serum aminotransferase levels are a characteristic diagnostic feature of acetaminophen hepatotoxicity, with values typically exceeding 3000–4000 IU/L.

A number of drugs are associated with the rare development of idiosyncratic drug-induced liver injury, which is not uncommonly associated with progression to acute liver failure. In some cases, eosinophilia or the presence of a rash, or both, suggests that hypersensitivity plays a role; however, in most cases, presumed idiosyncratic abnormalities in hepatic drug metabolism are likely the key pathophysiologic factors. Examples of drugs that have been implicated in idiosyncratic drug-induced liver injury resulting in acute liver failure include halothane, isoniazid, disulfiram, valproate, phenytoin, sulfonamides, methyldopa, propylthiouracil, and nonsteroidal anti-inflammatory drugs.

A small number of toxins have been associated with the development of acute hepatic failure, which in this setting is frequently accompanied by concomitant renal failure. Organic solvents, including the fluorinated hydrocarbons trichloroethylene and tetrachloroethane, have been associated with the development of acute liver failure. *Amanita phalloides,* the death cap mushroom, has been associated with the development of acute liver failure in association with renal failure, particularly in central Europe, where mushroom collecting and consumption is common. Liver transplantation has been used to successfully treat a handful of patients fortunate enough to be promptly referred to liver transplant centers.

Metabolic causes of acute liver failure include acute fatty liver of pregnancy and Reye's syndrome. Both of these syndromes are associated with microvascular fatty change rather than the more typical massive hepatic necrosis characteristic of other causes of fulminant hepatic failure. Acute fatty liver of pregnancy usually occurs in the third trimester and is characterized by the rapid onset of jaundice and encephalopathy, frequently accompanied by hypoglycemia. Even though the prothrombin time is markedly prolonged, the serum aminotransferase lev-

els are usually not elevated more than 1000 IU/L. Treatment consists of rapid delivery of the fetus (see Chapter 47).

A number of vascular events have also been associated with the development of acute liver failure (Table 35–2). Cardiac causes include myocardial infarction or cardiomyopathy associated with acute circulatory failure. In some cases, the underlying cardiac disease is not immediately apparent, and, thus, careful cardiovascular evaluation is appropriate in patients who initially have acute liver failure of uncertain cause. Hepatic venous outflow obstruction secondary to an acute form of Budd-Chiari syndrome or veno-occlusive disease has also rarely been associated with acute liver failure. Heat stroke with liver failure has been noted in miners as well as long-distance runners and is typically reversible.

Miscellaneous causes of acute liver failure include the aforementioned Wilson's disease and autoimmune hepatitis. Massive infiltration of the liver with metastatic tumor that spreads in an intrasinusoidal pattern has also rarely been associated with acute liver failure. The onset of fulminant hepatic failure may be the first clinical manifestation of hepatic metastasis, and hepatic imaging with ultrasonography or CT scanning may show only homogenous hepatomegaly. Finally, liver transplantation may be complicated by primary graft nonfunction and the rapid onset of acute liver failure, requiring retransplantation in the first few days after orthotopic liver transplantation.

The multiple causes of acute liver failure may follow a course characteristic of fulminant or subfulminant hepatic failure (Table 35–3). In 75% or more of cases, hepatitis A, B, D, and E; *Amanita phalloides* poisoning; acetaminophen overdose; and acute fatty liver of pregnancy are associated with a relatively short interval from the onset of jaundice to the development of hepatic encephalopathy (ie, fulminant hepatic failure). By contrast, patients with an indeterminate cause of acute liver failure, drug-induced liver injury, hepatic venous outflow obstruction, Wilson's disease, and autoimmune hepatitis more often have a subfulminant course. The other important distinction between fulminant and subfulminant hepatic failure

Table 35–3. Course of acute liver failure according to cause.

Predominantly fulminant hepatic failure:
Hepatitis A, B, D, and E
Amanita phalloides
Acetaminophen overdose
Acute fatty liver of pregnancy
Predominantly subfulminant hepatic failure:
Indeterminate or sporadic
Drug-induced liver injury
Budd-Chiari syndrome
Veno-occlusive disease
Wilson's disease
Autoimmune hepatitis

Table 35–4. Examples of survival rates of fulminant and subfulminant hepatic failure according to cause.[1]

Cause	Survival Rate (%)
Fulminant hepatic failure	
Acute hepatitis A	50–60
Acetaminophen overdose	50–55
Acute hepatitis B	40–50
Subfulminant hepatic failure	
Indeterminate or sporadic	25–30
Drug-induced liver injury	10–25

[1]In the absence of liver transplantation.

is the better survival rates of patients affected by fulminant as opposed to subfulminant hepatic failure (Table 35–4).

Clinical Findings

The essential clinical findings of acute liver failure include jaundice, hepatic encephalopathy, and coagulopathy. When severe, acute liver failure is also characterized by multiorgan failure, particularly cardiovascular and renal changes, multiple metabolic abnormalities, and an increased incidence of infection.

A. Symptoms and Signs: Acute liver failure often begins with nonspecific symptoms such as malaise or nausea, which are rapidly followed by jaundice and, over a variable period of time, changes in mental status. Hepatic encephalopathy is traditionally divided into four stages based on the mental state and the presence or absence of neurologic signs (Table 35–5). Stage 1 hepatic encephalopathy is characterized by mild confusion and mental slowness, with only subtle neurologic abnormalities. In stage 2, drowsiness is prominent and accompanied by personality changes and inappropriate behavior; asterixis and dysarthria are typically present. In stage 3, the patient sleeps most of the time. While arousable, the patient is unable to perform mental tasks

and is disoriented with respect to time or place. In stage 4, the patient is in coma and may or may not respond to painful stimuli. Hepatic encephalopathy itself is an important predictor of outcome; in patients with stage 4 coma, the survival rate is less than 20%.

On physical examination, characteristic abnormalities include changes in mental status, jaundice, and decreased or absent hepatic dullness on hepatic percussion.

B. Laboratory Findings: Laboratory findings that support the presence of acute liver failure include markedly elevated serum aminotransferases, hyperbilirubinemia, hypoprothrombinemia, and, when liver failure is particularly severe, hypoglycemia and metabolic acidosis. Other laboratory abnormalities that may be present include hyponatremia and respiratory alkalosis early in the course of illness. The hallmark laboratory abnormality is coagulopathy, which by definition in acute liver failure is associated with a prothrombin time or factor V level of less than 50% of normal.

Differential Diagnosis

The diagnosis of acute liver failure is typically straightforward, but the disease or disorder may be initially mistaken for gram-negative septicemia or a drug overdose. Once coagulopathy and hepatic encephalopathy supervene in the patient with markedly elevated serum aminotransferases, acute liver failure can be diagnosed with confidence.

The most important aspect of diagnosis in the setting of acute liver failure is the determination of the specific cause, since the pace of the illness and prognosis can be estimated based on the underlying condition (see Table 35–4). In addition, the approach to supportive therapy may vary according to the underlying etiologic diagnosis (eg, acetylcysteine for acetaminophen overdose), and determination of the cause of liver failure can predict the likelihood that orthotopic liver transplantation will be needed.

Table 35–5. Clinical stages of hepatic encephalopathy.

Stage	Mental State	Neurologic Signs
1	Mild confusion, euphoria, or depression; decreased attention; mental slowness; irritability; inverted sleep pattern	Incoordination; slight tremor; poor handwriting
2	Drowsiness; lethargy; deficits in analytic ability; personality changes; inappropriate behavior; intermittent disorientation	Asterixis; ataxia; dysarthria
3	Somnolent but arousable; unable to perform mental tasks; disorientation with respect to time or place; marked confusion; amnesia; fits of rage; incoherent speech	Hyperreflexia; muscle rigidity; fasciculations; Babinski's sign
4	Coma	Oculovestibular responses lost; response to painful stimuli lost; decerebrate posture

Complications

Life-threatening complications are common in patients with acute liver failure. Meticulous attention to detail in the management and anticipation of possible complications is critical to a successful outcome.

A. General Measures: All patients with acute liver failure should be managed in an intensive care unit to carefully watch for the unpredictable development of multiorgan failure. Because it is often difficult to predict which patients will recover and which will require orthotopic liver transplantation, patients should be transferred to a hospital with the capability of performing transplantation. Once at a transplant center, the patient is usually evaluated urgently by hepatologists, liver transplant surgeons, transplant coordinators, and anesthesiologists, with the goal of promptly assessing the patient's suitability for urgent transplantation. Once contraindications to urgent transplantation are excluded (Table 35–6), patients are often placed on the United Network for Organ Sharing (UNOS) transplant waiting list (see also Chapter 54). Intensive neurologic monitoring, usually including the direct measurement of intracerebral pressure and early treatment of cerebral edema, is critical to a successful outcome without permanent neurologic damage. If stage 3 or stage 4 hepatic encephalopathy develops, the patient is intubated for mechanical ventilation and UNOS status upgraded to the highest priority. Additional monitoring includes the placement of Swan-Ganz and intra-arterial catheters, a urinary catheter, and a nasogastric tube, with frequent gastric pH monitoring.

B. Hepatic Encephalopathy and Cerebral Edema: Hepatic encephalopathy and cerebral edema, although both having the similar clinical manifestation of changes in mental status, are likely caused by different pathogenic events. Accumulation of toxic substances in the central nervous system, particularly ammonia and endogenous benzodiazepine agonists, are postulated to mediate hepatic encephalopathy. Although hepatic encephalopathy is typically reversible and seldom fatal, cerebral edema is frequently lethal secondary to uncal herniation. In spite of a number of theories to explain the development of cerebral edema, its precise pathogenesis in acute liver failure remains poorly understood. Swelling of brain cells and disruption of the blood-brain barrier likely play contributory roles, however. Neurologic complications account for approximately 30% of the conditions that preclude orthotopic liver transplantation (Table 35–6). The overall prognosis for patients with grade 1 or grade 2 encephalopathy is usually good, while that for grade 3, and particularly grade 4, hepatic encephalopathy is much poorer. Cerebral edema is the leading cause of death in patients with grade 4 encephalopathy and is estimated to occur in approximately three-quarters of patients reaching this stage of cerebral dysfunction. Cerebral ischemia will occur if cerebral perfusion pressure (the difference between mean arterial pressure and intracerebral pressure) is not maintained at above 40 mm Hg.

The treatment of hepatic encephalopathy in the setting of fulminant hepatic failure is challenging. While lactulose is the cornerstone of treatment for chronic hepatic encephalopathy in patients with cirrhosis, it is less effective in patients with fulminant hepatic failure. In general, however, a trial of lactulose either orally (or by nasogastric tube, if necessary) or by rectal enemas is worthwhile. Lactulose is titrated to achieve two to four loose bowel movements daily. The effectiveness of antibiotics, such as neomycin or metronidazole, for hepatic encephalopathy secondary to fulminant hepatic failure is even less certain. Factors known to worsen hepatic encephalopathy such as gastrointestinal bleeding, hypokalemia, or sepsis should be identified and treated.

Cerebral edema is frequently manifested by hypertension, bradycardia, decerebrate rigidity and posturing, abnormal pupillary reflexes, and brain stem respiratory patterns and apnea. These clinical signs may occur late; therefore, it is generally preferred to monitor intracerebral pressure and institute therapy to maintain a pressure of less than 20 mm Hg at all times. CT scanning of the head is not a reliable way to estimate intracerebral pressure in fulminant hepatic failure, but CT scanning is often used to exclude other intracerebral problems, such as hemorrhage or other structural lesions, before proceeding with orthotopic liver transplantation.

In patients with fulminant hepatic failure, intracranial pressure is usually monitored with either subdural or epidural transducers. The risk of placement of intracerebral pressure transducers is hemorrhage, but the benefit appears to outweigh this risk. Epidural monitors are safer to place than subdural transducers, although their sensitivity may be lower. The goal of intracerebral pressure monitoring is to maintain the pressure at less than 20 mm Hg; a persistent pressure greater than 40 mm Hg and refractory to treatment precludes orthotopic liver transplantation. In addition, the cerebral perfusion pressure should be maintained above 50 mm Hg.

When cerebral edema develops on the basis of in-

Table 35–6. Contraindications to orthotopic liver transplantation for acute liver failure.[1]

Seropositivity for human immunodeficiency virus
Active alcohol or drug abuse
Advanced cardiopulmonary disease
Uncontrolled sepsis
Widespread thrombosis of portal and mesenteric veins
Irreversible brain damage
Sustained elevation of intracerebral pressure to > 50 mm Hg
Cerebral perfusion pressure < 40 mm Hg for > 2 hours
Improving hepatic function

[1]Modified from Muñoz SJ: Difficult management problems in fulminant hepatic failure. Semin Liv Dis 1993;13:395.

tracerebral pressure recordings or clinical signs, treatment with mannitol at a dosage of 0.5–1 g/kg is given by intravenous infusion over 5 minutes. Repeated doses of mannitol may be required to treat recurrent increases of intracerebral pressure. Mannitol should only be given if serum osmolality is less than 320 mosm/L. In patients who have renal failure, mannitol can only be given in combination with hemodialysis or continuous arteriovenous hemofiltration. Pentobarbital boluses of 100–150 mg intravenously every 15 minutes for 1 hour followed by a continuous infusion of 1–3 mg/kg/h can be given if mannitol fails to lower the intracerebral pressure.

Other useful therapies for the prevention or management of increases in intracerebral pressure include: disturbing the patient as little as possible; controlling agitation; elevating the head 20–30 degrees above the horizontal; providing moderate hyperventilation to a partial carbon dioxide pressure of 25–30 mm Hg; and administering intravenous barbiturate therapy.

C. Coagulopathy: In acute liver failure, there may be a number of abnormalities of coagulation. Decreased levels of factors II, V, VII, IX, and X account for prolongation of the prothrombin time and partial thromboplastin time. The patient's clinical condition and prognosis are best determined by serial measurements of prothrombin time and factor V levels. In fulminant hepatic failure, coagulopathy predisposes patients to bleeding from the gastrointestinal tract, venous access sites, and arterial lines. Hypoprothrombinemia should be corrected in part by administering fresh-frozen plasma before any invasive procedures are performed. In addition, active bleeding indicates that attempts at correcting coagulopathy should be made.

Thrombocytopenia is also common in fulminant hepatic failure, with platelet counts frequently less than 100,000/μL. The thrombocytopenia may be related to bone marrow suppression and low-grade disseminated intravascular coagulation. Clinical evidence of bleeding may necessitate the use of platelet transfusions if the platelet count is < 50,000/μL.

D. Renal Failure: Renal failure develops in approximately half of patients with fulminant hepatic failure and worsens the prognosis. The renal failure is oliguric and typically functional (ie, the hepatorenal syndrome), but acute tubular necrosis may also be found. Drug-induced nephrotoxicity should also be excluded. Any potentially nephrotoxic agent, such as aminoglycosides or contrast agents, should be avoided. Hypovolemia and hypotension should be corrected with intravenous colloids such as fresh-frozen plasma or albumin to achieve adequate cardiac filling pressures. Hemodialysis is frequently necessary for severe metabolic acidosis, hyperkalemia, or fluid overload, although some transplant centers prefer to use continuous arteriovenous he-

mofiltration. Other electrolyte abnormalities that are common and may require correction include hyponatremia, hypophosphatemia, hypocalcemia, or hypomagnesemia. Hepatorenal syndrome in the setting of fulminant hepatic failure can be reversed by orthotopic liver transplantation, and, thus, the development of renal failure should not exclude proceeding with transplantation.

E. Cardiovascular Abnormalities: Increased cardiac output and low systemic vascular resistance characterize the usual cardiovascular derangements in fulminant hepatic failure. Hypotension with poor organ perfusion may exacerbate hepatic failure, and lactic acidosis resulting from tissue hypoxia may also occur. Adequate replacement of volume to maintain blood pressure and infusion of dopamine may be required.

F. Hypoglycemia: Hypoglycemia is a common complication of severe fulminant hepatic failure. Hence, blood glucose levels should be monitored at least every 4 hours during all stages of hepatic encephalopathy. The pathophysiology of hypoglycemia is multifactorial, including impaired hepatic glucose release, impaired hepatic gluconeogenesis, and elevated serum insulin levels. All patients with fulminant hepatic failure should receive a continuous intravenous infusion of 10% dextrose. Treatment of hypoglycemia may occasionally require infusion of hypertonic glucose by central venous lines, with a reasonable goal of maintaining blood glucose levels at 60–200 mg/dL.

G. Infection: Patients with fulminant hepatic failure are at increased risk for a number of bacterial and fungal infections. Such infections will compromise a patient's eligibility for orthotopic liver transplantation; sepsis accounts for approximately 20% of conditions that contraindicate transplantation (Table 35–6). Bacteremia is a frequent problem because patients are often comatose and have numerous indwelling catheters, which increases the chance for infection. A number of recent prospective studies have shown that 80% or more of patients with fulminant hepatic failure have infection based on clinical assessment or culturing, with the respiratory and urinary tracts being the primary sites involved. The predominant infectious organisms are gram-positive streptococci, *Staphylococcus aureus,* and gram-negative organisms. As many as one-third of patients with fulminant hepatic failure develop fungal infections, primarily *Candida albicans.* These patients often have coexistent renal failure and have received antibiotics. Regular surveillance cultures and aggressive treatment of presumed or documented infection is critical to management. The role of empiric antibiotic therapy is uncertain. Prophylactic antifungal agents are more commonly used for patients with advanced hepatic encephalopathy, because of the relatively high incidence and level of morbidity of fungal infection.

Treatment

A number of proposed treatments, including corticosteroids, insulin, and glucagon, have no benefit in patients with fulminant hepatic failure. In particular, several controlled trials have failed to confirm any favorable effect from the use of corticosteroids. More recently, there has been interest in the use of prostaglandin analogs for the treatment of fulminant hepatic failure, with some early trials showing positive results. Recent controlled trials, however, have unfortunately shown no benefit from the use of prostaglandin analogs in patients with fulminant hepatic failure.

Historically, a number of aggressive therapies, such as repeated exchange transfusions, plasmapheresis, total body washout, and hemoperfusion through isolated primate livers, have either shown no benefit or been associated with a worse outcome. Charcoal hemoperfusion initially demonstrated promise in an uncontrolled trial, but a subsequent controlled trial in over 100 patients showed no improvement in survival rates with this therapy.

Because specific therapies have been ineffective, the two primary goals of therapy are: (1) to provide good supportive care in an intensive care unit; and (2) to assess whether orthotopic liver transplantation is indicated. An important approach to therapy is also to determine the cause of fulminant hepatic failure, because specific antidote therapy for certain conditions, such as acetaminophen and possibly mushroom poisoning, may be beneficial. H_2-receptor blockers are routinely given to prevent stress-induced ulceration and gastrointestinal hemorrhage. Pulmonary artery monitoring is helpful in the management of intravascular volume and optimal oxygenation. If the patient progresses to grade 3 or grade 4 hepatic encephalopathy, intubation with mechanical ventilation is begun, and consideration should be given to intracerebral pressure monitoring.

The only proven therapy for fulminant hepatic failure is orthotopic liver transplantation (see Chapter 54). For this reason, all patients should be transferred to a liver transplant center that is able to promptly assess patients and proceed with transplantation if indicated. A review of the published literature indicates that the outcome of transplantation is reasonably good, with 65–70% of patients surviving 1 year. It is important to note that this 1-year survival rate is approximately 10% less than the survival rate of patients undergoing orthotopic liver transplantation for end-stage liver disease. Before proceeding with transplantation, the patient must be promptly assessed for potential contraindications to transplantation (Table 35–6). Some of the obstacles to successful transplantation include safe transportation of a patient with cerebral edema to a transplant center, obtaining a reliable psychosocial assessment, securing funding on an urgent basis, and obtaining a suitable organ. In the setting of fulminant hepatic failure, marginal donors may be used and orthotopic liver transplantation may also be performed across ABO blood groups.

Alternative approaches to the treatment of hepatic encephalopathy remain experimental. Auxiliary heterotopic liver transplantation has been performed in emergency situations with good results. If the native liver recovers function, immunosuppression can be withdrawn and the heterotopic graft will undergo rejection and atrophy. A partial liver transplantation from a living relative, with implantation of a left lateral segment of the liver, has also been used for children and even young adults with fulminant hepatic failure. An extracorporeal human donor graft has even been used for temporary support for a few days if the organ is otherwise deemed not suitable for implantation at orthotopic liver transplantation.

Other methods of temporary liver support include various hepatic assist devices. The original approach was to transplant isolated hepatocytes, either alone or with pancreatic islets, into the spleen. Others have attached hepatocytes to various microcarriers and injected them into the peritoneal cavity. These approaches remain experimental and may or may not reach the level of clinical application. The use of hepatocyte growth factors also holds some interest as a straightforward approach to induce rapid hepatic regeneration.

Prognosis

The decision whether to proceed with orthotopic liver transplantation to treat/counter fulminant hepatic failure is difficult. The underlying cause of fulminant and subfulminant hepatic failure, as displayed in Table 35–4, is a major determinant of the likelihood of recovery and survival without transplantation. Perhaps the single most reliable guide to outcome is the stage of hepatic encephalopathy, with poor survival rates being expected in stage 3, and particularly stage 4, encephalopathy. In addition, Bernuau and colleagues have shown that factor V levels of less than 20% in patients under 30 years of age or less than 30% in older patients are an indication that failure to survive is likely when viral hepatitis is the cause of fulminant hepatic failure.

The most comprehensive experience with fulminant hepatic failure has been reported from King's College Hospital in London. Ongoing studies at this center have demonstrated an improvement in survival rates over the past 20 years due to better supportive care of patients with acute liver failure in intensive care units. A multivariate analysis of 588 patients seen at King's College Hospital over a 12-year period was used to develop criteria predicting death from fulminant hepatic failure and the need for orthotopic liver transplantation (Table 35–7). The cause of acute liver failure was important, with patients having acetaminophen overdose experiencing the best survival rates and patients with non-A, non-

Table 35–7. Prognostic indicators associated with adverse outcome and need for liver transplantation in fulminant hepatic failure.[1]

Fulminant hepatic failure secondary to acetaminophen overdose
  pH < 7.30, or
  Prothrombin time 6.5 (INR)[2] and serum
    creatinine > 300 µmol/L (3.4 mg/dL)
Fulminant hepatic failure secondary to viral hepatitis or drug reaction
  Prothrombin time 6.5 (INR), or
  Any 3 of the following variables:
    Cause is non-A, non-B hepatitis or drug reaction
    Age < 10 and > 40 years
    Duration of jaundice before encephalopathy > 7 days
    Serum bilirubin > 300 µmol/L (17.6 mg/dL)
    Prothrombin time 3.5 (INR)

[1]Data from O'Grady JG et al: Early indicators of prognosis in fulminant hepatic failure. Gastroenterology 1989;97:439.
[2]INR, international normalized ratio.

B hepatitis or idiosyncratic drug reactions having the worst survival rates. Other laboratory threshold values, particularly prothrombin times, were useful in predicting outcome. In this series, nearly all patients ultimately developed advanced stages of hepatic encephalopathy, which was not an independent prognostic variable. Thus, irrespective of the grade of encephalopathy, the presence of the adverse prognostic indicators shown in Table 35–7 should lead to the placement of a patient with fulminant hepatic failure on the list for orthotopic liver transplantation, if there are no contraindications.

Assessment of prognosis is critically important, so that orthotopic liver transplantation, with its lifelong requirement for immunosuppression and continuous care, can be avoided in patients who would otherwise recover from fulminant hepatic failure, while transplantation can expeditiously be carried out in patients who would otherwise die of acute liver failure. Proper application of transplantation has favorably altered the outcome of acute liver failure, which was dismal before the widespread availability of this procedure.

REFERENCES

Fingerote RJ, Bain VG: Fulminant hepatic failure. Am J Gastroenterol 1993;88:1000.

Lee WM: Acute liver failure. N Engl J Med 1993;329:1862.

Lidofsky SD: Liver transplantation for fulminant hepatic failure. Gastroenterol Clin North Am 1993;22:257.

Muñoz SJ: Difficult management problems in fulminant hepatic failure. Semin Liv Dis 1993;13:395.

Mutimer DJ, Elias E: Liver transplantation for fulminant hepatic failure. In: *Progress in Liver Diseases.* Vol 10. Boyer JL, Ockner RK (editors). Saunders, 1992.

Wright TL: Etiology of fulminant hepatic failure: Is another virus involved? (Editorial.) Gastroenterology 1993;104:640.

36

Viral Hepatitis

Bhupinder N. Bhandari, MD, & Teresa L. Wright, MD

The first cause of viral hepatitis was identified more than 20 years ago when hepatitis B virus (HBV) was shown to be the pathogen responsible for "serum hepatitis." Since then, there has been extensive characterization of properties of HBV and the host immune response to infection. Advances in molecular biology have resulted in the identification and sequence analysis of two viruses acquired by the fecal-oral route of transmission (hepatitis A virus, HAV, and hepatitis E virus, HEV) and two viruses acquired parenterally (hepatitis C virus, HCV, and hepatitis D virus, HDV). Other viruses which cause hepatitis (including cytomegalovirus, CMV) are discussed elsewhere (see Chapter 39). The pathogenesis, diagnosis and treatment of chronic viral hepatitis continues to be the focus of research. Sensitive and specific assays are available for all five forms (A to E) of viral hepatitis. Nevertheless, at least 5–20% of cases of acute and chronic hepatitis are cryptogenic in that they cannot be attributed to any of the known forms of viral hepatitis and do not appear to result from toxic, metabolic, or genetic conditions. These include 5–20% of cases of acute viral hepatitis, 10–20% of cases of chronic hepatitis, and approximately half the cases of fulminant hepatitis and hepatitis-associated aplastic anemia. Whether additional unidentified viruses cause acute or chronic liver disease is under intense investigation. This chapter will focus on clinical features of the five main viruses that cause acute and chronic hepatitis (Table 36–1).

GENERAL CONSIDERATIONS

Essentials of Diagnosis

Diagnostic tests for different clinical situations are summarized in Table 36–2. All infections other than HBV infection are diagnosed by detection of antibody (either IgM and/or IgG) rather than antigen. Antibodies or antigen in serum are usually detected by enzyme-linked immunoassay (ELISA) or radioimmunoassays.

Clinical Findings

A. Symptoms and signs: Symptoms of acute viral hepatitis are usually nonspecific with malaise, fatigue, nausea, anorexia and arthralgias. Fever, if present, is usually low-grade. With disease progression, pruritus, dark urine, scleral icterus, and jaundice may occur.

B. Laboratory Findings: In any acute viral hepatitis, serum transaminases are typically greater than 500 U/L and often greater than 1,000 U/L, with the ALT characteristically higher than the AST. Transaminase elevation starts in the prodromal phase and precedes the rise in bilirubin level. Serum alkaline phosphatase may be normal or only mildly elevated. Serum bilirubin is variably elevated, but albumin and prothrombin time should be normal unless there is significant impairment of hepatic synthetic function. In most instances bilirubin is equally divided between conjugated and unconjugated fractions; values above 20 mg/dL that persist late into the course of viral hepatitis are more likely to be associated with severe disease. Prolongation of the prothrombin time (greater than 3 seconds above control value) should raise concern and prompt close monitoring of the patient for worsening hepatic failure. Neutropenia and lymphopenia are transient and followed by a relative lymphocytosis. Hypoglycemia occurs occasionally in severe acute hepatitis. A mild and diffuse elevation of gamma globulin fraction is common. Liver biopsy is rarely necessary in acute viral hepatitis except when the diagnosis is questionable or when chronic hepatitis is suspected.

C. Imaging: Radiologic studies are rarely necessary unless biliary tract disease is suspected. In patients with profound intrahepatic cholestasis (such as occurs with hepatitis A infection), ultrasonography may be helpful in eliminating extrahepatic biliary tract obstruction.

Differential Diagnosis

Acute Viral Hepatitis: Infections with other viruses such as cytomegalovirus, infectious mononucleosis, herpes simplex, and coxsackieviruses can re-

Table 36–1. Properties and clinical charateristics of viruses.

	Hepatitis A	Hepatitis B	Hepatitis C	Hepatitis D	Hepatitis E
Size	27nm	42nm	32nm	36nm	27–34nm
Length	7.5kb	3.2kb	10kb	1.7kb	7.6kb
Genome	RNA	DNA	RNA	RNA	RNA
Incubation	14–49 days	14–84 days	14–160 days	21–42 days	21–63 days
Transmission	Fecal/oral (98%) Transfusion (2%)	IVDA (35%) Sexual (10%) Vertical (<5%) Transfusion (<5%) Needlestick (1%) Unknown (49%)	IVDA (35%) Sexual (10%) Vertical (rare) Transfusion (<5%) Needlestick (1%) Unknown (49%)	Parenteral	Fecal/oral
Vaccine	Available	Available	In development	None	None
Severity of acute illness	Usually mild Particularly in children	70% subclinical, 30% clinical, <1% severe	Usually subclinical <1% severe	Can be severe	May be severe— 30% mortality in pregnancy
Chronic infection	None	90% neonatal 50% infants 20% children <5% adults	>80%	5% with HBV coinfection 95% with HBV superinfection	None

sult in an acute viral hepatitis syndrome and elevated serum transaminases. Toxoplasmosis may also share clinical features with acute hepatitis. If HBsAg, anti-HBc, and IgM anti-HAV are negative, serological tests for these agents should be considered. Several drugs and anesthetic agents can produce a picture like acute hepatitis with cholestasis, and thus it is important to take a careful drug history. A past history of unexplained and repeated episodes of hepatitis raises the possibility of underlying chronic hepatitis. Alcoholic hepatitis is associated with a history of ethanol abuse, as well as with stigmata of alcoholism (see Chapter 40). In patients with alcoholic liver disease, serum transaminase levels rarely rise above 500 U/L, and typically, serum AST levels are greater than serum ALT levels. When abdominal pain is prominent, acute viral hepatitis may be confused with acute cholecystitis, common duct stone or ascending cholangitis. Careful clinical and radiological evaluation will assist in making the correct diagnosis and avoiding unnecessary surgery in such cases. Cholestatic viral hepatitis may be confused with ob-

structive jaundice due to pancreatic carcinoma or a common bile duct stone. Clinical features help to distinguish acute hepatitis from congestive hepatopathy and acute ischemic injury. Uncommonly inherited metabolic disorders like Wilson's disease mimic acute viral hepatitis.

Chronic Viral Hepatitis: When diagnosing chronic viral hepatitis, consideration should be given to autoimmune chronic active hepatitis, connective tissue disorders like systemic lupus erythematosis and rheumatoid arthritis, Wilson's disease, and primary biliary cirrhosis. Serology, biochemical testing, and liver histopathology helps in arriving at the correct diagnosis in most instances.

HEPATITIS A

Pathophysiology

Hepatitis A virus is an RNA virus which is transmitted by fecal-oral mode through ingestion of contaminated food (eg, shellfish) or water. The incu-

Table 36–2. Serologic diagnosis of viral hepatitis.

Significance	Anti-HAV IgM	HBsAg	HBeAg	Anti-HBc IgG	Anti-HBc IgM	Anti-HBs IgG	Anti-HCV IgM/IgG	Anti-HDV IgM	Anti-HEV IgM
Acute HAV	+	–	–	–	–	–	–	–	–
Acute HBV	–	+	+	–	+	–	–	–	–
Chronic HBV, active replication	–	+	+	+	–	–	–	–	–
Chronic HBV, quiescent	–	+	–	+	–	–	–	–	–
Resolved HBV	–	–	–	–	+	+	–	–	–
Post-vaccine immune	–	–	–	–	–	+	–	–	–
Chronic or recent HCV	–	–	–	–	–	–	+	–	–
Acute or chronic HDV	–	+	–	–	–	–	–	+	–
Acute HEV	–	–	–	–	–	–	–	–	+

bation period is 2–6 weeks and the phase when virus is present in serum is short (5–7 days); hence, parenteral transmission is rare. Infection is sporadic and associated with poor socioeconomic conditions, which can lead to epidemics. In several developing countries hepatitis A is endemic, with infection occurring in the majority of children before the age of 5 years. Improved socioeconomic conditions and sanitation has led to an increase in the mean age of infection in southern Europe. The liver cell damage probably results from cell mediated cytotoxicity. Serum neutralizing antibodies protect against HAV infection. The necroinflammatory changes are prominent in periportal areas and are accompanied by many plasma cells. In some cases, centrilobular cholestasis may be severe, particularly in adults. HAV antigen can be demonstrated by immunohistochemical staining as fine granules in the cytoplasm of hepatocytes and Kupffer cells.

Essentials of Diagnosis

Diagnosis of HAV infection depends on detection of antibodies (IgG for prior infection, IgM for recent infection). A positive anti-HAV result usually reflects total antibodies (both IgG and IgM) and cannot be used to distinguish between acute or prior exposure unless IgM is specified.

Anti-HAV IgM may persist for 6–12 months after acute infection. Hence, in a patient with acute transaminase elevation, presence of anti-HAV IgM, does not necessarily imply acute hepatitis A infection and may be represent hepatitis A infection within the prior year, with a superimposed, unrelated hepatitis.

Clinical Findings

Most cases of acute hepatitis are asymptomatic (particularly in children) or have nonspecific symptoms. When clinically apparent, patients present with jaundice, fatigue, and malaise. Uncommonly, HAV infection may result in a cholestatic picture.

Complications

Hepatitis A is rarely fulminant and never chronic. Systemic manifestations are uncommon and include cryoglobulinemia, nephritis, and leucytoclastic vasculitis. Concomitant meningoencephalitis has been reported in some patients. Cholestatic hepatitis with protracted cholestatic jaundice and pruritus can occur as a variant of acute hepatitis A. It has been suggested that in genetically susceptible individuals, HAV infection may trigger an autoimmune hepatitis. Hepatitis A may have a relapsing course, symptomatic for 6 months or more. The relapses are generally benign, with eventual complete resolution. Chronic infection never ensues, and complete recovery is the rule. Rarely (less than 1% of cases), fulminant hepatic failure with encephalopathy and coagulopathy results from acute infection. Such patients should be referred for consideration of liver transplantation. Once profound encephalopathy develops in elderly patients, mortality is high (up to 80%). In younger patients, the prognosis is better than in patients with fulminant liver failure of other causes.

Treatment

Treatment is largely supportive and consists of bed rest until jaundice subsides, a high caloric diet, discontinuation of potentially hepatotoxic medication and restriction of alcohol intake. Most cases do not require hospitalization, which is recommended for patients with advanced age, serious underlying medical conditions, or chronic liver disease, malnutrition, pregnancy, immunosuppressive therapy, hepatotoxic medication, severe vomiting that excludes adequate oral intake, and clinical and laboratory findings that suggest fulminant hepatitis. The occasional patient with fulminant hepatic failure, defined as the onset of encephalopathy within 8 weeks of the onset of symptoms, should be referred for consideration of liver transplantation (see Chapters 35, 54).

Prevention

Prevention of Hepatitis A is justified for public health reasons. General measures to prevent the spread of HAV include careful handwashing, safe water supply and proper sewage disposal. Immune globulin has been shown to be safe and effective in preventing HAV infection in both pre- and post-exposure situations (Table 36–3). If immediate protection is required, travelers should receive passive immunization with immunoglobulin as well as vaccine to confer protection. Passive immunization is by a single intramuscular dose of immune serum globulin of 0.02–0.06 ml/Kg. In post-exposure setting, immune serum globulin, if given within 10–14 days of exposure, has efficacy of about 85%, and usually aborts or reduces the severity of the HAV infection. The protection offered by immune serum globulin lasts only a few months. Human trials with inactivated whole HAV vaccines have shown a protective efficacy of 94–100% after 2–3 doses and only minor side effects. Such a vaccine is licensed in several countries, including the USA, and has recently become commercially available. Groups recommended to receive HA vaccine include travelers to areas endemic for hepatitis A, military personnel, and special populations, such as native Americans and Alaskans.

Prognosis

Virtually all previously healthy individuals recover completely without any clinical sequelae, and thus the prognosis is generally excellent and chronic liver disease does not occur. Recovery is slower in the elderly, and if fulminant hepatitis occurs, mortality in this patient group is high. Fortunately, fulminant hepatic failure is rare, and the overall case fatality rate with HAV infection is very low (about 0.1%).

Table 36–3. Post-exposure prophylaxis for HAV and HBV.

Post-exposure prophylaxis for HAV[1]	Treatment
• Acute exposure (household and sexual contacts) • Institutions (day-care centers) • Common source outbreaks	0.02 mL/kg within 2 weeks

Prevention of infection (75%)
Subclinical infection (15%)
Clinical infection (10%)

Post-exposure prophylaxis for HBV[2]	Treatment
• Acute HBV Sexual/needlestick	Anti-HBsIg plus vaccine; household, none

• Chronic HBV
  Sexual
  Household
  Casual contact
	
	Vaccine
	Vaccine
	None

[1]Pre-exposure prophylaxis when traveling to endemic areas (0.02 mg/kg subcutaneously 4–6 months).
[2]Dose of vaccine 20 mg intradermal, 3 at times; dose of anti-HBsIg 0.6 mg/kg IM; dose for neonates 0.5 ml plus HBV vaccine (0.5 ml within the first week, then at 1 month and 6 months).

HEPATITIS B

Pathophysiology

Hepatitis B virus is a DNA virus transmitted by blood, sexual or needle contact. In the United States, the most common modes of transmission are sexual and parenteral (horizontal spread), whereas in Asia, the most common mode is from mother to child (vertical spread). Injecting drug users are at high risk of also acquiring hepatitis C and D (see following sections).

HBV is a partially double-stranded DNA virus, which replicates through an RNA intermediate. Although HBV is strongly hepatotrophic, viral sequences, including HBV replicative intermediates, are present in extrahepatic tissues (lymph nodes, peripheral blood mononuclear cells). There are four open reading frames in HBV that encode four major proteins: (1) surface gene for hepatitis B surface antigen (HBsAg); (2) core gene for hepatitis B core antigen (HBcAg); (3) pol gene for the DNA polymerase, which catalyzes several steps in viral replication and assembly; and (4) the hepatitis B X gene for the X protein, which appears to up-regulate the replication of other viruses such as human immunodeficiency virus (HIV). HBsAg, the envelope protein of the virus that is excreted in excess as 20nm particles in serum, indicates ongoing infection. HBcAg, the protein found in the inner core of HBV, is not secreted into serum but is expressed on the hepatocyte surface. As such, it is the target of the host immune response to infection, playing an important role in the pathogenesis of HBV-induced liver damage. HBcAg can also be detected in the nuclei of hepatocytes. HBeAg is the secretory form of HBcAg, whose presence indicates active viral replication and increased infectivity. The C region has two initiation codons, and therefore two gene transcripts (pre-core and core), which result in two protein products (HBcAg and HBeAg). These polypeptides have considerable amino acid homology and immune cross-reactivity at the T cell level. Anti-HBc appears at onset of clinical hepatitis and may be the only marker detectable between disappearance of HBsAg and appearance of anti-HBs. Anti-HBe usually appears at the time of peak clinical symptoms and in combination with HBsAg, implies low viral replication and infectivity. Four antigenic subtypes of HBV exist (adw, ayw, adr, ayr), and there is geographic variation in the distribution of these subtypes.

Most damage from HBV infection is caused by host immune response. Cell-mediated response directed against cellular HBcAg is the primary cause of cell injury, with immune lysis of infected hepatocytes resulting in hepatitis. Hyperactive host response may lead to fulminant hepatitis, whereas a reduced host response increases the risk of chronic infection. In vertically acquired infection, the neonate is unable to mount an adequate immune response, which leads to a state of "tolerance" to the virus, which characterizes the asymptomatic carrier state.

In chronic hepatitis B, hepatocytes with ground glass cytoplasm are seen, particularly in patients with little or no necroinflammatory activity. HBcAg can be demonstrated in the hepatocyte nuclei and also the cytoplasm and cell membrane. HLA restricted cytotoxic T lymphocytes directed against the molecular complex of viral and histocompatibility antigens on the liver cell surface are the effector cells that mediate cell damage. Cytokine mediated cell injury and other mechanisms may also be involved in cell damage. HBeAg negative variants result from mutations in the pre-core region with failure of HBeAg synthesis, yet with continued viral replication. These mutant viruses have been associated with fulminant hepatitis and aggressive chronic disease.

Chronic HBV infection is strongly linked epidemiologically to the development of hepatocellular carcinoma (in up to 50% of patients with HBV-induced cirrhosis) (see Chapter 46). The mechanism of viral oncogenesis has been extensively studied. Viral integration into the host genome is required but no consistent sites of integration have been shown (eg, adjacent to a host tumor promotor or suppressor gene). Cell turnover associated with chronic inflammation likely contributes to the pathogenesis of hepatocellular carcinoma, as do environmental cofactors such as aflatoxins.

Essentials of Diagnosis

Diagnosis of HBV infection largely relies on the presence of hepatitis B surface antigen (HBsAg). Acute and chronic infections are distinguished by the presence of IgM and IgG antibodies to the inner hepatitis B core protein (anti-HBc). Acute HBV infection in the absence of HBsAg positivity (but anti-HBc IgM positive in the so-called "window period") is theoretically possible but rare. Presence of IgM anti-HBc indicates recent infection, although this marker may occasionally be present during acute reactivation of chronic infection. Hepatitis B e antigen (HBeAg) is a cleaved protein product of the hepatitis B core gene, which is indicative of active HBV replication. Antibodies to HBeAg (anti-HBe) are present in inactive or non-replicative HBV infection. Actively replicating mutant viruses (so-called "precore" mutants), with detectable HBV DNA in serum, have been reported in both acute and chronic HBV infection in the absence of HBeAg (anti-HBe positive). Antibodies to hepatitis B surface antigen (anti-HBs) indicate vaccine-induced immunity; antibodies to both core and surface proteins (anti-HBc and anti-HBs) indicate prior HBV infection. Interpretation of isolated anti-HBc (IgG) positivity is problematic since this may represent ongoing, low-level HBV infection, prior HBV infection, or a false-positive test. Typically anti-HBcore IgM is indicative of acute HBV infection and anti-HBcore IgG indicative of prior or resolving HBV infection. On occasion, acute flares of chronic HBV are associated with anti-HBcore IgM positivity.

Clinical Findings

The patient with acute HBV infection is infective for many weeks before clinical presentation. The incubation period is between 6 weeks and 6 months. Prodrome may include arthralgias and skin rash. Fatigue, anorexia, icterus, and alanine transaminase elevation correlate with anti-HBc appearance. Risk of chronicity is related to the age of acquisition: more than 90% in newborns, about 50% in early childhood, less than 5% in immunocompetent adults, and greater than 50% in immunocompromised adults such as transplant recipients, HIV-positive individuals, and patients with leukemia or leprosy.

Progression to chronic active hepatitis is suggested by the lack of complete resolution of anorexia, weight loss, and fatigue and persistent hepatomegaly, presence of bridging or multilobular hepatic necrosis on liver biopsy, persistence of HBsAg and aminotransferase, bilirubin, and globulin level elevations for at least 6 months after acute hepatitis. Extrahepatic manifestations include arthralgias, arthritis, Henoch-Schonlein purpura, angioneurotic edema, polyarteritis nodosa, glomerulonephritis, pleural effusions, pericarditis, and aplastic anemia.

Complications

Hepatitis B accounts for about 50% of fulminant hepatitis of viral cause (see Chapter 35). The diagnosis is suggested by decreasing liver size, rising bilirubin, an increasing prothrombin time, and signs of encephalopathy. Cerebral edema is common, and brain stem compression, GI bleeding, sepsis, respiratory failure, cardiovascular collapse, and renal failure are terminal events in this condition, which has a very high mortality. Survivors may have complete biochemical and histological recovery. In 5–10% of acute hepatitis B patients, a serum sickness-like syndrome with arthralgias, rash, angioedema, and rarely proteinuria and hematuria may develop in the prodromal phase. In children, hepatitis B may rarely present as anicteric hepatitis associated with a nonpruritic papular rash on the face, buttocks, and limbs. The risk of chronicity is influenced by age and immune responsiveness and is less than 5% in immunocompetent adults. Most patients with chronic infection have normal liver enzymes, no symptoms, are anti-HBe positive, and have normal or near normal liver histology. These "healthy" carriers seem to be immunologically tolerant to this virus and have an excellent prognosis. When there is a loss of tolerance with emergence of reactive T cell clones, hepatic inflammation and T cell-mediated liver damage may follow. Most patients with active liver disease have active viral replication and are HBeAg and HBV DNA positive. HBV DNA has been found integrated into chromosomal DNA of hepatocytes. Predominantly episomal HBV DNA is detectable in carriers with high levels of viral replication, with integrated HBV DNA detectable in those with less active viral replication. Patients with persistent active viral replication are at a greater risk of death from liver disease or hepatocellular carcinoma than those with inactive disease. The proportion of patients with integrated HBV DNA and anti-HBe positivity increases with the increasing age of the cohort.

The outcome in HBsAg-positive patients is also influenced by histological stage. Five-year survival rates in patients with early histological changes (chronic persistent hepatitis) are higher (97%) than in patients with chronic active hepatitis (85%). Development of cirrhosis is associated with a reduction in 5-year survival to about 50%. As noted above, HBsAg carriers have a several-fold increase in the risk of hepatocellular carcinoma. In regions where this viral infection is endemic, hepatocellular carcinoma is the leading cause of cancer-related death. Cirrhosis is present in more than 90% of HBV-related hepatocellular carcinoma, and the chronic inflammation and regenerative cellular proliferation associated with cirrhosis may predispose to cellular transformation and frank malignancy. Population- and clinic-based screening programs using serum α-fetoprotein and liver ultrasound have lead to identification of patients with small and potentially resectable tumors. It is not clear, however, that mortality from hepatocellular carcinoma is reduced by screening programs (see Chapter 46).

Uncommon complications of HBV infection include pancreatitis, myocarditis, atypical pneumonia, aplastic anemia, transverse myelitis, and peripheral neuropathy.

Treatment

In fulminant hepatitis, intensive care in a specialized unit likely reduces mortality, which approaches 80% (see Chapter 35). Protein intake should be restricted and oral lactulose or neomycin administered. Patients should be supported by maintaining fluid and electrolyte balance and cardiorespiratory function, controlling bleeding and managing other complications. Large corticosteroid doses, exchange transfusions, plasma perfusion, human cross-circulation, and porcine liver cross-perfusion have not proven effective. Orthotopic liver transplantation is being performed with increasing frequency, with good results. Thus, patients should be supported maximally until spontaneous recovery or until prognostic factors indicate worsening outcome necessitating transplantation. Patients transplanted for fulminant hepatitis B are at a lower risk of recurrence than those transplanted for chronic hepatitis.

Treatment of chronic hepatitis is aimed at reducing inflammation, symptoms, and infectivity. Recombinant alpha interferon converts 37% of patients from the replicative phase to non-replicative phase (ie, HBeAg negative) and is currently the only effective approved antiviral agent (Table 36–4). Effective treatment often triggers a flare of clinical hepatitis. Patients with active immune response are the best candidates for treatment. Their features include low serum HBV DNA levels, recent infection with high transaminases and active liver histology, and presence of at least some HBeAg producing wild type virions. Response to interferon is indicated by a loss of HBV DNA and HBeAg from the serum, normalization of serum alanine aminotransferase level, and improvement in liver histology. Interferon therapy is administered by injection; it is expensive and has some adverse effects. Major early adverse effects include a flu-like syndrome, fever, chills, malaise, muscle aches, and rigors. Later side effects include headaches, anorexia, and weight loss, hair loss, bone marrow depression (leukopenia and thrombocytopenia), and psychological effects (anxiety, depression, and irritability). Unusual adverse effects include seizures, acute psychosis, autoimmune reactions, thyroid abnormalities, proteinuria, cardiomyopathy, skin rashes, and bacterial infections. There is no evidence that antiviral therapy in acute hepatitis accelerates healing or clearance of virus or prevents progression to chronic disease. Nevertheless, in contrast to treatment of patients with HCV infection, those who do respond to interferon tend to have a long-term remission.

Liver transplantation has been employed as therapy for end-stage chronic HBV associated liver disease (see Chapter 54). One-year survival in patients transplanted for chronic HBV (50%) is poorer than in patients transplanted for alcoholic or cholestatic liver disease (90%) in most centers. Long-term survival is more likely in patients with evidence of HBV immunity (HBsAg negative, anti-HBs positive) than in HBsAg-positive patients with postnecrotic cirrhosis.

Table 36–4. Treatment with alpha interferon.

	Hepatitis B	Hepatitis C
Dose	5MU/d subcutaneously	3MU 3 times weekly subcutaneously
Duration	16 weeks	24 weeks
Selection criteria		
ALT	1.3XULN[1]	1.5XULN[1]
Serology	HBsAg (+), HBeAg (+)	Anti-HCV (+) (ELISA II)
WBC	≥1.5k/μL	≥1.5k/μL
Platelets	≥75k/μL	≥75k/μL
Absence of	Bilirubin ≤ 2.5 mg/dL	Bilirubin ≤ 2.5 mg/dL
decompensation	Albumin ≥ 3 g/dL	Albumin ≥ 3 g/dL
	Prothrombin time < 3 seconds prolonged	Prothrombin time < 3 seconds prolonged
Absence of	Uncontrolled cardiopulmonary disease	Uncontrolled cardiopulmonary disease
other diseases	Significant neuropsychiatric disease	Significant neuropsychiatric disease
	Renal insufficiency	Renal insufficiency

[1]ULN = upper limit of normal

Active pretransplant viral replication (HBeAg/or HBV DNA positive) is associated with a more aggressive posttransplantation course and a less favorable outcome. Reinfection is extremely common after transplantation, and the resulting hepatitis can be severe and is almost invariably chronic. The most effective approach to delaying and preventing recurrent HBV infection has been high dose immune globulin (anti-HBsIg) perioperatively and postoperatively. The use of high dose prophylactic hepatitis B immune globulin has resulted in prolonged survival following liver transplantation in those with and without active pretransplantation viral replication. Alpha interferon treatment in the peri-transplant period has been ineffective in preventing reinfection. Retransplantation has been tried in patients whose first graft failed because of HBV recurrence, but further infection is the rule unless specific precautions to prevent reinfection are taken. Low levels of HBV are demonstrable in liver, serum, and peripheral blood mononuclear cells by polymerase chain reaction, suggesting that long-term therapy is necessary to prevent overt posttransplantation recurrence.

Prevention

Hepatitis B vaccine is protective in over 90% of normal individuals. Recombinant vaccines have largely supplanted the original plasma-derived vaccine in most parts of the world. Common adverse effects are local reactions at the injection site (soreness, tenderness, pruritus, and swelling); serious adverse effects have not been reported (Table 36–5). For reasons that are unclear, a small percentage of healthy patients receiving HBV vaccine do not develop protective antibodies. Vaccination of those at high risk has been of only limited success, since compliance in even highly educated groups such as health-care workers has been poor. Despite the availability of an effective vaccine for more than a decade, the incidence of HBV infection in the USA has increased. Thus, the United States Public Health Service has recommended universal vaccination of all neonates and pre-pubertal teenagers. Protection is afforded against HBV surface antigenemia, clinically apparent Hepatitis B, and chronic infection. Currently, booster immunization is not recommended routinely. It can serve a useful role in the immunosuppressed persons who have lost detectable anti HBs or immunocompetent persons who sustain HBsAg inoculation after losing detectable antibody.

Prognosis

Ninety percent of patients with acute HBV infection have a favorable course and recover completely. Older persons and patients with diabetes mellitus and congestive heart failure may have a severe hepatitis with a prolonged course. Case fatality rate is low (0.1%), but increases with age and associated systemic illnesses. Patients presenting with ascites, ankle edema, and encephalopathy and those with prolonged prothrombin time, hypoglycemia, hypoalbuminemia and very high bilirubin levels have severe hepatocellular damage and should be hospitalized promptly. About 1–2% of normal, immunocompetent young adults remain chronically positive after acute infection. These patients may be asymptomatic carriers or may have chronic hepatitis with or without cirrhosis. Epidemiologic studies have established the link between HBV infection and hepatocellular carcinoma, although the mechanism of oncogenesis has not been elucidated.

Table 36–5. Individuals who benefit from Hepatitis B vaccine, by category.

Exposure Risk	Example
Professional	Health care workers (especially those exposed to blood, hemodialysis patients, and staff)
Relational/Familial	Spouses of infected persons and institutionalized persons Household and sexual contacts of HBsAg carriers
Nosocomial	Developmentally handicapped and institutionalized individuals Hemophiliacs and other patients who require repeated transfusion of blood products
Lifestyle	Parenteral drug users Individuals with multiple sex partners
Other	Persons traveling into areas of high endemicity

HEPATITIS C

Pathophysiology

Hepatitis C virus is a single-strand RNA virus. Its genome is fully characterized, encoding two structural proteins (core and envelope) and five nonstructural proteins (including a helicase and RNA polymerase, both of which are important in viral replication). Six major HCV genotypes, and many minor variants based upon divergence of nucleic acid sequence, have been recognized. There is considerable variation in geographic distribution of HCV genotypes, with certain genotypes having inherently greater replicative ability and increased resistance to interferon therapy. Hypervariability of regions of the HCV envelope proteins may be important in persistence of HCV infection, facilitating evasion of the host immune response. Levels of HCV in serum are much lower than levels of HBV, and HCV antigens are not detectable in blood.

HCV accounts for most post-transfusion hepatitis. HCV can be transmitted parenterally by blood transfusion and by needles as in injecting drug abusers.

Needlestick spread in health care workers inoculated with blood-contaminated needles has been confirmed by anti-HCV testing, but the seroconversion rate is low (approximately 4%), and this accounts for a very small proportion of HCV-infections (<1%). Sporadic HCV infection, in which the mode of transmission is unknown, is responsible for the vast majority of chronic NANB hepatitis. Sexual or vertical transmission can occur, but either is much less efficient than for HBV. Liver biopsies from patients with chronic HCV infection demonstrate micro- or macrovesicular steatosis (in 50%), bile duct damage (in 60%) and lymphocyte aggregates or follicles (in 60%). Immune-mediated damage is thought to produce hepatitis in HCV infection although the mechanism of cell injury is not fully understood. A direct cytopathic effect of HCV may also contribute to the damage in some situations.

Essentials of Diagnosis

HCV infection is diagnosed by presence of anti-HCV, which detects IgG antibodies to three different proteins in HCV, and may be present within 2 months of exposure. No anti-HCV IgM assays for acute infection are commercially available, but viral RNA can be detected directly (by polymerase chain reaction amplification, see below) within 2 weeks of exposure. Supplemental immunoblot assays have been approved to confirm the presence of anti-HCV (recombinant immunoblot assay or RIBA2).

Clinical Findings

A. Symptoms and Signs: Acute hepatitis C is typically mild and often not recognized clinically. Of all the hepatitis viruses, HCV is most likely to produce chronic infection. Following transfusion of HCV-infected blood (determined by a positive test for HCV antibodies by ELISA II immunoassay and recombinant immunoblot assay) hepatitis develops in approximately 80% of recipients. The chronic nature of this infection is underscored by the presence of detectable anti-HCV 4–6 years after transfusion in 83% recipients. About 20% of chronic HCV patients develop cirrhosis. Most of these patients are asymptomatic. Older age at infection, concomitant ethanol abuse, and HBV or HIV coinfection may be important aggravating factors. HCV is associated with hepatocellular carcinoma, although the mechanism of oncogenesis is unknown. Extrahepatic manifestations include membranoproliferative glomerulonephritis, leukocytoclastic vasculitis, and essential mixed cryoglobulinemia.

B. Anti-HCV Positive Test: The majority of anti-HCV-positive patients (by ELISA II) are infected with hepatitis C virus. In healthy blood donors (in whom the prevalence of infection is approximately 0.7%), positivity of a supplemental assay (RIBA2), is indicative of "true" infection. Conversely, a negative RIBA2 test in an anti-HCV positive blood donor likely represents a false-positive anti-HCV. Active HCV infection is present in the minority of anti-HCV-positive blood donors with an indeterminate RIBA2 result (approximately 20%). True HCV infection is present in almost all anti-HCV-positive patients with liver disease (elevated ALT) and a parenteral risk factor. In such situations, confirmation with RIBA2 or HCV RNA is rarely needed, and is indeed probably not warranted.

C. HCV-Autoimmune Hepatitis Overlap: Considerable confusion exists with regard to overlapping clinical and serological features of chronic HCV infection and autoimmune chronic active hepatitis (see Chapter 37). In patients with true autoimmune disease (steroid-responsive hepatitis, high titer autoantibodies, hypergammaglobulinemia, and other autoimmune features), first generation anti-HCV tests were frequently positive in the absence of true HCV infection (ie, in the absence of detectable HCV RNA). The incidence of "false-positive" anti-HCV tests fell when patients with autoimmune chronic active hepatitis were tested with second generation anti-HCV assays. Low titer autoantibodies (particularly antinuclear antibodies) are also frequently positive in patients with true HCV infection. The biochemical profile is similar in the two diseases, with elevation of serum alanine aminotransferase (ALT) usually exceeding that of the aspartate aminotransferase (AST), and with preservation of hepatic synthetic function (serum bilirubin, albumin, and prothrombin time) until liver disease is advanced. There are also overlapping histological features of these two entities. Patients with chronic active hepatitis of either viral or autoimmune origin, typically have disruption of the hepatic lobular architecture with inflammatory infiltrates (lymphocytes and plasma cells), hepatocyte necrosis, and bridging fibrosis. Features suggestive, but not pathognomonic, of HCV infection include lymphocytic infiltrates of bile ducts and steatosis. Distinction between autoimmune chronic active hepatitis and chronic HCV infection may be difficult, yet has important therapeutic implications.

Complications

Hepatitis C can lead to cirrhosis and hepatocellular carcinoma. The rate of progression to cirrhosis is slow. Commonly, the initial infection is subclinical and the consequences of infection are not apparent for many years. Once cirrhosis develops, however, patients are at increased risk of gastrointestinal bleeding (from portal hypertension), encephalopathy, life-threatening bacterial infections, and hepatorenal failure. Prior to the development of such complications, liver transplantation should be considered, although serological recurrence of HCV is the rule.

Treatment

Treatment of chronic HCV infection with 3 million units of alpha interferon, given subcutaneously three times a week, is FDA-approved and normalizes serum ALT in 50% of the patients (Table 36–4). Only about one-half of these patients continue to have normal ALT after stopping therapy. Long-term virologic remission is rare (< 5%). Presence of cirrhosis and high levels of pre-treatment HCV RNA are associated with a reduced responsiveness to interferon. Patients with clinically decompensated HCV-related liver cirrhosis (ie, decreased synthetic function or complications of portal hypertension) should be considered for liver transplantation. Recurrent HCV infection (determined by the presence of HCV RNA in serum) is common (more than 90% of patients with pre-transplantation infection). Unlike HBV, however, recurrence of HCV is typically associated with relatively mild disease (histologic hepatitis on biopsy in approximately 50% of patients, with cirrhosis in only 10% at 3 years).

In a young woman with liver disease, fatigue, high titer autoantibodies, and hypergammaglobulinemia, a trial of steroids is warranted if anti-HCV positive by ELISA, but not by RIBA. In a patient with liver disease, a parenteral risk factor, and detectable anti-HCV, interferon therapy should be considered even in the presence of low titer autoantibodies (see below). In patients with more striking autoimmune features, however, (eg, high titer autoantibodies, autoimmune thyroid disease), interferon should be avoided even if HCV infection is confirmed by supplemental assays (RIBA2). When in doubt, the physician should err on the side of not treating, because of a theoretical risk of aggravating autoimmune disease with an immune stimulant like interferon.

Prevention

Hepatitis C incidence can be reduced by blood donor screening for antibody to hepatitis C, although since transfusions account for only 5% of all cases of HCV infection in the USA, reduction in the incidence of post-transfusion HCV infection is unlikely to impact on the overall prevalence of disease. Vapor-heated clotting factor concentrates carry a very low, and possibly zero, risk of HCV transmission; chemical treatment of blood products to inactivate HCV is being pursued. Efficacy of standard immunoglobulin after needlestick, sexual, or perinatal exposure to HCV has not been determined and is not recommended. Currently there is no vaccine available for pre-exposure prophylaxis.

Prognosis

Following transfusion of HCV-infected blood or following acute community-acquired HCV infection, hepatitis develops and persists in more than 80% of recipients. Commonly, the initial infection is subclinical, and the consequences of infection are not apparent for many years. Acute hepatitis C is more often anicteric and less severe in the acute phase than acute hepatitis B. The case fatality rate is difficult to estimate but is extremely low. Fulminant hepatic failure does not appear to be a consequence of acute HCV infection in immunocompetent patients. Conversely, HCV infection may be a rare cause of fulminant hepatic failure of unknown etiology (so-called fulminant non-A non-B hepatitis).

Evaluation of blood transfusion recipients suggests that those who develop post-transfusion hepatitis have only a slightly increased long-term risk of liver related deaths (mean follow-up of 17 years) and no overall increased mortality. The slowly progressive nature of this disease is apparent from a retrospective study of HCV patients who had a prior parenteral exposure (blood transfusion) in which mean time to development of chronic hepatitis, cirrhosis, and hepatocellular carcinoma was 10, 21, and 29 years respectively. About 50% of patients with post-transfusion HCV infection have persistent transaminase elevations 1 year later. Although most of these patients are asymptomatic, a liver biopsy confirms chronic hepatitis in the majority. Cirrhosis develops in about 20% of patients with chronic post-transfusion hepatitis within 10 years of acute illness. The likelihood of chronic hepatitis is also about 50% after sporadic acute hepatitis C. Unfortunately, the natural history of HCV infection is not as well defined as for other causes of liver disease (eg, primary biliary cirrhosis), so that the timing of liver transplantation in these patients is more problematic. Transplantation should be considered in patients with biochemical evidence of deteriorating synthetic function or complications of portal hypertension (see Chapter 54).

HEPATITIS D

Pathophysiology

Hepatitis D virus is the smallest known animal RNA virus (1.7kB), which is replication-defective in that it is incapable of making its own envelope protein. For viral assembly, HDV uses excess surface protein of HBV (HBsAg) and thus in most instances, productive infection is only possible in patients who are also infected with HBV. Infection has been reported without HBV in liver transplant recipients. HDV inhibits HBV replication, thus patients with both HBV and HDV infection are usually HBeAg negative, anti-HBe positive. In experimental conditions, it has been possible to infect primary monolayer cells from woodchucks with HDV and to transfect cultured cells with cDNA clones of the entire HDV genome.

As with HBV, HDV is transmitted by parenteral or inapparent parenteral routes. HDV is most commonly found in patients with prior or ongoing parenteral drug use, or in their sexual contacts. In parts of the Mediterranean, HDV is endemic even in patients without known parenteral contact. In contrast to

HBV, the virus is believed to be directly cytopathic. Also unlike HBV, HDV infects only hepatocytes, with no extrahepatic sites of viral replication yet identified. In acute HDV infection, microvesicular steatosis and granular eosinophilic necrosis are often seen. In chronic hepatitis D, necroinflammatory activity is often severe but no specific histologic features are noted, and HDAg is readily demonstrated in nuclei and to a lesser extent, cytoplasm of hepatocytes.

Essentials of Diagnosis

HDV infection occurs only in the presence of HBV infection (HBsAg positive) and is detected by anti-HDV (IgM for acute or IgG for chronic infection).

Clinical Findings

Acute, simultaneous infection with HBV and HDV produces much more severe illness than HBV infection alone, and incidence of fulminant hepatitis is high. Hepatitis resulting from coinfection is self-limiting. Superinfection of an HBV carrier with HDV may also produce severe illness resulting in fulminant hepatitis, with survivors often developing chronic HDV infection with chronic active hepatitis.

Complications

Hepatitis D can be demonstrated in 30% of patients with acute fulminant hepatitis B and 70% of patients with fulminant hepatitis superimposed on chronic hepatitis B. Although chronic HBV infection is a well-recognized risk factor for the development of hepatocellular carcinoma, a similar association has not been clearly demonstrated for chronic HDV infection. A chronic healthy carrier state for HDV, similar to that noted with HBV, has been described. Labrea fever is an unusual form of delta hepatitis described from the Amazon basin in which fulminant hepatitis results in jaundice, fever, and black vomit.

Treatment

Alpha interferon (at doses of 9MU 3 times weekly) results in initial, but rarely sustained biochemical and virological response. Patients with decompensated cirrhosis resulting from chronic delta hepatitis are good candidates for liver transplantation, as risk of recurrent hepatitis is lower than that in patients with chronic HBV cirrhosis without HDV. Nevertheless, prophylactic peri- and postoperative anti-HB immunoglobulin should be given.

Prevention

Because of its requirement for chronic HBV infection, HDV infection can be prevented by vaccinating susceptible persons with hepatitis B vaccine. No effective vaccine is available for preventing Delta superinfection in HBsAg carriers.

Prognosis

In acute simultaneous HBV and HDV infection among drug addicts, the case fatality rate approaches 5%. In some outbreaks of severe delta superinfection in populations with a high HBV carrier rate, mortality is in excess of 20%. HDV superinfection can lead to fulminant hepatitis or progressive chronic active hepatitis and cirrhosis in patients with chronic hepatitis B.

HEPATITIS E

Pathophysiology

Hepatitis E virus (HEV) is an unenveloped spherical RNA virus; its genome has been cloned. Transmitted by the fecal-oral route, HEV is responsible for common source outbreaks. These outbreaks develop most frequently after rainy seasons of developing countries, where HEV is most commonly reported. HEV infection is rare in the USA except when imported by visitors from endemic areas. In acute infection, cholestasis with rosette formation of hepatocytes and polymorphonuclear leukocytes may be prominent. HEVAg is demonstrable in cytoplasm of scattered hepatocytes.

Essentials of Diagnosis

HEV infection is diagnosed by the presence of anti-HEV (both IgG and IgM), using ELISA for detection is expected to be available commercially in the near future.

New methods are under development for clinical use which directly detect the virus (by polymerase chain reaction amplification). Other tests to detect virus directly include hybridization assays as for HBV DNA.

Clinical Findings

Clinical course is similar to hepatitis A, but generally the infection is more severe. Persistent viremia and chronic liver disease have not been described.

Complications

Hepatitis E is associated with high mortality (10–20%) in pregnant women, particularly if they are in the third trimester.

Treatment

Treatment is largely supportive, and no effective vaccine is yet available.

Prevention

The only prophylactic measures against HEV infection that can be currently recommended are improved sanitation and sanitary handling of food and water. The efficacy of immunoglobulin for prevention of HEV infection remains to be evaluated. The lack of tissue culture system to grow HEV in vitro has prevented the development of an effective vaccine. Antigen preparations are being studied and there are prospects for recombinant subunit vaccines.

Prognosis

The case fatality rate is 1–2%, and up to 30% in pregnant women. HEV does not cause chronic liver disease.

REFERENCES

Alter HJ et al: Detection of antibody to hepatitis C virus in prospectively followed transfusion recipients with acute and chronic non-A, non-B hepatitis. N Engl J Med 1989;321:1494.

Choo-L et al: Isolation of a cDNA clone derived from a blood-borne non-A, non-B viral hepatitis genome. Science 1989;244:359.

Davis GL et al: Treatment of chronic hepatitis with recombinant interferon alpha. N Engl J Med 1989;321:1501.

Farci P et al: Treatment of chronic hepatitis D with interferon alfa-2a. N Engl J Med 1994;330:88.

Lemon SM: Type A viral hepatitis. New developments in an old disease. N Engl J Med 1985;313:1059.

Lok ASF, Ma OCK, Lau JYN: Interferon alfa therapy in patients with chronic hepatitis B infection. Gastroenterology 1991;100:756.

Ohto H et al: Transmission of hepatitis C virus from mothers to infants. N Engl J Med 1994;330:744.

Perillo RP et al: A randomized, controlled trial of interferon alfa-2b alone and after prednisone withdrawal for the treatment of chronic hepatitis B. N Engl J Med 1990;321:295.

Read AE et al: Hepatitis C in patients undergoing liver transplantation. Ann Intern Med 1991;115:282.

Samuel D et al and the investigators of the European concerted action on viral hepatitis study. Liver transplantation in European patients with the hepatitis B surface antigen. N Engl J Med 1993;329:1842.

Shapiro CN et al: Epidemiology of hepatitis A: Seroepidemiology and risk groups in the USA. Vaccine 1992;10(Suppl 1):S59.

Weissberg JI et al: Survival in chronic hepatitis B: An analysis of 379 patients. Ann Intern Med 1984;101:613.

Wright TL et al: Hepatitis C virus not found in fulmninat non-A, non-B hepatitis. Ann Intern Med 1991;115:111.

Chronic Nonviral Hepatitis

37

Albert J. Czaja, MD

Chronic nonviral hepatitis connotes an unresolving inflammation of the liver of unknown cause. The category of chronic nonviral hepatitis consists of autoimmune hepatitis, cryptogenic chronic hepatitis, autoimmune cholangitis, and autoimmune hepatitis with mixed features ("overlap syndromes"). Each entity lacks pathognomonic features, and, thus, the diagnosis is based on the exclusion of other similar conditions. Fortunately, a careful clinical history, a battery of laboratory tests, and expert examination of liver tissue can confidently secure the diagnosis in most instances (Table 37–1). Granulomatous hepatitis is not a true hepatitis but can be included within the category.

With the exception of autoimmune hepatitis, disease activity for at least 6 months is required to establish chronicity. By definition, patients lack serologic evidence of active infection with hepatitis B and C viruses. Although hereditary diseases (Wilson's disease, hemochromatosis, and α_1-antitrypsin deficiency), alcoholic and nonalcoholic steatohepatitis, bile duct diseases (primary biliary cirrhosis and primary sclerosing cholangitis), and drug-induced liver disease may at times resemble chronic nonviral hepatitis, each has pathogenic mechanisms, clinical and histologic findings, prognoses, and treatment strategies that warrant their separate classification.

AUTOIMMUNE HEPATITIS

Autoimmune hepatitis is a hepatocellular inflammation that is self-perpetuated by a presumed immunologic reaction against normal hepatocytic membrane protein. The disease implies the existence of a triggering factor (or factors), intrinsic impairment of host immunomodulating mechanisms, membrane expression of a target autoantigen, and expansion of cytotoxic T lymphocytes that infiltrate liver tissue and effect cell destruction. Unfortunately, the pathogenic mechanisms of autoimmune hepatitis are unclear and the precise nature of the putative immunologic reactions remains uncertain.

Diagnostic Studies

Autoimmune hepatitis is characterized by the presence in serum of autoantibodies directed against nuclear, cytosolic, or microsomal components of the hepatocyte (Table 37–2), hypergammaglobulinemia with predominant elevation of the immunoglobulin G fraction, and the presence of at least periportal hepatitis (piecemeal necrosis) on histologic examination (Figure 37–1). The disease typically responds to corticosteroid therapy, although such a response is not a requisite for diagnosis. Acute, even fulminant, presentations are recognized, and the diagnosis can be made at presentation without establishing 6 months of disease duration.

The definitive diagnosis of autoimmune hepatitis requires the following:

1. absence of markers of active viral infection, including those for cytomegalovirus and Epstein-Barr virus infection;
2. denial of parenteral exposure to blood or blood products;
3. absence of other etiologic factors such as excess alcohol consumption and drug use;
4. seropositivity for antinuclear antibodies, smooth muscle antibodies, or antibodies to liver/kidney microsome type 1 (anti-LKM1) at titers of at least 1:80;
5. total serum globulin, gamma globulin, or immunoglobulin G levels of greater than 1.5 times the upper limit of normal;
6. predominant serum aminotransferase elevations;
7. piecemeal necrosis with or without lobular hepatitis; and
8. no biliary lesions, granulomas, siderosis, copper deposits, or other histologic changes suggestive of a different cause.

A probable diagnosis of autoimmune hepatitis is justified if (1) serum gamma globulin levels are abnormal but not high; (2) autoantibody titers are less than 1:80; (3) antibodies other than conventional liver-related autoantibodies are present, such as anti-

Table 37–1. Differential diagnosis of chronic nonviral hepatitis and features that exclude the diagnosis.

Differential Diagnosis	Exclusionary Features
Chronic hepatitis B	HBsAg, HBeAg, hepatitis B virus DNA
Chronic hepatitis C	Antibodies to hepatitis C virus, recombinant immunoblot assay reactivity, hepatitis C virus RNA
Wilson's disease	Kayser-Fleischer rings, low ceruloplasmin level
Alpha₁-antitrypsin deficiency	Low alpha₁ level, MZ or ZZ phenotype
Hemochromatosis	Elevated serum ferritin, high transferrin saturation, hepatic iron index > 1.9
Alcoholic steatohepatitis	Fatty liver, Mallory bodies, regular alcohol excess
Nonalcoholic steatohepatitis	Fatty liver, Mallory bodies, alcohol abstinence
Primary biliary cirrhosis	Anti-M2 antibodies, florid duct lesion or interlobular duct damage
Autoimmune cholangitis	High-titer antinuclear antibodies, absent antimitochondrial antibodies, florid duct lesion or interlobular duct damage
Primary sclerosing cholangitis	Abnormal cholangiogram, fibrous obliterative cholangitis

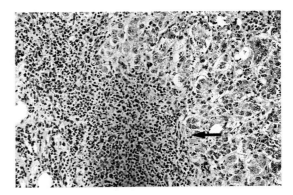

Figure 37–1. Piecemeal necrosis. Periportal hepatitis (piecemeal necrosis) is the histologic hallmark of autoimmune hepatitis but is not pathognomonic of the disease. It connotes disruption of the limiting plate of the portal tract by inflammatory infiltrate *(arrow)* (H&E; original magnification × 200).

bodies to soluble liver antigen or to asialoglycoprotein receptor (anti-ASGPR); and (4) risk factors such as previous alcohol use or exposure to hepatotoxic medications are present but not associated with perpetuation of current inflammatory activity.

Because autoimmune hepatitis is a syndrome comprised of many features that individually do not establish or preclude the diagnosis, a scoring system has been proposed to accommodate all manifestations of the disorder and grade the net strength of the diagnosis (Table 37–3). A scoring system theoretically permits the diagnosis of autoimmune hepatitis in individuals with inconsistent findings such as antimitochondrial antibody seropositivity, absence of immunoserologic markers, evidence of concurrent viral infection, or histologic features of bile duct damage if other, more characteristic features outweigh the isolated inconsistent findings. The validity of this scoring system has not yet been confirmed by prospective study.

Periportal hepatitis with or without lobular hepatitis is not specific for autoimmune hepatitis, but histologic examination is essential for the definitive diagnosis. Individual histologic findings such as moderate to severe piecemeal necrosis (Figure 37–1), lobular hepatitis (Figure 37–2), and plasma cell infiltration of the portal tracts (Figure 37–3) in the absence of portal lymphoid aggregates, steatosis, and bile duct injury can distinguish autoimmune hepatitis from chronic hepatitis C (Figure 37–4). Such patterns have a specificity of 81% and overall predictability of 62% for autoimmune hepatitis. Unfortunately, the sensitivity of these changes for the diagnosis is only 40%, and many patients with autoimmune hepatitis lack these characteristic findings.

Table 37–2. Autoantibodies pertinent to the diagnosis of autoimmune hepatitis.

Autoantibody	Autoantigens	Connotation
Antinuclear antibodies	Histones, centromere, ribonucleoproteins	Type 1 disease
Smooth muscle antibodies	Actin (F, G), tubulin, intermediate filaments	Type 1 disease
Anti-actin	Polymerized F actin	Type 1 disease
Anti–liver/kidney microsome type 1 (anti-LKM1)	Cytochrome P450IID6	Type 2 disease, hepatitis C virus infection
Anti-P450IID6	Cytochrome P450IID6 (254–271 motif)	Type 2 disease
Anti–liver cytosol 1 (anti-LC1)	Liver cytosol	Type 2 disease ("type 2a")
Anti–soluble liver antigen	Cytokeratins 8, 18	Type 3 disease, type 1 disease
Anti–liver-pancreas	Cytosolic noncytokeratins	Type 3 disease
Anti–human asialoglycoprotein receptor (anti-ASGPR)	Transmembrane hepatocyte glycoprotein	Autoimmune hepatitis (all types)

Table 37–3. Proposed scoring system for the diagnosis of autoimmune hepatitis prior to treatment.[1]

Features	Score
Male	0
Female	+2
Alkaline phosphatase:aminotransferase level ≥ 3	−2
< 3	+2
Globulin, γ globulin or IgG above normal > 2	+3
1.5–2	+2
1–1.5	+1
< 1	0
Antinuclear antibodies, smooth muscle antibodies, or anti-LKM1 titers > 1:80	+3
1:80	+2
1:40	+1
< 1:40	0
Other liver-related autoantibodies	+2
Antimitrochondrial antibodies present	−2
absent	0
IgM anti-HAV, HBsAg or IgM anti-HBc, or hepatitis C virus RNA	−3
Antibodies to hepatitis C virus or recombinant immunoblot assay reactivity	−2
Other markers of active viral infection	−3
Absence of all viral markers	+3
Hepatotoxic drugs or transfusions: Yes	−2
No	+1
Alcohol consumption (depending on amount)	0, −1, −2, +2
Concurrent autoimmune diseases (patient or relative)	+1
HLA-B8-DR3 or -DR4	+1
Piecemeal necrosis, lobular hepatitis, bridging	+3
Piecemeal necrosis without lobular or bridging changes	+2
Rosette formation	+1
Marked plasma cell infiltration	+1
Bile duct changes	−1 or −3
Incompatible findings	−3
Aggregate score: 10–15 = probable diagnosis	
>15 = definite diagnosis	

[1]Adapted from the recommendations of the International Autoimmune Hepatitis Group, Hepatology 1993;18:998.

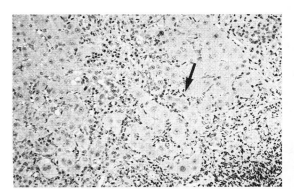

Figure 37–2. Lobular hepatitis. Prominent cellular infiltrates lining sinusoidal spaces in association with liver cell degenerative or regenerative changes connote lobular hepatitis **(arrow).** Moderate to severe lobular hepatitis can be present in autoimmune hepatitis, especially during relapse after corticosteroid withdrawal (H&E; original magnification × 200).

roiditis, Graves' disease, and rheumatoid arthritis. The presence of ulcerative colitis is compatible with the diagnosis, but it does compel cholangiography and expert histologic examination to exclude primary sclerosing cholangitis. Indeed, 42% of such patients have changes of primary sclerosing cholangitis and recalcitrance to corticosteroid therapy.

Twenty-five percent of patients with type 1 autoimmune hepatitis have cirrhosis at the time of presentation, indicating that the disease has an indolent but aggressive subclinical stage. Forty percent of patients may have an acute onset of symptoms that can be mistaken for an acute self-limited viral infection. Failure to recognize this presentation may needlessly delay institution of potentially life-saving therapy. Fortunately, such patients commonly have features

Subclassifications

Three subtypes of autoimmune hepatitis have been proposed based on immunoserologic markers, and a jargon has evolved to accommodate this proposal (Table 37–4). None of the subtypes has been officially endorsed, and treatment strategies are similar for each subtype.

A. Type I Autoimmune Hepatitis: Type 1 autoimmune hepatitis is characterized by the presence of smooth muscle antibodies or antinuclear antibodies, or both, in serum. It is the type found in the vast majority of patients with autoimmune hepatitis (Table 37–4). Antibodies to actin, especially the polymerized F-actin, support the diagnosis, and, in some regions, the disease is referred to as "anti-actin hepatitis."

Most patients (70%) with type 1 autoimmune hepatitis are women who are typically less than 40 years old. Seventeen percent of patients have concurrent immunologic diseases, including autoimmune thy-

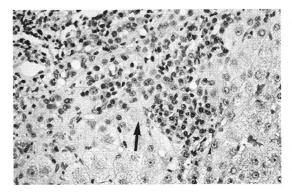

Figure 37–3. Plasma cell infiltration. Numerous plasma cells in groups or sheets in the portal tracts or as groups in the sinusoids characterize autoimmune hepatitis **(arrow)** (H&E; original magnification × 400).

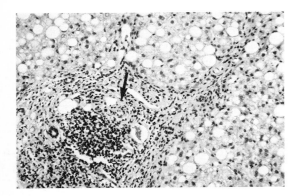

Figure 37–4. Portal lymphoid aggregate and steatosis. Densely packed small lymphocytes within a portal tract or a germinal center with surrounding small lymphocytes support the diagnosis of chronic hepatitis C *(arrow)*. Small, large, or mixed-size vacuoles of lipid within the cytoplasm of hepatocytes also typify chronic hepatitis C (H&E; original magnification × 400).

that suggest chronicity (eg, hypoalbuminemia, hypergammaglobulinemia, ascites, or cytopenia), and the appropriate therapeutic action can be undertaken promptly. In these cases, the "acute" onset of illness probably represents an exacerbation of long-standing, preexistent subclinical disease.

The target autoantigen of type 1 autoimmune hepatitis remains uncertain, and none of the autoantibodies that characterize the disorder are pathogenic. Viruses have been proposed as triggering agents, and isolated case reports have described higher than normal frequencies of measles virus genome in circulating peripheral blood cells of patients with the syndrome. Similarly, the development of autoimmune hepatitis has been linked to infections with hepatitis A or B virus or human immunodeficiency virus and

to treatment with recombinant interferon. The diversity of putative inciting agents, including drugs and environmental factors, suggests that these various agents trigger a final common pathogenic pathway.

Early studies indicated that intrinsic impairment of suppressor T cell function facilitated the unmodulated production of immunoglobulin G, which would bind to normal hepatocytic membrane protein and initiate an antibody-dependent, cell-mediated cytotoxic reaction that could result in autoimmune hepatitis. More recent hypotheses emphasize a cellular immunoreaction, in which a target autoantigen attracts CD4 lymphocytes, which then release cytokines to promote clonal expansion of cytotoxic, presumably CD8, lymphocytes that destroy the liver cells. Unfortunately, these elaborate hypotheses lack validation to date.

Hepatitis C virus has been the most thoroughly studied of the candidate triggering agents. Initial studies using first-generation immunoassays for the detection of antibodies to hepatitis C virus in serum indicated seropositivity in over 40% of patients. Subsequent studies recognized a high frequency of false seropositivity in such patients associated with the confounding effects of hypergammaglobulinemia on the assay. Second- and third-generation immunoassays and assessments by polymerase chain reactions for hepatitis C virus RNA in serum now indicate that hepatitis C virus infection is uncommon in type 1 autoimmune hepatitis (6–11%) and either an unimportant etiologic factor or, most likely, a coincidental finding.

B. Type 2 Autoimmune Hepatitis: Type 2 autoimmune hepatitis is characterized by the presence of anti-LKM1 in serum (Table 37–4). These antibodies are mutually exclusive of smooth muscle antibody or antinuclear antibody seropositivity (4% concurrence in adult patients), and they are detected by patterns of indirect immunofluorescence, which

Table 37–4. Subclassification of autoimmune hepatitis based on immunoserologic markers.

Feature	Type 1	Type 2	Type 3
Autoantibodies	Antinuclear antibodies, smooth muscle antibodies, anti-F actin	Anti-LKM1, anti-P450IID6	Antibodies to soluble liver antigen, antibodies to liver-pancreas
Age (years)	10–20 45–70	2–14 (adults, 4%)	30–50
Women (%)	70	89	90
Immune diseases (%)	17	34	58
Hypergammaglobulinemia	+++	+	++
Low serum IgA	–	+	–
Antinuclear antibodies ≥ 1:160 (%)	67	2	29
Smooth muscle antibodies ≥ 1:160 (%)	62	0	74
Anti-PDH-E2 (%)	5	0	14
Organ-specific antibodies parietal cell (%)	4	30	Uncertain
Steroid responsive	+++	++	+++
Develop cirrhosis (%)	45	82	75

demonstrate reactivity against the proximal tubule of the murine kidney and cytoplasm of the murine hepatocyte. An exuberant reaction against the renal tubule may obscure the distinction between proximal and distal tubular indirect immunofluorescence and suggest the possibility of antimitochondrial antibody seropositivity. Indeed, retrospective analyses have indicated that 27% of patients with autoimmune hepatitis and antimitochondrial antibody seropositivity are actually seropositive for anti-LKM1.

Type 2 autoimmune hepatitis afflicts mainly children (age 2–14 years) and is most prevalent in western Europe (France and Germany). The disease does occur in adults, but in the United States, such a presentation is rare (4% frequency). The clinical expression of the disease is different from that of type 1 autoimmune hepatitis, with a more aggressive behavior and higher frequencies of fulminant presentation and progression to cirrhosis (Table 37–4). Patients with type 2 autoimmune hepatitis have lower serum levels of gamma globulin (especially immunoglobulin A), lack antinuclear antibodies and smooth muscle antibodies in serum, more commonly have concurrent extrahepatic immunologic diseases such as vitiligo, insulin-dependent diabetes, and autoimmune thyroiditis, and more frequently are seropositive for organ-specific autoantibodies such as antibodies to parietal cells, islets of Langerhans, and thyroid than patients with type 1 disease (Table 37–4).

The cytochrome mono-oxygenase P450IID6 has been identified as the target autoantigen for this condition. The drug-metabolizing enzyme is expressed on the hepatocyte membrane surface of humans with the disease, and its expression can be modulated by tumor necrosis factor and interleukins. P450IID6 exhibits genetic polymorphism and is absent in 10% of individuals. Such genetic variability may explain regional differences in the prevalence of type 2 disease.

Antibodies to LKM1 recognize a short linear amino acid sequence of the P450IID6 antigen and are able to inhibit enzyme function in vitro, if not in vivo. Recombinant P450IID6 is available to map T and B cell epitopes, define cellular mechanisms of disease, and serve as the basis for an enzyme immunoassay for the detection of antibodies to P450IID6 (anti-P450IID6). Serum from patients with type 2 autoimmune hepatitis reacts at a very specific core amino acid motif of the recombinant antigen (amino acid sequence 254–271), and this reactivity distinguishes patients with type 2 autoimmune hepatitis from patients with nonspecific reactivity to other epitopes on the same antigen.

Hepatitis C virus has been implicated as a cause of type 2 autoimmune hepatitis. Surveys from Italy and Spain have indicated that as many as 86% of patients with anti-LKM1 seropositivity have antibodies to hepatitis C virus by first-generation immunoassays and that many of these patients have true hepatitis C virus infection by recombinant immunoblot assay

and polymerase chain reaction for hepatitis C virus RNA in serum. These observations have generated a proposal that type 2 autoimmune hepatitis be divided into subtypes 2a and 2b (Table 37–5). Patients with type 2a disease lack hepatitis C virus infection and have clinical profiles that resemble classic autoimmune hepatitis. Most are young women with high serum aminotransferase levels, high titers of anti-LKM1, and responsiveness to corticosteroids. In contrast, patients with type 2b disease have serologic evidence of true hepatitis C virus infection and have clinical profiles that reflect a chronic viral hepatitis. Patients are older and more commonly men than counterparts with type 2a disease. Titers of anti-LKM1 and serum aminotransferase activities are low. These patients are candidates for treatment with recombinant α-interferon. Interestingly, patients who are positive for anti-LKM1 and have hepatitis C virus infection are less frequently seropositive for anti-P450IID6 than patients without hepatitis C virus infection. Moreover, the antibodies to P450IID6 in anti-LKM1-positive patients react to epitopes other than the core amino acid 254–271 motif, suggesting that the antibodies in the two conditions are different. Antibodies to liver cytosol type 1 (anti-LC1) are present in many patients with anti-LKM1 who are uninfected with hepatitis C virus, and they may be useful in further distinguishing patients with type 2a disease from those with type 2b disease.

The high frequency of hepatitis C virus infection in patients with anti-LKM1 is not matched by a high frequency of anti-LKM1 in patients with chronic hepatitis C. Indeed, anti-LKM1 seropositivity is rare in chronic viral hepatitis, suggesting (1) that concurrent antibodies to hepatitis C virus and LKM1 in some patients are cross-reacting (molecular mimicry), (2) that the hepatitis C virus infection in those with anti-LKM1 is different than that in seronegative patients, or (3) that there are as yet unrecognized individual host differences in the expression of hepatitis C virus infection. Homologic characteristics have been described between the P450IID6 antigen, the hepatitis C virus genome, the GOR-47 antigen, and the herpes simplex virus; thus, cross-reacting antibodies may be generated by any of these antigens.

Table 37–5. Features of the subtypes of type 2 autoimmune hepatitis.

Type 2a	Type 2b
Hepatitis C virus absent	Heptatitis C virus present
Young	Old
Women	Men
High AST level	Low AST level
High-titer anti-LKM1	Low-titer anti-LKM1
Frequent anti-P450IID6	Rare anti-P450IID6
Reactive to 254–271 motif	Nonreactive to 254–271 motif
Anti–liver cytosol 1 present	Anti–liver cytosol 1 absent
Corticosteroid responsive	Interferon responsive

C. Type 3 Autoimmune Hepatitis: Type 3 autoimmune hepatitis is the newest and least established of the subtypes (Table 37–4). It is characterized by the presence of antibodies to soluble liver antigen in serum, which react against cytokeratins 8 and 18 within the cytoplasm of hepatocytes. Patients with type 3 autoimmune hepatitis are young and predominantly women (90%). Although these patients typically lack anti-LKM1, 74% have seropositivity for smooth muscle antibodies or antimitochondrial antibodies, indicating that seropositivity for antibodies to soluble liver antigen is not mutually exclusive of other immunoserologic markers. Indeed, 11% of patients with type 1 autoimmune hepatitis have antibodies to soluble liver antigen. Patients seropositive for this marker are indistinguishable from seronegative counterparts by either clinical and laboratory findings or by responsiveness to corticosteroid therapy.

Antibodies to soluble liver antigen occur only in patients with autoimmune hepatitis. It is uncertain, however, if they define a valid subtype of autoimmune hepatitis or represent a variant marker for type 1 disease. The greatest clinical value in testing for antibodies to soluble liver antigen may be in assessing patients with cryptogenic hepatitis. Eighteen percent of such patients are seropositive for these antibodies and can be reassigned to an autoimmune category.

Antibodies to liver-pancreas are directed against noncytokeratin cytosolic components of the hepatocyte, and, in this fashion, they are different from antibodies to soluble liver antigen (Table 37–2). They may coexist with markers of type 1 autoimmune hepatitis but can be the sole manifestations of autoimmunity in 33% of patients with cryptogenic hepatitis. Consequently, antibodies to liver-pancreas have been proposed as another marker for a type 3 autoimmune hepatitis.

Antibodies to asialoglycoprotein receptor (anti-ASGPR) are an important species of autoantibodies but do not yet define another subclassification of autoimmune hepatitis (see Table 37–2). Indeed, antibodies to human anti-ASGPR are present in all types of autoimmune hepatitis, occurring concurrently in 82% of patients with antinuclear antibodies or smooth muscle antibodies, or both, 67% of patients with anti-LKM1, and 67% of patients with antibodies to soluble liver antigen. The autoantibodies are directed against a transmembrane hepatocytic glycoprotein that can capture, display, and internalize potential antigens, induce T cell proliferation, and activate cytotoxic T cells. Antihuman anti-ASGPR occurs in 88% of patients with autoimmune hepatitis compared with frequencies of 7% in chronic hepatitis B, 8% in alcoholic liver disease, and 14% in primary biliary cirrhosis. Antihuman anti-ASGPR is an important diagnostic marker of autoimmune hepatitis and may be valuable in monitoring response to treat-

ment. Antibody reactivity correlates with inflammatory reactivity, and the antibodies disappear during successful therapy. Loss of these antibodies prior to drug withdrawal may identify patients who are less likely to relapse.

Genetic Predispositions

Human leukocyte antigens (HLA) DR3 and DR4 are independent risk factors for autoimmune hepatitis. Fifty-two percent of patients with type 1 autoimmune hepatitis have HLA-DR3 and 42% have HLA-DR4. HLA-B8 is in strong linkage dysequilibrium with HLA-DR3 (94% co-occurrence) and is present in 47% of patients. The HLA haplotype A1-B8-DR3 is found in 37% of individuals, and 11% are heterozygous for HLA-DR3 and HLA-DR4. Unfortunately, the predominant HLA haplotype of type 2 autoimmune hepatitis remains uncertain.

Recent studies have suggested that the HLA status influences the clinical expression of autoimmune hepatitis and its behavior (Table 37–6). Individuals with HLA-B8 are younger and have more active disease, as assessed by serum aminotransferase levels and histologic findings of confluent necrosis and cirrhosis, than counterparts without HLA-B8. Similarly, patients who are negative for HLA-A1 and positive for HLA-B8 relapse more frequently after corticosteroid withdrawal than patients with other haplotypes.

Patients with HLA-DR3 enter remission less frequently and deteriorate more commonly during corticosteroid therapy than counterparts with other HLAs, and they more frequently require liver transplantation (Table 37–6). In contrast, patients with HLA-DR4 are older and more commonly women than those with HLA-DR3. Additionally, they have higher serum levels of gamma globulin, a greater frequency of concurrent immunologic diseases, and a greater likelihood of entering remission during therapy than patients with HLA-DR3. The expression of smooth

Table 37–6. Comparisons between patients with autoimmune hepatitis based on HLA haplotype.

HLA-B8-DR3 Positive	HLA-DR4 Positive
Young (median age, 37 years)	Old (median age, 52 years)
Women, 68%	Women, 89%
Immune diseases, 27%	Immune diseases, 59%
Lower IgG levels	Higher IgG levels
Remission, 63%	Remission, 85%
Treatment failure, 32%	Treatment failure, 10%
Orthotopic liver transplantation frequently required	Orthotopic liver transplantation less frequently required
Less frequent smooth muscle antibody positivity	More frequent smooth muscle antibody positivity
Lower-titer antinuclear antibody	Higher-titer antinuclear antibody

muscle antibodies and a high titer of antinuclear antibodies has also been associated with HLA-DR4.

Further dissection of the genotypes of autoimmune hepatitis has indicated that the allele DRB3*0101, which encodes DR52a, and the DR4 subtype, DRB1*0401, are strongly associated with the disease (Table 37–6). Indeed, 81% of patients with autoimmune hepatitis possess either allele, and each is associated with a clinically distinct disease pattern. Patients with DRB1*0401 have less severe disease at presentation, relapse less frequently after corticosteroid withdrawal, and develop the disease later in life than counterparts with DRB3*0101. Since the alleles encode specific amino acid sequences in the DR β polypeptide that determine the ability of each class II molecule to bind and present antigens to T cells, these residues may influence the immunoreactivities of the effector cells and in turn the clinical manifestations and behavior of the disease. A strong dependence on genetic predispositions may also explain differences in disease frequency and severity in different geographic regions and ethnic groups.

Treatment

A. Corticosteroids: Prednisone alone or in combination with azathioprine induces clinical, biochemical, and histologic remission in 65% of patients with severe autoimmune hepatitis within 2 years. The benefit-risk ratio strongly favors therapy in these patients. The 5- and 10-year life expectancies after therapy for patients without cirrhosis at presentation exceed 90%, and are 80% and 65%, respectively, for patients with cirrhosis at presentation. Untreated disease of similar severity is associated with a 3-year mortality rate of 50% and a 10-year mortality rate of 90%.

In contrast to patients with severe disease, the benefit-risk ratio of corticosteroid therapy in patients with milder disease is unknown. Cirrhosis develops in only 49% of such patients within 15 years, and the 10-year mortality rate is only 10%. Periportal hepatitis progresses to cirrhosis in only 17% within 5 years, and spontaneous resolution of the disease occurs in 13–20%. This low potential for shortened immediate survival time must be balanced against the risk for treatment-related side effects. Cosmetic changes occur in 80% of patients after 1 year of continuous therapy, and the risk of extrahepatic cancer in pa-

tients receiving long-term treatment is 1.4-fold normal (95% confidence interval, 0.6- to 2.9-fold normal). Thus, the treatment decision must be highly individualized and tempered by the realization that in some patients, the treatment may be worse than the disease.

The absolute indications for corticosteroid therapy are incapacitating symptoms attributable to hepatocellular inflammation, sustained extreme elevations of serum aspartate aminotransferase (AST) and gamma globulin levels, or the presence on liver biopsy examination of bridging necrosis or multilobular collapse (Table 37–7). Relative indications for therapy are moderate symptoms or evidence of disease progression. Patients with less severe disease should be monitored closely for disease progression and exacerbation of inflammatory activity but not treated. Similarly, there is no role for corticosteroid therapy in the management of inactive cirrhosis with or without features of hepatic decompensation (Table 37–7).

Prednisone (20 mg/d), and prednisone (10 mg/d) in combination with azathioprine (50 mg/d), are maintenance regimens of comparable efficacy (Table 37–8). The combination regimen is preferred, because it is associated with fewer side effects than the higher-dosage regimen of prednisone alone (10% versus 44%). Postmenopausal women and patients with exogenous obesity, cushingoid features, labile hypertension, and brittle diabetes are ideal candidates for the combination schedule if azathioprine is not contraindicated by cytopenia, cancer, or the prospect of pregnancy. Prednisone alone is preferred in patients with severe cytopenia associated with hypersplenism and those who are pregnant or contemplating pregnancy. It is also appropriate for patients in whom a short treatment trial is proposed (3–6 months), since the advantages of combination treatment in reducing side effects are evident only after long-term use.

Treatment is continued until remission is evident on clinical, biochemical, and histologic findings; drug toxicity develops; deterioration (treatment failure) or death occurs; or abnormalities have not resolved after protracted (longer than 3 years) of therapy (incomplete response). Histologic improvements lag behind clinical and biochemical resolution by 3–6 months, and liver biopsy assessment is necessary to

Table 37–7. Indications for treatment of autoimmune hepatitis.

Absolute	Relative	None
Sustained serum AST ≥ 10-fold normal or ≥ 5-fold normal + gamma globulin level ≥ 2-fold normal	Moderate AST with gamma globulin elevation	Mild AST with or without gamma globulin elevation
Bridging necrosis or multilobular necrosis	Periportal hepatitis	Mildly active cirrhosis
Incapacitating symptoms	Mild to moderate symptoms	Minimal or no symptoms
	Relentless progression	Liver failure with mild or no inflammatory activity

Table 37–8. Treatment regimens for autoimmune hepatitis.

	Regimen I	Regimen II
Medication and daily dose	Prednisone 60 mg for 1 week Prednisone 40 mg for 1 week Prednisone 30 mg for 2 weeks Prednisone 20 mg until treatment end point	Prednisone 30 mg for 1 week Prednisone 20 mg for 1 week Prednisone 15 mg for 2 weeks Prednisone 10 mg until treatment end point Azathioprine 50 mg until treatment end point
Relative Indications	Severe cytopenia Pregnancy Concurrent neoplasm Short treatment trial Azathioprine intolerance	Postmenopausal women Osteoporosis Vertebral compression Brittle diabetes Cushingoid features Exogenous obesity Labile hypertension
Treatment end points	Remission Deterioration (treatment failure) Incomplete response after 3 years of continuous treatment Severe drug toxicity	Remission Deterioration (treatment failure) Incomplete response after 3 years of continuous treatment Severe drug toxicity

Table 37–9. Management of autoimmune hepatitis after a suboptimal response to conventional corticosteroid therapy.

Suboptimal Response	Treatment Options
Relapse First Multiple (≥ 2)	Original regimen Low-dosage indefinite prednisone; 2.5-mg dose reduction each month until mild symptoms or AST ≥ 5-fold normal, or both Indefinite azathioprine (2 mg/kg/d)
Treatment failure	Prednisone, 60 mg daily for 1 month, or prednisone, 30 mg daily, with azathioprine, 150 mg daily, for 1 month. Dose reductions each month of improvement by 10 mg for prednisone and 50 mg for azathioprine until conventional daily doses. Cyclosporine (5–6 mg/kg/d) (empiric therapy) Liver transplantation (if no response or progression despite therapy)
Incomplete response (after 3 years of continuous therapy)	Indefinite low-dosage prednisone as above Liver transplantation at first sign of decompensation
Severe drug toxicity	Dose reduction or drug withdrawal Improvisational drug management (low dosage, alternate days, or dose titration with prednisone or azathioprine alone)

establish histologic remission and prevent premature withdrawal of medication. Medication should always be withdrawn in a gradual, tapered fashion whenever a treatment end point is reached.

B. Management of Suboptimal Responses:

1. Relapse–Relapse occurs in at least 49% of patients within 6 months after drug withdrawal and is eventually seen in 74% within 3 years. Reinstitution of the original treatment regimen usually induces another remission, but the probability of relapse after retreatment exceeds 80%. Patients who relapse appear to progress to cirrhosis (38% versus 10%) and die from liver failure (14% versus 4%) more commonly than counterparts who sustain their remission after treatment. The only statistically significant consequence of relapse, however, is a higher frequency of corticosteroid-induced side effects (70% versus 21%).

Because relapse and retreatment are associated with a diminishing benefit-risk ratio, alternative therapies are appropriate for patients who relapse multiply (Table 37–9). Indefinite low-dosage therapy with prednisone or azathioprine is a treatment option. In the former strategy, the dosage of prednisone is reduced each month by decrements of 2.5 mg, until the lowest dose that will control symptoms and maintain serum aminotransferase levels below five-fold normal is achieved. In this fashion, 87% of patients can be managed satisfactorily on less than 10 mg of prednisone daily (median dose, 7.5 mg/d). Side effects that had accrued during conventional treatment improve during low-dosage maintenance therapy; new side effects do not develop; and survival time is unaffected. In the latter strategy, azathioprine (2 mg/kg/d) is administered indefinitely after corticosteroid withdrawal. Withdrawal myalgias and arthralgias can persist for up to 12 months, but biochemical and histologic features of inflammatory activity are usually controlled. The regimen does have the theoretic risks of teratogenicity and oncogenicity, which limit its general use.

2. Treatment failure–Treatment failure connotes clinical, biochemical, or histologic deterioration despite compliance with the treatment schedule. Progression to cirrhosis is not a treatment failure if the histologic features of inflammatory activity are improved. High doses of prednisone alone (60 mg/d), or prednisone (30 mg/d) in combination with azathioprine (150 mg/d), are able to induce clinical and biochemical improvement in 75% of patients within 2 years, but histologic remission occurs in only 20% (Table 37–9). Consequently, these patients become corticosteroid-dependent and are at risk for drug-related side effects and death from liver failure. Cyclosporine (5–6 mg/kg/d) has been used in these patients, with anecdotal success reported, although relapse after withdrawal is typical. These patients become dependent on cyclosporine and are at risk for its complications (hypertension, renal injury, cancer).

Liver transplantation is the preferred treatment for patients who deteriorate during therapy (Table 37–9) (see Chapter 54). The 5-year survival rate after transplantation is 92%. Recurrent disease after transplantation is rare, occurring only in individuals who are inadequately immunosuppressed or in those who are positive for HLA-DR3 but receive a graft from a donor who is negative for HLA-DR3. The decision to transplant must be based on failure to respond to corticosteroid treatment, as there are no findings at presentation that confidently predict survival rates before therapy. Patients with multilobular necrosis at presentation whose hyperbilirubinemia does not improve after 2 weeks of treatment invariably die, and they are candidates for expeditious transplantation. Patients who have required continuous corticosteroid therapy for at least 4 years become candidates for liver transplantation at the first sign of decompensation (usually ascites formation), since drug therapy is unlikely to produce a sustainable improvement.

3. Protracted treatment or incomplete response—Protracted treatment or incomplete response connotes failure to induce remission after 3 years of continuous therapy. Treatment extended beyond 3 years is associated with only a 7% probability of remission per annum, and the risk of drug-related side effects equals this likelihood. Empiric low-dosage corticosteroid therapy is an option in these patients, as efforts are best directed at preserving well being rather than inducing a sustained remission (Table 37–9).

4. Drug toxicity—Drug toxicity necessitates premature discontinuation of medication in 13% of patients. The major reasons for termination of therapy are intolerable obesity or cosmetic changes (47%), osteoporosis with vertebral compression (27%), brittle diabetes (20%), and peptic ulceration (6%). Therapy is individualized by reducing dosages to the lowest level possible to control manifestations of the liver disease and prevent worsening of the side effects (Table 37–9).

C. Promising Treatments:

1. FK-506—FK-506 is an immunosuppressive agent that has been used mainly to rescue patients with graft rejection after liver transplantation. Preliminary results from an open-labelled trial in a small group of patients with autoimmune hepatitis indicate that the drug can decrease serum aminotransferase and bilirubin levels after 3 months at an oral dose of 4 mg twice daily. Unfortunately, none of the patients was treated to clinical and biochemical remission; liver biopsy assessments were not performed to document possible drug-related improvements; and most patients developed abnormalities of serum creatinine and blood urea nitrogen levels. FK-506 still awaits comparison with prednisone in a prospective clinical trial.

2. Polyunsaturated phosphatidylcholine—Polyunsaturated phosphatidylcholine has been used successfully in conjunction with prednisone in the initial management of autoimmune hepatitis in some cases, but its role has not been established. A double-blind controlled trial has indicated that this combination can reduce histologic activity better than prednisone alone, presumably by modifying the hepatocyte membrane and blocking or altering the cytotoxic attack on the liver cell. The early reported success of this regimen has not been confirmed, and the combination cannot as yet be recommended as the initial approach to therapy. Similar results have been reported in a preliminary fashion using arginine thiazolidinecarboxylate as another "cytoprotective agent."

3. Ursodeoxycholic acid—Ursodeoxycholic acid administered daily for 2 months in doses of 250 mg, 500 mg, and 750 mg has reduced serum aminotransferase and gamma glutamyltransferase levels in some patients with chronic hepatitis, most of whom had viral disease. The efficacy of the medication in autoimmune hepatitis is unknown. The putative actions of ursodeoxycholic acid, including displacement of hydrophobic (highly detergent) bile acids from hepatocytes, prevention of their ileal absorption, protection of the hepatocyte membrane from noxious insults, and alteration of class I HLA expression on hepatocyte membranes, make it an appealing agent for further study in autoimmune hepatitis.

4. Brequinar and rapamycin—Brequinar, which inhibits B and T cell function, and rapamycin, which interferes with interleukin 2 activity, are other drugs that have putative actions of theoretic advantage to patients with autoimmune hepatitis but which have not been adequately studied.

CRYPTOGENIC CHRONIC HEPATITIS

Cryptogenic chronic hepatitis connotes active hepatocellular inflammation in the absence of epidemiologic risk factors for viral hepatitis, evidence of drug- or toxin-induced liver injury, viral markers, and autoantibodies. The designation does not include end-stage inactive cirrhosis that may have lost all distinguishing features. Cryptogenic chronic hepatitis is the second most common diagnosis (13%) in adults with chronic nonviral hepatitis after type 1 autoimmune hepatitis (80%).

Typically, patients with cryptogenic chronic hepatitis cannot be distinguished from patients with autoimmune hepatitis by age, gender, duration of illness, serum immunoglobulin levels, frequency of concurrent immunologic disorders, and histologic findings. Human leukocyte antigens B8 and DR3 occur as commonly in these patients as in autoimmune hepatitis and at a higher frequency than in counterparts with chronic viral hepatitis. Most importantly, these patients respond to corticosteroids to the same extent as patients with autoimmune hepatitis, with similar frequencies of remission (83% versus 78%) and treatment failure (9% versus 11%). Such patients should be selected for treatment by the same criteria and treated with the same regimens as patients with autoimmune hepatitis.

Because some patients with cryptogenic chronic hepatitis have antibodies to soluble liver antigen and liver-pancreas as well as the clinical and prognostic features of autoimmune hepatitis, this condition may be a form of autoimmune hepatitis that has escaped detection by conventional immunoserologic testing. Indeed, the designation "autoantibody-negative autoimmune hepatitis" has been proposed. Alternatively, cryptogenic chronic hepatitis may be either a standard type of autoimmune hepatitis in which the conventional immune markers are absent at the time of testing, a sporadic form of viral hepatitis that has eluded detection by second-generation immunoassays, or a hepatitis due to a virus that is not yet identified. Future investigations will undoubtedly diminish the significance of this category, but at present, symptomatic patients with severe disease should be treated with corticosteroids and monitored closely. Failure to improve within 3 months of therapy justifies corticosteroid withdrawal.

AUTOIMMUNE CHOLANGITIS

Autoimmune cholangitis is a chronic cholestatic hepatitis characterized by the presence of antinuclear antibodies (typically in high titer), absence of antimitochondrial antibodies (including antibodies against the M2 mitochondrial autoantigens), and features of chronic nonsuppurative destructive cholangitis on histologic examination (see also Chapter 51). Comparisons between patients with autoimmune cholangitis and primary biliary cirrhosis have emphasized that although both groups have many clinical, laboratory, and histologic similarities, the patients with autoimmune cholangitis are more commonly positive for antinuclear antibodies, have higher serum titers of smooth muscle antibodies, lower serum immunoglobulin M levels, and less serum AST activity than counterparts with primary biliary cirrhosis. Accordingly, a classification separate from primary biliary cirrhosis has been proposed. It is uncertain whether autoimmune cholangitis, idiopathic adulthood ductopenia, and small duct primary sclerosing cholangitis are separate entities.

The demonstration of bile duct changes indistin-

guishable from or compatible with primary biliary cirrhosis is essential for the diagnosis of autoimmune cholangitis. Duct destruction, paucity of interlobular bile ducts, granulomas, bile ductular proliferation, pseudoxanthomatous transformation of periportal hepatocytes, canalicular cholestasis, and fibrosis are within the spectrum of the disease. Primary sclerosing cholangitis (small duct and large duct varieties) and hepatitis C virus infection must be excluded in all patients.

Corticosteroid therapy has been of limited or no effectiveness in the management of this condition. Clinical and biochemical indices of inflammation may improve, but the histologic features are typically unchanged. Similarly, anecdotal experiences with ursodeoxycholic acid have indicated an inconsistent and incomplete response. Liver transplantation for the patient with advanced decompensated disease is an option, but results have not yet been reported.

AUTOIMMUNE HEPATITIS WITH MIXED FEATURES

Patients with autoimmune hepatitis can have concurrent features of viral infection, primary biliary cirrhosis, or primary sclerosing cholangitis. These mixed findings generate speculation about etiologic relationships; more importantly, they complicate treatment strategies. Recombinant α-interferon enhances display of HLA antigens on the hepatocyte membrane and reduces suppressor T cell function. Consequently, patients with viral markers and prominent autoimmune features may have exacerbation of their disease following α-interferon therapy. Additionally, α-interferon may increase the expression of a plethora of nonpathogenic autoantibodies, further confusing the diagnosis. Similarly, corticosteroids may fail to improve disease in patients with predominant viral features or those of primary sclerosing cholangitis. Indeed, corticosteroids in patients with predominant viral features may actually enhance the virus burden and make long-term management more difficult. To successfully manage these "overlap cases," the predominant disorder must be identified and then treated with the most appropriate regimen (Table 37–10).

Autoimmune Hepatitis With Viral Markers

Patients with autoimmune hepatitis may have serologic manifestations of an earlier viral infection, false-positive serologic tests for a current viral infection, or a coexistent true viral infection. Patients with autoimmune hepatitis who are negative for hepatitis B surface antigen (HBsAg) but have antibodies to HBsAg and hepatitis B core antigen (anti-HBc) have a serologic profile indicating previous hepatitis B virus infection and subsequent convalescence. These

Table 37–10. Management of autoimmune hepatitis with mixed features ("overlap syndromes").

Overlap Features	Treatment
Ancient viral infection	
HBsAg-negative, anti-HBsAg– and anti-HBc–positive	Corticosteroids
Isolated anti-HBc (IgM only negative)	Corticosteroids
False-positive viral markers	
Positive for antibodies to hepatitis C virus, recombinant immunoblot assay negative or indeterminate	Corticosteroids
Positive for antibodies to hepatitis C virus, negative for hepatitis C virus RNA	Corticosteroids
Isolated anti-HBc (IgM only negative)	Corticosteroids
True-positive viral markers	
Antinuclear antibodies or smooth muscle antibodies ≤ 1:160	α-Interferon
Antinuclear antibodies or smooth muscle antibodies ≥ 1:320	Corticosteroid trial (interferon if no response after 3 months)
Anti-LKM1 positive	Interferon
Primary biliary cirrhosis (positive for antimitochondrial antibodies, duct damage, or cholestasis)	Corticosteroid trial (ursodeoxycholic acid trial if no response after 3 months)
Primary sclerosing cholangitis (abnormal cholangiogram, duct damage, fibrous obliterative cholangitis)	Investigational treatment protocols

patients should be selected for treatment in accordance with the guidelines for uncomplicated autoimmune hepatitis. Similarly, patients with isolated seropositivity for anti-HBc or antibodies to hepatitis C virus whose specificity against hepatitis C virus–encoded antigens cannot be confirmed (ie, nonreactive or indeterminate) by recombinant immunoblot assay are considered to have false-positive viral markers and should be treated as patients with autoimmune hepatitis (Table 37–10).

Unfortunately, 38% of patients with chronic hepatitis B or C have seropositivity for antinuclear antibodies or smooth muscle antibodies, and it is in these patients that the viral and immunologic features must both be considered in implementing the optimal treatment. Importantly, such patients typically have low, nonspecific autoantibody titers and, rarely, multiple immunoserologic markers. In one study, there were no patients with antinuclear antibody titers of greater than 1:100 who were positive for antibodies to hepatitis C virus, while 64% with antinuclear antibody titers of less than 1:100 were positive for antibodies to hepatitis C virus. In another series, patients with chronic viral hepatitis more commonly had serum titers of smooth muscle antibodies or antinuclear antibodies of 1:80 or less compared with those

with autoimmune hepatitis (89% versus 16%); moreover, only 23% of patients with chronic viral hepatitis and autoantibody seropositivity had titers of 1:320 or higher. No patients with chronic viral hepatitis had concurrent smooth muscle antibody and antinuclear antibody positivity.

In contrast to those with viral markers, patients with autoimmune hepatitis without viral markers have a median titer of smooth muscle antibody seropositivity of 1:160 and antinuclear antibody seropositivity of 1:320. In these patients, the range of seropositivity may be as low as 1:40, but in such patients, there are usually additional immunoserologic findings that support the diagnosis of autoimmune hepatitis. In fact, only 6% of patients with autoimmune hepatitis have seropositivity for only one autoantibody measuring less than 1:80 in titer. Consequently, patients with true viral infection who have low titers of autoantibodies (< 1:320) should be considered as having viral predominant disease. These patients are candidates for α-interferon therapy (Table 37–10). Similarly, patients with anti-LKM1 and true hepatitis C virus infection have viral predominant disease and also are candidates for α-interferon therapy (Table 37–10). Experiences mainly from Italy have indicated that these patients tolerate antiviral treatment satisfactorily.

Rarely, true chronic viral infection is associated with antinuclear antibody or smooth muscle antibody titers of 1:320 or greater. The proper management of these unusual patients is uncertain. Individuals in whom a confident diagnosis of autoimmune hepatitis would have been made if viral markers had not been present should continue to be diagnosed as such even in the presence of viral markers. Accordingly, these patients should be treated with corticosteroids for a 3- to 6-month trial period under close observation. Improvement in all of the manifestations of the liver disease justifies continuation of the corticosteroid regimen, while lack of improvement compels a change to α-interferon therapy (Table 37–10). Over 50% of patients with true chronic hepatitis C and a high titer of antinuclear antibodies or smooth muscle antibodies respond to corticosteroid therapy, although relapse invariably follows corticosteroid withdrawal.

Autoimmune Hepatitis & Primary Biliary Cirrhosis

Patients with autoimmune hepatitis frequently have features of primary biliary cirrhosis but rarely are these features so pronounced that the diagnosis is in doubt. Indeed, 20% of patients with autoimmune hepatitis have seropositivity for antimitochondrial antibodies and 8% have antibodies to the E2 subunits of pyruvate dehydrogenase or branched-chain ketoacid dehydrogenase, or both. Typically, however, the titers of antimitochondrial antibodies in such patients are low (< 1:40) and only 12% have titers that exceed 1:160. Retesting may actually indicate the presence of anti-LKM1 rather than antimitochondrial antibodies in such patients, and histologic examination usually points in the correct direction. Similarly, serum alkaline phosphatase levels are increased in 81% of patients with autoimmune hepatitis but are greater than twofold normal in only 33% and more than fourfold normal in only 10%. In autoimmune hepatitis, it is rare for serum immunoglobulin M levels to exceed 6 mg/mL, histologic findings to suggest bile duct damage, or rhodanine staining to indicate the presence of hepatic copper, as is typical in primary biliary cirrhosis. Nevertheless, diagnostic confusion between autoimmune hepatitis and primary biliary cirrhosis may exist in rare patients; thus, it is still appropriate to try corticosteroids in an effort to establish the diagnosis based on treatment response (Table 37–10). In patients with autoimmune hepatitis who fail treatment, reconfirmation of the original diagnosis is always warranted, with reconsideration of the possibilities of primary biliary cirrhosis or primary sclerosing cholangitis. With continued refinement of the diagnostic criteria for autoimmune hepatitis, primary biliary cirrhosis, and autoimmune cholangitis, true "overlap" between these conditions may be reported less frequently.

Autoimmune Hepatitis & Primary Sclerosing Cholangitis

Clinical, biochemical, and histologic features of autoimmune hepatitis are present in 6% of patients with primary sclerosing cholangitis. In contrast, lymphoid, fibrous, and pleomorphic cholangitis suggestive of primary sclerosing cholangitis are found in 20% of patients with autoimmune hepatitis. Because both diseases have similar HLA haplotypes and autoantibodies to liver membrane protein, they may share pathogenic pathways, accounting for the similarities in clinical expression or concurrence of the disorders.

Hybrid conditions are especially common in children (even in the absence of ulcerative colitis) and in adults with autoimmune hepatitis and chronic ulcerative colitis. Cholangiography is necessary to establish the diagnosis in these instances. In adult patients with chronic ulcerative colitis, findings of primary sclerosing cholangitis are recognized in 42%. Such changes augur a poor response to corticosteroid therapy, and these patients are candidates for investigational treatment protocols (Table 37–10).

GRANULOMATOUS HEPATITIS

Hepatic granulomas are focal collections of epithelioid cells with surrounding lymphocytes that can occur anywhere within the liver (Figure 37–5). Most commonly, they are in or near portal tracts. Caseation necrosis and multinucleated giant cells

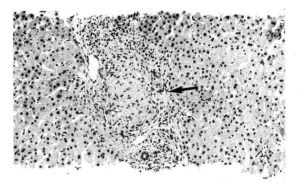

Figure 37–5. Noncaseating granuloma in idiopathic granulomatous hepatitis. The focal collection of epitheliod cells and surrounding lymphocytes is adjacent to a portal tract *(arrow)* (H&E; original magnification × 100).

may be components of the lesion, and clinical and biochemical manifestations may or may not be present. In some instances, the granulomas are isolated, unsuspected, serendipitous findings of uncertain clinical significance; in other instances, they may explain laboratory changes that reflect a focal infiltrative disorder of the liver characterized by prominent elevations of serum alkaline phosphatase and gamma glutamyltransferase levels. When the granulomas are the predominant histologic findings, the designation of granulomatous hepatitis is justified. Importantly, granulomatous hepatitis is not a true hepatitis and its classification as such reflects convention rather than conviction.

There are many causes of hepatic granulomas, including the following:

1. Infectious agents of bacterial, fungal, parasitic, and viral nature (tuberculosis, histoplasmosis, coccidioidomycosis, blastomycosis, brucellosis, Q fever, syphilis, schistosomiasis, tularensis, ascariasis, leprosy, Epstein-Barr virus, and cytomegalovirus)
2. Drugs (methyldopa, allopurinol, quinidine, phenytoin, hydrochlorothiazide, benzodiazepines, sulfonamides, and phenylbutazone)
3. Foreign bodies (beryllium, talc)
4. Immunologic reactions (primary biliary cirrhosis, inflammatory bowel disease, polymyalgia rheumatica, rheumatoid arthritis, Wegener's granulomatosis)
5. Sarcoidosis
6. Neoplasms (hairy-cell leukemia, Hodgkin's disease, melanoma, non-Hodgkin's lymphoma) (Table 37–11) (see also Chapter 45).

The most common causes of granulomatous hepatitis are tuberculosis (10–53% of cases) and sarcoidosis (12–55% of cases). Because granulomas are

Table 37–11. Common causes of granulomatous hepatitis.

Bacterial Agents
  Brucellosis
  Borreliosis
  Mycobacteria
  Salmonellosis
  Secondary syphilis
  Whipple's disease
Fungal Agents
  Actinomycosis
  Aspergillosis
  Blastomycosis
  Candidiasis
  Coccidioidomycosis
  Cryptococcosis
  Histoplasmosis
  Nocardiosis
Viral Agents
  Cytomegalovirus
  Epstein-Barr virus
  Human immunodeficiency virus-1
Parasitic Agents
  Amebiasis
  Ascariasis
  Giardiasis
  Toxoplasmosis
Rickettsial Agents
  Q fever
Drugs
  Allopurinol
  Cephalexin
  Chlorothiazide
  Chloropromazine
  Dapsone
  Diazepam
  Diltiazem
  Isoniazid
  Methyldopa
  Nitrofurantoin
  Oxacillin
  Phenylbutazone
  Phenytoin
  Quinidine
  Sulfasalazine
  Sulfonamides
Foreign Bodies
  Beryllium
  Silica
  Talc
  Thorium dioxide
Immune Diseases
  Crohn's disease
  Polymyalgia rheumatica
  Primary biliary cirrhosis
  Rheumatoid arthritis
  Sarcoidosis
  Ulcerative colitis
  Wegener's granulomatosis
Malignancies
  Hairy-cell leukemia
  Hodgkin's
  Melanoma
  Non-Hodgkin's lymphoma

common (2–35% of liver biopsy examinations), the frequency of idiopathic granulomatous hepatitis is high (30–50% of cases). Most likely, granulomas reflect a cell-mediated immunologic reaction against a variety of different antigens that are frequently undefinable.

Fever is present in up to 75% of patients with granulomatous hepatitis, and it may be relapsing or continuous in nature. In patients with idiopathic granulomatous hepatitis, activated mononuclear phagocytes within the granulomas probably release endogenous pyrogens, including interleukin 1, which affect hypothalamic thermoregulation. Nonspecific symptoms such as anorexia, fatigue, and malaise may also accompany the syndrome. Typically, liver biopsy examination is performed to evaluate the cause of fever rather than to assess the basis for abnormalities in hepatic chemistries. Multiple sections of the liver tissue sample are necessary to discover the lesions. Acid-fast and fungal stains are essential components of the tissue examination, although diagnostic findings are unusual and their absence is not exclusionary. Cultures of the liver tissue have a low yield for mycobacteria (< 10%), but results are better for fungi such as *Histoplasma capsulatum* (50% yield) and they should be performed. Portal hypertension may occur with extensive granulomatous infiltration of the liver, but this occurrence is rare. Cirrhosis is not an expected consequence of granulomatous hepatitis and may reflect a coincidence rather than a consequence.

The cause of granulomatous hepatitis must be sought in a thoughtful cost-effective fashion. The long list of etiologic possibilities (Table 37–11) can be shortened considerably by clinical assessment and a careful travel, drug, and occupational history. Specific etiologic factors can then be assessed by order of likelihood. Cultures of sputum, urine, gastric washings, and liver tissue for mycobacteria; serologic tests for fungi, Q fever, Epstein-Barr virus, cytomegalovirus, and toxoplasmosis; examination of stools for parasites; culture of liver tissue for fungi; blood cultures for bacteria; chest x-rays and imaging studies can then be tailored to the clinical situation.

Management is based on the cause of the condition and the severity of symptoms. Discontinuation of all medications and elimination of an infectious agent are obvious strategies. Patients with idiopathic disease can be observed or treated symptomatically. Such patients commonly have a benign prognosis and rarely manifest changes of tuberculosis, histoplasmosis, or sarcoidosis later in their course. Forty-one percent of patients with idiopathic granulomatous hepatitis may improve spontaneously within 1–12 months.

Febrile symptomatic patients warrant empiric therapy. Individuals with risk factors for tuberculosis or caseating hepatic granulomas should be treated with isoniazid (8 mg/kg/d) and ethambutol (15–25 mg/kg/d) for 8 weeks. If there has been no improvement with antituberculosis therapy, the medication can be discontinued and therapy with either indomethacin or prednisone (0.75–1 mg/kg/d) instituted. A response to antituberculosis treatment warrants the addition of pyridoxine (100 mg/d) to the regimen and continuation of therapy for 18 months. Symptomatic patients without risk factors for tuberculosis, negative cultures for mycobacteria, and no evidence of caseation can be treated directly with indomethacin or prednisone. Prompt defervescence and

symptomatic improvement should be expected in all such patients, and the dosage of medication can be withdrawn as tolerated in a gradual fashion. The duration of treatment is variable, ranging from 3 to 79 months. Close surveillance is indicated for emergence of the rare occult infection. Isoniazid (300 mg/d) and pyridoxine should be administered in conjunction with prednisone in those patients with positive tuberculin skin tests or a past history of tuberculosis.

REFERENCES

Bach N, Thung SN, Schaffner F: The histological features of chronic hepatitis C and autoimmune chronic hepatitis: A comparative analysis. Hepatology 1992;15:572.

Ben-Ari Z, Dhillon AP, Sherlock S: Autoimmune cholangiopathy: Part of the spectrum of autoimmune chronic active hepatitis. Hepatology 1993;18:10.

Bonkovsky H: Granulomatous hepatitis and hepatic granulomas. In: Medicine: For the Practicing Physician. Hurst JW (editor). Butterworths-Heinemann, 1992.

Czaja AJ: Autoimmune hepatitis: Current therapeutic concepts. Clin Immunother 1994;1:413.

Czaja AJ: Autoimmune hepatitis and viral infection. Gastroenterol Clin North Am 1994;23:547.

Czaja AJ: Chronic active hepatitis: The challenge for a new nomenclature. Ann Intern Med 1993;119:510.

Czaja AJ: Low dose corticosteroid therapy after multiple relapses of severe HBsAg-negative chronic active hepatitis. Hepatology 1990;11:1044.

Czaja AJ, Carpenter HA: Sensitivity, specificity and predictability of biopsy interpretations in chronic hepatitis. Gastroenterology 1993;105:1824.

Czaja AJ, Carpenter HA, Manns MP: Antibodies to soluble liver antigen, P450IID6, and mitochondrial complexes in chronic hepatitis. Gastroenterology 1993;105:1522.

Czaja AJ, Manns MP, Homburger HA: Frequency and significance of antibodies to liver/kidney microsome type 1 in adults with chronic active hepatitis. Gastroenterology 1992;103:1290.

Czaja AJ et al: Clinical and prognostic implications of human leukocyte antigen B8 in corticosteroid-treated severe autoimmune chronic active hepatitis. Gastroenterology 1990;98:1587.

Czaja AJ et al: Evidence against hepatitis viruses as important causes of severe autoimmune hepatitis in the United States. J Hepatol 1993;18:342.

Czaja AJ et al: Genetic predispositions for the immunological features of chronic active hepatitis. Hepatology 1993;18:816.

Czaja AJ et al: Hepatitis C virus infection as a determinant of behavior in type 1 autoimmune hepatitis. Dig Dis Sci [In press.]

Czaja AJ et al: The nature and prognosis of severe crypto-genic chronic active hepatitis. Gastroenterology 1993;104:1755.

Czaja AJ et al: Significance of HLA-DR4 in type 1 autoimmune hepatitis. Gastroenterology 1993;105:1502.

Desmet VJ et al: Classification of chronic hepatitis: Diagnosis, grading and staging. Hepatology 1994;19:1513.

Doherty DG et al: Allelic sequence variation in the HLA class II genes and proteins in patients with autoimmune hepatitis. Hepatology 1994;19:609.

Donaldson PT et al: Susceptibility to autoimmune chronic active hepatitis: Human leukocyte antigens DR4 and A1-B8-DR3 are independent risk factors. Hepatology 1990;13:701.

Homberg J-C et al: Chronic active hepatitis associated with antiliver/kidney microsome antibody type 1: A second type of "autoimmune" hepatitis. Hepatology 1987;7:1333.

Johnson PJ et al: Meeting Report: International Autoimmune Hepatitis Group. Hepatology 1993;18:998.

Lunel F et al: Liver/kidney microsome antibody type 1 and hepatitis C virus infection. Hepatology 1992;16:630.

Manns M et al: Characterization of a new subgroup of autoimmune chronic active hepatitis by autoantibodies against a soluble liver antigen. Lancet 1987;1:292.

Manns MP et al: LKM-1 autoantibodies recognize a short linear sequence in P450IID6, a cytochrome P-450 monooxygenase. J Clin Invest 1991;88:1370.

Poralla T et al: The asialoglycoprotein receptor as target structure in autoimmune liver diseases. Semin Liver Dis 1991;11:215.

Sartin JS, Walker RC: Granulomatous hepatitis: A retrospective review of 88 cases at the Mayo Clinic. Mayo Clin Proc 1991;66:914.

Yamamoto AM et al: Characterization of the anti-liver-kidney microsome antibody (anti-LKM1) from hepatitis C virus-positive and -negative sera. Gastroenterology 1993;104:1762.

Zoutman DE, Ralph ED, Frei JV: Granulomatous hepatitis and fever of unknown origin: An 11-year experience of 23 cases with three years' follow-up. J Clin Gastroenterol 1991;13:69.

Infections of the Liver

38

Ira S. Goldman, MD

BACTERIAL INFECTIONS

PYOGENIC LIVER ABSCESS

Pathophysiology

Pyogenic bacteria gain access to the liver by a variety of routes. Biliary tract disease currently accounts for the greatest percentage of cases, and may occur from either benign or malignant obstruction of the biliary tree with resultant cholangitis. Before antibiotics became available, seeding through the portal venous system occurred most frequently with appendicitis or diverticulitis. In childhood or infancy, pyogenic liver abscesses occur most frequently with umbilical vein infections. Infection via the hepatic artery may occur during bacteremia secondary to endocarditis, osteomyelitis, or other sources. Direct extension of infection from contiguous organs may permit bacteria to gain entry to the liver such as in pneumonia or subphrenic abscess. Penetrating injuries to the liver may directly seed bacteria into the organ. In almost one-half the cases of pyogenic liver abscess, no clear cause is ever found.

Pyogenic liver abscesses may be single or multiple; most single abscesses are located in the right lobe. Most abscesses of portal vein origin are single, whereas those of biliary tract origin are often multiple. The organisms recovered from pyogenic liver abscesses vary considerably. Approximately one-half are found to be due to infection with anaerobic organisms or mixed cultures of anaerobic and aerobic organisms. The most common organisms isolated include gram-negative enteric bacilli, anaerobic gram-negative bacilli, and microaerophilic streptococci (Table 38–1). *Escherichia coli* has been the organism most commonly isolated.

Essentials of Diagnosis
- Fever, malaise, hepatomegaly, right upper quadrant tenderness.
- Leukocytosis, elevated alkaline phosphatase and gamma-glutamyl transpeptidase (GGTP).
- Round or oval defects seen on ultrasound, CT scan, or MRI.

Clinical Findings

A. Symptoms and Signs: The clinical features of pyogenic liver abscess are often nonspecific and variable, but most often include fever, malaise, weight loss, and right upper quadrant abdominal pain. Hepatomegaly and right upper quadrant abdominal tenderness are the most common findings on physical examination. Jaundice is seen in approximately 25% of cases.

B. Laboratory Findings: Laboratory findings can be nonspecific and most often include leukocytosis and anemia, elevations of the alkaline phosphatase and GGTP, and hyperbilirubinemia in about 25% of cases. Aerobic and anaerobic culture of the abscess yields specific results in over three-quarters of pyogenic liver abscesses. Blood culture results are positive for the responsible bacteria in about one-half of cases.

C. Imaging: Routine chest x-rays are abnormal in almost 50% of patients with pyogenic liver abscess. Findings can include elevation of the diaphragm, air-fluid levels within a liver mass, or both. Ultrasonography detects pyogenic liver abscesses in 80–100% of cases. The characteristic appearance is a round or oval area within the liver that is less echogenic than the surrounding hepatic parenchyma. It may be difficult to image either abscesses that are high in the dome of the liver or multiple microabscesses. Computed tomography (CT) scanning reveals lesions that are less dense (lower attenuation values) than surrounding normal liver. Using intravenous contrast improves detection because an abscess does not enhance like surrounding normal liver parenchyma (Figure 38–1). Contrast-enhanced magnetic resonance imaging (MRI) has been used to demonstrate pyogenic abscesses, but CT scanning remains the imaging test of choice.

Table 38–1. Organisms cultured from pyogenic liver abscesses.

Aerobic	Anaerobic
Escherichia coli	Anaerobic streptococci
Klebsiella	Microaerophilic streptococci
Streptococcus viridans group	Bacteroides species
Staphylococcus aureus	Fusobacterium species
Enterococcus	Clostridium species
Proteus species	Actinomyces
Pseudomonas species	Eubacterium
Enterobacter	Propionibacterium
Listeria	
Yersinia	

(Adapted from Goldman IS, Farber BF, Brandborg LL: Bacterial and Miscellaneous Infections of the Liver. In: *Hepatology: A Textbook of Liver Disease*, 3/e. Zakim D, Boyer TD (editors). Saunders, 1995.)

Complications

Most complications of pyogenic liver abscess result from rupture or extension of the abscess into adjacent structures. In early series, pleuropulmonary involvement occurred in 15% of patients, while subphrenic abscess developed in about 3% of cases.

Treatment

If possible, a diagnostic aspiration under ultrasound or CT guidance should be performed before starting antibiotic therapy. Pyogenic liver abscesses can be effectively treated with antibiotics, alone or used in conjunction with percutaneous drainage. Significant coagulopathy or ascites are relative contraindications to percutaneous drainage, but in most other cases a percutaneous drainage should be attempted. When culture results from percutaneous aspiration are available, antibiotic choice can be specifically tailored to the sensitivities of the organism. Since growth in anaerobic cultures may take several days, however, it is advisable to continue anti-anaerobic coverage until all culture results are final. A large number of antibiotics can be used either singly or in combination as initial empiric therapy (Table 38–2). Antibiotic treatment before culture results are available should include coverage against gram-negative bacilli, microaerophilic streptococci, and anaerobic bacteria. The duration of antibiotic therapy varies, but should be given for at least 10–14 days intravenously, followed by a longer course of oral therapy lasting 6 or more weeks. The total duration of antimicrobial therapy may be guided by imaging studies. Open surgical drainage is reserved for those who do not respond to antibiotics and percutaneous drainage.

Prognosis

The mortality associated with untreated pyogenic liver abscess is extremely high. Multiple abscesses and polymicrobial infections are adverse risk factors. The recognition and diagnosis of pyogenic liver abscess is often delayed because the symptoms are nonspecific, adding to morbidity and mortality. Liver abscesses must be considered in patients with fever of unknown origin. Early use of ultrasound or CT imaging will detect abscesses that might otherwise go un-

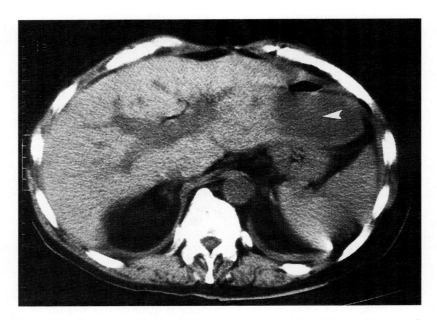

Figure 38–1. CT scan showing a large low-density (attenuation) mass in the left lobe of the liver *(arrow)*. Aspiration documented an *E coli* pyogenic liver abscess.

Table 38–2. Antibiotics used as empiric therapy for hepatic abscess.

- Second generation cephalosporin (cefoxitin, cefotetan), with or without aminoglycoside
- Broad spectrum penicillin (Timentin, ampicillin-sulbactam) with or without aminoglycoside
- Imipenem
- Third-generation cephalosporin plus metronidazole or clindamycin
- Clindamycin plus aminoglycoside

(Adapated from Goldman IS, Farber BF, Brandborg LL: Bacterial and Miscellaneous Infections of the Liver. In: *Hepatology: A Textbook of Liver Disease,* 3/e. Zakim D, Boyer TD (editors). Saunders, 1995.)

recognized. Even with prompt recognition and treatment, the mortality rate may be as high as 50%.

Barnes PF et al: A comparison of amebic and pyogenic abscess of the liver. Medicine 1987;66:472.

Barreda R, Roso P: Diagnostic imaging of liver abscess. Crit Rev Diagn Imaging 1992;33:29.

Stain SC et al: Pyogenic liver abscess: modern treatment. Arch Surg 1991;126:991.

LEPTOSPIROSIS

Leptospirosis in humans is caused by infection with a spirochete of the *Leptospira interrogans* complex, of which there are approximately 240 serotypes. The milder form of leptospirosis is usually anicteric, whereas the more severe and less common presentation, known as Weil's disease, is characterized by jaundice and severe systemic illness.

Pathophysiology

Leptospires are found in a number of both domestic and wild animals and are excreted in the urine. Humans are incidental hosts and are most often infected through contact with the urine of rodents, the most important vector for human exposure. Sewer workers, veterinarians, and slaughterhouse workers have occupational exposure, but disease may occur in patients in urban and suburban areas without such occupational risk. The organisms enter humans through a cut in the skin or via mucous membranes, and incubate for 5–20 days before clinical illness begins. Some patients have a biphasic illness. During the first, or leptospiremic phase, organisms can be isolated from the blood or cerebrospinal fluid. The first phase usually lasts 4–9 days, followed by a few days of symptomatic improvement. The second, or immune phase, is caused by the patient's immune response to the leptospiral infection. Any of the signs and symptoms of the first phase of illness may recur. In the immune phase, leptospires can no longer be isolated from the blood. In an usually severe form of leptospirosis, known as Weil's disease, there is profound hepatic, renal, and central nervous system dysfunction.

Essentials of Diagnosis

- Exposure history to infected animal tissue or urine.
- Abrupt onset of high fever, headache, myalgias, nausea, abdominal pain.
- Conjunctival suffusions may be present.
- May have biphasic illness; first phase lasting 4–9 days, followed by 1–3 days of defervescence, then recurrence of symptoms.
- Microscopic agglutination test and ELISA used to confirm the diagnosis.
- Weil's disease: jaundice, renal impairment, central nervous system dysfunction.

Clinical Findings

A. Symptoms and Signs: The first phase of illness is characterized by the abrupt onset of rapidly rising high fever, chills, severe myalgias, nausea, abdominal pain, headache, and malaise. The headache is often severe and constant. Conjunctival suffusions, arthralgias, rashes, cough, and evidence of hemorrhage may also be present. These symptoms usually last 4–9 days, after which there are a few days of clinical improvement with return of the temperature to normal. After another 1–3 days, fever recurs although not as high as initially. Headache is the most common symptom of this phase, though any of the symptoms may recur, especially myalgias and abdominal pain.

In Weil's disease, a severe form of leptospirosis occurring in 5–10% of cases, the illness is also biphasic, although the severity of illness may make this less evident. Jaundice and evidence of renal insufficiency may be seen as early as 2–3 days into the illness, and reach a peak during the second week of illness. Hypotension, bleeding, and confusion may be seen in Weil's disease.

B. Laboratory Findings: Leukocytosis is common. Mild forms of leptospirosis are characterized by minor elevations of the aminotransferases, alkaline phosphatase, GGTP, and a normal bilirubin. Weil's disease is characterized by hyperbilirubinemia that may reach 30 mg/dl or higher, and moderate elevations in the aminotransferases and alkaline phosphatase. The blood urea nitrogen and creatinine are high and renal insufficiency may become severe enough to cause anuria and require renal dialysis. The prothrombin time may be elevated. During the first phase of illness, diagnosis may occasionally be made by direct culture of the leptospires from blood or cerebrospinal fluid. Serologic tests including an IgM enzyme-linked immunospecific assay (ELISA) and the microscopic agglutination test are the most reliable ways to make the diagnosis. There should be a significant rise between the acute and convalescent antibody titers.

Treatment

Antibiotic treatment is most effective only when given within the first phase of illness, a time when the diagnosis is difficult to make. Doxycycline and penicillin G have both been shown to decrease the severity of infection when given early, but are ineffective once significant hepato-renal dysfunction has occurred. The treatment of Weil's disease is largely supportive, including renal dialysis.

Gollop JH et al: Rat-bite leptospirosis. West J Med 1993;159:76.
Jacobs R: Leptospirosis. West J Med 1980;132:440.
McClain JB et al: Doxycycline therapy for leptospirosis. Ann Intern Med 1984;100:696.
Shpilberg O et al: Long-term follow-up after leptospirosis. South Med J 1990;83:405.

HEPATIC CANDIDIASIS

Essentials of Diagnosis

- Immunocompromised patient; especially after bone-marrow transplantation, with prolonged periods of neutropenia, broad- spectrum antibiotic treatment.
- Fever, may have right upper quadrant abdominal pain.
- Elevated alkaline phosphatase and GGTP.
- Multiple low-attenuation areas in liver on CT scan, may have "halo" sign.

General Considerations

Involvement of the liver and spleen with *Candida* is an increasingly frequent complication of disseminated candidiasis. Infection usually occurs in patients with hematologic malignant tumors who have postchemotherapy neutropenia, and who have had prolonged treatment with broad-spectrum antibiotics. In some patients, empiric amphotericin treatment may have been given for prolonged fever. Spread is hematogenous from mucocutaneous sites throughout the body. Damage to the mucosa lining the gastrointestinal tract from chemotherapy may allow colonization with *Candida*, then dissemination via the portal vein to the liver.

Clinical Findings

A. Symptoms and Signs: Persistent fever is the hallmark of hepatic candidiasis, with fever spikes occurring in a random pattern. Right upper quadrant abdominal pain and tenderness are often found.

B. Laboratory Findings: Leukocytosis, after resolution of prior neutropenia, may be seen. Although the liver tests may be entirely normal, the alkaline phosphatase and GGTP are usually elevated. Mild elevations in the aminotransferases may be seen.

C. Imaging: Multiple, small 1–2 cm lesions may be seen throughout the liver and have been demonstrated with ultrasonography, CT scanning, and magnetic resonance imaging. CT scanning may show enhancing rings of increased attenuation surrounding low-attenuation abscesses ("halo" sign). Lesions are often also seen in the spleen (Figure 38–2).

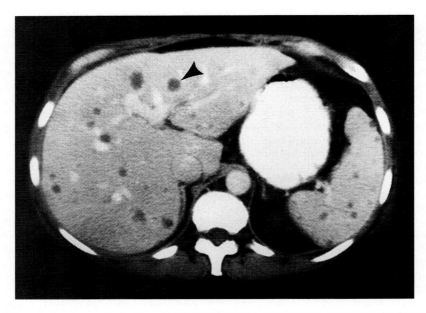

Figure 38–2. CT scan showing numerous low-density (attenuation) abscesses in the liver and spleen due to *Candida*. The arrow points to an abscess with an enhancing rim or "halo" sign, characteristic of hepatic candidiasis.

Diagnosis

Definitive diagnosis is difficult because cultures from percutaneously obtained aspirates are often negative, especially in patients who have received amphotericin. Laparoscopically directed biopsy, with culture and stain of aspirated material, may increase the diagnostic yield.

Treatment

Successful treatment of hepatic candidiasis is difficult and requires long periods of therapy with amphotericin B. Cumulative doses of greater than 4 g have been required. Fluconazole may be effective in some patients with chronic hepatic candidiasis who have not previously responded to amphotericin.

Flannery MT et al: Fluconazole in the treatment of hepatosplenic candidiasis. Arch Int Med 1992;152:406.

Gordon SC et al: Focal hepatic candidiasis with perihepatic adhesions; laparoscopic and immunohistologic diagnosis. Gastroenterology 1990;98:214.

Thaler M et al: Hepatic candidiasis in cancer patients: The evolving picture of the syndrome. Ann Intern Med 1988;108:88.

PARASITIC INFECTIONS OF THE LIVER

PROTOZOAN INFECTIONS

1. AMEBIC LIVER ABSCESS

Essentials of Diagnosis

- Right upper quadrant abdominal pain and tenderness, hepatomegaly, and fever are common.
- Leukocytosis and anemia are common. Liver tests may be normal or minimally elevated (especially the GGTP).
- Serologic tests positive in over 90% of cases; IgM ELISA available.
- Right hemidiaphragm often elevated on chest x-ray. Ultrasound, CT, or MRI demonstrates abscess.

General Considerations

Entamoeba histolytica is the only ameba responsible for liver abscesses, because of its ability to cause tissue invasion. The parasite exists as either a trophozoite or a cyst, the infective form. Up to 5% of the population of the United States may at some time be asymptomatic carriers of *E histolytica* cysts. Transmission occurs via the fecal-oral route.

Clinical Findings

A. Symptoms and Signs: Right upper quadrant abdominal pain is the most common symptom of an amebic liver abscess. Ten to 20 percent of patients either have had diarrhea prior to or at the time of diagnosis. Patients with pleuropulmonary complications may complain of a cough. Tender hepatomegaly and fever are the most common presenting signs on physical examination. About one-half of patients will have dullness or decreased breath sounds at the right lung base or right intercostal tenderness.

B. Laboratory Findings: Leukocytosis and anemia are the most consistent laboratory abnormalities. The aminotransferases, alkaline phosphatase, and GGTP may be normal or minimally elevated. Fewer than 10% of patients have an elevated bilirubin. Over 90% of patients have positive serologic tests. There are a number of currently available tests including ELISA, gel diffusion, indirect hemagglutination, and others. DNA probes for *E histolytica* are being developed as diagnostic tools. Due to variation in the sensitivity of serologic tests, using two of them in combination is helpful to confirm a diagnosis. When amebic abscesses are aspirated, the aspirate is usually reddish brown in color. The material is usually culture negative and may demonstrate amebic forms as well as necrotic material.

C. Imaging: Plain chest x-ray demonstrates elevation of the right hemi-diaphragm in 50% of patients. Amebic abscesses appear similar to pyogenic abscesses by ultrasonography, but are more commonly single than multiple. They are usually round or oval, located at the periphery of the right lobe, and may have enhancement of the rim. CT scanning is a more sensitive method for detecting hepatic amebic abscesses as well as extrahepatic extension. They appear as hypodense, round or oval lesions, and may have an enhancing wall or internal trabeculae. The diagnostic yield of MRI is similar to that of CT.

Complications

Pleuropulmonary complications are most common. Rupture of an abscess high in the dome of the right lobe through the diaphragm and pleura may lead to amebic empyema or consolidation of the right lung. Pleuritic chest pain, cough, and dyspnea are the most frequent symptoms of this complication. Left-sided perforations are less common. Rupture of an abscess into the peritoneum results in peritonitis and formation of an intra-abdominal abscess. Amebic abscesses of the left hepatic lobe may rarely perforate into the pericardium, which is associated with pericarditis, hypotension, and a high mortality rate.

Treatment

Metronidazole, 750 mg, given orally three times a day for 10 days, is the drug of choice. Following this, iodoquinol, an intestinal amebicide, is given at a dose of 650 mg orally, three times a day for 20 days. Elimination of amebae from the intestine decreases the risk of recurrent liver abscess. Therapeutic aspiration should be performed if the abscess is large and in danger of rupture, or there is no clinical response to medical therapy within a few days. Pleural effusions, if present, should be aspirated. Surgery is rarely needed except in cases with rupture of abscesses into the chest or peritoneum.

Prognosis

The mortality rate of an uncomplicated liver abscess is less than 1%. Pleuropulmonary complications raise the mortality rate to about 6%, and pericardial involvement to close to 50%.

Barreda R, Ross PR: Diagnostic imaging of liver abscess. Crit Rev Diagn Imag 1992;33:29.
Maltz G et al: Amebic liver abscess: a 15 year experience. Am J Gastroenterol 1991;86:704.
Reed SL: Amebiasis: An update. Clin Infect Dis 1992;14:385.

2. MALARIA

Essentials of Diagnosis
- High spiking fever, chills, headache, nausea.
- Tender hepatosplenomegaly.
- Mild elevations in the aminotransferases, alkaline phosphatase, and GGTP may be seen. Indirect bilirubin may be elevated in *Plasmodium falciparum* infection.
- Thick smear of blood shows parasites frequently; parasitized RBCs rarely seen on liver biopsy.

General Considerations

There are four species of *Plasmodium* that cause malaria in humans; *P falciparum, P vivax, P ovale, and P malariae*. When infected mosquitoes bite humans, saliva containing infectious sporozoites enter the bloodstream and are cleared by the liver. The sporozoites enter hepatocytes where asexual reproduction may occur. Periportal mononuclear infiltrates, Kupffer cell hyperplasia, iron deposition, and rarely, parasitized red blood cells, may be seen on liver biopsy.

Clinical Findings

A. Symptoms and Signs: High fever, with temperatures at times over 40°C, chills, headaches, and nausea are quite common presenting symptoms. The physical findings are nonspecific but may include tender hepatomegaly or splenomegaly. In severe forms of *P falciparum* malaria, signs of hepatic decompensation including encephalopathy, and jaundice may be seen.

B. Laboratory Findings: Mild leukocytosis as well as elevations of the aminotransferases, alkaline phosphatase, and GGTP are common. About 5% of those with *P falciparum* malaria have elevations of the serum bilirubin greater than 2 mg/dl. The liver

tests return to normal after treatment. Thick blood smears typically demonstrate parasitized red blood cells. Liver biopsy findings are nonspecific other than occasional parasitized red blood cells in hepatic sinusoids.

Treatment

Preventive treatment is recommended for all those traveling to endemic areas. There has been an increase in chloroquine-resistant *P falciparum* malaria, making both prophylactic and treatment regimens more complex. The Centers for Disease Control and Prevention (CDC), in Atlanta, Georgia, have telephone advice on current treatment programs available 24 hours a day.

Hollingdale M: Malaria and the liver. Hepatology 1985;5:327.
Mishra SK et al: Hepatic changes in *P falciparum* malaria. Ind J Malariol 1992;29:167.

HELMINTHIC INFECTIONS

1. ECHINOCOCCOSIS

Echinococcus in humans is caused by *E granulosus* and *E multilocularis*. These tapeworms live in the intestine of carnivores, which are definitive hosts, including dogs, cats, foxes, wolves, and other animals. Humans are the intermediate hosts of the larval stage (hydatid cyst) of the parasite; as are sheep, cattle, pigs, and other herbivores. *E granulosus* is found worldwide, but is most commonly seen in sheep-raising areas. In the United States, the disease is most commonly found in the Western states, Alaska, and the lower Mississippi valley. *E multilocularis* infection is different from *E granulosus* in that herbivores are not involved in the life cycle of infection. The definitive hosts are foxes, and rarely dogs or cats. The intermediate hosts are a number of rodent species. The definitive host becomes infected with tapeworms after eating the intermediate host. Humans become infected accidentally by ingesting *Echinococcus* eggs excreted in the feces of the definitive host. The disease is most common in parts of Alaska, Canada, Russia, and Europe.

Essentials of Diagnosis
- Exposure to dogs or foxes in sheep and cattle raising regions.
- Nonspecific symptoms, which may include right upper quadrant abdominal pain.
- Cystic mass in the liver, or rarely other organs on ultrasound, CT, or MRI.
- Positive echinococcal serology.

Pathophysiology

Echinococcus granulosus eggs are passed in the

stool of definitive hosts and are accidentally swallowed by humans or other animals (intermediate hosts). The outer shell of the egg is digested in the duodenum and the embryo is released. The embryo moves into the intestinal mucosa, enters small blood vessels, and is transported by the portal circulation until trapped in the microcirculation of the liver. Whereas most of the embryos are trapped by the liver, some larvae reach the lungs, spleen, brain, kidney, bone, and other organs. Although most of the embryos are destroyed by host defenses, surviving ones develop into the hydatid stage within several days while trapped in the microcirculation. The hydatid cysts have three layers and generally grow slowly, approximately one centimeter per year. The germinal layer, from which scoleces develop, is surrounded by the two outer layers. The life cycle is completed when a definitive host (dog) ingests infected tissue from the intermediate host (sheep). The adult worm develops in the intestine of the definitive host, where it sheds eggs in the intestinal lumen, to be then passed in the stool.

In *E multilocularis* infection, the germinal membrane is not surrounded by a cyst wall. Scoleces develop in an uncontrolled manner, invading adjacent tissue, much like a neoplasm. This continuous budding of the germinal membrane produces multiple small cavities, 2–5 mm, causing alveolar hydatid disease.

Clinical Findings

A. Symptoms and Signs: Echinococcal infection is generally asymptomatic until growth of the hydatid cyst enlarges to the point that it impinges on some other structure or becomes visible as an abdominal mass. Since the growth rate is only about one centimeter per year, clinical symptoms and signs may take 10 or more years to develop. Right upper quadrant abdominal pain and nausea may occur when the cyst is large. Abdominal masses, at times tender, may be found. Enlarging cysts may obstruct blood flow within the liver causing portal hypertension, or cause biliary obstruction with resultant jaundice or cholangitis. Cysts enlarging toward the abdomen may rupture into the peritoneal cavity, colon, or small intestine. Since the fluid in the cysts is highly antigenic, sudden rupture into the peritoneum may cause anaphylaxis and death.

B. Laboratory Findings: Routine laboratory tests are rather nonspecific. The liver tests are usually normal until the cyst has enlarged enough to cause jaundice from biliary obstruction. There may be a mild leukocytosis and eosinophilia, especially if a cyst has ruptured or is slowly leaking. Several serologic tests are available including ELISA, indirect hemagglutination, and indirect immunofluorescence. The ELISA and immunoblot assays are the most sensitive of these tests, however, false-positive reactions may occur with other parasitic infections. Tests to distinguish *E granulosus* from *E multilocularis* infection are being developed.

C. Imaging: Routine chest and abdominal x-rays may reveal cystic masses that occasionally are calcified around the rim. Ultrasonography, CT, MRI, or radionuclide scanning may also demonstrate echinococcal cysts. CT findings are those of a sharply delineated, low attenuation mass, with a rim that may enhance. The presence of daughter cysts within a cyst with a calcified rim is virtually pathognomonic of echinococcal disease. MRI may be more sensitive than CT in distinguishing echinococcal from epithelial cysts. Endoscopic retrograde cholangiopancreatography (ERCP) has been useful in demonstrating involvement of the common bile duct with hydatid disease.

E multilocularis infection resembles polycystic disease on ultrasound, CT, or MRI. There may be myriad small, 2–5 mm cystic areas, at times with calcified rims.

Complications

Continued growth of hydatid cysts cause problems because of their size and location. Biliary obstruction may cause cholangitis, especially with secondary bacterial infection. Rupture of a hepatic cyst into the biliary tree has been reported in various series to occur in 5–17% cases with liver involvement. Portal hypertension may result in esophageal varices, bleeding, and cirrhosis. Cyst rupture into the peritoneum may result in anaphylactic shock. Cysts may also rupture into the pleura, pulmonary parenchyma, or bronchi.

Treatment

Treatment of hepatic hydatid disease is primarily surgical, with considerable controversy as to the best type of surgical approach. The major objectives are to: (1) remove all parasitic material including the germinal membrane lining the cyst, (2) avoid spilling cyst contents, (3) close connections between cysts and other structures such as the biliary tree, and (4) manage the residual space remaining after cyst removal. The conservative surgical approach involves evacuating the cyst followed by cyst enucleation. Scolicidal agents such as hypertonic saline may cause sclerosing cholangitis resulting from their diffusion from the cyst into the biliary tree. Although the morbidity of this approach is low, recurrence rates may be as high as 10–30%. Those who favor the more aggressive approach of pericystectomy and partial hepatectomy argue that only the removal of the pericyst lining will result in complete cure. A pedicle of greater omentum (omentoplasty) is favored as the technique to close the cyst cavity. Albendazole is given preoperatively as prophylaxis against cyst spillage.

In a recent series of highly selected cases in which cysts were primarily fluid-filled and anechoic on ultrasonography, percutaneous ultrasound-guided drainage plus albendazole treatment was shown to be effective. ERCP has been used to extract daughter cysts from the common bile duct in both *E granulosis* and *E multilocularis* disease. When surgery is contraindicated or if patients have alveolar hydatid disease caused by *E multilocularis,* drug therapy is primary treatment. Albendazole, 400 mg orally twice a day for 28-day cycles, is the drug of choice since it achieves higher tissue and cyst levels than mebendazole. The drug is repeated in 28 cycles as needed, with a 1–2 week break between cycles. Albendazole causes elevation of the aminotransferases in up to two-thirds of treated patients. The liver tests should be monitored frequently.

Liver transplantation has been used successfully in otherwise unresectable alveolar hydatid disease caused by *E multilocularis.*

Akoglu M, Davidson BR: A rational approach to the terminology of hydatid disease of the liver. J Infect 1992;24:1.

Behrns KE, Van Heerden JA: Surgical management of hepatic hydatid disease. Mayo Clin Proc 1991;66:1193.

Gschwantler M et al: Combined endoscopic and pharmaceutical treatment of alveolar echinococcosis with rupture into the biliary tree. Gastrointest Endosc 1994;40:238.

Khuroo MS et al: Percutaneous drainage versus albendazole therapy in hepatic hydatidosis: a prospective, randomized study. Gastroenterology 1993;104:1452.

2. SCHISTOSOMIASIS

Pathophysiology

Human hepatic schistosomiasis is due to infection with the flukes *Schistosoma mansoni* or *S japonicum.* Humans are the definitive hosts and snails serve as intermediate hosts. *S mansoni* is found throughout the Middle East and Africa as well as parts of South America and the Caribbean. *S japonicum* has a more limited geographic distribution within Asia. There are differences between the two parasites in their patterns of egg laying in humans with resultant variation in disease responses to the parasites.

The schistosomal life cycle involving humans begins with the infective larvae (cercariae) from snails penetrating the skin or mucous membranes. They lose their tails and become schistosomulae which then migrate into the circulation. After many cercariae are destroyed by host defense mechanisms, those remaining mature to adult worms in various branches of the portal venous system. Within a month, these worms begin to lay eggs in the small terminal venules within the intestines. *S mansoni* lay eggs primarily in branches of the inferior mesenteric vein within the colon, whereas *S japonicum* deposit their eggs in the superior mesenteric vessels of the colon and small intestine. A pair of *S mansoni* worms

can release 1000 eggs per day; *S japonicum* worms can release up to three times that number. Some eggs develop to miracidia which may live in tissue for up to a month. Other eggs reach the bowel lumen and may appear in feces as early as 40 days after cercarial infection. Under proper conditions, these eggs hatch into miracidia which may find a snail host. Within the snail, a mother sporocyst develops giving rise to daughter sporocysts and cercariae. The life cycle is completed when the cercariae leave the snail, in water, where they survive for only a few hours unless they find an acceptable definitive host.

Adult worms are well-tolerated within humans, perhaps by incorporating human antigens into their lumens. Dead worms produce local inflammatory responses within terminal venules in the lung and liver resulting in necrosis and progressive fibrosis of these vessels. Most of the clinical manifestations of schistosomal disease result from the host's response to eggs trapped in tissues. This involves both circulating immune complexes and cell-mediated immune responses which are responsible for liver injury. These become more intense with repeated exposures to schistosomal antigens. Lymphocytes sensitized by cercarial antigens may stimulate collagen synthesis in areas such as the liver, where eggs are trapped. This has recently been shown to be a dynamic process under the control of fibrogenic cytokines. With increasing fibrosis, presinusoidal portal hypertension develops. Schistosomiasis-induced acquired lymphangiectasia and weakness in the portosystemic venous system may also promote the formation of gastric and esophageal varices.

Worm load influences the severity of the disease in conjunction with the host's response to the foreign antigens from these worms and eggs. *S japonicum* infection may be more severe than *S mansoni* infection because of the larger number of eggs trapped in the host's tissues.

Essentials of Diagnosis

- History of travel to an endemic area.
- Acute disease: fever, chills, nausea, diarrhea, myalgias, cough, hepatomegaly, mild splenomegaly, and mild leukocytosis with eosinophilia.
- Chronic disease: may be asymptomatic until late in disease. Diarrhea, hepatomegaly with significant splenomegaly, ascites, esophageal varices.
- Species specific ova found in stool.

Clinical Findings

A. Symptoms and Signs:

1. Acute schistosomiasis—Many patients infected with schistosomiasis remain asymptomatic. The initial symptom may be a pruritic, maculopapular rash caused by cercariae penetrating the skin. After a variable period of a few weeks to 2 months, patients develop anorexia, fatigue, headache, intermittent fevers, chills, myalgias, nausea, diarrhea, and cough. Both fevers and diarrhea may persist for 1–2 months. Hepatosplenomegaly along with generalized lymphadenopathy may be present. Red, edematous recto-sigmoid mucosa associated with small ulcerations and petechiae may be seen on sigmoidoscopic examination. An acute toxic reaction associated with severe abdominal pain, distention, jaundice, and even coma, has been seen rarely in endemic areas.

2. Chronic schistosomiasis—Chronic schistosomiasis is asymptomatic in the majority of patients, and it may take many months to years to develop the initial symptoms of abdominal pain, hepatosplenomegaly, and progressive weight loss and fatigue. Hepatosplenic schistosomiasis develops in about 10% of patients in endemic areas and may not occur until 5–15 years or longer after infection. Variceal bleeding and ascites may complicate the development of portal hypertension. Other stigmata of chronic liver disease are usually not present, or occur with terminal disease. Pulmonary hypertension and right sided congestive heart failure may complicate late stages of the disease. Large confluent schistosomal granulomas within the intestine or mesentery may be mistaken for colonic polyps or tumors. Central nervous system disease such as transverse myelitis, immune complex glomerulonephritis, and prolonged Salmonella infection are other complications of chronic schistosomiasis.

B. Laboratory Findings: In acute disease, eosinophilia is the most common laboratory abnormality seen. Routine liver tests are usually normal. With the development of chronic schistosomiasis, anemia and thrombocytopenia are seen, but eosinophilia is not a common feature. Low serum albumin and hypergammaglobulinemia are common. The aminotransferases are normal or minimally elevated.

The definitive diagnosis is generally made by finding ova in the stool. There are characteristic findings to distinguish between *S mansoni* and *S japonicum* eggs. Rectal biopsy with immediate examination of fresh tissue between two glass slides (crush prep) is a sensitive technique to demonstrate eggs or miracidia in tissue. Among the serologic tests available, ELISA is the screening test of choice. Immunoblot tests are used to confirm the diagnosis and distinguish between schistosome species.

C. Imaging: Ultrasonography of the liver may demonstrate characteristic findings of scarred portal tracts that appear as thick echogenic bands with central lucency. In advanced disease, with increasing fibrosis, this central lucency may disappear. There is a good correlation between ultrasonographic grading of hepatic fibrosis and clinical stage or endoscopic grading of size of esophageal varices. Characteristic CT and MRI findings have also been described, but these techniques are less useful for large-scale screening in endemic areas. Endoscopy and upper gastrointestinal series may be useful in demonstrating esophageal varices.

Treatment

Praziquantel is the drug of choice for both *S mansoni* and *S japonicum*. It is given at a dose of 20 mg/kg, three times a day for 1 day for *S japonicum*, and 20 mg/kg, twice a day for 1 day for *S mansoni*. Some reversal of fibrosis is possible with antihelminthic drugs provided the lesion is not advanced. Dizziness and headache are frequent, but transient side effects. Oxamniquine, 15 mg/kg as a single oral dose is an alternative treatment for *S mansoni*. Injection sclerotherapy has been the treatment of choice for managing esophageal varices. Propranolol may decrease portal pressure and reduce the risk of hemorrhage. Splenectomy is necessary in some patients to control thrombocytopenia and other effects of hypersplenism. Distal splenorenal shunt is the surgical treatment of choice for bleeding esophageal varices that have not responded to sclerotherapy.

Abdel-Wahab MF et al: Grading of hepatic schistosomiasis by the use of ultrasonography. Am J Trop Med Hyg 1992;46:403.

Aboul-Enein A, Arafa S, Sakr M: Pathogenesis of varices in schistosomal portal hypertension. Dig Dis Sci 1994;39:39.

DaSilva LC, Carrilho FJ: Hepatosplenic schistosomiasis. Pathophysiology and treatment. Gastroenterol Clin N Am 1992;21:163.

Tsang VCW, Wilkins PP: Immunodiagnosis of schistosomiasis. Clin Lab Med 1991;11:1029.

3. CLONORCHIASIS & OPISTHORCHIASIS

Clonorchiasis and opisthorchiasis are liver fluke infections with similar clinical, pathologic, and epidemiologic features. These diseases are found throughout Asia and Southeast Asia, but some studies have shown that up to 25% of Asian immigrants to the United States have active liver fluke infection.

Pathophysiology

Clonorchis sinensis, Opisthorchis felineus, and *Opisthorchis viverrini* are the three species of liver flukes that most commonly cause disease in humans. Humans, as well as other animals such as cats and dogs, are the definitive hosts. There are two intermediate hosts in the life cycle of these species, snails and fresh water fish. The adult liver flukes inhabit the bile ducts, gallbladder, and pancreatic ducts of humans or other animals where the eggs are shed, pass into the duodenum, and out into the stool. Snails ingest these eggs, miracidia develop into cercariae, and the free-swimming cercariae are shed into the water where they may penetrate the skin of freshwater fish. The parasite encysts in the muscles of fish where it becomes a metacercaria. Humans and other fish-eating animals acquire infection by eating raw or incompletely cooked fish. The parasites excyst in the definitive host's duodenum after action of digestive enzymes, migrate to the ampulla of Vater, and complete their life cycle in the bile ducts, pancreatic duct, and gallbladder. The worms may live for up to 30 years in the bile ducts of the definitive host. Adult worms begin to lay eggs within 3–4 weeks after initial infection of the definitive host.

Mechanical obstruction from worm burden, as well as potential injury from toxic metabolites of the worms, cause inflammation, thickening, and dilatation of the bile ducts. There may be secondary bacterial infection due to obstruction and bile stasis. Clonorchiasis predisposes patients to form intrahepatic gallstones, an uncommon finding in opisthorchiasis. Occasionally, ova, granulomas, and eosinophilic infiltrates are found within the hepatic parenchyma. Intrahepatic abscesses may form. Late disease may be complicated by secondary biliary cirrhosis and portal hypertension. There is an increased incidence of cholangiocarcinoma in these patients, although some authors have ascribed this to the high prevalence of hepatitis B in the same group of patients.

Essentials of Diagnosis

- Travel to an endemic area; history of eating raw or undercooked fish.
- Acute disease: asymptomatic with mild infection. Moderate disease causes fever, tender hepatomegaly, eosinophilia.
- Chronic disease: jaundice, tender hepatomegaly, enlarged gallbladder, eosinophilia. Dilated common or intrahepatic bile ducts on imaging studies.
- Definitive diagnosis based on finding ova in stool or duodenal aspirate.

Clinical Findings

A. Symptoms and Signs: Clinical presentation is dependent on the worm burden and duration of infection. Patients with light infection (under 100 worms) are usually asymptomatic, whereas moderate infection (up to 1000 worms) causes mild fever, nausea, anorexia, and occasionally tender hepatomegaly. In severe infection symptoms are due to the mass of worms present. Upwards of 10,000–20,000 flukes may be found in rare cases. Anorexia, right upper quadrant abdominal pain, hepatomegaly, enlargement of the gallbladder, and jaundice are common. If there is associated cholangitis, high fever, chills, and worsening jaundice are usually present. In late disease, secondary biliary cirrhosis may occur with portal hypertension and subsequent variceal bleeding.

B. Laboratory Findings: In early, mild disease the liver tests are usually normal. There is mild leukocytosis with eosinophilia. In moderate to severe cases, the alkaline phosphatase, GGTP, bilirubin, and aminotransferases are elevated. Low albumin and hypergammaglobulinemia may be found. Definitive diagnosis is made by finding characteristic ova in the stool or duodenal aspirate. Serologic testing has not been useful in diagnosis, since many parasites share similar group antigens, and the false positive rate of detection is quite high. DNA probes for diagnosis are being developed.

C. Imaging: Dilatation of the common bile duct, intrahepatic bile ducts, and gallbladder are best seen on ultrasonography. CT and MRI may also demonstrate bile duct or gallbladder dilatation, as well as cystic defects and abscesses. ERCP may be useful in demonstrating biliary strictures, cysts, or the flukes themselves.

Treatment

Praziquantel, 25 mg/kg three times a day for one day, is the drug of choice. Some authors advocate giving a second day of treatment for *C sinensis* infection.

Chan CW, Lam SK: Diseases caused by liver flukes and cholangiocarcinoma. Baillieres Clin Gastroenterol 1987;1:297.

Harinasuta T, Pungpak S, Keystone JS: Trematode infections. Opisthorchiasis, clonorchiasis, fascioliasis, and paragonimiasis. Infect Dis Clin North Am 1993;7:699.

Ona FV, Dytoc JN: Clonorchis-associated cholangiocarcinoma: a report of two cases with unusual manifestations. Gastroenterology 1991;101:831.

OTHER PARASITES

A number of other parasites are known to cause liver disease. American (Chagas' disease) and South American trypanosomiais, visceral leishmaniasis (Kala-Azar), strongyloidiasis, fascioliasis, capillariasis, ascariasis, toxocariasis, and toxoplasmosis are fairly uncommon and discussion of these illnesses is outside the scope of this chapter.

OTHER INFECTIONS

Liver involvement in syphilis had been described as occurring in 1–10% of cases. Although an increased incidence of *T pallidum* has been seen in association with HIV infection. Hepatic manifestations occur in the stage of secondary syphilis, often in association with other systemic manifestations such as rash, lymphadenopathy, and arthritis. The symptoms may mimic those seen in acute viral hepatitis. Elevations in the alkaline phosphatase and GGTP are common and persist longer than the elevations in the aspartate aminotransferase and alanine aminotransferase. Liver biopsy findings include Kupffer cell hyperplasia, focal necrosis of hepatocytes, and periportal inflammatory cell infiltrates. Spirochetes may be demonstrated with silver stains.

Lyme disease, caused by the spirochete *Borrelia burgdorferi,* is occurring with increasing incidence in a number of regions in the United States, particularly the northeast and Western states. Diagnosis is often made when the characteristic rash, erythema migrans, is seen in association with arthritis and a history of tick exposure. Acute hepatitis may rarely occur in early Lyme disease, with demonstration of *B burgdorferi* on liver biopsy. Liver test abnormalities, however, are fairly common, with elevations seen in up to 27% of cases. Elevation in the GGTP is the most common finding.

Liver test abnormalities may also rarely be seen in association with other infections such as in typhoid fever, shigellosis, brucellosis, Legionnaire's disease, Q fever or tuberculosis but will not be reviewed in detail in this chapter. Opportunistic infections seen in association with HIV infection are covered in Chapter 39.

Goellner MH et al: Hepatitis due to recurrent Lyme disease. Ann Intern Med 1988;108:707.

Kazakoff MA et al: Liver function test abnormalities in early Lyme disease. Arch Fam Med 1993;2:409.

Parcek SS: Liver involvement in secondary syphilis. Dig Dis Sci 1979;24:41.

LIVER DYSFUNCTION ASSOCIATED WITH SEPSIS

Liver test abnormalities and jaundice in association with bacteremia is an entity distinguishable from primary infection of the liver. Although initially described in infants and young children, cholestasis associated with sepsis is now recognized in both gram-negative and gram-positive infections. Elevations in the AST, ALT, and alkaline phosphatase are found in approximately 50% of patients who are bacteremic. These elevations are usually less than twice the upper limit of normal. Elevation of the bilirubin occurs less frequently, but may cause profound, and at times prolonged, jaundice. Liver biopsy is characterized by cholestasis without liver cell necrosis. Mild periportal inflammatory cell infiltration and Kupffer cell hyperplasia have been described. Dilation of the bile canaliculi has been demonstrated on transmission electron microscopy.

The mechanism of cholestasis associated with sepsis is not clear, but is probably multifactorial. Fever, hepatic hypoxia, bacterial endotoxins, and sepsis-induced cytokines may all play a role in causing hepatic dysfunction.

Oka Y et al: The mechanism of hepatic cellular injury in sepsis: an in vitro study of the implications of cytokines and neutrophils in its pathogenesis. J Surg Res 1993;55:1.

Sikuler E et al: Abnormalities in bilirubin and liver enzyme levels in adult patients with bacteremia. A prospective study. Arch Intern Med 1989;149:2246.

39

Liver & Biliary Disease in Patients With HIV Infection

Scott L. Friedman, MD

The liver and biliary tree are commonly involved by opportunistic infection or neoplasm in patients with human immunodeficiency virus (HIV) infection. In many cases, diagnosis of hepatic or biliary disease establishes the diagnosis of acquired immunodeficiency syndrome (AIDS) in a patient who is HIV-infected (Table 39–1). Involvement may occur as a result of pathogens unique to the immunocompromised state, infections common in both immunocompetent and immunocompromised patients, or heightened sensitivity to medications used to treat systemic complications of AIDS. In many cases, infection with HIV modulates the course of nonopportunistic liver disease. Some syndromes, in particular AIDS cholangiopathy (see below), are virtually unique to the HIV-infected population. The clinician must be aware of the broad differential diagnosis for hepatobiliary disease when evaluating a patient with HIV infection and right upper quadrant symptoms or abnormal liver tests, or both.

Essentials of Diagnosis

- Symptoms and signs alone unreliable; further evaluation required for specific diagnosis.
- Diagnosis often depends on level of immunocompromise.
- Hepatobiliary pathogens almost always present in late-stage HIV disease.
- Multiple infections common, especially in late-stage disease.

General Considerations

The clinical signs and symptoms alone rarely suggest a specific diagnosis, and some additional evaluation is almost always required in the symptomatic patient. Likely diagnoses may be stratified based on the extent of immunocompromise. For example, patients with well-preserved immune function, as manifested by normal or near-normal CD4 lymphocyte counts, are prone to bacterial infection, neoplasia, or drug-induced liver disease. In contrast, those with CD4 counts of less than 200/μL are additionally at risk for opportunistic infections with cytomegalovirus, fungi, atypical mycobacteria, and esoteric protozoa. In late-stage HIV disease, hepatobiliary pathogens (eg, cytomegalovirus and *Mycobacterium avium intracellulare*) are almost always part of systemic infection.

The evaluation should proceed from less to more invasive and is dictated by the severity and acuity of symptoms. Multiple infections are common, especially in late-stage immunocompromise. The clinician must discern nonpathogenic organisms from invasive pathogens. The main goal is identification of treatable infections or neoplasia. Failure to establish a specific cause for abnormal tests or persistent symptoms is not unusual in HIV disease. Clinicians must always individualize the need for invasive evaluation based on the overall clinical status.

Clinical Findings

A. Symptoms and Signs: Patients with liver or biliary abnormalities in HIV disease may be asymptomatic or may present with right upper quadrant discomfort, jaundice, or nonspecific symptoms such as malaise and anorexia. A common scenario is an asymptomatic patient with rising levels of transaminases or alkaline phosphatase; the next step is to decide how extensive further evaluation should be. In late-stage HIV disease, many common symptoms such as abdominal pain, weight loss, fevers, and wasting may be difficult to ascribe solely to hepatobiliary disease, because concurrent extrahepatic disease is almost always present.

B. Laboratory Findings:

1. ALT, AST, alkaline phosphatase–In general, right upper quadrant discomfort or abnormal liver tests reflect parenchymal liver disease or biliary tract disease, or both. The clinical presentation alone is rarely enough to distinguish between these two possibilities, although specific patterns of liver tests may provide useful clues. For example, disproportionate elevation of alkaline phosphatase compared with alanine aminotransferase (ALT) or aspartate aminotransferase (AST) suggests either biliary tract disease or lymphoma. If neither disorder is demonstrated, this pattern can be associated with *Mycobacterium avium* infiltration of the liver. In contrast, marked elevation of transaminases more commonly

Table 39–1. Hepatobiliary diseases that establish a diagnosis of AIDS.[1]

A diagnosis of AIDS can be made	
1. *Without* laboratory evidence of HIV infection (and assuming there are no other causes of immunosuppression)	And with *definite* evidence of cryptosporidiosis > 1 month; cytomegalovirus infection > 1 month; herpesvirus infection > 1 month; disseminated *M avium* or *M kansasii* infection
2. *With* laboratory evidence of HIV infection	And with *definite* evidence of disseminated nontubercular mycobacterial infection; extrapulmonary tuberculosis; recurrent *Salmonella* bacteremia; Kaposi's sarcoma; disseminated coccidioidomycosis; disseminated histoplasmosis; non-Hodgkin's lymphoma
3. *With* laboratory evidence of HIV infection	And with *presumptive* evidence of disseminated mycobacterial disease

[1]From 1987 revised CDC criteria.

reflects primary parenchymal disease, such as that due to use of certain drugs or infection with viruses or other opportunistic pathogens.

As noted above, the relative likelihood of particular diagnoses will be influenced by the extent of immunocompromise. Thus, the patient with abnormal liver tests but nearly normal CD4 counts is more likely to have disease due to an adverse drug reaction, hepatotrophic infection with hepatitis B or C virus, lymphoma, or nonopportunistic biliary disease, whereas in a patient with a CD4 count of less than 200/μL, one must additionally consider *Mycobacterium avium,* cytomegalovirus, bacillary peliosis hepatis, AIDS cholangiopathy, or opportunistic pathogens.

2. Liver biopsy–The role of liver biopsy in evaluating hepatobiliary disease in patients with HIV infection is not settled. Biopsy is indicated in symptomatic patients where a treatable hepatic complication is suspected and other less invasive measures, including imaging studies, blood and bone marrow cultures, and lymph node biopsy (if adenopathy is present), are not diagnostic. Coagulation studies must be normal before biopsy is considered; anecdotal reports describe instances of bleeding following biopsy despite normal values, although biopsy has been performed safely in almost all patients when appropriately indicated. When bleeding does occur, it might result from biopsy of a large peliotic lesion (see Differential Diagnosis, below) or unrecognized coagulopathy.

Several studies have suggested that liver biopsy rarely uncovers a diagnosis that is not already evident through other means. For example, biopsy might uncover *M avium* in a patient with late-stage infection that has already been identified through blood culture. Similarly, patients with suspected drug-induced liver disease would first benefit from a change in medication before biopsy is considered. In patients with presumed hepatitis B or C infection, biopsy should be considered only if confirmation of the diagnosis is likely to lead to a therapeutic trial with α-interferon or an investigational agent. Stable, moder-

ate abnormalities of liver tests (eg, AST or ALT < 250 IU/L) in a patient with no related symptoms are rarely an indication for liver biopsy in a patient with HIV infection. In any situation where liver biopsy is contemplated in this population, the clinician must determine that the liver disease is a more proximate cause of illness or death than other concurrent extrahepatic diseases; such an assessment requires sound clinical judgment and must consider the needs and wishes of the patient.

In contrast to blind liver biopsy with a conventional needle, directed fine-needle aspiration is useful in many patients with hepatobiliary disease, particularly if a coagulopathy is present. Abnormalities uncovered through abdominal imaging (see Imaging Studies, below), such as focal hepatic or intra-abdominal masses, must be sampled by directed aspiration and are suitable for cytologic studies, gram-stained smears, and cultures for acid-fast bacteria, viruses, and fungi. The procedure is associated with less risk of bleeding than conventional biopsy.

C. Imaging Studies: Abdominal imaging plays a critical role in the early evaluation of hepatobiliary disease in patients with HIV infection. Because concurrent pathologic changes are not unusual, imaging will identify both intrahepatic lesions and biliary tract abnormalities. Thus, any patient who is symptomatic and has elevated liver tests or right upper quadrant pain, or both, requires early imaging with abdominal ultrasound or CT scanning to identify regions of pathologic change. Findings of interest include focal or mass lesions of the liver, lymph node enlargement, intra- or extrahepatic bile duct dilatation, and gallbladder wall abnormalities. Imaging studies can also reveal findings consistent with chronic liver disease, including varices and ascites, as well as other intra-abdominal disorders such as pancreatic or peritoneal disease.

Patients with evidence of bile duct abnormalities, including dilatation or mass, typically require a contrast study of the biliary tree, either via endoscopic retrograde cholangiopancreatography (ERCP) or percutaneous transhepatic cholangiography (PTC). Patients with AIDS cholangiopathy (see Differential Diagnosis below) demonstrate either papillary stenosis or sclerosing cholangitis-like intrahepatic bile duct narrowing, or a combination of the two (Figure 39–1). Occasionally, long extrahepatic strictures may be seen. Normal ultrasound studies or CT scans do not conclusively exclude AIDS cholangiopathy; in one large series, imaging studies were normal in 25% of patients with disease ultimately proved by biliary contrast study.

Differential Diagnosis

A. Hepatic Parenchymal Disease: The differential diagnosis of hepatic parenchymal disease in patients with HIV infection is broad, and includes opportunistic infections, hepatitis virus infection, neoplasm, and adverse drug reaction (Table 39–2). Virtually any opportunistic infection can involve the liver; those more commonly seen are included below.

1. *Mycobacterium avium intracellulare* infection–M avium infection is the most common specific liver finding in autopsy series of AIDS patients. Typically, this is a late-stage infection, where the liver involvement is part of a systemic infection. The pathologic hallmark is the presence of poorly formed granulomas associated with large numbers of acid-fast bacilli within foamy histiocytes (Figure 39–1). Acid-fast smear of infected tissue usually reveals organisms, although distinction from *Mycobacterium tuberculosis* is not possible by smear alone. As indicated above, patients with *M avium* infection typically have systemic symptoms, including fever, lymphadenopathy, diarrhea, and night sweats. Associated bone marrow infiltration is common, and, thus, the diagnosis can often be established via bone marrow or lymph node examination prior to consideration of liver biopsy. Imaging studies may reveal diffuse intra-abdominal adenopathy. As noted in the preceding section, liver abnormalities typically include disproportionate elevation of serum alkaline phosphatase, with only modest elevations of bilirubin, AST, and ALT.

Table 39–2. Differential diagnosis of hepatic parenchymal disease in HIV infection.

More common
M avium intracellulare infection
Drug-induced disease, especially with sulfa, zidovudine
M tuberculosis infection
Bacillary peliosis hepatis
Lymphoma
Cytomegalovirus infection
Cryptococcosis, histoplasmosis
Kaposi's sarcoma
Hepatitis C virus infection
Hepatitis B or D virus infection
P carinii infection
Microsporidiosis
Less common

2. Drug reaction–Hepatotoxic drug reactions, particularly to sulfonamides, are common in HIV-infected individuals for unclear reasons. Sulfa intolerance is noted in up to 25% of patients in this setting and may be manifested as systemic allergy with or without elevations of AST and ALT. Eosinophilia is frequently noted. Abnormalities usually resolve upon withdrawal of the offending agent. Of great concern has been the emerging hepatotoxicity of nucleoside analogs, including zidovudine (AZT) and didanosine (DDI); some patients have developed progressive, fatal hepatic steatosis. Typically, the syndrome has occurred in patients who appear to be relatively well and has been ascribed to mitochondrial injury. In nonfatal cases, improvement following discontinuation of the antiviral agent has been observed, with no documented progression to chronic liver injury.

3. *Mycobacterium tuberculosis* infection–M tuberculosis infection is a growing concern, especially in inner-city populations, where intravenous drug use is common. Unlike *M avium* infection, *M tuberculosis* infection may occur before patients are markedly immunocompromised. Symptoms are those associated with tuberculous infection in immunocompetent individuals and include fever, cough, night sweats, and, occasionally, lymphadenopathy. Extrapulmonary tuberculosis, including liver disease, develops more commonly in HIV-infected patients, and may be manifested by abdominal pain, jaundice, or hepatosplenomegaly.

4. *Bacillary peliosis hepatis*–Bacillary peliosis hepatis is a recently described finding due to systemic infection with *Bartonella quintana* or *Bartonella henselae* (previously called *Rochalimaea* sp.), two newly described organisms closely related to other *Bartonella* species. In this lesion, bacilli are seen within dilated vascular (peliotic) spaces. Patients typically present with fever and elevated liver enzymes, often in association with cutaneous or bony involvement. The causative organism appears within amorphous clusters near dilated vascular spaces in the liver. These peliotic spaces may be micro- or macroscopic. Diagnosis is established by Warthin-Starry silver staining of infected tissue, chocolate agar culture, or polymerase chain reaction using specific primers.

5. Non-Hodgkin's lymphoma–Non-Hodgkin's lymphoma (now referred to as either large cell lymphoma or Burkitt's lymphoma, depending on the histologic findings) typically presents in extranodal sites, and occurs at all stages of HIV infection with equal frequency. The liver is among the more common extranodal sites; there may be focal hepatic lesions associated with pain, weight loss, night sweats, and a progressive rise in both alkaline phosphatase and transaminase levels. The lesion is typically identified by noninvasive imaging, and diagnosis can be established by an experienced pathologist using fine-needle aspiration and cytologic or conventional liver

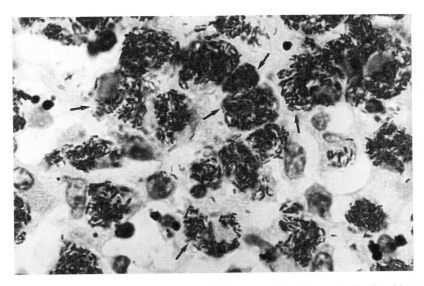

Figure 39–1. *Mycobacterium avium* complex in the liver. High-power photomicrograph of a liver biopsy specimen from a patient with late-stage HIV disease, in which tissue has been stained with an acid-fast stain, revealing large numbers of organisms within macrophages *(arrows)*. (Courtesy of Brian Herndier, MD.)

biopsy (Figure 39–2). The prognosis of non-Hodgkin's lymphoma is largely correlated with the stage of HIV infection and extent of immunocompromise (see Prognosis, below). Although not strictly an AIDS-defining diagnosis, advanced-stage Hodgkin's lymphoma, often with visceral involvement, is also seen with increased prevalence in all risk groups.

6. Cytomegalovirus infection—Cytomegalovirus infection of the liver has been documented in many patients with late-stage HIV infection, although luminal tract infection by cytomegalovirus is more common. As with other opportunistic infections, cytomegalovirus hepatitis is always part of systemic infection. Clinical findings with liver infection may include fevers and right upper quadrant pain in association with nonspecific elevations of transaminases. Infected tissue reveals typical viral inclusions, creating an owl's eye appearance within endothelial

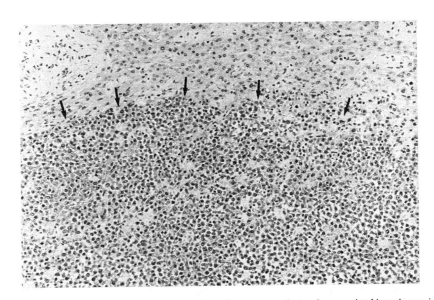

Figure 39–2. Non-Hodgkin's (large cell) lymphoma of liver. Low-power photomicrograph of lymphoma invading hepatic tissue. A monomorphic population of lymphocytes is evident *(arrows)* (hematoxylin & eosin stain). (Courtesy of Brian Herndier, MD.)

cells, macrophages, or hepatocytes. Mononuclear cell infiltration or neutrophils may be present.

7. Cryptococcal, coccidioidal, or histoplasmal infection–Cryptococcal, coccidioidal, and histoplasmal infections are usually seen in association with systemic disease. Liver involvement may be macro- or microscopic. *Candida* rarely infects the liver, despite its high prevalence in mucocutaneous sites. Hepatic *Candida* infections are confined to patients who are neutropenic, typically in response to systemic chemotherapy used to treat non-Hodgkin's lymphoma.

8. Kaposi's sarcoma–Kaposi's sarcoma, a neoplasm largely confined to homosexual men with HIV infection, can involve the liver. Hepatic lesions are usually asymptomatic; however, there have been reports of bleeding from lesions following liver biopsy.

9. Hepatitis C virus infection–Hepatitis C virus (HCV) frequently coinfects patients with HIV disease, particularly those who have been intravenous drug users. Unlike hepatitis B virus (HBV) infection (see below), the clinical course of HCV infection is often more aggressive in the setting of HIV—especially during advanced immunocompromise—than in immunocompetent hosts. HIV increases the cotransmissibility of HCV virus by sexual or perinatal transmission, although not because of an increase in HCV RNA levels.

10. Hepatitis B virus infection–HBV coinfection is also common in HIV disease, although its presence does not affect the overall survival rates of AIDS patients. Unlike HCV, symptomatic HBV disease is not common in HIV infection; this may reflect impairment of cytotoxic T cell function. Nonetheless, patients with coinfection by HBV and HIV have high levels of HBV DNA polymerase and surface antigen, making their body fluids highly infectious. Some patients with previous evidence of serologic clearance, manifested by positive HBsAb, have converted from surface antigen negative to positive following HIV infection. In HIV-positive patients without serological evidence of past or present HBV infection, vaccination is largely ineffective.

11. *Pneumocystis carinii* infection–Rare cases of *Pneumocystis carinii* or microsporidial infection in the liver have been reported. The presence of *P carinii* in extrapulmonary sites typically is seen in patients who have had inhalation therapy with a drug such as pentamidine, which fails to protect sites outside the airways.

12. HIV infection–Clear evidence for direct involvement of the liver by HIV has emerged. Typically, HIV is found within hepatic macrophages and occasionally sinusoidal endothelial cells. Infection of macrophages is not surprising given the propensity of the virus to infect the cell type in other organs. Nonetheless, infection of hepatic macrophages by HIV suggests that the liver may be a large reservoir of virus. Additionally, HIV infection of Kupffer's cells could result in impaired cell function, leading to the increased incidence of enteric bacteremias in this population. Despite the demonstration of HIV in liver, there is no discrete clinical syndrome of liver disease that has been ascribed to HIV alone.

B. Biliary Tract Disease: The differential diagnosis of biliary tract disease is dominated by a syndrome called AIDS cholangiopathy but also includes other opportunistic infections and neoplasms (Table 39–3).

1. AIDS cholangiopathy–AIDS cholangiopathy is a syndrome characterized by marked abnormalities of biliary ducts in patients with HIV disease of any stage. These abnormalities may include papillary stenosis, sclerosing cholangitis, or long extrahepatic strictures. The cause of this syndrome is uncertain, but in many cases it is associated with the presence of one or more organisms in the biliary epithelium, including microsporidium, cryptosporidium, or cytomegalovirus. Typical symptoms include right upper quadrant pain and fever, although the biliary changes may sometimes be asymptomatic. Laboratory abnormalities include marked elevation of alkaline phosphatase and modest elevation of AST and ALT. Jaundice is extremely unusual in this syndrome and should raise the possibility of an alternative or additional hepatobiliary disorder. Imaging studies are useful in evaluating AIDS cholangiopathy, as 75% of patients will have abnormal CT scans or ultrasound studies revealing ductal dilatation (see Imaging Studies, above).

2. Non-Hodgkin's lymphoma; Kaposi's sarcoma–Rare cases of non-Hodgkin's lymphoma or Kaposi's sarcoma have been reported in the biliary tree, reflecting the aggressive nature and unusual presentations of these neoplasms in this setting.

3. Cytomegalovirus cholecystitis–Acalculous cholecystitis due to gallbladder involvement by cytomegalovirus has been described, presenting as severe abdominal pain with or without peritonitis. Cytomegalovirus cholecystitis is not part of the AIDS cholangiopathy syndrome but should be suspected in any patient with clinical evidence of cholecystitis. Prolonged fasting (eg, in patients receiving total parenteral nutrition) may also lead to gallbladder distention and pain, although fasting has not been directly linked to acalculous cholecystitis in this population.

Table 39–3. Differential diagnosis of biliary tract disease in HIV infection.

AIDS cholangiopathy
Lymphoma
Kaposi's sarcoma
Acalculous cholecystitis (often due to cytomegalovirus)
Non-AIDS disorders, including gallstone disease

Treatment

Treatment of hepatobiliary abnormalities in patients with HIV infection is dictated by the specific findings uncovered during evaluation, the severity of immunocompromise, and the presence of concurrent underlying infections or neoplasms. Patients who are relatively active and at an earlier stage of disease are more likely to benefit from treatment than those who are wasted and profoundly immunosuppressed. Nonetheless, specific infections should be sought and treated appropriately.

A. Hepatic Disease:

1. Drug reaction–In view of the high rate and reversibility of adverse drug reactions in HIV-infected patients, any medication should be seen as potentially hepatotoxic and its discontinuation or substitution considered. Particularly culpable agents include sulfonamides and antiretrovirals.

2. *M avium* infection–For documented *M avium* infection, the goal is reduction in bacterial burden and relief of symptoms rather than complete eradication of the organism. Because of its prevalence, current recommendations for management of HIV disease include prophylactic use of antibiotics in patients with profound immunocompromise (CD4 count < 100/μL). In those with documented disease, multidrug regimens are required and typically include three to four of the following agents: clarithromycin, 500–1000 mg twice daily, or azithromycin, 500–1000 mg twice daily; rifampin, 10 mg/kg/d (maximum, 600 mg/d); ciprofloxacin, 750 mg twice a day, or ofloxacin, 400 mg twice a day; clofazimine, 100 mg/d; amikacin, 7.5 mg/kg/d intravenously.

3. *M tuberculosis* infection–Treatment of *M tuberculosis* in patients with HIV infection should include four drugs initially for 2 months while awaiting the results of sensitivity testing: isoniazid, 300 mg orally or intramuscularly; rifampin, 600 mg orally or intramuscularly; pyrazinamide, 15 mg/kg intramuscularly up to 1 g; and ethambutol, 15–25 mg/kg orally. This regimen is followed by isoniazid and rifampin twice weekly for 4–7 months for susceptible strains. An increasing prevalence of drug-resistant *M tuberculosis* infection is being seen, emphasizing the need to await culture and sensitivity results before finalizing therapy.

4. Bacillary peliosis hepatis–Bacillary peliosis hepatis responds to erythromycin, 500–1000 mg, four times per day, which is the drug of choice; parenteral administration may be required in severe cases. Responses to tetracycline, minocycline, or cephalosporin have also been documented; sulfonamides are ineffective. Long-term (ie, > 2 months) or chronic therapy is recommended in patients with HIV infection. Resolution of peliosis has been documented in several cases following antibiotic therapy.

5. Non-Hodgkin's lymphoma; Kaposi's sarcoma–Treatment options for Kaposi's sarcoma and non-Hodgkin's lymphoma include chemotherapy or radiation therapy. Although no improved survival rates have been documented following such regimens, some treatment is usually required because of the rapid growth of these tumors, particularly lymphomas. Chemotherapy is especially difficult to use in these immunocompromised patients, because most agents can further increase the susceptibility to infection, and also suppress the bone marrow. In patients with lymphoma and CD4 counts of less than 200/μL, chemotherapy is given in standard dosages combined with GM-colony stimulating factor (GM-CSF); more immunosuppressed patients require lower-dosage regimens. Novel immunologic and anticytokine therapies are currently under investigation but are not yet available for general use. Visceral symptomatic Kaposi's sarcoma is often treated with combination chemotherapy, including doxorubicin, bleomycin, or vincristine.

6. Cytomegalovirus infection–Cytomegalovirus infection is rarely localized only to the liver; patients with systemic cytomegalovirus disease involving the liver are treated with ganciclovir, 5 mg/kg intravenously every 12 hours for 10–14 days (induction), followed by 5–6 mg/kg for 5–7 days per week (maintenance). An alternative to ganciclovir in patients who do not respond is foscarnet, 60 mg/kg intravenously every 8 hours for 14 days, infused over 1 hour (induction), followed by 90–120 mg/kg/d intravenously as a 2-hour infusion (maintenance); dosages must be reduced in patients with impaired creatinine clearance. Vigorous hydration and careful monitoring of serum calcium levels are essential when using foscarnet, as life-threatening renal failure with hypocalcemia is a potential adverse reaction; the drug should not be used simultaneously with pentamidine. Patients with concurrent ocular cytomegalovirus infection must be treated chronically with either ganciclovir or foscarnet, whereas those with only visceral disease may be treated for 4–8 weeks. For recurrence, chronic maintenance therapy is appropriate. Chronic parenteral therapy usually requires placement of an indwelling venous catheter to permit outpatient administration.

7. Fungal infections–Visceral fungal infections involving the liver, including histoplasmosis, coccidiomycosis, candidiasis, and cryptococcosis, require parenteral therapy with amphotericin B, 0.6–0.8 mg/kg/d intravenously. The optimal duration of treatment has not been established but should be at least 2 weeks. Maintenance therapy with fluconazole, 200 mg/d orally, is recommended.

8. Hepatitis C infection–Treatment of chronic HCV infection is not usually indicated in patients with HIV infection, unless illness from this infection is significantly more severe than that of other underlying infections. α-interferon may reduce hepatic inflammation, but should only be considered in patients who are not already profoundly immunocompromised. The optimal dosage and duration of therapy in this setting is not established. Use of α-interferon in patients with coinfection by HBV and HIV is not indicated, except in the context of experimental trials.

9. P carinii infection–Those rare cases of *P carinii* infection involving the liver will respond to oral therapy with dapsone and trimethoprim in mild cases. Severely ill patients require parenteral therapy for 14–21 days with pentamidine, 3–4 mg/kg/d intravenously, or trimethoprim, 15 mg/kg/d, and sulfamethoxazole, 100 mg/kg/d.

B. Biliary Tract Disease:

1. AIDS cholangiopathy–Effective therapy of AIDS cholangiopathy is confined to patients with papillary stenosis, whose pain is improved in at least 50% of cases by endoscopic sphincterotomy. In all patients, the syndrome is associated with progressive elevation of alkaline phosphatase, possibly reflecting progressive intrahepatic biliary lesions. Trials of medical therapy with ursodeoxycholic acid are under way, but its efficacy is still unproved.

2. Acalculous cholecystitis–Acalculous cholecystitis is usually a surgical emergency. In otherwise stable patients, cholecystectomy is indicated, but patients are often too ill to tolerate laparotomy. In this circumstance, cholecystotomy by a percutaneous catheter or minilaparotomy may be feasible. Evidence or strong suspicion of cytomegalovirus infection as an underlying cause may necessitate use of ganciclovir or foscarnet.

Prognosis

The prognosis in the patient with HIV infection is dictated almost entirely by the extent of immunocompromise and severity of wasting, and not by the nature of specific lesions in the liver or biliary tract. Indicators of long-term disease progression (several months to years) in HIV infection include serum CD4 lymphocyte counts, CD4:CD8 lymphocyte ratios, measurements of β_2-microglobulin, and hemoglobin, and the erythrocyte sedimentation rate. These parameters are less useful for indicating short-term disease activity, because some fluctuation, particularly of the CD4 count, is common. Severe wasting also portends a reduced survival time. In one study, patients with serum albumin of less than 2 g/dL had a dramatically reduced mean survival rate, compared with those whose albumin was greater than 3 g/dL.

REFERENCES

Adal KA, Cockerell CJ, Petri WA: Cat scratch disease, bacillary angiomatosis, and other infections due to *Rochalimaea*. N Engl J Med 1994;330:1509.

Cappell MS: Hepatobiliary manifestations of the acquired immunodeficiency syndrome. Am J Gastroenterol 1991;86:1.

Cappell MS, Schwartz MS, Biempica L: Clinical utility of liver biopsy in patients with serum antibodies to the human immunodeficiency virus. Am J Med 1990;88:123.

Cello JP: Acquired immunodeficiency syndrome cholangiopathy: Spectrum of disease. Am J Med 1989;86:539.

Centers for Disease Control: Revision of the CDC surveillance case definition for acquired immunodeficiency syndrome. MMWR 1987;36:3s.

Cohen PT, Sande MA, Volberding PA (editors): The AIDS knowledge base: A textbook on HIV disease from the University of California, San Francisco, and the San Francisco General Hospital. Massachusetts Medical Society, Little Brown, 1994.

Eyster ME et al: Heterosexual co-transmission of hepatitis C virus (HCV) and human immunodeficiency virus (HIV). Ann Intern Med 1991;115:764.

Eyster ME et al: Natural history of hepatitis C virus infection in multitransfused hemophiliacs: Effect of coinfection with human immunodeficiency virus. J AIDS 1993;6:602.

Freiman JP et al: Hepatomegaly with severe steatosis in HIV-seropositive patients. AIDS 1993;7:379.

Friedman SL (guest editor): AIDS: A review for the hepatologist. Semin Liv Dis 1993;12:103.

Herndier BG, Kaplan KD, McGrath MS: Pathogenesis of AIDS lymphomas. AIDS 1994;8:1025.

Housset C et al: Immunohistochemical evidence for human immunodeficiency virus-1 infection of liver Kupffer cells. Hum Pathol 1990;21:404.

Housset C et al: Interactions between HIV-1, hepatitis delta virus and hepatitis B virus infections in 260 chronic carriers of hepatitis B virus infection. Hepatology 1992;15:578.

McDonald JA et al: Effect of human immunodeficiency virus (HIV) infection on chronic hepatitis B hepatic viral antigen display. J Hepatol 1987;4:337.

Perkocha L et al: Clinical and pathological features of bacillary peliosis hepatis in association with human immunodeficiency virus infection. N Engl J Med 1990;323:1581.

Scharschmidt BF et al: Hepatitis B in patients with HIV infection: Relationship to AIDS and patient survival. Ann Intern Med 1992;117:837.

Schmitt MP, Steffan AM, Gendrault JL: Multiplication of human immunodeficiency virus in primary cultures of human Kupffer cells: Possible role of liver macrophages infection in the physiopathology of AIDS. Res Virol 1990;141:143.

Slater L: *Rochalimaea henselae* causes bacillary angiomatosis and peliosis hepatis. Arch Intern Med 1992;152:602.

Small PM et al: Treatment of tuberculosis in patients with advanced human immunodeficiency virus infection. N Engl J Med 1991;324:289.

Wilkins MJ et al: Surgical pathology of the liver in HIV infection. Histopathology 1991;18:459.

Alcoholic Liver Disease

40

Jacquelyn J. Maher, MD

Essentials of Diagnosis

- History or strong suspicion of heavy ethanol use (40–80 g/d for at least 1 year).
- Mild to moderate elevation of hepatic transaminases (< 500 IU/L, with AST:ALT ratio > 2).
- Liver biopsy with steatosis; Mallory bodies; ballooning degeneration of hepatocytes; neutrophilic infiltrate; with or without pericellular fibrosis.

General Considerations

Excessive alcohol consumption can lead to several abnormalities in the liver, ranging from steatosis, to alcoholic hepatitis, to hepatic fibrosis and cirrhosis. These terms are based largely on histologic status; they infer a spectrum of increasing disease severity, although clinically there can be significant overlapping among these disorders. Steatosis represents a purely biochemical disturbance in hepatocytes. It does not connote true liver injury, and is completely reversible with abstinence. Hepatitis and fibrosis, by contrast, are serious disorders characterized by hepatic inflammation, necrosis, and scarring. In many patients, alcoholic hepatitis precedes fibrosis, although the two lesions often occur together and may arise from different pathophysiologic mechanisms. Hepatic fibrosis, if unchecked, ultimately leads to irreversible cirrhosis.

There is little doubt that chronic ethanol ingestion plays a key role in the development of liver disease. Countries from around the world report a direct correlation between cirrhosis-related mortality rates and per capita ethanol consumption; in the United States, cirrhosis represents the ninth leading cause of death, with most patients suffering from alcoholic liver disease. Over 900,000 persons in the United States are estimated to have cirrhosis; at least 40% and perhaps as many as 90% of these individuals consume ethanol chronically.

Figure 40–1 provides vivid proof of a cause-and-effect relationship between alcohol consumption and mortality rates from cirrhosis. This graph, which depicts the age-adjusted death rates from cirrhosis in the United States from 1910 to 1984, demonstrates a sharp decline in cirrhosis-related mortality rates after the enactment of Prohibition in 1916 and a gradual increase following its repeal in 1932. Similar observations have been made recently in Finland, where loosening of restrictions on the sale of low-alcohol beer led to a rapid rise in ethanol consumption and a 100% increase in mortality rates from cirrhosis over a 20-year period.

Alcoholic liver disease develops only after prolonged periods of abuse. Epidemiologic studies indicate that individuals must consume a "threshold" dose of ethanol, amounting to 80 g/d for 10–20 years, before they exhibit signs of liver injury (80 g of ethanol is equivalent to eight 12-oz beers, 1 L of wine, or one-half pint of distilled spirits). Virtually 100% of individuals who achieve this threshold have hepatic steatosis; alcoholic hepatitis, on the other hand, occurs in only 35% of patients, and only 10–15% develop cirrhosis. It is important to note that this threshold dose of ethanol predicts the *onset* of liver injury but not the *extent* of liver damage. The low incidence of serious liver injury in alcoholics, along with the poor correlation between the amount of ethanol consumed and disease severity, suggests that hereditary or environmental factors, or both, interact with ethanol to produce alcoholic liver disease.

Pathophysiology

Ethanol has been described as an idiosyncratic hepatotoxin in humans because it does not reproducibly cause liver damage even in heavy drinkers. A number of different mechanisms have been proposed by which ethanol induces liver disease; to date, no single theory is considered predominant. The following section describes how chronic ethanol ingestion (in the absence of hereditary or environmental cofactors) might produce liver damage.

A. Ethanol Metabolism in the Liver: Ethanol metabolism is essential to the development of alcoholic liver injury. In the liver, ethanol is oxidized primarily by the cytosolic enzyme alcohol dehydrogenase (ADH). ADH converts ethanol to acetaldehyde, which is then oxidized to acetate (primarily in mito-

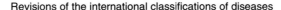

Revisions of the international classifications of diseases

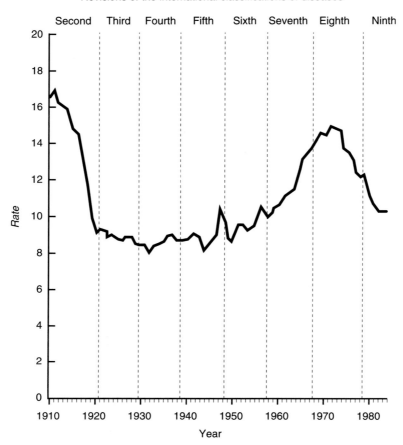

Figure 40–1. Age-adjusted death rates of liver cirrhosis: Death Registration States, 1910–1932, and United States, 1933–1984. (Death rates per 100,000 population.) (Reproduced, with permission, from Grant BF, Dufour MC, Harford TC: Epidemiology of alcoholic liver disease. Semin Liver Dis 1988;8:12.)

chondria) by aldehyde dehydrogenase (ALDH). Both ADH-mediated ethanol oxidation and ALDH-mediated acetaldehyde oxidation are coupled to the reduction of NAD^+ to NADH (Figure 40–2).

Alternate pathways of ethanol metabolism also exist in the liver. In alcoholics, ethanol can be oxidized in microsomes by the cytochrome P4502E1; this mixed-function oxidase is greatly induced by chronic ethanol consumption. In both alcoholics and nonalcoholics, ethanol can also be metabolized in peroxisomes by catalase, although this is considered a minor pathway in relation to ADH and P4502E1. P4502E1-mediated ethanol metabolism in alcoholics is particularly relevant to liver injury because it leads to formation of reactive oxygen intermediates (see following discussion). P4502E1 has a much higher K_m for ethanol than does ADH; thus, even in alcoholics, ADH metabolizes much of the ethanol reaching the liver, with P4502E1 contributing to its metab-

olism only when blood levels are high. Both ADH and P4502E1 are present in highest concentration near terminal hepatic venules; this may account in part for the centrizonal distribution of alcoholic liver injury.

Recent studies indicate that ADH is present in the stomach and intestine as well as the liver. A significant amount of ingested ethanol is metabolized by the gastric enzyme (referred to as "first-pass" metabolism of ethanol). This is important when considering hepatotoxicity, because the elimination of ethanol in the stomach limits the amount reaching the portal circulation and ultimately the liver. Gastric ADH activity is lower in women than in men; consequently, women are predisposed to higher blood ethanol levels than men after alcohol ingestion. This may contribute to their increased susceptibility to alcoholic liver disease.

B. Direct Toxic Effects of Ethanol (Table 40–1):

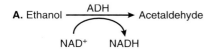

A. Ethanol $\xrightarrow{\text{ADH}}$ Acetaldehyde

NAD$^+$ NADH

B. Acetaldehyde $\xrightarrow{\text{ALDH}}$ Acetate

NAD$^+$ NADH

C. Ethanol + O_2 + H^+ $\xrightarrow{\text{P4502E1}}$ Acetaldehyde + H_2O

NADPH   NADP$^+$

Figure 40–2. *A:* Oxidative metabolism of ethanol. Ethanol is oxidized to acetaldehyde by alcohol dehydrogenase (ADH). ***B:*** Acetaldehyde is then metabolized to acetate by aldehyde dehydrogenase (ALDH). Both reactions are accompanied by the conversion of NAD$^+$ to NADH. ***C:*** In alcoholics, cytochrome P4502E1 can also contribute to ethanol metabolism. This reaction uses oxygen and NADPH, producing NADP$^+$ and H_2O.

1. Alteration of lipid and carbohydrate metabolism–The reduction of NAD$^+$ to NADH that accompanies ethanol oxidation shifts the redox state of hepatocytes. The excess NADH alters several NAD$^+$-dependent processes, particularly those involved in intermediary metabolism. The redox shift enhances triacylglycerol synthesis in hepatocytes; at the same time, it inhibits β-oxidation of fatty acids, resulting in esterification and storage as triglyceride. The end result is hepatic steatosis.

A high NADH:NAD$^+$ ratio also causes disturbances in gluconeogenesis by limiting the availability of several intermediates in the gluconeogenic pathway (oxaloacetate, pyruvate, and dihydroxyacetone-phosphate) and by inhibiting the activity of key enzymes involved in glucose production. Together, these alterations can result in profound hypoglycemia, particularly in alcoholics with underlying carbohydrate malnutrition.

2. Oxidative stress–Metabolism of ethanol by cytochrome P4502E1 gives rise to oxygen-derived free radicals, including the superoxide ion radical (O_2^-) and the hydroxyl radical (*OH). These reactive oxygen species, particularly the hydroxyl radical, can interact with cellular proteins, lipids, or DNA to begin a chain reaction of peroxidation that results in cell injury or death. ADH-mediated ethanol oxidation may also promote free radical production in liver cells by a different mechanism. In this case, the high NADH:NAD$^+$ ratio resulting from ethanol oxidation promotes mobilization of iron from ferritin, which can then react with H_2O_2 to produce hydroxyl and superoxide radicals. The resultant oxidative stress can lead to hepatocellular injury.

Other metabolic processes linked to ethanol metabolism may also promote oxidative stress in the liver. Acetaldehyde oxidation, for example, yields acetate; in high concentrations, acetate promotes conversion of pyridine nucleotides to purines in liver cells, which are then catabolized by xanthine oxidase in a reaction that generates oxygen radicals. Acetaldehyde oxidation itself can potentially lead to free radical production, if catalyzed by alternate pathways from ALDH (such as aldehyde oxidase or xanthine oxidase). Neutrophils and Kupffer cells, which produce superoxide upon activation, can be stimulated by chronic ethanol ingestion and provide an additional source of oxygen radicals.

The oxidative stress induced in the liver by ethanol metabolism can be exacerbated by a concomitant decrease in the liver's ability to defend against free radical attack. Chronic ethanol ingestion leads to a reduction in hepatic glutathione, a nonprotein thiol that plays a key role in protection against oxidative injury. Ethanol affects mitochondrial levels of glutathione preferentially; this renders cells particularly susceptible to oxidative injury because mitochondria represent a major site of H_2O_2 production and because these organelles lack alternative mechanisms of antioxidant defense. This combination of enhanced oxidant stress and impaired antioxidant de-

Table 40–1. Putative mechanisms of alcoholic liver injury.

Direct toxic effects of ethanol	
Oxyradical formation —————————▶	Peroxidation of membrane lipids
Acetaldehyde-protein adduct formation ————▶	Altered enzyme function; altered protein trafficking
Disturbance of intermediary metabolism ————▶	Fatty liver; hypoglycemia
Immune responses to ethanol	
Cytokine production ——————————▶	Hepatocellular necrosis; neutrophil infiltration
Autoimmune responses to hepatocellular proteins ——▶	Hepatocellular necrosis; ? fibrosis
Mechanisms of fibrosis	
Oxyradical formation	
Lipid peroxidation	
Local production of transforming growth factor-β	▶ Lipocyte (stellate cell) activation
Extracellular deposition of acetaldehyde-protein adducts (?)	

fense in alcoholics may contribute importantly to alcoholic liver injury.

Despite the fact that ethanol metabolism is known to alter both oxidant production and antioxidant defense in liver cells, it remains uncertain whether the *amount* of oxidative stress generated by ethanol in vivo is sufficient to promote hepatic damage. Studies in rats suggest that peroxidative injury may only become important when ethanol is consumed with large amounts of polyunsaturated fat. Animals may be protected to a degree from ethanol-induced oxidative injury because their diets are replete with antioxidant vitamins. The role of oxidative stress in human alcoholic liver injury is being actively investigated.

3. Acetaldehyde effects—Acetaldehyde is a highly reactive compound that may directly promote hepatocellular injury and necrosis. One means by which acetaldehyde can provoke cellular damage is by reacting with lysine residues on cellular proteins to form acetaldehyde-protein adducts. Adduct formation may interfere with the catalytic activity of lysine-dependent enzymes; it may also have profound effects on protein transport processes in hepatocytes, such as glycoprotein secretion and receptor-mediated endocytosis. The latter may result from interactions between acetaldehyde and tubulin. In vitro, acetaldehyde reacts readily with lysine residues on tubulin; acetaldehyde-modified tubulin does not assemble properly into microtubules, and in vivo, this could slow microtubule-dependent processes such as protein trafficking. Acetaldehyde has been linked to protein secretory abnormalities in hepatocytes, which represent the major event underlying hepatocellular swelling ("ballooning"). Whether the effect of acetaldehyde is mediated through adduct formation with tubulin remains unproved. Finally, some evidence suggests that acetaldehyde-protein adducts serve as "neoantigens," provoking an immune response that may contribute to hepatocellular injury (see following discussion).

C. Immune and Inflammatory Mechanisms of Alcoholic Liver Injury (Table 40–1):

1. Cytokine production—Interleukin-1, interleukin-6, and tumor necrosis factor-α are all associated with alcoholic liver injury. These compounds have a broad range of metabolic effects on liver cells, and with excessive alcohol use, they may provoke clinical manifestations of hepatitis such as fever, altered nutrient metabolism, and ascites. Over 75% of patients with alcoholic hepatitis have increased levels of interleukin-1, interleukin-6, and tumor necrosis factor-α in plasma; interleukin-6 and tumor necrosis factor-α levels correlate with the degree of hepatic inflammation, whereas interleukin-1 levels are similar in patients with both active alcoholic hepatitis and inactive alcoholic cirrhosis. Despite the fact that all three cytokines can contribute to the symptoms of alcoholic hepatitis, only tumor necrosis factor-α has been implicated as a true mediator of liver injury.

Several observations point to tumor necrosis factor-α as a mediator of hepatocellular injury in alcoholics. In experimental animals, ethanol feeding stimulates hepatic expression of tumor necrosis factor-α mRNA before inducing hepatocellular necrosis and inflammation; similarly, in alcoholic patients, circulating tumor necrosis factor-α levels increase during periods of hepatic inflammation and correlate with a poor prognosis. These findings coincide with other data indicating that tumor necrosis factor-α has cytotoxic potential toward hepatocytes.

Another cytokine with a presumptive role in alcoholic liver disease is interleukin-8. Interleukin-8 is not directly toxic to liver cells but may cause liver damage by recruiting neutrophils to the hepatic parenchyma and promoting their release of proteolytic enzymes and superoxide. Neutrophil chemoattractants are of particular interest to the pathogenesis of alcoholic liver disease because the neutrophilic infiltrate of alcoholic hepatitis distinguishes it from many other types of liver disease.

Interleukin-8 is elevated in the plasma of patients with acute alcoholic hepatitis. It has also been identified by immunohistochemical studies in the livers of alcoholics, although it is uncertain whether this signifies local production of interleukin-8 or merely uptake of the cytokine from plasma. Recent studies suggest that hepatocytes produce interleukin-8 in response to ethanol oxidation. Ethanol metabolism by liver cells also leads to production of an arachidonic acid metabolite that is chemotactic for neutrophils. The role of this compound in alcoholics in vivo, as well as its efficacy in comparison with interleukin-8, is still unknown.

2. Immune responses to altered hepatocellular proteins—Chronic ethanol ingestion may lead to autoimmune liver injury by inducing cellular or humoral responses to various proteins. The targets of these immune responses are hepatocellular proteins altered in vivo by ethanol, such as acetaldehyde-protein adducts or Mallory bodies (see following section, "Histology"). Antibodies directed against these compounds can be found in the serum of alcoholic patients; in some cases, they are used as markers of alcohol consumption. It remains controversial, however, whether autoantibodies actually contribute to alcoholic liver injury. One problem related to the immune theory of alcoholic liver injury is that most of the autoantibodies identified to date in alcoholics are directed against *intracellular* proteins. This makes it difficult to envision how the antibodies reach their target antigens and lead to cytotoxicity. Antibodies directed against plasma membrane antigens may more readily provoke liver injury; recent studies have identified antibodies against membrane antigens, including LMA and P450ZE1. Ongoing studies are searching for other acetaldehyde-protein adducts that could lead to liver injury by an autoimmune mechanism.

Cell-mediated immune responses to acetaldehyde-protein adducts or Mallory bodies may also lead to alcoholic liver injury. In vitro, acetaldehyde-modified liver membranes stimulate neutrophils to degranulate and produce superoxide; likewise, Mallory bodies, when incubated with lymphocytes in culture, induce activation and cytokine production. Whether the same cell-mediated responses occur in alcoholics in vivo is unknown.

D. Mechanisms of Fibrosis (Table 40–1): The deposition of excess connective tissue in the liver may be mediated by some of the same compounds that induce hepatocellular injury in alcoholics. The main effectors of fibrosis are hepatic lipocytes (Ito cells, stellate cells, fat-storing cells), which are mesenchymal liver cells that reside in the space of Disse. Acetaldehyde and lipid aldehydes both promote collagen synthesis by lipocytes; these compounds may either be produced by lipocytes (which have a modest capacity to oxidize ethanol) or released from hepatocytes during ethanol metabolism. Transforming growth factor-β may also be an important stimulus to hepatic fibrosis in alcoholics; this fibrogenic cytokine is produced by Kupffer's cells in response to chronic ethanol ingestion, and is a potent inducer of lipocyte collagen synthesis. Oxyradicals are toxic to lipocytes; in low concentrations they may stimulate collagen production.

Friedman SL: The cellular basis of hepatic fibrosis: Mechanisms and treatment strategies. N Engl J Med 1993;328:1828.

Klassen LW et al: Detection of reduced acetaldehyde protein adducts using a unique monoclonal antibody. Alcohol Clin Exp Res 1994;18:164.

Lieber CS: Biochemical factors in alcoholic liver disease. Semin Liver Dis 1993;13:136.

Maher JJ: Hepatic fibrosis caused by alcohol. Semin Liver Dis 1990;10:66.

McClain C et al: Cytokines and alcoholic liver disease. Semin Liver Dis 1993;13:170.

Cofactors Implicated in Alcoholic Liver Disease

In an effort to explain why only a small proportion of alcoholics develop serious liver disease, confounding variables have been sought that might contribute to end-organ damage in the large population at risk. Numerous cofactors have been implicated in the pathogenesis of alcoholic liver disease, including inherited differences in ethanol metabolism, nutritional abnormalities (eg, protein-calorie malnutrition, antioxidant depletion, and iron overload), and concomitant infection with hepatitis viruses. One or more of these variables is often present in alcoholics with liver disease (Table 40–2).

A. Hereditary Factors: A number of investigators have attempted to identify subpopulations of alcoholics at high risk for liver disease by examining their histocompatibility antigen profiles. Although several antigens of the A and B classes are more

Table 40–2. Cofactors implicated in the pathogenesis of alcoholic liver disease.

Cofactor	Means of Enhancing Liver Injury
Inherited variations in ADH, ALDH	Rapid ethanol oxidation Slow acetaldehyde elimination
Female gender	Diminished gastric ethanol metabolism
Nutrition	Enhanced lipid peroxidation via (1) Antioxidant depletion (2) Increased iron stores (3) (?) Increased polyunsaturated fat
Viral hepatitis	(?) Enhanced viral replication
Cigarette smoking	(?)

common in patients with liver injury than in those without injury, none has proved to be a reliable predictor of disease risk. More recently, investigators have focused on inherited differences in ethanol and acetaldehyde *metabolism* as potential contributors to alcoholic liver injury. Variations in ethanol metabolism may be caused by genetic polymorphisms of ADH, ALDH, or cytochrome P4502E1. ADH is a homodimeric enzyme with at least three alleles encoding the hepatic enzyme; studies suggest that variations in ADH phenotype among individuals can result in three- to 10-fold differences in the ethanol elimination rate. Interestingly, it appears that individuals with the most rapid elimination rates may be at higher risk of alcoholic liver disease. ALDH polymorphisms have also been linked to alcoholic liver injury, but in this case, the allele that results in slow acetaldehyde elimination appears to be responsible. The ALDH2*2 allele, which is present in about 50% of Chinese and Japanese persons, is completely inactive toward acetaldehyde. Patients homozygous for ALDH2*2 experience a severe flushing reaction after drinking ethanol and generally avoid ethanol completely. Patients heterozygous for ALDH2*2, however, occasionally abuse ethanol, and these individuals develop liver injury more frequently and with lower alcohol intake than patients with a normal ALDH phenotype.

B. Gender: Women are more susceptible to alcoholic liver injury than men. Studies suggest that women who consume 80 g/d of ethanol begin to display signs of liver disease after as short a time as 10 years; women consuming smaller quantities of ethanol can also develop liver injury over longer periods of time (eg, 40 g/d of ethanol for 20 years). This predisposition to alcoholic liver disease is unexplained. Some have attempted to connect the increased risk to gastric ethanol metabolism, which is slower in women than in men; this means that in women, a larger proportion of ingested ethanol escapes gastric metabolism and enters the portal circulation. The relative paucity of gastric ADH in women explains why they display higher blood ethanol levels than men after drinking similar quantities of ethanol; it may not fully explain their predisposition to alcoholic liver injury. Behavioral scientists argue that the higher blood ethanol levels achieved in women should act as a negative stimulus to further ethanol consumption, and thus limit the total dose of ethanol consumed.

C. Nutrition: The role of nutrition in the pathogenesis of alcoholic liver injury is quite controversial. Studies in baboons indicate that ethanol can induce liver injury despite adequate protein-calorie and vitamin nutrition; clinical studies, however, suggest that alcoholic liver injury correlates strongly and inversely with nutritional status. Despite the fact that malnutrition portends a poor prognosis in alcoholic hepatitis, it remains to be determined whether it is a precipitating factor in the development of alcoholic liver disease. Malnutrition could facilitate alcoholic liver injury by several mechanisms. Depletion of antioxidant vitamins could lead to enhanced oxidative stress in the livers of alcoholics; vitamins A and E in particular are known to be depleted by chronic ethanol consumption. A diet high in polyunsaturated fat may also enhance the risk of alcoholic liver injury by permitting the accumulation in the liver of substrates for ethanol-induced lipid peroxidation. Chronic ethanol ingestion enhances absorption of iron from the gut and increases hepatic iron stores. Given the importance of iron in free radical production during the metabolism of ethanol and acetaldehyde, it too provides a means of enhancing ethanol-induced oxidative liver injury.

D. Viral Hepatitis: There is general agreement among all investigators that hepatitis C virus infection contributes importantly to liver injury in alcoholics. Roughly 18–25% of alcoholics are infected with this virus. In some instances, infection has been reported to correlate strongly with the presence of advanced liver disease (40% of cirrhotics are positive for hepatitis C virus as compared with 25% with nonfibrotic liver injury). This is not the case in all series; curiously, it seems to hold true in Europe but not in the United States. Two groups from the United States find a constant percentage of hepatitis C virus seropositivity in alcoholics with a broad range of disease severity. They admit, however, that alcoholics infected with hepatitis C virus appear to develop liver injury at a younger age and with a lower cumulative intake of ethanol than those who are not infected.

Hepatitis B virus infection also increases the incidence of chronic liver injury in alcoholics. Epidemiologic data suggest that hepatitis B poses an additive, rather than synergistic, risk of liver injury in combination with alcohol. Hepatitis C and alcohol may be a more serious combination; basic scientific studies indicate that alcohol enhances hepatitis C virus replication.

E. Excess Hepatic Iron: Alcoholics with liver disease frequently exhibit increased serum iron saturation, and liver biopsy may reveal quantitative iron

levels as high as 5000 μg/g of dry liver weight. These abnormalities are likely due to increased intestinal absorption of dietary iron or increased hepatic uptake of transferrin-bound iron, or both. In the setting of ethanol oxidation, iron catalyzes several reactions that lead to free radical production (see previous section, "Pathophysiology"); excess iron can enhance these processes and lead to oxidative liver injury. It is interesting to note that patients with hereditary hemochromatosis, who progressively accumulate hepatic iron with age, develop cirrhosis at an early age if they also abuse alcohol.

F. Cigarette Smoking; Coffee Drinking: Alcoholics who smoke more than one pack of cigarettes per day have three times the risk of cirrhosis as those who do not smoke. By contrast, alcoholics who consume four or more cups of coffee daily have a fivefold lower incidence of cirrhosis than those who do not drink coffee. The reason for the synergistic effect of smoking and the protective effect of coffee is uncertain; the effect of coffee is unrelated to caffeine, as tea drinking does not afford the same benefit.

Bosron WF, Ehrig T, Li TK: Genetic factors in alcohol metabolism and alcoholism. Semin Liver Dis 1993;13:126.

Caldwell SH et al: Hepatitis C infection by polymerase chain reaction in alcoholics: False-positive ELISA results and the influence of infection on a clinical prognostic score. Am J Gastroenterol 1993;88:1016.

Frezza M et al: High blood alcohol levels in women: The role of decreased gastric alcohol dehydrogenase activity and first-pass metabolism. N Engl J Med 1990;322:95.

Klatsky AL, Armstrong MA: Alcohol, smoking, coffee, and cirrhosis. Am J Epidemiol 1992;136:1248.

Mendenhall CL et al: Protein-calorie malnutrition associated with alcoholic hepatitis. Veterans Administration Cooperative Study Group on Alcoholic Hepatitis. Am J Med 1984;76:211.

Mendenhall CL et al: Relevance of anti-HCV reactivity in patients with alcoholic hepatitis. Veterans Administration Cooperative Study Group #275. Gastroenterol Jpn 1993;28(Suppl 5):95.

Nalpas B et al: Association between HCV and HBV infection in hepatocellular carcinoma and alcoholic liver disease. J Hepatol 1991;12:70.

Stal P, Hultcrantz R: Iron increases ethanol toxicity in rat liver. J Hepatol 1993;17:108.

Clinical Findings

The term alcoholic hepatitis is used to describe the acute clinical manifestations of alcoholic liver disease. In order for this diagnosis to be made, patients should have a significant history of ethanol consumption (approximately 80 g/d of ethanol, preferably for 1 year or more), along with signs or symptoms of active liver injury. Because alcoholics frequently underestimate or deny active alcohol consumption, the only accurate estimation of recent drinking habits may come from family members or acquaintances, who should be interviewed whenever possible. Patients who meet diagnostic criteria for alcoholic hepatitis can exhibit a wide range of disease severity. As shown below, features such as encephalopathy, hyperbilirubinemia, and hypoprothrombinemia are good predictors of advanced injury. Stratification of patients according to the severity of illness is useful for predicting prognosis and planning therapy. The clinical use of the term alcoholic hepatitis is more broad than the histologic use; in fact, patients with clinical alcoholic hepatitis may have a combination of steatosis, inflammation, and fibrosis on biopsy. In contrast to histologic findings in the liver, the clinical features of alcoholic hepatitis correlate reliably with patient outcome.

A. Symptoms and Signs: The most common clinical manifestation of alcoholic liver disease is hepatomegaly. Liver enlargement can be detected in more than 75% of patients who are actively drinking, and is observed consistently at all stages of liver injury. Hepatomegaly is related in part to the accumulation of fat within liver cells; this may explain its presence even in patients with mild disease. Hepatocyte swelling, rather than steatosis, is believed to be the major cause of liver enlargement in moderately or severely ill patients.

1. Mild disease—The symptoms of mild alcoholic liver disease are vague, with anorexia and weight loss predominating (Table 40–3). These symptoms are present in only one-third of patients, making a history of heavy ethanol consumption important for establishing a diagnosis. Ascites is detectable in 30% of patients; this may be due to hepatomegaly and resultant "acute" portal hypertension, even in the absence of cirrhosis. Altered mentation may be indicative of hepatic encephalopathy. Fewer than one-fourth of patients with mild alcoholic liver injury complain of abdominal pain.

2. Moderate to severe disease—Patients with moderate to severe alcoholic liver disease exhibit different signs and symptoms, with jaundice, ascites, and encephalopathy predominating (Table 40–3). Jaundice is a good predictor of disease severity, as it is present in 100% of patients with mild to moderate

disease but only 17% of patients with mild disease. Ascites is detectable in over three-fourths of patients, and encephalopathy in over half. Another important feature of alcoholic hepatitis is fever, which is present in roughly 25% of patients and does not necessarily predict infection. Diffuse abdominal pain is distinctly uncommon, and should raise concern about concurrent peritonitis.

B. Laboratory Findings: Derangements can be found in both the hematologic and biochemical profiles of alcoholics (Table 40–4). Patients with alcoholic hepatitis are often anemic (average hematocrit 36%); over three-fourths exhibit macrocytosis (mean corpuscular volume $102mm^3$). Leukocytosis is also common in alcoholic hepatitis, particularly in patients with moderate to severe disease.

Hepatic transaminases are only modestly elevated in alcoholic hepatitis; regardless of disease severity, aspartate aminotransferase (AST) and alanine aminotransferase (ALT) rarely exceed 500 IU/L. Elevations significantly greater than 500 IU/L should raise concern about other or concurrent causes of liver injury (eg, drug toxicity or ischemia).

The ratio of AST to ALT is helpful in distinguishing alcoholic from nonalcoholic liver disease. Patients with alcoholic hepatitis often have an AST:ALT ratio of more than 2; this is in contrast to patients with viral hepatitis, in which the ratio is commonly less than 1 (Figure 40–3). An AST:ALT ratio between 1 and 2 is not diagnostic of alcoholic liver disease; such ratios can be seen in patients with nonalcoholic hepatitis and postnecrotic cirrhosis. A ratio of more than 3 is very suggestive of alcoholic liver injury.

It is important to note that active drinkers who develop acute nonalcoholic liver injury will often display elevated AST:ALT ratios in serum. A classic example of this phenomenon is acetaminophen poisoning, which in alcoholics causes AST elevation in marked disproportion to ALT. The reason for the discrepancy is that chronic alcohol consumption, even in the absence of liver disease, alters the proportion

Table 40–3. Clinical manifestations of alcoholic liver disease.[1]

Sign or Symptom	MIld Disease (%)	Moderate to Severe Disease (%)
Hepatomegaly	84	80–95
Jaundice	17	100
Ascites	30	79–86
Anorexia	39	57–60
Encephalopathy	27	55–70
Alcohol withdrawal	36	15–30
Weight loss	37	8–28

[1]Excerpted from Mendenhall CL. Alcoholic hepatitis. Clinics in Gastroenterology 1981;10:417–441.

Table 40–4. Laboratory abnormalities in alcoholic liver disease.[1]

Laboratory Test	Mild Disease	Moderate Disease	Severe Disease
Hematocrit	38	36	33
WBC (thousand)	8	11	12
AST (mU/ml)	84	124	99
ALT (mU/ml)	56	56	57
Alkaline phosphatase (IU/ml)	166	276	225
Bilirubin (mg/kl)	1.6	13.5	8.7
Prothrombin time (sec over control)	0.9	2.4	6.4
Albumin (g/dl)	3.7	2.7	2.4

[1]Excerpted from Mendenhall CL. Alcoholic hepatitis. Clinics in Gastroenterology 1981;10:422.

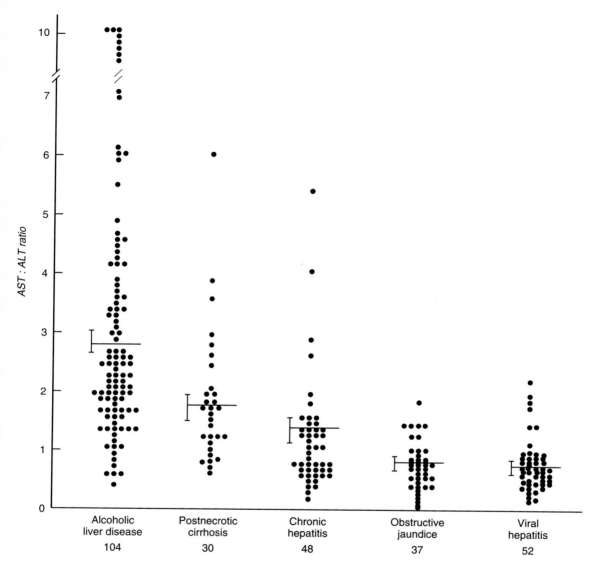

Figure 40–3. AST:ALT ratios in alcoholic and nonalcoholic liver disease. (Reproduced, with permission, from Cohen JA, Kaplan MM: The SGOT/SGPT ratio: An indicator of alcoholic liver disease. Dig Dis Sci 1979;24:835.)

of AST to ALT in hepatocytes. Consequently, when active drinkers contract acute liver disease, they are prone to release more AST than ALT into the circulation. This tendency is present regardless of the cause of the acute liver injury.

The laboratory parameters that are most useful in predicting the severity of alcoholic liver injury are bilirubin levels, prothrombin time, and perhaps albumin levels. The first two have been used to formulate a "discriminant function" (defined as [4.6 × (prothrombin time-control)] + bilirubin); when the result is greater than 32, a mortality rate of 50% can be predicted within 1 month. Similar criteria were used to subdivide alcoholic patients into the mild, moderate,

and severe disease categories displayed in Tables 40–3 and 40–4. Of note is that the level of serum bilirubin, once a value of 5 mg/dL has been reached, does not correlate with disease severity. The prothrombin time increases progressively with worsening illness.

Other laboratory tests have been evaluated as markers of alcohol consumption or alcoholic liver injury but are not yet used in clinical practice. These include mitochondrial AST, carbohydrate-deficient transferrin, and serum markers of connective tissue metabolism such as collagen propeptides and tissue inhibitor of metalloproteinase. Carbohydrate-deficient transferrin appears to be useful for detecting recent ethanol consumption; the collagen propeptides, despite their relationship to collagen metabolism, distinguish patients with alcoholic hepatitis more reliably than those with alcoholic fibrosis. The overall objective in searching for new parameters is to develop reliable noninvasive methods for diagnosing alcoholism and alcoholic liver injury.

C. Imaging Studies: There are no characteristic radiographic features of alcoholic liver disease. The most common finding is hepatic steatosis, detectable by increased echogenicity on sonography or by extremely low attenuation of the liver on CT scan.

Histology

Ideally, a diagnosis of alcoholic liver disease should be based on histologic findings. In practice, many physicians dispense with liver biopsy when clinical clues strongly suggest alcohol-related illness. If alcoholic liver disease is suspected on the basis of clinical and laboratory information, the diagnosis is correct in approximately 90% of cases. Liver biopsy is still quite useful, however, in distinguishing other types of liver injury that often coexist in alcoholics (eg, chronic hepatitis in patients coinfected with hepatitis C virus). Liver biopsy is helpful in determining the extent of fibrosis in patients with good synthetic function. In the early stages of alcoholic liver injury, perivenular fibrosis can portend progression to hepatic fibrosis and ultimately cirrhosis. Cardinal features of alcoholic liver injury that can be recognized with light microscopic studies include steatosis, ballooning of hepatocytes, Mallory bodies, an inflammatory infiltrate in which neutrophils are prominent, and fibrosis. The first four features are frequently observed together, while fibrosis may be absent, mild, or extensive.

Steatosis, which connotes the presence of fat droplets in hepatocytes, is present in almost 100% of patients with alcoholic liver injury. Alcoholic steatosis is most prominent in pericentral zones, but in severe cases exhibits a panlobular distribution. The classic pattern of alcoholic steatosis is macrovesicular, with the large fat droplets pushing hepatocyte nuclei into an eccentric position. Despite this, a recent survey showed that alcoholic steatosis often is both macrovesicular and microvesicular. In microvesicular steatosis, small fat droplets fill the hepatocyte cytoplasm but leave the nucleus in a central position. This pattern of steatosis has also been termed "alcoholic foamy degeneration."

Ballooning degeneration of hepatocytes describes marked cell swelling, with a pale, often granular appearance of the cytoplasm. This pattern is not unique to alcoholic liver disease but can also be observed in many conditions that result in hepatocellular necrosis. Like steatosis, ballooning degeneration in alcoholic liver injury is most prominent pericentrally. In association with ballooned hepatocytes, one may see acidophil bodies, which are small, densely eosinophilic structures that represent apoptotic hepatocytes. Hepatocyte ballooning can be detected in over 75% of patients with clinical alcoholic liver injury.

Mallory bodies are crescent-shaped, eosinophilic structures that often wrap around the nucleus of hepatocytes. They represent a condensation of intermediate filaments, particularly cytokeratins, within the cytoplasm of hepatocytes. Mallory bodies are found in 76% of patients undergoing biopsy for alcoholic liver disease; they can be distinguished by periodic acid–Schiff (PAS) staining from enlarged mitochondria, which can also be present in alcoholics (mitochondria stain positive; Mallory bodies stain negative). Because Mallory bodies are seen in patients with primary biliary cirrhosis and Wilson's disease as well as alcoholic liver disease, and can be induced by drugs such as griseofulvin or amiodarone, their presence is not diagnostic of alcoholic liver injury.

Neutrophils are often present in the livers of alcoholics and are commonly found in the pericentral zones, adjacent to fatty or ballooned hepatocytes. Neutrophils are rarely found in nonalcoholic liver disease. Mononuclear cell infiltrates can also be observed pericentrally in alcoholics; at times, the pattern suggests chronic active hepatitis, which may reflect infection with hepatitis C or B virus.

Fibrosis in alcoholic liver injury begins with deposition of connective tissue around the terminal hepatic venule. As the lesion progresses, connective tissue extends into the hepatic parenchyma, surrounding hepatocytes in a "chicken-wire" fashion. Pericellular fibrosis is quite delicate and may be detectable only with special stains such as the Masson trichrome stain. In advanced fibrosis, bridging is common, involving central or portal veins, or both. Cirrhosis connotes distortion of the parenchyma into nodules, usually less than 1 cm in size, that are completely surrounded by bands of connective tissue. Moderate to severe fibrosis can be detected in roughly half of patients with alcoholic liver injury.

For diagnostic and investigational purposes, liver histologic findings in alcoholics can be arranged in categories such as fatty liver, alcoholic hepatitis, cirrhosis, and cirrhosis with alcoholic hepatitis. Histologic classification of patients with alcoholic hepatitis, however, does not always correlate well with the severity of clinical disease.

Differential Diagnosis

A. Nonalcoholic Steatohepatitis: Patients who do not abuse ethanol can develop liver disease that is clinically and histologically indistinguishable from alcoholic hepatitis. This entity is termed nonalcoholic steatohepatitis, and occurs in patients who are obese, diabetic, or taking medications such as estrogens, diethylstilbestrol, glucocorticoids, or amiodarone (see Chapter 45). It has also been reported after jejunoileal bypass surgery and in patients receiving total parenteral nutrition. Nonalcoholic steatohepatitis affects women predominantly (81%); it is often asymptomatic (77%) and is discovered only by elevation of hepatic transaminases. Patients do not commonly have an exaggerated AST:ALT ratio (> 3 in only 32% of cases). On histologic examination, they tend to have less severe inflammation and less fibrosis than patients with alcoholic liver disease.

B. Hemochromatosis: In patients who display high serum iron saturations and have siderosis on liver biopsy, there may be some difficulty in distinguishing alcoholic liver disease from hereditary hemochromatosis. Differentiation can be made by measuring hepatic iron levels and calculating a "hepatic iron index" ([μg hepatic iron divided by 58] divided by age in years). An index of greater than 2 indicates hereditary hemochromatosis (see Chapter 41).

Cohen JA, Kaplan MM: The SGOT/SGPT ratio: An indicator of alcoholic liver disease. Dig Dis Sci 1979;24:835.

Diehl AM et al: Relationship between pyridoxal 5′-phosphate deficiency and aminotransferase levels in alcoholic hepatitis. Gastroenterology 1984;86:632.

French SW et al: Pathology of alcoholic liver disease. Veterans Administration Cooperative Study Group 119. Semin Liver Dis 1993;13:154.

Mendenhall CL: Alcoholic hepatitis. Clin Gastroenterol 1981;10:417.

Complications

The complications of alcoholic liver disease are similar to those encountered in nonalcoholic chronic liver disease. Ascites, gastrointestinal hemorrhage, and encephalopathy are related to portal hypertension; coagulopathy and hypoalbuminemia arise from hepatocellular dysfunction. Hypoglycemia can occur in malnourished patients who are actively drinking; it may also be a sign of overt liver failure.

There is some uncertainty as to whether alcoholic cirrhosis predisposes patients to hepatocellular carcinoma. Although 80% of all patients with hepatocellular carcinoma have underlying cirrhosis, some studies suggest that the risk is borne primarily by patients with postnecrotic cirrhosis and those with hereditary diseases such as hemochromatosis. Others suggest that alcohol is a risk factor for hepatocellular carcinoma, even when it is separated from cofactors such as viral hepatitis. At present, there is no strong indication for screening patients with alcoholic cirrhosis for hepatocellular carcinoma if they do not also have hepatitis C infection.

Treatment

The mainstay of treatment for alcoholic liver disease is abstinence. Abstinence substantially improves the survival time of patients, even those with cirrhosis and portal hypertension at the time of diagnosis (see following section, "Prognosis"). For patients with severe alcoholic hepatitis, whose short-term mortality rate is high, pharmacologic therapy has been tried as an adjunct to abstinence and general supportive care. The utility of certain drugs in the treatment of alcoholic hepatitis is discussed below.

A. Corticosteroids: Patients with severe alcoholic hepatitis, judged either by a discriminant function of more than 32 (see Laboratory Findings above) or by the presence of encephalopathy, benefit from methylprednisolone (32 mg intravenously) or prednisolone (40 mg orally) administered daily for 28 days. Short-term survival rates in treated patients increase from 63% to over 90%. The salutary effect of corticosteroids has been confirmed in numerous clinical trials. Finding adequate candidates for treatment can be difficult; corticosteroids are not recommended for patients with active gastrointestinal hemorrhage, infection, or renal insufficiency. The long-term effect of corticosteroids on liver injury and survival rates is unknown.

B. Nutrition: Nutritional supplements, provided either by the enteral or parenteral route, have been studied as adjuncts to the care of patients with severe alcoholic hepatitis. For the most part, these treatments consist of conventional amino acids, with some protocols substituting branched-chain amino acids and others adding lipid. Alcoholic patients treated with nutritional supplements often display more rapid normalization of biochemical liver tests (AST, bilirubin, albumin) than those receiving standard hospital diets. Such therapy has little or no effect on survival rates. Conventional amino acid preparations are tolerated well by most patients, even those with advanced cirrhosis. They should be the first choice for therapy, with branched-chain amino acids being reserved for patients who develop encephalopathy in response to routine formulas.

C. Propylthiouracil: This drug is advocated for alcoholic hepatitis based on evidence that liver injury is related to a "hypermetabolic state," with increased hepatic oxygen consumption. Controlled trials of propylthiouracil suggest that it significantly increases the survival rates of patients with alcoholic liver injury (87% as compared with 75% at 2 years). Despite this, clinical use of this drug has not expanded, perhaps because of concerns about hypothyroidism or speculation that differences between experimental and control patients were not attributable to the drug (they occurred early, before the expected antithyroid effect of propylthiouracil in euthyroid patients). Clinical trials of this drug in alcoholic liver disease are ongoing.

D. Colchicine: Colchicine (1 mg/d orally for 30 days) is of no benefit in the treatment of acute alcoholic hepatitis. Long-term treatment of cirrhotic patients with colchicine (1 mg/d for up to 14 years), on the other hand, has been reported to significantly improve patient survival rates. To date, the benefit of colchicine has been demonstrated in only one clinical trial. This study has been criticized on several counts, including a high dropout rate, poor documentation of compliance, and uncertainty as to whether deaths in the placebo group were attributable to liver disease. For these reasons, colchicine is not widely used in the treatment of alcoholic liver disease.

E. Polyunsaturated Lecithin: This compound, extracted from soybeans, has been shown to prevent hepatic fibrosis in alcohol-fed baboons. It supposedly acts by stimulating collagenase activity in hepatic lipocytes (stellate cells), thus down-regulating the net amount of collagen deposited by these same cells in alcoholic liver injury. A trial of polyunsaturated lecithin in human alcoholics is currently under way.

F. Liver Transplantation: Transplantation is an option for some patients with end-stage alcoholic liver disease, provided that a defined period of abstinence (preferably 6 months or longer) precedes the surgery (see Chapter 54). Although the ethics surrounding transplantation in alcoholics are quite controversial, reports suggest that the rate of recidivism

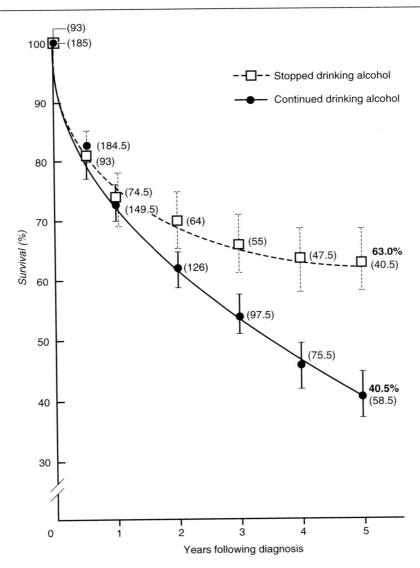

Figure 40–4. Five-year survival rates in patients with alcoholic cirrhosis as a function of ethanol intake. Even in the setting of irreversible hepatic fibrosis, patients who abstain from ethanol *(open squares)* have a significantly better prognosis than those who continue to drink *(closed circles)*. (Reproduced, with permission, from Powell WJ, Klatskin G: Duration of survival in patients with Laennec's cirrhosis: Influence of alcohol withdrawal, and possible effects of recent changes in general management of the disease. Am J Med 1968;44:406.)

in transplanted patients is low (6.7% for patients with > 6 months' abstinence preoperatively). The long-term survival rate of alcoholic patients undergoing transplantation is comparable to that of nonalcoholic patients (60% at 3–5 years).

G. Other Drugs (Cytokine Antagonists; Antioxidants): Based on a growing understanding of the contribution of cytokines and oxidant stress to alcoholic liver injury, therapies such as anticytokine antibodies, cytokine receptor antagonists, and antioxidants are currently under study. To date, their efficacy in alcoholic liver injury is unproved.

Akriviadis EA et al: Failure of colchicine to improve short-term survival in patients with alcoholic hepatitis. Gastroenterology 1990;99:811.

Imperiale TF, McCullough AJ: Do corticosteroids reduce mortality from alcoholic hepatitis? A meta-analysis of the randomized trials. Ann Intern Med 1990;113:299.

Kumar S et al: Orthotopic liver transplantation for alcoholic liver disease. Hepatology 1990;11:159.

Lieber CS et al: Phosphatidylcholine protects against fibrosis and cirrhosis in the baboon. Gastroenterology 1994;106:152.

Orrego H et al: Long-term treatment of alcoholic liver disease with propylthiouracil. Part 2. Influence of drop-out rates and of continued alcohol consumption in a clinical trial. J Hepatol 1994;20:343.

Schenker S, Halff GA: Nutritional therapy in alcoholic liver disease. Semin Liver Dis 1993;13:196.

Prognosis

The outcome of patients with alcoholic liver disease is dependent upon several variables, including (1) the clinical severity of liver injury at diagnosis; (2) the extent of irreversible liver damage (ie, cirrhosis) at diagnosis; and (3) subsequent drinking behavior. Patients with severe alcoholic hepatitis (determined clinically by indices such as the discriminant function) have an estimated mortality rate of 50%; the overall mortality rate of alcoholic hepatitis is roughly 17%. Even in the absence of acute alcoholic hepatitis, alcoholic cirrhosis alone has a negative effect on survival rates (30% mortality rate within 3–5 years, as opposed to an 18% mortality rate in those without cirrhosis). When clinical and histologic parameters are monitored together, cirrhosis with alcoholic hepatitis clearly emerges as the most ominous combination. Patients with both cirrhosis and alcoholic hepatitis have a 5-year mortality rate of approximately 60%.

Abstinence dramatically improves the survival rates of patients with alcoholic liver disease, even if cirrhosis is present at the time of diagnosis. Figure 40–4 demonstrates that patients with alcoholic cirrhosis have a 5-year survival rate approaching 65% with abstinence; if drinking continues, the survival rate drops to 40.5%.

Chedid A et al: Prognostic factors in alcoholic liver disease. Veterans Administration Cooperative Study Group. Am J Gastroenterol 1991;86:210.

Goldberg S et al: Veterans Administration Cooperative Study on Alcoholic Hepatitis. IV. The significance of clinically mild alcoholic hepatitis: Describing the population with minimal hyperbilirubinemia. Am J Gastroenterol 1986;81:1029.

Niemela O et al: Markers of fibrogenesis and basement membrane formation in alcoholic liver disease: Relation to severity, presence of hepatitis, and alcohol intake. Gastroenterology 1990;98:1612.

Orrego H et al: Prognosis of alcoholic cirrhosis in the presence and absence of alcoholic hepatitis. Gastroenterology 1987;92:208.

Powell WJ, Klatskin G: Duration of survival in patients with Laennec's cirrhosis: Influence of alcohol withdrawal, and possible effects of recent changes in general management of the disease. Am J Med 1968;44:406.

Metal Overload Diseases

41

Paul C. Adams, MD

HEMOCHROMATOSIS

Pathophysiology

Hemochromatosis, a genetic disease arising out of Northern Europe, is now recognized as one of the most common autosomal recessive diseases, occurring in 1 in 300 persons in the white population. The cause remains elusive. The hemochromatosis locus has been localized to an area of chromosome 6 closely linked to the HLA complex (6p21.3), but the gene product is unknown. An intestinal defect affecting iron absorption is the most likely cause. Recent studies have described several new iron-binding and regulatory proteins in the intestine and liver in hemochromatosis patients, but the role of these proteins in the pathogenesis of the disease remains to be determined. The progressive accumulation of iron probably results in oxidative damage to parenchymal organs.

Clinical Findings

A. Symptoms and Signs: Because the signs and symptoms of hemochromatosis are nonspecific and occur at a late stage of the disease, patients that would benefit the most from early therapeutic intervention are often undetected. The classic description of "bronze diabetes" is a late and uncommon presentation of the disease that is seen in less than 10% of patients. The clinical presentation of 93 hemochromatosis patients was recently reviewed at the author's center. Abdominal pain (16%), joint pains (11%), and weakness (9%) were prominent features that brought the patient to the physician. Impotence was present in 38% of male patients. Manifestations of liver disease (84%), arthritis (11%), and diabetes (2%) were the signs that led the physician to the diagnosis.

1. Hepatic disease–Hepatomegaly is one of the most common physical signs in this condition. The extent of liver damage depends on the age and sex of the patient. Signs of chronic liver disease can insidiously develop over many years.

2. Articular disease–Arthritis is one of the most common symptoms associated with hemochromatosis. Although chondrocalcinosis is also associated with the disease, a degenerative osteoarthritis involving the metacarpophalangeal joints is the most common articular manifestation. Nonspecific anti-inflammatory therapy is the treatment of choice.

3. Endocrine disease–Diabetes is a late complication of the disease. Early studies implied that iron deposits damaged the pancreatic islet cells, but more detailed studies on insulin metabolism have shown that many hemochromatosis patients have high insulin levels, with insulin resistance similar to that of most patients with type II diabetes. Iron depletion therapy does not usually affect the diabetes.

Endocrine dysfunction is also usually manifested as impotence, which is related to pituitary hypofunction, although testicular atrophy can also occur. Hypothyroidism is a less common endocrine manifestation. Testosterone therapy is often ineffective in the treatment of impotence.

4. Cardiac disease–Cardiac disease is one of the less common presenting features, although some young males may present with life-threatening cardiomyopathy. Future genetic studies may demonstrate that this unusual but dramatic presentation may be a mutation of a more common hemochromatosis gene. Cardiac biopsy of patients in transplantation centers has also led to inadvertent discovery of the disease. Iron depletion can lead to marked improvement in cardiac function. Cardiac arrhythmias have also been described, particularly during major surgery.

B. Laboratory Findings:

1. AST and ALT–Mild abnormalities in aspartate aminotransferase (AST) and alanine aminotransferase (ALT) have been described in 65% of patients. The mean elevation in AST is typically less than 100 IU/L in both cirrhotic and noncirrhotic patients, however. Hemochromatosis is not associated with extensive liver inflammation and hepatocyte necrosis. Thus, the patient with marked elevations in AST and ALT in association with increased serum ferritin or transferrin saturations (or both) is unlikely to have hemochromatosis alone but rather some other inflammatory disease.

2. Serum ferritin and transferrin—Patients can be readily screened for hemochromatosis with serum ferritin and transferrin saturation (serum iron per total iron-binding capacity). Serum iron alone is an unreliable marker for the disease. The transferrin saturation is usually abnormal at a young age, and the ferritin saturation rises progressively with age. Females will have a lower serum ferritin level because of menstruation. In the author's series, the mean serum ferritin level at the time of diagnosis in male probands was 2911 μg/L and in females 1499 μg/L. The combination of serum ferritin and transferrin saturations has a sensitivity of 94% and a specificity of 86% but only within a known hemochromatosis family. Serum ferritin can be elevated in both acute and chronic inflammation as well as in certain tumors (Table 41–1). Extreme elevations (> 100,000 μg/L) can be seen in malignant histiocytosis, and this has led to speculation that macrophages are the source of serum ferritin. Heterozygous patients do not develop progressive iron overload, although 10–15% may have minor elevations in serum ferritin or transferrin saturations (or both) (Figure 41–1).

3. Iron staining—The liver biopsy is the "gold standard" for the diagnosis of hemochromatosis. Iron staining shows excess parenchymal iron deposition. At advanced stages of the disease, there may be portal fibrosis, cirrhosis, bile duct iron deposition, and hepatocellular carcinoma. Iron-free foci may represent a premalignant lesion. The hepatic iron concentration can be measured from the paraffin block by means of atomic absorption spectrophotometry; this is a more accurate method of assessing the degree of iron loading than iron staining. Hemochromatosis patients will have at least twice as much iron as patients with alcoholic siderosis of the same age. This has been expressed as the hepatic iron index ((μmol/g)/age) and is usually greater than 2 in homozygotes.

4. HLA typing—HLA typing has been used as a surrogate genetic test for hemochromatosis because of the close linkage between the hemochromatosis gene and the HLA complex. HLA typing predicts the risk of developing iron overload in siblings, whereas serum ferritin levels are directly related to the degree of iron overload. Although HLA-A3 is seen in 75% of hemochromatosis patients, it should not be used as a diagnostic test for hemochromatosis. HLA typing is most valuable in the investigation of siblings of a proband case. HLA-identical siblings nearly always

already have or will develop iron overloading. Siblings that share one HLA haplotype will be heterozygotes, and siblings that share no haplotypes are extremely unlikely to develop iron overloading. The cost effectiveness of HLA typing depends on the age of the proband and is most useful in a young family. Patients are often most concerned about their children, who will be carriers but will not develop iron overload unless the patient's spouse is an occult heterozygote. Children can be readily screened for the disease as teenagers by means of serum ferritin and transferrin saturation.

C. Population Screening for Hemochromatosis: Because hemochromatosis is a common disease that can be detected by simple blood tests, some have advocated screening of the general population for this disease. Widespread screening has been studied in blood donors and in inpatient and outpatient clinics using serum ferritin and transferrin saturations. Selective screening strategies in arthritis and diabetes clinics have also been studied. Because patients who are diagnosed in the precirrhotic stage of the disease have survival rates similar to those of the general population, early diagnosis and therapy based on these relatively inexpensive screening tests can be highly advantageous to the individual patient. The lack of specificity of the blood tests will result in some patients without the disease undergoing liver biopsy and some patients with the disease remaining undetected, depending on the threshold used to pursue further investigations. For the primary care physician, it would be reasonable to screen all patients with any symptoms, abnormal liver enzyme, or a family history of the disease using serum ferritin and transferrin saturation.

Patients with cirrhosis of the liver are at risk for hepatocellular carcinoma. In a collected series of 649 cirrhotic hemochromatosis patients, hepatocellular carcinoma was described in 18.5%. This is similar to the prevalence in other types of cirrhosis such as that of hepatitis B and C and suggests that cirrhosis is the major risk factor rather than iron overload. Although screening studies for hepatocellular carcinoma in hemochromatosis patients with alpha-fetoprotein measurements and ultrasound have led to earlier detection, the therapeutic options of resection, chemoembolization, and transplantation are often not curative.

D. Imaging Studies: Abdominal imaging (CT and MRI scanning) can detect moderate to severe iron overload. The current lack of sensitivity of available imaging methods limits their usefulness in the detection of early disease, and these studies do not alleviate the need for diagnostic liver biopsy. It has been estimated that up to 40% of hemochromatosis patients would be missed because of the lack of sensitivity of these methods, but the occasional patient will be identified when scanning is done for another abdominal problem.

Table 41–1. Causes of elevated serum ferritin levels.

Hereditary hemochromatosis
Chronic hepatitis
Alcoholic liver disease
Histiocytosis
Hepatocellular carcinoma
Hyperthyroidism
Adult Still's disease
Chronic inflammation

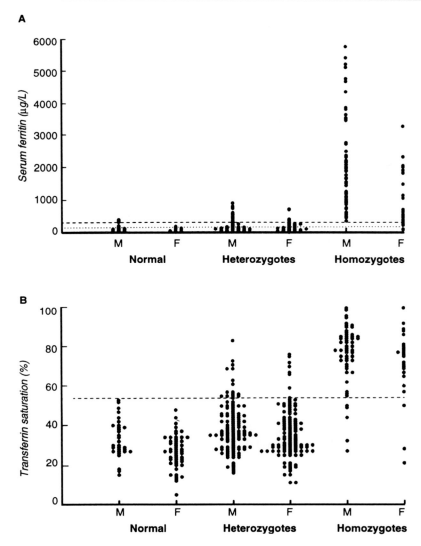

Figure 41–1. **A:** Serum ferritin in normal patients, putative heterozygotes and putative homozygotes for hemochromatosis (M = male, F = female). The reference range was 15–200 µg/L for females and 30–350 µg/L for males. The dotted lines represent the upper limit of normal in males (-------) and females (·····). **B:** Transferrin saturation (%) in normal patients, putative heterozygotes and putative homozygotes for hemochromatosis (M = male, F = female). The reference range was 20–55%. The dotted line represents the upper limit of the reference range. (Reproduced, with permission, from Adams PC: Am J Hematol 1994;45:147.)

Differential Diagnosis

Confusion persists about the differential diagnosis of iron overload, particularly in a patient who consumes alcohol heavily. In an era of intensive diagnostic evaluations, it is alarming to note that in many major centers in the United States, hemochromatosis is diagnosed initially at the time of liver transplantation.

As previously noted, hemochromatosis is strongly suggested by a marked elevation in the serum ferritin and transferrin saturation. The two major problems associated with these tests are the failure to order

them in the first place and the misinterpretation of mild abnormalities. A typical clinical presentation that often creates confusion is a middle-aged patient with a mild elevation in serum ferritin (< 1000 µg/L), a borderline elevation in serum transferrin, significant alcohol consumption, and no family history of hemochromatosis. The clinical diagnosis is alcoholic liver disease, but the elevated iron levels raise the possibility of hemochromatosis. A concomitant rise in the erythrocyte sedimentation rate or C-reactive protein level suggests that the ferritin elevation may be secondary to inflammation rather than iron overload. If the clinical suspicion for hemochromatosis is low, it is reasonable to reassess the serum ferritin at a later date. Homozygotes for hemochromatosis will have a progressive rise in serum ferritin levels of 50–100 µg/L/year. A rising ferritin level is an indication for percutaneous liver biopsy.

At a center where hemochromatosis is a common diagnosis, there is usually little doubt from the biopsy about the diagnosis. An older patient with cirrhosis from hemochromatosis has such marked iron staining that the diagnosis can be made by gross inspection of the slide without using the microscope! At centers where there are fewer cases of hemochromatosis and many cases of alcoholic liver disease, biopsies with characteristic features of alcoholic liver disease (fat, Mallory's hyaline bodies, and polymorphonuclear infiltration) (Figure 41–2) and mild to moderate iron deposition on staining still create some diagnostic confusion. Although alcoholic liver disease can coexist with hemochromatosis, in the author's experience, the relationship between alcoholism and hemochromatosis has been overemphasized, and the hemochromatosis literature historically has erroneously included patients who actually have alcoholic siderosis rather than hemochromatosis. The hepatic iron index can be useful in differentiating alcoholic siderosis from hereditary hemochromatosis (Table 41–2). This index has not been extensively validated in other nonalcoholic liver diseases in the differential diagnosis of hepatic iron overload (eg, thalassemia, transfusional iron overload, and porphyria cutanea tarda) and following portacaval shunting (Table 41–3).

Another strategy in the alcoholic patient is to investigate siblings with serum ferritin and transferrin saturation and HLA typing. If an HLA-identical sibling who does not drink alcohol has normal ferritin and transferrin saturations, this strongly suggests alcoholic siderosis rather than hemochromatosis in the proband case. Alcoholic siderosis should also be reconsidered in an older patient who becomes anemic (< 10 g/dL) after less than 10 venesections have been done, because in a patient with hemochromatosis, the number of venesections required usually increases with age. An increasing number of patients with chronic hepatitis (hepatitis B or C or idiopathic hepatitis) have been found to have elevated ferritin and transferrin saturation with mild elevations in hepatic iron concentration. Some of these patients may be heterozygous for hemochromatosis, and this could be confirmed if a true genetic test became available.

Treatment

A. Venesection: The goal of therapy is to deplete iron stores to prevent any further tissue damage. Patients begin a program of weekly venesections of approximately 500 mL. The author determines the hemoglobin at the time of each venesection and proceeds with the next venesection if the hemoglobin is

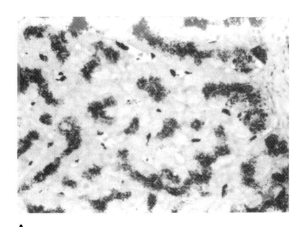

A

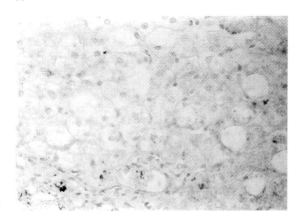

B

Figure 41–2. Comparative liver biopsies from a patient with **(A)** hereditary hemochromatosis and **(B)** alcoholic siderosis. The degree of iron overload is much greater in the hemochromatosis patient. The alcoholic patient of a similar age has much less stainable iron, iron in Kupffer cells and hepatocytes, polymorphonuclear infiltrates, and fat. (Photomicrographs courtesy of J Frei.)

greater than 10 g/dL. A mild anemia (10–12 g/dL) is common throughout therapy and stimulates erythropoiesis and iron mobilization. Serum ferritin levels are monitored every 3 months, and venesections are continued until the level is approximately 50 µg/L. Young patients can often tolerate two venesections per week, whereas elderly patients may tolerate only one venesection every 2 weeks. The duration of therapy depends on the age of the patient and the iron burden at the time of diagnosis. Weekly venesection therapy can last for as long as 3 years in an older male proband or as little as a few months in a young female.

Following depletion of iron stores, patients can begin a maintenance program of 3–4 venesections per year on a lifelong basis. The interval between vene-

Table 41–2. Differentiation between hereditary hemochromatosis and alcoholic siderosis.[1]

Clinical Feature	Hemochromatosis	Alcoholic Siderosis
Serum ferritin (15–350 µg/L)	> 1500 µg/L[2]	< 1500 µg/L
Liver pathologic findings	Hepatocyte iron	Fatty change, Mallory's hyaline bodies, polymorphonuclear leucocytes, hepatocyte and Kupffer cell iron
Hepatic iron (< 35 µmol/g)	200–800 µmol/g	40–100 µmol/g
Iron index (iron/age)	> 2	< 2
Sibling investigation	Positive	Negative

[1]Reproduced, with permission, from Adams PC: Can J Diagnosis 1993;10:132.
[2]Serum ferritin in hemochromatosis is dependent on the age and sex of the patient. The example shown would be typical for a 50-year-old male patient.

sections can be adjusted based on an annual serum ferritin measurement. An alternative approach is to follow the serum ferritin level annually and restart weekly venesections when it becomes abnormal.

B. Chelation Therapy: Chelation therapy with deferoxamine is reserved for the patient with iron overload secondary to iron-loading anemia, and oral iron chelators have shown promise in children with thalassemia. Despite iron depletion, many of the symptoms such as arthritis, impotence, and diabetes do not improve.

C. Liver Transplantation: Liver transplantation is indicated for patients with end-stage liver disease (see Chapter 54). Preliminary data suggest that hemochromatosis patients have a higher mortality rate following transplantation than other cirrhotic patients because of concomitant cardiac disease and a higher incidence of infection. Initial studies also suggest gradual reaccumulation of iron in the transplanted liver. The inadvertent transplantation of a hemochromatosic liver into a normal recipient resulted in complete mobilization of the excess hepatic iron within the first year following transplantation. This is compelling evidence against an intrahepatic defect

Table 41–3. Differential diagnosis of hepatic iron overload.[1]

Hereditary hemochromatosis
Alcoholic siderosis
Transfusional siderosis
Thalassemia
Sideroblastic anemia
Porphyria cutanea tarda
Bantu siderosis
Portacaval shunting

[1]Reproduced, with permission, from Adams PC: Can J Diagnosis 1993;10:132.

being the primary metabolic abnormality in hemochromatosis.

Prognosis

Cirrhosis is the major clinical factor influencing long-term survival rates, and patients with cirrhosis at the time of diagnosis are 5.5 times more likely to die than noncirrhotic patients. Diagnosis and venesections prior to the development of cirrhosis will prevent this complication. Patients that are noncirrhotic at the time of diagnosis have an estimated survival rate that does not differ from age- and sex-matched members of the normal population (Figure 41–3). Survival rates at 5, 10, and 20 years have been found to be 87%, 81%, and 71%, respectively, in the author's series, with a mean follow-up period of 8.1 years (range of 0–31 years).

Adams PC: Hepatocellular carcinoma in hereditary hemochromatosis. Can J Gastroenterol 1993;7:37.

Adams PC: Prevalence of abnormal iron studies in heterozygotes for hereditary hemochromatosis: An analysis of 255 heterozygotes. Am J Hematol 1994;45:146.

Adams PC, Kertesz AE: Human leucocyte antigen typing in siblings in hemochromatosis: A cost model. Hepatology 1992;15:263.

Adams PC, Kertesz AE, Valberg LS: Clinical presentation of hemochromatosis: A changing scene. Am J Med 1991;90:445.

Adams PC, Kertesz AE, Valberg LS: Rate of iron reaccumulation in hereditary hemochromatosis: Implications for venesection therapy. J Clin Gastroenterol 1993;16:207.

Adams PC, Speechley M, Kertesz AE: Long-term survival analysis in hereditary hemochromatosis. Gastroenterology 1991;101:368.

Adams PC et al: Transplantation of haemochromatosis liver into donor: Evidence against an inherited intrahepatic defect. Gut 1991;32:1082.

Bonkovsky HL et al: Usefulness and limitations of laboratory and hepatic imaging studies in iron-storage disease. Gastroenterology 1990;99:1079.

Deugnier YM et al: Preneoplastic significance of hepatic iron-free foci in genetic hemochromatosis: A study of 185 patients. Hepatology 1993;18:1363.

Edwards CQ, Kushner JP: Screening for hemochromatosis. N Engl J Med 1993;328:1616.

Farrell FJ et al: Outcome of orthotopic liver transplantation in patients with hemochromatosis. Gastroenterology 1993;104:A900.

Hramiak I, Finegood D, Adams PC: Insulin sensitivity in hemochromatosis. AASLD Meeting, Chicago, November 1992. Hepatology 1992;16:232A.

Kowdley K et al: Prevalence of primary liver cancer and survival in hereditary hemochromatosis patients undergoing orthotopic liver transplantation. Hepatology 1993;18:57A.

Lin E, Adams PC: Biochemical liver profile in hemochromatosis: A survey of 100 patients. J Clin Gastroenterol 1991;13:316.

Olivieri NF et al: Comparison of the oral iron chelator L1 and desferrioxamine in iron-loaded patients. Lancet 1990;336:1275.

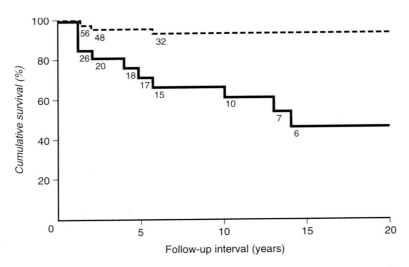

Figure 41–3. Cumulative survival (%) in 27 cirrhotic and 58 noncirrhotic patients. Numbers on the graph refer to the numbers of patients in each group at risk for each follow-up interval after death and censoring. Survival rates were significantly reduced in cirrhotic patients as compared with noncirrhotic patients (p < 0.004; log-rank test). (Reproduced, with permission, from Adams PC et al: Gastroenterology 1991;101:370.)

Olynyk J et al: Determination of hepatic iron concentration in fresh and paraffin-embedded tissue: Diagnostic implications. Gastroenterology 1994;106:674.

Summer KM, Halliday JW, Powell LW: Identification of homozygous hemochromatosis subjects by measurement of hepatic iron index. Hepatology 1990;12:20.

WILSON'S DISEASE

Pathophysiology

Wilson's disease (hepatolenticular degeneration) is a hereditary disorder of copper metabolism. It is an autosomal recessive condition with a prevalence of approximately 1 in 30,000. Patients with Wilson's disease progressively accumulate dietary copper, which eventually becomes toxic to the liver, brain, kidney, eye, and other organs. Studies of the biliary excretion of radiolabeled copper in these patients have demonstrated decreased excretion of the copper and its accumulation in hepatic lysosomes. A transport defect from lysosomes to bile or in the bile canalicular membrane has been postulated as a primary defect in this condition. The gene for Wilson's disease has recently been identified on the long arm of chromosome 13 (pWD, 13q14.3). A genetic defect in a copper-transporting adenosinetriphosphatase (ATPase) has been predicted based on sequence homology to a known gene (Mc1) in another copper transport disorder (Menke's disease). Already, four independent mutations of the gene for Wilson's disease have been described, and this may account for different phenotypic expressions of the disease in American, Sicilian, and Russian patients.

Clinical Findings

A. Symptoms and Signs: Because Wilson's disease is a systemic metabolic disorder, the initial manifestations may not be related to the liver. In a study of patients in the United States, the predominant clinical manifestation was hepatic in 42%, neurologic in 34%, psychiatric in 10%, renal in 1%, and hematologic or endocrine in 12%.

1. Hepatic disease–The signs and symptoms of chronic liver disease appear at an earlier age than the neurologic symptoms. Most patients will have features of cirrhosis or chronic active hepatitis. Some patients with fulminant hepatic failure are seen for the first time as candidates for liver transplantation. Fulminant hepatic failure can also be seen if chelation therapy is inadvertently discontinued in a patient with known Wilson's disease. The diagnosis should be suspected in any young patient (< 40 years of age) with cirrhosis of unknown cause, particularly if it is associated with hemolysis and neurologic findings. Although this is often considered a childhood disease, asymptomatic patients have been described in the sixth decade. Hepatocellular carcinoma is an uncommon complication of the cirrhosis in Wilson's disease in contrast to hemochromatosis.

2. Neurologic disease–The most common neurologic findings are dysarthria, tremor, incoordination, and ataxia. Deterioration in schoolwork or athletic prowess may be an initial clue in a child, and late findings have included dystonia, spasticity, rigidity, and seizures. These findings are more commonly noted in adolescence or early adulthood. Although excess copper is distributed throughout the brain, the basal ganglia are particularly affected.

3. Ophthalmologic disease–An important physical finding is the presence of a Kayser-Fleischer ring, which is a deposition of excess copper in Descemet's membrane of the cornea (Figure 41–4). Although this may be grossly visible, a careful ophthalmologic examination by a specialist is recommended. Sunflower cataracts can also be detected during this examination. The Kayser-Fleischer ring is always present in patients with neurologic symptoms. It has rarely been described in non-Wilson's disease patients with chronic cholestasis. Neither the Kayser-Fleischer ring nor the cataracts usually affect visual acuity.

4. Systemic manifestations–Hemolytic anemia may be the presenting complaint and is likely related to the rapid release of hepatic copper, causing oxidative damage to red blood cells. Many patients have bone and joint abnormalities, including osteoarthritis, osteoporosis, osteomalacia, polyarthritis, and chondrocalcinosis. Patients may have proximal or distal renal tubular acidosis, leading to aminoaciduria and a low serum uric acid level. Cardiac, skin, and endocrine abnormalities have also been described in Wilson's disease.

B. Laboratory Findings: Although copper overloading is the characteristic feature of Wilson's disease, the serum copper level is usually not elevated and is an unreliable marker of the disease. The urinary copper level is markedly elevated in patients with Wilson's disease, and a 24-hour urinary collection for copper is an important diagnostic test. Most patients will excrete more than 1.6 μmol (100 μg)/24 hours. Serum ceruloplasmin, a circulating copper-binding protein, is typically low in Wilson's disease; the basis for this is unknown. Most patients will have a serum ceruloplasmin measurement of less than 1.5 μmol/L (200 mg/L) at the time of diagnosis. Because ceruloplasmin may rise with inflammation, it may sometimes increase into the low normal range in Wilson's disease. Features that may be discrete clues to the diagnosis are the presence of a Coomb's negative hemolytic anemia and hypouricemia (renal tubular defect) (Table 41–4).

Liver enzymes (AST, ALT) are only slightly elevated, with AST higher than ALT. Another clue may be the relatively modest elevation in serum alkaline phosphatase despite a high bilirubin level. These findings are less reliable in the setting of fulminant hepatic failure. A liver biopsy is important to establish the diagnosis and determine the degree of liver injury. It is imperative to realize that the histologic features of Wilson's disease are often nonspecific and may be described as idiopathic chronic active hepatitis. Histochemical staining for copper may be unreliable. **Hepatic copper concentration is the "gold standard" for diagnosis, as determined by atomic absorption spectrophotometry.** Hepatic copper can be measured in a sample excised from a paraffin block if the diagnosis had not been initially considered. Hepatic copper concentrations can range from 4 to 47 μmol/g dry weight (250–3000 μg).

C. Imaging Studies: Although radiocopper studies to assess copper metabolism and excretion have provided information about the pathogenesis of

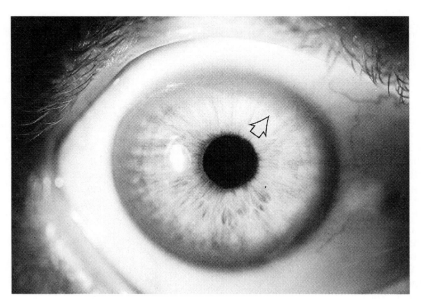

Figure 41–4. Kayser-Fleischer ring. The deposition of copper can be seen as a dark homogenous ring obscuring visualization of the peripheral iris **(arrow)**. It is best viewed by slit lamp examination. (Photograph courtesy of C Canny.)

Table 41–4. Laboratory diagnosis of Wilson's disease.

High hepatic copper concentration
Low serum ceruloplasmin
High urinary copper
Low serum uric acid
Hemolytic anemia

Table 41–5. Therapies for Wilson's disease.

Penicillamine
Triethylene tetramine
Zinc
Liver transplantation

the disease, the short half-life of the isotope and the cost have limited the use of this test to research centers with a special interest in this disease.

Abdominal imaging contributes no specific information in Wilson's disease but may reveal related findings, including hepatosplenomegaly and abnormalities suggesting portal hypertension.

MRI and CT scanning of the head have demonstrated abnormalities in the brain stem, cerebellum, and cerebrum in advanced disease, but these do not correlate with the clinical findings.

Differential Diagnosis

The most common differential diagnosis considered in the patient with Wilson's disease is idiopathic chronic active hepatitis. Indian childhood cirrhosis is an unusual condition associated with micronodular cirrhosis with a high hepatic copper concentration. The role of genetic and environmental factors in the pathogenesis of this condition is not clearly established. Any chronic cholestatic liver disease (primary biliary cirrhosis, sclerosing cholangitis, arteriohepatic dysplasia) can be associated with hepatic copper accumulation, but the clinical features (jaundice, pruritus, bile duct abnormalities) and degree of copper overloading can usually distinguish these patients from patients with Wilson's disease.

Treatment

Chelation therapy is the primary treatment for Wilson's disease. Penicillamine (1–2 g/d orally) is administered on a lifelong basis. Because this drug has considerable toxicity, patient compliance is a problem, and withdrawal of the drug may precipitate liver failure and hemolysis. Fever, skin rashes, leukopenia, thrombocytopenia, and proteinuria can occur within the first few weeks of therapy. During the first 2 months of therapy, complete blood counts, serum creatinine levels, and urinalysis should be monitored weekly and then decreased to monthly for the next 6 months. Twenty-four-hour urinary copper determinations can be performed to monitor efficacy and compliance with therapy. Neurologic disease may also worsen after initiation of penicillamine therapy. An alternative chelator is triethylene tetramine (trientine). Oral zinc has been advocated as an alternative to inhibit intestinal copper absorption but should not be considered as the primary treatment of choice (Table 41–5).

Clinical improvement depends on the stage of the disease at the time of initiation of therapy. Patients who present with advanced decompensated cirrhosis or acute fulminant hepatic failure should proceed directly to liver transplantation after which the metabolic defect and neurologic symptoms often but not always improve.

Prognosis

In general, the prognosis of Wilson's disease is determined by how early the diagnosis is established and when chelation treatment is initiated. Even patients with chronic active hepatitis, cirrhosis, or neurologic findings, however, may have an excellent long-term prognosis if appropriately treated. A long-term retrospective study of 51 patients reported that the long-term survival rates of treated patients were similar to an age- and sex-matched control group. In another study, 20 patients with chronic active hepatitis due to Wilson's disease were followed for up to 25 years and had an excellent prognosis for up to 25 years if they were compliant with chelation therapy. A retrospective study of 127 patients with a mean follow-up period of 12 years demonstrated a 15-year survival rate of 74% in treated patients, which was less than the predicted survival rate of 99%. A long-term follow-up study of the effects of chelation therapy on neurologic disorders in 137 patients showed complete resolution in 42%, with clinical improvement in an additional 26%.

Brewer GJ, Yuzbasiyan-Gurkan V: Wilson's disease. Medicine 1992;71:139.

Friedman LS: Zinc in the treatment of Wilson's disease: How it works. Gastroenterology 1993;104:1566.

Sallie R et al: Failure of simple biochemical indexes to reliably differentiate fulminant Wilson's disease from other causes of fulminant hepatic failure. Hepatology 1992;16:1206.

Scheinberg IH, Sternlieb I: Major Problems in Internal Medicine. Vol 23. Wilson's Disease. Saunders, 1984.

Schilsky ML, Scheinberg IH, Sternlieb I: Liver transplantation for Wilson's disease: Indications and outcome. Hepatology 1994;19:583.

Schilsky ML, Scheinberg IH, Sternlieb I: Prognosis of Wilsonian chronic active hepatitis. Gastroenterology 1991;100:762.

Scolapio JS et al: Survival in Wilson's disease is less than expected: An analysis of 127 patients followed long term. Gastroenterology 1994;106:A863.

Sternlieb I: The outlook for the diagnosis of Wilson's disease. J Hepatol 1993;17:263.

Stremmel W et al: Wilson's disease: Clinical presentation, treatment and survival. Ann Intern Med 1991;115:720.

Tanzi RE et al: The Wilson disease gene is a copper transporting ATPase with homology to the Menkes disease gene. Nature 1993;5:344.

Thuomas KA et al: Magnetic resonance imaging of the brain in Wilson's disease. Neuroradiology 1993;35:134.

Walshe JM, Yealland M: Chelation therapy for neurological Wilson's disease. Q J Med 1993;86:197.

Yarze JC et al: Wilson's disease: Current status. Am J Med 1992;92:643.

42

Hepatic Porphyrias

D. Montgomery Bissell, MD

GENERAL CONSIDERATIONS

Pathophysiology

The porphyrias comprise a group of diseases that are subdivided into acute (neurologic) and chronic (cutaneous) forms. While genetically distinct, all types of porphyria represent disturbances in the formation of heme, an essential component of hemoglobin and cellular cytochromes. Because the pathway of heme formation is well understood, it serves as a logical framework for viewing the porphyrias. Porphyrins are darkly colored compounds (Greek *porphyos,* purple) that are either intermediates or side products of heme formation. They are detectable in urine or feces, but excretion normally represents less than 1% of the daily flux through the pathway. Porphyria denotes markedly increased excretion of porphyrins or porphyrin precursors, in association with symptoms.

A. The Pathway of Heme Formation: The formation of heme, investigated in the 1940s, was one of the first biosynthetic pathways elucidated through the use of radioisotopic tracers. It was proved that all of the carbons in heme are supplied by the amino acid glycine and by succinic acid, a Krebs cycle intermediate (Figure 42–1). These simple precursors combine to form α-aminolevulinic acid (ALA), the first intermediate committed to heme synthesis. The reaction is catalyzed by ALA synthase and is normally rate-limiting for the pathway as a whole. ALA synthase is subject to negative regulation by heme, which ensures that the flow of precursors into the pathway matches the need of the cell for new heme formation. In the second reaction, two molecules of ALA condense to form porphobilinogen (PBG), a five-membered ring with acetic and propionic side chains. Both ALA and PBG are colorless and water soluble. In the next reaction, four molecules of PBG are linked to create a linear tetrapyrrole in a reaction catalyzed by PBG deaminase. The first porphyrin of the pathway (uroporphyrinogen) uses another enzyme, uroporphyrinogen synthase, which cyclizes the linear tetrapyrrole. As indicated in Figure 42–1, the true intermediates of the pathway,

up to protoporphyrin, are porphyrinogens, which are reduced porphyrins. The corresponding porphyrins are side products of the pathway and are irreversibly oxidized: They cannot reenter the pathway and must be excreted into either bile (and thence to feces) or urine. Such leakage from the pathway normally is minimal, although porphyrins are detectable in the urine and feces of healthy individuals. A marked increase in porphyrin excretion suggests a disturbance in the flow of heme precursors along the pathway.

The conversion of uroporphyrinogen, first into coproporphyrinogen and then into protoporphyrinogen, requires two enzymes (Figure 42–1), which mediate a progressive decarboxylation of the original acetic and propionic side chains of uroporphyrinogen. As shown, this gives rise to a series of intermediates, named according to the number of carboxyl side chains on the porphyrin nucleus. Of these, the most important, quantitatively, are octacarboxyporphyrin, otherwise known as uroporphyrin, and tetracarboxyporphyrin, known as coproporphyrin. The hepta-, hexa-, and pentacarboxyporphyrins are minor.

The progressive decarboxylation of uroporphyrinogen leads to compounds with reduced water solubility and a change in their principal route of excretion: Uroporphyrin is excreted almost entirely in urine (as its name implies), coproporphyrin in both urine and feces, and protoporphyrin entirely in feces. In the final step of the pathway, iron is inserted into protoporphyrin forming heme; the reaction is catalyzed by heme synthase (ferrochelatase).

The pathway traverses both the mitochondrial and cytosolic compartments of the cell. It starts in the mitochondrion, with ALA synthase, then moves to the cytosol, where the next three enzymes are located (PBG synthase, PBG deaminase, and uroporphyrinogen synthase), returning to the mitochondrion, where coproporphyrinogen oxidase and heme synthase are located. Most of the newly synthesized heme then is exported to the cytosol for combination with globin (in erythropoietic cells) or apocytochromes (in other nucleated cells) (Figure 42–1). A small fraction is degraded to bile pigment.

B. Enzyme Defects in Porphyria: The por-

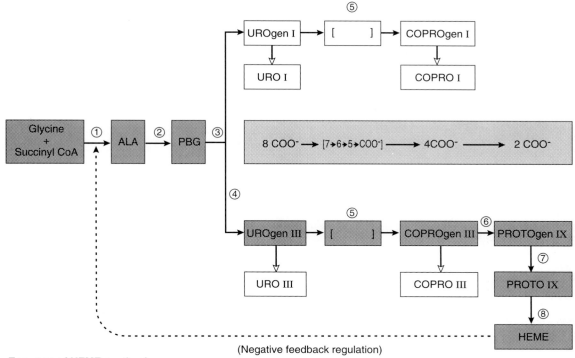

Enzymes of HEME synthesis

① ALA synthase
② PBG synthase
③ PBG deaminase
④ UROgen III synthase
⑤ UROgen decarboxylase
⑥ COPROgen oxidase
⑦ PROTOgen oxidase
⑧ HEME synthase (ferrochelatase)

Figure 42–1. The pathway of heme synthesis. The solid arrows indicate the flow of metabolites in the normal situation. The dashed arrows indicate side pathways, which normally are minor but increase in porphyria. (Reproduced, with permission, from Bissell DM: The Porphyrias. In: *The Molecular and Genetic Basis of Neurological Disease.* Rosenberg R et al (editors). Butterworth Heinemann, 1992.)

phyrias represent hereditary or acquired defects in one of the enzymes of heme synthesis. The most important result from genetic deficiencies. The enzyme defect appears to create a partial block to the flow of heme precursors, with spillover of intermediates to excretory routes. The pattern of metabolic intermediates reflects the site of the block and is diagnostic for each type of porphyria (Figure 42–2).

C. Classification of the Porphyrias: Porphyrias are usually grouped as erythropoietic or hepatic, according to the principal source of excess porphyrin or porphyrin precursors. In genetic porphyria, the enzyme defect is present in all tissues. Heme synthesis, however, does not occur much in tissues other than the bone marrow, where it serves hemoglobin

production, and in the liver, where it is required for synthesis of microsomal heme proteins. Among the latter, the cytochrome P-450 family is present in high concentration and turns over rapidly, requiring a substantial level of ongoing heme synthesis. This classification is presented in Table 42–1. Clinically, the porphyrias can be grouped according to their presentation: acute (neuropsychiatric) or chronic (cutaneous). There is overlap, however, with some types being cutaneous and chronic but on occasion also acute.

D. Pathogenesis of Symptoms in Acute Porphyria: Most attacks are induced by drugs (see below). The inducers usually are compounds that elicit new synthesis of hepatic cytochrome P-450. In-

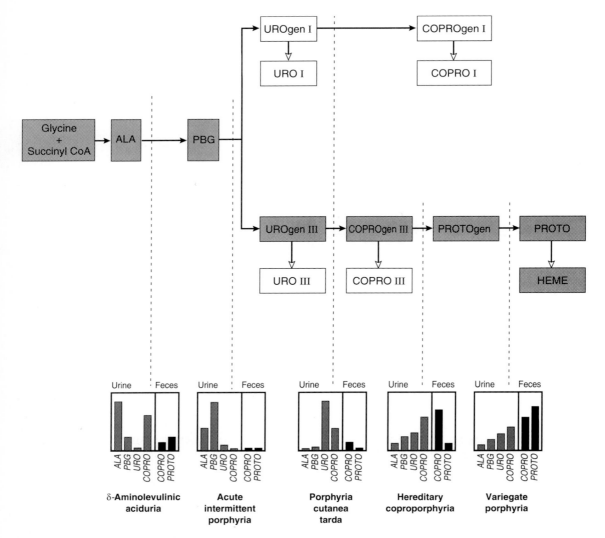

Figure 42–2. Urinary and fecal excretion of heme precursors associated with genetic hepatic porphyria. The vertical dashed lines indicate the point in the pathway at which an enzyme deficiency exists (see Figure 42–1 for a list of enzymes). Each defect gives rise to a unique excretory pattern of heme precursors. The "I" and "III" refer to isomers of porphyrin: only the III series are intermediates in heme formation. For the patterns associated with the individual acquired or erythropoietic porphyrias, see text. (Reproduced, with permission, from Bissell DM: The Porphyrias. In: *The Molecular and Genetic Basis of Neurological Disease.* Rosenberg R et al (editors). Butterworth Heinemann, 1992.)

duction of cytochrome P-450 entails a demand for heme synthesis, to which the liver reacts with an increase in ALA synthase, the rate-limiting enzyme of the pathway. In porphyria, where an inherited or acquired enzyme deficiency exists distal to ALA synthase, the affected enzyme limits the flow of precursors, resulting in heme production failing to meet the demand. As precursors prior to the block accumulate, an acute attack ensues.

All of the acute-attack porphyrias have in common overproduction of ALA and PBG, although it remains unclear whether such overproduction directly underlies symptoms. ALA bears a structural resemblance to the inhibitory neurotransmitter γ-aminobutyric acid (GABA), and may act as a GABA analog in vivo.

E. Pathogenesis of Symptoms in Cutaneous Porphyria: While the precursors ALA and PBG are colorless, porphyrins are purple and fluorescent and, at a sufficient concentration in skin, photosensitizing. This effect has been proved by the finding that the "action spectrum" of photocutaneous injury (with a peak at about 400 nm) corresponds exactly to the wavelength at which a porphyrin is ex-

Table 42–1. Classification of the prophyrias.[1]

Type	Enzyme Defect	Inheritance	Clinical Type
Hepatic porphyria			
Acute intermittent porphyria	PBG deaminase	Dominant	Acute, neurologic
Hereditary coproporphyria	COPROgen oxidase	Dominant	Acute, neurologic (+ cutaneous)
Variegate porphyria	PROTOgen oxidase	Dominant	Acute, neurologic (+ cutaneous)
δ-ALAuria	PBG synthase	Recessive	Acute, neurologic
Cutanea tarda	UROgen decarboxylase	Dominant (+ acquired?)	Chronic, cutaneous
Lead intoxication	PBG synthase + COPRO oxidase	(Acquired)	Neurologic
"Toxic" porphyria	UROgen decarboxylase	(Acquired)	Cutaneous
Erythropoietic porphyria			
Congenital erythropoietic porphyria	UROgen synthase	Recessive	Cutaneous
Protoporphyria	Heme synthase	Dominant	Cutaneous (+ hepatic)

[1]PBG, porphobilinogen; COPROgen, coproporphyrinogen; PROTOgen, protoporphyrinogen; UROgen, uroporphyrinogen; δ-ALA, δ-aminolevulinic acid.

cited to its reactive form. In variegate porphyria and protoporphyria, the inherited deficiency appears to be both necessary and sufficient for porphyrin overproduction. On the other hand, the clinical expression of porphyria cutanea tarda clearly requires environmental factors as well as a deficiency in uroporphyrinogen decarboxylase (Table 42–2). Such factors include a moderate level of iron overload, which is present in virtually all patients with porphyria cutanea tarda, as indicated by transferrin saturation in excess of 50% and stainable iron on liver biopsy. The basis for the excess iron is controversial. It does not correlate with clinical liver disease and, therefore, cannot be viewed merely as secondary to hepatic pathologic changes, nor can it be attributed solely to alcohol ingestion. Studies of genetic markers for hemochromatosis have led investigators to postulate that some persons with porphyria cutanea tarda also are heterozygous for hereditary hemochromatosis and accumulate iron for this reason.

In addition to moderately increased iron stores, alcohol abuse and liver disease (often mild) are common in porphyria cutanea tarda. Estrogens and a small number of other drugs play a role in some patients. Sensitivity to inducers of heme synthesis (such as barbiturates) is *not* a factor, however. Finally, porphyria cutanea tarda appears to occur with unexpectedly high frequency in patients with HIV infection, usually with manifest AIDS. The reason for this association is unknown.

Table 42–2. Environmental factors in porphyria cutanea tarda.

Iron overload; dietary iron supplements
Alcohol
Estrogens
Chronic liver disease
Acquired immunodeficiency syndrome

Diagnostic Screening Tests

Cutaneous lesions, in porphyrias displaying them (see Table 42–1), are characteristic and should immediately suggest the diagnosis. The "neurologic" syndrome, on the other hand, often takes the form of complaints (nausea, abdominal pain, constipation) that occur commonly in the general population. As in other unusual diseases, the "classical" clinical presentation of abdominal pain, psychosis, and dark urine in a young female is seldom seen. More often, porphyria comes under consideration only after other diagnostic possibilities have been exhausted. In such patients, accurate laboratory evaluation is the key to diagnosis. Various "screening" tests are available, but have important limitations.

A. Urinary ALA and PBG; Watson-Schwartz Test: For the evaluation of pain and neurologic symptoms, the appropriate tests are for urinary ALA and PBG, the porphyrin precursors. In all of the acute porphyrias, these are elevated, although in ALAuria and lead poisoning, only the ALA is increased. The Watson-Schwartz test, in which urine is mixed with Ehrlich's reagent (dimethylaminobenzaldehyde in hydrochloric acid), is a rapid qualitative test for PBG and suitable for emergency room use provided it is performed correctly. If no pink color forms, the test is negative. Importantly, however, formation of a pink color is positive *only* if the color proves resistant to extraction with n-butanol (ie, remains in the aqueous phase). Thus, the extraction step is critical to a correct interpretation of the test. Color that is present initially but extractable is due to urobilinogen or certain medications and unrelated to porphyria.

B. Porphyrin Screening: Cutaneous symptoms are evaluated with measurement of porphyrins (not porphyrin precursors) in urine, stool, or blood. The choice of sample depends on the pattern of porphyrin overproduction in the disease under consideration. In porphyria cutanea tarda, for example, the salient change is increased uroporphyrin, and urine analysis is performed. In variegate porphyria, protoporphyrin is increased, and a stool analysis is appropriate (Figure 42–2).

A "porphyrin screen" is useful for rapid assessment of cutaneous disease. Because it reflects total porphyrins irrespective of type, quantitative analysis of individual porphyrins is needed to ascertain the type of porphyria. With a complete profile of heme precursors in urine and feces (and, occasionally, in blood), virtually all porphyrias can be typed (Figure 42–2). Notably, persons with symptoms exhibit markedly abnormal porphyrin excretion. For example, in acute neurologic attacks, the amount of PBG in urine exceeds 30 mg/d (normal < 2 mg/d) and ranges up to 200 mg/d. For porphyria cutanea tarda with cutaneous symptoms, urine uroporphyrin exceeds 500 μg/d (normal < 50 μ/d). In short, in persons with symptoms, the laboratory abnormalities are not subtle.

A pattern of porphyrin excretion frequently encountered in clinical practice is an isolated, usually minor increase in urine coproporphyrin. As a rule, rather than signifying a hereditary porphyria, this is nonspecific, associated with a variety of acute and chronic illnesses, including acquired liver disease. The only specific diagnostic considerations are lead poisoning and asymptomatic hereditary coproporphyria. Diagnosis of the latter requires analysis of fecal coproporphyrin, which is elevated only in the hereditary condition.

Genetic Diagnosis

The acute-attack (neurologic) porphyrias are inherited in an autosomal dominant manner, except for α-ALAuria, in which a double defect in the gene for PBG synthase is required for the expression of clinical disease. All porphyrias are viewed as rare, although their prevalence is relatively high in certain inbred populations. Acute intermittent porphyria is found in 1 in 1000 persons in northern Scandinavia; variegate porphyria is present in as many as 1 in 300 South Africans of Dutch ancestry. In the latter case, the gene has been traced back to the original group of Dutch settlers who emigrated to the Cape area in the late seventeenth century; the story is recounted by Dean (see references). Investigation of the molecular defects in families with acute intermittent porphyria indicates the presence of several mutations, all leading to inactive or unstable PBG deaminase. Because there appears to be no predominant mutation, molecular diagnosis is not currently in use except for screening individual large kindreds.

With regard to the cutaneous porphyrias, two types of porphyria cutanea tarda are postulated: one is clearly genetic, involving a partial deficiency of uroporphyrinogen decarboxylase. In a second type, the deficiency is expressed only in the liver and appears to be detectable only prior to treatment. The latter defect may be acquired, but because a genetic lesion has not been excluded, this form is termed "sporadic" porphyria cutanea tarda. For clinical purposes, the distinction is unimportant. All porphyria cutanea tarda is eminently treatable, and for this reason genetic analysis usually is not pursued. A third condition that can be grouped with porphyria cutanea tarda is hepatoerythropoietic porphyria, in which uroporphyrinogen decarboxylase is profoundly decreased. Although this is suggestive of homozygous porphyria cutanea tarda, the molecular defects identified to date have not been found in familial porphyria cutanea tarda.

Protoporphyria is autosomal dominant but with more than one subtype. Many carriers appear to be asymptomatic. The affected enzyme is heme synthase (ferrochelatase).

ACUTE INTERMITTENT PORPHYRIA

Acute intermittent porphyria is an acute hepatic porphyria with no cutaneous manifestations.

Clinical Findings

A. Symptoms and Signs: The principal symptoms are shown in Table 42–3. Pain is typical, often in the abdominal region but sometimes involving the back or extremities. It may be diffuse, deep, and achy or may be localized, mimicking a surgical abdomen. Indeed, a history of recurrent abdominal pain with negative laparotomy should suggest the diagnosis. Porphyric symptoms have a characteristic course, increasing over a period of days rather than hours. Many patients will report chronic constipation that worsens at the onset of an attack. A family history should be sought but is often absent because of the infrequency of acute attacks in genetic carriers. Many attacks occur in the setting of an inducing drug; thus, a review of medications is particularly important. Attacks can occur also as a result of decreased caloric intake, either because of intercurrent illness, such as influenza, or an attempt at rapid weight reduction. Elective surgery can be the setting for an acute attack because of the routinely imposed

Table 42–3. Presentation of acute porphyria: percentage of patients with symptom or sign.[1]

Symptom	%	Sign	%
Abdominal pain	90	Tachycardia	83
Vomiting	80	Hypertension	55
Constipation	80	Motor neuropathy	53
Pain in limbs	51	Pyrexia	38
Pain in back	50	Leukocytosis (> 12,000)	20
Confused state	32	Bulbar involvement	18
Seizures	12	Sensory loss	15
Diarrhea	8	Cranial nerve involvement	9

[1]Modified from Eales M: Porphyria as seen in Cape Town: A survey of 250 patients and some recent studies. S Afr J Lab Chem Med 1963;9:151.

preoperative fasting and the use of barbiturates for induction of anesthesia.

Attacks are more frequent in women than in men and have a peak incidence between age 20 and 40 years. Although reported, attacks are rare prior to puberty. Female sex hormones may predispose women to acute attacks and account also for the virtual absence of symptoms prior to puberty; oral contraceptives have been implicated in some cases. Cyclical premenstrual exacerbations can occur that resolve with the onset of menses. The effect of pregnancy is unpredictable.

The physical findings of acute porphyria are, for the most part, consistent with a neuropathic process (Table 42–3). None is diagnostic, however. A clue to the examining physician may be the impression that symptoms are out of proportion to the physical findings. Psychosis is part of the classic description but usually is not overt. More commonly, patients exhibit an "hysterical" affect, which can be misconstrued as drug-seeking behavior. Weakness, when present, is initially proximal and, in a patient with abdominal pain, should suggest the diagnosis. Seizures can occur early and represent a particular risk in that use of phenytoin and related drugs may aggravate the attack and cause rapid progression of porphyria. Fever suggests a coexisting infection, a setting in which acute attacks may occur in the absence of an inducing drug.

B. Laboratory Findings: Minor abnormalities in blood urea, liver transaminases, and thyroxine have been reported. The most important finding, when present, is hyponatremia. It appears to result in at least some patients from inappropriate secretion of antidiuretic hormone, and it can develop rapidly, particularly with aggressive administration of dextrose-in-water as initial therapy (see below). The diagnostic finding in acute porphyria is marked elevation of urinary (or serum) PBG. The Watson-Schwartz test is a rapid qualitative test for PBG; as noted above, the butanol extraction is critical for eliminating false positives. It should be confirmed by quantitative assay of PBG, which is available in many commercial laboratories. Quantitative urine porphyrins are needed for establishing the type of porphyria. In addition to the major porphyrins (uroporphyrin and coproporphyrin), many laboratories report the intermediate forms (hepta-, hexa-, and pentacarboxyporphyrins). The latter provide no additional diagnostic information and are best ignored, being usually present in such low concentrations that accurate measurement is difficult.

C. Genetic Diagnosis: Because prevention of attacks plays a large role in management, identification of asymptomatic carriers (eg, first-degree relatives of an index case) is important. While quantitative assay of urine PBG is appropriate as the initial screening test, there is a significant false-negative rate (estimated at 30% of the healthy carrier popula-

tion). Therefore, the urine test is supplemented by assay of erythrocyte PBG deaminase, which is less than normal in most affected individuals regardless of symptoms. In some carriers, however, values fall in the low-normal range, and in one genetic variant, the enzyme in erythrocytes is normal but in liver is deficient. Nonetheless, the combination of urinary PBG and erythrocyte PBG deaminase identifies at least 90% of carriers. Molecular diagnosis is a research procedure (discussed above).

D. Prenatal Testing: Although this is feasible by analysis of amniotic cells, it is not pursued because of the low probability of acute attacks, particularly if carriers are identified prospectively. This assumes, of course, that parents will have their offspring evaluated at the appropriate time and will ensure that those who are carriers understand how to avoid attacks (see below). Such testing can be deferred until well beyond infancy, in that symptoms of any sort are exceedingly rare prior to puberty.

Differential Diagnosis

Cholestasis, appendicitis, or other acute abdominal process can resemble porphyria. Such conditions should be excluded rigorously in patients manifesting fever and leukocytosis, which are not regularly part of a porphyric attack. Hereditary tyrosinemia has many features of acute porphyria, including increased urinary ALA, but it presents in childhood. Finally, the symptoms of lead intoxication may mimic those of acute porphyria, including abdominal pain and altered mental status. Urinary excretion of ALA and coproporphyrin is increased, presumably reflecting an inhibitory effect of lead on PBG synthase and coproporphyrinogen oxidase, respectively. Unlike acute porphyria, PBG is normal; erythrocyte protoporphyrin may be elevated. The diagnosis is confirmed by blood lead determination; assay of PBG synthase also has been used.

Treatment

The approach to an acute attack is outlined in Table 42–4. Carbohydrate reverses the fasting state, which according to experimental evidence sensitizes the liver to porphyria-inducing chemicals. The goal is to give 400–500 g/d, orally if possible. If intravenous administration is necessary, careful monitoring of serum electrolytes, particularly sodium, is essential. Pain relief usually requires opiates such as meperidine. There is little risk of addiction for a patient with a bona fide acute porphyric attack, although caution is indicated where the diagnosis is in doubt. Chlorpromazine has been used, but sedation may be its principal effect.

For women who experience premenstrual exacerbations of porphyria, suppression of the ovulatory cycle may provide relief. Peptide analogs of luteinizing-hormone releasing hormone (LHRH) are the preferred agents; unlike estrogen-based drugs, these have no demonstrable porphyria-inducing activity. Known genetic carriers of acute porphyria may experience intermittent somatic complaints but without the expected elevation of urinary PBG. Such patients often do not respond to hematin and most likely have an unrelated condition. In the absence of a specific diagnosis, empiric therapy should be tried (with due regard for hazardous drugs); opiates are inappropriate.

When seizures occur in acute porphyria, their management poses a problem in that virtually all first-line anticonvulsants are contraindicated (Table 42–5). Diazepam will provide short-term suppression while the attack is brought under control with hematin (see below); intravenous magnesium sulfate also has been used. For chronic seizures in porphyrics, bromide is the only treatment that clearly is safe and also effective. Although this therapy was eclipsed 50 years ago by the discovery of phenytoins (Dilantin and others), it has been reintroduced for problems such as refractory childhood epilepsy. Close monitoring of serum bromide levels is essential, and side effects are frequent.

Hematin represents the only specific therapy for acute porphyria. In theory, it corrects heme deficiency, which is the fundamental metabolic defect in the disease ("hematin" refers to heme in aqueous solution). Although not evaluated in controlled trials, its efficacy is supported by substantial clinical experience. Hematin should be given early to all patients presenting with neurologic signs and otherwise to those whose symptoms fail to respond within 48 hours to the measures outlined in Table 42–4. It is provided as a dry powder (Panhematin, Abbott Laboratories, Chicago), to be reconstituted immediately prior to infusion. In general, 1.5 mg/kg (or 100 mg) every 24 hours is effective. This can be given every 12 hours in urgent circumstances. Urinary excretion of PBG is monitored to ensure that the patient has received an effective dose; a decrease to approximately 10% of prehematin levels should occur within 48 hours. A symptomatic response follows that is often dramatic, with the requirement for pain medication decreasing rapidly and disappearing on the fourth or fifth day of treatment. Side effects of hematin are minor. The solution is slightly alkaline and, if infused

too rapidly or into a small vein, causes a local chemical phlebitis. It also causes transient anticoagulation and should be given cautiously, if at all, to patients at risk of bleeding or receiving anticoagulant therapy.

Prevention of Attacks

Once an index diagnosis is established, screening of first-degree relatives is performed to identify latent carriers by the procedures outlined above (see Genetic Diagnosis). Because the gene is inherited as an autosomal dominant, those family members not identified as carriers (50%, on average) are normal and will not pass on the condition to their children. The vast majority of carriers will remain asymptomatic if they avoid drugs that precipitate acute attacks (Table 42–5). They are advised also to avoid fasting and fad diets. On the other hand, there is no convincing evidence that a diet rich in carbohydrates prevents attacks, and obesity is an unwanted side effect.

Prognosis

The most ominous development in acute porphyria is a motor neuropathy, which can progress to respira-

Table 42–4. Initial management of acute prophyric attacks.

1. Suppress seizures, if present, with intravenous diazepam.
2. Ensure that patient is receiving no porphyria-inducing drugs.
3. Provide pain relief.
4. Monitor electrolytes, particularly hyponatremia.
5. Initiate a 24-hour urine collection for porphobilinogen.
6. Administer carbohydrate.
   If neurologic signs are present, or if the above regimen fails to produce a symptomatic response within 48 hours, then:
7. Administer intravenous hematin.

Table 42–5. Unsafe and safe drugs in porphyria.[1]

	Unsafe	Believed To Be Safe
Anticonvulsants:	**Barbiturates** **Carbamazepine** Clonazepam **Ethosuximide** **Hydantoins** **Phenytoin** Primidone Valproic acid	Bromides Diazepam Magnesium sulfate
Hypnotics or sedatives:	**Barbiturates** Chlordiazepoxide Ethchlorvynol **Gluthethimide** **Meprobamate** **Methyprylon**	Chloral hydrate Chlorpromazine Diphenhydramine Lithium Lorazepam Meclizine Trifluoperazine
Other drugs:	**Alpha-methyldopa** Danazol **Diclofenac** **Ergot preparations** Estrogens **Griseofulvin** Imipramine **Pentazocine** **Pyrazinamide** **Sulfonamides** **Sulfonylureas**	ACTH Allopurinol Aminoglycosides Aspirin Atropine Codeine Colchicine Dexamethasone Furosemide Ibuprofen Insulin Meperidine Morphine Naproxen Penicillins Warfarin

[1]The agents in **bold print** have been implicated repeatedly in acute attacks. For the other "unsafe" compounds, the clinical information is anecdotal but supported by tests in experimental animals or in vitro.

tory paralysis. Prior to the advent of modern intensive care and the use of hematin, the mortality rate in such attacks approached 50%. The outlook is much improved now. Neurologic deficits resolve slowly but, as a rule, completely. Although psychosis is a component of the acute presentation, it resolves promptly as the attack subsides. There is no evidence of long-term or progressive psychiatric disease.

HEREDITARY COPROPORPHYRIA

Hereditary coproporphyria is an acute hepatic porphyria; because circulating porphyrins are increased, cutaneous manifestations occur in about 30% of cases. This type appears to be expressed clinically less frequently than is acute intermittent porphyria. Population surveys have not been done, and the prevalence of the carrier state is unknown.

Clinical Findings
A. Symptoms and Signs: The acute attack is indistinguishable from that of acute intermittent porphyria (see Table 42–4). The cutaneous manifestations, when present, may be chronic and resemble those of porphyria cutanea tarda (see below).

B. Laboratory Findings: In acute attacks, urinary PBG is elevated as in acute intermittent porphyria. The diagnostic finding in carriers is elevation of fecal coproporphyrin as well as urine coproporphyrin.

C. Genetic Diagnosis: Carriers usually are identified by analysis of urine and feces. Although a blood test for coproporphyrinogen oxidase is available commercially, the results should be confirmed with conventional analysis.

Treatment & Prognosis
Treatment and prognosis are the same as for acute intermittent porphyria.

VARIEGATE PORPHYRIA

Variegate porphyria is an acute hepatic porphyria, with chronic cutaneous manifestations in most genetic carriers.

Clinical Findings
A. Symptoms and Signs: Acute attacks are identical to those in acute intermittent porphyria. The cutaneous manifestations are chronic in many affected persons and are similar to those in porphyria cutanea tarda (see below).

B. Laboratory Findings: Urinary PBG is elevated in attacks, as in acute intermittent porphyria, but may be normal otherwise. In persons with cutaneous disease only or in asymptomatic individuals, the diagnosis relies on an elevation of fecal protoporphyrin.

C. Genetic Diagnosis: The affected enzyme is protoporphyrinogen oxidase, a mitochondrial enzyme. Its assay is a research procedure at present. Carriers are identified by analysis of urine and feces.

Treatment & Prognosis
Acute attacks are handled as in acute intermittent porphyria and have a similar prognosis. There is no satisfactory treatment for the cutaneous manifestations other than protective clothing. Topical sunscreens are ineffective.

δ-AMINOLEVULINIC ACIDURIA

This type of porphyria involves deficiency of the second enzyme in heme synthesis, PBG synthase. It is recessively inherited and is rare. Acute attacks are similar to those in acute intermittent porphyria, and there is no cutaneous component. The pattern on urinalysis is increased urinary ALA, with normal PBG and increased coproporphyrin. The findings are similar to those of lead intoxication (see below), which must be excluded.

PORPHYRIA CUTANEA TARDA

Porphyria cutanea tarda is a chronic hepatic type, with cutaneous manifestations only; acute attacks do not occur.

Clinical Findings
A. Symptoms and Signs: Patients typically fail to relate their cutaneous problem to sun exposure, complaining mainly of "fragile skin." Seemingly trivial contact to the back of the hand produces an ulcer or sloughing of skin. The problem can be disabling for mechanics and others who require heavy use of the hands. They may report dark-colored (usually brownish) urine, which is due to porphyrins. The photosensitizing effects of porphyrins in the skin are manifest initially as blisters that range in size from milia to 1–2 cm, typically on the dorsa of the hands or on the face. These eventually open, leaving shallow ulcerations. With chronic injury, pigmented or depigmented scars are present as well as increased hair growth, which is noticeable mainly on the face. Sclerodermatous plaques can occur.

B. Laboratory Findings: The hallmark of the disease is markedly increased urine uroporphyrin. The presence of skin disease implies uroporphyrin excretion of at least 500 μg/24 hours, and values in the range of 1500–3000 μg/24 hours are not unusual. Urine PBG is normal or minimally elevated; fecal coproporphyrin and protoporphyrin are normal, and this distinguishes porphyria cutanea tarda from hereditary coproporphyria and variegate porphyria.

Assay of uroporphyrinogen decarboxylase is not usually available.

Pathologic changes in the liver in porphyria cutanea tarda are those of the associated liver disease (commonly due to alcohol abuse). In addition, a uroporphyrin hepatopathy has been described. The accumulation of uroporphyrin renders the tissue fluorescent under long-wave ultraviolet excitation.

Differential Diagnosis

A. Tumor-Associated Porphyria: Hepatic tumors may overproduce porphyrins in quantities sufficient to cause manifestations similar to those of porphyria cutanea tarda. The pattern in urine differs from that of porphyria cutanea tarda, however. For this reason, tumor screening of patients with the typical laboratory findings of porphyria cutanea tarda is not advocated.

B. Bullous Dermatosis of Hemodialysis: Patients with chronic renal failure on hemodialysis may have bullous lesions indistinguishable from those of porphyria cutanea tarda. The cause of the problem is unclear. Plasma porphyrins are minimally elevated in most cases, even though uroporphyrin is not effectively dialyzed.

C. Toxic Porphyria: In the late 1950s, an outbreak of cutaneous porphyria occurred in Turkey that was attributable to contamination of grain with hexachlorobenzene, a fungicide. This prompted experimental studies of halogenated aromatic hydrocarbons, several of which caused a uroporphyria in animals. Dioxin was among the most potent and, moreover, was of interest as a known contaminant of herbicides such as Agent Orange, which had been used in Vietnam. Detailed evaluation of Vietnam veterans and other exposed groups over a 20-year time span, however, has failed to produce convincing evidence of either porphyria or a subclinical state consistent with chemical porphyria. It would appear that environmental exposure to dioxin (with mainly cutaneous absorption) is less risky to humans than was suggested by studies of animals given the compound systemically.

Treatment

Alcohol, estrogen, and dietary iron supplements should be discontinued (see Table 42–2). While this step alone may lead to improvement, iron-depletion therapy hastens recovery in virtually all patients. This is best accomplished by venesection at the rate of 500 mL weekly or biweekly, with monitoring of the hemoglobin level, until transferrin saturation drops below 40%. Follow-up consists of an annual check of urine uroporphyrin and iron status, with resumption of phlebotomy as indicated. For patients unable to tolerate phlebotomy, continuous subcutaneous infusion of desferrioxamine is effective, albeit expensive. Chloroquine is an alternative, causing depletion of uroporphyrin apparently by complexing with it in the liver. It should be used at low doses (eg, 125 mg chloroquine base, twice weekly), however, to minimize the risk of adverse hepatic reactions.

Topical transparent sunscreens offer little or no protection from light-induced damage.

Prognosis

Virtually all patients respond to iron depletion, although the period of treatment required to produce a response can vary from a few weeks to 6 months or more. Provided the responsible environmental factors (notably alcohol) have been eliminated, the remission may be long lasting.

CONGENITAL ERYTHROPOIETIC PORPHYRIA

This is a rare, recessively inherited disease in which levels of blood and urine uroporphyrin are massively elevated. Photocutaneous lesions are evident from an early age, beginning usually in infancy. The relevance to gastroenterology is that some cases are relatively mild and may present in adulthood with cutaneous disease resembling that of porphyria cutanea tarda. Activated charcoal by mouth is an experimental therapy that has proved beneficial in a few patients. It presumably binds porphyrin in the intestine, preventing its enterohepatic recirculation and thus decreasing the total body burden. Iron-depletion therapy is of no value.

PROTOPORPHYRIA

Protoporphyria is a chronic cutaneous porphyria; in most cases, the excess porphyrin originates from the bone marrow, but in some it comes at least in part from the liver.

Clinical Findings

A. Symptoms and Signs: The cutaneous disease involves an immediate edematous, urticarial reaction to sunlight, distinct from the blistering that occurs in porphyria cutanea tarda. Repeated exposure produces cutaneous thickening and fibrosis. Because circulating protoporphyrin is excreted essentially entirely into bile, relatively high levels may accumulate in the liver. Such deposition appears to be the basis for a hepatopathy that is rare but can progress rapidly to portal hypertension and a fatal outcome. Jaundice heralds hepatic decompensation. About 10% of patients have protoporphyrin-containing gallstones.

B. Laboratory Findings: The characteristic abnormality is elevation of erythrocyte and fecal protoporphyrin, with little, if any, change in the other heme precursors. Circulating erythrocytes may be fluorescent. Anemia usually is not present. The accumulation of protoporphyrin in hepatocytes gives rise to birefringent inclusions under polarizing light. The best predictor of liver disease appears to be a plasma protoporphyrin level in excess of 100 μg/dL.

C. Genetic Diagnosis: Direct assay of the deficient enzyme, heme synthase, is not usually available. In some families, carriers can be identified by their fluorescing erythrocytes, but others lack this finding.

Treatment & Prognosis

Individuals with worrisome levels of plasma protoporphyrin should have tests of liver function and needle biopsy, if necessary, to assess the activity of the liver disease. Cholestyramine or activated charcoal has been used to trap protoporphyrin in the intestine and facilitate its excretion. Anecdotal reports suggest some benefit of this approach. Red cell transfusion reduces protoporphyrin production by way of suppressing erythropoiesis but is cumbersome. Oral administration of β-carotene alleviates the cutaneous symptoms, apparently by quenching active oxygen, which mediates the light-induced damage. A noticeable yellowing of the skin occurs as a cosmetic side effect.

are genetic and represent deficiency of a specific enzyme of the pathway. The "acute-attack" (neurologic) types have clinical features in common, including increased urinary excretion of ALA and PBG. Cutaneous porphyria results from overproduction of porphyrins, which are photosensitizing. The specific diagnosis is determined from the pattern of porphyrin intermediates in blood or excreta.

Management is tailored to the type of porphyria. The only specific treatment for acute attacks is hematin, which should be considered for any patient with objective neurologic signs and for those whose symptoms fail to respond to conservative measures. The most prevalent of the cutaneous porphyrias, porphyria cutanea tarda, is effectively treated by iron depletion, while the cutaneous symptoms in protoporphyria respond to administration of β-carotene. Toxic (acquired) porphyria occurs following intensive exposure to some halogenated hydrocarbons and resembles porphyria cutanea tarda. It appears, however, to be a rarity in Western Europe and North America under current standards of environmental safety.

SUMMARY

The porphyrias are a group of diseases involving disturbances in heme synthesis. The most important

REFERENCES

Anderson KE: LHRH analogues for hormonal manipulation in acute intermittent porphyria. Semin Hematol 1989;26:10.

Bissell DM: Haem metabolism and the porphyrias. In: *Wright's Liver and Biliary Disease.* Millward-Sadler GH, Arthur MJP (editors). Balliere Tindall, 1992.

Bissell DM: Treatment of acute hepatic porphyria with hematin. J Hepatol 1988;6:1.

Bloomer JR: The liver in protoporphyria. Hepatology 1988;8:402.

Dean G: Pursuit of a disease. Sci Am 1957;196:133.

Edwards CQ et al: HLA-linked hemochromatosis alleles in sporadic porphyria cutanea tarda. Gastroenterology 1989;97:972.

43

Complications of Chronic Liver Disease

Jaquelyn F. Fleckenstein, MD, & Anna Mae Diehl, MD

The complications of chronic liver disease are multiple and highly variable in presentation. Patients may be asymptomatic, with only incidentally detected laboratory test abnormalities, or may have florid features of hepatic parenchymal failure and portal hypertension. The clinical features of chronic liver disease are usually most evident when it has progressed to **cirrhosis,** which results when the normal liver "architecture" is replaced with fibrosis and regenerating nodules of various sizes. Fibrogenesis and regeneration are components of the wound healing response triggered by various types of chronic liver injury. The cellular basis of these components has been the subject of several recent reviews (see "References" at the end of this chapter) and will not be detailed here. Table 43–1 lists the most common causes of cirrhosis.

The complications of cirrhosis can be categorized as consequences of portal hypertension or parenchymal failure. The neoplastic complications of chronic liver disease are beyond the scope of this chapter (see Chapter 46).

CONSEQUENCES OF PARENCHYMAL FAILURE

Pathophysiology

When liver cells die, the remaining hepatocytes quickly compensate by increasing their metabolic efficiency and by replicating to restore lost liver mass. This regenerative response is necessary for survival after liver injury, because no artificial liver support apparatus is currently available, except in experimental protocols. Extensive liver damage usually occur before the hepatic regenerative capacity is overwhelmed, and clinical evidence of liver dysfunction therefore indicates extreme damage. Current therapy, aside from liver transplantation, has little impact on mortality rates once liver disease becomes clinically overt. This happens when substances that are normally synthesized by the liver are deficient, while toxic products normally cleared by the liver accumulate. Clinical features of parenchymal failure are summarized in Table 43–2.

Clinical Findings

A. Symptoms and Signs: Symptoms of parenchymal failure are typically vague and nonspecific, such as malaise, anorexia, fatigue, and weakness (see Chapter 34). Several signs of parenchymal failure (eg, edema and coagulopathy) result from reduced plasma concentrations of proteins that are synthesized by the liver (eg, albumin, fibrinogen, and coagulation factors), and the severity of these deficits is commonly used to estimate the severity of liver dysfunction.

1. Hypoalbuminemia–The clinical consequences of hypoalbuminemia result from reduced plasma oncotic pressure, which permits the drainage of fluid from the vascular space and promotes tissue edema. As previously noted, the degree of hypoalbuminemia is often used to gauge the severity of liver disease. This is an imperfect indicator of liver function, however, because the plasma concentration of albumin is also affected by nutritional and fluid status and possible renal losses (ie, albuminuria).

2. Coagulopathy–Another clinically important consequence of impaired hepatic protein synthesis is coagulopathy, which is common in advanced liver disease because all clotting factors except factor VIII are synthesized by the liver. The severity of coagulopathy, as evidenced by the magnitude of prolongation of prothrombin and partial thromboplastin times, provides another marker of the severity of hepatic parenchymal dysfunction. Like hypoalbuminemia, however, coagulopathy at best provides only an estimate of parenchymal failure, because several other conditions can also cause coagulopathy. For example, less severe forms of liver disease and other conditions that decrease bile flow (cholestasis) can lead to vitamin K malabsorption, with failure to activate vitamin K-dependent procoagulants. Fortunately, the coagulopathy of vitamin K deficiency is easily distin-

COMPLICATIONS OF CHRONIC LIVER DISEASE / 559

Table 43–1. Causes of cirrhosis.

Autoimmune hepatitis
Alcohol-induced liver injury
Drug- or toxin-induced liver injury
Viral hepatitis B, C, or D
Metabolic diseases
   α_1-antitrypsin deficiency
   Wilson's disease
   Hemochromatosis
Vascular derangements
   Chronic right heart failure
   Budd-Chiari syndrome
Biliary cirrhosis
   Primary biliary cirrhosis
   Biliary cirrhosis secondary to chronic large bile duct
     obstruction
   Primary sclerosing cholangitis
   Biliary atresia
   Congenital paucity of intrahepatic ducts
Cryptogenic disease

guished from that of liver failure because only the former responds to treatment with parenteral vitamin K. Other causes of coagulopathy that must be distinguished from liver failure in cirrhotic patients include coagulopathies associated with sepsis and hepatocellular carcinoma. Consumptive coagulopathy associated with sepsis can be distinguished from the coagulopathy of liver failure by factor VIII levels, which are decreased in sepsis but not in liver failure. The coagulopathy that sometimes complicates hepatocellular carcinoma is due to the production of inactive forms of fibrinogen; this situation may be impossible to distinguish from the dysfibrinogenemia associated with advanced parenchymal liver failure.

3. Jaundice–Jaundice is an additional sign of parenchymal failure; the extent of hyperbilirubinemia indicates the severity of liver disease. Jaundice occurs in parenchymal failure because the hepatocyte's ability to excrete conjugated bilirubin into bile be-

Table 43–2. Common clinical features
of parenchymal failure.

Symptoms and Signs	Laboratory Abnormalities
Weakness	Hyperbilirubinemia
Malaise	Prolonged prothrombin and partial
Anorexia	thromboplastin times
Fatigue	Hypoalbuminemia
Pruritus	Hyperammonemia
Easy bleeding or	Elevated creatinine or blood urea
bruising	nitrogen
Edema or ascites	
Jaundice	
Cachexia	
Feminization (gyne-	
comastia, testicular	
atrophy, palmar	
erythema, spider	
telangiectasias)	
Clubbing	
Encephalopathy	

comes impaired and the retained conjugated bilirubin "regurgitates" back into the bloodstream. Decreased excretion of bilirubin into bile (ie, cholestasis) also changes the composition of bile and limits its ability to detoxify lipid-soluble wastes. The latter is thought to contribute to the pruritus that often complicates chronic cholestasis. Like the other signs of parenchymal failure, jaundice is not specific. Any condition that causes overproduction of bilirubin (eg, hemolysis), decreased hepatic uptake or conjugation of bilirubin (eg, Gilbert syndrome), or mechanical obstruction of the flow of bile into the intestine (eg, obstructing choledocholithiasis or pancreatic cancer) can cause jaundice in the absence of cirrhosis.

4. Cachexia–Cachexia is another important measure of parenchymal dysfunction. Although it is not a specific marker of advanced liver disease, cachexia has great prognostic significance in patients with cirrhosis. Many factors doubtlessly contribute to cachexia in cirrhotic patients, including (1) anorexia; (2) malabsorption of nutrients because of intestinal edema and decreased bile flow; (3) reduced hepatic stores of many water-soluble vitamins and trace elements; (4) impaired hepatic and muscle intermediary metabolism as a result of increased circulating levels of proinflammatory cytokines; and (5) altered balance of many hormones that normally maintain metabolic homeostasis (eg, insulin, insulinlike growth factor, glucagon, thyroid hormones).

5. Renal failure–Renal failure is a devastating complication of hepatic parenchymal failure. The pathogenesis of kidney dysfunction secondary to hepatic failure is poorly understood but clearly involves the action of circulating factors that reversibly compromise renal perfusion and glomerular function. Anuria with consequent uremia, volume overload, and acid-base and electrolyte imbalance can prove fatal, unless dialysis is employed. Indeed, renal failure secondary to "hepatorenal syndrome" is often one of the terminal events in patients with parenchymal hepatic failure who cannot undergo liver transplantation. Paradoxically, the failing kidneys will function normally if transplanted into a recipient with normal liver function. Because systemic hypotension with secondary renal hypoperfusion may contribute to accelerated renal dysfunction in patients with liver failure, therapeutic efforts are usually directed toward optimizing renal blood flow by (1) treating underlying sepsis; (2) avoiding concurrent use of nonsteroidal anti-inflammatory drugs (NSAIDs); (3) restoring intravascular volume losses that occur from hemorrhage, diuretics, or cathartics; and (4) maintaining tissue perfusion with combinations of inotropic and vasodilatory agents. No specific pharmacologic therapy has yet been identified that can restore renal function in patients with hepatic parenchymal failure. Preliminary studies suggest that the potent vasoconstrictor endothelin-1 may play a role.

6. Other findings—Other clinical features of cirrhosis may occur, at least in part, because parenchymal failure limits the efficiency of hepatic enzyme systems responsible for detoxification of hormones, cytokines, and drugs. Prolonged half-lives of the parent substance or extrahepatic metabolism of these agents to biologically active intermediates may contribute to "feminization" (gynecomastia female pattern of hair distribution), autonomic neuropathy, osteodystrophy, encephalopathy, hepatopulmonary syndrome, and renal dysfunction in patients with cirrhosis. Once again, it is important to recognize that none of these are specific indicators of parenchymal failure, because many may also ensue from direct toxic actions on peripheral tissues (eg, alcohol testicular toxicity, iron toxicity in the hypothalamus and pituitary, toxin-induced renal damage) in the absence of cirrhosis.

Treatment

Other than liver transplantation, there is no specific curative therapy for hepatic parenchymal failure. Rapid progress is being made in the use of hepatic assist devices (ie, artificial liver) for short-term support, but none are yet approved for use. Consequently, treatment strategies focus on palliating disabling symptoms and preventing the progression of disease-related complications.

A. Coagulopathy: Efforts to correct coagulopathies should be reserved for patients who are actively bleeding or about to undergo procedures associated with a high risk of significant bleeding. In such circumstances, treatment with fresh-frozen plasma may improve the coagulation status. Typically, however, large amounts of fresh-frozen plasma are required, and this may precipitate problems related to overexpansion of intravascular volume, in addition to increasing the risk of viral infection contracted from contaminated blood products. Prothrombin complex concentrates should be avoided, because they contain activated procoagulants that may not be cleared by the diseased liver.

B. Hypoalbuminemia: Hypoalbuminemia seldom requires treatment. One exception may be the use of intravenous albumin supplements to maintain intravascular volume after large-volume paracentesis in nonedematous patients with renal insufficiency (see the following discussion, "Ascites"). If albumin is administered in this setting, 6–8 g should be given for every liter of ascites removed. Half of the albumin is usually infused immediately following the paracentesis and the remainder 6 hours later.

C. Jaundice: There is no specific therapy for jaundice resulting from parenchymal failure. Care should be taken to exclude potentially reversible causes of hyperbilirubinemia in this population. Noninvasive imaging studies (eg, ultrasound) are useful in excluding most causes of bile duct obstruction that would benefit from mechanical decompression. Pruritus as a result of chronic cholestasis can be a disabling symptom of advanced liver disease and is often difficult to palliate. Potential treatments for pruritus are listed in Table 43–3. (See also Chaper 51.)

CONSEQUENCES OF PORTAL HYPERTENSION

Pathophysiology

Portal hypertension is a serious complication of cirrhosis, contributing to many of the complications of chronic liver disease. As shown in Figure 43–1, the portal vein is derived from the splenic vein and large mesenteric veins. As such, it carries blood draining from the splanchnic circulation to the liver. The liver is the main site of resistance to portal blood flow and acts as a distensible vascular network with low resistance. Portal venous pressure is therefore normally low (5–10 mm Hg), and portal hypertension is defined as pressure that exceeds 10 mm Hg.

Changes in pressure in the portal vein are regulated by **Ohm's law,** which states that changes in pressure (P1–P2) along a blood vessel are a function of the interaction of blood flow (Q) and vascular resistance (R), where (P1–P2) = Q × R. Increased resistance to portal blood flow can develop anywhere along the venous system, eg, in the portal vein or its tributaries before blood reaches the liver (prehepatic obstruction), in the vascular spaces within the liver (intrahepatic obstruction), or in the veins or vascular compartments that receive the portal blood flow after it exits the liver (posthepatic obstruction). Examples of prehepatic and posthepatic portal hypertension are listed in Table 43–4. Intrahepatic obstruction, however, is much more complex and can occur at multiple sites in the liver. Occlusion of small portal vein branches within portal triads (presinusoidal obstruction) may complicate liver diseases in which there is extensive portal and periportal inflammatory infiltration or fibrosis. Alternatively, portal blood flow may be impeded by narrowing of the hepatic sinusoids because of collagen deposition or occlusion of the sinu-

Table 43–3. Treatments for pruritus associated with cholestasis.

Standard clinical practice
   Cholestyramine (1 package before meals)
   Ursodeoxycholic acid (300 mg twice daily)
   Phenobarbital (30 mg at bedtime)
   Rifampicin (150 mg twice daily)
Experimental options
   Opioid receptor antagonists (naloxone, propiphol)
   Plasmapheresis

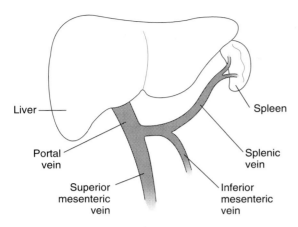

Figure 43–1. Anatomy of the normal portal vein.

soids by contractile cellular elements (sinusoidal obstruction). Finally, portal blood flow may be obstructed at the level of the terminal hepatic venules, because of toxin-induced occlusion of these vessels (postsinusoidal obstruction). Table 43–4 includes examples of various intrahepatic causes of portal hypertension. It is important to recognize that although cirrhosis is a major cause of portal hypertension, portal hypertension can occur in the absence of cirrhosis.

Pressure in the portal vein can be measured directly or indirectly. Direct measurement is performed by inserting a catheter into the portal vein (via laparotomy) or one of its branches (by percutaneous, transhepatic cannulation of the intrahepatic portal vein branch and advancement of the cannula into the main portal vein). Direct measurement within the portal vein is the most reliable way to estimate portal pressure when blood flow is obstructed before it reaches the liver. Portal vein pressure is estimated by indirect methods based on the assumption that the pressure across the sinusoidal bed within the liver has equalized, so that the pressure in the small tribu-

Table 43–4. Causes of portal hypertension.

Prehepatic obstruction of portal venous flow
   Splenic vein thrombosis
   Portal vein thrombosis
Intrahepatic obstruction of portal venous flow (in addition to cirrhosis)
   Presinusoidal: schistosomiasis, sarcoidosis, congenital hepatic fibrosis
   Sinusoidal: alcoholic fibrosis, sickle cell crisis, infiltration of the liver with myeloid elements in myelofibrosis
   Postsinusoidal: alcohol-induced perivenular fibrosis, veno-occlusive disease from antineoplastic agents
Posthepatic obstruction of portal venous flow
   Right heart failure
   Constrictive pericarditis
   Budd-Chiari syndrome
   Hepatic vein webs

taries of the portal vein (which deliver blood to the sinusoids) equals the pressure in the small branches of the hepatic vein (which carry blood away from the sinusoids). A catheter is inserted into an antecubital or femoral vein and advanced with fluoroscopic guidance into the hepatic vein. By "wedging" the catheter into a small branch of the hepatic vein, the pressure in the hepatic sinusoids (and, thus, indirectly in the portal vein) is recorded. The wedged hepatic venous pressure (WHVP) is then subtracted from the pressure that is freely recorded in the hepatic vein (free hepatic venous pressure [FHVP]) to normalize for the effect of intra-abdominal pressure. Thus, portal pressure is estimated by recording the pressure gradient between FHVP and WHVP. This procedure is extremely safe and simple and is the most common method used to measure portal pressure; however, it may not be accurate if portal blood flow is blocked before it enters the sinusoids. In such cases, the hepatic venous pressure gradient would underestimate the severity of portal hypertension. To avoid confusion in this circumstance, another indirect method, which records the pressure in the splenic pulp, can be used to measure portal vein pressure. This method is rarely used, however, because percutaneous puncture of the spleen carries a significant risk of bleeding (1–2% of patients) and the technique has no method to normalize for intra-abdominal pressure.

Clinical Findings

When portal blood flow is obstructed (either inside or outside of the liver), blood begins to pool in the vascular beds that normally empty into the portal vein. Congestion of omental tissues contributes to the pathogenesis of ascites. Sequestration of blood in the spleen causes splenomegaly and hypersplenism, with secondary thrombocytopenia, neutropenia, and anemia. Eventually, a collateral circulatory system (ie, varices) develops to decompress the portal bed by diverting portal blood flow into systemic veins. These collateral veins can become quite prominent in the esophagus, stomach, and distal intestine. Increased flow through such esophagogastric and hemorrhoidal varices can lead to vessel rupture, with devastating hemorrhage. If extensive variceal collaterals develop, significant amounts of portal blood flow are shunted away from the liver and portal pressure may fall to within the normal range. The end result, however, is the liver is deprived of portal blood and must rely increasingly on hepatic artery blood. This dependence impairs the liver's capacity to regenerate and causes it to atrophy. Hepatic arterial dependence also makes the liver more vulnerable to changes in systemic blood pressure and increases the risk of hepatic ischemia during hypotension. In addition, portovenous shunting diverts blood draining the intestines away from the liver and delivers it "prematurely" into the systemic circulation, compromising hepatic clearance of gut-derived products and contributing to hepatic encephalopathy and sepsis. Many physical findings in cirrhotic patients are caused by portal hypertension (Table 43–5). Thus, detection of these signs in a patient with liver disease suggests that cirrhosis has developed.

Because many portal hypertension complications present significant threats to survival in cirrhotic patients, they have been the focus of considerable diagnostic and therapeutic efforts. The following sections briefly summarize current knowledge about the pathogenesis, diagnosis, and treatment of each of these clinically important complications.

CLINICAL COMPLICATIONS OF PORTAL HYPERTENSION

1. GASTROINTESTINAL BLEEDING

Gastrointestinal bleeding is a serious, yet relatively rare, complication of portal hypertension. As few as one-third of cirrhotic patients have varices. While many potential sources of bleeding (eg, peptic ulcers, portal hypertensive gastropathy, portovenous collaterals) may coexist in cirrhotic patients, the most clinically significant hemorrhage typically occurs when dilated venous collaterals (varices) rupture.

Esophageal, gastric, and hemorrhoidal collaterals have the highest propensity to bleed profusely, although varices can form in many other locations (eg, in surgical scars, ostomies, and the umbilical vein). Esophageal and gastric varices are connections between the coronary and short gastric veins and the azygous vein. Hemorrhoidal varices are the result of connections between the portal system and the middle and superior hemorrhoidal veins.

A threshold portal pressure gradient of at least 12 mm Hg (ie, WHVP minus FHVP) is necessary for esophageal varices to develop; however, they may not form even if the pressure gradient is greater than 12 mm Hg. Other factors that appear to play a role in the development of esophageal varices are the extent of other collateral routes of drainage and permissive conditions (eg, lower esophageal sphincter pressure) for blood flow into the esophageal collateral system.

Once varices have formed, they usually do not bleed. In fact, the risk of an index episode of bleeding has been estimated to be no greater than 30% per year. The risk of variceal rupture is more directly dependent on the wall tension of the varix than on the portal pressure. **Wall tension** is determined by the diameter of the varix and its wall thickness, as well as the pressure within its lumen. Hence, large, thin-walled veins within the esophagus are at greatest risk of rupture. Although vessel wall thickness appears to be important in determining which collaterals rupture, erosion from without (eg, resulting from esophagitis or nasogastric tube placement) is much less of a threat to variceal integrity than rupture of the vessel wall as a result of elevations in intravascular (ie, portal) pressure. Consequently, there is little evidence that prophylactic antipeptic therapy decreases the risk of bleeding from esophageal varices. On the other hand, treatment with β-blockers, which diminish portal venous pressure, decreases the initial risk of bleeding in patients with alcoholic cirrhosis and large esophageal varices. The dose of β-blockers used to prevent index bleeding from varices (ie, for prophylaxis) is adjusted to reduce the heart rate by 25% (see the following discussion). Other treatments to prevent index bleeding from varices, such as prophylactic endoscopic sclerotherapy or portosystemic shunt, have proved too toxic to justify widespread use in patients who have never had bleeding episodes.

Hemorrhage from varices is a dramatic event, with painless hematemesis, melena, or hematochezia; bleeding is rarely insidious or chronic. Signs of hemodynamic instability (hypotension, tachycardia) are common. The risk of dying from variceal bleeding is variable and depends on the severity of hemorrhage and the underlying liver disease. Patients with severely decompensated liver disease have at least a 50% chance of dying after hospitalization with a hemodynamically significant variceal hemorrhage. Furthermore, once varices have bled, they are at high risk (70–80%) of bleeding again, particularly within the first few weeks to months following the index hemorrhage.

Once the patient is hemodynamically resuscitated, the source of gastrointestinal bleeding must be identified by upper endoscopy. Endoscopy is essential because nonvariceal sources of gastrointestinal bleeding are also common in cirrhotic patients, and both short- and long-term management differ markedly, depending on the source of bleeding. Optimal resuscitation requires intensive monitoring of the patient's blood loss and moving the patient into an intensive care unit. Following hemodynamic stabilization and airway protection, the source of bleeding should be identified endoscopically.

Active bleeding from a varix, adherent clot on a varix, or signs of redness or thinning of a varix wall (dubbed "red or blue wale signs") in the absence of other identifiable bleeding sources implicate varices as the source of hemorrhage. Treatment of variceal bleeding can be divided into acute management of active or recent bleeding and therapies to prevent delayed rebleeding (Figure 43–2).

Table 43–5. Signs of portal hypertension.

Splenomegaly ("hypersplenism" with thrombocytopenia, leukopenia, anemia)
Variceal collaterals (esophagogastric, hemorrhoidal, abdominal wall)
Ascites
Hepatic encephalopathy (hyperammonemia)
Hepatopulmonary syndrome

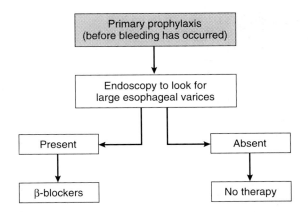

Figure 43–2. Primary prophylaxis for gastrointestinal bleeding resulting from portal hypertension.

Management of Acute Variceal Bleeding

Figure 43–3 shows a protocol for managing active gastrointestinal bleeding resulting from portal hypertension.

A. Endoscopic Sclerotherapy: Endoscopic control of hemorrhage by sclerotherapy or banding is considered the optimal technique for acute management of variceal bleeding. Sclerosants (eg, ethanolamine oleate, sodium tetradecyl, or sodium morrhuate) are injected into or around varices in 1–2 mL increments. The technique is successful in arresting bleeding in more than 90% of patients and decreases the risk of early rebleeding from 70% in untreated patients to 30–40%. This is associated with a short-term improvement in mortality rates. Approximately 20% of patients experience side effects associated with sclerotherapy including chest pain, fever, bacteremia, pleural effusion, acute esophageal ulceration with or without bleeding, and delayed development of esophageal strictures.

B. Variceal Banding: Because of local complications with sclerotherapy, variceal banding is evolving as an attractive alternative. The technique requires placing a rubber band ligature directly over the bleeding varix guided by an endoscope. The effectiveness of this techniques in controlling bleeding equals endoscopic sclerotherapy, with fewer ulcerations and pulmonary complications. Moreover, recurrent bleeding in the acute setting (within 48 hours) can be managed with further attempts at banding; this is unlike sclerotherapy because administration of the sclerosant must be limited.

C. Drug Therapy: Efforts to arrest bleeding by administering pharmacologic agents such as vasopressin or somatostatin analogs, which promote splanchnic vasoconstriction, are less successful than endoscopic sclerotherapy. If pharmacologic agents are used, octreotide (a somatostatin analog) is given

intravenously at 50 µg/h, and vasopressin is given intravenously at 0.3 u/min, with titration to a maximum of 0.9 u/min. Vasopressin, unlike somatostatin, may precipitate tissue ischemia when administered in high dosages, but adjunctive therapy with nitroglycerin (preferably intravenously) may minimize some of these side effects and is often helpful. These treatments are usually reserved for patients in whom definitive endoscopic therapy must be delayed or has been unsuccessful.

D. Variceal Tamponade: In patients with persistent and uncontrolled hemorrhage, mechanical tamponade of actively bleeding varices with specially designed nasogastric tubes (eg, Minnesota or Sengstaken-Blakemore tubes) is necessary. These tubes contain balloons, which, when inflated, apply pressure directly to the esophageal wall or gastric cardia, or both. Care should be used during tube placement because malpositioning or overinflation can result in esophageal or gastric rupture. The risk of esophageal rupture can be reduced by inflating only the gastric and not the esophageal balloon. Endotracheal intubation protects the airway thereby reducing the risk of aspiration. Balloon tamponade is a temporary maneuver that prevents hemorrhage while more definitive treatments to decompress the portal system are being arranged. It should never be used for more than 24 hours.

E. Surgical Portosystemic Shunts: Traditionally, portal decompression has been accomplished by creating surgical shunts that direct portal blood from the portal vein or its tributaries (the splenic vein or inferior mesenteric vein) into the inferior vena cava or its tributaries (the renal vein). Surgically created portosystemic shunts (eg, portacaval, mesocaval, splenorenal shunts) remain the most effective means to arrest active variceal bleeding and prevent recurrent hemorrhage. However, acute portosystemic shunting is rarely performed, because perioperative rates of complications and death are extremely high when it is done emergently in actively bleeding cirrhotic patients. Esophageal transection with or without devascularization is another surgical approach that is sometimes used to control variceal hemorrhage; however, it is also associated with high perioperative rates of complications and death.

F. TIPS: Recent advances in invasive radiology have made nonsurgical construction of portosystemic shunts feasible and attractive. Transjugular intrahepatic portosystemic shunting (TIPS) is an angiographic technique in which the portal vein is cannulated via the transjugular route through the liver, and then an expandable stent is inserted to construct an intrahepatic shunt between the portal circulation and the left hepatic vein. TIPS is an effective means of arresting variceal bleeding for patients in which sclerotherapy has failed, but its long-term efficacy and safety relative to other management options for acute variceal hemorrhage have not yet been established.

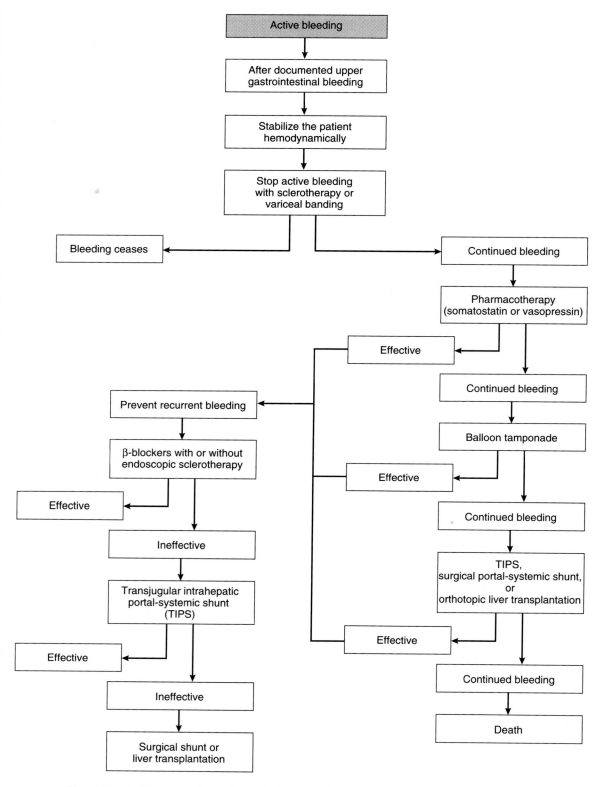

Figure 43–3. Management of active gastrointestinal bleeding resulting from portal hypertension.

Treatments to Prevent Delayed Rebleeding From Varices

A. Endoscopic Sclerotherapy: Because endoscopic sclerotherapy is effective in arresting esophageal variceal bleeding and preventing early rebleeding, its efficacy in preventing delayed rebleeding from varices has also been evaluated. Long-term control of variceal hemorrhage by sclerotherapy requires periodic endoscopy (ie, every 2–4 weeks initially; then, every 2–3 months) to detect and obliterate recurrent varices. The effectiveness of sclerotherapy appears to diminish over time, as esophageal varices are obliterated and replaced by gastric and intestinal collaterals that are less easily eradicated. Repeated sclerosis also increases the incidence of treatment-related complications, especially esophageal stricture.

B. Drug Therapy: While pharmacologic therapy appears inferior to sclerotherapy for the acute management of variceal bleeding, it may be more advantageous than endoscopic sclerotherapy when used chronically. Indeed, several trials indicate that treatment with β-blockers (eg, propranolol, nadolol), which reduce the heart rate by 25%, decreases the risk of delayed rebleeding from varices. In addition, β-blockers lower the pressure in gastric collaterals and, thus, unlike sclerotherapy, can reduce the risk of bleeding from gastric varices and portal hypertensive gastropathy. Consequently, β-blockers are often used alone or as adjunctive therapy in patients who are undergoing chronic sclerotherapy. The major obstacle to chronic β-blocker therapy appears to be patient acceptance. Dosages sufficient to achieve adequate β-blockade are often associated with lethargy, depression, and symptomatic bradyarrhythmias.

C. TIPS: TIPS has been suggested as an alternative strategy to prevent delayed variceal rebleeding. Because TIPS is relatively noninvasive and decompresses the entire portal system, it offers the theoretic advantage of being more effective than sclerotherapy and less risky than portosystemic shunt surgery. Emerging evidence suggests that this optimism may have to be tempered because of the high rate of shunt occlusion (approximately 50% per year), with reemergence of symptomatic portal hypertension, and a risk of encephalopathy.

D. Surgical Portosystemic Shunts: Apart from liver transplantation, surgically constructed portosystemic shunts remain the most effective means to prevent delayed rebleeding from varices. Because "selective" (ie, mesocaval and distal splenorenal) shunts divert only a portion of the portal blood flow away from the liver, they are preferable to "total" (portacaval) shunts. Thus, they achieve adequate portal decompression without excessive risk of hepatic encephalopathy. Although the risk of shunt occlusion and rebleeding is extremely low in selective shunts (< 10% at 5 years) and the incidence of refractory encephalopathy is acceptable (also < 10%), elective shunt surgery is seldom performed in patients who are candidates for liver transplantation. This is because it does not prevent death from other complications of advanced cirrhosis and may make subsequent transplant surgery more difficult. Surgical decompression remains an option for selected patients with well-preserved parenchymal function who have failed other efforts to prevent recurrent portal hypertensive bleeding.

2. HEPATIC ENCEPHALOPATHY

Another complication of portal hypertension is hepatic encephalopathy, a neuropsychiatric disorder characterized by changes in personality, cognition, motor function, or level of consciousness. Hepatic encephalopathy is usually reversible and results when products that are usually metabolized (or detoxified) by the liver escape into the systemic circulation. It is usually due to parenchymal failure and portal hypertension caused by cirrhosis, but may also occur in individuals with normal livers and spontaneous or surgically constructed portosystemic shunts.

Pathophysiology

Although the precise pathophysiology of hepatic encephalopathy is unknown, four major classes of neuroactive substances have been implicated: (1) ammonia; (2) false neurotransmitters derived from amino acid imbalance; (3) γ-aminobutyric acid (GABA); and (4) endogenous ligands of the benzodiazepine receptor. The potential importance of these putative mediators is supported by some evidence but refuted by other observations. While current dogma favors a primary role of endogenous benzodiazepine receptor ligands in the pathogenesis of hepatic encephalopathy, it is increasingly recognized that each of the other mediators may variably contribute.

Clinical Findings

Hepatic encephalopathy may be virtually asymptomatic (ie, subclinical) or present as recurrent or chronic cognitive or motor disorders. Altered mentation or level of consciousness can range from subtle personality changes to lethargy to coma. The spectrum of motor disorders is also quite broad, ranging from asterixis to spastic paralysis. A schema has been developed to grade the clinical severity of hepatic encephalopathy (Table 43–6).

Fortunately, subclinical hepatic encephalopathy is the most common form of hepatic encephalopathy and occurs in 50–80% of patients suffering from cirrhosis. It is recognized only if psychometric tests are performed, but associated subtle deficits in visual and motor coordination may contribute to work and traffic accidents. Recurrent attacks of clinically overt changes in mental status are the next most common presentation of hepatic encephalopathy in cirrhotic

Table 43–6. Stages of hepatic encephalopathy.

Stage	Consciousness	Cognition	Behavior	Motor Function	Psychometric Tests
0–1	Normal	Normal	Normal	Normal	Slow
1	Abnormal sleep	Attention	Moody	Dyscoordination	Very slow
2	Lethargic Ataxia Dysarthria	Memory	Dysinhibition	Asterixis	Poor
3	Confusion Delirium Semi stupor Incontinence	Disoriented Incoherent Amnesia Rigidity	Bizarre Anger Paranoia Seizures	Abnormal reflexes Nystagmus Babinski reflex	
4	Coma	None	Absent	Oculocephalic or oculovestibular response, decorticate or decerebrate posture, dilated pupils	

patients; these attacks are usually precipitated by identifiable factors (Table 43–7). The neurologic deficits may progress over time. Correction of the precipitating factors typically permits patients with recurrent bouts of overt encephalopathy to return to subclinical states of the disorder. Chronic hepatic encephalopathy is much more difficult to manage because variable degrees of mental status alteration occur in the absence of any identifiable precipitating cause. A few patients with chronic disease develop a severe motor disorder known as **hepatocerebral degeneration.** Unremitting spastic paralysis ensues in rare patients with this disorder.

Because the manifestations of hepatic encephalopathy are so variable, it should be suspected as a potential cause of essentially any neuropsychiatric abnormality in a cirrhotic patient. This disorder has no apparent clinical or laboratory abnormalities, and it remains a diagnosis of exclusion. Other disorders that may masquerade as hepatic encephalopathy must be excluded in the workup of patients with suspected disease (Table 43–8).

Treatment

Treatment of hepatic encephalopathy (Table 43–9) is derived from efforts to control the generation of putative neuroactive toxins. Because gut-derived, nitrogenous products may serve as a source of ammonia, lactulose is administered orally to decrease ammoniagenesis by enteric flora and reduce ammonia

absorption from the gastrointestinal tract. Other drugs, including neomycin and metronidazole, have also been used for this purpose. All of these agents have some toxicity. Common side effects of lactulose include flatulence and diarrhea and, less commonly, acidosis and hypernatremia. Neomycin can cause serious ototoxicity and nephrotoxicity. Dysgeusia and painful peripheral neuropathy may complicate therapy with metronidazole. Because lactulose has the most acceptable treatment-related side-effects, it is the mainstay of therapy.

Dietary intake of protein is restricted when lactulose therapy fails. However, it is important to understand that dietary protein deprivation (< 70 g/d) eventually results in increased catabolism of muscle protein, which not only provides an alternative ammonia source but also exacerbates the general cachexia associated with cirrhosis. Efforts to maintain nitrogen balance and restore the normal plasma ratios of branched-chain to aromatic amino acids by administering branched-chain-enriched amino acid

Table 43–7. Precipitating factors for recurrent hepatic encephalopathy.

Gastrointestinal bleeding
Infection (especially spontaneous peritonitis)
Excessive dietary protein intake
Constipation
Overdiuresis
Electrolyte abnormalities (decreased potassium, increased or decreased sodium)
Azotemia
Sedative use
Hepatic insults (viral infection, toxic damage, surgery, hepatocellular carcinoma)

Table 43–8. Differential diagnosis of hepatic encephalopathy.

Intracranial lesions
  Hemorrhage
  Infarct
  Tumor
  Abscess
Infections
  Meningitis
  Encephalitis
  Sepsis
Metabolic encephalopathies
  Hyperglycemia or hypoglycemia
  Uremia
  Acidosis
  Electrolyte imbalances
Alcohol-related disorders
  Intoxication
  Withdrawal
  Wernicke's encephalopathy
Drug toxicity (sedatives or other psychoactive drugs)
Postictal encephalopathy
Primary neuropsychiatric disorders

Table 43–9. Treatments for hepatic encephalopathy.

Agents that decrease gut absorption of nitrogenous products
   Lactulose
      30–120 mL/d orally (goal is 2–4 soft bowel movements
        per day)
      Can be administered by enema if oral intake is
        impossible
   Neomycin
      1–2 g orally 4 times a day alone or with lactulose
   Metronidazole
      250 mg orally 3 times a day alone or with lactulose or
        neomycin
Dietary protein restriction
   Sometimes necessary for acute management of refractory
      hepatic encephalopathy
   Should attempt to maintain at least 70-g protein diet chron-
      ically
Intravenous amino acids
   Branched-chain enriched formulations are expensive and
      usually ineffective
Benzodiazepine receptor antagonists (eg, flumazenil)
   Transient benefits; this remains an experimental therapy

formulations are generally ineffective at improving hepatic encephalopathy and are expensive. Recently, flumazenil, an intravenously administered benzodiazepine receptor antagonist, has shown some effectiveness at transiently improving refractory encephalopathy, but it has little practical usage at present.

3. ASCITES

The accumulation of ascites is often one of the first signs of decompensated chronic liver disease and implies the presence of both portal hypertension and some degree of hepatic parenchymal failure. The importance of both portal hypertension and parenchymal failure in the pathogenesis of cirrhotic ascites is suggested by observations that clinically significant ascites is relatively unusual in patients with either acute liver failure or noncirrhotic portal hypertension.

Pathophysiology

Portal hypertension and consequent hypoperfusion of hepatocytes with portal blood appears to initiate the exchange of signals between the liver and the kidney that result in enhanced renal reabsorption of sodium and water. This, in turn, expands the plasma volume and increases the flow of blood into the portal vein. When resistance to that blood flow is relatively fixed because of hepatic fibrosis, pressure in the system only rises further, without marked improvement in hepatocyte perfusion. Undampened signals to increase renal salt and water retention persist and lead to marked overexpansion of intravascular volume. Increased hydrostatic pressure forces fluid out of the vascular space and leads to tissue edema. This is exacerbated by hypoalbuminemia,

which decreases oncotic pressure. At first, most of the extravasated fluid can be returned to the vascular fluid by increased lymphatic flow. Eventually, however, the lymphatic capacity is overwhelmed, and excess fluid in the extracellular tissue space begins to "weep" into the peritoneal cavity, forming ascites. Coincidentally, collateral venous channels begin to open in an effort to decompress the engorged portal system, and some of the circulating blood volume begins to pool in the splanchnic bed. These two events result in a relative diminution in circulating blood volume, which appears to jeopardize perfusion of other vital organs (eg, kidney, heart, and brain). This triggers a cascade of compensatory events, including the release of sympathetic neurotransmitters and activation of the renin-angiotensin system, to maintain hemodynamic stability in the systemic circulation. Renal retention of salt and water continues to increase, and this only exacerbates the problem by further increasing portal blood flow in the face of fixed and elevated resistance to flow. In addition, splanchnic arteriolar dilatation may independently stimulate sodium and free water retention by increasing sympathetic tone. A vicious cycle ensues, and for a while, perfusion within the kidney remains balanced because of the renal production of vasodilatory cytokines. In time, renal compensation fails and perfusion of cortical nephrons declines. This impairs glomerular filtration and results in functional renal failure (ie, **hepatorenal syndrome**). It is important to recognize that in cirrhosis, renal function is disturbed long before the first drop of ascites forms and that the mechanisms that drive ascites formation change as portal hypertension and parenchymal failure progress.

Clinical Findings

Large amounts of ascites are easily detected on physical examination. Smaller amounts or loculated fluid collections are harder to recognize without imaging modalities such as ultrasound, CT, or MRI. New-onset ascites should always be evaluated with diagnostic paracentesis to help determine its cause. **The most useful parameter to classify ascites is the serum-ascites albumin gradient,** which is calculated by subtracting the ascites albumin concentration from the serum value. A gradient of greater than 1.1 g/dL is consistent with ascites secondary to portal hypertension. Gradients of less than 1.1 g/dL are associated with other causes of ascites such as pancreatitis, bile peritonitis, malignant chylous ascites, or chronic infections such as tuberculosis. In ascites with a low gradient, further evaluation should be done. An ascitic fluid amylase value greater than the serum amylase value is diagnostic of pancreatic ascites, and, similarly, a bilirubin level of ascitic fluid higher than that of serum is consistent with bile ascites. A triglyceride level of over 200 mg/dL or higher than the serum triglyceride level suggests chylous ascites, and cytologic studies and gram-stained smears are needed to evaluate for cancer and infection.

Treatment

Treatment of clinically apparent ascites is important because the accumulation of large amounts of fluid in the peritoneal space is not only uncomfortable but also compromises ventilation, increases the risk of ruptured umbilical hernias, impedes venous return, and serves as a source of infection. Treatment of ascites varies as liver disease progresses.

A. Diuresis: Initially, most patients with ascites will be improved by reducing dietary sodium or by gentle diuresis, or both. Treatment with aldosterone antagonists is preferable initially because of their long duration of action (> 72 hours in cirrhotics) and potassium-sparing effects. In patients with normal serum creatinine levels, aldactone can be safely started at a dose of 50 mg/d and then incrementally increased by 50 mg every 3–4 days to achieve a rate of weight loss that equals about 0.5 lb/d. If a dose of 300 mg of aldactone is reached without satisfactory diuresis, then it is likely that sodium reabsorption is so avid proximally that sufficient sodium is not reaching the distal nephron, the site of aldactone action. Such avid sodium retention does not usually occur until cirrhosis is quite advanced, and, in that case, a diuretic such as furosemide or hydrochlorothiazide, or both, is added to decrease sodium reabsorption at more proximal parts of the nephron. A reasonable starting dose of furosemide is 20–40 mg/d; this may be increased by 20-mg increments every third day, if diuresis is inadequate. It is seldom necessary to use more than 100 mg/d. In such cases, the addition of low doses of hydrochlorothiazide (25 mg/d) to the diuretic regimen often effect satisfactory diuresis.

Patients who fail to respond to diuretics after an aggressive regimen of dietary salt restriction and high doses of aldactone and furosemide plus hydrochlorothiazide are considered refractory to diuretic therapy. Fortunately, this occurs in a minority of cirrhotic patients with ascites and usually implies the presence of advanced liver disease. More often, high doses of diuretics cannot be employed because of diuretic-associated toxicities; notable in this regard are potentially life-threatening acid-base and electrolyte disturbances, ototoxicity, and painful gynecomastia.

B. Paracentesis: Patients who fail diuretic therapy are candidates for mechanical removal of ascites. This is usually accomplished by large-volume paracentesis. Ten or more liters of ascitic fluid can be safely removed in a single setting with little need for plasma volume-expanding agents, unless the patient has renal insufficiency or little peripheral edema. Intravenous administration of albumin (6–8 g per liter of ascites removed) is the most widely used volume expander. One-half of the albumin is usually infused

at the end of the paracentesis and the remainder 6 hours later. The acute risks of large-volume paracentesis are low and mainly include bleeding and infection. Repeated large-volume paracenteses are inconvenient for both patient and physician and can result in significant depletion of total body protein stores.

C. Shunts: Other techniques to mobilize diuretic-resistant ascites include peritoneojugular shunts, TIPS, and surgical portosystemic shunts. Of these, TIPS appears to have the most acceptable risk-to-benefit ratio. A few reports also suggest that TIPS may be useful in treating hepatic hydrothorax (or pleural ascites), a complication of advanced cirrhosis that is notoriously refractory to both diuretics and large-volume paracentesis.

D. Treatment of Hyponatremia: Advanced cirrhosis, particularly in conjunction with aggressive efforts to mobilize ascites, is frequently complicated by hyponatremia. Severe hyponatremia (< 115 mEq/L) can provoke hemolysis, encephalopathy, and seizures and, therefore, demands therapy. However, treatments that increase free water excretion are usually ineffective in this setting, and rapid overcorrection of this problem by administering hypertonic saline can lead to cortical demyelination. Thus, the best strategy is to guard against the development of significant hyponatremia by judicious monitoring of serum electrolytes, followed by appropriate restriction of free water intake and discontinuation of diuretics until the serum sodium value reaches 130 mEq/L.

4. SPONTANEOUS BACTERIAL PERITONITIS

Pathophysiology

Spontaneous bacterial peritonitis is a common complication of cirrhotic ascites, with a high mortality rate. By definition, it is caused by a single organism, without an identifiable intra-abdominal source. It is a different entity than polymicrobial bacterial peritonitis, which is often associated with a perforated viscus. Spontaneous bacterial peritonitis is usually ascribed to peritoneal seeding after bacteremic episodes or possible translocation of gut-derived bacteria; impaired reticuloendothelial cell clearance of portal blood bacteremias may also contribute. Patients with low levels of total protein in their ascitic fluid (< 1.5 g/dL) are at increased risk for developing spontaneous bacterial peritonitis because of reduced ascitic complement levels and opsonic activity.

The most frequent causative organism is *Escherichia coli,* but other coliforms, *Klebsiella,* pneumococci, and *Enterococcus* are also common.

Clinical Findings

Fever, worsening jaundice, abdominal pain, and confusion are the most common clinical findings of spontaneous bacterial peritonitis, although the patient may be asymptomatic. Abdominal tenderness is present in approximately 50% of patients, but its absence does not rule out the diagnosis of spontaneous bacterial peritonitis. Ascitic fluid features are as listed below. Gram-stained smears of ascitic fluid are not helpful, because they are rarely positive. All cirrhotic patients with ascites who are admitted to an inpatient unit should be considered for diagnostic paracentesis to rule out spontaneous bacterial peritonitis. Unless the patient has disseminated intravascular coagulation or primary fibrinolysis, paracentesis with a small-gauge needle can be carried out safely, despite abnormalities in coagulation.

The diagnosis of spontaneous bacterial peritonitis requires analysis of the peritoneal fluid (via paracentesis) and should not be made presumptively. Ascitic white blood cell counts of greater than 500/μL with more than 50% PMNs (ie, total neutrophil count > 250/μL) establishes the diagnosis; leukocyte counts greater than 300/μL raise suspicion for spontaneous bacterial peritonitis but are not definitive. If grossly bloody fluid is present, the PMN count should be corrected before the diagnosis of peritonitis is considered. Both blood cultures (positive in approximately 25% of patients) and peritoneal fluid cultures should be done. The technique of directly injecting peritoneal fluid into bone culture vials at the bedside increases the yield of positive cultures.

Imaging studies are not helpful in diagnosing spontaneous bacterial peritonitis (unless perforated viscus is suspected), and diagnostic paracentesis should be performed immediately whenever the condition is suspected, even if clinical peritonitis is absent.

Treatment

A high level of suspicion and early therapy are the most important aspects of therapy. Antibiotic therapy should be instituted in all patients with ascitic fluid counts of greater than 500/μL with 50% neutrophils (or 250/μL absolute neutrophil counts), regardless of culture results. Initially, broad-spectrum intravenous antibiotics are the treatment of choice. Currently, cefotaxime or a similar third-generation cephalosporin is the most widely used antibiotic in the empiric therapy of peritonitis. Treatment should continue for at least 5 days or, optimally, until the ascitic fluid PMN count normalizes.

Prophylactic therapy with daily oral quinolone therapy (norfloxacin, 400 mg at bedtime) may decrease the incidence of gram-negative spontaneous bacterial peritonitis and should be considered for cirrhotic patients with low ascitic protein concentrations (< 1 g/dL). Orthotopic liver transplantation should be considered in all patients who have survived spontaneous bacterial peritonitis and are otherwise suitable transplantation candidates (see Chapter 54).

Prognosis

There is a high mortality rate in patients with spontaneous bacterial peritonitis, with approximately 40% dying during the index hospitalization. Many patients in whom the infection clears die from other complications of liver disease. Recurrence of peritonitis within 1 year is common. A low ascitic fluid protein concentration is the best predictor of recurrence.

5. HEPATOPULMONARY SYNDROME

Portal hypertension may be complicated by the development of arteriovenous fistulas and bronchial varices in the lungs. This is associated with variable degrees of right-to-left shunting of blood, with subsequent oxygen desaturation. Usually, such pulmonary vascular abnormalities result in relatively subtle clinical manifestations, but occasional patients experience exertional dyspnea and markedly reduced diffusing capacity on pulmonary function testing. These abnormalities are improved, but not entirely reversed, by supplemental oxygen. Liver transplantation appears to reverse the syndrome in some patients.

REFERENCES

Friedman SL: The cellular basis of hepatic fibrosis: Mechanisms and treatment strategies. N Engl J Med 1993;328:1828.

Genecin P, Groszman R: Portal Hypertension. In: *Diseases of the Liver,* 7th ed. Schiff L, Schiff E (editors). Lippincott, 1993.

Gines P et al: Comparison of paracentesis and diuretics in the treatment of cirrhotics with tense ascites: Results of a randomized study. Gastroenterology 1987;93:234.

Laine L et al: Endoscopic ligation compared with sclerotherapy for the treatment of bleeding esophageal varices. Ann Intern Med 1993;119:1.

Lind CD et al: Incidence of shunt occlusion or stenosis following transjugular intrahepatic portosystemic shunt placement. Gastroenterology 1994;106:1277.

Michalopolous GK: Liver regeneration: Molecular mechanisms of growth control. FASEB J 1991;4:176.

The North Italian Endoscopic Club for the Study and Treatment of Esophageal Varices: Prediction of the first variceal hemorrhage in patients with cirrhosis of the liver and esophageal varices: A prospective multicenter study. N Engl J Med 1988;319:983.

Poynard T et al: Beta-adrenergic-antagonist drugs in the prevention of gastrointestinal bleeding in patients with cirrhosis and esophageal varices: An analysis of data and prognostic factors in 589 patients from four randomized clinical trials. N Engl J Med 1991;324:1532.

Rector WG Jr (editor): *Complications of Chronic Liver Disease.* Mosby-YearBook, 1992.

Rossle M et al: The transjugular intrahepatic portosystemic stent-shunt procedure for variceal bleeding. N Engl J Med 1994;330:165.

Runyon B: Care of patients with ascites. N Engl J Med 1994;330:337.

Schiff ER (editor): Management of Difficult Problems in Hepatology. Semin Liver Dis 1994;13:317–435.

Wong F, Blendis L: Hepatorenal Disorders. Semin Liver Dis 1994;14:1–105.

Drug-induced Liver Disease

44

Nathan M. Bass, MD, PhD

Liver injury may be produced by a large variety of chemical substances, including medicinal agents, industrial toxins, and natural products. More than 800 different drugs have been implicated. Drugs are estimated to be responsible for up to 5% of hospital admissions for jaundice and as many as 10% of all cases investigated for liver disease. The problem of drug-induced liver disease assumes an even greater significance in patients over 50 years of age, in whom the combination of increased susceptibility to adverse drug reactions and greater exposure to therapeutic drugs plays a role. The type of injury produced is extremely varied, and may mimic the entire spectrum of hepatobiliary disorders. The degree of severity of liver disease produced is also highly varied. Many drugs cause subclinical liver injury manifested only as abnormal serum liver enzyme tests, which rapidly reverse upon withdrawal of the drug. At the other extreme, drugs can initiate progressive, chronic liver disease as well as acute, fulminant hepatic failure. A relatively small proportion of drugs causes predictable, dosage-dependent toxic injury to the liver; the vast majority of injuries occur as unexpected reactions to a therapeutic dosage of a drug. The understanding of the molecular mechanisms involved in drug-induced liver disease as well as the determinants of individual susceptibility that underlie the idiosyncratic nature of most cases has increased greatly over the past 2 decades, but much remains unknown.

MECHANISMS OF DRUG-INDUCED LIVER DISEASE

The central role played by the liver in the clearance and biotransformation of chemicals is fundamental to its susceptibility to drug-induced injury. A key concept in this type of injury is that the parent drug or chemical is rarely responsible for producing the injury. Rather, a metabolite derived from the parent drug as a result of biotransformation by the hepatic drug-metabolizing enzymes is usually more di-

rectly responsible for producing an injurious effect upon liver structure and function.

Role of Hepatic Drug Metabolism

Most drugs are lipophilic in nature (ie, they are readily soluble in lipids such as body fat and cell membranes but poorly soluble in water). The hepatic drug-metabolizing enzymes are responsible for rendering these agents more water soluble, thus permitting their efflux into the plasma and excretion in the urine, or elimination via the canalicular secretory apparatus into the bile. Hepatic metabolism of drugs and toxins is catalyzed by three classes of enzymes: oxidoreductases, hydrolases, and transferases. The oxidation-reduction and hydrolytic reactions, usually referred to as phase 1 reactions, tend to increase the polarity or water solubility of a molecule, often through the generation of metabolically active moieties, such as hydroxyl groups, in the parent compound. By contrast, the transferases catalyze synthetic reactions, referred to as phase 2 (ie, conjugation) reactions, in which polar compounds including acetate, amino acids, sulfate, glucuronic acid, and glutathione are covalently attached to the drug (Figure 44–1). Phase 2 reactions often employ as substrates drugs that have been metabolized via phase 1 reactions, and this further increases the water solubility of the drug. Many compounds, however, can be metabolized by phase 2 reactions without first having undergone phase 1 metabolism. As discussed below, phase 1 reactions may result in the generation of metabolites that are far more chemically reactive and hence potentially damaging to the cell. The importance of phase 2 reactions in such instances is in rendering these reactive phase 1 metabolic products relatively inert, commonly via the attachment of a polar compound (eg, glutathione) to the reactive chemical group generated by the phase 1 reaction on the parent drug.

The superfamily of cytochrome P-450 enzymes, which are located in the endoplasmic reticulum, is the most important family of hepatic phase 1 drug-metabolizing enzymes. There is a tremendous diver-

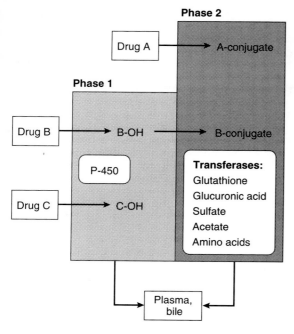

Figure 44–1. Pathways of hepatic drug metabolism. A, B, and C represent three different drugs. Drugs may undergo primary phase 2 biotransformation (A) or initial phase 1 and subsequent phase 2 metabolism (B). Drug C is secreted from the hepatocyte following phase 1 metabolism only.

sity of individual P-450 gene products. These comprise several structurally related subfamilies that are contained in about 10 distinct gene families in mammals. The P-450 isoenzymes that are important in drug metabolism belong largely to families 1, 2, and 3 (Table 44–1). It is the presence of multiple distinct, yet related, P-450 enzymes in the hepatocyte that allows the liver to perform oxidative metabolism on a

Table 44–1. Examples of hepatic cytochrome P-450.

P-450[1]	Substrates	Reaction Type	Inducers
1A2	Caffeine	*N*-demethylation	Hydrocar-
	Theophylline	*N*-demethylation	bons in ciga-
			rette smoke
2B1	Testosterone	Hydroxylation	Phenobarbital
2C9	Tolbutamide	Hydroxylation	None
	Ticrynafen[2]	Hydroxylation	identified
2D6	Debrisoquin	Hydroxylation	None
	Perhexiline		identified
2E1	Acetaminophen		Ethanol
	Ethanol		Isoniazid
3A	Erythromycin	*N*-demethylation	Rifampin
	Cyclosporine		Anticonvulsants
	Ketoconazole		Glucocorticoids

[1]The number/letter/number P-450 nomenclature designates family/subfamily/individual gene product.
[2]This uricosuric diuretic was withdrawn because of its severe hepatotoxicity.

vast array of xenobiotics and natural substances. Three important properties of the P-450 system have a direct bearing on the mechanisms of drug-induced liver disease:

A. Genetic Heterogeneity: Each of the P-450 proteins identified to date appears to be a unique gene product, with genetic heterogeneity or polymorphism in its expression. This accounts, in part, for the wide range of individual human differences in the ability to perform P-450 metabolism on some drugs.

B. Variations in Specific P-450 Enzyme Activity: These variations occur in a given individual largely as a result of enzyme induction. Many factors, including chemicals, drugs, hormones, and nutritional factors, induce cytochrome P-450 in expression patterns that are highly specific for a particular inducer (Table 44–1). Induction of a particular P-450 enzyme substantially increases the oxidative metabolism of drugs that are substrates of that specific enzyme. As a consequence, there is an increased rate of elimination of the drug and, in certain instances, an increased rate of formation of reactive and potentially toxic intermediate metabolites.

C. Competitive Inhibition: Drugs that share the same P-450 specificity for their biotransformation (Table 44–1) may competitively inhibit this biotransformation. This important type of drug interaction can lead to substantial blood and tissue accumulation of drugs metabolized by P-450. For example, patients undergoing organ transplantation who receive both the immunosuppressive drug cyclosporine and the antifungal agent ketoconazole markedly accumulate cyclosporine as a result of ketoconazole inhibition of P-450-3A. Drug interactions at the level of P-450 biotransformation may also reduce the rate of formation of toxic intermediates generated by specific P-450 enzymes and thus offer a potential therapeutic strategy. For example, in mice, 8-methoxypsoralen prevents acetaminophen-induced hepatotoxicity via the inhibition of P-450, with a marked reduction in the formation of reactive acetaminophen intermediates generated by P-450.

Predictable & Unpredictable Hepatotoxicity

Conventionally, drugs with the potential for producing liver injury are divided into predictable, or direct, hepatotoxins and unpredictable, or idiosyncratic, hepatotoxins. Typically, direct hepatotoxins produce liver damage in a predictable, dosage-dependent fashion, whereas idiosyncratic hepatotoxins produce damage in an unpredictable manner, usually while being administered within an accepted therapeutic range. Although there are several excellent examples of drug-induced liver injury that support this categorization, the division is often somewhat arbitrary. For example, although direct hepatotoxins, such as acetaminophen and carbon tetrachloride, will produce liver injury in all individuals who ingest a sufficient quantity, there is substantial variation among individuals in susceptibility to injury in the submassive dosage range. Also, there are numerous examples of drugs commonly viewed as idiosyncratic hepatotoxins that will produce milder levels of liver damage in a larger proportion of patients and often in a dosage-related manner. Table 44–2 compares some of the essential features of direct and indirect drug-induced liver disease.

Molecular Mechanisms of Drug-induced Hepatocellular Injury

Most direct hepatotoxins that produce serious liver disease require activation to reactive electrophiles or free radicals via the cytochrome P-450 system (Table 44–3 and Figure 44–2). Others undergo repeated cycles of enzymatic bioreduction, followed by oxidation by molecular oxygen (redox cycling), a process that results in the generation of large amounts of reactive oxygen species, including superoxide anion radical and hydrogen peroxide. Both electrophiles and free radicals can form covalent adducts with cellular macromolecules, including proteins, lipids, and nucleic acids, and this leads to disruption of their function. In the case of proteins, binding to thiol groups by electrophilic compounds inactivates enzymes and disrupts membrane cation transporters. One of the more devastating effects of the latter is the collapse of calcium compartmentation in the mitochondria and endoplasmic reticulum. This results in an influx of calcium into the cytoplasmic and nuclear compartments, with activation of phospholipases and nucleases and, eventually, cell death.

The so-called covalent-binding hypothesis of cellular injury by drugs has stressed the importance of the covalent modification of cellular macromolecules by reactive drug intermediates in the production of cellular damage. In some experimental models, however, the extent of covalent binding of drug intermediates to cellular proteins does not correlate with the

Table 44–3. Mechanisms of drug-induced hepatotoxicity.

Mechanism	Example
Conversion to reactive intermediates:	
Electrophiles producing covalent adducts with tissue macromolecules	Acetaminophen
Electrophiles acting as oxidants	Acetaminophen
Free radicals producing lipid peroxidation	Carbon tetrachloride
Redox cycling with production of reactive oxygen species	Nitrofurantoin
Alteration of membrane physical properties	Estrogens
Inhibition of membrane enzymes	Chlorpromazine
Interference with hepatic uptake processes	Rifampin
Impairment of cytoskeletal function	Chlorpromazine
Formation of insoluble complexes in bile	Chlorpromazine

severity of cellular necrosis, and this brings into question the importance of this mechanism. The specificity of the proteins attacked by a particular reactive intermediate may be more significant than the amount of covalent modification per se. In addition, oxidative processes are of fundamental importance in the pathogenesis of cell damage. For example, the reactive electrophile produced by the P-450 metabolism of acetaminophen, in addition to forming covalent adducts with key cellular proteins, may also act as a cellular oxidant, producing oxidation of protein thiol groups. Free radicals are, in general, more reactive than electrophiles and attack lipids, proteins, or nucleic acids closer to the vicinity of their formation. Lipid peroxidation initiated by free radical attack on polyunsaturated fatty acids leads to the formation of free lipid radicals, which are subsequently oxidized by molecular oxygen to form lipid peroxy radicals. These can initiate a further cycle of lipid peroxidation. In this manner, lipid peroxidation may proceed in a chain reaction, amplifying the injurious effects of the original free radicals. Certain solvents such as carbon tetrachloride, in addition to producing liver damage via free radical formation, may in native form cause an early, direct disruption of cellular membranes. Alteration of the physical properties of cell membranes and inhibition of membrane enzymes are also important mechanisms in the hepatotoxicity produced by drugs such as estrogens and chlorpromazine.

Drugs that cause unpredictable hepatotoxicity often form covalent adducts with cellular proteins in experimental models; this raises the question of why these drugs produce liver disease in only a minority of patients. There clearly exist other, often poorly understood, host factors in the production of liver disease by these agents (Table 44–4). In some instances (eg, the idiosyncratic acute hepatitis caused by isoniazid), the reactive metabolite responsible for the liver injury is overproduced only in some individuals. Other types of idiosyncratic hepatic drug reactions

Table 44–2. Predictable and unpredictable hepatotoxins.

Characteristic	Predictable	Unpredictable
Dosage-dependence	Invariable	Unusual
Latent period[1]	Hours to days	Weeks to months
Dependence on host factors	Low	High
Histologic findings	Zonal necrosis Steatosis	Necrosis Cholestasis Granulomas Duct lesions
Systemic features	Multiorgan toxicity	Drug allergy
Examples	Acetaminophen Aspirin Carbon tetrachloride	Approximately 800 therapeutic agents

[1]The interval between starting the drug and the onset of the hepatotoxic reaction.

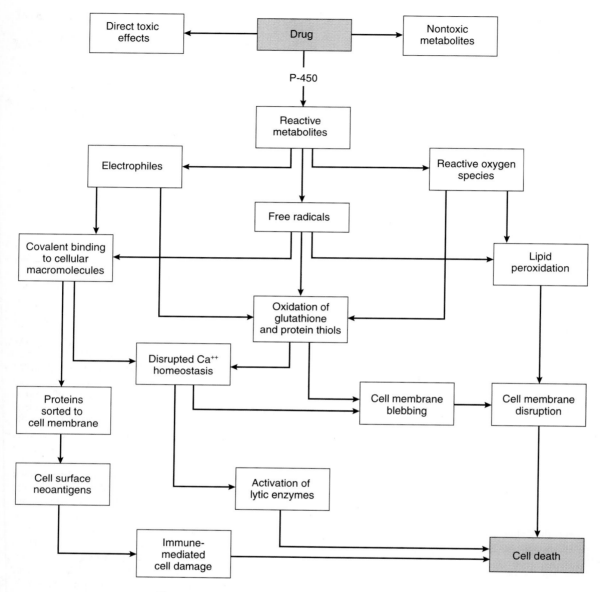

Figure 44–2. Mechanisms of drug-induced hepatotoxicity.

are accompanied by marked immunologic or hypersensitivity phenomena, including fever, rash, eosinophilia, serum sickness syndrome, and even the emergence of classic autoimmune serologic markers. In these instances, immunologic processes play a major pathogenic role. Thus, in liver disease produced by halothane, diclofenac, and ticrynafen (tienilic acid, a uricosuric diuretic withdrawn from use because of its hepatotoxicity), there is strong evidence for a mechanism in which reactive intermediates of these drugs form covalent adducts with specific microsomal proteins, including the cytochrome P-450 enzymes involved in their biotransformation. The adduct-modified microsomal proteins are next transported to the plasma membrane, where they are expressed as neoantigens that are recognized as foreign by the immune system, and this elicits an immune-mediated attack upon the liver. For example, patients who developed hepatitis after taking the diuretic ticrynafen demonstrated a high incidence of circulating anti-liver-kidney microsome (anti-LKM$_2$) autoantibodies that recognize epitopes specific to cytochrome P-450-2C9, the major P-450 enzyme involved in the metabolism of ticrynafen. Anti-LKM$_2$ autoantibodies are highly specific for drug-induced autoimmunelike chronic hepatitis, and differ

Table 44–4. Host factors as determinants of individual susceptibility to hepatotoxicity.

Host Factor		Increased Susceptibility
Age:	Older adults	Isoniazid, NSAIDs
	Infancy	Valproic acid
Sex:	Female	Isoniazid, halothane, zidovudine
	Male	Amoxicillin-clavulanic acid
Race:	Black	Isoniazid
	Asian	Isoniazid
Renal insufficiency:		NSAIDs, methotrexate
Hypoalbuminemia:		Aspirin, methotrexate
Preexisting liver disease:		Isoniazid, acetaminophen, methotrexate
Obesity:		Halothane, methotrexate
HIV positive or AIDS:		Oxacillin, trimethoprimsulfamethoxazole
Other drugs:	Alcohol	Acetaminophen, NSAIDs, methotrexate
	Isoniazid	Acetaminophen
	Anticonvulsants	Acetaminophen, valproic acid
	Rifampin	Isoniazid
Genetic polymorphism or defect:		
	Slow acetylators	Isoniazid
	P-450-2D6	Perhexiline maleate
	Urea cycle	Valproic acid
	Mitochondrial β-oxidation	Valproic acid, aspirin
	Uridine diphosphate glucuronosyl transferase	Acetaminophen

from the anti-LKM$_1$ antibody characteristic of idiopathic type 2 autoimmune hepatitis, which, by contrast, reacts specifically with P-450-2D6 (see Chapter 37).

Cellular Defenses Against Toxic Injury

Liver cells possess several important defenses against drug-induced injury. Most important is the tripeptide glutathione, which is present in millimolar concentration intracellularly. Glutathione provides a reactive thiol group that forms conjugates with electrophilic compounds, either spontaneously or catalyzed by the glutathione S-transferases, which are abundantly present in the cytosol of liver cells. The resulting conjugates are excreted in the bile. Glutathione also performs a major antioxidant function by maintaining the reduced state of protein thiols in the cell. Glutathione, as a substrate for glutathione peroxidases, reduces both hydrogen peroxide and organic hydroperoxides such as polyunsaturated fatty hydroperoxides, which arise during lipid peroxidation. Finally, along with vitamin E, carotenoids, and ascorbic acid, glutathione scavenges free radicals within the cell. Superoxide dismutase disposes of the superoxide radical, while catalase, along with the glutathione peroxidases, also prevents accumulation of hydrogen peroxide in the cell. Impairment of the above defenses may constitute an important factor in determining individual sus-

ceptibility to toxic liver injury. Thus, impairment of glutathione synthesis and its depletion in the hepatocyte is implicated in the marked susceptibility to the toxicity of acetaminophen, and possibly other medications, in chronic alcoholics, patients with acquired immunodeficiency syndrome (AIDS), and malnourished individuals (Table 44–4).

Determinants of Individual Susceptibility to Toxic Liver Damage

A variety of host factors—some more definite than others—determine individual susceptibility to both direct and indirect hepatotoxins (Table 44–4). The variation in individual susceptibility to drug-induced liver injury depends both on the production of a toxic derivative of a drug and on the effectiveness of the defenses responsible for its elimination. Thus, for a drug to cause liver injury, a given set of conditions affecting toxic species production or removal, or both, must exist. For drugs regarded as predictable hepatotoxins, the necessary conditions exist in most persons, whereas for idiosyncratic hepatotoxins, the necessary conditions rarely coexist. Induction of cytochrome P-450 enzymes, as discussed above, may markedly increase the rate of toxic species production and the risk of liver damage. Well-recognized examples include induction of P-450-2E1 by chronic exposure to alcohol and anticonvulsant medication, which leads to enhanced acetaminophen toxicity, and increased isoniazid toxicity due to coadministration of rifampin. Depletion of glutathione in patients with AIDS may explain their increased susceptibility to drug toxicity from agents including oxacillin and sulfa drugs. Decreased plasma protein binding that leads to increased tissue levels of a drug may be the underlying reason for the association of hypoalbuminemia with an increased risk of toxicity from aspirin and methotrexate. The increased susceptibility of the elderly to hepatotoxicity from a number of drugs, especially the nonsteroidal anti-inflammatory drugs (NSAIDs), may depend on several age-related changes in hepatic enzyme activities and pharmacokinetics, including reduced hepatic blood flow and mass and prolonged drug half-lives.

Specific inborn errors of metabolism that are phenotypically subtle or quiescent may reveal themselves as a marked susceptibility to particular types of liver dysfunction with certain drugs. For example, congenital abnormalities of the mitochondrial β-oxidation and urea cycles may cause increased susceptibility to hepatic dysfunction, with microvesicular fat infiltration in children exposed to aspirin (Reye's syndrome) or valproic acid. In many other varieties of idiosyncratic drug-induced liver injury, abnormal production or elimination of toxic drug metabolites resulting from genetic polymorphisms in drug-metabolizing enzymes is likely to play a key role. Examples include the greater apparent susceptibility to isoniazid and possibly sulfonamide hepatotoxicity in individuals with a slow acetylator phenotype (deficient N-acetyltransferase), and an association between the poor-metabolizer phenotype for debrisoquin hydroxylation (which is a result of a defect in P-450-2D6 gene expression) and hepatotoxicity from perhexilene maleate. Also, deficient glucuronidation in individuals with Gilbert syndrome may impose an increased susceptibility to acetaminophen hepatotoxicity. Similarly, the lymphocytes of individuals (and their first-degree relatives) who have sustained hepatic damage with phenytoin or amineptine are abnormally susceptible to in vitro damage from P-450-generated metabolites of these drugs; this points to a defect in defenses against these reactive metabolites.

The concept of "metabolic idiosyncrasy" in hepatic drug toxicity emphasizes the accumulation in susceptible individuals of a particular reactive intermediate, with production of cellular damage via either the covalent or oxidative disruption of protein structure and function. However, as discussed above, both metabolic and immunologic processes play a prominent role in some types of idiosyncratic hepatotoxicity. In such instances, the generation of drug hapten neoantigens by reactive metabolites appears to be of significance. Neoantigen formation on the hepatocyte surface by certain drugs occurs far more commonly than liver injury produced by these drugs. This suggests that immunologic rather than metabolic idiosyncrasy is the main determinant of liver damage developing after exposure to these drugs. For example, probably all individuals exposed to halothane produce adducts of trifluoroacetic acid (a highly reactive intermediate produced by the oxidative hepatic biotransformation of halothane) with hepatic microsomal proteins, which can be expressed on the hepatocyte surface membrane. Only the sera of patients afflicted with halothane hepatitis contain antibodies directed against these hepatic trifluoroacetylated proteins, however; this suggests the existence of a defect in immunologic tolerance to these drug-induced neoantigens. "Molecular mimicry" may also be an important component of halothane hepatitis. Recent studies have demonstrated that the unmodified E2 subunit of pyruvate dehydrogenase reacts strongly with the sera of patients who had developed halothane hepatitis. This subunit, which is the major autoantigen recognized by the M2 antimitochondrial antibodies characteristic of primary biliary cirrhosis, contains lipoic acid as a prosthetic group. Lipoic acid mimics the epitopic structure of the N-ε-trifluoroacetyl-L-lysine moiety common to the trifluoroacetylated proteins arising after halothane exposure. Thus, the recognition of the pyruvate dehydrogenase E2 subunit by halothane hepatitis sera results from a form of molecular mimicry, in which a normal hepatic protein is rendered autoantigenic after sensitization by drug-induced neoantigens. The molecular basis for such immuno-

logic idiosyncrasy is poorly understood. An association of particular "autoimmune" HLA alleles (eg, HLA-B8) with a susceptibility to drug-induced autoimmunelike hepatitis is an attractive possibility but currently lacks experimental support.

CLINICAL & MORPHOLOGIC PATTERNS OF DRUG-INDUCED LIVER INJURY

Drugs produce a wide variety of clinical and histologic patterns of liver injury. The two most common types of injury are termed hepatocellular, or cytotoxic, and cholestatic. Some drugs produce more than one pattern of damage (eg, oral contraceptives may cause cholestasis, adenoma, sinusoidal dilatation, or peliosis hepatis) (Table 44–5).

Drug-induced liver injury is designated **hepatocellular injury** if the alanine aminotransferase (ALT)

Table 44–5. Patterns of drug-induced liver disease.

Category	Examples
Zonal necrosis	Acetaminophen, carbon tetra-chloride
Hepatitis	
Viral hepatitis-like reaction	Halothane, isoniazid, phenytoin, diclofenac
Focal hepatitis	Aspirin, oxacillin
Chronic hepatitis	
Autoimmune hepatitis-like reaction	Methyldopa, dantrolene, diclofenac
Viral hepatitis-like reaction	Isoniazid, halothane
Cholestasis	
Noninflammatory cholestasis	Estrogens, androgenic and anabolic steroids
Inflammatory cholestasis	Amoxicillin-clavulanic acid, piroxicam
Ductal cholestasis	Flucloxacillin, thiabendazole
Sclerosing cholangitis	Floxuridine
Steatosis	
Macrovesicular fatty liver	Ethanol, corticosteroids
Microvesicular fatty liver	Tetracycline, valproic acid, didanosine
Phospholipidosis	Amiodarone, perhexiline maleate
Pseudoalcoholic hepatitis	Amiodarone, perhexiline maleate, nifedipine
Granulomas	Phenylbutazone, allopurinol, quinidine
Firbrosis	Methotrexate, hypervitaminosis A
Vascular lesions	
Hepatic vein thrombosis	Estrogens
Veno-occlusive disease	Anticancer agents, azathioprine
Peliosis hepatis	Androgenic and anabolic steroids, estrogens
Hepatic arteritis	Allopurinol, floxuridine
Nodular regenerative hyperplasia	Azathioprine, anticancer agents
Tumors	
Adenoma	Estrogens
Hepatocellular carcinoma	Estrogens, androgenic and anabolic steroids
Angiosarcoma	Vinyl chloride, thorium dioxide

level is increased to more than twice the upper limit of normal, or if the ratio of ALT to alkaline phosphatase is equal to or greater than 5, where both enzymes are expressed as multiples of the upper limit of normal. Liver injury is designated **cholestatic injury** when the alkaline phosphatase level is increased to twice the upper limit of normal, or when the ratio of ALT to alkaline phosphatase is less than or equal to 2. Mixed patterns of injury are common, and are characterized by elevations in both ALT and alkaline phosphatase levels to greater than twice the upper limit of normal for these enzymes, with the ratio of ALT to alkaline phosphatase greater than 2 but less than 5. The specific morphologic patterns of liver injury that are recognized in drug-induced hepatotoxicity are summarized in Table 44–5 and are discussed briefly below.

Zonal Necrosis

The typical injury caused by most direct hepatotoxins is liver cell necrosis largely confined to a particular zone of the liver lobule. Centrilobular or perivenous necrosis is typical of carbon tetrachloride, acetaminophen, and *Amanita* mushroom toxins. This pattern is explained by the greater abundance of P-450 drug-metabolizing enzymes in the centrizonal region and possibly also the relative hypoxemia of this region. Periportal zonal necrosis is much rarer and is produced by allyl alcohol and yellow phosphorus. In severe cases of liver injury by zonal toxins, the necrosis may extend further throughout the liver lobule and may progress to submassive or massive necrosis. Extremely high levels of serum aminotransferase are typical with this type of injury, which may also result in severe disturbance of liver cell function or even fulminant hepatic failure.

Hepatitis

The term hepatitis connotes a morphologic pattern of drug-induced liver damage in which hepatocellular necrosis with accompanying inflammatory cell infiltrates is prominent. Three patterns of drug-induced hepatitis are commonly encountered:

A. Viral Hepatitis-like Reactions: This is a common pattern of hepatotoxicity produced by idiosyncratic hepatotoxins. The pathologic features resemble those of acute viral hepatitis, with diffuse hepatocellular necrosis, acidophil bodies, and variable inflammatory infiltration. In severe cases, the lesion may progress to bridging, submassive or massive liver necrosis, and fulminant liver failure. Drugs producing this type of injury pattern include halothane, isoniazid, ketoconazole, and phenytoin.

B. Focal Hepatitis (Nonspecific Hepatitis): Scattered foci of liver cell necrosis with mononuclear cell infiltrates may result from many forms of drug injury, including those due to aspirin and oxacillin. This is usually a mild type of injury that resolves completely upon discontinuation of the drug.

C. Chronic Hepatitis: Ongoing hepatocellular injury with features of chronic hepatitis both temporally and histologically has been associated with many drugs, including amiodarone, dantrolene, diclofenac, isoniazid, methyldopa, nitrofurantoin, hydralazine, phenytoin, propylthiouracil, sulfonylureas, and sulfonamides. This type of lesion is characterized by a chronic, progressive process leading to cirrhosis in some instances. The clinical, serologic, and histologic features resemble those of autoimmune hepatitis most closely when oxyphenisatin, nitrofurantoin, or ticrynafen is the offending drug. With other drugs such as isoniazid, the manifestations are more like those of chronic viral hepatitis.

Cholestasis

In drug-induced cholestatic liver injury, the symptoms of pruritus and jaundice may be prominent; an elevated serum alkaline phosphatase level is the dominant biochemical finding (see beginning of this section). There are at least four distinct forms of cholestatic drug-induced liver injury:

A. Noninflammatory (Bland) Cholestasis: This is caused principally by estrogens and 17α-substituted androgenic and anabolic steroids. There is impairment of bile secretion by the hepatocytes, with little or no evidence of hepatocellular necrosis or parenchymal inflammation.

B. Inflammatory Cholestasis: This pattern of injury, sometimes referred to as cholestatic hepatitis, is characterized by significant hepatocellular necrosis and portal lobular inflammation, and prominent cholestasis. Systemic symptoms include rash, fever, and athralgias. Agents that typically cause inflammatory cholestasis include phenothiazines, amoxicillin-clavulanic acid, sulfonylureas, propylthiouracil, and erythromycin estolate. The prognosis is usually favorable.

C. Ductal Cholestasis: This lesion is characterized by progressive destruction of the small bile ducts, producing a clinical syndrome similar to that of primary biliary cirrhosis. Profound cholestasis may persist for months to years before resolving, or progress to secondary biliary cirrhosis. This "vanishing bile duct syndrome" is a variant of the cholestatic injury produced by chlorpromazine, carbamazepine, sulfonylureas, and flucloxacillin.

D. Sclerosing Cholangitis: This is a unique type of drug-induced liver injury that has followed intrahepatic arterial infusion chemotherapy with floxuridine. The lesion, in many respects, resembles the diffuse ductal strictures of primary sclerosing cholangitis and results from ischemic duct injury secondary to a drug-induced chemical arteritis.

Steatosis (Fatty Liver)

Triglyceride accumulation in hepatocytes may occur as a major or associated manifestation of hepatotoxicity. Two main patterns of fat accumulation in the liver are recognized:

A. Macrovesicular Steatosis (Large-droplet Fatty Liver): Fat droplets coalesce to form large vacuoles, which may occupy most of the hepatocyte volume. In spite of the dramatic appearance of this type of fat infiltration, it is usually associated with little disturbance in liver cell function. This pattern of injury is typically produced by corticosteroids, alcohol, and other direct hepatotoxins. It resembles the fatty liver seen in systemic conditions such as obesity and poorly controlled diabetes mellitus.

B. Microvesicular Steatosis (Small-droplet Fatty Liver): This pattern is less commonly encountered and is seen in association with tetracycline, valproic acid, and didanosine hepatotoxicity and hypoglycin poisoning (Jamaican vomiting sickness). While distinct in some features, this type of hepatotoxicity is similar to the rare systemic disorders of Reye's syndrome (which in many cases appears to be related to aspirin usage) and acute fatty liver of pregnancy. Mitochondrial dysfunction appears to be an important factor common to the different causes of microvesicular steatosis. The fat is deposited in small droplets throughout the liver cell, producing a foamy appearance under conventional light microscopy. It is usually associated with a profound disturbance of hepatocellular function and may produce a picture of fulminant hepatic failure. The distinction between the clincopathologic entities of macro- and microvesicular steatotic liver injury may sometimes not be that clear. For example, alcoholic liver damage may produce a mixed pattern of macro- and microvesicular steatosis, often with profound hepatic dysfunction. Also, the nucleoside analog zidovudine has been implicated in several cases of liver disease characterized by hepatomegaly and macrovesicular steatosis, in which profound hepatic dysfunction occurred, with fatal lactic acidosis.

C. Phospholipidosis: A distinctive type of hepatic phospholipid accumulation resembling the inherited disorders of phospholipid metabolism, Niemann-Pick disease and Tay-Sachs disease, occurs following the use of certain drugs, including amiodarone, perhexiline maleate, and 4,4'-diethylaminoethoxyhexestrol. The lesion results from lysosomal phospholipid storage secondary to inactivation of lysosomal phospholipases by these drugs.

Pseudoalcoholic Hepatitis (Steatonecrosis)

A liver lesion resembling the typical histologic finding of alcoholic hepatitis, with hepatocellular necrosis, neutrophil inflammatory infiltrates, fatty change, fibrosis, and Mallory bodies, can be seen in some patients treated with amiodarone, perhexilene maleate, or nifedipine. Progression to cirrhosis occurs in some instances.

Granulomas

Medications may account for up to a third of cases of granulomatous hepatitis (see Chapter 37). Drug-induced granulomas are typically noncaseating and are often associated with granulomas in other tissues and prominent systemic features of hypersensitivity and systemic vasculitis. Commonly responsible agents include quinidine, allopurinol, phenytoin, phenylbutazone, hydralazine, and sulfonamides.

Fibrosis

Some agents will produce an increase in collagen deposition, with minimal or absent features of necrosis or inflammation. This type of fibrosis may progress to cirrhosis and portal hypertension, although the latter may also occur as a result of portal fibrosis, even in the absence of cirrhosis. This type of injury has been observed following chronic administration of methotrexate and also with prolonged ingestion of high dosages of vitamin A, inorganic arsenicals, thioguanine, and azathioprine.

Vascular Lesions

Direct damage to the hepatic vascular endothelium may be the basis for the wide variety of vascular lesions caused by toxins and medications. Hepatic veno-occlusive disease, first recognized as a result of the ingestion of bush teas containing hepatotoxic pyrrolizidine alkaloids, is now seen most commonly in patients treated with azathioprine as an immunosuppressive agent and in patients receiving combination chemotherapy for bone marrow transplantation. Oral contraceptives may cause focal sinusoidal dilatation. Both contraceptives and anabolic steroids may lead to peliosis hepatis, a more striking lesion characterized by extrasinusoidal blood-filled spaces. Nodular regenerative hyperplasia, a lesion associated with hyperviscosity syndromes and vasculitic diseases, has also been linked to azathioprine and antineoplastic drugs.

Tumors

Neoplastic lesions have in some cases been ascribed to prolonged exposure to certain drugs or toxins. These tumors include hepatic adenoma and hepatocellular carcinoma associated with either oral contraceptives or androgenic-anabolic steroids, and angiosarcoma caused by exposure to vinyl chloride monomer, thorium dioxide, or arsenic.

SPECIFIC DRUGS CAUSING LIVER INJURY

Acetaminophen

Hepatotoxicity from this widely used analgesic is most commonly seen as a result of intentional or accidental overdosage, but toxicity even in the therapeutic range is increasingly encountered in chronic alcoholics. The mechanism of acetaminophen-induced liver necrosis has been extensively studied (Figure 44–3). When taken in therapeutic dosages,

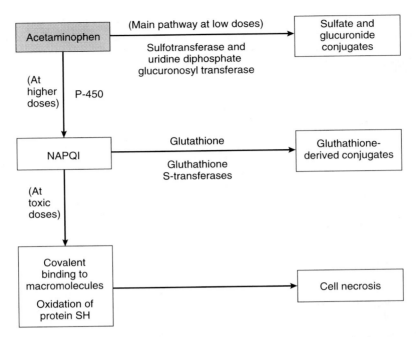

Figure 44–3. Mechanism of acetaminophen-induced hepatotoxicity. At usual therapeutic dosages, acetaminophen is metabolized predominantly by conjugation reactions. The capacity of these pathways becomes saturated at higher dosages of acetaminophen, leading to greater diversion of the drug to the P-450-mediated pathway that generates the reactive electrophile N-acetyl-p-benzoquinone imine (NAPQI), which subsequently undergoes phase 2 conjugation with glutathione. After ingestion of acetaminophen at toxic dosages, NAPQI formation leads to glutathione depletion, allowing the electrophile to exert damaging effects within the cell via covalent binding to cellular macromolecules and via the oxidation of protein thiol groups.

acetaminophen is eliminated mainly via hepatic conjugation with sulfate and glucuronic acids. A small proportion of the drug undergoes biotransformation via cytochrome P-450-2E1 to a reactive metabolite, N-acetyl-p-benzoquinone imine (NAPQI), which subsequently undergoes phase 2 conjugation with glutathione. When a large dose of acetaminophen is ingested, usually more than 10–15 g in an adult, the capacities of the glucuronidation and sulfation pathways of elimination become saturated, and a greater proportion of the drug is directed toward the P-450-mediated formation of NAPQI. As more NAPQI is formed, glutathione is rapidly consumed at a rate faster than the ability of the glutathione synthetic pathway to replenish hepatic stores. When the glutathione pool available for NAPQI conjugation is critically depleted, the reactive metabolite arylates hepatic macromolecules, leading to the formation of protein thiol adducts, with subsequent alteration in protein function. Among the most important of these are membrane-associated calcium pumps, damage to which results in disruption of intracellular calcium homeostasis. In particular, mitochondrial calcium homeostasis is believed to play an important role in the subsequent events that occur leading to liver cell necrosis following acetaminophen overdosage.

In chronic alcoholics, severe hepatocellular necrosis has been observed with acetaminophen taken at doses of 2–6 g/d for several days. The markedly increased susceptibility of alcoholics to acetaminophen hepatotoxicity is the result of two major processes. The first is induction of cytochrome P-450-2E1 by alcohol, which increases the flux of acetaminophen through this pathway and hence the rate of formation of NAPQI. The second is the depletion of hepatic glutathione stores as a result of both consumption of glutathione and inhibition of its synthesis. Other factors that may increase susceptibility to acetaminophen toxicity include starvation (depletion of glutathione) and concurrent treatment with drugs that induce cytochrome P-450 (eg, phenobarbital). Acetaminophen is a classic zonal toxin, producing necrosis in the perivenular (zone 3) region of the liver lobule, corresponding to the predominant region of cytochrome P-450-2E1 expression.

In the first few hours following acetaminophen overdosage, patients may develop nausea and vomiting. These symptoms are followed by a relatively asymptomatic phase lasting approximately 24 hours, following which clinical and laboratory signs of liver damage become evident. Serum aminotransferase levels often rise to more than 5000–10,000 U/L. Severe liver injury may lead to progressive liver failure, with encephalopathy, coagulopathy, hypoglycemia, and acidosis. Acute renal failure may also develop as a sequela of direct acetaminophen toxicity.

The plasma level of acetaminophen is the most reliable means for assessing prognosis following an overdosage (Figure 44–4). Levels in excess of 200 mg/L at 4 hours, 100 mg/L at 8 hours, or 50 mg/L at 12 hours after ingestion are predictive of severe liver damage and indicate that treatment with acetylcysteine is needed. Although often useful, plasma levels of acetaminophen should not be relied upon exclusively in deciding whether to administer this antidote. When uncertainty exists regarding the quantity of acetaminophen ingested or the time interval between ingestion and presentation, it is prudent to treat with N-acetylcysteine. In patients presenting very early after an overdosage, oral administration of activated charcoal may help to reduce further absorption of the drug. N-acetylcysteine, which is a highly effective antidote, should be administered without delay. Its efficacy is based upon stimulation of endogenous glutathione synthesis. In patients who receive N-acetylcysteine within 16 hours of acetaminophen overdosage, severe liver injury is rarely observed. The initial dose is 140 mg/kg orally, followed by a maintenance dose of 70 mg/kg every 4 hours for 48–72 hours. In the United Kingdom, an intravenous formulation of N-acetylcysteine is available that is given in an initial dose of 150 mg/kg over 15 minutes in 200 mL of 5% dextrose, with subsequent doses of 50 mg/kg administered at 4-hour intervals thereafter, to a total dose of 300 mg/kg. Although it is clear that the hepatoprotective effect of N-acetylcysteine is greatest if it is given within the first 16 hours following an overdosage, there is evidence to suggest that later administration, even up to 36 hours following ingestion, may afford some benefit. Patients who survive acute acetaminophen toxicity recover fully, without evidence of progressive or residual liver damage. Among those who develop fulminant hepatic failure, recovery is still the rule, although advanced encephalopathy, severe coagulopathy, and acidosis are associated with a poor outcome. In this circumstance, expedited referral for liver transplantation is indicated.

Amiodarone

This iodinated benzofuran used in the treatment of refractory arrhythmias can produce an unusual form of liver injury. Subclinical liver damage with mild increases in serum aminotransferase levels is seen in up to 20% of patients who receive this drug. However, 1–3% of patients develop a more severe liver injury that histologically resembles acute alcoholic hepatitis, with steatosis, focal necrosis, fibrosis, polymorphonuclear leukocyte infiltrates, and Mallory bodies. This lesion may progress to a micronodular cirrhosis, portal hypertension, and liver failure. Hepatomegaly is common, but jaundice is rare. Evidence of liver damage may persist for several months after the drug is discontinued. On electron microscopy, most patients receiving amiodarone demonstrate unusual lysosomal morphologic characteristics, with concentric, electron-dense myeloid bodies resulting from phospholipid accumulation. This acquired phospholipidosis results from the fact that amiodarone concentrates in lysosomes and inhibits lysosomal phospholipases. This effect of the drug is seen in most patients who receive it, and appears to bear little relationship to the risk of development of pseudoalcoholic hepatitis with amiodarone.

Chlorpromazine

This drug, as well as other phenothiazines, may produce a cholestatic reaction in up to 1% of patients after 3–5 weeks of treatment. Symptoms of fever, anorexia, nausea, upper abdominal pain, rash, and arthralgias may be present at the onset. Pruritus and jaundice soon follow, and eosinophilia is commonly present. Liver biopsy reveals cholestasis with canalicular bile plugs and prominent portal inflammation with a cellular infiltrate consisting of

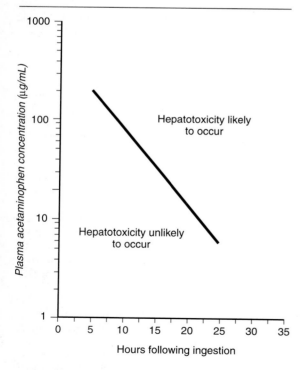

Figure 44–4. The Rumack-Matthew nomogram showing the relationship between the plasma acetaminophen concentration at various times after ingestion and the likelihood of liver damage. (Adapted, with permission, from Rumack BH, Matthew H: Acetaminophen poisoning and toxicity. Pediatrics 1975;55:871.)

mononuclear, polymorphonuclear, and eosinophilic leukocytes, with variable focal liver cell necrosis. Symptoms usually subside over a period of weeks following discontinuation of the drug, but, rarely, a syndrome of prolonged cholestasis resembling primary biliary cirrhosis may occur.

Cocaine

Cocaine is a dosage-dependent hepatotoxin in mice, producing acute hepatic necrosis via P-450-dependent formation of chemically reactive metabolites. In humans, the use of cocaine as a recreational drug has been associated with both abnormal liver tests and occasionally significant hepatic necrosis. A direct causal role for cocaine in these cases has been difficult to substantiate. Many cocaine users with abnormal liver function tests are intravenous-injecting drug users with a high probability of hepatitis C virus infection, and, therefore, the presence of this virus in an individual who has concomitant ethanol abuse is likely to account for most chronic test abnormalities. Instances of acute hepatic necrosis in cocaine abusers have usually been associated with a multisystem disorder in which profound hypotension and disseminated intravascular coagulation have been prominent. The histologic findings have typically included zone 3 and zone 2 necrosis; this suggests that shock and hypotension leading to impaired hepatic oxygenation were primarily responsible for the hepatic damage. In some instances, however, the presence of microvesicular fat on liver histologic studies has implicated cocaine more directly.

Erythromycin

A cholestatic reaction with components of inflammation and necrosis of liver cells may result from the use of the lauryl sulfate salt of propionyl erythromycin (erythromycin estolate). It is also occasionally associated with the ethylsuccinate, lactobionate, and propionate salts of this antibiotic. Hepatotoxicity typically presents as an acute syndrome of right upper quadrant pain, fever, and variable cholestatic symptoms. The clinical picture may closely mimic that of acute cholecystitis or cholangitis and has resulted in surgical exploration in some instances. The prognosis is usually excellent, but the reaction typically recurs if the drug is readministered. The prognosis is uniformly excellent for the cholestatic reaction observed with oral erythromycin preparations, but fulminant hepatitis has resulted from the intravenous administration of this antibiotic.

Halothane

This halogenated alkane anesthetic rarely causes a viral hepatitis-like reaction, which in severe cases has progressed to fatal massive hepatic necrosis. Cross-sensitization may occur between halothane, methoxyflurane, and enflurane, although hepatic injury appears to be less common with the latter two

anesthetic agents. Isoflurane appears to have the least hepatotoxic potential of all halogenated alkane anesthetic agents in current use. Susceptibility to halothane hepatitis is increased in older persons, women, and obese individuals, and severe reactions are more likely after previous or multiple exposures to this anesthetic. Symptoms typical of viral hepatitis occur 7–10 days after anesthesia, but this interval may shorten considerably after repeated exposure. Symptoms at the onset include severe fever, chills, and sweats, followed by jaundice. Features of hypersensitivity such as rash and eosinophilia are less frequent. The course may progress to fulminant hepatic failure within days, with a high mortality rate. Some patients develop a more protracted course, with either slow recovery or evolution into progressive liver failure. Halothane is metabolized along two pathways, which result in different mechanisms of liver damage. In the presence of high oxygen tension, oxidative biotransformation yields trifluoroacetic acid, which, as described in the previous section, "Mechanisms of Drug-induced Liver Disease," forms adducts with microsomal proteins that are sorted to the hepatocyte membrane. These trifluoroacetic acid-protein adducts act as neoantigens that trigger humoral and cell-mediated immune responses leading to hepatocellular necrosis. At low oxygen tension, biotransformation occurs along a reductive pathway that yields a free radical metabolite capable of producing necrosis directly.

Isoniazid

A mild increase in aminotransferase levels is observed in up to 20% of individuals taking isoniazid for single-drug chemoprophylaxis within the first few weeks of therapy. These abnormalities subside in most patients, despite continued administration of the drug. About 0.6% of patients receiving isoniazid develop significant liver injury, which follows a viral hepatitis-like pattern. The onset is usually within 2–3 months after commencing the drug, and initial symptoms are often nonspecific, with malaise and anorexia preceding signs of liver disease. Clinical features of hypersensitivity are distinctly unusual. The liver disease may present as an initially mild acute process but may progress to a subacute or chronic hepatitis or fatal massive liver necrosis. Older individuals are far more susceptible to severe isoniazid liver injury, the incidence of which increases significantly after age 35 years and probably exceeds 2% among individuals over age 50 years. Isoniazid appears to injure the liver through a toxic metabolite, the formation of which may be increased in individuals with a slow-acetylator phenotype. Both hydrazine and toxic derivatives of monoacetylhydrazine formed during the metabolism of isoniazid have been implicated in the mechanism of hepatotoxicity. The formation of the nontoxic derivative diacetylhydrazine from monoacetylhydrazine may be impaired in slow acetylators, thus favoring the formation of more toxic derivatives of monoacetylhydrazine via cytochrome P-450-mediated metabolism. Induction of P-450 by rifampin may account for a severe form of isoniazid hepatitis in patients receiving both drugs.

Patients receiving isoniazid should be followed at regular intervals and advised to report intercurrent symptoms. If these are associated with evidence of disturbed liver function, the drug should be discontinued pending further evaluation. Because minor liver abnormalities are a common and transient finding, particularly in the early course of isoniazid treatment, routine monitoring of liver tests in patients taking the drug is not usually recommended, except in those over age 35 years. In these individuals, given the increased risk-to-benefit ratio of isoniazid chemoprophylaxis, a conservative approach to chemoprophylaxis is warranted, along with appropriate monitoring of liver function tests. A fourfold or increasing elevation in serum aminotransferases in this older age-group should be regarded as potentially serious and may justify discontinuation of the drug, particularly since the prognosis is closely related to the severity of hepatic dysfunction at the time of presentation.

Methotrexate

Chronic treatment of patients with psoriasis and rheumatoid arthritis with methotrexate may rarely lead to significant fibrosis and cirrhosis. Concomitant alcohol consumption, diabetes, obesity, and impaired renal function may all increase the risk of methotrexate-induced hepatic fibrosis. In most patients, the disease is subclinical and nonprogressive. The insidious development of fibrosis due to methotrexate means that routine tests of liver function are often normal and therefore unsuitable for patient monitoring. Instead, liver biopsy must be considered once the total dose exceeds 1.5 g. For patients receiving chronic treatment with methotrexate, both the need for and the timing of a liver biopsy is debated, however. The presence of significant disease on liver biopsy is considered a relative contraindication to continued use of the drug.

Methyldopa

As with isoniazid, patients taking methyldopa have minor, apparently inconsequential abnormalities in liver function in up to 6% of cases. Clinically overt hepatotoxicity is much less common and usually presents as acute viral hepatitis or chronic hepatitis within 20 weeks after the drug is started. The Coombs' test is often positive but does not correlate with the occurrence of hepatic injury. Furthermore, clinical manifestations of drug hypersensitivity are unusual. Injury usually abates when the drug is discontinued, but full recovery may be delayed by months; progression to a fatal outcome despite discontinuation of the drug has been reported.

Penicillins

Penicillin G and ampicillin have little hepatotoxic potential. Amoxicillin is also considered safe, but when it is in combination with the β-lactamase inhibitor clavulanic acid, its use has resulted in delayed cholestatic liver injury presenting up to several weeks after treatment has ended. Elderly males are most frequently affected. Jaundice is a consistent feature, and histologic studies of the liver show cholestasis with minimal necrosis or inflammation. Hypersensitivity manifestations are unusual. The clinical course has been benign in most cases, with complete recovery within 4–6 months. A less benign course has accompanied flucloxacillin treatment in some individuals. This drug appears to target the biliary epithelium selectively to produce a form of idiosyncratic cholestatic liver injury that has affected several hundred individuals to date. Older patients treated for longer than 2 weeks seem to be at particular risk, with the onset of jaundice and pruritus usually 1–3 weeks after cessation of therapy. Although resolution of clinical symptoms usually occurs within 2 months, abnormalities in serum liver enzymes may persist for months to years. In a minority of patients, the injury has pursued a progressive course characterized by bile duct damage and depletion of intralobular bile ducts (vanishing bile duct syndrome), with the ultimate development of secondary biliary cirrhosis over several years.

Phenytoin

This anticonvulsant has rarely been associated with a severe, viral hepatitis-like liver injury with pronounced hypersensitivity features. The onset is usual within 6 weeks of starting the drug and is characterized by malaise, fever, lymphadenopathy, and a striking rash. Leukocytosis, atypical lymphocytosis, and eosinophilia may be present. Histologic studies of the liver resemble acute viral hepatitis but with greater abundance of eosinophils. Progression to liver failure and death has ensued. In spite of the marked hypersensitivity features that characterize phenytoin hepatotoxicity, a toxic metabolite may participate in its pathogenesis. Phenytoin is partly converted in the liver to highly reactive arene oxides, and a genetically determined impairment in detoxifying these reactive intermediates may underlie individual susceptibility to hepatotoxicity.

Valproic Acid

This medium branched-chain fatty acid used principally in the treatment of petit mal epilepsy may produce hepatotoxicity that is occasionally fatal. Infants and young children are at appreciably higher risk. There is an incidence of 10–40% of transient, slight increases in serum aminotransferase levels after several weeks of therapy. Severe liver injury occurs more rarely, with clinical and histologic features reminiscent of Reye's syndrome, although with a greater frequency of jaundice. Histologically, the lesion is characterized by centrilobular necrosis, small-droplet fat infiltration, and bile duct injury. The mechanism of valproate-induced liver injury is uncertain, but available evidence suggests that a valproate metabolite impairs the mitochondrial oxidation of long-chain fatty acids. Underlying inherited abnormalities in mitochondrial β-oxidation or urea synthesis may predispose to this form of hepatotoxicity.

ENVIRONMENTAL & INDUSTRIAL HEPATOTOXINS

Botanical Hepatotoxins

A diverse range of naturally occurring substances derived from plants or fungi may cause liver damage, usually in a dosage-dependent manner. These substances may be ingested in medicinal herbal teas or remedies or, as in the case of *Amanita* mushroom poisoning, accidentally ingested. *Amanita* species contain a variety of hepatotoxic cyclopeptides, including α-amanitine and phalloidin. The onset of symptoms is delayed for up to 24 hours after ingestion of the mushrooms, with abdominal pain and profuse watery diarrhea that may lead to profound dehydration being prominent initially. Over the subsequent 48 hours, gastrointestinal symptoms subside but liver test abnormalities become marked, with progression to fulminant hepatic failure. Liver transplantation has been life-saving in severe cases. Liver damage from *Amanita* mushroom poisoning is characterized by fatty change and zone 3 necrosis.

Among hepatotoxic principals derived from plants, the pyrrolizidine alkaloids present in *Senecio, Heliotropium, Crotalaria,* and *Symphytum* (comfrey) species are the best known and have been responsible for outbreaks of veno-occlusive disease, largely in developing countries. Poisoning with pyrrolizidine alkaloids may present acutely or more chronically, with features of hepatic venous outflow obstruction (ie, portal hypertension and ascites) and variable features of hepatocellular failure.

Herbal remedies are increasingly being recognized as potential hepatotoxins. In France, a number of cases of toxic hepatitis recurring on rechallenge have been attributed to drinking tea brewed from the wall germander *(Teucrium chamaedrys)*. The onset of symptoms has occurred 3–18 weeks after initial ingestion of this remedy, which has been taken for weight reduction. Jaundice has been common, with histologic features of hepatocellular necrosis, particularly in zone 3.

Industrial Hepatotoxins

Industrial solvents and other compounds used in the manufacturing industries have given rise to liver disease ranging from asymptomatic elevation of serum aminotransferase levels to fulminant hepatic failure and hepatic cancer. The best known and most extensively characterized of these compounds is carbon tetrachloride; its use has been abandoned because of its extreme hepatotoxic potential. Carbon tetrachloride is a classic, direct hepatotoxin, which produces a dosage-dependent hepatocellular necrosis most severe in zone 3. Other solvents that have been more recently implicated in cases of hepatotoxicity include 2-nitropropane, 1,1,1-trichloroethane, and dimethylformamide.

DIAGNOSIS & MANAGEMENT OF DRUG- & TOXIN-INDUCED LIVER INJURY

It is often difficult to establish a causal relationship between the use of a drug and a liver injury, because drugs may produce abnormalities similar to those of other common hepatic disorders. Also, hepatotoxicity often occurs in patients who are receiving multiple therapeutic agents. Because of the severity of hepatic damage and dysfunction that may accompany many types of drug-induced liver disease, early diagnosis is essential and will rely on a thorough drug history, including details of recent and past exposure to therapeutic agents. Exposure to hepatotoxic drugs in the form of combination over-the-counter and prescription formulations should not be overlooked. For example, severe hepatic necrosis can occur from acetaminophen contained in over-the-counter preparations such as Nyquil, or in combination with other analgesics such as hydrocodone, propoxyphene, and oxycodone. Details of the patient's occupation and work environment should be routinely obtained, and information about the use of herbal preparations and "traditional" medications should be sought. From a practical point of view, no histologic or clinical features specific for drug-induced liver disease exist, although zonal necrosis on liver biopsy is highly suggestive of a toxic cause. Accordingly, the diagnosis of drug-induced liver disease will ultimately depend upon a history of exposure, consistent clinical, laboratory and, in select cases, liver biopsy findings, and resolution of the liver injury after the presumed toxin is discontinued. In instances where a single agent is involved, the diagnosis may be relatively straightforward. Conditions are far more complex when several drugs are being used. The role of a particular drug in the causation of idiosyncratic liver injury can often be established through rechallenge with the drug, but this is rarely justified because of the risk of severe or even fatal liver injury. Usually, it is not necessary to incriminate the responsible drug unambiguously by rechallenge, because alternative agents are often available.

The most important initial step in managing drug-induced liver disease is to discontinue the implicated drug, with supportive care of acute hepatitis and hepatic failure as required. In the case of severe drug-induced liver failure, urgent liver transplantation may be life-saving. Specific drug treatment is limited to the administration of acetylcysteine for acetaminophen overdosage. In general, corticosteroids have no established value in the treatment of drug-induced liver disease, although they may suppress the marked systemic hypersensitivity features associated with certain idiosyncratic reactions (eg, allopurinol, diclofenac, and azulfidine-induced liver disease). Management of protracted drug-induced cholestasis is similar to that for idiopathic chronic cholestatic liver diseases such as primary biliary cirrhosis. Basic principles of management include the alleviation of pruritus with cholestyramine, supplementation with fat-soluble vitamins, and, ultimately, liver transplantation for cases that progress to secondary biliary cirrhosis.

REFERENCES

Bass NM, Ockner RK: Drug-induced liver disease. In: *Hepatology: A Textbook of Liver Disease,* 3/e. Zakim D, Boyer TD (editors). Saunders, 1995.

Bénichou C et al: Criteria of drug-induced liver disorders: Report of an international consensus meeting. J Hepatol 1990;11:272.

Bissuel F et al: Fulminant hepatitis with severe lactic acidosis in HIV-infected patients on didanosine therapy. J Intern Med 1994;235:367.

Dalton TA, Berry RS: Hepatotoxicity associated with sustained-release niacin. Am J Med 1992;93:102.

Davies MH et al: Antibiotic-associated acute vanishing bile duct syndrome: A pattern associated with severe, prolonged, intrahepatic cholestasis. J Hepatol 1994;20:112.

DeLeve LD, Kaplowitz N: Glutathione metabolism and its role in hepatotoxicity. Pharm Ther 1991;52:287.

Døssing M, Sonne J: Drug-induced hepatic disorders: Incidence, management and avoidance. Drug Safety 1993;9:441.

Eichelbaum M, Kroemer HK, Mikus G: Genetically determined differences in drug metabolism as a risk factor in drug toxicity. Toxicol Lett 1992;64–65(Special No.):115.

Farrell GC: *Drug-Induced Liver Disease.* Churchill-Livingstone, 1994.

Freiman JP et al: Hepatomegaly with severe steatosis in HIV-seropositive patients. AIDS 1993;7:379.

Gholson CF, Warren GH: Fulminant hepatic failure associated with intravenous erythromycin lactobionate. Arch Intern Med 1990;150:215.

Hagley MT, Hulisz DT, Burns CM: Hepatotoxicity associated with angiotensin-converting enzyme inhibitors. Ann Pharmacother 1993;27:228.

Henry JA, Jeffreys KJ, Dawling S: Toxicity and deaths from 3,4-methylenedioxymethamphetamine ("ecstasy"). Lancet 1992;340:384.

Kaplowitz N, Berk PD (editors): Recent Advances in Drug Metabolism and Hepatotoxicity. Vol 10. Semin Liver Dis, Thieme, 1990.

Kassianides C et al: Liver injury from cyclosporine A. Dig Dis Sci 1990;35:693.

Larrey D et al: Hepatitis associated with amoxicillin-clavulanic acid combination: Report of 15 cases. Gut 1992;33:368.

Levinson JR, Gordon SC: Liver diseases in the elderly. Clin Geriat Med 1991;7:371.

Lewis JH, Zimmerman HJ: Drug-induced liver disease. Med Clin North Am 1989;73:775.

Neuberger JM: Halothane and hepatitis: Incidence, predisposing factors, and exposure guidelines. Drug Safety 1990;5:28.

Perry MC: Chemotherapeutic agents and hepatotoxicity. Semin Oncol 1992;19:551.

Rabinovitz M, Van Thiel DH: Hepatotoxicity of nonsteroidal anti-inflammatory drugs. Am J Gastroenterol 1992;87:1696.

Rigas B: The evolving spectrum of amiodarone hepatotoxicity. Hepatology 1989;10:116.

Rosenberg WM et al: Dextropropoxyphene-induced hepatotoxicity: A report of nine cases. J Hepatol 1993;19:470.

Roy AK, Mahoney HC, Levine RA: Phenytoin-induced chronic hepatitis. Dig Dis Sci 1993;38:740.

Salpeter SR: Fatal isoniazid-induced hepatitis: Its risk during chemoprophylaxis. West J Med 1993;159:560.

Sanchez MR et al: Retinoid hepatitis. J Am Acad Dermatol 1993;28:853.

Thomas SHL: Paracetamol (acetaminophen) poisoning. Pharmacol Ther 1993;60:91.

Wysowski DK et al: Fatal and nonfatal hepatotoxicity associated with flutamide. Ann Intern Med 1993;118:860.

The Liver in Systemic Disease

45

Brent A. Neuschwander-Tetri, MD

Because the liver serves multiple metabolic and immunologic functions, it is frequently involved in systemic diseases or diseases primarily affecting other organ systems. This involvement can be trivial or substantial, and the spectrum of the clinical sequelae ranges from minor pathologic findings to life-threatening liver dysfunction. An awareness of these associations is essential for anticipating and appropriately evaluating liver abnormalities in patients with systemic disease.

The unique circulatory anatomy of the liver accounts, in part, for its response to systemic disease. The low sinusoidal hydrostatic pressure within the liver prevents the loss of massive quantities of fluid through the fenestrated hepatic endothelium into the perisinusoidal space of Disse. The endothelial fenestrations promote intimate contact between the hepatocyte cell membrane and circulating plasma proteins such as albumin, which transports fatty acids from peripheral storage sites to the liver. Although it is important for the function of the liver, this high-capacitance, low-pressure vascular tree makes the liver particularly sensitive to blood flow obstruction occurring anywhere between the hepatic central vein and the left ventricle.

The liver must also handle a wide variety of metabolic stresses. It is exposed to the entire mesenteric blood flow, which is not only enriched with physiologic fuels and metabolic precursors but is also laden with potentially antigenic food components, ingested toxins, and by-products of colonic flora metabolism. To handle some of these products, there is active scavenging by resident hepatic macrophages, also known as Kupffer cells. Like many macrophages, Kupffer cells may release potent cytotoxic agents, and these factors have the capability of injuring the other cells of the liver.

Although the liver is complex in its functions, it has a limited number of ways in which the response to injury or metabolic abnormalities is expressed clinically (Table 45–1). The most important implication of these responses is their potential reversibility or irreversibility. The extreme consequence of

chronic liver injury, cirrhosis (severe fibrosis with regenerative nodules), is usually irreversible (see Chapter 43). Most other liver abnormalities are potentially reversible if effective therapy for the underlying disorder is available. Therefore, the management of patients with liver abnormalities as a consequence of extrahepatic diseases should be focused on preventing irreversible liver injury while treating the underlying disease.

CARDIAC DISEASE

1. LOW-FLOW STATES & SHOCK LIVER

Essentials of Diagnosis

- A sudden rise in serum aminotransferases after a period of systemic hypotension, followed by rapid normalization after restoration of normal perfusion.
- Recurrent transient increases of serum aminotransferases that correlate with episodes of poor systemic perfusion in the patient with marginal left ventricular function.
- Concomitant ischemic injury of the kidneys and central nervous system after a prolonged period of hypotension.

General Considerations

Although the liver is relatively protected from ischemic injury by virtue of its dual blood supply, acute low-flow states caused by hemorrhagic or cardiogenic shock lead to severe ischemic liver injury. After an isolated episode of hypoperfusion severe enough to cause liver injury, evidence of renal and central nervous system ischemic injury are usually seen as well. In the patient with marginal left ventricular output and evidence of ischemic liver injury, altered mental status and evidence of renal insufficiency are usually evident. Acute left heart failure in a patient with long-standing right heart failure is also a classic setting for the development of ischemic liver injury.

Table 45–1. Clinical manifestations of liver injury.

Hepatocellular death
  Acute (acetaminophen overdose, shock, viral hepatitis)
  Chronic (viral hepatitis, venous obstruction)
Hepatocellular dysfunction
  Global dysfunction (acute fatty liver of pregnancy, alcohol)
  Cholestasis (drugs, sepsis, parenteral nutrition)
  Fibrosis (alcohol, viral hepatitis, genetic hemochromatosis, biliary obstruction)
Bile duct injury (primary biliary cirrhosis, allograft rejection)
Vascular injury (veno-occlusive disease, ischemia and reperfusion injury)

Clinical Findings

A. Symptoms and Signs: The symptoms and signs are usually dominated by sequelae outside of the liver such as altered mentation and hypotension. The presence of stigmata of chronic liver disease suggests preexisting liver disease.

B. Laboratory Findings: Serum aminotransferase levels may rise to more than 100 times the upper limit of normal with severe ischemic liver injury. With injury of this severity, the prothrombin time will be elevated and the bilirubin levels will rise 1–5 days after the insult. With less severe injury, the aminotransferase elevations will be less pronounced yet characteristic in the rapidity with which they rise after the initial insult (over 1–2 days). Typical of ischemic injury is the rapid normalization of aminotransferase measurements with the restoration of adequate perfusion. Only after toxin-induced liver injury (eg, with acetaminophen) is such prompt normalization of aminotransferase levels also seen. This prompt biochemical resolution corresponds to the rapid elimination rate of circulating aminotransferases ($T_{1/2}$ of AST, 12–24 hours; $T_{1/2}$ of ALT, 36–48 hours).

C. Liver Biopsy: The rapid improvement in serum aminotransferases after resolution of the precipitating event allows the diagnosis of ischemic injury to be made on a clinical basis, and biopsy is rarely, if ever, needed. Persistent aminotransferase elevations should raise the possibility of ongoing injury due to other causes such as viral hepatitis or drug toxicity.

Differential Diagnosis

Dramatic, acute elevations of aminotransferases can be seen in hepatitis due to drug reactions, toxins (eg, the mushroom toxin, α-amanita), and hepatitis A, B, or D virus infections. Prompt resolution of aminotransferase elevations does not occur in infectious hepatitis; this development suggests toxin exposure or ischemia as the most likely diagnosis as the clinical course evolves during the first week. In the setting of circulatory collapse, ischemic hepatitis can thus be diagnosed on a clinical basis.

Complications

The remarkable regenerative capacity of the liver promotes the return to normal liver function after a substantial acute ischemic insult. Irreversible hepatic necrosis is unusual, and death in the setting of ischemic liver usually occurs from multiorgan failure.

Treatment & Prognosis

Optimization of cardiac output and removal of precipitants to hypoperfusion, where possible, is the required treatment for ischemic liver injury. When recurrent hepatic ischemia is caused by severe left ventricular failure, efforts to reduce cardiac afterload pharmacologically can further compromise organ perfusion and thus perpetuate ongoing liver injury, as evidenced by persistently fluctuating aminotransferase elevations. When this happens, the outlook is poor, unless definitive therapy for the failing heart can be provided. On the other hand, potentially avoidable liver injury caused by other factors such as drugs should be considered when the aminotransferase elevations persist despite well-preserved cardiac function.

2. CONGESTIVE HEPATOPATHY

Essentials of Diagnosis

- Jugular venous distention should be evident.
- Hepatomegaly and ascites can develop.
- Jaundice can develop with a normal or near normal alkaline phosphatase measurement.

General Considerations

Congestive hepatopathy can present in any patient with impeded blood flow across the heart. The specific predisposing conditions include constrictive pericarditis, tricuspid insufficiency, severe right ventricular failure, cor pulmonale, mitral stenosis, and severe left ventricular failure. In patients with left ventricular failure, a mixed picture of hepatic congestion and a low-flow state leading to ischemic liver injury can be present (see preceding section). Unrecognized chronic congestion of the liver may in some circumstances lead to cirrhosis ("cardiac cirrhosis"), although this sequela is rarely observed in current clinical practice.

Clinical Findings

A. Symptoms and Signs: Patients will occasionally complain of aching right upper quadrant pain, likely due to stretching of the liver capsule (Table 45–2). Those with severe left ventricular failure often have prominent symptoms of pulmonary vascular congestion (eg, orthopnea). Hepatomegaly is a frequent but not essential finding. Jugular venous distention is an important physical finding that suggests congestive hepatopathy as an explanation of bilirubin and liver enzyme elevations. This physical finding is especially important in the patient without recognized heart disease who presents with jaundice

Table 45–2. Clinical features of congestive hepatopathy and ischemic liver injury.

	Congestive Hepatopathy	Ischemia
Clinical setting	Blood flow obstruction between right atrium and aorta	Systolic hypotension
Symptoms	Right upper quadrant pain	
Signs	Jugular venous distention; hepatomegaly; ascites; lower extremity edema	Altered mentation due to CNS hypoperfusion
Laboratory findings	Elevated bilirubin, elevated prothrombin time, alkaline phosphatase and aminotransferase < four times upper limit of normal	Rapid rise and fall of aminotransferases

or ascites and may have constrictive pericarditis. Manual pressure on the distended liver during physical examination can measurably increase the jugular venous pressure (hepatojugular reflex), although this finding does not imply that the liver is pathologically congested. Ascites may be present and reflects the elevated sinusoidal pressure within the liver.

B. Laboratory Findings: Bilirubin levels and prothrombin time are typically elevated out of proportion to the true degree of liver dysfunction. Additionally, a normal or only minimally elevated alkaline phosphatase measurement helps to differentiate hyperbilirubinemia caused by hepatic congestion from biliary obstruction (see Chapter 34). Fluctuating aminotransferase elevations suggest intermittent underperfusion causing episodic ischemic injury. Evaluation of ascitic fluid demonstrates a high serum to ascites albumin gradient (serum albumin minus ascites albumin > 1.1 mg/dL), a finding characteristic of portal hypertension. Yet, the total protein concentration is high, and this is unusual in chronic liver disease (see Chapter 43). Low protein content of both serum and ascites suggests the progression of congestive hepatopathy to cirrhosis and impaired liver synthetic function. Other causes of liver disease must be excluded routinely; in patients with congestive heart failure, diagnostic considerations include genetic hemochromatosis as well as viral hepatitis and other less common causes of chronic liver disease.

C. Liver Biopsy: The diagnosis of congestive hepatopathy is usually made on clinical grounds without the need for liver biopsy. The patient undergoing evaluation for heart transplantation may require liver biopsy, however, to rule out otherwise silent cirrhosis, which would adversely affect the likelihood of a successful transplant outcome.

Grossly, the liver has a "nutmeg" appearance because of the pericentral congestion. Histologically, sinusoidal dilatation and congestion is evident, accompanied by hepatocyte atrophy.

Treatment

Treatment of the underlying cause of the hepatic congestion is indicated when possible. For the patient with heart failure, this usually includes afterload reduction and use of digitalis and diuretics. Recognizing constrictive pericarditis as a cause of congestive hepatopathy can lead to definitive treatment, which may save the liver from permanent damage. Similarly, correcting severe valvular dysfunction can alleviate hepatic congestion and avoid further liver injury.

Prognosis

The prognosis is determined by the severity of the underlying cardiac disease. Because an elevated prothrombin time and the presence of jaundice do not necessarily imply end-stage liver disease, these findings should not preclude definitive surgical correction of the responsible cardiac abnormality.

Arcidi JM, Gorre GW, Hutchins GM: Hepatic morphology in cardiac dysfunction: A clinicopathologic study of 1000 subjects at autopsy. Am J Pathol 1981;104:159.

Dunn GD et al: The liver in congestive heart failure: A review. Am J Med Sci 1973;265:174.

BUDD-CHIARI SYNDROME

Essentials of Diagnosis

- Disease can develop acutely or chronically.
- Acute progression is characterized by right upper quadrant pain, hepatomegaly, and ascites.
- Indolent progression is characterized by the development of ascites, varices, jaundice, and liver failure.
- Imaging of hepatic blood flow and liver biopsy are needed to confirm the diagnosis.

General Considerations

Hepatic congestion can occur with obstruction of blood flow at any level from the centrilobular vein to the aortic valve. Budd-Chiari syndrome should be thought of as obstructed venous blood flow between the hepatic venules and the right atrium; congestive hepatopathy (arbitrarily) connotes obstruction between the right atrium and the aortic valve, with transmission of elevated pressure back to the liver. By comparison, the term hepatic veno-occlusive disease is used to describe the nonthrombotic occlusion of central veins and their immediate tributaries within the liver. Veno-occlusive disease will cause many of the hepatic manifestations also seen with congestive hepatopathy and Budd-Chiari syndrome, but because it has its own set of predisposing conditions, it differs clinically in its course and response to therapy (see Chapter 49).

Pathophysiology

Budd-Chiari syndrome is a disease with many similarities to congestive hepatopathy in its hepatic manifestations but a conceptually different pathogenesis and spectrum of predisposing diseases. Whereas congestive hepatopathy classically describes venous congestion transmitted from the cava and right atrium, Budd-Chiari syndrome is a disease of intrahepatic venous congestion caused by obstruction of blood flow within the liver. Truly a syndrome rather than a specific disease, this disorder can result from obstruction of either large- or small-caliber veins. Recognized predisposing factors are numerous but can be categorized as prothrombogenic, mechanical, infectious, or due to a variety of other diseases (Table 45–3) that lead to obstruction of hepatic venous outflow. Myeloproliferative disorders account for about a third of cases.

Clinical Findings

A. Symptoms and Signs: Right upper quadrant abdominal pain and hepatomegaly are characteristic of Budd-Chiari syndrome and should prompt further investigation. The absence of jugular venous distention is a key finding that differentiates it from congestive hepatopathy (see preceding section). Ascites is frequently present and may contribute to ab-

Table 45–3. Predisposing factors to venous outflow obstruction (Budd-Chiari syndrome).

Hypercoagulable states
  Myeloproliferative disorders
  Polycythemia vera
  Oral contraceptives
  Postpartum status
  Paroxysmal nocturnal hemoglobinuria
  Lupus anticoagulant
  Antithrombin III deficiency
  Protein C deficiency
  Essential thrombocytosis
Mechanical disorders
  Membranous septae
  Congenital abnormalities of hepatic venous system
  Tumors: renal cell carcinoma, hepatocellular carcinoma,
    Wilms' tumor, adrenal carcinoma, leiomyosarcoma
  Infections: amebic abscess, hydatid cysts, aspergillosis
  Adult polycystic disease
Collagen vascular diseases
  Systemic lupus erythematosus
  Mixed connective tissue disease
  Sjögren's syndrome
  Behçet's disease
Miscellaneous
  Ulcerative colitis
  Syphilis
  α-1-antitrypsin deficiency
  Sarcoidosis
  Trauma

dominal pain and a sensation of fullness. The presence of severe lower extremity edema and distended abdominal veins suggests concomitant obstruction of the inferior vena cava. Hepatic encephalopathy is a terminal manifestation.

B. Laboratory Findings: The alkaline phosphatase and aminotransferase measurements may be elevated (< 10 times the upper limit). The bilirubin levels and prothrombin time are elevated with progression of disease to severe liver injury. Analysis of the ascites would be expected to reveal a difference between serum and ascites albumin of more than 1.1 g/dL, although this has not been directly demonstrated in clinical studies.

C. Imaging Studies: Establishing the patency of the hepatic venous outflow is a cornerstone of diagnosing Budd-Chiari syndrome. Pulsed Doppler ultrasound has proved useful in this regard, although a normal study should not be relied on too heavily if the clinical suspicion for Budd-Chiari syndrome is high. MRI can also be used to assess hepatic blood flow. Dynamic abdominal CT scanning with intravenous contrast material will show delayed drainage of contrast material from involved sections of the liver and can reveal rapid drainage from the caudate lobe, which has direct venous drainage to the inferior vena cava. When these indirect measures of hepatic blood flow are equivocal, retrograde hepatic angiography can be performed to directly assess the localization and extent of venous outflow obstruction.

D. Liver Biopsy: Liver biopsy is essential to confirm the diagnosis of Budd-Chiari syndrome. Centrilobular sinusoidal dilatation occurs early in the disease and may not be uniform throughout the liver. Similar to congestive hepatopathy, hepatocyte atrophy is present and can progress to the point of complete dropout of cell plates surrounding the central vein. Congestion of sinusoids with blood and accumulation of red cells within the subendothelial space confirm the presence of congestion and differentiate the lesion from other causes of sinusoidal dilatation. Organized thrombus within central veins and sublobular veins can also be seen in about one-half of the cases and distinguish Budd-Chiari syndrome from congestive hepatopathy. Late in the disease, progression to cirrhosis is evident, with extensive fibrosis involving the centrilobular regions.

Differential Diagnosis

There is nothing in the clinical presentation and no changes in serum biochemical findings that are specific for Budd-Chiari syndrome. The approach to the patient with right upper quadrant pain, hepatomegaly, and modestly elevated liver enzymes should include evaluation of a variety of infectious and metabolic causes (see Chapter 34). A high index of suspicion for this disease is required to guide the diagnostic evaluation to the correct conclusion. The diagnosis is typically established by imaging studies to assess blood flow and a liver biopsy when the absence of significant coagulopathy or ascites permits.

Complications

Patients with acutely developing Budd-Chiari syndrome can succumb rapidly to liver failure. Those with a more indolent form of the disease can develop esophageal varices, hepatic encephalopathy, and the hepatorenal syndrome. None of these complications is an impediment to liver transplantation.

Treatment

Treatment of Budd-Chiari syndrome is tailored to the specific cause, if one can be identified. Vascular malformations such as membranous webs are amenable to surgical or radiologic dilation. Anticoagulation has a role in preventing the progression of disease early in its course. When the patient's symptoms are related to portal hypertension rather than liver insufficiency, decompression of the liver vasculature can be accomplished surgically and, in selected patients, by transjugular intrahepatic portosystemic shunting. When liver insufficiency dominates the clinical picture, liver transplantation should be considered as an option. Anticoagulation therapy following transplantation may be required in these patients to prevent recurrence of the disease.

Prognosis

Without definitive therapy, most symptomatic patients with Budd-Chiari syndrome will die of liver failure or its complications in months to several years after diagnosis. Asymptomatic patients diagnosed during evaluation of liver enzyme abnormalities develop significant functional vascular collaterals and have a much better outlook.

Asherson RA, Khamashta MA, Hughes GRV: The hepatic complications of the antiphospholipid antibodies. Clin Exp Rheum 1991;9:341.

Dilawari JB et al: Hepatic outflow obstruction (Budd-Chiari syndrome): Experience with 177 patients and a review of the literature. Medicine 1994;73:21.

Hadengue A et al: The changing scene of hepatic vein thrombosis: Recognition of asymptomatic cases. Gastroenterology 1994;106:1042.

Knoop M et al: Treatment of the Budd-Chiari syndrome with orthotopic liver transplantation and long-term anticoagulation. Clin Transplant 1994;8:67.

Kohli V et al: Management of hepatic venous outflow obstruction. Lancet 1993;342:718.

SARCOIDOSIS

Essentials of Diagnosis

- Noncaseating granulomas on liver biopsy.
- Elevated serum angiotensin-converting enzyme activity usually present.
- Negative antimitochondrial antibody.

General Considerations

Pulmonary disease typically predominates in the patient with sarcoidosis. Liver involvement is found in most patients (60–95%) but is rarely significant in terms of liver function or impedance to blood flow. Cirrhosis and portal hypertension thought secondary to sarcoidosis have been described in older studies, but a contributory role of currently identifiable causes of chronic hepatitis and cirrhosis such as hepatitis C was not excluded.

Pathophysiology

Sarcoidosis is a systemic disease of unknown cause manifested by noncaseating granulomas involving lymph nodes, lungs, liver, heart, and many other organs.

Clinical Findings

A. Symptoms and Signs: Active sarcoidosis manifested by fever and arthralgias is predictive of liver involvement, although the involvement is usually asymptomatic. In rare cases, portal hypertension manifested as ascites and esophageal varices has been documented. Similarly, significant cholestasis with jaundice and pruritus is an unusual complication that can develop. None of the signs and symptoms are specific for sarcoidosis, and the diagnosis is based on laboratory and histologic findings.

B. Laboratory Findings: Serum alkaline phosphatase levels are often elevated and can be as high as 25 times the upper limit of normal. When alkaline phosphatase measurements are elevated, primary biliary cirrhosis must be excluded by measuring the antimitochondrial antibody titer. It is normal in sarcoidosis and elevated in 95% of patients with primary biliary cirrhosis (see Chapter 51). The aminotransferases can be moderately elevated (up to five times the upper limit) in sarcoidosis, but synthetic function is preserved, as indicated by a normal prothrombin time.

C. Imaging Studies: The liver on CT scanning is typically unremarkable. In 10% of patients, intrahepatic nodules and hepatomegaly may be seen.

D. Liver Biopsy: The granulomas of sarcoidosis are typically found in the portal tracts, although they can also be found throughout the parenchyma. Bile duct injury should suggest primary biliary cirrhosis, although an unusual variant of hepatic sarcoidosis can cause progressive bile duct loss.

Differential Diagnosis

Although sarcoidosis is one of the most common causes of hepatic granulomas, a large number of other diseases can also be responsible for granulomas found on liver biopsy (see Chapter 37). Thus, the diagnosis of hepatic sarcoidosis is based on establishing sarcoid involvement of other organs and excluding other causes of hepatic granulomas.

Treatment

Therapy with corticosteroids is effective for active sarcoidosis involving other organs (eg, pulmonary sarcoidosis) but is not indicated for asymptomatic hepatic involvement. Hepatic granulomas remain after corticosteroid therapy, despite resolution of systemic symptoms.

Prognosis

Because functionally significant liver disease attributable to sarcoidosis is rare, the prognosis of patients is usually determined by the extent of other organ involvement and the response to corticosteroid therapy. Patients with portal hypertension due to cirrhosis have irreversible structural changes within the liver and are unlikely to have improved liver function following treatment with corticosteroids.

Hercules DM, Bethlem NM: Value of liver biopsy in sarcoidosis. Arch Pathol Lab Med 1984;108:831.

James DG, Sherlock S: Sarcoidosis of the liver. Sarcoidosis 1994;11:2.

Murphy JR et al: Small bile duct abnormalities in sarcoidosis. J Clin Gastroenterol 1990;12:555.

Pereira-Lima J, Schaffner F: Chronic cholestasis in hepatic sarcoidosis with clinical features resembling primary biliary cirrhosis: Report of two cases. Am J Med 1987;83:144.

Valla D et al: Hepatic sarcoidosis with portal hypertension: A report of seven cases with a review of the literature. Q J Med 1987;63:531.

Warshauer DM et al: Abdominal CT findings in sarcoidosis: Radiologic and clinical correlation. Radiology 1994;192:93.

ULCERATIVE COLITIS & CROHN'S DISEASE

Essentials of Diagnosis

- Jaundice and symptomatic liver dysfunction suggest cirrhosis, primary sclerosing cholangitis, or liver disease unrelated to inflammatory bowel disease.
- An elevated alkaline phosphatase level necessitates evaluation for primary sclerosing cholangitis or cholangiocarcinoma.
- Aminotransferase elevations are not specific and warrant evaluation for other causes of liver injury.

General Considerations

Hepatic manifestations of varying severity can be found in nearly all patients with ulcerative colitis and Crohn's disease at the time of autopsy. Clinically evident biochemical abnormalities are much less common and warrant further evaluation when detected. The presence of hepatic abnormalities in patients with ulcerative colitis and Crohn's disease is not related to the severity or duration of inflammatory bowel disease. Nonetheless, in those patients who do have liver involvement, biochemical evidence of liver injury can fluctuate with disease activity.

Pathophysiology

The major hepatobiliary complications of inflammatory bowel disease are listed in Table 45–4. The pathophysiology of these liver abnormalities remains unclear. A postulated role for abnormal permeability of the inflamed gut mucosa and exposure of the liver to toxic bacterial products has been proposed. However, the development of the most important complication, primary sclerosing cholangitis, despite disease remission or surgical colectomy, suggests that other etiologic factors play a role (see Chapter 51). A primary defect in cellular immunity may predispose the epithelia of the gut, biliary tract, and liver to damage by unregulated inflammation and thus explain the independent development of disease in these tissues.

Clinical Findings

A. Symptoms and Signs: Most patients with inflammatory bowel disease are asymptomatic from the standpoint of liver disease. The presence of jaundice or pruritus suggests primary sclerosing cholangitis, although biliary obstruction from gallstones or the development of cholangiocarcinoma must also be considered. Hepatomegaly and splenomegaly can be found but are unusual on physical examination. Progression of sclerosing cholangitis to cirrhosis is characterized by worsening jaundice and the development of portal hypertension with ascites and esophageal varices. Fever, rigors, and right upper quadrant pain may signal bacterial cholangitis in the patient with sclerosing cholangitis or the develop-

Table 45–4. Prevalence of hepatobiliary complications of inflammatory bowel disease.

	Ulcerative Colitis	Crohn's Disease
Primary sclerosing cholangitis	5–10%[1]	< 1%[2]
Cholangiocarcinoma[3]	< 1%[4]	< 1%[4]
Hepatic steatosis	6%	4%
Chronic hepatitis[5]	?	?
Cirrhosis[5]	< 1%	< 1%
Gallstones	—	< 1%[6]
Hepatic granulomas	—	< 1%[7]
Amyloidosis	—	< 1%[7]
Liver abscess	Rare	Rare

[1]In patients with primary sclerosing cholangitis, ulcerative cholitis can be found in 90%, although it may be clinically quiescent.

[2]Ten percent of patients with primary sclerosing cholangitis have Crohn's disease.

[3]Cholangiocarcinoma only occurs in the presence of primary sclerosing cholangitis.

[4]Cholangiocarcinoma develops in 10% of patients with primary sclerosing cholangitis.

[5]The prevalence of chronic hepatitis and cirrhosis in inflammatory bowel disease is unknown when hepatitis C is excluded as a cause.

[6]Significant ileal disease or ileal resection is a risk factor for developing gallstones.

[7]Complication can regress with resection of involved bowel.

ment of a liver abscess in the patient with Crohn's disease. Cholangitis is particularly common if there has been previous surgical revision of the biliary tract or recent ductal manipulation during cholangiography.

B. Laboratory Findings: Mild elevations of the serum aminotransferases and alkaline phosphatase commonly occur in both ulcerative colitis and Crohn's disease but cannot be used to predict the severity of liver involvement. Rigorous evaluation of other causes of chronic hepatitis should always be undertaken with the first presentation of biochemical evidence of liver disease in the patient with inflammatory bowel disease to exclude drugs, viral infection, and metabolic causes as contributing factors. An elevated alkaline phosphatase level suggests sclerosing cholangitis, although this biochemical marker can be normal in the early stages of primary sclerosing cholangitis. Hyperbilirubinemia should also raise the possibility of sclerosing cholangitis, although endstage liver disease or other types of liver disease such as drug toxicity from sulfasalazine or viral hepatitis, must be excluded.

C. Imaging Studies: Primary sclerosing cholangitis is diagnosed by visualization of the intrahepatic and extrahepatic bile ducts, generally by ERCP, revealing bile duct strictures and beaded dilatations. Making the distinction between benign strictures of primary sclerosing cholangitis and cholangiocarcinoma can prove difficult radiologically. Brush cytologic studies of the biliary duct at the time of ERCP are helpful, and endoscopic intraductal ultrasound is a new imaging modality that may also be contributory.

D. Liver Biopsy: Over one-half of all patients with inflammatory bowel disease have abnormal liver biopsies. Macrovesicular fatty liver (steatosis) is a common finding when bowel disease is active and there is biochemical evidence of liver disease (ie, elevated aminotransferase, alkaline phosphatase, or bilirubin levels). Varying degrees of hepatitis characterized by portal and lobular infiltrates with mononuclear inflammatory cells can be found in patients with inflammatory bowel disease. At this time, it is unknown whether inflammatory bowel disease can directly cause these abnormalities or if they are only seen with concomitant primary sclerosing cholangitis or one of the causes of chronic hepatitis such as hepatitis C (see Chapter 34). Sclerosing cholangitis should be considered in patients with ulcerative colitis or Crohn's disease and an elevated alkaline phosphatase level. The diagnosis of primary sclerosing cholangitis is confirmed by imaging of the bile ducts (see preceding section) because there are no pathognomonic findings of this disorder on liver biopsy. Pericholangitis is a term once commonly used to describe the inflammatory cells within the portal triad in patients with both Crohn's disease and ulcerative colitis as well as other intra-abdominal inflammatory processes. It probably describes the histologic sequelae of primary sclerosing cholangitis as well as other diseases such as chronic viral hepatitis C and thus has not proved to be useful diagnostically or prognostically. Bile duct proliferation is common, as it is in any chronic portal-based inflammatory process. Intrahepatic bile duct cell injury is not a feature of inflammatory bowel disease, and its presence suggests primary biliary cirrhosis. Varying degrees of fibrosis, including cirrhosis, can be found in a small percentage of patients with ulcerative colitis or Crohn's disease.

Hepatic amyloidosis is an infrequent but well-documented complication of active Crohn's disease and is due to the deposition of a poorly soluble fragment of serum amyloid A protein (see following section).

Differential Diagnosis

Because of the potential for severe liver disease as a consequence of inflammatory bowel disease, patients should be evaluated at least annually. Those found to have elevated liver enzymes should be further evaluated in the same manner as any other patient, ruling out viral hepatitis, drug toxicity, and other causes. Diagnostic considerations in the patient with an elevated alkaline phosphatase or bilirubin measurement include primary sclerosing cholangitis, cholangiocarcinoma, or common bile duct stones. Gallstone disease, which is relatively common in the general population, is more common in patients who have had ileal resection because of alterations in the bile salt pool.

Complications

Primary sclerosing cholangitis is the major complication of inflammatory bowel disease. Although it can slowly progress in a benign fashion for a decade or more, cholangiocarcinoma eventually develops in about 10% of patients, and biliary cirrhosis with liver failure eventually develops in most, if not all, patients over time.

The natural history of chronic hepatitis and cirrhosis developing in the patient with inflammatory bowel disease is less certain because of the possibility of other contributory factors such as hepatitis C. Those with chronic hepatitis C infection may be treatable with α-interferon, although this therapy must be undertaken cautiously, because it may promote a flare-up of the underlying bowel disease.

Treatment

Although biochemical evidence of liver disease can fluctuate with disease activity, treatment of the bowel disease with corticosteroids and salicylates does not clearly improve the outcome from associated liver disease. Similarly, surgical resection of involved bowel does not improve sclerosing cholangitis or fatty liver. For the patient with severe deterioration of liver function, liver transplantation is an effective option. The presence of cholangiocarcinoma as a complication of primary sclerosing cholangitis precludes transplantation because of the high likelihood of recurrent tumor.

Prognosis

How the presence of liver disease in patients with ulcerative colitis and Crohn's disease affects the overall outcome depends on the nature of the liver disease. Steatosis is a benign lesion. Primary sclerosing cholangitis is an indolent disease, but death from liver failure or cholangiocarcinoma is inevitable over time. When the diagnosis is established early (as is often the case with the evaluation of asymptomatic elevations of alkaline phosphatase by ERCP), it may be 10–20 years before impaired liver function becomes clinically significant. The natural history of chronic hepatitis in patients with inflammatory bowel disease is less clear. Whether it is a risk factor for cirrhosis in the absence of primary sclerosing cholangitis and hepatitis C is currently unknown.

Broome U et al: Liver disease in ulcerative colitis: An epidemiological and follow-up study in the county of Stockholm. Gut 1994;35:84.

Rankin GB: Extraintestinal and systemic manifestations of inflammatory bowel disease. Med Clin North Am 1990;74:39.

Schrumpf E et al: Hepatobiliary complications of inflammatory bowel disease. Semin Liver Dis 1988;8:201.

Wewer V et al: Prevalence of hepatobiliary dysfunction in a regional group of patients with chronic inflammatory bowel disease. Scand J Gastroenterol 1991;26:97.

Vakil N et al: Liver abscess in Crohn's disease. Am J Gastroenterol 1994;89:1090.

DIABETES MELLITUS

Essentials of Diagnosis

- Hepatomegaly is an occasional finding and is due to hepatic steatosis.
- Serum aminotransferases and alkaline phosphatase are normal or within four times the upper limit of normal.

Pathophysiology

The liver is adversely affected by several of the metabolic derangements of diabetes mellitus. Episodic hyperglycemia, increased fatty acid delivery from peripheral stores in times of hypoglycemia, and insufficient insulin all participate in the hepatic complications. For example, the accumulation of fat in the liver of the type I diabetic reflects poor glucose control. During periods of insulin deficiency, peripheral fat stores are mobilized, and the free fatty acids released into the circulation are taken up by the liver for conversion to alternative energy forms (eg, ketone bodies). Fatty acids that do not undergo mitochondrial β-oxidation in the liver are recycled back into triglycerides and transported to the peripheral stores by very low density lipoproteins. Any interference in the complex process of synthesizing and secreting triglycerides from hepatocytes is manifested histologically as steatosis. In the type II diabetic, obesity is the primary cause of fatty liver due to ongoing oversupply of the liver with fatty acids from peripheral stores. Although the accumulation of fat in the liver can cause biochemical evidence of liver injury, diabetes itself rarely, if ever, is a cause of cirrhosis. Impaired liver function caused by other factors (eg, chronic viral or alcoholic cirrhosis) can unmask latent diabetes by increasing peripheral insulin resistance. Thus, an overrepresentation of diabetes in cirrhotic patients cannot be interpreted as the former causing the latter.

Clinical Findings

A. Symptoms and Signs: Hepatomegaly is occasionally detectable on physical examination and can be a source of vague right upper quadrant pain. Patients with stigmata of chronic liver disease must be further evaluated for causes apart from diabetes (eg, chronic viral hepatitis, hemochromatosis).

B. Laboratory Findings: The serum alkaline phosphatase and aminotransferase levels may be mildly elevated but cannot be used to distinguish steatosis alone from coexisting inflammation or fibrosis.

C. Liver Biopsy: Hepatocyte glycogen stores are nearly always increased, and glycogen nuclei (clear vacuoles within hepatocyte nuclei) are frequently present. Macrovesicular (large cytoplasmic droplet) steatosis is found in about one-half of type II diabetics and a minority of type I diabetics. In the presence of steatosis, the finding of inflammatory cells (neutrophils and mononuclear leukocytes) within the parenchyma and portal triads suggests the development of nonalcoholic steatohepatitis.

Differential Diagnosis

There are no specific tests for liver abnormalities in diabetes. Aminotransferase elevations in a diabetic should be evaluated as in any other individual, ruling out viral and metabolic causes as well as alcohol abuse. An elevated alkaline phosphatase level should be further evaluated with sonographic study of the biliary tree. Iron studies (serum iron, transferrin, ferritin) are indicated in any adult new-onset diabetic to rule out hemochromatosis, because of its association with both liver disease and diabetes.

Complications

It is debatable whether diabetes itself can lead to inflammatory cell infiltration into the liver, fibrosis, or even cirrhosis. Nonalcoholic steatohepatitis, a type of liver disease sometimes found in diabetics, is found in obese and otherwise metabolically normal patients as well. Nonetheless, diabetes is one risk factor for developing this disease, which is characterized by foci of neutrophils and mononuclear inflammatory cells within the liver parenchyma and portal triads, as well as varying degrees of fibrosis.

Treatment

There are no specific therapies proven effective for the liver abnormalities in diabetics. Nonetheless, maintenance of euglycemia in the type I diabetic and weight reduction in the overweight type II diabetic are recommended, based on the current understanding of the pathogenesis of the liver abnormalities in these patients.

Prognosis

Hepatic steatosis in the absence of inflammation or fibrosis in the diabetic is not associated with any adverse outcomes. The degree to which it predisposes to nonalcoholic steatohepatitis, liver fibrosis, and cirrhosis is unknown, and specific therapies for these latter sequelae have not been established.

Bacon B et al: Nonalcoholic steatohepatitis: An expanded clinical entity. Gastroenterology 1994;107:1103.

Falchuk KR, Conlin D: The intestinal and liver complications of diabetes mellitus. Adv Intern Med 1993;38:269.

Petrides AS et al: Pathogenesis of glucose intolerance and diabetes mellitus in cirrhosis. Hepatology 1994;19:616.

Powell EE et al: The natural history of nonalcoholic steatohepatitis: A follow-up study of forty-two patients for up to 21 years. Hepatology 1990;11:74.

Wanless IR, Lentz JS: Fatty liver hepatitis (steatohepatitis) and obesity: An autopsy study with analysis of risk factors. Hepatology 1990;12:1106.

OBESITY

Essentials of Diagnosis

- Hepatomegaly is often present but can be difficult to appreciate on examination.
- Stigmata of chronic liver disease should raise the suspicion of other causes of liver disease.
- Serum aminotransferase and alkaline phosphatase measurements are often mildly elevated (< four times the upper limit of normal).
- Liver biopsy invariably demonstrates steatosis.
- Inflammation, fibrosis, and eventually cirrhosis attributable to obesity can also occur.
- Alcohol abuse must be excluded as a cause of liver disease.

Pathophysiology

Fatty infiltration of the liver is a nearly invariable finding in the morbidly obese patient (> 20% above ideal body weight) and can be associated with inflammatory changes and varying degrees of parenchymal fibrosis. It is uncertain whether the accumulation of fat within hepatocytes causes the inflammation and fibrosis found in a small percentage of obese patients.

Clinical Findings

A. Symptoms and Signs: Fatty infiltration is generally asymptomatic, although some patients may complain of right upper quadrant discomfort, possibly due to capsular swelling. Chronic liver disease, if present, rarely has clinical manifestations until quite advanced. Physical examination can reveal hepatomegaly, which is commonly present but difficult to detect.

B. Laboratory Findings: Elevated serum aminotransferase and alkaline phosphatase levels can be mildly elevated (< four times the upper limit) and normalize with weight loss to ideal body weight. Unlike alcoholic liver disease, where aspartate aminotransferase (AST) is characteristically higher than alanine aminotransferase (ALT), in obese patients with elevated aminotransferases due to fatty infiltration, the ALT is usually higher than the AST. Gamma-glutamyl transpeptidase is typically not elevated. This serves as another important feature that distinguishes the hepatic steatosis of obesity from the steatosis associated with alcohol abuse.

C. Imaging Studies: Fatty infiltration of the liver is revealed as a diffusely echogenic liver on sonography and a homogeneously low density liver when compared with the spleen on CT scanning. Sonographically echodense liver parenchyma is also seen in patients with hepatitis in the absence of steatosis.

D. Liver Biopsy: Hepatic steatosis is almost invariably found in the morbidly obese patient. Less common but more worrisome are the findings of inflammation (up to a third of patients) and fibrosis or even cirrhosis (1–5% of patients). This histologic appearance mimics alcoholic hepatitis and has been termed nonalcoholic steatohepatitis to emphasize this similarity (see Chapter 43 and Chapter 40).

Differential Diagnosis

The obese patient with an enlarged fatty liver cannot be assumed to have benign steatosis of obesity until other causes have been ruled out. Alcohol abuse, diabetes, and drug toxicity must all be considered as contributing factors. Persistently elevated aminotransferases (> 6 months) with a negative evaluation for viral, autoimmune, or metabolic causes (see Chapter 34), should be further evaluated by liver biopsy, especially if no response to weight loss occurs.

Complications

Fatty infiltration of the liver per se does not necessarily lead to any adverse outcomes. The presence of inflammation and fibrosis on biopsy are worrisome, however, and should provide an impetus for weight reduction.

Treatment

Weight loss is effective in reducing hepatic steatosis, inflammation, and even fibrosis.

Prognosis

The prognosis of fatty liver alone is benign. When inflammation and fibrosis are evident on liver biopsy, however, the progression to cirrhosis may be possible over time. Although the true risk of this progression has not been defined, weight reduction should be aggressively pursued.

Bacon B et al: Nonalcoholic steatohepatitis: An expanded clinical entity. Gastroenterology 1994;107:1103.

Nanji AA, French SW, Freeman JB: Serum alanine aminotransferase to aspartate aminotransferase ratio and degree of fatty liver in morbidly obese patients. Enzyme 1986;36:266.

Palmer M, Schaffner F: Effect of weight reduction on hepatic abnormalities in overweight patients. Gastroenterology 1990;99:1408.

Ranlov I, Hardt F: Regression of liver steatosis following gastroplasty or gastric bypass for morbid obesity. Digestion 1990;47:208.

Silverman JF et al: Liver pathology in morbidly obese patients with and without diabetes. Am J Gastroenterol 1990;85:1349.

SICKLE CELL DISEASE

Essentials of Diagnosis

- Severe right upper quadrant pain with nausea, often in the setting of a typical crisis.
- Tender hepatomegaly.
- Markedly elevated aminotransferases and profound hyperbilirubinemia in severe crises.
- Differentiating hepatic crisis from ascending cholangitis and acute cholecystitis requires rapid clinical assessment and diagnostic imaging.

Pathophysiology

The obstruction of sinusoidal blood flow by sickled erythrocytes can cause acute episodes of severe ischemic injury or recurrent subclinical episodes of injury. Concomitant hemolysis further contributes to hyperbilirubinemia during episodes of severe hepatic crisis.

Clinical Findings

A. Symptoms and Signs: Severe right upper quadrant pain characterizes hepatic crisis and can be associated with other symptoms of sickle crisis such as back and joint pain and fever. Tender hepatomegaly is usually detectable.

B. Laboratory Findings: The biochemical evidence of liver injury in sickle crisis reflects a combination of ischemic injury and hemolysis, with markedly elevated aminotransferases (> 10 times the upper limit of normal), elevated prothrombin time, and profound hyperbilirubinemia (can exceed 50 mg/dL). Leukocytosis is also frequently seen and does not necessarily signify cholangitis or cholecystitis.

C. Imaging Studies: Cholelithiasis with radiopaque calcium bilirubinate gallstones is common in sickle cell disease. Thus, sonography should be performed to rule out acute biliary obstruction as a cause of right upper quadrant pain and jaundice. If doubt persists about the patency of the common bile duct, ERCP should be performed. Sonography is also useful for detecting acute cholecystitis as a cause of right upper quadrant pain. Radionuclide scanning can effectively exclude cholecystitis if it shows normal filling of the gallbladder. This imaging modality is ineffective in the presence of severe hepatocellular dysfunction, however.

D. Liver Biopsy: Hepatic sickle crisis is characterized by focal hepatocellular necrosis due to ischemic injury. Sinusoidal congestion and engulfed red blood cells within sinusoidal macrophages can also be seen during a crisis, as well as in baseline states in sickle cell disease. Cirrhosis is evident in up to 20% of patients at autopsy and may reflect the repeated ischemic insults or transfusion-acquired hepatitis C.

Differential Diagnosis

The constellation of symptoms and laboratory findings in hepatic crisis is distinctive and readily suggests the diagnosis. Fever and leukocytosis may suggest infection but can also be attributed to hepatic crisis after appropriate exclusion of other potential causes. Acute drug toxicity and viral hepatitis must be excluded by reviewing the patient's history and obtaining viral serologic studies (see Chapter 34). Hepatitis A in the patient with sickle cell disease can lead to fulminant hepatitis, which is an otherwise unusual complication of acute hepatitis A. Other important diagnostic considerations include choledocholithiasis and acute cholecystitis. These are difficult to distinguish from hepatic crisis on clinical grounds alone, and the biliary tree must be imaged sonographically in patients with hepatic crisis. The patient without right upper quadrant pain but abnormal aminotransferases should be evaluated for other causes of liver disease, especially hepatitis C acquired from repeated blood transfusions.

Complications

Fulminant liver failure as a consequence of hepatic crisis can occur but is rare. Previous cocaine use predisposes to more severe liver injury during hepatic crisis and should be sought in the patient's history. Progressive chronic liver injury due to either repeated acute injury or coexisting transfusion-related viral hepatitis is probably the cause of the 20% incidence of cirrhosis in these patients. Transfusion-associated hemosiderosis is found on biopsy, but the role of iron accumulation in chronic liver injury has not been established.

Treatment

Treatment of hepatic crisis is no different from the treatment of sickle crisis in general, with transfusion, hydration, analgesia, and optimization of hemoglobin oxygenation. Acetaminophen-containing analgesics should be avoided because of their hepatotoxic potential.

Hassell KL, Eckman JR, Lane PA: Acute multiorgan failure syndrome: A potentially catastrophic complication of severe sickle cell pain episodes. Am J Med 1994;96:155.
Pearson HA: The kidney, hepatobiliary system, and spleen in sickle cell anemia. Ann NY Acad Sci 1989;565:120.

COLLAGEN VASCULAR DISEASES

Essentials of Diagnosis

- Hepatomegaly is an occasional finding in many forms of collagen vascular diseases.
- Liver enzymes are usually normal or mildly elevated (< four times the upper limit).
- Hepatic artery vasculitis in a patient with systemic lupus erythematosus or polyarteritis nodosa can cause fatal hepatic infarction or aneurysm rupture, presenting as severe right upper quadrant pain.

General Considerations

Liver involvement is common but usually mild in patients with systemic lupus erythematosus, polyarteritis nodosa, rheumatoid arthritis, Felty's syndrome, Sjögren's disease, polymyalgia rheumatica, or adult Still's disease. Although there can be serologic overlapping of these diseases with primary liver diseases such as primary biliary cirrhosis and chronic autoimmune hepatitis, the appropriate diagnosis can usually be made on clinical grounds. The historical use of the term "lupoid hepatitis" to refer to autoimmune liver disease has sometimes led to confusion. This entity is completely distinct from systemic lupus erythematosus (see Chapter 37).

Clinical Findings

A. Symptoms and Signs: Hepatomegaly can be found on examination, but symptoms referable to liver involvement are unusual. A notable exception is the rupture of an intrahepatic arterial aneurysm in patients with polyarteritis nodosa or systemic lupus erythematosus. This catastrophic complication can lead to severe right upper quadrant pain, shock, and death.

B. Laboratory Findings: Mild elevations (< four times the upper limit of normal) of the serum aminotransferases and alkaline phosphatase of liver origin are frequent. Substantial elevations of bilirubin and aminotransferases are rare and should guide the investigation toward other causes such as drug toxicity, autoimmune liver disease, and viral hepatitis.

C. Imaging Studies: Abdominal CT scanning is indicated in patients with systemic lupus erythematosus or polyarteritis nodosa who have severe right upper quadrant pain, in order to rule out hepatic infarction or rupture of an arterial aneurysm. Active vasculitis of the hepatic artery can be further pursued in the patient with right upper quadrant pain, fever, and an elevated sedimentation rate by angiography.

D. Liver Biopsy: Liver biopsy should be performed when there is clinical suspicion of significant liver dysfunction (physical findings, elevated bilirubin, elevated prothrombin time). Hepatic steatosis is not typically present and when evident may be the result of corticosteroid therapy. Periportal inflammation and liver fibrosis occur in a small fraction of patients with collagen vascular diseases. Nodular regenerative hyperplasia is an unusual histologic finding that is sometimes seen in patients with Felty's syndrome. Secondary hepatic amyloidosis (see following section) may develop in patients with uncontrolled rheumatoid arthritis.

Differential Diagnosis

Drug-induced hepatotoxicity must be excluded in the patient with significant liver enzyme elevations. Nonsteroidal anti-inflammatory drugs can cause liver injury, and fulminant hepatitis has been described in patients treated with aspirin and nonsteroidal anti-inflammatory agents for collagen vascular diseases.

Treatment

Active vasculitis of the hepatic artery should be treated with corticosteroids. The patient with severe right upper quadrant pain should be evaluated for surgical or radiologic intervention to prevent exsanguinating hemorrhage from a ruptured aneurysm. Otherwise, specific treatment for the hepatic manifestations of collagen vascular diseases have not been identified.

Ilan Y, Ben-Chetrit E: Liver involvement in giant cell arteritis. Clin Rheumatol 1993;12:219.
Leggett B: The liver in systemic lupus erythematosus. J Gastroenterol Hepatol 1993;8:84.
Matsumoto T et al: The liver in systemic lupus erythematosus: Pathologic analysis of 52 cases and review of the Japanese Autopsy Registry Data. Hum Pathol 1992; 23:1151.
Zimmerman H: Hepatotoxicity. Disease-a-Month 1993; 39:747.

AMYLOIDOSIS

Essentials of Diagnosis

- Fatigue, weight loss, and peripheral edema can be long-standing before the diagnosis is considered.

- Hepatic involvement is frequent, but liver-specific symptoms are rare.
- Hepatomegaly, peripheral edema, macroglossia, peripheral neuropathy, skin capillary fragility, and congestive heart failure are found with varying frequency.
- Fat, skin, or rectal biopsies are preferable to liver biopsy to establish the diagnosis.

General Considerations

The shared feature of all forms of amyloidosis is the perivascular deposition of protein fragments folded in the highly stable and insoluble β-pleated sheet configuration. This configuration is responsible for the birefringent microscopic appearance observed under polarized light and is a common internal structural arrangement of many proteins. Molecular techniques have identified many of the protein fragments that cause amyloidosis, as well as the function of the intact proteins from which the fragments are derived. With this new information, a rational approach to treatment is now possible for many forms of amyloidosis.

There are two common types of amyloidosis, and their prevalence varies depending on the population studied. One type, caused by the deposition of excessively produced immunoglobulin light chain fragments has been termed primary, or AL, amyloidosis. This light chain excess can result from monoclonal expansion of a plasma cell or B-cell line, either as multiple myeloma or a subclinical myeloid cell dyscrasia. The disease may respond to cytotoxic therapy. The other common type of amyloidosis has been termed secondary, or AA amyloidosis and is caused by the perivascular deposition of fragments of a protein called serum amyloid A. This protein is an apolipoprotein synthesized by the liver that circulates in the plasma bound to high-density lipoprotein. Like C-reactive protein, it is one of the acute phase reactants that responds most robustly to inflammation (100- to 1000-fold increase). This type of amyloidosis is associated with lymphomas and chronic inflammatory states, including untreated inflammatory bowel disease, rheumatoid arthritis, osteomyelitis, tuberculosis, leprosy, and familial Mediterranean fever.

Mutations of genes encoding several other proteins have also been recognized to cause deposition of specific protein fragments, which appear microscopically as perivascular amyloid. These include transthyretin, β-amyloid protein P, apolipoprotein A1, procalcitonin, and β-2 microglobulin. Establishing the molecular identities of the proteins causing these types of amyloidosis is important. For example, the thyroxin-binding protein transthyretin is susceptible to point mutations, which lead to its deposition as amyloid. Clinically, this particular form of amyloidosis causes fatal neurologic and cardiac complications. Because transthyretin is synthesized by the liver, identification of this disease early in its course and

treatment with liver transplantation has proved effective in preventing an otherwise fatal outcome.

Pathogenesis

The term amyloidosis connotes an etiologically diverse group of diseases sharing the common feature of perivascular accumulation of protein folded in the stable β-pleated sheet configuration.

Clinical Findings

A. Symptoms and Signs: Liver deposition of amyloid protein has been associated primarily with light chain disease (primary amyloidosis) and serum amyloid A disease (secondary amyloidosis). The clinical presentation of amyloidosis was defined before the identification of specific types of amyloidosis by molecular techniques. Thus, our understanding of each type of amyloidosis may evolve with further elucidation of the diverse pathogenetic mechanisms.

In general, nonspecific complaints of fatigue, unintentional weight loss, edema, and dyspnea are long-standing by the time the diagnosis is considered. Symptoms due to liver dysfunction are generally not present, even in advanced disease. Occasionally, ascites occurs, but congestive heart failure and nephrotic protein loss may be contributory factors. Rarely, hepatic involvement can cause cholestasis with associated pruritus.

Hepatomegaly is a common finding on examination. Dependent edema is also frequent and may reflect associated congestive heart failure or nephrotic syndrome. Macroglossia, although an infrequent finding, can be helpful in suggesting the diagnosis. Skin fragility (sloughing, purpura, easy bruisability), carpal tunnel syndrome, and peripheral neuropathy may be seen.

B. Laboratory Findings: Serum alkaline phosphatase levels are usually mildly elevated (< four times normal), and the aminotransferases are normal or mildly elevated (< four times normal). Coagulation abnormalities may be present, associated with reduced levels of factors IX and X, due to their binding to the amyloid proteins.

C. Imaging Studies: Imaging of the liver by CT scanning or sonography can identify hepatomegaly. A nuclear liver-spleen scan is generally not required but may show patchy uptake of tracer material consistent with inhomogeneous liver involvement.

D. Liver Biopsy: The diagnosis of hepatic amyloidosis is confirmed by the finding of eosinophilic protein within the subendothelial space of Disse, which exhibits green birefringence when stained with Congo red. The site of amyloid protein within the liver does not establish the type of amyloidosis. Hepatocyte atrophy is commonly found, possibly caused by compromised transfer of oxygen and nutrients from the vascular space to the cell. Cirrhosis is not a feature. Performing a liver biopsy may be associated with an increased risk of bleeding due to deficient clotting factors and capillary abnormalities. Therefore, biopsies must be undertaken cautiously, especially in the patient with a history of purpura, which suggests capillary fragility.

Complications

The liver generally tolerates the accumulation of perivascular protein well compared to the heart and central nervous system, and patients typically present with dysfunction of organs other than the liver. Occlusion of the sinusoidal space can lead to clinically evident portal hypertension in a minority of cases.

Treatment

Specific therapies for each type of amyloidosis are evolving as individual pathogenetic mechanisms are elucidated. Cytotoxic therapy has been successful for the paraproteinemia of primary immunoglobulin light chain amyloidosis, even in the absence of multiple myeloma. For secondary amyloidosis, treatment of the underlying inflammatory disorder is the mainstay of therapy. Colchicine is beneficial in preventing amyloidosis in patients with familial Mediterranean fever and in some patients with other chronic inflammatory diseases. Familial amyloidosis caused by dominant mutations of the transthyretin gene have now been successfully treated with liver transplantation. These new therapeutic options emphasize the need to make an early and accurate diagnosis of amyloidosis.

Benson M, Wallace M: Amyloidosis. In: The Metabolic Basis of Inherited Disease, 6th ed. Scriver C et al (editors). McGraw-Hill, 1989.

Buck F, Koss M: Hepatic amyloidosis: Morphological differences between systemic AL and AA types. Hum Pathol 1991;22:904.

Gertz M, Kyle R: Primary systemic amyloidosis: A diagnostic primer. Mayo Clin Proc 1989;64:1505.

Rienhoff H et al: Molecular and cellular biology of serum amyloid A. Mol Biol Med 1990;7:287.

Mass Lesions & Neoplasia of the Liver

Douglas R. LaBrecque, MD

Rapid advances in medical technology over the past two decades have greatly increased the ease and accuracy of diagnosing hepatic tumors. The wide availability of ultrasonography and computed axial tomography (CT) has also increased the serendipitous identification of asymptomatic benign liver masses, a situation that leads to anxiety for patients, frustration for physicians, and increased expense. Nonetheless, distinguishing benign from malignant masses is always essential.

The liver is the major site of blood borne metastases from within the abdomen and a very common site of metastases from tumors above the diaphragm. It is the most frequent site of metastatic disease in patients who die from neoplasia; 36–42% of patients dying from primary extrahepatic tumors have liver metastases. Metastatic liver tumors are up to 40 times more common than primary hepatic tumors. The most frequent mass found in the liver, however, is a benign hemangioma, which occurs in 7% or more of patients. Thus, when a mass is unexpectedly discovered on ultrasound or CT, the clinician's goal is to establish a diagnosis efficiently and with the least risk and expense to the patient.

HEPATOCELLULAR CARCINOMA

Pathophysiology

A number of factors have been associated with the pathogenesis of hepatocellular carcinoma, including physical, chemical, infectious, and metabolic/hereditary causes (Table 46–1). The rodent liver is one of the most successful models of chemical carcinogenesis and has contributed a great deal to our current understanding of the common steps in the pathogenesis of malignant transformation. This multi-step model of hepatocarcinogenesis (Figure 46–1) includes four steps. **Initiation** occurs when an infection or chemical exposure produces a fixed genetic change that makes the initiated cell responsive to promotion. During **promotion,** hepatocyte necrosis, inflammation with production of cytokines and growth factors; or exposure to specific chemicals (anabolic steroids,

alcohol, iron) leads to liver regeneration and active or inactive cirrhosis. This "fixes" the genetic defect, preventing the liver from eliminating the cell with its altered genome. **Progression** occurs when these "growth advantaged" malignant cells are stimulated to produce microscopic foci of hepatocellular carcinoma by clonal expansion. Phenobarbital and other chemicals are particularly effective in producing progression. Ultimately, continued growth stimulation and clonal expansion of the malignant cells leads to one or more macroscopic foci of hepatocellular carcinoma and clinically apparent cancer. Most explanations of hepatocellular carcinogenesis attempt to recapitulate these steps and generally no single agent is felt to be sufficient acting alone to induce hepatocellular carcinoma.

A. Risk Factors
1. Physical and Chemical Agents:
a. Radiation—Ionizing radiation causes liver tumors in mice, but does not appear to be a significant factor in the development of human hepatocellular carcinoma. Long-term follow-up of those who survived the atomic bombing of Nagasaki and Hiroshima has not demonstrated an increase in hepatocellular carcinoma, although veno-occlusive disease and the Budd-Chiari Syndrome do increase following radiation exposure. The low rate of cell turnover in the adult liver with the limited opportunity for fixation of genetic alterations may account for such failure. Long-term continuous exposure to radiation, however, can produce tumors in the human liver. The unfortunate use of **thorotrast,** one of the original radiologic contrast agents and the radionuclide of choice from the late 1920s to the mid-1950s, has produced hemangiosarcomas and even hepatocellular carcinomas. This alpha radiation emitter has a biologic half-life of approximately 400 years, and well over 50,000 adults remain at risk for the development of hepatocellular carcinoma.

b. Chemical carcinogenesis—Everything consumed by mouth traverses the liver before reaching the systemic circulation because of the liver's unique anatomic position and its dual blood flow; this occurs via the portal drainage of the abdominal viscera.

Table 46–1. Risk factors for development of hepatocellular carcinoma.

Definite	Possible
Chronic Hepatic B virus infection	Oral contraceptives
Chronic Hepatitis C virus infection	Androgenic/anabolic steroids
Aflatoxin	α_1-antitrypsin deficiency
Cirrhosis	Ataxia telangiectasia
Hereditary tyrosinemia	Alcohol
Vinyl chloride monomer*	
Thorotrast*	

*Primarily hemangiosarcomas

Compounds that enter the body via other routes also find their way to the liver, which receives 25% of the cardiac output. Over 12,350,000 unique chemical compounds have been identified, and this total grows by more than 11,500 each week as new compounds are synthesized or found in the environment. Over 90,000 are in regular use, including some 800 as food additives. In animal models, more than 3,000 chemicals are known to be carcinogenic and, as noted above, the rodent liver has been the standard model used to delineate the multi-step model of hepatic carcinogenesis. Despite the overwhelming evidence of carcinogenicity of such chemicals, and the massive daily exposure of the human liver to chemicals in general, only two chemicals are clearly documented human hepatic carcinogens: aflatoxin and vinyl chloride monomer. The former, a contaminant of foodstuffs, eg, nuts and grains, is produced by the mold *Aspergillus flavus*. It contaminates food stored for long periods in a hot or humid environment and is

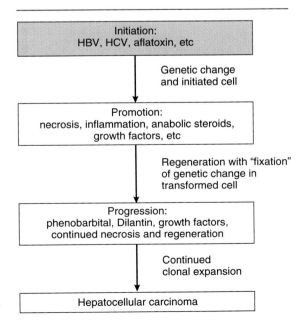

Figure 46–1. Multistep pathogenesis of hepatocellular carcinoma.

clearly associated with hepatocellular carcinoma, particularly as a cofactor with the hepatitis B virus in many sections of Africa and Southeast Asia. Aflatoxin is the most powerful human hepatocarcinogen known. Vinyl chloride monomer induces angiosarcomas in animal models as well as in industrial workers manufacturing polyvinyl chlorides.

3. Viral infections–There are many examples of virus-induced tumors in animal models. In most cases, the viral genome becomes incorporated into the host cells' genetic material either directly, if it is a DNA virus, or following reverse transcriptase production of a DNA copy if it is an RNA virus. The viral material, inserted into the host cell genome, may then act as a mutagen, a promoter to alter gene expression to produce new proteins, particularly oncogenes, or cause over-expression of normal genes which lead to malignant transformation. The hepatitis B virus has the strongest association with the development of hepatocellular carcinoma, and hepatitis B viral DNA has been found integrated into the genome of the host DNA in up to 80% of hepatocellular carcinoma patients who are hepatitis B carriers. The site of viral integration does not appear to be a critical determinant of hepatocellular carcinoma development. Risk of hepatocellular carcinoma is particularly high in patients with lifelong HBV infection resulting from perinatal exposure, as is typical in Asia and Africa. In contrast to HBV, hepatitis C (HCV), which is also strongly associated with hepatocellular carcinoma, is unlikely to exert its effect by inserting into the host cell genome, since it is an RNA virus and lacks reverse transcriptase activity. Nonetheless, HCV increases the risk of hepatocellular carcinoma. In Japan, where 70% of hepatocellular carcinoma patients are HCV-positive, patients with chronic hepatitis C are three times more likely to develop hepatocellular carcinoma than those with chronic hepatitis B. Unlike in hepatitis B, however, HCV-related hepatocellular carcinoma only occurs after the development of cirrhosis, and it may be the continuous necro-inflammatory reaction with subsequent regeneration that ultimately produces the tumor (see following section, "Cirrhosis").

4. Parasitic infection–Chronic schistosomiasis often occurs in patients who also have chronic active hepatitis B with cirrhosis; thus, hepatocellular carcinoma is common in these patients, as well. In pure hepatosplenic schistosomiasis, however, portal fibrosis is the primary lesion, and the parenchyma is relatively undamaged. In contrast, oriental cholangiohepatitis, caused primarily by the liver fluke, *Clonorchis sinensis*, has a strong association with the development of cholangiocarcinoma.

5. Cirrhosis–A common denominator in most cases of hepatocellular carcinoma is the presence of cirrhosis. In some cases, such as hepatitis C, the necro-inflammatory reaction and continuous regeneration may ultimately "fix" the mutation, leading to malignant transformation and unrestrained growth. In other cases, such as hereditary hemochromatosis, in which 3–27% of patients develop hepatocellular carcinoma, tumor develops only in patients who are cirrhotic (see Chapter 41). The life-long risk of developing hepatocellular carcinoma is reduced to that of the normal population if timely phlebotomy is performed before the development of cirrhosis.

Cirrhosis, however, is only one of many cofactors for developing hepatocellular carcinoma. In Western industrialized countries, where hepatocellular carcinoma is uncommon, 80–90% of patients who develop hepatocellular carcinoma will have underlying cirrhosis, typically in older individuals. In contrast, in Africa, where chronic hepatitis B and aflatoxin exposure are common cofactors, hepatocellular carcinoma occurs at an earlier age, and only 60–70% of patients have underlying cirrhosis. A combination of chronic hepatitis B infection with cirrhosis increases the risk of developing hepatocellular carcinoma by at least fourfold over those who are hepatitis B negative. Virtually any form of cirrhosis is a risk factor, but the overall rates may vary from 40–50% in those with hepatitis B to 5–15% in those whose with alcoholic cirrhosis. The highest rate is found in hereditary tyrosinemia (see following section, "Genetics"). Cirrhosis most likely increases the susceptibility for developing hepatocellular carcinoma in patients who are exposed to one or more additional cofactors, which then trigger the transformation of normal parenchymal cells into malignant ones. In addition to "fixing," the malignancy-inducing mutation may continue its damage and provoke a necro-inflammatory reaction, and may also provide the appropriate growth stimuli to expand microfoci of transformed cells into clinically significant ones.

6. Drugs and alcohol–In the Western industrialized world, hepatocellular carcinoma is most commonly associated with alcohol. The lifetime risk of developing hepatocellular carcinoma appears to be about 15% in alcoholic cirrhosis, which persists even after ceasing alcohol ingestion. In one study, 55% of patients who had stopped drinking showed hepatocellular carcinoma at autopsy.

As noted in the section on chemicals, many drugs act as initiators, promotors or progression factors in the development of hepatocellular carcinoma in animals. Surprisingly few have a proven role in human hepatocellular carcinoma. A possible exception are **anabolic steroids** and **estrogens,** which likely contribute to hepatocellular carcinoma, hepatic adenomas, and hemangiomas (see below). Phenobarbitol and diphenylhydantoin are among the most potent promoters and inducers in animals, but have shown no association with hepatocellular carcinoma in humans. Similarly, tolazamide, oxytetracycline and aminopyrine have not been established as hepatic carcinogens in humans, despite their metabolism to carcinogenic nitrosamines.

7. Genetics–Hereditary tyrosinemia has the clearest association with the development of hepatocellular carcinoma. Close to 40% of patients in one study developed hepatocellular carcinoma despite good dietary control. The best recognized and most striking association between a hereditary disease and hepatocellular carcinoma is hereditary hemachromatosis. As previously discussed, however, progression to cirrhosis is required before patients acquire the risk of hepatocellular carcinoma. Tumors have also been reported in association with α_1-antitrypsin deficiency and ataxia telangiectasia. Most other associations have not been borne out by more careful study, and convincing evidence of a genetic predisposition to the development of hepatocellular carcinoma is lacking. Familial clustering of hepatocellular carcinoma is seen in patients with chronic hepatitis B, but this is probably related to vertical and horizontal transmission of the hepatitis B. Differences between ethnic and geographic groups have been discussed above, and are probably more environmental than genetic. The association with Fanconi's anemia is probably related to the androgens used to treat the anemia rather than the underlying disease.

8. Summary–The precise pathogenesis of hepatocellular carcinoma is most likely multifactorial, representing the end of a multi-step process in which more than one factor must interact with the liver before hepatocellular carcinoma develops.

B. Epidemiology: The incidence of hepatocellular carcinoma varies dramatically worldwide, ranging from 150 cases per 100,000 population per year in areas such as Taiwan, Mozambique, and Southeast China to a low of 3–7 cases per 100,000 population in North and South America, North and Central Europe, and Australia (see following discussion, "General Considerations"). Intermediate rates from 5–20 cases per 100,000 population per year are found in Japan, the Middle East, and European countries bordering on the Mediterranean.

While these generalities hold true, marked differences can be seen within the same geographic area. Native black South Africans and native Maori males in New Zealand have attack rates 28 and 7 fold greater than whites in their respective countries. Blacks in southern California have an attack rate 4 times greater than that of whites. Although these findings suggest racial and/or genetic factors, environmental differences may play an even bigger role. It is commonly found, for example, that when natives move from areas with a high attack rate to one with a low attack rate, the incidence falls as they adopt the Western lifestyle. In contrast, individuals who move from highly developed countries to developing lands tend to retain their low attack rate, possibly because they maintain their original lifestyle rather than that of their adopted country. Hepatocellular carcinoma is considerably more common in males (8:1 in areas of high incidence and 2:1 to 3:1 in areas of low incidence).

General Considerations

The liver is comprised of several cell types, including hepatocytes, biliary epithelium, vascular endothelium, Kupffer cells, stellate (Ito) cells, lymphoid cells and neuroendocrine cells. Any of these cells may give rise to malignant or benign tumors (Table 46–2). Ninety to ninety-five percent of all primary liver tumors, however, are hepatocellular carcinomas which arise from the parenchymal cell.

Although hepatocellular carcinoma is an uncommon tumor in the Western world, where it represents only 0.5–2.0% of all cancers, and has an annual incidence of only 3–5 cases per 100,000 population in the United States, hepatocellular carcinoma has an attack rate as high as 150 per 100,000 population in areas of Sub-Saharan Africa and Southeast Asia. Worldwide, it is the most prevalent visceral neoplasm and may be the single most common cancer overall.

Essentials of Diagnosis

- Frequently asymptomatic with normal or minimally abnormal liver tests.
- Elevated α-fetoprotein in 50% or more of hepatocellular carcinomas.
- Physical examination may reveal rock-hard hepatomegaly, tender hepatomegaly, signs of chronic liver disease or be completely normal.
- Presence of a bruit or friction rub over the liver strongly suggests liver tumor.
- Imaging studies key to diagnostic evaluation.
- Biopsy usually necessary to confirm and differentiate malignant growths.

Clinical Findings

A. History: Risk factors described previously (see "Pathogenesis") should be elicited in the history. These include known HBV or HCV infections, high-risk activities which would expose the patient to hepatitis B or C; travel in countries where ingestion of raw fish could lead to liver fluke infection; a family history of metabolic diseases, prior liver disease or liver cancer; known inflammatory bowel disease; primary sclerosing cholangitis or congenital biliary anomaly; ingestion of medications such as oral contraceptives or anabolic androgenic steroids; or exposure to environmental carcinogens such as vinyl chloride monomer.

B. Symptoms and Signs: Often, the patient with hepatocellular carcinoma has no symptoms or signs of liver disease. Rapid, unexplained weight loss, or the finding of a hepatic bruit or friction rub on physical examination, strongly suggest underlying tumor. Stigmata of chronic liver disease also point to the liver as the possible site of a tumor. Severe right upper quadrant pain, shoulder pain or an acute abdomen might indicate hemoperitoneum resulting from the rupture of hepatocellular carcinoma or hepatocellular adenoma. Jaundice is uncommon unless the patient has extremely advanced liver disease, tumor compressing the biliary tree, or a primary tumor of the biliary tree. Hypertension with diarrhea, flushing or vasomotor abnormalities suggests carcinoid syndrome, which frequently metastasizes to the liver.

Findings on palpation of the liver may vary from entirely normal to a large, rock-hard organ; the latter strongly suggests tumor. A distended, very tender liver suggests possible hemorrhage into hepatocellular carcinoma, hepatic adenoma or hemangioma, or could result from tension on the liver capsule due to a large, rapidly expanding mass. If clinical signs of liver disease are evident, including ascites, splenomegaly, abdominal collateral vessels, spider angiomata and jaundice, hepatocellular carcinoma is more likely. Invasion of the portal and hepatic veins, which occurs frequently with hepatocellular carcinoma, may also produce portal hypertension in the absence of frank cirrhosis.

C. Clinical Presentation: The clinical presentation of hepatocellular carcinoma varies dramatically throughout the world. In developing countries with a high incidence of hepatocellular carcinoma, the disease occurs most often in younger individuals between the ages of 20 and 50, and almost always presents as a massive tumor which is easily diagnosed. Right upper quadrant or epigastric pain, sometimes radiating to the right shoulder, is a common presentation. As noted previously, a dramatic increase in the pain usually indicates hemorrhage into the tumor or hemoperitoneum. Marked weakness and rapid weight loss often accompany these complaints, and patients are frequently aware of the recent development of a right upper quadrant mass or swelling. Cirrhosis is only present in between 40 and 50% of these younger patients, thus, signs of chronic liver disease may be absent.

In contrast to developing nations, hepatocellular carcinoma in Western countries usually develops insidiously. Patients are older, usually 50–70 years of age. Fatigue, weight loss, right upper quadrant pain, abdominal swelling (from ascites), or a change in a previously stable cirrhosis, usually herald hepatocellular carcinoma. Despite the frequently mild complaints, it is discouraging how often large and multiple tumors are found at the time of presentation. When this occurs, death frequently follows diagnosis within a few months. In these patients, signs of liver disease are common due to the advanced stage of the underlying cirrhosis. Spider angiomata, palmar erythema, prominent muscle wasting that may have become much more noticeable shortly before diagnosis, and marked fatigue are common complaints.

Hepatocellular carcinoma must always be suspected in a patient with rapid and dramatic change in a previously stable cirrhosis. On routine visits, liver size, (both and right and left lobes), the presence or absence of ascites, numbers of spider angiomata, and degree of palmar erythema, as well as status of nutrition, muscle mass, and presence or absence of jaundice, should be recorded. Significant or rapid changes in any of these parameters, as well as the development of new symptoms or signs, should prompt the immediate search for possible development of hepatocellular carcinoma.

A number of **paraneoplastic syndromes** may also develop in the patient with hepatocellular carcinoma. Hypoglycemia, erythrocytosis, hypercholesterolemia, or a combination may be the only presenting signs or symptoms of hepatocellular carcinoma in approximately 4–5% of patients.

D. Laboratory Findings: Most striking in hepatocellular carcinoma is how often patients have completely normal laboratory findings. Transaminases (AST, ALT) are most often normal or only minimally elevated. Alkaline phosphatase (AP) and gamma-glutamyl transferase (GT) are the most frequently abnormal tests, but are rarely more than 2–3 fold elevated. Lactate dehydrogenase (LDH) can be markedly and disproportionately elevated in patients with metastatic liver disease, particularly those of hematogenous origin.

The most useful and specific liver test commonly available is the α-fetoprotein, which is elevated in 70–90% of patients with hepatocellular carcinoma. It is also frequently elevated, however, in patients with very active hepatocellular necrosis and some tumors metastatic to the liver. Thus, α-fetoprotein is most useful when it is either extremely high (greater than 300–500 nanograms per ml), is newly elevated, or is steadily rising. Other tests are either not readily available or not particularly helpful.

E. Imaging Studies: The greatest advances in the diagnosing of hepatocellular carcinoma are attributable to technological improvements in real time ultrasonography (Figure 46–2A), computerized axial tomography (CT) (Figure 46–2B), and magnetic resonance imaging (MRI) (Figures 46–2D and 46–2E). Hepatic angiography (Figure 46–2F) is probably still the single most accurate technique, but it is invasive, requires exposure to contrast media and high doses of radiation, and is expensive. At the other extreme, ultrasound is readily available and significantly less expensive but is unable to clearly distinguish malignant masses from other hyper- and hypoechoic masses. The combination of liver ultrasound and dynamic bolus CT, in which rapid images of the lesion in question are taken following a bolus injection of contrast material, is usually sufficient to produce a reliable diagnosis. CT arterioportography (CTAP), however, in which a CT is performed during arterial portography, is considerably more sensitive in identifying lesions which may be missed by regular ultrasonography or CT, and is quite helpful in mapping out the lesion or lesions for the surgeon prior to attempted resection (Figures 46–3A and 46–3B). The limitation of this technique is the frequency of false positives in the patient with severe underlying cirrhosis, in whom most of the bolus is shunted around the liver due to portal hypertension. In that situation, the new, high-resolution fast-spin echo magnetic resonance imaging, with or without contrast, is superior, although much more expensive. By far, the most sensitive and accurate technique is intra-operative ultrasonography, which provides the surgeon with the best delineation of tumor extension when resection is considered or attempted.

Imaging studies combined with biochemical tests will usually allow one to distinguish between a malignant and benign mass. In most cases, however, tissue diagnosis will be needed and ultrasound or CT-guided fine needle aspiration cytology (if an experienced hepatocytologist is available) or directed core biopsy will be required. Because the histology of well differentiated hepatocellular carcinoma and hepatic adenomas can so closely mimic normal hepatic histology, it may be necessary to request outside consultation from a highly experienced hepatopathologist to rule out malignancy. Usually, though, the use of appropriate imaging studies, plus testing for α-fetoprotein is sufficient. In fact, in a cirrhotic patient with another risk factor such as hepatitis C, hepatitis B, hemochromatosis, or alcohol, the presence of a typical lesion on ultrasound and CT imaging, plus a high or rapidly rising α-fetoprotein may be sufficient to make the diagnosis without histologic verification.

F. Hepatocellular Carcinoma Surveillance: Because hepatocellular carcinoma has such a dismal prognosis and surgical resection remains the only curative option, it is of vital importance to discover the tumor when it is as small as possible. As discussed above, most patients do not present with clinical disease until they already have massive or multiple tumor nodules. Thus, attempts have been made to identify patients at high risk for the development of hepatocellular carcinoma, and follow them closely via periodic ultrasound and α-fetoprotein studies. This issue is controversial and recommendations vary, but studies in Japan, China, and among American Eskimos have clearly shown that close surveillance every 6 months significantly increases the identification of resectable lesions in populations at high risk. Similar data have not yet been produced to document the utility of such a program, particularly its cost-effectiveness, in low-risk populations.

Differential Diagnosis

Hepatocellular carcinoma must be distinguished from all of the other malignant and benign masses noted in Table 46–2.

Complications

Deaths from hepatocellular carcinoma occur for a variety of reasons, but most often because of liver failure. Severe hemorrhage from tumor rupture or variceal bleeding, severe hypoglycemia, sepsis or bacterial peritonitis, are also frequent terminal

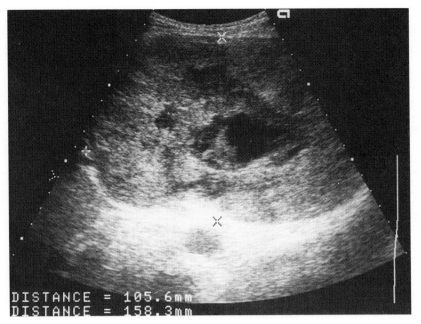

A

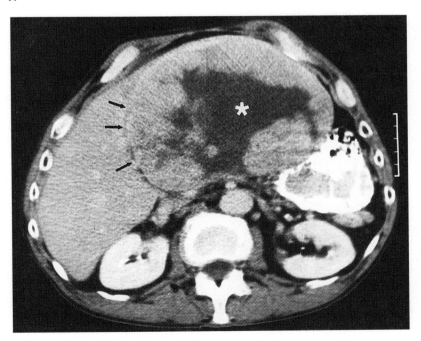

B

Figure 46–2. Imaging of Hepatocellular Carcinoma by Multiple Modalities. *A:* A 66-year-old male former alcoholic complained of a painless mid-abdominal mass. α-fetoprotein was negative. Ultrasound showed a 10.5 × 15.8 cm hyperechoic mass in the left lobe of the liver with central hypodense areas due to fluid or necrosis (edges marked by Xs). ***B:*** CT with contrast of the same patient shows a large hepatocellular carcinoma occupying virtually the entire left lobe of the liver and penetrating the right lobe. Note that the tumor is almost isodense with the normal liver ***(small arrows along border)*** and, were it not for the hypodense center (*) caused by tumor necrosis, the tumor could have been easily overlooked.

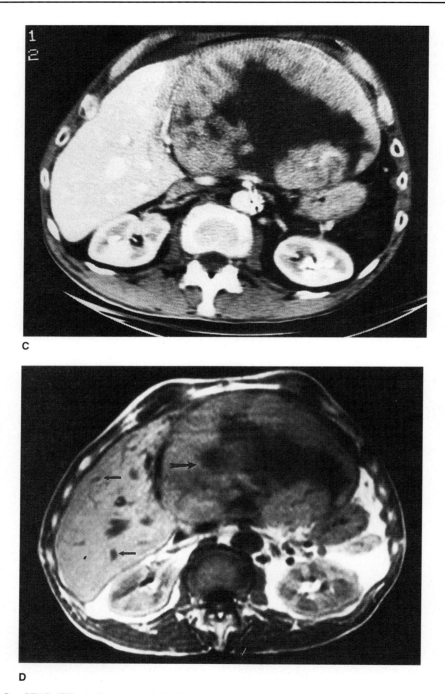

C

D

Figure 46–2 *C:* CTAP (CT arterioportography) of same patient shows dramatic difference in density between normal liver and tumor, highlighting the low-density tumor around the necrotic center and readily delineating the border between normal and neoplastic tissue. ***D:*** Axial MRI of same patient. The decreased intensity on the T_1 weighted images ***(large arrow)*** indicates fluid in the center of the mass. Note similar low intensity of vessels in the right lobe ***(small arrows).***

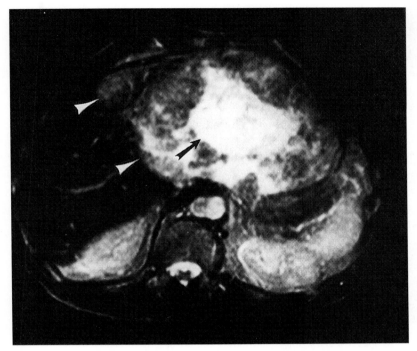

E

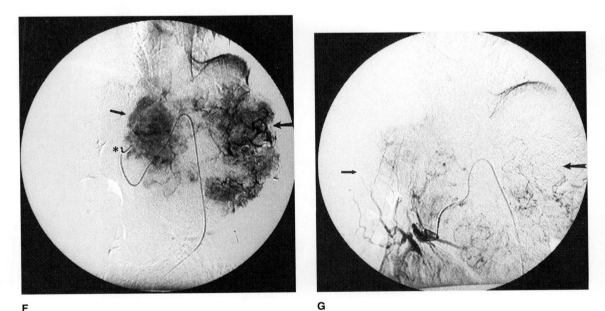

F

G

Figure 46–2. *E:* T$_2$ weighted axial MRI shows a marked increase in signal intensity in the center of the mass *(arrow)*, indicative of central tumor necrosis. The signal intensity of the tumor itself is also greater than that of the normal right lobe due to its increased vascularity *(**white arrowheads at edge of the tumor**). **F:*** Angiogram catheter can be seen selectively placed in the left hepatic artery(*) of the same patient where it supplies the tumor. The hepatocellular carcinoma demonstrates a typical bizarre vascular pattern resulting from tumor neovascularity *(**large arrow**)* and a tumor blush *(**small arrow**). **G:*** Angiogram with the same projection as Figure 46–2F following embolization with Gelfoam. Note the almost complete absence of blood flow in the tumor *(**large arrow**)* with good flow to the right lobe *(**small arrow**).*

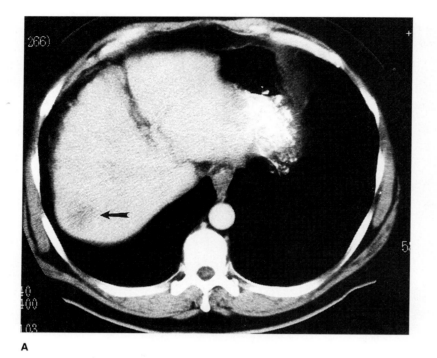

A

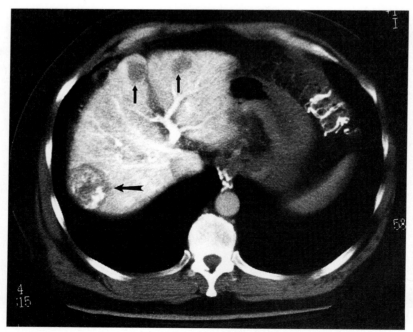

B

Figure 46–3. Sensitivity of CTAP vs CT. **A:** Regular CT with contrast shows area of slightly decreased density in the lower right lobe of the liver **(arrow).** **B:** CTAP in the same plane as **A** makes the lesion in the right posterior lobe obvious and identifies two additional anterior lesions **(arrows).**

Table 46–2. Simple classification of major liver tumors.

Malignant	Benign
Epithelial	**Epithelial**
Hepatocellular Carcinoma	Hepatocellular adenoma
Fibrolamellar Carcinoma[1]	Focal nodular hyperplasia
Hepatoblastoma[2]	Nodular regenerative hyperplasia
Cholangiocarcinoma	Bile duct adenoma
Biliary cystadenocarcinoma	Biliary cystadenoma
Carcinoid Tumor	Intrahepatic biliary papillomatosis
Mesodermal	**Mesodermal**
Hemangiosarcoma	Hemangioma (cavernous hemangioma)
Epithelial hemangioendothelioma	Infantile hemangioendothelioma[2]
Undifferentiated (embryonal) sarcoma[2]	
Embryonal rhabdomyosarcoma[2]	
Lymphoma	
Other sarcomas, rare tumors,	
and mixed tumors	

Tumor-like
Peliosis hepatis
Simple cyst
Mesenchymal hamartoma[2]
Hepatic Abscess

[1]An important histologic variant of hepatocellular carcinoma with a significantly better prognosis.
[2]Occurs in infants and children.

events. Many patients with hepatocellular carcinoma suffer from debilitating ascites, and marked palliation can be provided by repeated large volume paracentesis. Standard diuretic therapy is of limited benefit in these patients. The ascites is usually transudative and lacks direct evidence of hepatocellular carcinoma, which rarely metastasizes to the peritoneum; thus, malignant cells are not often found in the ascites. Direct extension of the tumor to the diaphragm or surrounding areas is uncommon, but two-thirds or more will expand directly into the hepatic vascular system or the vena cava, which may accelerate the accumulation of ascites. At autopsy, almost one-half of the cases will show metastases, most often in the portal, pancreatic and para-aortic lymph nodes. The lung is the next most common site of metastasis, with occasional metastases to the adrenal, bone, and myocardium.

Treatment

A. Medical Approaches: Despite many innovative and complex approaches to treating hepatocellular carcinoma (Table 46–3), hepatocellular carcinoma remains remarkably resistant to cure. Of chemotherapeutic agents, only doxorubicin (Adriamycin) has shown a better than 20% response rate. There have been virtually no cures with chemotherapy given systemically, either as a single agent or in combination. Site-directed chemotherapy via intra-arterial perfusion has shown only a modest increase in response rate by allowing delivery of larger doses of chemotherapeutic agents directly to the tumor site. More promising, but primarily for short- or long-term palliation, is embolizing the vessels feeding the tumor with gel foam (Figures 46–2F and 46–2G) or

Lipiodol, an oily substance that becomes trapped in the tumor (Figure 46–4A). An extension of these two approaches, known as chemoembolization, combines embolization of the tumor vessels with chemotherapy, thus producing a combination of anoxic necrosis with high local concentrations of trapped chemotherapeutic agents. For small tumors, less than 5 cm and preferably less than 3 cm in size, percutaneous ethanol, acetic acid and even hot saline injections have proved beneficial in improving 3- to 5-year survival. Encapsulation of Adriamycin in liposomes, and a variety of attempts to target the tumor with

Table 46–3. Therapeutic options for HCC.

Generally accepted modalities
1–3 nodules, <5 cm in diameter
  (1) Surgical resection
  (2) Percutaneous ethanol injection
  (3) Chemoembolization with or without liver transplantation*
>3 nodules or >5 cm in diameter
  (1) Percutaneous ethanol injection
  (2) Chemoembolization with or without liver transplantation
Experimental modalities
  1. Surgical resection with adjuvant chemotherapy
  2. Liver transplantation with or without chemoembolization before transplant with or without adjuvant chemotherapy*
  3. Immunotargeting with mono- or polyclonal antibodies to α-fetoprotein, ferritin or "tumor associated antigens"
    a. Monoclonal antibodies alone
    b. Antibodies conjugated to chemotherapeutic agents
    c. Antibodies conjugated to ^{131}I, ^{125}I, ^{90}Y, ^{99m}Tc (radioimmunodetection and therapy)

*Liver transplantation with its many multi-modal approaches is clearly still experimental but is listed in both categories because of its widespread use and availability.

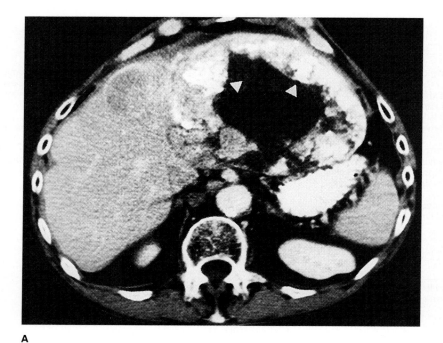

A

B

Figure 46–4. **A:** CT shows lipiodal trapped in the tumor of patient in Figure 46–2 following chemoembolization of the tumor *(arrow heads).* **B:** CT shows a normal liver 1 year following chemoembolization and transplantation of patient in Figure 46–2.

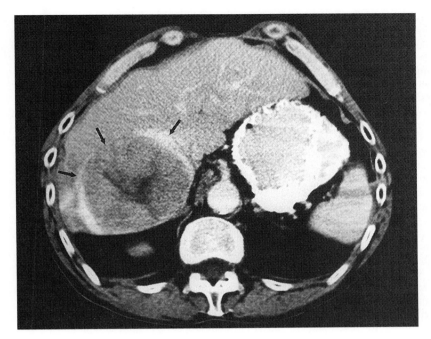

C

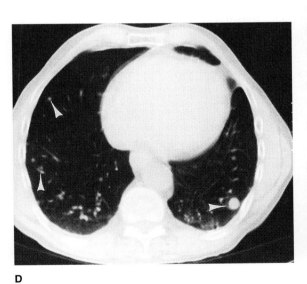

D

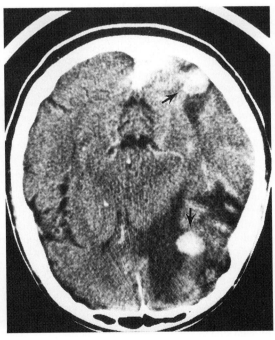

E

Figure 46–4. *C–E:* CT 6 months later (18 months post transplantation) shows tumor recurrence in right lobe of transplanted liver. Note rim enhancement of this hypervascular lesion *(arrows)* and hypodense necrotic center. Boney metastases (not shown) and lung metastases were also apparent *(arrow heads) (D)*. Two months later the patient developed slurring speech and an ataxic gait. Brain metastases were found in the right frontal and right parieto-occipital lobes *(arrows, [E])*.

monoclonal antibodies, or antibodies to molecules produced in high concentration by the tumor (α-feto-protein, ferritin) have also been used experimentally, but to date have either been used only in animals, or have shown no significant improvement over other modalities when used in humans.

B. Surgical Approaches: The only potentially curative technique currently available is surgical resection. Cure is likely, however, only for single nodules less than 3 cm in size. Larger nodules or the presence of multiple nodules make recurrence almost inevitable. Liver transplantation, which removes the entire liver, and with it all intrahepatic micrometastases, was originally theorized as the ideal way to treat hepatocellular carcinoma. Most patients, however, showed rapid recurrence in the transplanted organ (Figure 46), presumably due to the presence of localized micrometastases outside the liver bed, and the decreased immunosurveillance caused by the immuno-compromised status of the post-transplant patient (see Chapter 54). Thus, in most transplant centers hepatocellular carcinoma is a relative contraindication to liver transplantation. Liver transplantation may be worth reconsidering, however, and is once again enjoying a surge of interest, as investigators combine the modalities of neoadjuvant chemoembolization and post-transplant adjuvant chemotherapy in patients who have no evidence of tumor outside the liver itself. Such approaches can improve survival rates to levels of 50% over 3 years and 30% over 5 years, but the best results are obtained in patients with small tumors and limited numbers of nodules, the same patients who do best with chemoembolization, percutaneous ethanol injection, or surgical resection alone (Figures 46–4 A–E).

C. Other Treatment Considerations: The use of historical or untreated controls, or controls treated with only systemic chemotherapy, makes it difficult to evaluate rigorously the range of treatments currently available. Controlled trials will be necessary to determine whether any of the more aggressive treatments offers an advantage over a simple resection or chemoembolization. Meanwhile, the limitations on treatment remain (1) the lack of highly effective chemotherapeutic agents; and (2) the poor surgical candidacy of the majority of patients with hepatocellular carcinoma due to the large size of the tumor at presentation or the severity of the underlying cirrhosis. The major complication following liver resection in such patients is hepatic failure. In addition, when the native liver remains in place, the likelihood of new tumors developing remains high. This is because the risk factors for hepatocellular carcinoma due to cirrhosis and continued necro-inflammatory change—as well as any other predisposing conditions such as hepatitis B or C—remain unchanged. At present, the most reasonable approach is to identify patients at high risk for developing hepatocellular carcinoma, follow them carefully in hopes of identifying very early lesions, and consider resection of small lesions by a surgeon well trained in hepatic surgery. Any other approaches should be considered only as part of clinical trials so that useful data will be developed to improve future therapy. Prevention of hepatocellular carcinoma by aggressive universal immunization against hepatitis B on a worldwide basis, eliminating food contamination by aflatoxin and other hepatocarcinogenic toxins, reducing alcoholism, and careful screening of blood products will have the greatest effect on hepatocellular carcinoma incidence by eliminating the major factors contributing to its pathogenesis.

Prognosis

The overall prognosis for hepatocellular carcinoma remains very poor. Mean survival after diagnosis of large tumors is less than 6 months, if left untreated. Small tumors have a considerably better prognosis, with one study showing 90% survival at 3 years for tumors smaller than 3 cm; another found 63% survival at 3 years in patients with tumors less than 5 cm in size, and Child-Pugh Class A (compensated) cirrhosis. Currently, no adequate staging system takes into account all prognostic factors identified in individual studies, and virtually all studies use historical or no controls at all.

OTHER MALIGNANT TUMORS

1. FIBROLAMELLAR HEPATOCELLULAR CARCINOMA

This important variant of hepatocellular carcinoma is characterized by its occurrence primarily in younger patients between the ages of 20 and 40 in the absence of cirrhosis. It has no gender predominance or known risk factors, and α-fetoprotein is usually normal. Over one-half of the tumors occur in the left lobe, making it particularly amenable to surgical resection. Histologically, this carcinoma is characterized by monotonous benign-looking cells with extremely rare mitoses, and the presence of fibrous bands that traverse the tumor in a lamellar fashion dividing it into cords and nodules. Prognosis is considerably better than that for hepatocellular carcinoma, and long-term survival is frequent with either resection or liver transplantation.

2. MINUTE OR ENCAPSULATED HEPATOCELLULAR CARCINOMA

This unusual variant accounts for 10% of the hepatocellular carcinoma cases in Japan, and is found almost exclusively in Southeast Asia. This slow-growing tumor, usually only 3–5 cm in diameter, has a thick fibrous capsule. Well differentiated histologically, it rarely invades the vascular system. No risk factors are known, and only 50% are α-fetoprotein positive. Because of its small encapsulated nature and the lack of vascular invasion, it has a very high surgical cure rate.

3. HEPATOBLASTOMA

This rare liver tumor of infancy presents almost exclusively before 3 years of age, and most often before 2 years of age. It is the most common liver tumor of infants, but is the cause of only 0.2–5.8% of childhood malignant growths. Two-thirds are solitary, most often in the right lobe of the liver. Presentation is usually unexplained abdominal swelling, and the tumor may already be large at the time of birth. Associated findings may include anorexia, diarrhea, vomiting, abdominal pain, irritability, weight loss, and failure to thrive. Tumor rupture may produce hemoperitoneum. A variety of associated congenital anomalies have been noted, including hemihypertrophy, talipes, macroglossia, right diaphragmatic defect, Meckel's diverticulum, cardiac and renal malformations, and polyposis coli. Approximately twice as many males are affected as females. α-fetoprotein levels are increased in 80–90% of patients, but routine liver tests are usually normal or show only minor abnormalities. Ectopic production of human chorionic gonadotropin may produce precocious puberty, in addition to osteopenia with fractures, hypoglycemia and isosexual precocity. Cystathioninuria has been reported. Metastases may be noted to the lung. The lesion is avascular on angiography and frequently shows calcification. Because of its large size and aggressive growth (mean 10–12 cm, range 3–20 cm), hepatoblastoma is rapidly fatal in most cases. Surgical resection should be performed immediately if possible. If not, aggressive chemotherapy may debulk the tumor sufficiently to allow curative surgery. A combination of chemotherapy and radiotherapy following surgery may improve prognosis.

4. ANGIOSARCOMA

Although the most common mesenchymal tumor of the liver, fewer than 25 cases occur in North America each year, and the attack rate is 0.14–0.25 cases per million. Four out of five cases occur in males, generally in their sixth or seventh decades. Thorotrast and vinyl chloride monomer have been the most carefully documented causes of this tumor, but it has also been associated with arsenic and potassium arsenite ("Fowler's solution"), which was previously used to treat psoriasis. Also implicated have been radium, inorganic copper, and phenylethylhydrazine. Workers exposed to polyvinyl chloride have a 400-fold greater risk of developing angiosarcoma, but the incidence of this tumor has been decreasing with better manufacturing controls and the declining number of patients alive who received thorotrast.

Abdominal pain or discomfort, abdominal swelling, rapidly progressive liver failure, malaise, weakness, weight loss, anorexia, and vomiting can all be presentations of the disease. One-half of the patients have splenomegaly, and 25% have jaundice and ascites, which may be blood-tinged. Low platelets are found in 50% of patients, and 15% will present with hemoperitoneum. There is no association with hepatitis B or other viruses, and α-fetoprotein and CEA are normal. Hepatic arteriography demonstrates displacement of hepatic arteries by tumor, with a tumor blush and "puddling" during the mid-phase of arteriography. Because of tumor necrosis, central enhancement may not occur. Liver biopsy is generally avoided because of the high risk of hemorrhage. Life expectancy from the time of diagnosis is 6 months, with 50% or more of the patients dying of liver failure. To date, no successful therapy has been found.

5. CHOLANGIOCARCINOMA

(See also Chapter 52.) Cholangiocarcinoma is an uncommon disease in the Western world, with an incidence of 2–2.8 per 100,000 population per year. Incidence is much higher in the Far East, however, because of the frequency of biliary parasites. Cholangiocarcinoma is associated with a variety of liver and biliary tract diseases, including: (1) inflammatory bowel disease, even in the absence of sclerosing cholangitis; (2) congenital biliary anomalies including choledochal cysts, polycystic liver disease, and Caroli's disease; (3) Oriental cholangiohepatitis (*Clonorchis sinensis*); (4) chemical exposure, including thorotrast, benzidine, 3'3 dichlorobenzidine, and *m*-toluenediamide. The best recognized of these associations is that with primary sclerosing cholangitis. Seven to fifteen percent of patients coming to liver transplant for sclerosing cholangitis are found to have cholangiocarcinoma, the diagnosis frequently being made only after the liver has been removed.

Pathophysiology

One-half or more of the tumors occur at the confluence of the right and left hepatic ducts (Klatskin tumor). Another 21% are in the mid and 21% in the distal common bile duct. Five percent are diffuse. Most are adenocarcinomas that arise from the biliary epithelium, and there is a heavy, fibrous reaction to the tumor. This strong desmoplastic reaction, along with the presence of inflammation, may make it difficult to diagnose from brushings, or even full thickness biopsies, as the tumor cells may be sparse and well separated.

Essentials of Diagnosis

- 3:1 male to female ratio.
- Most frequent in sixth and seventh decades.
- Presentation with jaundice most often when tumor is located at the bifurcation of the right and left hepatic ducts (Klatskin tumor).
- Weight loss, diarrhea, and acholic stool in 60–75% of cases.
- Epigastric distress with weight loss common.
- Elevated alkaline phosphatase, and gamma glutamyl transferase uniformly present; bilirubin elevated only if total or near total obstruction at the bifurcation or the common duct.
- Anorexia and fat malabsorption common if jaundice present.
- Bacterial cholangitis usually only in late-stage disease or if a stent is in place.

Clinical Findings

A. Symptoms and Signs: Symptoms and signs depend on the location of the tumor (at the bifurcation of the right and left hepatic duct, or more distal) and the degree of obstruction. Patients with unilateral bile duct obstruction may have a normal bilirubin. If there is significant obstruction, jaundice, acholic stools, dark urine, and pruritus may be present. Anorexia, epigastric distress, weight loss and diarrhea are also present in up to 60–70% of cases. Bacterial cholangitis is uncommon, except late in the disease when total or near total obstruction has occurred.

B. Laboratory Findings: Mild to marked elevations in alkaline phosphatase, and gamma glutamyl transferase are uniformly found. Bilirubin may be normal, unless significant obstruction is present. Transaminases (AST and ALT) are generally minimally abnormal. α-fetoprotein is negative, but CA19-9 and CEA are frequently positive, although not pathognomonic.

C. Imaging Studies: Ultrasound may demonstrate dilated intrahepatic ducts if a Klatskin lesion is present and extrahepatic duct dilation will occur to the level of obstruction if there is a distal obstruction. CT scan will not demonstrate a mass lesion until late in the disease, but can confirm the dilated ducts. Angiography is indicated only if surgical resection is contemplated, because vascular invasion is a contraindication to surgical resection. Endoscopic retrograde cholangiopancreatography (ERCP) or percutaneous transhepatic cholangiography (PTC) will demonstrate the biliary obstruction at the site of the tumor and allow brushings for cytology examination. A good cytology specimen will be positive in approximately 75% of cases.

Differential Diagnosis

Cholangiocarcinoma must be differentiated from all other biliary obstructive lesions. Particularly problematic is the differentiation from primary sclerosing cholangitis, which increases the risk of cholangiocarcinoma. ERCP and PTC are the most useful in ruling out other causes of cholestasis and attempting to document the presence of malignancy. Even good cytological brushings, however, will be negative in the presence of tumor at least 25% of the time.

Complications

Patients most often die of liver failure because of the development of biliary cirrhosis, although sepsis, cholangitis, and metastatic destruction of the liver can also occur.

Treatment

Curative resection is rarely possible because of the advanced stage of disease at which patients present. Liver transplantation has been equally disappointing as a result of the 100% recurrence rate of cholangiocarcinoma following transplantation. There is no effective chemotherapy at the present time. Very aggressive approaches to unresectable tumor are currently attempted in only a few centers, utilizing external beam radiotherapy, brachyradiotherapy with iridium 192 implants placed by ERCP, and combinations of the above with liver transplantation. Not enough patients have been reported at the present time to establish the long-term efficacy of such approaches. Significant palliation can be produced by dilation and stenting of strictures when resection is not possible. Endoscopic stent placement provides an advantage over externally drained stents because the former maintains biliary enteric continuity, and should be possible in 85% of cases when a well trained endoscopist is available. The stent tends to become obstructed over time, and many centers routinely exchange the stents at least every 4 to 6 months on an outpatient basis.

Prognosis

Five-year survival is only 4–10%. Patients die from liver failure or infectious complications due to problems with biliary drainage. Anorexia, malaise, and inanition frequently accompany end-stage disease. Local invasion of the portal vein and hepatic artery may also produce the standard complications of portal hypertension, ascites, and variceal bleeding.

NONMALIGNANT (BENIGN) EPITHELIAL TUMORS

Nonmalignant hepatic masses can range from simple cysts and hemangiomas to hepatocellular adenomas and focal nodular hyperplasia. Although all are benign in growth characteristics, some can produce significant morbidity and even mortality if inaccurately diagnosed and left untreated. Others can lead to unnecessary, costly and sometimes mischievous interventions when they would be better left alone.

1. HEPATOCELLULAR ADENOMA

Hepatocellular adenomas are benign epithelial cell tumors that were extremely rare in the United States prior to 1954; only two were found in 50,000 autopsies at the Los Angeles County General Hospital prior to that time. Since 1970, however, there has been a dramatic rise that has been attributed to the common use of estrogens in oral contraceptives. The estimated current incidence is 3–4 per 100,000 users per year.

Pathophysiology

Estrogen exposure is the major risk factor for the development of hepatocellular adenoma, and the risk correlates with the dose and duration of estrogen ingestion. Hepatocellular adenomas have been identified in men taking anabolic androgenic steroids, which can be aromatized to estrogens, indicating a possible common pathway. This benign tumor has also been reported in patients with glycogen storage disease type 1, tyrosinemia and galactosemia. When it occurs in association with a metabolic disease, hepatocellular adenoma is primarily a male disease with a high risk of malignant transformation. An unrelated condition, **multiple hepatocellular adenomatosis,** presents with multiple adenomas, usually more than four, scattered among the hepatic lobes. It is not associated with other liver diseases or estrogen intake.

Essentials of Diagnosis

- 60% with history of oral contraceptive use.
- 90% solitary lesions.
- Liver tests normal or minimally abnormal.
- Regression after discontinuing hormonal therapy.
- Anabolic androgenic steroids and certain metabolic diseases also risk factors.
- Complications of intra-tumor hemorrhage and hemoperitoneum from tumor rupture.
- Resection required in most cases.

Clinical Findings

A. Symptoms and Signs: Patients may present in crisis due to rupture of an adenoma with intra-abdominal hemorrhage; with complaints of right upper quadrant pain due to intra-tumor hemorrhage; after noting a palpable mass; or, most frequently, following the incidental finding of a liver mass during an ultrasound or CT examination performed for another purpose.

B. Physical Examination: There are usually no findings on physical examination. A palpable and sometimes tender mass may be noted in the right upper quadrant. When hemoperitoneum is present, findings typical of an acute abdomen and possibly shock, depending on the severity of the hemorrhage, will predominate.

C. Laboratory Findings: Laboratory findings are not helpful and are most often normal. Minor elevations of alkaline phosphatase, gamma GT, or transaminases may be noted. α-fetoprotein is normal.

D. Imaging Studies (Table 46–4): Ultrasound and CT examinations will usually identify the lesion without difficulty. Because of its lack of phagocytic Kupffer cells (hepatic macrophages), hepatocellular adenoma will present as a defect on nuclear medicine sulfur colloid scan. There are no diagnostic findings on ultrasound or CT. The lesion is hypervascular, which can be noted on MRI. Angiography may demonstrate large peripheral vessels with centrifugal flow; central avascular scars may be present due to internal hemorrhage. Some adenomas, however, will be hypovascular.

Differential Diagnosis

Hepatocellular adenoma must be differentiated from malignant lesions (Table 46–5). It is most often solitary, and frequently quite large, often greater than 10 cm in size. Histologically, it may also be difficult to differentiate from normal liver and from highly differentiated hepatocellular carcinoma. Adjacent normal hepatocytes should be distinguishable from the "neohepatocytes" of the tumor. Failure to find portal tracts or bile ducts is a particularly useful histological difference. Giant cell formation, cholestasis, alcoholic hyaline, and α_1-antitrypsin inclusions may also be found.

Complications

Up to one-third of patients may present with acute hemoperitoneum, requiring emergent resection or hepatic artery ligation. This is the major risk, although occasional progression to hepatocellular carcinoma has been noted, primarily in those related to underlying metabolic disorders.

Treatment

The majority of hepatocellular adenomas should be resected if possible. Controversy exists concerning smaller lesions in patients on oral contraceptives, as the tumors will usually regress with discontinuation of the oral contraceptives. If the adenoma is not surgically removed, close follow-up should be maintained to rule out an increase in size or malignant transformation. Estrogens and pregnancy should be avoided. Pregnancy can be successfully carried out if no recurrence is noted following successful resection of a hepatic adenoma.

Prognosis

Prognosis is excellent with discontinuation of estrogens and resection.

2. FOCAL NODULAR HYPERPLASIA

Focal nodular hyperplasia is the most common benign hepatic tumor, other than vascular tumors. In

Table 46–4. Imaging techniques and hepatic masses.

Technique	Discussion
Ultrasound	Noninvasive, low cost, readily available; with Doppler imaging, also provides information on vascular patency and volume and direction of flow; sensitivity to 1 cm; ideal screening technique; diagnostic for simple cysts; unable to convincingly determine cause of solid or mixed masses; excellent technique for guided biopsy; marked obesity or bowel gas interfere with the examination; generally the screening test of first choice.
CT	Radiation and contrast exposure; readily available and provides "normal anatomy" for non-radiologist; sensitivty to 1 cm; nearly isodense lesions may be missed because of volume averaging or timing of imaging to contrast injection; will screen for extrahepatic lesions simultaneously, thus identifying metastatic disease beyond the liver.
Dynamic bolus CT	Increased radiation exposure (must first localize lesion and then take multiple timed images); used mostly for characterizing the enhancement pattern of hepatic masses; correctly identifies 2/3 of hemangiomas.
CTAP	Invasive, requiring placement of angiography catheter for bolus injection; superior delineation of anatomic location of lesions to help with surgical planning; more sensitive than standard CT and will often save unnecessary surgery by identifying additional tumor nodules not noted on standard CT or ultrasound; may produce increase in false-positive findings in presence of severe cirrhosis.
MRI	Noninvasive but expensive; excellent biplanar images with sensitivity to 1.0 cm; more accurate than CTAP in the presence of severe cirrhosis; problems identifying lesions near the diaphragm due to cardiac motion-induced artifacts; provides additional information on vascular supply and patency.
Angiography	Most invasive with high-contrast dose and high radiation exposure; most expensive (along with MRI); provides most accurate information on vascular supply, patency and flow, including vascular pressures, if needed.
Radionuclide scanning	Minimally invasive, less costly (except for ultrasound) and readily available; less sensitive (2 cm minimum); primarily useful to distinguish hepatic adenomas from focal nodular hyperplasia (due to the lack of Kupffer cells for colloid uptake in the adenomas) and identifying hemangiomas (with the ^{99m}Tc tagged RBC-SPECT study).

CT, computerized axial tomography
CTAP, CT arterioportography
MRI, fast spin echo magnetic resonance imaging
RBC-SPECT, ^{99m}Technetium-tagged red blood cell study utilizing single photon emission computerized tomography

one large series from the University of Southern California, approximately 8% of all primary hepatic tumors were focal nodular hyperplasia.

Pathogenesis

Focal nodular hyperplasia has been described either as a benign tumor, a hamartoma, or a manifestation of liver regeneration. Most likely it develops because of a congenital vascular malformation with subsequent cellular hyperplasia and possibly hepatocellular metaplasia. Its association with oral contraceptive agents is unclear, and it occurs almost equally in men, children and women not on oral contraceptive agents, thus making the association considerably weaker than for hepatic adenomas.

Essentials of Diagnosis

- 2/3 to 3/4 discovered incidentally.
- 90% solitary lesion.
- Normal laboratory studies.
- Occasionally pain due to rupture or hemorrhage.
- "Spoked-wheel" appearance on hepatic angiography.
- Not premalignant, and generally no therapy required.
- Avoid oral contraceptives and pregnancy.

General Considerations

This is not believed to be a premalignant lesion,

and is most often discovered incidentally and best left alone.

Clinical Findings

A. Symptoms and Signs: The vast majority of these benign tumor-like lesions are found incidentally. If symptoms or signs are present, most commonly a mass has been noted in the upper abdomen. Pain is occasionally present, usually in association with hemorrhage into the nodule or rupture. Hemorrhage most often occurs in women taking oral contraceptives.

B. Laboratory Findings: Laboratory findings are almost always normal. α-fetoprotein is normal.

C. Pathology and Imaging: Findings on imaging studies are better understood when correlated with the histologic findings. Focal nodular hyperplasia is usually found subcapsular as a single lesion less than 5 cm in size. The characteristic finding is a central fibrous scar with fibrous septae radiating to the periphery of the lesion. Early reports described this as "focal cirrhosis," and large arterial vessels with fibromuscular hyperplasia, as well as multiple bile ductules travel along the septae. Kupffer cells are present, providing another means to differentiate it from hepatocellular adenomas. Ultrasound and CT readily identify the lesion, but have no characteristic findings, although the central scar is often noted on

Table 46–5. Common hepatic mass lesions.

	Hepatocellular Carcinoma	Metastatic Carcinoma	Hepatocellular Adenoma	Focal Nodular Hyperplasia	Cavernous Hemangioma	Simple Cyst
Incidence/100,000[1]	1–4800[2]	3–20	8–4	3–4	410–7500	170
Solitary	20–40%	5–10%	90%	90%	90%	
Coexisting liver disease	HBV, HCV, cirrhosis	Uncommon in cirrhotic liver	None	None	None	None
Pathogenesis	HBV, HCV, alcohol, aflatoxin, cirrhosis	Hematogenous, lymphatic or direct spread	Estrogens, anabolic steroids	Congenital, possibly estrogens	Congenital, estrogens	Congenital
Imaging[3]	Ultrasound, CT	Ultrasound, CT, CTAP	Ultrasound, CT, 99mTc	Ultrasound, CT, MRI, 99mTc	Dynamic bolus CT, 99mTc-RBC-SPECT scan	Ultrasound, CT
α-fetoprotein	>300–500 ng/ml	Normal	Normal	Normal	Normal	Normal
Diagnosis[4]	FNAB or core biopsy	FNAB or core biopsy	Imaging, biopsy	Imaging, biopsy	Imaging	Imaging
Treatment	"Curative resection" or ethanol injection if solitary, <5.0 cm; ?transplantation +/- chemoembolization	"Curative resection" if <3.0 cm and 3 or fewer nodules	Discontinue estrogens/androgens; resect if possible, especially if large; otherwise periodic imaging	Discontinue estrogens; periodic imaging	Surgical resection only if symptomatic or >10.0 cm; discontinue estrogens; periodic imaging	No treatment unless symptomatic

[1]From autopsy series
[2]Varies with geographic origin
[3]Most useful imaging technique with which to obtain a diagnosis
[4]Definitive test required for confident diagnosis
CT, computerized axial tomography
Dynamic bolus CT, Rapid sequential CT images taken at plane of the mass, with delayed images up to 20 minutes
CTAP, Computerized axial tomography arterioportogram
MRI, Fast spin echo magnetic resonance imaging
99mTC, 99mTechnetium-labelled sulfur colloid scan
RBC-SPECT, 99mTechnetium-tagged red blood cell study utilizing single photon emission computerized tomography
FNAB, Fine needle aspiration biopsy for cytology.

CT. The same scar will be hyperdense on MRI T_2 weighted images, and such findings should suggest focal nodular hyperplasia. Angiography may demonstrate the hypervascular lesion with a hypovascular central scar and vessels radiating towards the center in a "spoked-wheel" fashion.

Differential Diagnosis

This lesion must be differentiated from all other benign and malignant mass lesions of the liver (see Table 46–5). Usually, the characteristic imaging findings are sufficient to make the diagnosis. In as many as two-thirds of cases, when the lesion is found incidentally at surgery, it is biopsied and the histology is characteristic.

Treatment

No treatment is necessary because the lesion is rarely symptomatic and there is no convincing evidence of malignant predisposition. On the rare occasion when pain or hemorrhage occurs, surgical resection is appropriate.

Prognosis

Prognosis is excellent, and, other than the rare case of abdominal crisis from rupture and hemorrhage, focal nodular hyperplasia is unlikely to produce morbidity or mortality. As noted, there is no clear predisposition to malignancy. However, it is probably best to avoid the use of oral contraceptives, and most authorities do not recommend pregnancy.

3. NODULAR REGENERATIVE HYPERPLASIA

This unusual and uncommon condition is characterized by nodules of hyperplastic hepatocytes surrounded by compressed and distorted adjacent hepatocytes, giving a superficial appearance of cirrhosis, although no fibrosis is present. The hyperplastic hepatocytes are arranged in plates more than one-cell thick and the lesion is best demonstrated on reticulin stain.

Pathogenesis

What causes this lesion is unclear, but it is felt to involve occlusion of multiple intrahepatic portal vein branches, producing local ischemia and atrophy with subsequent compensatory regeneration of surrounding hepatocytes leading to compression of adjacent lobules. A possible association with arterial or portal venous inflammation, or both, has been suggested, and the assistance of a pathologist has always been required for diagnosis. Although usually idiopathic, nodular regenerative hyperplasia has often been reported in association with rheumatoid arthritis, Felty's syndrome, subacute bacterial endocarditis, CRST syndrome, and the long-term use of certain drugs (corticosteroids and oral contraceptives). It has also

been noted in association with hematologic diseases such as myeloma, polycythemia vera, and myelofibrosis. Hereditary hemorrhagic telangiectasia, polyarteritis nodosa, diabetes mellitus, and the toxic oil syndrome have also been reported associations.

Clinical Findings

A. Symptoms and Signs: Nodular regenerative hyperplasia is rarely recognized other than as an incidental finding. Occasionally, development of portal hypertension or its complications will lead to the diagnosis.

B. Laboratory Findings: Laboratory tests are normal, unless the patient develops portal hypertension. Laboratory abnormalities related to associated diseases are frequently present and may lead to the suggestion of nodular regenerative hyperplasia, when the primary disease has been diagnosed. α-fetoprotein is normal.

C. Imaging Studies: Ill-defined nodules may be noted on ultrasound or CT, but they have no defining characteristics, and histology is required for diagnosis.

Differential Diagnosis

Nodular regenerative hyperplasia must be distinguished from focal nodular hyperplasia, hepatocellular adenoma, and hepatocellular carcinoma, as well as cirrhosis (see Table 46–5). Histology is required to make this distinction.

Complications

Portal hypertension, if present, may require the standard therapy for ascites, bleeding varices, or hepatic encephalopathy, although all of these are uncommon. Most often the treatment is directed at the underlying associated disease. On rare occasion, nodular regenerative hyperplasia can lead to liver failure, and patients have required liver transplantation. Rupture of the liver has also been a rare event. As with the other benign conditions discussed above, patients are advised not to use contraceptive steroids.

4. OTHER UNCOMMON CONDITIONS

Anabolic Steroid-Associated Hepatocellular Adenoma

C-17 alkylated forms of anabolic steroids have been reported as potential inducers of a variety of liver problems, including peliosis hepatis, hepatocellular adenoma, and possibly cholangiocarcinoma and hepatocellular carcinoma. **Peliosis hepatis** is a condition in which multiple small, dilated, blood-filled cavities, with no supporting stroma develop. These cavities usually do not have any lining endothelium. They are less than 5–10 mm in diameter and are associated with the use of anabolic steroids as well as estrogenic compounds. Cavities also may be a precursor to hemangiosarcoma in patients exposed to vinyl chloride monomer. For the past 20–30 years, increasing numbers of hepatocellular adenomas have been reported in patients taking anabolic steroids, but this remains an infrequent occurrence.

Seventy-five percent of cases occur in males regardless of age, but particularly in adolescents. Hepatomegaly and pain are the usual presenting symptoms, although hemoperitoneum may occur. It is rare for tumors to be noted unless patients have been taking steroids for more than 40–80 months. Laboratory studies are not helpful, and α-fetoprotein is normal. If α-fetoprotein is elevated, underlying cholangiocarcinoma or hepatocellular carcinoma should be suspected.

Multiple small tumors or numerous small nodules are the usual finding, although they can range up to 11 cm. Tumor nodules usually resolve with discontinuation of steroid therapy, but may persist. Clearly documented progression to hepatocellular carcinoma has not been demonstrated, although long-term follow-up without development of tumor after 10–15 years of use, has been reported. Overall prognosis is generally excellent and more dependent on the underlying condition than the benign tumors associated with it.

Micro-Regenerative Nodules

Micro-regenerative nodules related to prior submassive hepatic necrosis or cirrhosis are occasionally noted. They contain normal portal areas, as well as hyperplastic hepatocytes and lack neoplastic characteristics or potential.

Partial Nodular Transformation

This extremely rare condition may be related to nodular regenerative hyperplasia. Nodules of hyperplastic hepatocytes up to 4 cm in size are found in the perihilar area in association with portal hypertension. A marked reduction in the number and size of portal vein branches is found, and is most likely the cause of the portal hypertension rather than compression by the nodules. Cavernous transformation of the portal vein may also be found.

OTHER LIVER MASSES & TUMOR-LIKE CONDITIONS

1. HEPATIC CYSTS

(See Chapter 53.) As many as 0.17% of livers at autopsy will have incidental small cysts, with a similar prevalence also noted on ultrasound scans. Classic hepatic cysts have a thin, poorly cellular, fibrous wall, lined by a single cuboidal epithelium, and contain clear fluid. Ultrasound examination demonstrates no internal echos and through transmission of the sound waves (Figure 46–5A).

With these findings, there is essentially no differential diagnosis. Abscesses, hepatocellular carcinoma, metastases, hematomas, and echinococcal cysts should not be confused with a simple cyst, because the latter will ordinarily have a variety of irregular internal echos and distinct, well-defined borders. Cysts also show a sharply demarcated, smooth wall and water density interior on CT; however, in cysts that are smaller than 2 cm, volume averaging may make them difficult to identify on CT. MRI is rarely necessary to distinguish simple cysts, and generally no treatment is required. On occasion, hemorrhage into the cyst or superinfection of the cyst will require percutaneous drainage, surgical excision or enucleation.

2. BILIARY CYSTADENOMA

This benign epithelial cystic tumor is multilocular and has a dense fibrous capsule that clearly separates it from the surrounding liver parenchyma. It is relatively rare and found most frequently in young women. Presenting symptoms and signs include abdominal pain, a large palpable mass, or both. Differentiation is primarily from a simple cyst and is usually not difficult because of the unilocular nature of simple cysts and the very thin, diaphanous wall of simple cysts, both of which are readily appreciated on imaging studies. The distinction is important, because up to 25% of biliary cystadenomas are, or may become, malignant. Thus, in contrast to simple hepatic cysts, biliary cystadenomas should be resected.

3. CAVERNOUS HEMANGIOMA

Among hepatic masses, hemangiomas probably present the greatest diagnostic challenge and present the most difficulty for the clinician and radiologist. Occurring in up to 7% of the population, they are generally benign, and require no therapy but may prove quite difficult to distinguish from malignant growths.

Essentials of Diagnosis
- 85% asymptomatic.
- Dynamic bolus CT scan is diagnostic study of choice.
- Confirmation usually possible with MRI or tagged red blood cell (SPECT) study.
- Follow-up imaging study at 3–6 months.
- Avoid estrogenic hormones and pregnancy.
- Large (greater than 10 cm) cavernous hemangiomas should be resected if possible.

General Considerations
These benign blood-filled mesenchymal tumors have a normal endothelial cell lining, with a thin fi-

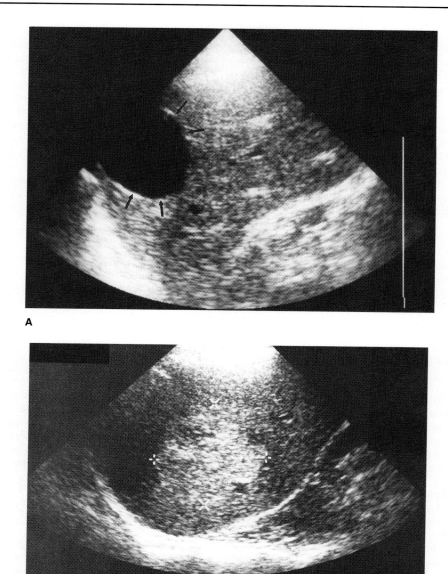

Figure 46–5. Imaging of an Hepatic Cyst and an Hemangioma. *A:* A benign hepatic cyst is clearly seen on this ultrasound image. The cyst is completely anechoic with a sharply defined, thin wall. Compare with the mixed hyper and hypochoic areas in 2A (hepatocellular carcinoma) and the hyperchoic mass in 5B (cavernous hemangioma). ***B:*** A 5 cm × 5 cm hyperechoic mass is readily seen on this ultrasound image. The edges of the mass are marked with crosses. Color Doppler ultrasound (not shown) revealed virtually no flow, strongly suggesting a diagnosis of cavernous hemangioma.

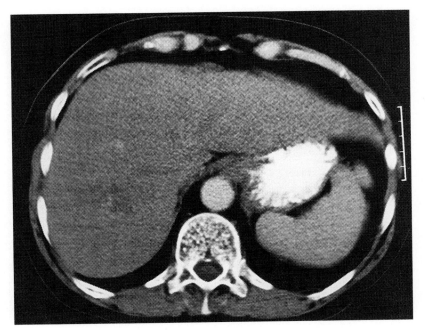

C

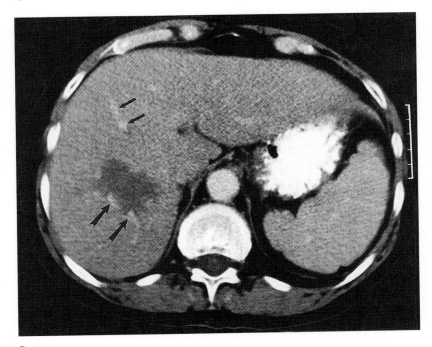

D

Figure 46–5. *C–D:* Diagnosis was confirmed by a dynamic bolus CT. Just before injection of the contrast bolus *(C),* the hemangioma is virtually indiscernible from the normal liver. Within 20 seconds of injecting the bolus *(D),* the hypodense hemangioma is readily apparent with some puddling of contrast at the periphery of the lesion *(large arrows)*; blood vessels are easily identified *(small arrows)*.

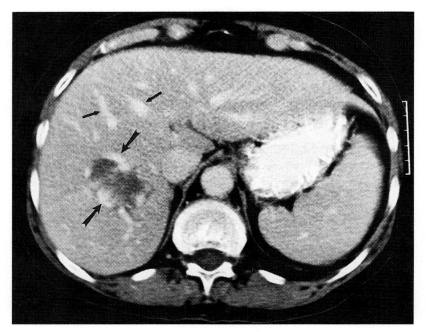

E

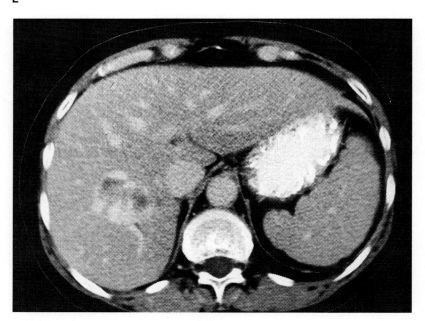

F

Figure 46–5. *E–F:* The puddling of contrast at the periphery is more apparent by 1 minute and blood vessels are more apparent **(E)**; at 5 minutes **(F),** the lesion has begun filling in from the periphery but a hypodense core is still apparent.

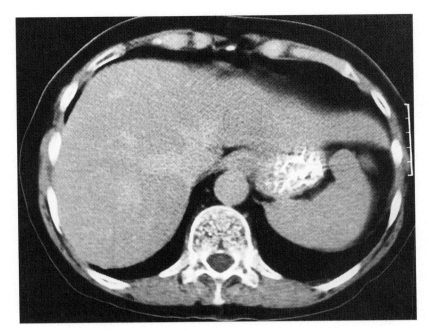

G

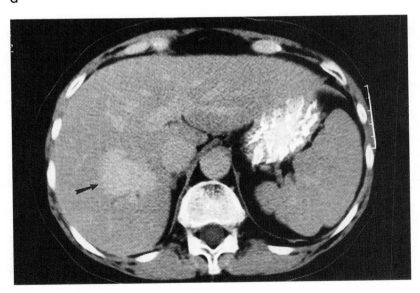

H

Figure 46–5. **G–H:** By 18 minutes **(G),** the entire lesion is isodense with the liver parenchyma and cannot be discerned; 1 minute later **(H),** the lesion is hyperdense compared to the rest of the liver as the contrast agent drains more slowly from the hemangioma **(large arrow).**

brous stroma producing multiple cavernous spaces. Usually solitary, they range in size from 2 mm to greater than 20 cm. More than 85% are asymptomatic, and are picked up incidentally by ultrasonography or CT performed for other reasons.

Clinical Findings

A. Symptoms and Signs: Fewer than 15% of patients have any complaints. The most common symptom is pain, often sharp, and usually related to hemorrhage into the hemangioma. An abdominal crisis may occur if there is rupture of the hemangioma. The patient's worst symptoms on presentation are usually concern and frustration, as the possibility of a malignant growth has frequently been raised due to the findings on ultrasound and CT, but no certain diagnosis has yet been made (Figure 46–5B). Laboratory findings are of no help, other than ruling out other possible diagnoses. Thus, negative α-fetoprotein and CEA tests are useful indirect evidence that the patient does not have an hepatocellular carcinoma.

B. Imaging Studies: The most readily available and generally reliable test is the dynamic bolus CT scan. In this study, the lesion is first identified on CT scan, and sequential cuts are taken of the same area over at least a 20-minute interval following bolus contrast injection. With a cavernous hemangioma, the lesion, which is usually hypodense to start, is seen to fill-in from the periphery, gradually become isodense with the surrounding liver, and then hyperdense as the contrast puddles within the hemangioma on delayed scans (Figures 46–5 C–H). Approximately one-third of cases will not meet all of these criteria. In those cases, a fast-spin echo MRI is quite sensitive and specific, demonstrating a low-signal intensity on T1-weighted images, and a very high signal intensity on T2-weighted images. Specificity of MRI ranges from 92–100%. [99m]Technetium-tagged red blood cell studies utilizing single photon emission computerized tomography (SPECT), are equally sensitive and specific. If the radionuclide study is available, it is often less expensive than MRI.

Differential Diagnosis

In most cases, diagnosis can be confidently made by the finding of a hyperechoic, well-defined lesion on ultrasound (Figure 46–5A) and confirmed by a dynamic bolus CT scan, MRI, or tagged red cell SPECT study. On occasion, however, the diagnosis is still unclear because of problems in distinguishing the lesion from an abscess, focal fatty infiltration, or malignant growth. This problem is particularly difficult if the patient has an existing or prior malignant tumor. In such cases, fine needle aspiration biopsy is generally safe, as long as there is sufficient hepatic parenchyma between the lesion and the liver surface to tamponade any potential hemorrhage. Even with a negative needle aspiration cytology, however, a malignant growth can be missed; hence, suspect masses should be followed up at 3–6 month intervals to be certain that the lesion is not enlarging.

Complications

Most hemangiomas are benign and asymptomatic and require no treatment. Large (> 10 cm) cavernous hemangiomas should be resected if possible because of the high risk of rupture with hemorrhagic crisis. Symptomatic hemangiomas, usually due to hemorrhage into the hemangioma, should also be resected, because they will usually hemorrhage again.

Prognosis

Prognosis is excellent. Estrogenic compounds should be avoided and pregnancy should be discouraged if the hemangioma cannot be resected.

METASTATIC TUMORS

The most common neoplasms in the liver are metastatic. Approximately 40% of patients with primary or extrahepatic tumors have evidence of hepatic metastases at the time of death (Table 46–6).

Pathophysiology

The liver's unique dual blood supply provides blood-borne access to the liver from all organs of the body, especially the visceral organs of the abdomen (via the portal vein). The lymphatic system and direct extension from other organs also serve as sources of metastatic liver disease.

Essentials of Diagnosis

- Jaundice rare and laboratory studies frequently normal, despite extensive liver involvement.
- Symptoms include malaise, fatigue, weight loss, hepatic pain, and right upper quadrant distension or mass.
- Rock-hard hepatomegaly in approximately 1/3 of patients
- Hepatic friction rub or bruit suggest tumor.

Table 46–6. Frequency of tumor metastasis to liver[1].

Primary Tumor	Percent with Liver Metastasis
Gallbladder	77.6
Pancreas	70.4
Unknown primary	57.0
Colon	56.0
Breast	53.2
Melanoma	50.0
Ovary	48.0
Stomach	44.0
Bronchogenic	41.8

[1]Data derived from Craig JR, Peters RL, Edmondson HA: Tumors of the Liver and the Intrahepatic Bile Ducts. Washington DC: Armed Forces Institutes of Pathology, 1989:257.

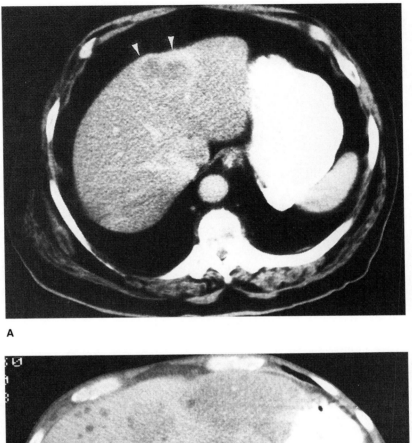

A

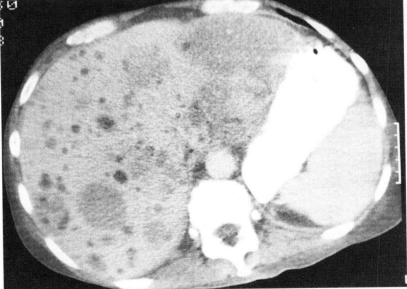

B

Figure 46–6. Metastatic and Hematologic Malignancies in Liver. *A:* Rim enhancement of hypodense liver metastasis from lung cancer is present on this CT following contrast injection *(arrow heads).* *B:* 54-year-old white male with hepatomegaly. Numerous hypodense areas of varying size could represent tumor, candidiasis, or microabscesses. In this case, liver tissue was replaced by infiltrating chronic lymphatic leukemia.

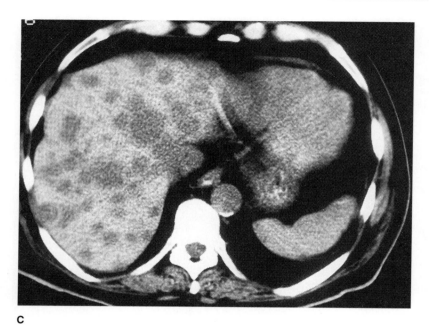

C

Figure 46–6. **C:** 67-year-old male renal transplant patient with similar CT performed without contrast. His lesions were due to lymphoma.

- Alkaline phosphatase, gamma GT, and 5'nucleotidase most likely liver test abnormalities.
- AST and ALT rarely elevated.
- Disproportionately increased LDH a possible indicator of malignant growth, particularly hematogenous.

General Considerations

Metastatic liver disease is frequently the first sign of liver tumor elsewhere and in many cases the primary tumor cannot be identified. Unexplained malaise, fatigue, and weight loss should always prompt a consideration of occult malignant growth and any biochemical liver abnormalities should prompt the use of imaging studies.

Clinical Findings

A. Symptoms and Signs: Most patients have no signs of underlying liver disease and jaundice is rare until late in the disease, unless the biliary tree is obstructed. Symptoms are nonspecific, although severe malaise and weight loss should suggest underlying tumor. The presence of a hepatic friction rub or bruit should strongly suggest underlying tumor.

B. Laboratory Findings: Laboratory studies are often remarkably normal despite massive infiltration of the liver by tumor. Alkaline phosphatase, gamma GT, and 5' nucleotidase are most often elevated, but the transaminases (ALT, AST) rarely so. A disproportionate rise in the LDH should strongly suggest the possibility of underlying malignant growths

when other causes for LDH elevation (hemolysis, muscle necrosis) have been eliminated. This is a particularly common finding in patients with infiltration of the liver by tumors of hematogenous origin (lymphomas and leukemias).

C. Imaging Studies: Any of the imaging techniques currently available will usually demonstrate metastatic lesions. Ultrasound (see Figures 46–2A and 46–5A) and CT (Figures 46–6 A–C) are generally the most useful, because they will distinguish cystic from solid lesions. CT may also show areas of low attenuation within the tumor, suggesting hemorrhage and necrosis (Figures 46–2B and 46–6A). Unenhanced CT, without contrast, is particularly helpful, especially with vascular neoplasms such as carcinoid and islet cell tumors which may be isodense with the normal liver and missed entirely if scans are not taken immediately after peak enhancement has occurred.

Differential Diagnosis

Metastatic liver tumors must be distinguished from primary liver tumors and benign conditions. A tissue diagnosis is virtually always required and this is best obtained under ultrasound or CT guidance. A single pass blind liver biopsy in a patient with multiple metastatic lesions will be positive in 40–50% of patients. A second pass at a slightly different angle along with cytology and a touch preparation of the specimen will improve the yield to 60–70%. Use of CT or ultrasound-guided biopsy, however, will increase the yield to 90–95%. Fine needle aspiration cytology is frequently sufficient to diagnose the general class of metastatic tumor and point the direction for further evaluation to identify the primary tumor. A general diagnosis of adenocarcinoma, squamous cell carcinoma, or undifferentiated carcinoma, however, with no clear indication of the primary tumor's location, may be the best the pathologist can provide.

Treatment & Prognosis

The finding of multiple metastatic lesions is generally a very poor prognostic sign, although it varies, depending on the type of tumor found. Making a tissue diagnosis is always worthwhile, because certain tumors are remarkably responsive to therapy; thus, significant palliation—and occasionally cure—can be obtained. Surgical resection of isolated metastases, if fewer than three in number, can provide sig-

nificant long-term palliation in certain tumors, particularly adenocarcinoma of the colon, if all other disease has been resected. Often a single metastasis is the first evidence of tumor recurrence and surgical removal will provide another prolonged period of disease-free survival. Resection has also shown some success with carcinoid tumors and long remissions have been noted with breast cancer, malignant melanoma, and occasionally, sarcoma. Such an approach, however, is applicable to only 5–10% of patients. In most cases, until more successful chemotherapeutic regimens become available, the prognosis will remain poor. Liver transplantation is not an option except in certain limited research protocols which are investigating the use of aggressive chemoembolization followed by transplantation to treat selected cases of carcinoid tumor and sarcomas.

REFERENCES

Bennett WF, Bova JG: Review of hepatic imaging and a problem oriented approach to liver masses. Hepatology 1990;12:761.

Bismuth H, Chiche L: Surgery of hepatic tumors. In: *Progress in Liver Diseases,* vol. 11. Boyer JL, Ockner RK (editors). Saunders, 1993.

Bottles K, Cohen MB: An approach to fine needle aspiration biopsy diagnosis of hepatic masses. Diagn Cytopathol 1991;7:204.

Bruix J et al: Phase II study of transarterial embolization in European patients with hepatocellular carcinoma: Need for controlled trials. Hepatology 1994;20:643.

Chen M-F et al: Postoperative recurrence of hepatocellular carcinoma: Two hundred five consecutive patients who underwent hepatic resection in 15 years. Arch Surg 1994;129:738.

Cherqui D et al: Multimodal adjuvant treatment and liver transplantation for advanced hepatocellular carcinoma: A pilot study. Cancer 1994;73:2721.

Craig JR, Peters RL, Edmondson HA: Tumors of the liver and intrahepatic bile ducts. In: *Atlas of Tumor Pathology,* 2nd series. Armed Forces Institute of Pathology, 1989.

Farmer DG et al: Current treatment modalities for hepatocellular carcinoma. Ann Surg 1994;219:236.

Gordon JW: Transgenic mouse models of hepatocellular carcinoma. (Editorial.) Hepatology 1994;19:538.

Jenkins RL, Johnson LB, Lewis WD: Surgical approach to benign liver tumors. Semin Liver Dis 1994;14:178.

Kato Y et al: Risk of hepatocellular carcinoma in patients with cirrhosis in Japan: Analysis of infectious hepatitis viruses. Cancer 1994;74:2234.

LaBrecque DR: Neoplasia of the liver. In: *Liver and Biliary Diseases.* Kaplowitz N (editor). Williams & Wilkins, 1996 (in press).

McMahon BJ et al: Hepatocellular carcinoma in Alaskan Eskimos: Epidemiology, clinical features, and early detection. In: *Progress in Liver Diseases,* vol. 9. Popper H, Schaffner F (editors). Harcourt Brace Jovanovich, 1990.

Miller WJ et al: Malignancies in patients with cirrhosis: CT sensitivity and specificity in 200 consecutive transplant patients. Radiology 1994;193:645.

Novell JR, Hilson AJW: Iodine-131-lipiodol for hepatocellular carcinoma: The benefits of targeting. (Editorial.) J Nucl Med 1994;35:1318.

Oka H et al: Prospective study of α-fetoprotein in cirrhotic patients monitored for development of hepatocellular carcinoma. Hepatology 1994;19:61.

Ravikumar TS et al: Intraoperative ultrasonography of liver: Detection of occult liver tumors and treatment by cryosurgery. Cancer Detect Prev 1994;18:131.

Ringe B et al: Surgical treatment of hepatocellular carcinoma: Experience with liver resection and transplantation in 198 patients. World J Surg 1991;15:270.

Rizzi PM et al: Accuracy of radiology in detection of hepatocellular carcinoma before liver transplantation. Gastroenterology 1994;107:1425.

Sato M et al: Well-differentiated hepatocellular carcinoma: Clinicopathological features and results of hepatic resection. Am J Gastroenterol 1995;90:112.

Schwartz ME: Primary hepatocellular carcinoma: Transplant versus resection. Semin Liver Dis 1994;14:135.

Sheiner PA, Brower ST: Treatment of metastatic cancer to the liver. Semin Liver Dis 1994;14:169.

Shouval D, Adler R: Tumor site-directed therapy for hepatocellular carcinoma using monoclonal antibodies against hepatoma-associated antigens. In: *Progress in Liver Diseases,* vol. 11. Boyer JL, Ockner RK (editors). Saunders, 1993.

Summary of a workshop on screening for hepatocellular carcinoma. MMWR 1990;39:619.

Tabor E, DiBisceglie AM, Purcell RH (editors): *Etiology, pathology, and treatment of hepatocellular carcinoma in North America.* Gulf Publishing, 1991.

Tang ZY et al: Surgery of small hepatocellular carcinoma: Analysis of 144 cases. Cancer 1989;64:536.

Tsai JF et al: Hepatitis B and C virus infection as risk factors for liver cirrhosis and cirrhotic hepatocellular carcinoma: A case-control study. Liver 1994;14:98.

Venook AP: Treatment of hepatocellular carcinoma: Too many options? J Clin Oncol 1994;12:1323.

Wahlstrom HE: Liver transplantation for hepatocellular carcinoma: Is it worth it? (Editorial). Mayo Clin Proc 1994;69:599.

Wong PYN et al: Clinical course and survival after liver transplantation for hepatitis B virus infection complicated by hepatocellular carcinoma. Am J Gastroenterol 1995;90:29.

Liver Disease in Pregnancy

47

Rebecca W. Van Dyke, MD

Interactions between the pregnant state and liver disease will be reviewed in this chapter. The discussion will be divided into three areas: (1) the effects of pregnancy on the liver and liver function, (2) the effects of common liver diseases when they occur during pregnancy, and (3) a review of liver diseases unique to the pregnant state.

EFFECTS OF PREGNANCY ON THE LIVER

CHANGES IN LIVER BIOCHEMICAL TESTS

Most liver functions are not affected by a normal pregnancy. In spite of a large increase in blood volume in late pregnancy, hepatic blood flow does not change; however, levels of serum albumin fall by 10–60% because of dilution, and this decrease is not a sign of liver disfunction. Plasma concentrations of acute phase reactant proteins are increased in pregnant women and women receiving oral contraceptives. Because of an increase in triglyceride flux and fatty acid metabolism during pregnancy, hepatic production of lipoproteins is increased, as are levels of plasma triglycerides, cholesterol, and phospholipids. Biochemical tests of liver injury, including aspartate aminotransferase (AST) and alanine aminotransferase (ALT), remain normal throughout pregnancy; however, serum alkaline phosphatase and leucine aminopeptidase activities rise progressively, owing to placental synthesis and release of these enzymes. At term, over one-half of women have alkaline phosphatase levels that exceed the upper limit of normal. These values, however, are rarely greater than twofold normal. Although these modest increases in serum enzyme activities do not indicate biliary tract disease, serum alkaline phosphatase levels that are increased to more than three to five times the upper limit of normal, or a consistent increase in serum aminotransferase measurements, is a reliable indicator of hepatobiliary disease during pregnancy and should prompt further investigation.

CHOLESTASIS

Normal pregnancy is associated with a progressive, albeit mild, decline in hepatic transport of bile salts and other organic anions (eg, bilirubin) and in the formation of hepatic bile. This mild cholestasis is probably a result of elevated estrogen levels. Serum levels of bile salts rise gradually throughout pregnancy, although in most women, values do not exceed the upper limit of normal, even at term. A subset of women, probably those susceptible to development of intrahepatic cholestasis of pregnancy (see discussion later in this chapter), exhibit serum bile acid levels late in pregnancy that are twofold or threefold the upper limit of normal. In most women, this degree of cholestasis is of no clinical significance; however, changes in bile formation during pregnancy predispose women to the formation of gallstones.

GALLSTONE FORMATION

Pregnancy appears to predispose patients both to the formation of gallstones and to the manifestation of clinical symptoms. The risk of developing cholesterol gallstones is related epidemiologically to the female gender, the use of exogenous female steroid hormones, and the number and frequency of pregnancies; these factors probably reflect the effects of estrogens on cholesterol metabolism. Exposure to estrogens increases hepatic secretion of cholesterol, decreases hepatic secretion of bile acids, and increases cholesterol saturation in gallbladder bile. Exposure to high levels of progesterones, particularly late in pregnancy, is associated with impairment of gallbladder emptying. This change in gallbladder motility, combined with increased biliary cholesterol saturation, contributes to the formation of biliary sludge and to cholesterol stones. In recent studies, ultrasound examinations have documented the development of biliary sludge in approximately one-third of women during normal pregnancy, and by the time of delivery, 10–12% of women have gallstones. Most of the biliary sludge disappears during the postpartum period, but only one-third of small stones resolve. Studies of both men and women exposed to high levels of estrogens suggest that estrogen use also accelerates development of symptoms in patients with preexisting gallstones. During pregnancy, biliary colic occurs in up to one-third of women with existing stones and usually responds to conservative medical management.

Because pregnancy is a predisposing factor in gallstone formation, acute cholecystitis is a common cause of nonobstetric surgery during pregnancy, occurring in one to eight cases per 10,000 pregnancies. The diagnosis of biliary colic or acute cholecystitis is relatively straightforward, based on the clinical history, physical examination, and ultrasound examination. Treatment for biliary colic is usually conservative; because most patients will experience spontaneous resolution of symptoms, cholecystectomy may be deferred until after delivery. Patients with frequent recurrences of biliary colic during pregnancy or those who develop acute cholecystitis may undergo cholecystectomy if symptoms are truly intractable or clinical deterioration occurs following conservative management. Laparoscopic cholecystectomy has been employed successfully during the first and second trimesters.

HEPATIC ADENOMA

Hepatic adenomas are uncommon estrogen-sensitive neoplasms. Enlargement with development of symptoms (abdominal pain, nausea, and vomiting) and rupture has been reported, albeit rarely, during pregnancy, presumably related to increased estrogen levels. Screening for adenomas in all pregnant women is not indicated; however, for patients previously known to have small adenomas, the size of the tumors can be monitored during pregnancy by ultrasonography. If adenomas grow rapidly and become large, thereby increasing the risk of rupture, termination of pregnancy or early delivery should be considered. Elective surgical resection of large adenomas to prevent their growth and rupture during a future pregnancy should be considered in women with known adenomas who wish to bear children.

HYPEREMESIS GRAVIDARUM

Hyperemesis gravidarum is not a liver disease per se, but the liver may be involved in women with severe hyperemesis who require hospitalization for de-

hydration. In 10–30% of these women, liver dysfunction and jaundice have been noted. Clinical signs include jaundice, dark urine, occasional pruritus, mild hyperbilirubinemia, and moderate increases in serum transaminases (up to two to three times normal levels). On rare occasions, values of aminotransferase activity up to 10–20 times the upper limit of normal have been noted. Alkaline phosphatase activities are elevated above the level expected for pregnancy in only a few patients. These modest changes in liver biochemical tests are usually of little clinical significance and resolve rapidly as vomiting is controlled and dehydration and malnutrition are reversed.

LIVER DISEASES OCCURRING DURING PREGNANCY

ACUTE VIRAL HEPATITIS

Any of the acute viral hepatitides may occur during pregnancy; moreover, viral hepatitis is the most common cause of jaundice during pregnancy in the United States. For most of the hepatitis viruses (A, B, C, and D), the disease has no demonstrable detrimental effect on the mother or the pregnancy in well-nourished women. In Asia and India, where the waterborne hepatitis E virus (HEV) is endemic and women are often poorly nourished, the infection is associated with a high frequency of fulminant hepatic failure and maternal and fetal death. During epidemics of HEV infection, pregnant women exhibit much more clinically significant disease, and rates of fulminant hepatic failure and death approach 15–20%. Rates of spontaneous abortion and fetal demise are also high. This may reflect a unique and as yet unknown interaction between HEV and pregnancy.

Viral hepatitis in well-nourished women in the USA has little effect on the fetus, although some epidemiologic studies suggest a minor increase in fetal and perinatal mortality rates. The most important risk factor is vertical transmission of the virus to the fetus or newborn infant, particularly when infection occurs during the third trimester. Vertical transmission of hepatitis B virus (HBV) has been studied extensively and is common when a chronically infected mother with high levels of viral replication (as indicated by detectable HBV DNA and hepatitis B e antigen [HBeAg] in the serum) gives birth. At the time of delivery, the rate of transmission of HBV from such a mother to her offspring is more than 50%. Most of the infected children fail to clear the virus and become lifelong HBV carriers. Vertical transmission from a mother with acute hepatitis B or with chronic hepatitis B but lesser degrees of viral replication is less frequent but still possible. Vertical transmission of HBV may be prevented if the newborn infant of a woman with hepatitis B surface antigen (HBsAg) in her blood is treated immediately after delivery with one intramuscular dose of hepatitis B immune serum globulin and the first of three injections of hepatitis B vaccine (Table 47–1). Thus, current recommendations are to screen all pregnant women during the third trimester for HBsAg and prepare to treat their offspring at birth, if necessary.

Vertical transmission of hepatitis C virus (HCV) is uncommon. It has been observed more frequently when mothers are also infected with the human immunodeficiency virus (HIV). No immunoprophylaxis is currently available. Vertical transmission of HAV, hepatitis D virus (HDV), HEV, and other non-A, non-B viruses occurs rarely, if at all.

HERPES SIMPLEX HEPATITIS

Herpes simplex hepatitis is rare in healthy adults, but over one-half the reported cases have been pregnant women. The mortality rate in this group is at least 50%. Typical clinical features include a 4- to 14-day history of fever, systemic symptoms typical of viral infection, and abdominal pain. Laboratory findings include high aminotransferase levels (> 1000 IU/L), liver synthetic failure as documented by an increased prothrombin time, and a modest degree of hyperbilirubinemia (serum levels typically < 3 mg/dL). Liver biopsy may be diagnostic, revealing typical intranuclear inclusions. Liver, vaginal, cervical, or throat cultures for HSV are often positive.

Immediate therapy with acyclovir can successfully treat both mother and infant. Thus, pregnant women who have symptoms and signs of severe viral hepatitis should be evaluated aggressively for HSV, with immediate institution of acyclovir, based on the clinical presentation, biopsy, or positive culture results. Vertical transmission of HSV to the fetus in utero or the infant after delivery can occur, and infants should be monitored closely and treated appropriately.

CHRONIC HEPATITIS & CIRRHOSIS

The effect of chronic hepatitis or cirrhosis on the mother and fetus is related primarily to the degree of liver dysfunction and portal hypertension. Women with mild chronic hepatitis and normal liver synthetic function have normal fertility rates and tolerate pregnancy well. Women with severe active chronic hepatitis or cirrhosis have reduced fertility rates and rarely become pregnant. If pregnancy does occur, liver biochemical tests, including serum bilirubin, alkaline phosphatase, and serum transaminase measurements, may worsen, although in a number of women these tests return to baseline values after delivery. For women with known cirrhosis, mortality rates as high as 10% have been reported, primarily because of liver failure or variceal hemorrhage, or both. It is unknown whether these rates are higher than would be expected if the women were not pregnant. Bleeding from esophageal varices is common during pregnancy in women with cirrhosis or extrahepatic portal vein thrombosis. Bleeding occurs in 18–30% of these women and in up to 50% of women known to have portal hypertension. This probably reflects, in part, the expansion of intravascular volume that takes place during the second and third trimesters. Bleeding from esophageal varices is not precipitated by vaginal delivery.

With the advent of sclerotherapy, bleeding episodes can be managed, and prophylactic elective portosystemic shunts or prophylactic sclerotherapy do not seem to be justified. Mothers and babies have survived pregnancies complicated by one or more episodes of variceal bleeding, managed either by sclerotherapy or therapeutic portosystemic shunting, although the numbers of such cases are small. The mortality rate from episodes of variceal hemorrhage is lower in women with extrahepatic portal vein thrombosis, because liver function is usually normal.

Fetal outcome is compromised in the face of severe maternal chronic hepatitis or cirrhosis. Pregnancies in such women are associated with a high rate of spontaneous abortion, stillbirth, and perinatal death. Surviving fetuses are phenotypically and developmentally normal, however.

Table 47–1. Prevention of vertical transmission of hepatitis B.

Test all women in the third trimester of pregnancy for HBsAg	
Administer prophylaxis within hours of delivery to all infants of HBsAg-positive women	
Hepatitis B immune globulin	0.5 mL intramuscularly[1]
Hepatitis B vaccine	0.5 mL intramuscularly,[1] with follow-up doses at 1 and 6 months
Test and vaccinate other family members of HBsAg-positive women	

[1]Dosage recommendations should be checked using current manufacturer's specifications.

LIVER DISEASES UNIQUE TO PREGNANCY

INTRAHEPATIC CHOLESTASIS OF PREGNANCY

Intrahepatic cholestasis of pregnancy (**pruritus gravidarum; cholestasis of pregnancy**) is an uncommon and usually benign cholestatic disorder that appears late in pregnancy. The syndrome disappears rapidly after delivery but often recurs either during subsequent pregnancies or with the use of oral contraceptives.

Pathophysiology

Intrahepatic cholestasis of pregnancy is thought to reflect a genetic predisposition to the cholestatic effects of estrogens. It frequently affects female relatives of index cases. The syndrome has been identified in up to three generations in some families. Female relatives also have a much higher incidence of cholestasis after taking oral contraceptives. Both male and female family members of women with intrahepatic cholestasis of pregnancy have an increased sensitivity to the cholestatic effects of estrogens, as assessed by sulfobromophthalein excretion tests. In Scandinavia and Chile, the disorder is seen in up to 5% of pregnancies, but it is much less common in the USA.

Clinical Findings

A. Symptoms and Signs: Intrahepatic cholestasis of pregnancy can present at any age and any degree of parity (Table 47–2). Seventy percent of cases present during the third trimester. The major clinical feature is intense pruritus, which often prevents sleep and leads to skin excoriations, minor skin infections, and depression. The onset of pruritus is usually at 28–30 weeks. In approximately 25% of patients with more severe cholestasis, jaundice is also seen. Nausea, vomiting, abdominal pain, and hepatomegaly are observed in a few patients.

B. Laboratory Findings: Laboratory features are those of cholestasis, with alkaline phosphatase levels more than twofold the upper limit of normal, a mild hyperbilirubinemia averaging 3 mg/dL, and modest elevations of transaminases (usually, 100–200 IU/L; rarely, as high as 1000 IU/L). Serum bile acid levels are markedly elevated but rarely measured. In women with severe, long-lasting cholestasis, vitamin K deficiency and steatorrhea may occur, with modest elevation of the prothrombin time.

Differential Diagnosis

The history, physical examination, and laboratory tests should reliably differentiate intrahepatic cholestasis of pregnancy from acute viral hepatitis, acute fatty liver of pregnancy, or preeclamptic liver disease. The histologic appearance of the liver on a biopsy specimen is usually diagnostic, showing intense intrahepatic cholestasis with little inflammation or hepatocellular necrosis; however, biopsy is rarely necessary, because the diagnosis can usually be made on the basis of the clinical findings.

Treatment & Prognosis

Intrahepatic cholestasis of pregnancy is a self-limited entity that rapidly resolves after delivery. In rare instances, cholestasis may persist for several weeks into the postpartum period; however, the pruritus usually disappears within 24–48 hours. Patients with severe pruritus may respond to oral cholestyramine or phenobarbital, which may be used during pregnancy. Hypnotics may be helpful, as nocturnal pruritus may be severe. Vitamin K administration near the time of delivery is indicated in patients with steatorrhea and an elevated prothrombin time. Several additional therapeutic agents have been suggested, including S-adenosyl-L-methionine (SAME) and ursodeoxycholic acid (UDCA). SAME has been tested in two controlled clinical trials, with opposite outcomes. UDCA has been tested only in small, uncontrolled studies, but it is known to be helpful in chronic cholestatic liver diseases. These small studies have reported improvement in both symptoms and laboratory values. Oral dexamethasone, which may suppress fetal-placental estrogen production for a prolonged period, has been given for 7 days to a small number of women, with reported long-term reduction in pruritus and in abnormal laboratory test results. For severely symptomatic women, a short trial of UDCA or dexamethasone may be considered, although neither agent has been tested extensively for safety during pregnancy.

The prognosis of intrahepatic cholestasis of pregnancy for mothers is excellent. The prognosis for the fetus may not be as benign; several studies from Scandinavia suggest a significant increase in fetal distress during late pregnancy and labor, premature labor, and neonatal death. Although other studies have not clearly documented an increased risk of fetal illness and death, experts have recommended close monitoring of women and fetuses during the third trimester. Monitoring is particularly important if (1) the onset of intrahepatic cholestasis of pregnancy occurs before 32 weeks, (2) the pregnancy is multiple, (3) clinical jaundice occurs, or (4) there was a previous stillbirth. In these circumstances, pro-

Table 47–2. Clinical findings in intrahepatic cholestasis of pregnancy.

Incidence	~ 0.5 to ~ 3% of pregnant women
Onset	Third trimester (median onset, 29 weeks)
Symptoms and signs	
Pruritus	100%
Jaundice	25%
Nausea and vomiting	5–50%
Abdominal pain	10–25%
Laboratory findings	
Alkaline phosphatase	2- to 5-fold increase
Bilirubin	1–4 mg/dL
Aminotransferases	3- to 4-fold increase
Serum bile salts	5- to 10-fold increase
Prothrombin time	Modest increase in 20% of patients

visions for early delivery should be made if signs of fetal distress develop.

ACUTE FATTY LIVER OF PREGNANCY

Acute fatty liver of pregnancy is a rare, sporadic disease that occurs in late pregnancy and is associated with acute liver failure and considerable risk of maternal and fetal illness and death.

Pathophysiology

Acute fatty liver of pregnancy is characterized by infiltration of hepatocytes with microvesicular droplets of fat, a histologic picture strikingly similar to that seen in Reye's syndrome, Jamaican vomiting sickness, valproic acid hepatotoxicity, and acyl-CoA dehydrogenase deficiency, a group of diseases known as the **hepatic microvesicular steatoses.** Although most cases of acute fatty liver of pregnancy are sporadic and nonrecurrent, genetic abnormalities in fatty acid oxidation (in either the mother or the fetus) may predispose at least some women to its development. In a normal pregnancy, hepatic metabolism of triglycerides and fatty acids increases greatly. Impairment of mitochondrial β-oxidation of fatty acids (resulting from the combined effects of estrogens, genetic abnormalities in acyl-CoA dehydrogenases, inflammatory cytokines, and/or drugs such as salicylates or tetracycline) may, in rare instances, cause significant impairment of β-oxidation. Impaired β-oxidation may in turn lead to elevated hepatic levels of potentially toxic free fatty acids and liver injury.

Clinical Findings

A. Symptoms and Signs: The onset of acute fatty liver of pregnancy is usually in the third trimester (at approximately 35 weeks), although onset as early as 26 weeks and as late as the immediate postpartum period has been reported (Table 47–3). The early clinical signs are nonspecific and include nausea, fatigue, malaise, vomiting, and right upper quadrant or epigastric pain. Fever, headache, diarrhea, and myalgias are seen in some patients. Clinical signs of liver disease may ensue within days. Physical findings may be minimal but include right upper quadrant tenderness. Jaundice, edema, ascites, and hepatic encephalopathy signal liver failure. Signs and symptoms of preeclampsia, such as hypertension and proteinuria, are seen in at least one-fifth of cases.

Although patients with mild degrees of liver damage are described, the characteristic clinical course of acute fatty liver of pregnancy is rapid progression to liver failure. This clinical course is similar to fulminant hepatic failure, which can occur in patients with acute viral hepatitis. These severely affected individuals exhibit all of the complications of fulminant he-

Table 47–3. Clinical findings in acute fatty liver of pregnancy.

Incidence	1 in 13,000 pregnancies
Onset	Third trimester (median onset, 35 weeks)
Symptoms and signs	
Nausea and vomiting	80%
Abdominal pain	60%
Hypertension, proteinuria, and edema	20–25%
Jaundice	90%
Encephalopathy	70%
Hypoglycemia	25%
Ascites (modest)	50%
Laboratory findings	
Alkaline phosphatase	2- to 5-fold increase
Bilirubin	2–30 mg/dL
Aminotransferases	5- to 20-fold increase
Prothrombin time	Marked increase in severe disease to > 20 seconds
Platelet count	Decrease late in severe disease with evidence of disseminated intravascular coagulation
Serum uric acid	Modest elevation in most patients

patic failure, including hypoglycemia, coagulopathy, hepatic encephalopathy, and cerebral edema.

B. Laboratory Findings: Laboratory abnormalities include evidence of liver damage but with only modest elevations of alkaline phosphatase and serum transaminase values. Transaminase levels are relatively low, averaging 200–300 IU/L, but values up to and exceeding 1000 IU/L have been reported. Serum bilirubin levels are characteristically elevated; however, the range of values reported is broad, from normal to 36 mg/dL. Evidence of liver failure is frequent, as exemplified by a rising prothrombin time. Hematologic studies suggest the presence of disseminated intravascular coagulation in severely affected patients. Nucleated red blood cells, red blood cell fragments, and thrombocytopenia may be present. The white blood cell count is usually elevated, in the range of 12,000–46,000/μL. Serum uric acid levels universally are mildly elevated, and renal function is usually impaired, with serum creatinine averaging 3 mg/dL.

Differential Diagnosis

Disorders most commonly confused with acute fatty liver of pregnancy include acute viral hepatitis and preeclamptic liver disease, such as the HELLP syndrome (see following discussion). Both of the latter disorders are characterized by intense hepatocellular necrosis and are most readily distinguished from acute fatty liver of pregnancy by high levels of serum aminotransferase activity. Acute fatty liver of pregnancy is typified by relatively modest increases in serum aminotransferase levels, even with the development of fulminant liver failure. Other distinguishing features include early evidence of thrombocytopenia and disseminated intravascular coagulation in preeclamptic liver disease, and serologic evidence of viral infection in acute viral hepatitis. Liver biopsy may be diagnostic, especially if fat staining is done on frozen sections of tissue to identify microvesicular steatosis; however, in severe cases, coagulopathy may be a contraindication for liver biopsy.

Treatment & Prognosis

Acute fatty liver of pregnancy resolves spontaneously and rapidly after delivery. Therefore, treatment is based on prompt delivery as well as supportive care for the complications of liver failure. Patients with mild disease—no evidence of impaired liver synthetic function (as monitored by the serum prothrombin time), and no evidence of fetal distress—can be monitored closely. In these patients, contingency plans for rapid delivery by induction of labor or cesarean section should be made in the event that maternal hepatic function deteriorates or fetal distress is observed. For patients who present with severe liver involvement and liver synthetic failure (as exemplified by an increased prothrombin time), rapid induction of labor or delivery via cesarean section should be undertaken promptly.

Although treatment by rapid delivery has never been studied in a controlled clinical trial, maternal and fetal outcomes in acute fatty liver of pregnancy have improved since this approach has been used. Patients should be followed by both the appropriate obstetric and neonatal services and a physician experienced in the care of patients with fulminant hepatic failure. Because acute fatty liver of pregnancy usually resolves spontaneously after delivery, evaluation for liver transplantation for severely affected women is usually not necessary. Overall, maternal and fetal mortality rates of approximately 50% have been reported. Maternal mortality rates of 15% and infant mortality rates of 40% have been reported in more recent series in which mild cases were identified and rapid delivery undertaken. The high rate of fetal mortality in this disorder probably reflects not only maternal decompensation and premature delivery but maternal disseminated intravascular coagulation with fibrin deposition in the placenta, leading to placental infarcts and fetal asphyxia.

PREECLAMPTIC LIVER INJURY

Preeclampsia, characterized by hypertension, proteinuria, and edema in the third trimester of pregnancy, is not primarily a liver disease, but the liver may be involved in severe cases. The two best characterized hepatic syndromes observed in women with preeclampsia or eclampsia include HELLP syndrome (named for the laboratory features of *h*emolysis, *e*le-vated *l*iver enzymes, and *l*ow *p*latelet count) and acute hepatic rupture.

Pathophysiology

Preeclampsia is thought to arise from abnormalities in placental perfusion, leading to maternal endothelial activation, sensitivity to endogenous pressor agents, hypertension, intense vasoconstriction, and progressive endothelial damage resulting in fibrin and platelet deposition and a picture resembling that of disseminated intravascular coagulation. Renal involvement occurs in virtually all affected women, but hepatic involvement can be seen in at least 10% of patients. Hepatic disease is marked by deposition of fibrin along hepatic sinusoids, ischemic necrosis (either focal or confluent), and periportal and portal tract hemorrhage, with little or no inflammation. In cases with severe confluent liver necrosis, large intrahepatic hematomas may form and rupture.

1. HELLP SYNDROME

HELLP syndrome was first defined by Louis Weinstein in 1982. As previously mentioned, the syndrome is an acronym for the characteristic laboratory features of *h*emolysis, *e*levated *l*iver enzymes, and *l*ow *p*latelet count. HELLP syndrome probably represents the middle of the spectrum of liver involvement in preeclampsia (ie, the point at which clinically significant liver necrosis and disseminated intravascular coagulation occurs, but not confluent necrosis).

Clinical Findings

A. Symptoms and Signs: Patients with HELLP syndrome exhibit the signs or symptoms of preeclampsia, including hypertension, proteinuria, and edema (Table 47–4). Patients are usually in their first pregnancy, and the onset commonly occurs at around 33 weeks. Nonspecific signs or symptoms such as nausea, vomiting, epigastric and right upper quadrant pain, headache, and hepatic tenderness are often, although not invariably, present.

B. Laboratory Findings: The diagnosis is suggested by the characteristic laboratory features, primarily thrombocytopenia. A platelet count of less than 100,000/μL is required to make the diagnosis. Fibrinogen levels are modestly decreased. Evidence of disseminated intravascular coagulation and intravascular hemolysis may be found in many patients, if sensitive tests are employed such as those for fibrin degradation products, *d*-dimer levels, and morphologic studies of red blood cells. Abnormal clotting times, measured by both the prothrombin time and partial thromboplastin time, are common. Liver involvement is typified by moderate elevations of serum transaminases, typically in the range of 200–500 IU/L, although values up to several thousand international units per liter are reported in se-

Table 47–4. Clinical findings in HELLP syndrome.

Incidence	~ 1% of all pregnancies, especially first pregnancies ~ 10% of women with pre-eclampsia
Onset	Third trimester (median onset, 33 weeks)
Symptoms and signs	
Hypertension, proteinuria and edema	100%
Headache	60%
Nausea and vomiting	35%
Abdominal pain	80%
Hepatic tenderness	~ 100%
Laboratory findings	
Thrombocytopenia	100%, early onset
Abnormal morphologic studies of RBCs	Frequent (fragments, schistocytes)
Prothrombin time	Modest increase
Fibrin degradation products	Increased early
Aminotransferases	5- to 20-fold increase
Alkaline phosphatase	Normal or modest increase (2-fold)
Bilirubin	Low, unless extensive hemolysis and hepatic necrosis occur
Serum creatinine	Mild increase

vere cases. Serum bilirubin levels are commonly, but modestly, elevated, in part reflecting the degree of intravascular hemolysis. Impaired renal function is virtually universal, as indicated by increases in serum blood urea nitrogen and creatinine levels. Complications include bleeding due to the underlying coagulopathy, progressive hepatic hemorrhage, and development of hepatic rupture (see following discussion), and, rarely, fulminant hepatic failure.

Differential Diagnosis

HELLP syndrome can be differentiated from acute viral hepatitis and acute fatty liver of pregnancy (Table 47–5) by the early appearance of thrombocytopenia and evidence of disseminated intravascular coagulation. The transaminase values are often as high as those seen in acute viral hepatitis and much higher than those typically seen in acute fatty liver of pregnancy. Liver biopsy can be diagnostic but is usually not indicated, because of the patient's underlying coagulopathy. Differentiation of HELLP syndrome from acute fatty liver of pregnancy may be difficult, because some cases appear to reflect an overlap syndrome, with features of both acute fatty liver of pregnancy and preeclamptic liver disease. In such cases, laboratory values may represent a combination of those typical for each disease, and liver biopsy may show both microvesicular fatty infiltration and evidence of fibrin deposition and hepatocyte necrosis. Because the treatment for both entities is virtually identical, differentiation of acute fatty liver of pregnancy from HELLP syndrome may not be essential.

Treatment & Prognosis

Preeclampsia resolves spontaneously and rapidly after delivery, and the clinical signs or symptoms of HELLP syndrome usually resolve within 24–48 hours. Thus, the principal treatment for this disorder is rapid identification of HELLP syndrome and ur-

Table 47–5. Differential diagnosis of acute liver disease in pregnancy.

	Viral Hepatitis	Biliary Tract Disease	Intrahepatic Cholestasis of Pregnancy	Acute Fatty Liver of Pregnancy	HELLP Syndrome
Time of onset	Variable	Variable	Third trimester	Third trimester	Third trimester
Nausea and vomiting	Yes	Variable	Rare	Yes	Occasionally
Abdominal pain	Variable	Variable	Rare	Yes	Yes
Associated with preeclampsia	No	No	No	Occasionally	Yes
Cholestasis	Mild to marked	Marked	Marked	Modest and late	Mild or absent
Transaminase elevation	High	Low	Low	Modest	Modest to high
Coagulopathy	Rare and late	No	No	Common but late	Early, thrombocytopenia; late, disseminated intravascular coagulation
Hepatic failure	Variable	No	No	Yes	Rare
Hepatic ultrasound or CT scan	Nonspecific	Dilated bile ducts	Normal	No change or low density	Areas of infaction and necrosis
Liver biopsy	Inflammatory infiltrate, spotty hepatocyte necrosis	Cholestasis, variable inflammation	Cholestasis	Microvesicular fatty infiltration	Patchy hemorrhagic necrosis, fibrin deposition

gent vaginal or abdominal delivery, if necessary. In patients with mild liver involvement and mild coagulopathy, the maturity of the fetus should be assessed and its well-being closely monitored. Delivery may be cautiously postponed if the lungs are not mature. In all other cases, it is preferable to move toward rapid delivery. The peak of thrombocytopenia may not occur until 1–2 days following delivery, but platelet counts should return to normal within 72 hours. In rare cases in which thrombocytopenia persists for more than 72 hours after delivery, exchange transfusions have been suggested as a potential therapy.

Because the clinical outcome for both mother and fetus is worse in women with preeclampsia who also develop HELLP syndrome, some investigators advocate screening all women with preeclampsia, especially those with abdominal pain, for this syndrome, using laboratory tests for liver injury and coagulation parameters. Those with HELLP syndrome should undergo close monitoring and rapid delivery, as previously outlined.

Maternal prognosis is related to the severity of liver involvement and coagulopathy. In those with no bleeding complications, the outcome is excellent. Fetal outcome is not as good; retardation of intrauterine growth is common and sudden death can occur because of rapid changes in placental blood flow. The chances of fetal survival are clearly better when prompt delivery is instituted. The maternal mortality rate is 2.5% or less, although the fetal mortality rate may be as high as 40–50%. The recurrence rate of preeclampsia or HELLP syndrome is only 3.4% of monitored pregnancies.

2. HEPATIC RUPTURE

Clinical Findings

Hepatic rupture in pregnancy was first described in 1844, and is due to confluent hepatic necrosis from preeclamptic liver disease. It is reported in 1–77 of every 100,000 deliveries, and in 1–2% of women with preeclampsia.

A. Symptoms and Signs: Hemorrhage may occur up to 48 hours after delivery in women with severe liver necrosis. Virtually all patients have clinical and histologic features of preeclampsia, and most would satisfy the criteria for HELLP syndrome. Contained intrahepatic hemorrhage is more common than free rupture into the peritoneal cavity. Both types of rupture are heralded by the sudden onset of abdominal pain, usually in the right upper quadrant. Clinical findings include hepatic tenderness, diffuse abdominal pain, peritoneal findings, chest and shoulder pain, and shock. These signs and symptoms are seen in a variety of intra-abdominal catastrophes, including rupture of hepatic adenoma, abruptio placentae, perforated viscus, and intestinal infarction.

B. Diagnostic Studies: Diagnosis is based on clinical suspicion, laboratory or clinical evidence of preeclampsia, and imaging of the liver. Abdominal CT is the most sensitive test for either contained or free hepatic rupture. MRI can identify intrahepatic hematomas but is more sensitive for chronic, rather than acute, hematomas.

Treatment & Prognosis

Patients with free hepatic rupture require immediate treatment to survive. Angiographic embolization of bleeding arterioles has been attempted in a limited number of cases with some success, but only in patients with rupture limited to one portion of the liver. Most patients with free rupture who survive have undergone emergency surgery, with drainage and packing of the ruptured areas. The outcome appears to be better in patients treated with drainage and packing than in those who undergo lobectomy. Women with contained hepatic hematomas, diagnosed by abdominal CT or another radiologic procedure, may do well without surgery if they receive adequate hemodynamic support and are followed closely. If there is suspicion of free rupture, the threshold for investigation with exploratory laparotomy should be low. Overall, the maternal and fetal mortality rates for acute hepatic rupture are high (> 50%). The mortality rate is lower in women with contained hematomas; in such individuals, the hematomas gradually resolve over several weeks. Recurrences of acute hepatic rupture have not been reported but are possible, as preeclampsia and liver involvement may recur in subsequent pregnancies.

REFERENCES

Everson GT: Pregnancy and gallstones. (Editorial.) Hepatology 1993;17(No 1):159.

Freund G, Arvan DA: Clinical biochemistry of preeclampsia and related liver diseases of pregnancy: A review. Clin Chim Acta 1990;191:123.

Gleicher N (editor): *Principles and Practice of Medical Therapy in Pregnancy.* Appleton & Lange, 1992.

Martin JN Jr et al: The natural history of HELLP syndrome: Patterns of disease progression and regression. Am J Obstet Gynecol 1991;164:1500.

Riely CA: Acute fatty liver of pregnancy. Semin Liver Dis 1987;7:47.

Riely CA, Abell TL (editors): Gastrointestinal and Liver Problems in Pregnancy. Vol 21 of: Gastroenterol Clin North Am. Saunders, 1992.

Van Dyke RW: The liver in pregnancy. In: *Hepatology,* 2/e. Zakim D, Boyer TD (editors). Saunders, 1995.

Varma RR: Course and prognosis of pregnancy in women with liver disease. Semin Liver Dis 1987;7:59.

Pediatric Liver Disease

48

Victoria R. Masakowski, MD, PhD, & Joel E. Lavine, MD, PhD

NORMAL LIVER ANATOMY & FUNCTION

Pediatrics is unique in the diversity of its patient population, with the passage from birth to adolescence marked by profound growth and development. Many liver diseases present primarily in the pediatric age group, when rapid diagnosis and treatment can prevent death or significant morbidity. Chronic liver disease in children presents an additional challenge to the practitioner: enabling the affected child to achieve optimal growth and to lead as normal a lifestyle as possible.

ANATOMY & DEVELOPMENT

The liver originates as a diverticulum of endodermal cells arising from the primitive foregut within the first weeks following conception. By the third week of gestation, the diverticulum divides into the solid cranial pars hepatica, destined to become the liver, and the hollow, caudal pars cystica, which will become the gallbladder and extrahepatic biliary ducts. The lumen of these ducts becomes occluded with endodermal cells, but is normally recanalized by the seventh week. By the sixth week, bile canaliculi form between the hepatoblasts, with duct formation occurring by the ninth week. After 3 months, the intra- and extrahepatic biliary structures have joined, with initiation of bile formation and bile excretion into the duodenum, giving meconium its characteristic color. Failure of either recanalization of the nascent extrahepatic biliary ducts at week 7, or joining of the intra- and extrahepatic biliary drainage systems at week 12, results in malformation or atresia of the biliary tree, with consequent derangement of normal bile metabolism. The exact cause of these anatomic malformations is unknown.

Pediatric hepatic anatomy is identical to the adult.

The liver is composed of right, left, quadrate, and caudate lobes. The left and right hepatic ducts join outside the porta hepatis to form the common hepatic duct. The gallbladder is united with this system via the cystic duct, which becomes the common bile duct after joining with the common hepatic duct. The common bile duct ends in the papilla of Vater, where it is also united with the pancreatic duct to form the ampulla of Vater, circumscribed by the sphincter of Oddi. The latter regulates secretion of bile into the duodenum.

At the cellular level, hepatocytes are specialized in their concentration of drug and toxin metabolizing enzymes located in the smooth endoplasmic reticulum. In the newborn period, these enzymes, including the glucuronyl transferases involved in bilirubin metabolism, have reduced activity. This leads to inefficient and sometimes insufficient metabolism of drugs and endogenous toxins such as bilirubin, especially when the newborn is stressed (eg, sepsis, hemolysis). This decreased enzymatic activity predisposes the neonate to a common sign of illness, hyperbilirubinemia.

FUNCTION

The fetal liver is relatively inactive, relying on the maternal liver to perform its chores via the placenta. As gestation nears completion, the fetus prepares for birth and cessation of this dependency by stockpiling glycogen and lipids, substances critical for survival in the immediate postnatal period. The primary functions of the postnatal liver include: (1) conversion of nutrients to storage forms that are readily accessible; (2) synthesis of proteins (including albumin and clotting factors); (3) synthesis of bile acids, key in intestinal fat absorption; and (4) toxin disposal, including excretable derivatives of bilirubin and ammonia. These functions develop rapidly after birth, with closure of the ductus venosus, maturation of microsomal enzymes, and use of the gastrointestinal tract (stimulation of bile secretion).

Storage of Nutrients

The liver plays a primary role in glucose homeostasis. After a meal, it replenishes depleted glycogen stores with surplus glucose; in the fasting state, the liver must break down the glycogen to supply energy to the body. With depletion of the glycogen stores in a prolonged fast (longer than 8–12 hours), the liver must synthesize glucose from amino acids supplied through muscle breakdown (gluconeogenesis). This capacity is utilized from birth, as the newborn infant compensates for the loss of maternal support by mobilizing greater than 90% of stockpiled glycogen in the first 2 hours of life.

Synthetic Function

The fetal liver possesses full synthetic function by 3 months gestation. Albumin is quantitatively the most important plasma protein synthesized by the liver. Others include coagulation factors (fibrinogen, II, V, VII, IX, and X). Of these, factors II, VII, IX, and X depend on vitamin K as a cofactor. Vitamin K is synthesized in the gut by colonic flora.

Newborns initially have sterile gastrointestinal tracts, and thus require exogenous vitamin K supplementation at birth to prevent hemorrhagic disease of the newborn. The prothrombin time, often used as a gauge of hepatic synthetic function in fulminant hepatic failure, depends on the presence of factors II, V, VII, and fibrinogen.

Bile Acids & Fat Absorption

The newborn absorbs dietary fat inefficiently because of immaturity in production and intestinal reabsorption of bile acids. Not only is the neonatal bile acid pool smaller than the adult; the composition differs as well. The fetal liver contains more chenodeoxycholic acid than cholic acid, while in the term infant and adult, these ratios are reversed. Fetal livers also contain bile acids not found in the adult liver. There are few endogenous secondary bile acids in the neonatal liver, because the intestine is sterile at birth and secondary bile acids are formed by the action of colonic bacteria on primary bile acids. A small amount can be transplacentally acquired from the maternal supply. Newborns are also prone to excessive fecal bile acid losses that result from poor reabsorption. In the adult, enterohepatic circulation of bile acids occurs via three mechanisms: (1) passive jejunal absorption, (2) active absorption in the distal ileum, and (3) passive colonic transport. In the neonate, all reabsorption is passive. There is also impaired hepatic uptake of bile acids from the circulation. This leads to increased serum bile acid levels in the neonate, a useful indicator of hepatic dysfunction. This immaturity of the newborn bile acid system not only results in inefficient fat absorption, but also in inefficient absorption of fat soluble vitamins (A, D, E, and K) and a tendency towards cholestasis.

Toxin Clearance

Postnatally, the liver must assume many of the detoxification functions previously handled by the placenta. Mono-oxygenase and conjugative microsomal enzymes are central to the conversion of hydrophobic metabolites to hydrophilic derivatives more readily excreted in bile and poorly reabsorbed from the intestine. While these microsomal enzymes are minimally active antenatally, their maturation is triggered at birth. The importance of the liver in detoxification, and the impact immaturity of these systems may have on the individual, is illustrated best by the following examination of bilirubin metabolism in the neonate.

Once the placental clearance of bilirubin is abolished, there is an immediate need for an alternative clearance mechanism. Bilirubin is predominantly a breakdown product of heme; neonates are burdened with an increased load (greater than twice that accommodated by adults) because of a reduced erythrocyte life span (80–90 days) and greater contributions from non-heme sources of bilirubin. Substrate load is further augmented by prematurity, hypoxia, acidosis, sepsis, hypoglycemia, inherited defects of conjugation, and hemolysis from conditions such as ABO-fetal-maternal blood group incompatibility or red cell enzymopathies.

Bilirubin must be conjugated for excretion, because it is insoluble in water at pH less than 7.8. The liver conjugates bilirubin by transfer of one or two glucuronic acid residues from uridine diphosphoglucuronic acid (UDPGA); this reaction is catalyzed by a specific microsomal glucuronyl transferase. In neonates, conjugation is hindered by lack of UDPGA (which may be conserved by forming monoglucuronides rather than diconjugates), and by an incompletely developed bilirubin uridine diphosphate (UDP) glucuronyl transferase activity. Conjugated bilirubin is excreted in the adult feces as a nonabsorbable urobilinogen derivative formed by intestinal microorganisms. In neonates, bacterial conversion is inhibited by lack of the appropriate colonic flora. Also, newborn stool and colonic mucosa contains active β-glucuronidase which hydrolyzes bilirubin glucuronide to absorbable free pigment. Thus in the neonate, enterohepatic shunting of bile may further contribute to substrate load for an already taxed system. Bilirubin travels in plasma attached to proteins with a high affinity for hydrophobic compounds, such as albumin. Drugs such as sulfonamides, salicylates, or organic anions such as fatty acids may reduce the affinity of albumin for bilirubin, leading to segregation in hydrophobic environments such as plasma membranes, meninges, adipose tissue, and the brain. **Kernicterus** is the term applied to bilirubin staining of the basal ganglia. This causes a toxic encephalopathy which can result in death or permanent sequelae ranging from cerebral palsy and mental retardation to mild cognitive impairment.

A final mechanism contributing to inefficient

bilirubin clearance involves neonatal vascular anatomy. At birth, the blood supply to the left lobe of the liver changes from the highly oxygenated umbilical venous blood to portal venous blood. Flow via the hepatic arteries is minimal. The ductus venosis remains patent for several days, creating a potential shunt away from the liver which would contribute to delayed plasma bilirubin clearance.

With all of these mechanisms contributing to delayed and inefficient bilirubin clearance by the neonatal liver, it is not surprising that jaundice is a frequent presenting sign in the neonatal period. Jaundice refers to the yellow staining of the skin, sclerae, and deeper tissues from excess serum bile pigments. It can be cholestatic, resulting from an excess of conjugated bile due to the impedance of normal flow in the biliary system; or non-cholestatic, reflecting an increase in the absolute amount of serum bile without an associated decrease in bile flow. The majority of cases of non-cholestatic jaundice result from an abundance of unconjugated bilirubin, effectively trapping the excess bilirubin within the circulation. Two presentations of neonatal hyperbilirubinemia reflect the temporary inefficiency of neonatal hepatic excretion of bilirubin as outlined above. **"Physiologic" jaundice,** common between the second and sixth days of life, is non-cholestatic and predominantly results from non-conjugated bilirubin, which accumulates before adequate maturation of the UDP glucuronyl transferase conjugation system is achieved. **Breast milk jaundice** is another type of unconjugated hyperbilirubinemia sometimes confused with physiologic jaundice. Breast milk jaundice is often characterized by more pronounced hyperbilirubinemia (15–20 mg/dL) which persists for longer, up to 2–3 weeks. The breast milk component causing the problem is undefined. Theories have included agents such as 3-alpha-20-beta-pregnanediol or free fatty acids. Often many of the siblings within a family are affected. Cessation of breastfeeding leads to immediate diminution of the bilirubin level.

Although most neonatal jaundice is benign, jaundice can be the first clue to significant underlying hepatic pathology. The key is to pursue a logical, stepwise evaluation guided by clinical presentation and persistence of symptoms. An algorithm for a sample approach to this problem is presented in Figure 48–1.

LIVER DISEASES PRESENTING IN CHILDHOOD: AN ETIOLOGIC CLASSIFICATION

Common presenting signs and symptoms of pediatric liver disease include jaundice, hepatomegaly, coagulopathy, encephalopathy, or elevation of liver enzymes or waste products such as ammonia; this represents a relatively limited repertoire to herald a wide array of diseases. To most efficiently review the spectrum of pediatric liver disease, we will categorize by cause rather than by symptom into the following groups: anatomic abnormalities; infections; metabolic defects; toxin exposure; vascular anomalies; and oncologic problems.

ANATOMIC ABNORMALITIES

Pathophysiology

Most anatomic anomalies occur in the biliary tract. There are several points in gestation at which malformations are believed to arise, including failure of recanalization of the occluded ducts at 7 weeks, and failure of the intra- and extrahepatic drainage systems to join, occurring at the close of the first trimester.

General Considerations

Biliary tract malformations are divided into disorders of **intrahepatic** and **extrahepatic** ducts. Diagnosis must include determination of the exact location and type of malformation and an estimation of surgical correctability. Rapid diagnosis is essential to prevent irreversible hepatic damage.

Differential Diagnosis

1. Disorders of intrahepatic bile ducts
   a. congenital hepatic fibrosis
   b. intrahepatic paucity of bile ducts
      1. syndromic (Alagille's)
      2. non syndromic
   c. Caroli's disease
2. Disorders of extrahepatic bile ducts
   a. extrahepatic biliary atresia (EHBA)
   b. choledochal cyst
   c. extraluminal compression resulting from extrinsic compression (cyst, tumor)
   d. spontaneous perforation of extrahepatic bile ducts
   e. intraluminal obstruction (stones)

Clinical Findings

A. Symptoms and Signs: It is difficult to establish the primary cause from clinical presentation alone, although there are some diagnostic clues. Intrahepatic lesions can be silent until fibrosis leads to cirrhosis and portal hypertension, heralded by the development of hepatomegaly or variceal bleeding. This is often the case with **congenital hepatic fibrosis,** an autosomal recessive disorder, unless associated renal anomalies facilitate earlier detection of the occult disease, or the less common presentation with abdominal pain and cholangitis spurs investigation. Intrahepatic paucity of ducts can be associated with

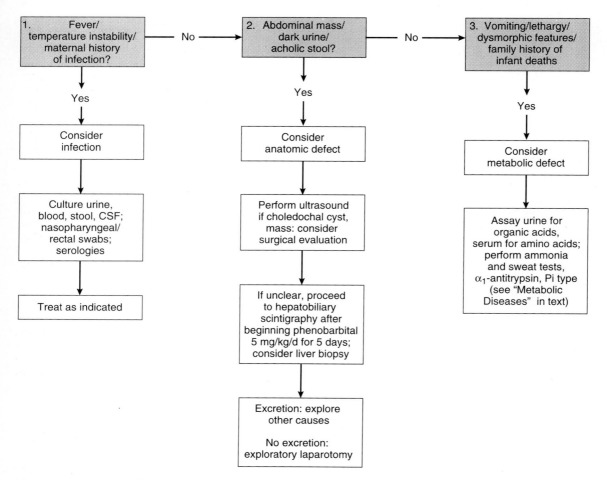

Figure 48–1. Evaluation of hyperbilirubinemia in the neonate. In a neonate older than 7 days with a direct bilirubin of greater than 4 mg/dL, consideration of possible pathologic causes should be initiated. In the sample approach outlined below, the physician *AIMs* towards the diagnosis, in recognition of the three major etiologic groups: *A*natomic, *I*nfectious, and *M*etabolic. Also consider potential contributory toxic effects of medications and parenteral nutrition.

jaundice and pruritus. With **Alagille's syndrome**, diagnosis is facilitated by recognition of the characteristic constellation of signs, including a typical facial appearance with deeply set, widely spaced eyes, a small, pointed chin and a flat nasal bridge. Other associations include a cardiac murmur, often caused by peripheral pulmonic stenosis, atrial septal defect, or Tetralogy of Fallot; butterfly anomalies of the vertebrae; and ocular anomalies (posterior embryotoxon). **Nonsyndromic paucity of interlobular bile ducts** also exists. Another intrahepatic defect is **Caroli's disease**, a congenital cystic malformation of the biliary tract often associated with autosomal recessive polycystic kidney disease. There is a female predominance. A common presentation is recurrent abdominal pain, icterus, emesis, and hepatomegaly.

Anomalies of the extrahepatic biliary tree are less subtle in presentation. Impedance of bile flow,

whether the result of stasis from a cystic dilatation, absence or diminution of ducts, or the occlusion of ducts by extrinsic masses or intrinsic stones, results in progressive jaundice and cholestasis. **Choledochal cysts** usually present as abdominal masses (exclusion of other causes, specifically tumors, can often be performed with imaging studies—see below). Choledochal cysts are congenital cystic dilatations of the biliary tree, and as such form a continuum with Caroli's disease (see also Chapter 53). There is again a female predominance, as well as a high incidence among those of Asian heritage. The five types of cysts are presented schematically in Figure 48–2. Choledochal cysts account for 2–5% of cases of extrahepatic neonatal cholestasis.

Spontaneous perforation of the extrahepatic ducts, although rare, presents as sudden jaundice, abdominal distension from ascites, and acholic (white)

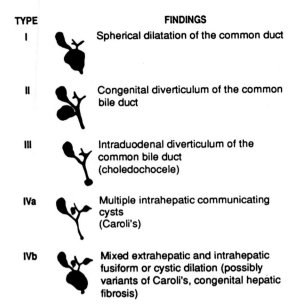

TYPE	FINDINGS
I	Spherical dilatation of the common duct
II	Congenital diverticulum of the common bile duct
III	Intraduodenal diverticulum of the common bile duct (choledochocele)
IVa	Multiple intrahepatic communicating cysts (Caroli's)
IVb	Mixed extrahepatic and intrahepatic fusiform or cystic dilation (possibly variants of Caroli's, congenital hepatic fibrosis)

Figure 48–2. Schematic representation of types of cystic dilatations of the biliary tract. Types I-III are extrahepatic. (Reproduced, with permission, from Hathaway WE et al (editors): *Current Pediatric Diagnosis & Treatment,* 11/e. Appleton & Lange, 1993.)

stools in the absence of hepatomegaly in a previously healthy newborn. The ascitic fluid is bilious if sampled; extravasation of fluid often stains the umbilicus and scrotum green, an important diagnostic clue.

Diagnosis of **extrahepatic biliary atresia (EHBA)** remains the greatest challenge. Presenting as progressive jaundice, pruritus, and hepatomegaly in a neonate with acholic stools and dark urine, it cannot be readily distinguished from other entities with similar presentations, including idiopathic neonatal (giant cell) hepatitis. **Giant cell hepatitis** is a nonspecific reaction of the neonatal liver to a variety of insults, including infections or metabolic anomalies, although in the vast majority of cases a cause cannot be identified (see Figure 48–3A for histology). EHBA occurs with a frequency of 1 in 15,000 live births. Its cause remains obscure, with both environmental and genetic factors implicated in pathogenesis. There are several cases in the literature of concordance in twins, although there is a greater number of discordant twins. A "2-hit" phenomenon has been hypothesized, where manifestation of EHBA is dependent on a genetic vulnerability with subsequent exposure to unknown precipitants (eg, toxins, ischemia, infection). Ten percent of neonates with EHBA have an associated vascular anomaly.

B. Laboratory Findings: Laboratory findings are not specific in disorders of the biliary system. Bilirubin is usually elevated if jaundice is present. The predisposition of the newborn to cholestasis is exacerbated if there is mechanical impedance to flow as described above; this can result in higher elevations in serum bile acids. Markers of biliary tract irritation, including alkaline phosphatase and γ-glutamyl transferase (GGT), may be elevated but are not helpful diagnostically. Transaminases may be slightly elevated as well, but synthetic function is usually preserved at presentation.

C. Imaging: Radiologic studies are key to the diagnosis of anatomic malformations. Sonographic imaging can identify the presence or absence of a gallbladder (often absent in EHBA) as well as the presence of cysts or dilatations, stones, or inhomogeneity in the surrounding hepatic parenchyma. Figure 48–4 illustrates a sonogram of a choledochal cyst. Estimations of the caliber of the biliary tract are readily made; this can be helpful when a proximal dilatation has occurred, but the offending obstruction has passed. Doppler flow studies can detect the early development of portal hypertension with reversal of flow in key vessels such as the portal vein.

Direct imaging of the biliary tree with contrast agents can be performed via intraoperative or percutaneous cholangiogram, or by endoscopic retrograde cholangiography (ERC) with cannulation of the ampullae and injection of radiopaque dye. Figure 48–5 illustrates a fluoroscopic view of a percutaneous cholangiogram revealing a choledochal cyst.

Hepatobiliary scintigraphy is also a useful technique, especially in the diagnosis of EHBA. Utilizing intravenous injection of one of several common radiolabeled tracers, including ^{99}mTc diethyliminodiacetic acid (DIDA) and ^{99}mTc p-isopropylacetanilidoiminodiacetic acid (PIPIDA), the scan estimates both integrity of the hepatic parenchyma via visualization of its ability to concentrate tracer, and patency of the biliary drainage system, as the tracer is accumulated in the gallbladder and excreted into the small intestine in normal controls within 4 hours of administration. EHBA is likely if after hepatic uptake the gallbladder is not visualized and if no intestinal excretion occurs on delayed images. Hepatobiliary scans can also be helpful in the diagnosis of choledochal cysts. Figure 48–6 illustrates examples of several hepatobiliary scans.

Liver Biopsy: The liver biopsy is diagnostic in congenital hepatic fibrosis, with characteristic dense bands of fibrous tissue containing distorted bile ducts (Figure 48–3B). In Caroli's disease, biopsy reveals normal hepatic parenchyma with an abundance of dilated channels lined by biliary epithelium. In EHBA, biopsy reveals cholestasis, giant cell transformation of the hepatocytes, and proliferation of bile ductules with a paucity of interlobular ducts (Figure 48–3C).

Complications/Treatment/ Prognosis

The options for treatment of anatomic abnormalities depend on the diagnosis. For congenital hepatic

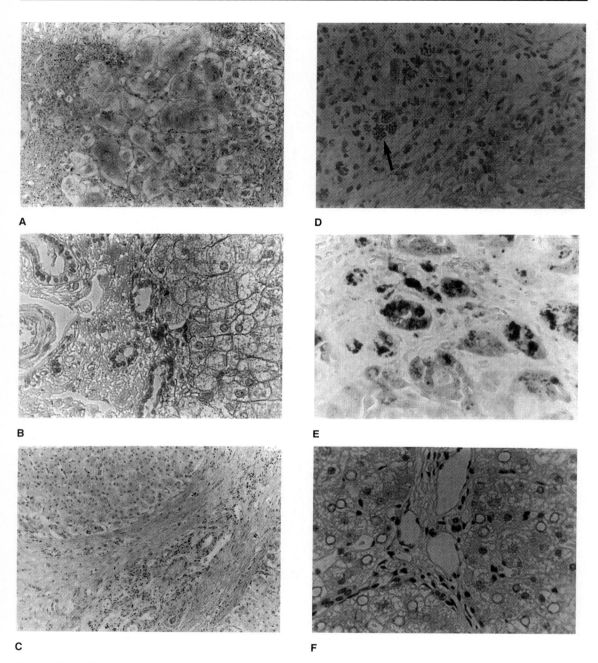

Figure 48–3. Characteristic histology in six examples of pediatric liver disease. **A:** Neonatal giant cell hepatitis. Note central cluster of multinucleated hepatocytes with ballooning degeneration. Autopsy specimen from a 2 month old infant with fulminant hepatic failure of unknown etiology. Magnification: 100×. Hematoxylin and eosin stain. **B:** Congenital hepatic fibrosis. There is a broad fibrous septum which occupies a significant percentage of the biopsy. Multiple cystically dilated tortuous bile ducts can be seen within the septum. Hepatocytes appear normal. From a 2-year-old presenting with portal hypertension and hematemesis. Magnification: 400×. Hematoxylin and eosin stain. **C:** Biliary atresia. Extension of portal tract by fibrosis, with proliferation of bile ducts characteristic of biliary atresia. Macro/micronodular cirrhosis is evident. Wedge biopsy from liver excised prior to transplant in an 8-month-old child following Kasai portoenterostomy, with recurrent episodes of cholangitis, growth failure, and progressive jaundice. Magnification: 100×. Hematoxylin and eosin stain. **D:** α_1-antitrypsin deficiency. Note diffuse hepatocellular disarray with ballooning, steatosis, and fibrosis. Intracytoplasmic inclusions resistant to diastase confirm the diagnosis *(arrowhead)*. Magnification: 400×. Diastase-treated PAS stain. **E:** Neonatal hemochromatosis. Hematoxolin and eosin stained sections show marked architectural disarray,

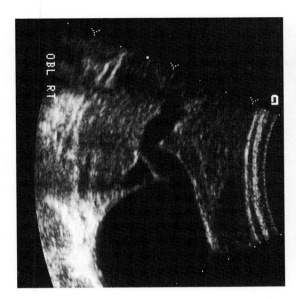

Figure 48–4. Ultrasonographic view of choledochal cyst; with cystic dilatation of common duct discernible as lucent area at bottom. (Courtesy of Carlo Buonomo, MD, Children's Hospital, Boston.)

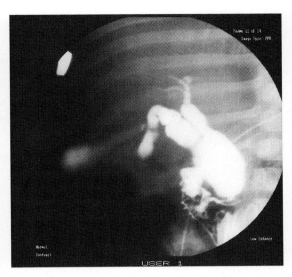

Figure 48–5. Fluoroscopic view of percutaneous cholangiogram demonstrating large spherical dilatation of the common duct typical of a choledochal cyst. (Courtesy of Carlo Buonomo, MD, Children's Hospital, Boston.)

fibrosis, Alagille's syndrome, and Caroli's disease, treatment is supportive. Supportive measures include treatment of the consequences of cholestasis, including pruritus, jaundice, malabsorption, steatorrhea, and fat soluble vitamin deficiency (Table 48–1). There is an increased risk of cholangitis with Caroli's disease, presenting as fever without other source, and progressive jaundice. Treatment requires several weeks of broad spectrum intravenous antibiotics. Progression of fibrosis to cirrhosis can lead to the complication of portal hypertension, with consequent development of varices and an associated risk of spontaneous hemorrhage. Bleeding varices can be treated with sclerotherapy or banding. If cirrhosis or complications of portal hypertension progress to end stage hepatic failure, transplantation becomes an option (Section III).

Extrahepatic biliary abnormalities are treated surgically. Cystic dilatations of the biliary tract are excised with subsequent portojejunal anastomosis. Spontaneous perforation of the bile ducts requires surgical repair. Obstruction or ductal dilatation due to intraluminal causes (ie, retained stone, constriction) can often be remedied via ERC with sphincterotomy or stent placement. Without operative intervention, the natural history of EHBA is progressive cirrhosis resulting in death by 12–18 months. Treatment was revolutionized in 1959 by the development of the Kasai portoenterostomy procedure, in which an intestinal conduit is anastomosed to the transected ductal remnants at the liver hilum, with drainage of bile established via the remaining intrahepatic bile ductules. The procedure has the best chance of reestablishing bile flow if performed by an experienced surgeon on a patient less than 2 months of age, and before the patient has accumulated significant fibrosis. Although a successful procedure relieves the immediate biliary obstruction, its effect on long-term outcome is variable, as the mechanism of the underlying disease remains unknown. The vast majority of patients go on to develop chronic liver disease requiring transplantation despite the portoenterostomy. The Kasai procedure does, however, allow time for patient growth and development. Transplantation is

hepatocellular damage, and micro/macronodular cirrhosis. Diffuse intracellular iron deposition, evident here, was mirrored in salivary gland biopsies. From a neonate presenting with fulminant hepatic failure. Magnification: 400×. Iron stain. *F:* OTC deficiency/Reye's-like syndrome. Note moderate fibrosis of the portal tract in the center with bridging; prominent microvesicular steatosis; hepatocyte disarray, and glycogenated nuclei. This biopsy is from a previously healthy 14-year-old boy presenting with encephalopathy and hyperammonemia after taking aspirin during a viral illness. Although initially diagnosed as Reye's syndrome, urinary orotic acid levels were elevated, and the hepatic fibrosis was suggestive of a chronic phenomenon. Enzymatic analysis of liver tissue revealed a deficiency in ornithine transcarbamylase. Magnification: 400×. Hematoxylin and eosin stain.

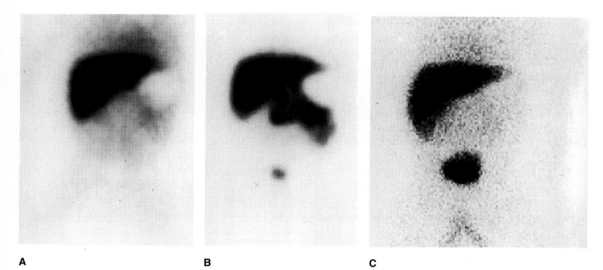

A **B** **C**

Figure 48–6. Hepatobiliary scintigraphy. **A, B:** Normal study. **A:** Initial view confirming uniform, facile uptake and concentration of the tracer by healthy hepatic parenchyma. **B:** Excretion of tracer into the duodenum *(arrow)* at 15 minutes. A small amount of tracer is visible in the bladder, an alternative route of excretion. **C:** View at 60 minutes from a patient with EHBA; although the hepatic parenchyma concentrated the tracer well, there is no visible excretion. (Courtesy of Carlo Buonomo, MD, Children's Hospital, Boston.)

technically easier in an older child, and donor organs are more readily available for recipients who weight more than 15 kg. Portoenterostomy and liver transplantation are thus complementary approaches to treating EHBA.

INFECTIOUS DISEASES

Pathophysiology

Infections involving the liver can be caused by bacterial, viral, fungal, or protozoal organisms. Primary hepatic infections are caused by hepatotropic viruses (for example, the hepatitis viruses A through E) or by parasites with an affinity for the liver (including *Entamoeba* and *Echinicoccus*). **Liver abscesses** are rare in children. The liver may also be

secondarily affected by agents causing disseminated infection. Examples include CMV, adenovirus, brucellosis (unpasteurized dairy products), leptospirosis (animal urine), and perihepatitis associated with pelvic inflammatory disease (Fitz-Hugh-Curtis Syndrome). Route of infection varies, especially in the neonatal period, and can be congenital (transplacental), perinatally acquired (ascending infection with ruptured membranes, swallowed blood, or other fluid at delivery), and postnatally acquired (breast milk, hospital personnel). Older children and adolescents are more prone to fecal-oral, parenteral (blood products, injecting drug abuse), or sexual modes of transmission. Liver abscesses, often polymicrobial, result from ascending infection via the portal system (pancreatitis, omphalitis); spread from contiguous structures (cholangitis); systemic bacteremia (via the he-

Table 48–1. Sequelae of chronic cholestasis, with suggested management.

Symptom	Pathophysiologic Findings	Treatment
Jaundice	Obstructed biliary tract, decreased bile flow	Phenobarbital
Pruritus	Increased serum bile acids or their metabolites	Cholestyramine, nalaxone, rifampin
Malabsorption steatorrhea	Reduced enteric bile acids, with diminished micelle formation and consequent fat malabsorption	Medium-chain triglyceride oil, vitamins A, D, E, K
Malnutrition	Steatorrhea, anorexia, early satiety	Increase calories
Ascites	Portal hypertension, fluid overload, low serum oncotic pressure	Fluid and salt restriction, diuretics, paracentesis
Bleeding	Varices, coagulopathy from factor deficiency and thrombocytopenia	Vitamin K, fresh-frozen plasma, cryoprecipitate
Encephalopathy	Decreased clearance of neurotoxins	Lactulose, neomycin, dietary protein restriction, plasmapheresis

patic artery–cystitis, endocarditis, osteomyelitis); or direct inoculation (trauma, surgery, transplantation).

Infections generally cause hepatic damage in two ways: either via direct toxic/cytopathic effect, as in the case of herpes simplex virus (HSV) infection or endotoxin release; or via immune-mediated damage, as with cirrhosis from chronic hepatitis B infection. Immunocompromised individuals have a heightened susceptibility to hepatic infection; examples include fungal infection of the liver in a neutropenic oncology patient, or *Mycobacterium avium-intracellulaire* hepatic infection in a pediatric AIDS patient. Neonates are also functionally more susceptible to infection because of immune immaturity.

General Considerations

Presenting signs and symptoms of infection can be myriad yet subtle, and include nonspecific systemic manifestations such as persistent fever, malaise, or lethargy in addition to more localizing signs of hepatic involvement, including right upper quadrant pain, jaundice, or elevated transaminases. Important history to assist in diagnosis includes maternal exposures and medications in the case of a neonate; or in an older child, age of onset, recent diet, travel history, pets, or pica. Once an infection has been identified, specific treatment can be prescribed.

Differential Diagnosis

1. Viral
   a. hepatitis A–E
   b. rubella
   c. cytomegalovirus (CMV)
   d. herpes simplex virus (HSV)
   e. human immunodeficiency virus (HIV)
   f. adenovirus
   g. Epstein-Barr virus (EBV)
   h. enterovirus (Coxsackie, echovirus)
2. Bacterial
   a. *Escherichia coli*
   b. *Listeria monocytogenes*
   c. *Treponema pallidum* (syphilis)
3. Protozoal/Parasitic
   a. *Toxoplasma gondii* (toxoplasmosis)
   b. *Entamoeba histolytica* (amebiasis)
   c. *Toxocara cani* (toxocariasis)
   d. *Echinococcus granulosis* (hytatid disease)
   e. *Schistosoma mansoni/japonicum* (schistosomiasis)
4. Fungal

Clinical Findings

A. Signs and Symptoms: Presentation varies depending on the age of the child and the particular infection in question. **Congenital infections** often present with vomiting, lethargy, temperature instability, anorexia, jaundice, and hepatomegaly. Associated malformations can provide important additional diagnostic clues to congenital infections; these in-

clude microcephaly, intracranial calcifications (toxoplasmosis, CMV), hydrocephalus (toxoplasmosis), cataracts, congenital heart disease, sensorineural hearing deficit (rubella), and growth failure, whether intrauterine (CMV, rubella) or postnatal (HIV). **Bacterial infections in the neonate** often have a more abrupt onset (48–72 hours post-delivery) with shock and disseminated intravascular coagulopathy. Bacterial infections can also be secondary to an underlying metabolic disorder such as galactosemia, known to predispose to *E coli* infections. **Liver abscesses** can present in a variety of ways, with fever, nausea, vomiting, malaise, weight loss, abdominal pain, right upper quadrant tenderness, and jaundice. These symptoms can be part of fulminant sepsis or a smoldering nonspecific illness, or can follow abdominal trauma, surgery, or immunocompromise. Liver abscesses, more common in children with sickle cell disease as liver or intestinal infarcts resulting from sickling can serve either as a nidus for abscess formation or allow ascension of organisms such as *Salmonella*. Immunocompromised patients, including those with malignancy, AIDS, or X-linked chronic granulomatous disease, are also more prone to liver abscesses, with common agents including *Candida*, *Mycobacterium avium-intracellulaire*, or gram-negative enteric bacteria.

TORCH infections result from a group of organisms causing similar devastating congenital infections, affecting 0.5–2.5% of all births. They include *t*oxoplasmosis, *r*ubella, *c*ytomegalovirus, *h*erpes virus, and usually syphilis and HIV ("*o*ther"). Toxoplasmosis, caused by the obligate intracellular organism *Toxoplasma gondii*, can be transmitted transplacentally if an acute infection occurs during gestation. The earlier in the pregnancy infection occurs, the more devastating the outcome. The fetus is protected, however, by pregestational maternal antibodies to toxoplasma. Rubella and syphilis are rare in the era of vaccination and antibiotics, which makes them all the more difficult to diagnose when they do occur. Cytomegalovirus affects 2% of all live births, and unlike toxoplasmosis, maternal immunity does not prevent virus reactivation or control spread, although infants infected in utero by maternal CMV reactivation are less likely to demonstrate significant sequelae.

The **hepatitis viruses (A–E)** share similarities in clinical presentation despite their diverse genetic origins. Hepatitis A (HAV) is endemic in many developing countries. In the United States, populations at risk include day care workers, international travelers to known endemic areas, and those with known contact with a hepatitis A-positive individual or with contaminated food or water. Transmission is fecal-oral. Anicteric infection in children is more common, and 90% of infected children younger than 5 years of age are asymptomatic. These children are highly infectious, nevertheless, with virus particles shed in feces concurrent with transaminase elevation and peak of anti-HAV IgM. These asymptomatic children serve as a reservoir for adult infection. There is life-long immunity established after infection, with no chronic phase.

Hepatitis B virus (HBV) infection is endemic in the Far East, Africa, and Southeast Asia. In the United States, it affects approximately 300,000 people yearly. Unlike hepatitis A, up to 10% of those infected with HBV go on to develop chronic infection with complications of cirrhosis and hepatic failure, and increased risk of primary hepatocellular carcinoma. Similar to hepatitis A, childhood infection with HBV can be asymptomatic, leading to underestimation of numbers infected yearly. Transmission can be perinatal, parenteral, or sexual. In utero transmission is rare. Risk of perinatal transmission is highest if maternal infection occurs in the third trimester; if the mother is HBeAg positive, there is a 70–90% chance of transmission. Although occasionally the neonate develops fulminant hepatic failure, the more usual clinical scenario is chronic infection, defined as failure to clear HBsAg and persistently elevated transaminases for at least 6 months.

Hepatitis C (HCV) is the most common cause of non-A, non-B hepatitis, although little is known regarding its effects or prevalence in childhood. Transmission is parenteral, although there is evidence for infrequent vertical transmission. One percent of adult blood donors in the USA possess antibodies to HCV. Presentation may be asymptomatic, or characterized by mild jaundice and malaise in the setting of elevated transaminases. Diagnosis is based on detection of antibodies to HCV. High risk children include those with a significant blood product requirement: hemophiliacs, cancer survivors, transplant recipients, and patients with thalassemia or undergoing dialysis.

Parasitic infections affecting the liver have been infrequent in the United States, but this is changing with the increase in immigration from endemic countries and the prevalence of international travel. Amebiasis results from ingestion of cysts in feces or contaminated meat or water. Liver involvement occurs when activated trophozoites invade the gut mucosa and are directed by the portal blood to form a solitary abscess in the right lobe. Ingestion of infected cat or dog feces leads to toxocariasis, typical in toddlers with sandboxes and a tendency towards pica. Symptoms are variable in toxocariasis and infections are often asymptomatic, unless the inoculum is large or a significant allergic response is generated.

B. Laboratory Findings: Clues to hepatic involvement include elevation of transaminases, bilirubin, alkaline phosphatase, and gamma glutamyl transferase. More problematic is identifying the specific etiologic agent. In the neonatal period, infections are the prime suspect for any unusual symptom. Maternal history; bacterial cultures from blood, urine, and cerebrospinal fluid (CSF); viral cultures

from urine, CSF and rectal and nasopharyngeal swabs are often diagnostic. Serologic testing is also important, including maternal and infant TORCH titers, IgM anti-HAV, anti-HCV IgG, and detection of HBsAg. In older children, stool ova and parasite testing may be informative. Liver biopsies can often be supportive if not diagnostic, as with identification of acidophilic intranuclear inclusions in HSV infection. Biopsy cultures may also be informative.

C. Imaging: Imaging studies, specifically ultrasonography and computed tomography, are useful for characterizing the location and size of hepatic abscesses. These can be solitary right lobe lesions (amebiasis, hytatid disease) or multiple disseminated lesions more common with fungal or mycobacterial infection.

Complications/Treatment/ Prognosis

Bacterial infections are effectively treated with broad spectrum antibiotics that are narrowed once specific etiologic agents are identified. Abscesses need surgical drainage if antibiotic therapy is incompletely effective. Effective antiviral therapies are more limited and lack the specificity of antibiotics. Ganciclovir and foscarnet for CMV infection can be supplemented by globulin preparations containing high titers against the virus. Acyclovir is used with varicella as well as herpes simplex infections.

Prevention of hepatitis A infection is accomplished by avoidance of infected persons and tainted food or water, and by delivery of gamma globulin for passive transient protection from pooled antibodies. Recently, a safe, formalin-inactivated vaccine has proven efficacious in several clinical trials in the United States and Thailand. Greater than 95% of children are protected after one dose. Current recommendations call for immunization of travelers to endemic countries, and of military recruits, food handlers, and day care workers or sewage workers.

The risk of developing chronicity after HBV infection is up to 90% for those infected at less than 1 year of age, with a 25% lifetime risk of end-stage complications such as cirrhosis or primary hepatocellular carcinoma. Some children who are HBeAg positive as well as HBV DNA positive clear their infection before reaching adulthood. Some, however, progress to cirrhosis by the time of initial liver biopsy. The best treatment is prevention, with education about the risks of intravenous drug abuse and unprotected sexual activity. The widely available recombinant vaccine containing surface antigen elicits formation of protective antibodies in greater than 95% of those vaccinated. Initial attempts to target at-risk populations failed to significantly reduce the number of HBV infections.

It is crucial to note that new guidelines established by the American Academy of Pediatrics and the Advisory Committee on Immunization Practices call for

universal immunization at birth regardless of the HBV status of the mother, with booster doses at 1 and 6 months. If the mother is HBsAg positive, hepatitis B immune globulin (HBIG) should be given in addition to the vaccine; this combination prevents infection in the newborn.

Treatment of chronic HBV infections with alpha interferon appears efficacious in children (although interpretation of success is complicated by the rate of spontaneous improvement). Children adopted from other countries where HBV infection is endemic and horizontal transmission is known to occur pose an important risk to adoptive families, whose members should be serologically screened and vaccinated. The risk is associated only with repetitive, intimate contact, however; classmates at school or day care are not at risk unless the infected child exhibits aggressive behavior such as biting, or has a bleeding disorder.

The natural history of hepatitis C infection in children is largely unknown, but an estimated 50% of HCV-positive adults progress to cirrhosis. The only available treatment is alpha interferon, shown to be beneficial in transaminase reduction and viral clearance in a minority of patients.

METABOLIC DEFECTS

Pathophysiology

As might be expected from its diverse yet essential roles in glucose homeostasis, protein and lipid synthesis, and detoxification, the liver is the primary organ affected by a wide range of metabolic derangements, many of which initially manifest in infancy and childhood. These abnormalities include defects in carbohydrate, protein and amino acid metabolism; fatty acid oxidation; bilirubin conjugation and bile acid synthesis; and copper transport. In most cases the exact biochemical defect has been characterized; in some, the actual genetic defect has been identified as well. Careful study of these experiments of nature has contributed substantially to the understanding and appreciation of the complexities of normal liver function.

Glycogen storage disorders represent a series of enzymatic defects in the pathways devoted to glycogenolysis or gluconeogenesis in the liver. Galactosemia and hereditary fructose intolerance are characterized by defects in the ability to metabolize galactose and fructose respectively. **Abnormalities of protein metabolism** include enzymatic defects in the urea cycle, the principal mechanism for disposal of waste nitrogen. Enzymatic defects in fatty acid oxidation are exposed during periods of prolonged fasting or increased energy demands, when glycogen is no longer available and metabolism of fats provides the major energy source. **Defects in lipid metabolism** also lead to a variety of lysosomal storage defects, including Wolman's disease, cholesterol ester storage disease, Gaucher's disease, and Niemann-Pick disease. α_1-antitrypsin deficiency is another storage defect, in which a defective protease inhibitor accumulates as diastase-resistant glycoprotein in hepatocytes, interfering with their normal function (Figure 48–3D). **Disorders of bilirubin metabolism** include the Crigler-Najjar syndromes, in which a deficiency of UDP glucuronyl transferase results in a profound unconjugated hyperbilirubinemia. **Defects in bile acid synthesis** are rare and extremely difficult to accurately diagnose, given the protean number of enzymatic steps involved. At least one bile acid synthesis defect is attributable to absence of functioning peroxisomes (Zellweger's syndrome). Both cystic fibrosis and Wilson's disease result from defects in ion transport; in cystic fibrosis, there is a defective chloride channel, the cystic fibrosis transmembrane regulator (CFTR), whereas in Wilson's disease, copper accumulation occurs because of a defective copper transporter, a P-type ATPase. The pathophysiology of **neonatal hemochromatosis** remains obscure, but this disorder results in progressive and almost invariably fatal hepatic insufficiency, with significant hepatic (as well as extrahepatic) iron deposition (see Figure 48–3E). The defect responsible for the decreasingly prevalent **Reye's syndrome** has never been identified, although possible candidates have included toxic exposures (aspirin, insecticides) or unusual presentations of fatty acid or urea cycle defects, manifest under conditions of starvation and stress from illness (see Figure 48–3F).

General Considerations

Although individually rare, these conditions collectively comprise a significant proportion of chronic liver disease in children. Initial clinical manifestations are often nonspecific. It is important, however, to suspect possible metabolic disease whenever repeated episodes of vomiting, lethargy, hyperammonemia, or hypoglycemia occur. This is especially of note during the neonatal period, when prompt diagnosis and treatment can prevent death or crippling sequelae. Although many metabolic diseases present nonspecifically, some present in ways that provide unique clues to the appropriate diagnosis. For example, persistent jaundice and unconjugated hyperbilirubinemia suggest Crigler-Najjar syndrome; the temporal association of symptom onset and introduction of fructose to the diet suggests hereditary fructose intolerance. Diagnosis is usually confirmed by the lack of demonstrable enzymatic activity in liver or other tissue; by demonstration of the accumulation of a toxic metabolite in blood, urine or liver; or by identification of the abnormal genotype (cystic fibrosis) or phenotype (α_1-antitrypsin deficiency).

Differential Diagnosis

1. Disorders of carbohydrate metabolism

   a. glycogen storage disorders
   b. galactosemia
   c. hereditary fructose intolerance
2. Disorders of protein or amino acid metabolism
   a. tyrosinemia
   b. urea cycle defects
      (1) ornithine transcarbamylase deficiency (OTC)
      (2) argininosuccinic aciduria
      (3) carbamyl phosphate synthetase deficiency (CPS)
3. Disorders of fatty acid oxidation
   a. medium chain acyl-CoA dehydrogenase deficiency (MCAD)
   b. long chain acyl-CoA dehydrogenase deficiency (LCAD)
   c. primary carnitine deficiency (systemic)
4. Disorders of bilirubin and bile acid metabolism
   a. Crigler Najjar Types I and II
   b. bile acid synthesis defects
      (1) cerebrotendinous xanthomatosis
      (2) cerebrohepatorenal syndrome (Zellweger's)
      (3) 3β-hydroxysteroid dehydrogenase/isomerase deficiency
      (4) Δ^4-3-oxosteroid 5β-reductase deficiency
5. Disorders of storage
   a. α_1-antitrypsin deficiency
   b. lysosomal storage
      (1) Wolman's disease
      (2) cholesterol ester storage disease
6. Disorders of ion transport
   a. cystic fibrosis
   b. Wilson's disease
7. Idiopathic metabolic disorders
   a. neonatal hemochromatosis
   b. Reye's syndrome

Clinical Findings

A. Signs and Symptoms: The diagnosis of a metabolic defect involves pattern recognition based on clinical presentation and history, as well as a high index of suspicion. Metabolic disease must be considered as part of the differential diagnosis in any situation involving unexplained lethargy, poor feeding, recurrent vomiting, hypoglycemia, hyperbilirubinemia, or hyperammonemia, especially in a neonate. Suspicion must remain high even into adolescence, as teenagers can present with mental status changes (Wilson's disease), hyperammonemia in the setting of a viral illness (Reye's or Reye's-like syndrome, urea cycle defects) or with cryptogenic cirrhosis (α_1-antitrypsin deficiency). Other important clues include parental consanguinity, unexplained sibling deaths or deaths ascribed to SIDS or Reye's syndrome.

The **glycogen storage diseases (GSD)** are a heterogenous group of disorders involving derangements in glucose or glycogen metabolism. Although there are more than 10 forms, not all have liver disease as a primary component. Type I, or Von Gierke's disease, is the most common as well as the most severe GSD, involving an enzyme important in gluconeogenesis. Type Ib differs from Ia in that the enzyme in question, glucose-6-phosphatase, cannot be detected in fresh tissue but is released when tissue microsomes are disrupted. Long-term complications in addition to growth failure include the formation of hepatic nodules potentially associated with adenoma or hepatocellular carcinoma, as well as the development of renal failure. Type III GSD (Cori's disease, limit dextrinosis) results from an autosomal recessive defect in a debrancher enzyme important in glycogenolysis. It presents with hepatomegaly, hypoglycemia and growth failure, with later complications of hepatic fibrosis, cardiomyopathy, and muscle weakness related to undegradable glycogen in these tissues. In GSD Type IV, a deficiency in a brancher enzyme results in formation of a glycogen similar to a plant starch. Hepatomegaly, growth failure and splenomegaly develop soon after birth, with fibrosis quickly progressing to cirrhosis as a result of the foreign glycogen. Type VI GSD results from a defect in phosphorylase, and presents with marked hepatomegaly and growth failure.

Other disorders of carbohydrate metabolism include **galactosemia**, a deficiency of galactose-1-phosphate uridyl transferase resulting in an inability to tolerate dietary galactose. This defect is perhaps best known for its association in the neonatal period with frequent infections, notably *E coli* urinary tract infections. **Fructose intolerance** can take three forms: fructokinase deficiency, causing benign essential fructosuria; and the more serious fructose 1-6 diphosphatase and fructose-1-phosphate aldolase deficiencies. The latter results in hereditary fructose intolerance characterized by vomiting, hypoglycemia, jaundice, hepatomegaly, reducing substances in the urine, and a metabolic acidosis upon exposure to fructose. The toxic effects on liver, intestine and kidney are related to sequestration of phosphate as fructose-1-phosphate, with a consequent decrease in intracellular stores of phosphate and ATP. Fructose 1,6 diphosphatase deficiency has a similar presentation without jaundice.

Disorders of protein or amino acid metabolism present in the neonatal period after initiation of feeding. These defects include the urea cycle defects as well as hereditary tyrosinemia. The latter is a defect in fumaryl acetoacetic acid hydrolase (FAH), leading to increased serum and tissue concentrations of tyrosine. There are two phenotypes; in the acute form, vomiting, jaundice, hepatomegaly, anemia, hypoglycemia, and metabolic acidosis develop within the first few months of life. A renal Fanconi syndrome is also often part of the clinical picture, with glycosuria, phosphaturia, hypercalcuria and renal bicarbonate wasting leading to hypophosphatemia and a hypochloremic metabolic acidosis. The chronic form has a much more indolent course, with slowly progressive cirrhosis complicated by a 37% incidence of hepatocellular carcinoma.

The **urea cycle defects** as a group impair the functioning of the primary pathway for waste nitrogen excretion via ammonia detoxification. Whereas many liver diseases result in secondary hyperammonemia because of generalized impairment of liver metabolism, the urea cycle defects represent a primary derangement in this specific pathway. Clinical hallmarks include hyperammonemia often leading to vomiting, lethargy, and other CNS effects including coma, seizures, and apnea. Ornithine transcarbamylase (OTC) deficiency is the most common urea cycle defect, affecting 1 out of every 50,000 births. It is the only X-linked defect, with classic presentation being a catastrophically ill male neonate with hyperammonemic coma and respiratory failure. Female carriers have variable penetrance due to unfavorable lyonization of the affected X chromosome; their symptoms can include episodic vomiting, aversion to high protein foods, headaches, intermittent lethargy, seizures and hepatomegaly. They are prone to hyperammonemia during acute illnesses or following other precipitants such as excessive protein ingestion, surgery, or vaccine administration (myolysis). There is also a small subgroup of males with milder late-onset OTC deficiency due to a less severe gene defect or mosaicism; it is easy to misdiagnose these late-onset atypical presentations as Reye's syndrome if careful diagnostic evaluations are not conducted. The second most common urea cycle defect is argininosuccinic aciduria, an autosomal recessive deficiency of argininosuccinic acid lyase leading to accumulation of argininosuccinic acid (ASA) in blood, urine, and tissues. Carbamyl phosphate synthetase deficiency has an almost identical presentation to OTC deficiency, with a severe, usually fatal neonatal onset as well as a milder form apparent in the first year (with 10–25% residual enzyme activity).

Fats supply energy to the body during prolonged fasts when glycogen stores have been depleted. **Fatty acid oxidation defects** present with persistent vomiting, cardiomegaly, hepatomegaly, hypotonia, developmental delay, and sometimes seizures in the setting of decreased food intake (gastroenteritis) or increased energy demands (fever). Medium chain acyl-CoA dehydrogenase deficiency (MCAD) specifically presents as recurrent episodes of illness in the first 2 years of life, with prolonged fasting leading to vomiting, lethargy, hypoglycemia and often coma and death. The risk of mortality exceeds 50% for affected individuals from 15–26 months of age. Long chain acyl-CoA dehydrogenase deficiency presents similarly, but with a more severe involvement manifest at a younger age, with more pronounced cardiac and skeletal muscle involvement. Carnitine is responsible for ferrying long chain fatty acids into mitochondria for oxidation. Synthesized in the liver, car-

nitine is transported via the serum into muscle, where it is present in high concentrations. Primary carnitine deficiency is an autosomal recessive defect affecting the carnitine uptake mechanism. Systemic manifestations include weakness, cardiomyopathy, and episodic hepatic encephalopathy with hypoglycemia and hypoketosis.

Some presentations of metabolic diseases are unique, as with the persistently elevated total bilirubin levels without any detectable conjugates in serum or bile seen in an otherwise healthy infant with **Crigler Najjar syndrome**. Crigler Najjar types I and II are distinguished by responsiveness to phenobarbital. As type I involves a total absence of the conjugating enzyme UDP glucuronyltransferase, phenobarbital is of little efficacy in reducing the unconjugated pool. Type II, by contrast, is defined by responsiveness to phenobarbital, supporting the existence of at least a small pool of partially functioning enzyme.

Bile acids serve vital roles in the elimination of cholesterol, promotion of bile flow, and facilitation of fat and fat-soluble vitamin absorption. **Derangements in bile acid synthesis** result in significant illness, as seen in four of the known syndromes involving such defects. Cerebrotendinous xanthomatosis is a lipid storage disease presenting with progressive neurologic compromise, ataxia, and xanthomatous lesions in the brain and tendons. Its biochemical abnormalities include reduced synthesis of primary bile acids and markedly elevated cholestanol levels. **Cerebrohepatorenal or Zellweger's syndrome** is a disorder of reduced or absent peroxisomes. The resulting interference with β-oxidation of fatty acids causes abnormal bile acid synthesis (among many other defects). Two of the other known disorders of bile acid synthesis are associated with neonatal cholestasis and familial giant cell hepatitis. 3β-hydroxysteroid dehydrogenase/isomerase deficiency is characterized by jaundice, acholic (white) stools, dark urine, cholestasis, hepatocellular damage, and fat soluble vitamin malabsorption. No chenodeoxycholic or cholic acids are detectable in the plasma. Hepatoxicity is thought to result from impaired bile flow or direct toxic effect of the mutant bile acid species synthesized. Δ^4-3-oxosteroid 5β-reductase deficiency presents in a similar fashion with cholestasis and increased urinary bile acid secretion. Interestingly, in addition to giant cell transformation on liver biopsy, the bile canaliculi are noted to be small with few microvilli, suggesting a possible role for adequate bile acid concentration in normal morphologic development.

α_1-antitrypsin deficiency has a broad range of clinical manifestations, including primary lung disease (emphysema) in addition to isolated liver involvement. A missense mutation leads to retention of this protease inhibitor in the endoplasmic reticulum, resulting in accumulation of diastase-resistant glycoprotein deposits in periportal hepatocytes (Figure 48–3D) and consequent interference with normal hepatocyte function. Cirrhosis frequently develops. This secretory defect results in diminished serum α_1-AT levels. The natural history and prevalence of this defect has been well documented in the Swedish cohort studies of Sveger; 20% of those carrying the PiZZ phenotype develop liver disease in childhood. Newborns can present with cholestasis, failure to thrive, and hepatosplenomegaly; alternatively, silent progression to cirrhosis or portal hypertension also occurs. There is evidence for increased intracellular aggregate formation of defective protein in settings of stress or fever, as with intercurrent illnesses. Some of those afflicted with the defective gene remain asymptomatic until lung disease, exacerbated by smoking, develops in middle age.

Two other storage diseases involve defects in the same enzyme, acid lipase, which is important in degradation of lipoproteins. **Wolman's disease** is an autosomal recessive defect presenting in the newborn period with abdominal distension, hepatosplenomegaly, ascites, anemia, widespread lipid storage, and bilateral adrenal calcification, an essentially pathognomonic finding. Liver biopsy reveals marked accumulation of lipid within lysosomes. Stored lysosomal fat is also found in intestinal mucosa, vascular endothelium, spleen, lymph nodes, bone marrow and circulating leukocytes. Death occurs before 6 months of age in 90% of patients. **Cholesterol ester storage disease** results from a deficiency of the same enzyme, and is thought to represent a milder allelic variant. Often the only presenting symptoms are hepatomegaly and hyperlipidemia. Birefringent crystals of cholesterol esters can be demonstrated within lysosomes on liver biopsy.

Cystic fibrosis can present as cholestasis in infancy related to inspissated bile, with hepatomegaly related to protein malabsorption and fatty infiltration, or with biliary cirrhosis in the adolescent (20% of adolescents with CF have cirrhosis). Gallbladder anomalies are also frequently found in these patients. The cirrhosis may be asymptomatic (apart from hepatosplenomegaly) or present as ascites or variceal bleeding. The underlying defect involves mutations in the chloride channel protein, CFTR. **Wilson's disease** also results from an ion (copper) transport defect (see Chapter 41). A defective P-type ATPase similar to the protein defective in Menke's disease is responsible for the toxic accumulation of copper in brain (neuropsychiatric symptoms), eyes (Kayser-Fleischer rings), kidneys, and liver. The absorption of copper is normal. Wilson's disease is among the most difficult of the metabolic defects to accurately diagnose given its range of presentation, from mild lethargy and malaise, abdominal pain, jaundice, and decreased school performance, to outright psychosis or fulminant hepatic failure.

Neonatal hemochromatosis is an uncommon idiopathic liver disease characterized by early fulminant hepatic failure in the setting of extensive intra- and extrahepatic iron deposition. The iron is readily detectable in both hepatocytes and in additional sites such as salivary glands by staining of tissue sections (Figure 48–3E). No specific defect has been identified.

Rarely diagnosed today, **Reye's syndrome** was first described in 1963 in Australia, and was characterized by a severe encephalopathy, marked cerebral edema, and diffuse fatty infiltration of the viscera, especially the liver. Onset was innocuous, 2–5 days after the start of a viral illness, with a resurgence of malaise and emesis that would progress quickly. In addition to the characteristic viral prodrome, there was frequently association with recent aspirin consumption. This association fueled today's practice of using acetaminophen as an antipyretic in the pediatric age group, especially in children with varicella. The cause of Reye's syndrome has never been elucidated, and the frequency has decreased to almost zero. It is conjectured that many cases represented previously undiagnosed metabolic derangements existing as forme frustes or partial defects uncovered by conditions of stress, fasting, fever, etc. Candidate categories include urea cycle defects, especially late onset male or carrier female OTC deficiencies, or fatty acid oxidation defects.

B. Laboratory Findings: Demonstration of deficient enzyme activity in a liver biopsy sample or cultured skin fibroblasts is a frequent key to diagnosis in many metabolic diseases. Histologic examination of the liver biopsy itself can also yield important diagnostic clues, such as the abnormal glycogen deposition seen in many of the GSD, or the birefringent lysosomal cholesterol ester crystals in the cholesterol ester storage diseases.

A few unique approaches deserve special mention. One of the earliest diagnostic clues to the presence of a fatty acid oxidation defect is the presence of a low serum glucose (<50) in the absence of urinary ketones. Although easily and rapidly performed using commercially available "on the spot" blood sugar estimator sticks and urine dipsticks, these results reveal the central problem in this disorder, the inability to break down fats for energy during prolonged fasts with exhausted glycogen storage.

Two urea cycle defects, OTC deficiency and CPS deficiency, have extremely similar presentations. Prior to enzyme assay of affected tissue to identify the precise defect, a diagnostic clue can be provided by measurement of urinary orotic acid. This substance is elevated in OTC deficiency but not in CPS deficiency.

Unique technology is utilized to diagnose suspected bile acid synthesis defects: fast atom bombardment-mass spectrometry, FAB-MS. In concert with gas chromatography (GC-MS), FAB-MS facilitates identification of abnormal bile acid metabolites in urine samples. In healthy individuals, there is negligible urinary bile acid excretion, but this changes in conditions of cholestasis, as in bile acid synthesis defects.

C. Liver Biopsy: For many metabolic diseases, it is the enzymatic assay rather than characteristic histology which makes liver biopsy diagnostic. Percutaneous needle biopsies often provide insufficient material for enzymatic assay, necessitating an open wedge biopsy.

Complications/Treatment/ Prognosis

In addition to the dietary restrictions traditionally used to treat many metabolic diseases, including galactosemia, fructose intolerance, and tyrosinemia, there are increasing numbers of innovative pharmacologic therapies with a design based on a comprehensive understanding of the affected biochemical pathways. These therapies usually facilitate alternative enzymatic pathways, or block the synthesis of precursors which become toxic in excess. Examples include therapies for urea cycle defects and tyrosinemia. For urea cycle defects, treatment involves not only a restriction of protein intake (decreasing nitrogen load), but also the use of sodium benzoate and phenyl acetate to divert nitrogen from urea synthesis to other waste products (hippurate and phenylacetyl glutamine). Long-term prognosis in these disorders still depends on the severity of hyperammonemic crises, and the rapidity with which the metabolic derangement is normalized. Hereditary tyrosinemia has traditionally been treated with dietary restriction of tyrosine, phenylalanine, and methionine. Recently, 2-(-2-nitro-4-trifluromethyl-benzoyl)-1,3-cyclohexanedione (NTBC) has been successfully utilized in this disorder. This compound acts to block tyrosine metabolism proximal to the enzymatic defect by inhibition of 4-OH phenylpyruvate dioxygenase. It is unclear whether use of this substance in conjunction with the dietary restrictions will lessen the high (37%) incidence of hepatocellular carcinoma in individuals with the chronic form of this disease.

Other metabolic diseases treated pharmacologically include Wilson's disease (use of penicillamine as a copper chelator) and cystic fibrosis and the bile acid synthesis defects (oral bile acids, which stimulate bile flow and inhibit synthesis of potentially toxic novel bile acids). While the first line therapy for Crigler-Najjar type I disease remains phototherapy, there has been investigation into use of metalloporphyrin injections as a means of inhibiting de novo bilirubin production. As with urea cycle defects and the risks of long-term sequelae from repeated episodes of hyperammonemia, the risk of kernicterus with permanent neurologic deficit or even death remains high in Crigler-Najjar type I disease, even after the patients have reached adulthood.

Liver transplantation is almost always an option, if the disease condition is confined to the liver, or if the key systemic proteins are hepatically synthesized. Correctable examples include the urea cycle defects, Crigler-Najjar type I, hereditary tyrosinemia and some of the bile acid synthesis deficiencies. Difficulties arise in choosing the optimal timing for the transplant. The procedure must be performed prior to accrual of irreversible effects of the underlying disease; yet, the child must be old enough so that the risks of the transplant itself are minimized. Liver transplantation is not necessarily curative if other areas of primary disease exist in the body, such as with cystic fibrosis (depending on extent of lung involvement) or lysosomal defects such as Gaucher's disease. Although a patient with Gaucher's disease was reported to experience temporary resolution of symptoms after an orthotopic liver transplant, symptoms returned within 2 years as Gaucher cells infiltrated the allograft.

Antenatal diagnosis is possible for many of these diseases. This may be beneficial from a therapeutic point of view, eg, by permitting initiation of appropriate dietary restrictions during pregnancy to prevent accrual of damage in utero. Antenatal diagnosis also allows the option of abortion if, after extensive genetic counseling, this choice is desired by the mother.

TOXINS*

Pathophysiology

The liver plays a primary role in detoxification of a variety of endogenous and exogenous substances, including bilirubin and various drugs. The role can be viewed as a balance between two processes:

- Activation. A compound is altered to an unstable or reactive intermediate by one of the cytochrome p450 enzymes or an inducible mono-oxygenase;
- Detoxification. The usually hydrophobic intermediate is transformed to a hydrophilic compound suitable for excretion in urine or bile.

These processes place the liver at considerable risk should there be an imbalance of activation and detoxification, with an excess of reactive intermediates. The activated metabolites can be directly hepatotoxic, or can act as neoantigens, eliciting an autoimmune response with the potential for significant toxicity of its own. Damage is primarily hepatocellular, often concentrated in zone 3, the location of many of the drug metabolizing enzymes.

Toxicity related to total parenteral nutrition (PN) represents a special, more complex situation. Most reports of PN-associated cholestasis have been in the pediatric age group, where 65% of cases are in

---

*See Chapter 44.

neonates with a birth weight of less than 2000 g. By contrast, adults receiving parenteral nutrition are more likely to present with a reversible steatosis sometimes accompanied by cholestasis; only 15% have histologically significant lesions related to PN usage. Risk factors associated with the development of PN cholestasis in a neonate include prematurity, sepsis, lack of enteral stimulation, a history of hypoxia or abdominal surgery, and duration of PN use greater than 2 weeks. The pathophysiology remains obscure but is likely of multifactorial cause, related to the immaturity of neonatal bile secretion resulting in an overall decrease in bile flow, to the frequent simultaneous use of multiple potentially hepatotoxic drugs in sick premature neonates, and to the frequent co-existence of sepsis or urinary tract infection, with associated endotoxin release also acting as a hepatotoxin. Additional factors include an increase in the proportion of potentially toxic secondary bile acids (lithocholate) in the bile acid pool. The solutions used in parenteral nutrition have also been implicated, with hepatic damage attributed to lack of tyrosine, cysteine, or taurine (found in high levels in breast milk); toxicity of photodegraded tryptophan; and excessive caloric contributions of dextrose or amino acids.

General Considerations

The possibility of toxin-induced damage should be included in the differential diagnosis of any pediatric liver disease. Such instances are probably less common than in the adult population, due to use of fewer simultaneous medications and absence of many hormonal and noxious influences contributing to the development of hepatotoxicity (obesity, ethanol abuse). In addition to being a less frequent occurrence, manifestations of toxin-mediated hepatic damage differ in children, because of developmental changes and maturation occurring in the detoxification systems; this further complicates facile diagnosis. Important information to gather when considering toxin-mediated liver damage includes a complete list of medications including over-the-counter preparations; the dosage of medications given; and the timing of initiation and discontinuation of the medications in relation to onset of hepatic pathology.

Differential Diagnosis (partial list)

1. Antipyretics
   a. acetaminophen
   b. acetylsalicylic acid
2. Anticonvulsants
   a. phenytoin
   b. carbamazepine
   c. phenobarbital
   d. valproate
3. Antibiotics
   a. sulfonamides
   b. erythromycin
   c. isoniazid
4. Immunomodulators
   a. cyclosporine
   b. methotrexate
5. Miscellaneous
   a. halothane
   b. parenteral nutrition

Clinical Findings

A. Signs and Symptoms: The range of presentation of toxin induced liver damage is broad, from mild transaminase elevation to fulminant hepatic failure. The extent of hepatocellular damage determines the degree of transaminase elevation or cholestasis. Hypersensitivity or autoimmune reactions lead to more systemic manifestations, including fever, rash, and eosinophilia.

For cholestasis associated with parenteral nutrition, diagnosis is suggested by the presence of a rising conjugated hyperbilirubinemia in a neonate on parenteral nutrition for greater than 2 weeks.

B. Laboratory Findings: In general, laboratory findings reflect underlying hepatocellular damage, with increased transaminases, hyperbilirubinemia, cholestasis, and coagulopathy, depending on the extent and duration of damage. Eosinophilia suggests a hypersensitivity reaction. With PN-associated cholestasis, the serum bile salt concentrations will be increased, as will the proportion of lithocholate in the pool. Rising conjugated bilirubin and elevated GGT are also important diagnostic clues.

C. Imaging: Diagnostic imaging is generally not helpful with diagnosis, although steatosis can be demonstrated on ultrasound or computed tomography.

D. Liver Biopsy: Most biopsies with toxin-associated pathology demonstrate focal necrosis, with concentration of hepatocellular damage in zone 3. Microvesicular steatosis is a frequent finding in valproate toxicity, as is eosinophilic infiltration in erythromycin associated toxicity. Biopsy characteristics supportive of but not pathognomonic for TPN cholestasis include early steatosis and periportal inflammation, progressing to cholestasis, fibrosis, and widening of the portal tracts with bile duct proliferation, giant cell transformation, and eventual cirrhosis. TPN cholestasis is a diagnosis of exclusion; other potential causes of cholestasis, especially infection, metabolic defects or biliary tract obstruction, must be considered.

Complications/Treatment/ Prognosis

In most cases, discontinuation of the offending medication is sufficient and will result in cessation of symptoms and reversal of damages excepting fibrosis. Treatment of PN-associated cholestasis is more complex, not only because the cause is unknown but because most patients receiving PN are extremely ill with limited nutritional options. Compromises include concurrent initiation of small amounts of enteral feeding, limitation of calories delivered as dextrose or amino acids (not to exceed 3.5 g/kg/d), and allowing several hours per day free from nutrient infusion ("cycling"). Phenobarbital and ursochenodeoxycholic acid may minimize cholestasis by facilitating bile flow.

VASCULAR DISORDERS*

Pathophysiology

The liver receives a dual vascular supply, with both hepatic and portal veins supplying blood to the extensive network of sinusoids bathing the hepatic parenchyma. Unimpeded blood flow is needed to sustain the liver and to allow successful performance of its myriad functions, including detoxification of waste products and metabolism of drugs, dissemination of synthesized proteins, and maintenance of glucose homeostasis. Because its function is so closely dependent on its vascular supply, the liver is susceptible to a variety of vascular insults. These can be arbitrarily divided on an anatomical basis into pre-, intra-, and posthepatic problems.

Portal hypertension can be of pre-, intra-, or posthepatic cause (see Chapter 43). Prehepatic causes are a result of portal vein occlusion, whether from a congenital malformation such as a web; or a result of infection or instrumentation in the neonatal period. Intrahepatic portal hypertension is usually a result of cirrhosis impeding blood flow. As described in the previous sections, cirrhosis can be the end result of numerous hepatic derangements, including those of anatomic, infectious, metabolic, toxic causes. Posthepatic portal hypertension results from hepatic vein or inferior vena cava thrombosis (Budd-Chiari syndrome), a rare finding in children.

The liver as a vascular organ is subject to damage from sudden changes in cardiac output, even if transient. **Decreased cardiac output** with consequent ischemia can lead to hepatocellular damage indicated by elevated transaminases as well as cholestasis. The extent of damage is determined by the duration of the ischemic episode. Right-sided heart failure (cor pulmonale), often associated with end-stage lung disease in cystic fibrosis, can lead to hepatomegaly from passive congestion of the liver.

Other intrahepatic vascular disturbances include **veno-occlusive disease** (VOD), characterized by the triad of an enlarged, tender liver; ascites or unexplained weight gain; and jaundice (with or without elevated transaminases) (see Chapter 49). Although the precise cause is unknown, this disorder frequently follows allogeneic bone marrow transplantation, with associated factors of high dose chemotherapy, total body irradiation, or graft versus host disease. The clinical picture mimics the result of ingestion of pyrrolizidine alkaloids (Jamaican bush tea), which leads to occlusion of small hepatic veins and hepatocyte congestion and necrosis.

Differential Diagnosis

1. Prehepatic
   a. portal hypertension secondary to portal vein thrombosis
      (1) congenital anomalies
      (2) omphalitis
      (3) UVC placement
   b. ischemia
2. Intrahepatic
   a. portal hypertension secondary to cirrhosis
      (1) biliary atresia
      (2) infectious disease with chronic sequelae
      (3) metabolic diseases
      (4) toxins
   b. VOD
3. Posthepatic
   a. portal hypertension secondary to hepatic venous or IVC occlusion (Budd-Chiari)
      (1) congenital anomalies
      (2) trauma
      (3) tumor
      (4) clotting abnormality
   b. passive congestion

Clinical Findings

A. Signs and Symptoms: The presentation of portal hypertension can often be dramatic, heralded by gastrointestinal bleeding from esophageal or gastric varices. If due to post- or intrahepatic causes, there can be significant hepatomegaly with or without splenomegaly. The latter often results in sequestration of white blood cells and platelets within the enlarged spleen (hypersplenism), leading to neutropenia and thrombocytopenia. The liver is normal size in prehepatic portal hypertension. Passive congestion and veno-occlusive disease often present with hepatomegaly.

B. Laboratory Findings: In cases of suspected vascular disease, especially portal hypertension, it is important to obtain a complete blood count with differential and platelets, coagulation studies, and liver function tests. If hemorrhage is present, a type and cross in preparation for a possible transfusion is indicated. Prehepatic causes of portal hypertension are often associated with normal lab values.

C. Imaging: Ultrasonography with Doppler is the most facile way to confirm a suspected diagnosis of portal hypertension. In addition to detection of reversed or hepatofugal flow, the presence of clots and the caliber of vessels can be assessed. The hepatic parenchyma can be examined as well. Computed tomography with and without contrast can detect fixed vascular anomalies such as cavernous transformation

*See Chapters 43, 45.

of the portal vein. It is also useful in the evaluation of hemangiomas of the liver. The newer technique of MR angiography is becoming popular as a substitute for traditional angiography in documenting hepatic vasculature. Invasive angiography may be necessary to document vascular anatomy prior to operative procedures, or to assess intravascular or intrasplenic pressure.

D. Liver Biopsy: Biopsy is not a useful diagnostic technique in portal hypertension except to assess the presence or extent of cirrhosis. Findings consistent with passive congestion or ischemia are supportive but not illuminating as to cause. Histopathologic lesions in VOD may be helpful in demonstrating central venous congestion, centrilobular hemorrhage, and necrosis with minimal inflammatory response.

Complications/Treatment/Prognosis

Treatment of portal hypertension depends on presentation. Gastrointestinal hemorrhage requires transfusion followed by endoscopy for diagnosis and possible treatment with sclerotherapy or banding. Agents to lower portal pressure (eg, vasopressin, somatostatin) may also be useful in decreasing variceal bleeding. Ascites requires a low-salt diet and use of diuretics such as spironolactone or furosemide. For intrahepatic causes of portal hypertension, it is important to treat the cause of the cirrhosis. Congenital webs or other anomalies require surgical repair. Persistent variceal bleeding with continued hepatic deterioration is an indication for liver transplantation. Treatment for the remainder of vascular defects discussed is supportive. Hepatic damage from transient ischemia is reversible if the episode was isolated.

NEOPLASTIC DISORDERS*

Pathophysiology

Primary liver tumors represent the third largest group of abdominal neoplasms in children. One-third are benign, with the most common being mesenchymal hamartomas and hemangioendotheliomas. Two-thirds are malignant, and include hepatoblastoma, hepatocellular carcinoma, and metastases. Common childhood tumors metastatic to the liver include Wilms, stage IV neuroblastoma, and leukemia. A literature survey of primary pediatric liver tumors revealed hepatoblastoma to be the most common (43%), followed by hepatocellular carcinoma (23%), hemangiomas/hemangioendotheliomas (13%), and mesenchymal hamartomas (6%).

Hemangiomas are the most common benign liver tumors. They usually present within the first six months of life, grow rapidly for the first year, then gradually involute over 5–8 years. Cavernous heman-

giomas are often asymptomatic and small, but capillary hemangiomas, or hemangioendotheliomas, are large, frequently multiple, and often hemodynamically significant. Intrahepatic lesions are often accompanied by cutaneous ones. Hemangiomas often result in congestive heart failure and consumptive coagulopathy (Kasabach-Merritt syndrome). Mesenchymal hamartomas arise from mesenchymal rest cells of the portal tract. A usual patient would be a male under two years old. The lesions usually consist of large septated cysts filled with mucoid material and lined by flattened biliary epithelium.

Hepatoblastomas are of mesodermal origin, and are formed from incompletely differentiated hepatocytes. They usually present at less than 3 years of age. They occur more frequently in males, in the right lobe, and are generally large and multinodular. The cellular components can be diverse; most recapitulate a stage of normal fetal hepatic development. This variety complicates evaluation, because treatment and prognosis are tightly linked to histology. The worst prognosis is associated with tumor composed of small undifferentiated cells. There is a broad spectrum of genetic alterations associated with hepatoblastomas. In the tumor itself, trisomy 2, trisomy 20, and various translocations and partial deletions have been documented. There is a clear association with familial adenomatous polyposis, with a 1000-fold increased incidence of hepatoblastoma in children from affected families compared to the general population.

Hepatocellular carcinoma (HCC) occurs more frequently in older children, with an increased frequency in males. The spectrum of cell types involved is similar to the adult presentation. Hepatocellular carcinoma has a much higher incidence in chronic carriers of HBV and in various metabolic disorders, including the glycogen storage diseases, type I tyrosinemia, and α_1-antitrypsin deficiency. The reason for the high association between chronic hepatitis B infection and HCC remains an area of active investigation. Likely, certain foci of cells with particular HBV integrations and chromosomal rearrangements are selected for their growth advantage and resistance to HBV-directed immune attack.

General Considerations

Once an abdominal mass has been identified, swift and accurate diagnosis is imperative, because many liver tumors will have already grown to considerable dimensions. The primary decisions center around the questions of benign or malignant, resectable or nonresectable. Imaging studies are vital to characterization of the mass, revealing diagnostic clues in addition to important information concerning vascularity and hence resectability.

Differential Diagnosis

1. Benign tumors
   a. hemangiomas, cavernous

---

*See Chapter 46.

   b. hemangioendotheliomas
   c. mesenchymal hamartomas
2. Malignant tumors
   a. hepatoblastoma
   b. hepatocellular carcinoma
3. Metastatic
   a. neuroblastoma
   b. Wilms

Clinical Findings

A. Signs and Symptoms: The most frequent presentation is an asymptomatic abdominal mass. It is often discovered by the primary physician during a routine "well-child" check-up, or by a parent during bath time or play. Masses often grow to sizable proportions prior to discovery. Other common features include abdominal pain, anorexia, weight loss, vomiting, diarrhea, and jaundice with or without pruritus, if tumor growth causes impedance of bile flow. In cases of large hemangioendotheliomas or vascular or mesenchymal hamartomas, the presentation can involve congestive heart failure as well as hepatomegaly. With hemangioendotheliomas, there are also often cutaneous lesions or a bruit audible on auscultation of the liver.

B. Laboratory Findings: As with any disruption of normal hepatic architecture, transaminase elevation and hyperbilirubinemia may accompany tumor growth. Anemia can sometimes be found in association with hepatoblastoma, as can thrombocytopenia with hemangioendotheliomas (Kasabach-Merritt syndrome). Substances which can be used as tumor markers to aid in diagnosis and to follow efficacy of therapeutic regimens include: α-fetoprotein, elevated in 80–90% of hepatoblastoma patients and 60–90% of those with hepatocellular carcinoma; serum ferritin, almost universally elevated in cases of hepatocellular carcinoma; and descarboxyprothrombin, also elevated in HCC.

C. Imaging: As with primary vascular anomalies, radiologic imaging is essential for diagnosis of liver masses. Ultrasonography is especially useful for delineation of cystic lesions or for guidance of fine needle aspirates. Computed tomography with and without contrast is best for lesions that are exceptionally small or difficult to assess by ultrasound; for documentation of metastases; and for preoperative assessment of vascular involvement. Figure 48–7 illustrates an hepatoblastoma on CT scan with contrast. Magnetic resonance angiography (MRA) is becoming the best noninvasive way of accurately imaging tumor vascularity and potential encroachment on hepatic vessels. Therapeutic angiography can be used to selectively embolize vessels supplying a hemangioendothelioma.

Complications/Treatment/ Prognosis

The major therapeutic goal for liver neoplasms is

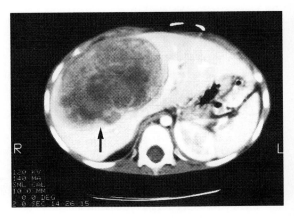

Figure 48–7. CT scan of the liver with contrast. Note the large, circumscribed hepatoblastoma **(arrow).** Necrotic areas are visible within the tumor. The portal vein is displaced. (Courtesy of Carlo Buonomo, MD, Children's Hospital, Boston.)

complete excision. The staging mechanism reflects this goal, with stage I consisting of complete resection; stage II, microscopic residual tumor; stage III, gross residual tumor; and stage IV, metastatic disease. The primary barriers to excision include size, location and vascularity of the tumor. If the tumor is too large for resection at presentation, an attempt at tumor reduction with chemotherapy or radiotherapy is made. Hepatoblastoma has proven responsive to doxorubicin as well as to regimens including vincristine, cyclophosphamide, 5-fluorouracil, and cisplatinum. HCC responds poorly to chemotherapy, however; only 10–25% are resectable, and post-resection adjuvant chemotherapy cures less than one-third of patients. Liver transplantation for HCC is generally unsuccessful because of rapid re-infiltration of the allograft with tumor. Perhaps the best tool to combat HCC is prevention of chronic HBV infection using aggressive vaccination, and careful surveillance in clinical situations known to predispose to HCC (ie, tyrosinemia).

The treatment of hemangiomas also depends on presentation. As described earlier, the natural history of these benign tumors involves rapid growth over the first year of life with subsequent gradual involution. Treatment in an attempt to reduce the size of lesions becomes important in the case of large or multiple lesions compromising vital structures or their function. For lesions localized to the liver, resection or selective embolization is possible. For disseminated lesions, treatment in the past has involved radiation, cyclophosphamide, or more recently, steroids to accelerate the rate of involution. Research at Boston Children's Hospital has documented the efficacy of subcutaneous interferon alpha 2a in life-threatening cases which have failed steroid therapy.

Benign mesenchymal hamartoma need be excised only if symptomatic.

PEDIATRIC LIVER TRANSPLANTATION

(See also Chapter 54.)

Liver transplantation has become an important therapy for a number of previously fatal pediatric diseases including metabolic derangements such as tyrosinemia and ornithine transcarbamylase deficiency. Approximately 350 children annually receive liver transplants in the United States.

The three major indications for transplantation in a pediatric patient are:

- primary progressive liver disease resulting in failure without intervention (acute idiopathic hepatic failure, biliary atresia, sclerosing cholangitis);
- primary static liver disease with morbidity significant enough to overshadow the risks of transplantation (refractory pruritus, absolute growth failure);
- metabolic disease.

Lesser indications include liver disease secondary to systemic illness primarily affecting another organ system (cystic fibrosis), or primary hepatic malignancy (hepatocellular carcinoma). Indications for transplantation at Children's Hospital, Boston, from 1983–1994 are shown in Table 48–2. As in most series, biliary atresia is the most frequent indication.

Table 48–2. Frequency of liver transplantation for various disorders.[1]

Disorder	Number	% of Total
Biliary atresia	38	52.8
Hepatic failure	12	16.7
Metabolic disease	8	11.1
Tyrosinemia	2	2.7
Carbamyl phosphate synthetase deficiency	1	1.3
Ornithine transcarbamylase deficiency	1	1.3
α_1-antitrypsin deficiency	3	4.1
Neonatal hemochromatosis	1	1.3
Neonatal hepatitis	4	5.5
Cryptogenic cirrhosis	3	4.1
Congenital hepatic fibrosis	2	2.7
Hepatitis C virus	1	1.3
Cystic fibrosis	1	1.3
Micronodular cirrhosis	1	1.3
Chronic active hepatitis	1	1.3
Cholestasis associated with parenteral nutrition	1	1.3
Total	72	100

[1]Data courtesy of Susan Treacy, RN and Liver Transplant Coordinator, Children's Hospital, Boston, 1984–1993.

The second most common indication is acute failure, with third place occupied by the metabolic diseases as a group.

Timing of transplantation is obviously critical. Technically, liver transplantation is easier in an older child, and donor organs easier to obtain. Older children are also less likely to have growth problems. Delaying transplantation can be hazardous, however. Chronic liver disease can itself lead to growth failure because of a variety of reasons including fat and fat-soluble vitamin malabsorption, early satiety, and anorexia (see Table 48–1 for treatment options). Some complications, such as variceal hemorrhage, spontaneous bacterial peritonitis or recurrent cholangitis, can be life-threatening. In the case of metabolic diseases, the passage of time increases the chances of accumulation of central nervous system damage from recurrent episodes of hyperammonemia or hyperbilirubinemia, or of development of hepatocellular carcinoma. Attempts to develop methods to aid in prediction of optimal timing of transplantation have not been successful. In the case of chronic failure, quantitation of a first-pass metabolite of lidocaine, monoethylglycinexylidide (MEGX), appears to correlate with hepatic function, but this test remains investigational.

Once the difficult decision to proceed with transplant has been made, timing ultimately is controlled through the ranking system of the United Network for Organ Sharing (UNOS). This system is necessary because of the severe shortage of cadaveric donor organs, most acute in the pediatric age group. Pediatric donors commonly arise from accident victims, with the most frequent susceptible age range being toddlers and school age children. Most children waiting for a liver are less than 2 years of age and less than 30 kg. Innovative graft surgery has helped to lessen the impact of this critical shortage. Approaches include the use of reduced-size cadaveric organs, in which a large organ is custom-trimmed to accommodate the recipient's size, and living-related donor transplants, in which a portion of the donor's left lobe (or left lateral lobe) is resected. This latter procedure ensures graft quality and has enabled transplants to be performed electively, before the deterioration of the child's health. Donors are usually parents who are carefully screened and evaluated to minimize risk. Additionally, auxiliary transplants are being developed for the treatment of transient insults or metabolic diseases, where temporary support or minimal auxiliary function is sufficient to augment native liver function.

The central goal of the pediatrician caring for a child with liver disease is to optimize their growth and development. While liver transplantation often represents the cure for underlying disease, it brings new problems as well. For example, immunosuppression is required for successful graft maintenance, but predisposes to infection as well as to secondary malignancy (posttransplant lymphoproliferative disease associated with EBV infection). Additionally, these medications contribute to transplant-associated growth failure, especially during the first 6 months, when regimens are most stringent. Transplantation at less than 2 years of age results in poor growth. There are also a variety of factors leading to poor oral intake, including nausea from medications or infections, gastric dysmotility, and persistent malabsorption. With children, behavioral factors are important as well, with frequent noxious stimuli such as suc-

tioning or intubation leading to residual oral aversion and refusal to feed.

Despite these potential complications, it is important to emphasize that the vast majority of pediatric transplant recipients grow and develop normally in a fashion that would not have been possible without the transplant. In some centers, survival rates as high as 80–90% have been reported. Many children lead fully normal lives with regular school attendance and normal maturation into adulthood.

REFERENCES

Becht MB et al: Growth and nutritional management of pediatric patients after orthotopic liver transplantation. Gastroenterol Clin North Am 1993;22:367.

Burton BK: Inborn errors of metabolism: The clinical diagnosis in early infancy. Pediatrics 1987;79:359.

Codona-Franch P, Bernardo O, Alvarez F: Long-term follow-up of growth in height after successful liver transplantation. J Pediatr 1994;124:368.

Finegold MJ: Tumors of the liver. Semin Liver Dis 1994;14:270.

Knisely AS: Iron and pediatric liver disease. Semin Liver Dis 1994;14:229.

Kocoshis SA et al: Pediatric liver transplantation: History, recent innovations, and outlook for the future. Clin Pediatr 1993;32:386.

Mowat AP: Selected developments in pediatric hepatology. Curr Opin Gastroenterology 1993;9:423.

Peter G et al (editors): *1994 Red Book: Report of the Committee on Infections and Diseases,* 23/e, Elk Grove Village: American Academy of Pediatrics, 1994.

Romero R, Lavine JE: Viral hepatitis in children. Semin Liver Dis 1994;14:289.

Treem WR: Inherited and acquired syndromes of hyperammonemia and encephalopathy in children. Semin Liver Dis 1994; 14:236.

Whitington PF, Alonzo EM, Piper JB: Pediatric liver transplantation. Semin Liver Dis 1994;14:303.

49

Hepatic Complications of Bone Marrow Transplantation

George B. McDonald, MD

Hepatic diseases are common in marrow and peripheral blood stem cell transplantation recipients. Diagnoses are often difficult, as the marrow transplantation milieu is complex and patients are susceptible to toxic, infectious, and immunologic liver diseases, sometimes concurrently.

HEPATOBILIARY DISEASES IN CANDIDATES FOR MARROW TRANSPLANTATION

FUNGAL INFECTION IN THE LIVER

Patients who are candidates for transplantation and have a history of granulocytopenia, fever, and fungal sepsis may have fungal abscesses in the liver. These should be identified and treated before transplantation, if possible; if not, intravenous amphotericin should be given throughout the transplantation procedure until the fungal lesions have resolved.

HEPATIC METASTASES

Liver involvement with tumor is common in patients who are undergoing transplantation for a malignant disorder, and this is not a contraindication to transplantation. It is important to be sure that filling defects seen on liver imaging tests do not represent abscesses rather than metastases.

HEPATITIS

Elevated serum transaminase levels are common before transplantation because of a high frequency of viral hepatitis B and C infections (from prior blood products) and because of drug toxicity. Hepatitis predisposes patients to fatal veno-occlusive disease of the liver. Viral hepatitis B and C infections may rarely cause fulminant hepatitis after transplantation, but the usual course is asymptomatic viral replication after conditioning therapy, followed by mild hepatitis after day 60, followed by chronic hepatitis.

GALLSTONES

Asymptomatic gallstones can be watched throughout the transplantation process, but symptomatic biliary disease (biliary colic, cholecystitis, or common duct stones) is an indication for surgical correction before the start of conditioning therapy.

LIVER DISEASES IN THE FIRST 100 DAYS AFTER TRANSPLANTATION

The approach to hepatic diseases after transplantation starts with a review of the individual patient's risk factors for these diseases (Table 49–1). The differential diagnosis becomes more manageable if certain diseases can be dismissed on the basis of a low probability that they are present. The timing of liver dysfunction in relation to conditioning therapy, marrow or stem cell infusion, and immune system reconstitution is also useful in constructing a list of likely diagnoses.

VENO-OCCLUSIVE DISEASE OF THE LIVER

Veno-occlusive disease is the most common cause of jaundice in the first few weeks following marrow or stem cell infusion. Its toxicity may limit the dosages of cytoreductive drugs for patients with cancer who are candidates for transplantation.

Cytoreductive therapy ("conditioning therapy") given before marrow or stem cell infusion may cause

Table 49–1. Overview of liver diseases commonly seen in marrow transplantation patients.

Hepatic Disease After Transplantation	Risk Factors	Timing
Veno-occlusive disease	High-dosage conditioning regimens: total body irradiation dose > 13 Gy; busulfan/ cyclophosphamide; BCNU/cyclophosphamide/ VP-16; regimens that contain cytarabine or thiotepa Elevated serum transaminase levels before cytoreductive therapy Persistent fever before and during cytoreductive therapy Mismatched or unrelated donor allogeneic marrow Second conditioning regimen and transplantation	Onset from before marrow infusion to day +20 posttransplantation Onset differs with various regimens of cytoreductive therapy
Fungal liver disease	Pretransplantation filling defects in liver Fungal colonization or infection Veno-occlusive disease or graft-versus-host disease of liver Granulocytopenia	During granulocytopenia, usually before day 50
Cholangitis lenta	Persistent fever Sepsis syndrome	During sepsis, usually before day 50
Acute graft-versus-host disease	Allogeneic marrow donor, especially HLA-mismatched or unrelated donor Lack of prophylactic immunosuppressive drugs (cyclosporine, methotrexate)	Onset day +20–60 Note "hyperacute graft-versus-host disease" in patients who do not receive prophylactic drugs
Biliary sludge disease	Minimal oral intake Prolonged parenteral nutrition Conditioning therapy Use of medications that precipitate in bile (cyclosporine, ceftriaxone)	Found on ultrasound by day +10 Symptoms by day +20–35
Drug- or TPN-induced liver injury	Known hepatotoxic drug Prolonged, noncyclic TPN ± sepsis	At any time
Bacterial infection of the liver	Prior infection with *M tuberculosis* Prior BCG vaccination	Early, during granulocytopenia Later, during immunosuppression
Epstein-Barr virus lymphoproliferative disease	T-lymphocyte depleted marrow Acute graft-versus-host disease High-dosage, prolonged immunosuppressive therapy	Later, usually day +50–100
Malignant cells in the liver	Pretransplantation malignant disease Transplantation in leukemic relapse	Day +50–100
Nodular regenerative hyperplasia	High burden of chemotherapy before transplantation High-dosage cytoreductive therapy for marrow transplantation Signs of veno-occlusive disease before day 20	Day +50–100
Acute viral hepatitis	Evidence of active or latent viral infection before transplantation (herpes simplex virus, varicella-zoster virus, hepatitis B or C virus, cytomegalovirus) Restitution of cell-mediated immunity after transplantation (hepatitis B or C virus) Exposure to adenovirus	For herpesviruses and adenovirus, day +30–100 For hepatitis viruses, after immune reconstitution, day +60–120

widespread damage to zone 3 of the liver acinus (the area surrounding the central veins). This damage includes injury to endothelial cells lining the sinusoids and venules, hepatocyte necrosis, occlusion of venular walls with thrombotic material, and, in severe cases, fibrosis of hepatic venules and sinusoids. Risk factors for the development of severe veno-occlusive disease are the intensity of the conditioning regimen (higher-dosage regimens are more likely to cause severe disease) and factors individual to each patient, such as the presence of hepatitis before transplantation, persistent fever during conditioning therapy,

and the degree of mismatching between patient and marrow donor. Patients who receive a second dose of conditioning therapy, particularly adults, are also predisposed to severe veno-occlusive disease.

Clinical Findings

A. Symptoms and Signs: The triad of painful hepatomegaly, weight gain caused by fluid retention, and jaundice is present in most patients with veno-occlusive disease. These signs follow the start of cytoreductive therapy by 1 to 14 days, depending on the drugs used. The onset is usually within 7–14 days of the start of regimens that include busulfan plus cyclophosphamide, cyclophosphamide plus total body irradiation, or carmustine (BCNU) plus cyclophosphamide plus etoposide. In some cases, the onset is before day 0, the day of marrow infusion. The clinical onset develops later with regimens that include cytarabine or those with multiple alkylating agents (eg, busulfan plus melphalan plus thiotepa).

Hepatomegaly and weight gain are the initial manifestations, followed by jaundice 4–7 days later, on average. The onset can be abrupt, with severe abdominal pain from rapid hepatic enlargement. In some cases, the onset is insidious and the diagnosis not apparent until day 15–30, when ascites and jaundice are noted.

B. Diagnostic Studies: In patients with a classic presentation, biopsy may not be necessary. If the clinical presentation is atypical or other liver diseases are present simultaneously with veno-occlusive disease, accurate diagnoses can be achieved with transvenous liver biopsy and measurement of the hepatic venous pressure gradient (> 10 mm Hg is highly predictive of veno-occlusive disease in this setting).

Serum transaminase and alkaline phosphatase levels are usually normal or minimally elevated; in some patients, however, transaminase levels can exceed 1000 IU/L. Platelet counts are lower than expected in patients with severe veno-occlusive disease, probably because of rapid consumption.

Differential Diagnosis

Hepatomegaly can be seen with tumor or fungal infiltration of the liver, hepatic vein obstruction (Budd-Chiari syndrome), right heart failure, or constrictive pericarditis. Jaundice in the early posttransplantation period can be caused by persistent septicemia (cholangitis lenta), liver injury due to drug toxicity or total parenteral nutrition, or acute graft-versus-host disease. Ascites can also result from the spreading of intraperitoneal tumor or pancreatitis.

Complications

Veno-occlusive disease is a major risk factor for renal failure, cardiac enlargement, respiratory insufficiency, septicemia, neurologic symptoms, and intestinal bleeding. The cause of death in patients with severe veno-occlusive disease is usually not fulminant hepatic failure but rather multiorgan failure. Fungal liver infections are more frequent in patients with severe veno-occlusive disease.

Treatment & Prognosis

Several approaches have been used to prevent veno-occlusive disease. Using lower dosages of conditioning therapy will result in less disease, but the risk of recurrence of the underlying cancer is then increased. Some centers use liver shielding during total body irradiation for patients at high risk for severe veno-occlusive disease. When busulfan is part of the conditioning regimen, individualized dosages based on pharmacokinetic measurements from the first dose result in less veno-occlusive disease. Some centers use prophylactic heparin infusions, because microthromboses are part of the histologic findings in veno-occlusive disease; evidence supporting this treatment is contradictory, however.

Treatment of established veno-occlusive disease is largely supportive. Minimizing the amount of retained fluid will lessen cardiac and pulmonary congestion and the volume of ascites. Limiting sodium intake and increasing urinary sodium excretion with diuretics will accomplish this goal, but in patients with severe veno-occlusive disease, it is often difficult to maintain a negative sodium balance without resorting to hemodialysis or hemofiltration. Uncontrolled experience with thrombolytic therapy suggests a role for this treatment in patients with severe veno-occlusive disease. Fatal bleeding has been described in marrow transplantation patients who have received thrombolytic therapy. Liver transplantation has been undertaken in some patients with severe veno-occlusive disease, but there are no reports of long-term survivors.

Of patients who develop veno-occlusive disease, 75% recover spontaneously, usually by day 30–40 following transplantation, and 25% have a more severe illness associated with multiorgan failure and death. Patients whose course will be severe can be identified soon after the clinical onset, because they gain weight more rapidly and become more deeply jaundiced than those who recover.

FUNGAL LIVER INFECTION

Fungal liver abscesses are sequela of fungal infections of the bloodstream. *Candida* species are the usual cause, but unusual fungi and molds can also be seen. Major risk factors include granulocytopenia, colonization or superficial infection with fungi, deep fungal infection (particularly bloodstream infections), and the presence of severe liver disease caused by veno-occlusive disease and graft-versus-host disease. The most common portal of entry for fungi is the intestine, which allows yeast forms to pass directly into the portal circulation.

Fungal infection isolated to the liver occurs in less than 10% of marrow transplantation patients; most infected patients have fungal lesions in other organs (spleen, kidneys, lungs) as well. The presence of widespread visceral infection is a result of heavy colonization with fungi in a patient whose granulocyte counts are low.

Fungal liver abscesses may be found incidentally at surgery and autopsy, usually in patients who are receiving high-dosage prednisone for treatment of acute graft-versus-host disease.

Clinical Findings

A. Symptoms and Signs: Persistent fever may be the only sign. Hepatomegaly and pain in the liver are signs of extensive fungal infiltration.

B. Diagnostic Studies: In marrow transplantation patients, the diagnosis of fungal infection is difficult because of a high frequency of liver dysfunction and fever that is unrelated to infection, and the unreliability of imaging studies (CT, X-ray, and ultrasound studies are only 20–30% sensitive). If imaging studies are positive, however, fungal abscesses will be found more than 90% of the time. Diagnosis is often based on evidence of persistent colonization with fungi or prior fungal sepsis and a compatible clinical picture. Definitive diagnosis requires study of liver tissue via fine-needle aspiration or open biopsy.

Serum alkaline phosphatase levels rise progressively in the presence of untreated infection. Signs and symptoms of fungal infection and positive culture results of the intestine, spleen, kidneys, lungs, and heart point to liver infection.

Differential Diagnosis

The differential diagnosis of painful hepatomegaly includes veno-occlusive disease, right heart failure, and tumor infiltration. A common problem is deciding whether a defect on CT scanning, X-ray, or ultrasound studies represents fungal infection, tumor in the liver, or a preexisting lesion such as a liver cyst, hemangioma, or focal fibrosis, and whether the defect is related to signs and symptoms.

Complications

If the diagnosis is not made and the patient not treated, *Candida* lesions may coalesce and grow into the biliary ducts and gallbladder. *Aspergillus* and *Mucor* species may invade the hepatic veins to cause Budd-Chiari syndrome and may extend beyond the liver capsule. These are rare events.

Treatment & Prognosis

Prevention of fungal liver infection is based on four strategies: prevention of colonization with fungi, prompt treatment of superficial fungal infections (especially those involving the oropharynx and esophagus), treatment of fungal bloodstream infections with intravenous amphotericin, and restoration of granulocyte function. Fluconazole has proved to be effective in preventing visceral infections caused by *Candida albicans* in marrow transplantation patients, but there may be emergence of *Candida* species resistant to this agent. Oral, nonabsorbable antifungal agents (nystatin, clotrimazole, amphotericin) and new transplantation strategies to restore granulocyte counts more rapidly may affect the current problem with visceral fungal infection. Fungal liver abscesses are treated with intravenous amphotericin. The end-point of therapy may be ill-defined, because filling defects seen on imaging studies may persist despite eradication of fungal elements from the liver.

Treatment is usually successful if granulocyte counts return to normal and immunosuppressive drug dosages can be minimized. Patients with fungal liver infection almost never die because of liver infection; rather, they die because of the persistence of the underlying diseases that led to the infection. In rare patients, the liver fungi become encapsulated by fibrous material and cause no clinical signs or symptoms, despite the presence of viable fungi within these lesions. Immunosuppressive drugs may activate such lesions.

CHOLANGITIS LENTA (CHOLESTASIS CAUSED BY SEPSIS)

Jaundice may develop after prolonged fever or infection distant from the liver. Although earlier reports implicated bacterial cell wall components and endotoxin, recent evidence points to the inflammatory response, particularly the cytokine interleukin-6, as leading to cholestatic liver injury.

Clinical Findings

A. Symptoms and Signs: Cholangitis lenta is probably a common cause of mild jaundice in febrile marrow transplantation patients but an unusual cause of severe jaundice. It occurs after fungal or bacterial infections.

The presentation is usually that of hyperbilirubinemia that follows persistent fever or sepsis syndrome by days or weeks. Liver synthetic function is preserved, and there is no evidence of liver failure.

B. Diagnostic Studies: There may be elevation of serum alkaline phosphatase levels and a rise in total serum bilirubin levels to 15 mg/dL when cholangitis lenta occurs in isolation. When it occurs in patients who already have liver dysfunction, serum bilirubin levels may rise to more than 50 mg/dL. Liver biopsy shows either pericentral canalicular cholestasis or periportal ductular cholestasis, but the portal inflammation often seen with this condition in septic patients may be absent in marrow transplantation patients. In many cases, this diagnosis is made in retrospect.

Differential Diagnosis

The diseases that lead to isolated hyperbilirubinemia in this setting include hemolytic anemia, veno-occlusive disease of the liver, graft-versus-host disease, drug-induced cholestasis (especially with cyclosporine), and liver injury related to total parenteral nutrition.

Complications

There are no complications from this form of cholestasis per se. If graft-versus-host disease is mistaken for sepsis-related cholestasis and high-dosage immunosuppressive therapy is begun in error, the patient may have an adverse course.

Treatment & Prognosis

There is no specific treatment other than treatment of the underlying infection. Patient outcomes are related to immune competence and control of the underlying infection.

ACUTE GRAFT-VERSUS-HOST DISEASE

Graft-versus-host disease results from infusion of alloimmune lymphoid cells into a host that is unable to reject them. Epithelial cells of small bile ducts, hepatocytes in zone 1 of the liver acinus, and periductular glandular epithelial cells are the target cells of graft-versus-host disease. Necrosis of target cells in the liver occurs by apoptosis, or programmed cell death, a result of cell-to-cell interaction between lymphoid cells and target cells. The molecular events leading to apoptosis in graft-versus-host disease are not well understood. Release of cytokines, both locally and systemically, is a cause of tissue damage and symptoms.

Clinical Findings

A. Symptoms and Signs: In the marrow transplantation setting, hepatic graft-versus-host disease occurs exclusively in recipients of allogeneic marrow or stem cell infusions, often in conjunction with the development of a skin rash and intestinal symptoms (nausea, vomiting, anorexia, diarrhea, and pain) caused by acute graft-versus-host disease. Diagnosis of acute disease is frequently made on clinical grounds, that is, the onset or worsening of jaundice in proximity to skin and gut symptoms, plus the exclusion of infectious causes of this clinical picture. Hepatic graft-versus-host disease can develop without apparent skin and gut disease, but this is unusual. The average time of onset of acute graft-versus-host disease is day 19; it may be earlier if the patient has not received prophylactic medications or later if prophylaxis has been effective.

B. Diagnostic Studies: Progressive elevations of serum bilirubin, transaminases (usually ≤ 10 times the upper limit of normal), and alkaline phosphatase (2–10 times normal) are characteristic. Liver biopsy may be needed to determine whether graft-versus-host disease is present. Histologic findings of acute disease include necrosis and dropout of epithelial cells of small bile ducts, mild hepatocyte necrosis, and cholestasis. In severe cases, one sees portal areas devoid of recognizable small bile ducts.

In recipients of allogeneic marrow, particularly when there is an HLA-mismatched or unrelated donor, liver graft-versus-host disease is always under consideration in the jaundiced patient. The diagnosis of hepatic graft-versus-host disease is not difficult when it develops in skin, gut, and liver at day 19 following transplantation. Recognition of graft-versus-host disease in the liver can be difficult when a patient already has significant liver disease (eg, veno-occlusive disease and cholangitis lenta) at the time graft-versus-host disease starts, or when the onset of graft-versus-host disease is concurrent with the onset of sepsis and multiorgan failure.

Total serum bilirubin and alkaline phosphatase measurements usually rise in parallel, but in some cases, early elevations of transaminase enzymes or only alkaline phosphatase are seen. Skin lesions, gut symptoms, and fever are present in typical cases. The liver may be slightly enlarged and tender. The disease is primarily cholestatic; in the early phases of graft-versus-host disease, liver failure and ascites are absent. Bilirubin elevations occur rapidly when graft-versus-host disease develops in the presence of veno-occlusive disease. When hemolysis or renal failure develops in patients with graft-versus-host disease, the level of serum bilirubin may exceed 50–60 mg/dL.

Differential Diagnosis

From day 7–20, the differential diagnosis includes veno-occlusive disease, cholangitis lenta, fungal liver infection, and liver injury caused by drugs. After day 20, veno-occlusive disease becomes less of a consideration but can obscure the onset of graft-versus-host disease of the liver if present previously. From day 20–60, cholangitis lenta, fungal liver infection, liver injury caused by drugs, extrahepatic obstruction caused by biliary sludge, and viral infections with herpes viruses or adenovirus are considerations. After day 60, engraftment is usually more advanced and infections less common, but viral hepatitis B and C may appear after restoration of cell-mediated immunity. At all times, the major difficulty is determining which combination of liver disorders is present, not which single disease.

Complications

Hepatic graft-versus-host disease, while prognostically important, is not a common cause of liver failure. The complications relate both to the destruction of target organs and the severe immunosuppression that results from the disease itself and the medications used to treat it. The most common cause of death is infection. Prolonged, unremitting hepatic graft-versus-host disease may lead to portal hypertension and ascites.

Treatment & Prognosis

Prevention of graft-versus-host disease is important because treatment of severe multisystem graft-versus-host disease is usually futile. Prevention strategies include better donor-host genetic matches, depletion of donor T lymphocytes, and pharmacologic modulation of the grafted marrow with drugs (usually combinations of cyclosporine, methotrexate, prednisone, FK-506 (tacrolimus), and antilymphocyte antibodies).

Treatment of acute graft-versus-host disease is usually with prednisone, 2 mg/kg/d, in addition to the prophylactic medications being given. The approach to treatment failures varies among centers; some increase the prednisone dosage to 4–8 mg/kg/d, and others give antithymocyte globulin. Experimental therapies under current study include modulation of cytokine effects and targeting of putative lymphoid effector cells with specific antibodies. Because hepatic graft-versus-host disease is primarily a cholestatic process, ursodiol can be given at 12–15 mg/kg/d.

Treatment of acute graft-versus-host disease is successful 50–75% of the time, depending on the degree of donor-host genetic disparity and the success of delivery of prophylactic drugs. Persistent hepatic involvement with graft-versus-host disease is an independent predictor of a fatal outcome, usually from sepsis. Acute disease is a risk factor for chronic graft-versus-host disease of the liver.

BILIARY SLUDGE DISEASE

The combination of cytoreductive therapy, prolonged gallbladder stasis resulting from the patient's inability to eat, and increased biliary excretion of precipitable material (calcium bilirubinate, cyclosporine, antibiotics) leads to a 60–70% prevalence of sonolucent gallbladder sludge by day 14. The exfoliation of mucus-containing cells from the gallbladder mucosa caused by cytoreductive therapy may provide nucleating material. Symptoms may result when gallbladder sludge is lodged in the cystic duct, common bile duct, or ampulla of Vater.

Clinical Findings

A. Symptoms and Signs: Postprandial epigastric pain, nausea, and vomiting are typical symptoms of the passage of common bile duct sludge; they may last for 7–10 days before resolution. Jaundice is unusual, but transient increases in liver enzymes may occur. Acute pancreatitis is heralded by the onset of steady abdominal pain.

B. Diagnostic Studies: Ultrasound studies of the gallbladder in asymptomatic patients will often reveal sludge and thickening of the gallbladder wall. A careful history is therefore more useful than ultrasound in deciding when symptoms are caused by biliary sludge. The diagnosis of cholecystitis in the marrow transplantation setting may also depend on the history and physical findings, unless gallbladder imaging gives unequivocal evidence of mucosal necrosis, perforation, or gas in the gallbladder wall. The diagnosis of common bile duct obstruction and pancreatitis depends on demonstrating common bile duct dilatation and elevations of pancreatic amylase and lipase enzymes.

Because so many patients have gallbladder sludge after transplantation, the usefulness of gallbladder imaging as a diagnostic tool in patients with vague symptoms is questionable. The eventual elimination of sludge from the gallbladder, brought on by eating, sometimes leads to biliary symptoms and pancreatitis. In most patients, these are transient problems that are not life-threatening.

Differential Diagnosis

The abrupt onset of abdominal pain during the period from day 20–35 can be due to acute graft-versus-host disease, infectious enteritis, liver abscess, intestinal perforation, or acute pancreatitis. Cholecystitis may also be caused by infections (cytomegalovirus, fungal invasion) and pancreatitis by viral infections and drug toxicity.

Complications

Although severe symptoms can occur, most patients have a self-limited illness. Acute cholecystitis is a relatively unusual event, despite the presence of sludge. Acute pancreatitis occurs sporadically; some cases are severe, especially if extensive retroperitoneal bleeding occurs because of thrombocytopenia.

Treatment & Prognosis

Supportive care and analgesia usually suffice, because the gallbladder empties itself of most of its sludge with continued eating. The duration of symptoms is 1–10 days.

The prognosis is usually good, although cholecystitis and pancreatitis can present problems.

LIVER INJURY INDUCED BY DRUG TOXICITY OR TOTAL PARENTERAL NUTRITION

The major drug toxicity is caused by cytoreductive therapy (see veno-occlusive disease, above). Other drugs may cause hepatotoxicity in a dose-dependent manner (methotrexate, cyclosporine), but the dosages used in the transplantation setting seldom cause clinically evident liver damage. Cyclosporine interferes with canalicular excretion of bile at the cellular level at therapeutic doses. The reactions to other drugs are idiosyncratic (see Chapter 44).

Clinical Findings

The usual guilt-by-association diagnosis of drug-induced liver injury is difficult to prove in a setting where there are so many other causes of hepatic disease (Table 49–2). High blood levels of cyclosporine may give some insight into unexplained serum aspartate aminotransferase (AST) or alanine aminotransferase (ALT) elevation. Transient elevations of AST may follow use of methotrexate. Drugs that are known to cause idiosyncratic injury can be discontinued in problematic cases. Liver histologic studies are seldom helpful in this setting.

Table 49–2. Drugs that may cause liver injury in the marrow transplant setting.

Drug	Pattern of Liver Injury	Diagnostic Features
Cytoreductive therapy	Venular lesions, hepatocyte necrosis, fibrosis	Hepatomegaly, weight gain, jaundice
Cyclosporine	Cholestasis (pharmacologic doses), hepatocyte necrosis (high blood levels)	Hyperbilirubinemia, elevated serum transaminases (high blood levels)
Methotrexate	Hepatocyte necrosis	Transient elevations in transaminase enzymes
Biologicals (antithymocyte globulin, interleukin-2, interferon-alpha, anti-T-lymphocyte antibodies)	Hepatocyte necrosis	Elevations in transaminase enzymes
Trimethoprim-sulfamethoxazole	Cholestasis or hepatocyte necrosis	Elevations of transaminase enzymes, alkaline phosphatase
Mezlocillin	Hepatocyte necrosis	Elevations of transaminase enzymes
Fluconazole, itraconazole	Hepatocyte necrosis	Elevations of transaminase enzymes
Ceftriaxone	Gallbladder sludge	Biliary symptoms

Evidence of hepatocyte necrosis and cholestatic liver disease can be seen in serum liver enzymes. With some medications such as trimethoprim-sulfamethoxazole, anorexia and nausea may accompany liver toxicity.

Differential Diagnosis

All of the liver disorders discussed in the preceding sections must be considered.

Complications

In general, drugs are an uncommon cause of severe liver disease in the transplantation setting. Continued use of a toxic drug, however, may cause progressive liver damage.

Treatment & Prognosis

The treatment is discontinuation of the offending drug. Unless a toxic drug is continued despite ongoing liver injury, the outcome is usually good.

LIVER INFECTION WITH BACTERIA

Bacteria reach the liver via the bloodstream or the bile ducts. Mycobacteria may exist in the liver in a latent form before transplantation and become active while immunosuppressive therapy is being given.

Clinical Findings

A. Symptoms and Signs: Pyogenic bacterial abscesses present with fever and painful hepatomegaly. There is usually a history of septicemia or biliary infection. Mycobacterial infections are activated from latency and present in a more subtle manner, with fever, anorexia, and hepatomegaly.

B. Diagnostic Studies: Liver abscesses are identified by imaging tests showing characteristic lesions in the liver parenchyma; directed needle aspiration may be necessary to identify the organism. Mycobacterial infections cause granulomas in the liver but seldom gross abscesses; skin tests before transplantation may or may not identify patients at risk,

depending on the level of immunity. Liver biopsy is needed for diagnosis of mycobacterial infection, unless the organisms are found elsewhere (marrow, lungs).

Pyogenic bacterial liver abscesses are rare in the transplantation setting, probably because of empiric use of antibiotics for fever. Mycobacterial infections (*M tuberculosis, M avium* complex, bacille Calmette-Guérin) are likewise rare, because screening before transplantation identifies most patients at risk.

Differential Diagnosis

Bacterial liver abscesses are greatly outnumbered by fungal lesions, which usually involve the kidneys and spleen as well as the liver. Lesions seen on liver imaging studies that could be confused with abscesses include cysts, hemangiomas, and tumor nodules. Mycobacterial infections have a broader differential diagnosis that encompasses cholestatic liver diseases such as graft-versus-host disease, cytomegalovirus hepatitis, and liver injury caused by drugs.

Complications

Pyogenic infections are usually a manifestation of granulocytopenia and uncontrolled sepsis, which is the usual cause of death. Unrecognized mycobacterial infections cause inanition and marrow failure.

Treatment & Prognosis

Broad-spectrum antibiotics are used to treat bacterial infection. Antimycobacterial therapy depends on the organism identified by biopsy.

Uncontrolled bacterial infections are fatal. Mycobacterial infections can be effectively treated if host immunity recovers.

EPSTEIN-BARR VIRUS LYMPHOPROLIFERATIVE DISEASE

This is a disease seen in patients who have received prolonged immunosuppressive therapy, usually to treat acute graft-versus-host disease, and in recipients of T-lymphocyte depleted donor marrow. Epstein-Barr virus infection of lymphoid cells transforms them into immunoblasts that infiltrate tissues.

Clinical Findings

A. Symptoms and Signs: Liver involvement is characterized by rapidly progressive hepatomegaly and abdominal pain. Infiltration of other organs occurs in parallel. Fever is common.

B. Diagnostic Studies: The diagnosis is suggested by the clinical situation and clinical findings. Liver imaging tests may show a diffuse infiltrative process. Tissue biopsy of affected organs (eg, liver, intestine, lymph nodes, lungs) is required for diagnosis. The morphologic characteristics of the infiltrative process are usually diagnostic, although there can be difficulty in differentiating an intense inflammatory response from this lymphoma-like process.

Differential Diagnosis

Rapidly progressive infiltrative liver lesions are unusual; the only common cause is recurrent malignant tumors. Unrecognized fungal infection and fatty liver could be mistaken for lymphoproliferative disease.

Complications

This is usually a progressive, lymphoma-like illness that leads to death.

Treatment & Prognosis

Until recently, discontinuation of immunosuppressive drugs was the only treatment that could be offered, and that was usually unsuccessful. Successful treatment with infusion of donor T cells has been reported. This form of therapy may in turn cause severe acute graft-versus-host disease.

Most cases have been rapidly fatal, except for those treated with donor T cell infusions.

MALIGNANT CELLS IN THE LIVER

When conditioning therapy given to eradicate malignant cells is not successful, recurrent tumor may involve the liver, whether or not there was liver involvement at the start of therapy. In rare instances, there may be contamination of autologous marrow or peripheral blood stem cells with tumor cells; infusion of these cells following conditioning therapy may lead to liver seeding.

Recurrent tumor in the liver should be considered when the original malignant tumor involved the liver or when the indication for transplantation was a leukemia with a propensity to recur.

Clinical Findings

Progressive hepatomegaly, elevation of serum alkaline phosphatase measurements, and signs of portal hypertension may be early indications of recurrent

tumor in the liver. There may also be evidence of recurrent tumor in the marrow and other organ systems.

Clinical signs and symptoms lead to imaging studies (CT or MR) that show filling defects if the tumor burden is large. Directed needle aspiration cytology or biopsy is useful if positive; however, recurrent tumor in the liver may be microscopic and focal. Detection of tumor cells in other sites (particularly marrow) makes the identification of liver tumor of little additional value.

Differential Diagnosis

Most recurrences of tumor occur beyond day 50. The differential diagnosis includes fungal liver infection, graft-versus-host disease, constrictive pericarditis, Epstein-Barr virus lymphoproliferative disease, nodular regenerative hyperplasia, and persistent veno-occlusive disease.

Complications

Rapid growth of tumor may result in portal hypertension and ascites, but liver metastases are not the usual cause of illness in patients with recurrent malignant tumors.

Treatment & Prognosis

No treatment is available in most cases. The outcome is poor.

NODULAR REGENERATIVE HYPERPLASIA

The pathogenesis of nodule formation in the liver is unknown, but most authors speculate that vascular injury precedes the formation of hyperplastic nodules. This lesion has been described following conventional chemotherapy as well as after marrow transplantation.

Nodular hyperplasia is probably not a major cause of clinical liver disease in marrow transplantation patients but can be found at autopsy. It could be responsible for signs of portal hypertension that are seen months after transplantation.

Clinical Findings

Portal hypertension, hepatorenal syndrome, and ascites, occurring months after transplantation, can be due to nodular regenerative hyperplasia. Esophageal varices are rare.

Inspection of the surface of the liver is useful, as there are multiple small nodules (usually < 5 mm in diameter) diffusely present in the liver. Imaging studies may fail to detect nodularity. Definitive diagnosis requires a large liver biopsy; the nodules are encircled by bands of collapsed reticulin. Reticulin and antitrypsin staining may be useful.

Differential Diagnosis

Veno-occlusive disease is the major cause of portal hypertension after transplantation. Cirrhosis of the liver has a similar appearance on gross inspection, but histologic studies show fibrosis rather than collapsed reticulin.

Complications

It is difficult to define a symptom complex or complications that result from nodular regenerative hyperplasia alone in these patients.

Treatment & Prognosis

Portacaval shunts are often curative in non-marrow transplantation patients whose portal hypertension is problematic. The overall prognosis is good, because liver function is preserved.

ACUTE VIRAL HEPATITIS

Hepatitis viruses B and C can be transmitted from marrow donors but more commonly have been acquired from previously given blood products. These viruses replicate after conditioning therapy and circulate in high titers immediately following transplantation, but do not appear to cause liver injury until after the immune system is reconstituted. Some of the viruses that infect the liver in the transplantation setting cause hepatocyte necrosis in the absence of lymphocytes (eg, adenovirus, varicella-zoster virus, herpes simplex virus). Cytomegalovirus causes microabscesses in the liver and can infect the biliary epithelium. Epstein-Barr virus may cause a lymphoma-like illness (see above).

The viral infections that cause fulminant hepatitis usually occur soon after conditioning therapy has ablated the immune system, or during immunosuppressive treatment of acute graft-versus-host disease. Fortunately, effective prophylaxis with acyclovir and ganciclovir has almost eliminated infection with herpes group viruses in this setting, leaving adenovirus as the most common cause of fulminant viral hepatitis. Despite high viral titers, the hepatitis viruses B and C do not appear to be a cause of hepatitis in the first 30–60 days following transplantation.

Clinical Findings

Table 49–3 shows the major diagnostic features of infection with the most frequent viral causes of liver injury. Because most of these infections are caused by reactivation of latent viruses, it is important to review pre-bone-marrow-transplant serologic studies (herpes simplex virus, cytomegalovirus, varicella-zoster virus, hepatitis B or C virus) to identify these latent viruses; however, false-negative serologic findings can be seen in immune-deficient transplantation candidates and false-positive findings in patients who are receiving immune globulin. Diagnosis of pre-bone-marrow-transplant infection with hepatitis B or C virus may require detection of hepatitis B

virus DNA or hepatitis C virus RNA. Posttransplantation infection with adenovirus, herpes simplex virus, or varicella-zoster virus is heralded by rapid rises in serum transaminases to over 1000 IU/L, with clinical deterioration and death in 2–10 days in severe cases. Although these viruses commonly cause hepatic necrosis as part of a disseminated disease, liver involvement can be the initial presentation. Liver biopsy and immunohistologic searching for viral antigens in liver tissue comprise the ultimate diagnostic test. Almost all cases of posttransplantation hepatitis B and C can be predicted by examining the pre-bone-marrow-transplant hepatitis virus status of both patient and donor. Rarely, hepatitis B virus is present in the liver in the absence of serum antigen, antibody, or DNA. Posttransplantation determination of hepatitis B virus antigens and DNA and hepatitis C virus RNA is reliable, but antibody detection is inaccurate.

Differential Diagnosis

Other diseases that present with transaminase elevation before day 60 are veno-occlusive disease (where the serum AST may rarely rise to 2000–10,000 IU/L), acute graft-versus-host disease (where the serum AST may range to 1200 IU/L in severe cases), liver injury caused by drugs, and liver ischemia related to septic shock or low cardiac output states. Severe veno-occlusive disease and graft-versus-host disease are usually clinically obvious, but their presence does not preclude a viral infection. The differential diagnosis of hepatitis after day 60 is narrower; it includes flare-ups of acute graft-versus-host disease during attempts at tapering immunosuppressive therapy, de novo onset of chronic graft-versus-host disease (see below), and liver injury caused by drugs. Discerning the cause of rising liver enzymes following the tapering of doses of immunosuppressive drugs can be difficult when both graft-versus-host disease and hepatitis B or C are present, because all of these diseases respond similarly. Higher alkaline phosphatase levels and more extensive bile duct destruction on liver biopsy favor graft-versus-host disease.

Complications

Fulminant hepatitis and death are major but rare complications of viral liver infection. Viral hepatitis in a liver already affected by veno-occlusive disease or graft-versus-host disease may also lead to a fatal outcome. Reactivation or acquisition of hepatitis B or C leads to chronic hepatitis in high frequency among patients, but a small number of fulminant cases has also been described.

Treatment & Prognosis

Prevention of viral infection is outlined in Table 49–3. Effective prophylaxis is limited to those viruses that are sensitive to acyclovir or ganciclovir.

Table 49–3. Viruses that infect the liver in marrow transplantation patients.

Virus	Presentation in Transplantation Patients	Diagnosis	Prevention	Treatment
Adenovirus	Fulminant hepatitis	Rapidly rising transaminases Gut, lung, urinary infection Viral cultures Liver histologic studies and culture	None for latent infection Hand washing, avoidance of infected visitors, for primary infection	None proved Ribavirin and ganciclovir have antiviral activity Immune globulin, donor T lymphocyte infusions may be effective
Varicella zoster virus	Fulminant hepatitis	Rapidly rising transaminases Skin lesions Abdominal pain common Viral cultures Liver histologic studies and culture	Acyclovir	Acyclovir
Herpes simplex virus	Fulminant hepatitis	Rapidly rising transaminase levels Skin lesions Viral cultures Liver histologic studies and culture	Acyclovir	Acyclovir
Cytomegalovirus	Mild abnormalities of liver enzymes	Cytomegalovirus disease usually obvious in lungs, gut Viral cultures Liver histologic studies (microabscesses)	Ganciclovir, for latent infection Cytomegalovirus seronegative blood products ± ganciclovir, for primary infection	Ganciclovir Foscarnet
Hepatitis B virus	Acute hepatitis, rarely fulminant	Pre-BMT presence of hepatitis B virus or anti-HBVc or hepatitis B–positive donor Transaminase elevations after day 60 HBsAg, hepatitis B virus DNA Liver histologic studies	Infusion of marrow from donor immune to hepatitis B virus	None proved
Hepatitis C virus	Acute hepatitis, rarely fulminant	Pre-BMT presence of hepatitis C virus RNA or hepatitis C–positive donor Transaminase elevations after day 60 Hepatitis C virus RNA Liver histologic studies	Treatment of donor with IFN α pre-BMT	None proved

There is evidence that transplantation of marrow from a donor who is immune to hepatitis B virus (because of vaccination or prior exposure) will allow a hepatitis B virus-infected patient to clear the virus. A clinical suspicion of fulminant viral hepatitis caused by varicella-zoster virus or herpes simplex virus should lead to empiric acyclovir therapy before the final diagnosis is available. Adenovirus hepatitis may be treated with ribavirin, ganciclovir, immune globulin, or donor T cell infusions, but clinical experience with these agents is limited. Hepatitis B or C that appears following tapering of immunosuppressive drugs can be treated by increased dosages of these drugs, which may slow the course of hepatitis. There is little published experience with this strategy or with interferon-α therapy in this setting.

Adenovirus, herpes simplex virus, and varicella-zoster virus hepatitis may be fatal unless diagnosed and treated early. Cytomegalovirus hepatitis is usually seen only with disseminated cytomegalovirus disease, and the liver disease is almost never severe. Posttransplantation hepatitis B and C are frequently asymptomatic or clinically mild, but fulminant cases have been reported. There is a high frequency of chronic hepatitis and cirrhosis among long-term survivors of transplantation who are infected with hepatitis B or C virus.

LIVER DISEASES IN LONG-TERM MARROW TRANSPLANTATION SURVIVORS

With increasing intervals from the day of transplantation, the prevalence of liver dysfunction is reduced and the differential diagnosis of liver disease narrows (Table 49–4).

CHRONIC GRAFT-VERSUS-HOST DISEASE

Chronic graft-versus-host disease of the liver can be an insidious process leading to prolonged cholestasis, or an abrupt process that rapidly destroys small bile ducts. Chronic disease affects many organs in the body and is associated with profound immunodeficiency; unless recognized and treated aggressively, it can lead to death.

Chronic graft-versus-host disease may follow acute graft-versus-host disease, or may appear after acute disease has resolved, or may appear de novo. Chronic graft-versus-host disease has many autoimmune features and is caused by abnormalities of both cellular and humoral immunity only in recipients of allogeneic donor marrow infusions.

Clinical Findings

A. Symptoms and Signs: Although liver involvement can be seen as an isolated finding, it is more common to find dry eyes, oral mucositis, and skin involvement, along with liver disease. In the early phases, elevated serum alkaline phosphatase levels may be the only abnormality, but most patients become jaundiced unless treated. Patients who have a rapid, de novo onset may have elevated serum transaminase levels initially.

Table 49–4. Overview of liver diseases in long-term survivors of marrow transplantation.

Hepatic Disease	Risk Factors
Chronic graft-versus-host disease	Allogeneic marrow graft recipient Prior acute graft-versus-host disease Unrelated or mismatched marrow donor
Chronic viral hepatitis	Serologic or virologic evidence of hepatitis B or C virus before or after transplantation Hepatitis C virus RNA–positive marrow donor Hepatitis B virus–seropositive marrow donor
Malignant cells in the liver	Pretransplantation malignant disease Transplantation in leukemic relapse Secondary cancer

B. Diagnostic Studies: Elevations of serum alkaline phosphatase and bilirubin are characteristic of liver involvement with chronic graft-versus-host disease. When these are seen in a patient with clinically obvious lacrimal gland, oral, and skin involvement, a clinical diagnosis can be made. Definitive diagnosis requires liver biopsy. Histologic features include abnormal, small bile ducts (leading to ductopenia), lymphoid infiltration of the epithelium, and cholestasis.

Differential Diagnosis

Viral hepatitis C may mimic mild chronic graft-versus-host disease, because both diseases cause mild elevations of serum transaminase measurements and histologic abnormalities of small bile ducts; both may also respond to immunosuppressive therapy with decreased levels of serum liver enzymes. Serum alkaline phosphatase elevations are likely to be higher in chronic graft-versus-host disease, especially if the disease is severe. Cholestatic liver injury caused by drugs, biliary tract disease, and, rarely, granulomatous hepatitis should also be considered. When de novo chronic graft-versus-host disease develops rapidly, acute viral hepatitis is also included in the differential diagnosis (varicella zoster virus, herpes simplex virus, hepatitis B and C viruses).

Complications

If left untreated, chronic graft-versus-host disease of the liver may progress to severe cholestatic liver injury and eventually cirrhosis. Immunodeficiency associated with chronic graft-versus-host disease and its treatment predispose patients to fatal bacterial infections.

Treatment & Prognosis

Immunosuppressive therapy, usually with prednisone and cyclosporine, is standard. Other drugs that are in current trials include FK-506 (tacrolimus) and thalidomide. Ursodiol may play a role in modulating the severity of cholestatic injury.

Immunosuppressive therapy is usually successful in damping the activity of this chronic inflammatory disease. Some patients, however, require therapy indefinitely; in others, dosages of immunosuppressive drugs can be tapered without flare-ups of chronic graft-versus-host disease.

CHRONIC VIRAL HEPATITIS

The pathophysiology of hepatitis is discussed in Chapter 36, Viral Hepatitis. In marrow transplantation patients, persistent hepatitis B and C infections are common when chronic graft-versus-host disease is present or immunosuppressive drugs are being given. Some patients who were chronically infected with hepatitis B virus before transplantation have cleared virus after receiving marrow from a donor who was immune to hepatitis B virus.

The prevalence of chronic viral hepatitis in patients who underwent transplantation before 1991 is high but has been reduced considerably since the advent of effective hepatitis C screening of blood products.

Clinical Findings

The presentation and laboratory findings of chronic hepatitis are discussed in Chapters 36 and 37. There may be progression of chronic hepatitis to cirrhosis in marrow transplantation patients over a period of 10–15 years.

Measurement of viral antigens (HBs, HBc) and nucleic acids (hepatitis B virus DNA, hepatitis C virus RNA) is reliable, even when patients are immunodeficient or receiving immune globulin. Liver biopsy is needed when both viral hepatitis and chronic graft-versus-host disease are under consideration. The histologic distinction between hepatitis C and chronic graft-versus-host disease is difficult, because both diseases cause lymphoid infiltration and abnormalities of small bile ducts. Immunosuppressive therapy may alter the histologic appearance of hepatitis C virus infection. In some patients, chronic viral hepatitis and chronic graft-versus-host disease coexist.

Differential Diagnosis

Chronic graft-versus-host disease and drug-induced liver injury are usually the only other considerations.

Complications

Chronic viral hepatitis may lead to cirrhosis. Some of the extrahepatic manifestations could be confused with the autoimmune manifestations of chronic graft-versus-host disease.

Treatment & Prognosis

Although it is known that chronic viral hepatitis may lead to cirrhosis in long-term survivors of marrow transplantation, the frequency of and time to onset of cirrhosis have not been defined in this population.

There is no published experience with antiviral agents in marrow transplantation patients with chronic hepatitis B or C virus. α-Interferon appears to be ineffective in patients who have chronic graft-versus-host disease or who are receiving immunosuppressive therapy. The presence of residual liver iron (from prior transfusions) may affect a patient's response to interferon. Liver transplantation should be considered if incipient liver failure develops.

MALIGNANT CELLS IN THE LIVER

The liver may be a site of recurrence of the original malignant tumor or the appearance of a secondary malignant tumor. The latter is usually lymphoid in origin. The clinical findings and differential diagnosis are the same as during the first 100 days following transplantation (see preceding section).

Some patients with recurrent or secondary cancers have undergone second transplantations; most of the successes with this approach have been in children. The prognosis is poor.

REFERENCES

Bearman SI: The syndrome of hepatic veno-occlusive disease after marrow transplantation. Blood 1995;85:3005.

Flomenberg P et al: Increasing incidence of adenovirus disease in bone marrow transplantation patients. J Infect Dis 1994;169:775.

Forman SJ, Blume KG, Thomas ED (editors): *Bone Marrow Transplantation,* 1/e. Blackwell, 1994.

Johnson JR et al: Hepatitis due to herpes simplex virus in marrow-transplantation recipients. Clin Infect Dis 1992;14:38.

Kanamori H et al: Case report: Fulminant hepatitis C viral infection after bone marrow transplantation. Am J Med Sci 1992;303:109.

Martin PJ et al: A retrospective analysis of therapy for acute graft-versus-host disease: Initial treatment. Blood 1990;76:1464.

McDonald GB et al: Veno-occlusive disease of the liver and multiorgan failure after bone marrow transplantation: A cohort study of 355 patients. Ann Intern Med 1993;118:255.

Papadopoulos EB et al: Infusions of donor leukocytes to treat Epstein-Barr virus–associated lymphoproliferative disorders after allogeneic bone marrow transplantation. N Engl J Med 1994;330:1185.

Rossetti F et al: Fungal liver infection in marrow transplantation patients: Prevalence at autopsy, predisposing factors, and clinical features. Clin Infect Dis 1995;20:801.

Shuhart MC et al: Marrow transplantation from hepatitis C virus seropositive donors: Transmission rate and clinical course. Blood 1994;84:3229.

Shulman HM et al: Utility of transvenous liver biopsies and wedged hepatic venous pressure measurements in sixty marrow transplant recipients. Transplantation 1995;59:1015.

Shulman HM et al: Veno-occlusive disease of the liver after marrow transplantation: Histologic correlates of clinical signs and symptoms. Hepatology 1994;19:1171.

Snover DC et al: Nodular regenerative hyperplasia of the liver following bone marrow transplantation. Hepatology 1989;9:443.

50 Gallstones

Ira M. Jacobson, MD

Cholelithiasis is one of the most common gastrointestinal diseases seen in clinical practice. Most patients with gallstones are asymptomatic. The clinical manifestations of gallstones can include episodic pain, acute inflammation, or obstructive jaundice, cholangitis, and pancreatitis, complications resulting from gallstone migration into the common bile duct.

The clinical approach to gallstones has undergone major revision recently because of the development of laparoscopic cholecystectomy. As a result, pharmacologic and other nonoperative approaches have been relegated to a secondary role. Moreover, the widespread availability of endoscopic retrograde cholangiopancreatography (ERCP) in recent years has dramatically decreased the need for surgical removal of common bile duct stones.

Classification

Gallstones are usually classified as cholesterol or pigment stones, but this is an oversimplification for two reasons. First, stones containing only one component or the other are uncommon. Second, pigment stones can themselves be divided into two major groups with different pathogeneses: Black pigment stones consist of polymers of bilirubin with large amounts of mucin glycoproteins, while calcium salts of unconjugated bilirubin (calcium bilirubinate) make up the chief component of brown pigment stones.

Most gallstones in patients in the United States and Europe are cholesterol rich, often containing mucin glycoproteins in layers alternating with cholesterol crystals. Even cholesterol-rich stones usually contain some degree of bilirubin-derived material, however. A large proportion of gallstones in Asian patients are pigment stones, especially brown pigment stones rich in calcium bilirubinate. These may originate in the gallbladder but may also form as primary bile duct stones. As outlined below, the composition of gallstones in a particular patient can often be linked to specific epidemiologic risk factors.

Pathogenesis

A. Cholesterol Stones: The three main constituents of normal bile are cholesterol, bile salts, and phospholipids, over 90% of which is lecithin. Most biliary cholesterol is derived from de novo hepatic synthesis rather than secretion of dietary cholesterol. The primary bile acids, chenodeoxycholic acid and cholic acid, are secreted into the bile after conjugation in the liver with taurine or glycine. The conjugated primary bile acids are reabsorbed in the terminal ileum via the enterohepatic circulation, and a small proportion is deconjugated by bacteria in the distal bowel. The deconjugated bile acids may themselves be reabsorbed, or they may be dehydroxylated by colonic bacteria, forming the secondary bile acids deoxycholic acid and lithocholic acid. These, in turn, also undergo partial absorption. Bile acids within the enterohepatic circulation down-regulate hepatic bile acid synthesis.

Normally insoluble in aqueous solution, cholesterol depends for its solubility in bile on the formation of mixed micelles containing aggregates of cholesterol, bile acids, and lecithin. Micelle formation is based on the ability of lipid molecules to align themselves so that their hydrophilic regions form the external environment and their hydrophobic regions the internal environment. In addition to micelles, phospholipids and cholesterol in bile form spherical bilayers, or vesicles, in which hydrophobic portions are aligned inward and hydrophilic groups outward. With increasing concentrations of cholesterol in vesicles, the vesicles fuse into multilamellar forms. Cholesterol crystals form on the surface of these multilamellar vesicles, and subsequently nucleate into the solid form.

Essential to cholesterol gallstone formation is the hepatic synthesis of bile with supersaturated cholesterol concentrations. In patients with equivalent degrees of supersaturation, bile will form cholesterol crystals at variable rates; this indicates the existence of other factors that contribute to stone formation. Biliary proteins, including mucous glycoproteins, appear to play a role as promoters of the nucleation of cholesterol crystals. An additional role has been ascribed to impaired gallbladder motility in patients with supersaturated bile, leading to stasis and the promotion of gallstone formation. Other postulated contributing factors for cholesterol gallstone formation include altered gallbladder synthesis of prostaglandins and excessive biliary calcium concentrations.

A precursor to the formation of stones in some patients is biliary sludge, consisting of viscous mucoproteins containing cholesterol crystals. Such sludge may be visible sonographically and may be the only abnormality in patients presenting with biliary pain, pancreatitis, or cholangitis. Since sludge may be a transient finding, particularly in fasting patients, its specificity is somewhat limited. Recent publications have emphasized, however, that sludge is pathogenic in some patients with biliary-related illnesses, particularly pancreatitis, that would otherwise be classified as "idiopathic." When sludge is not visible on sonographic studies in such patients, some investigators collect gallbladder bile by duodenal intubation after stimulating the gallbladder contractility with cholecystokinin. The bile is then analyzed under the light microscope for cholesterol crystals, which, if found, purportedly establish a causal relationship sufficient to warrant cholecystectomy. The value of this approach is not universally accepted, however.

B. Pigment Stones: Black pigment stones form primarily in the gallbladder in patients with cirrhosis or chronic hemolytic diseases such as sickle cell anemia. Brown pigment stones, on the other hand, may form either in the gallbladder or the bile duct; primary bile duct stones are usually of this type. Bacterial infection, the usual cause for the formation of primary bile duct stones, leads to deconjugation of bilirubin by bacterial β-glucuronidases. The deconjugated bilirubin then binds with calcium to form insoluble calcium bilirubinate, which in turn becomes the nidus for primary duct stone formation. Primary bile duct stones are particularly common in Asia, where bacterial contamination of the bile may be attributable to biliary parasites such as *Clonorchis* or other factors not well understood. Brown pigment stones may also form primarily in the gallbladder; this may occur in patients receiving total parenteral nutrition, who commonly have gallbladder stasis.

Epidemiologic Findings

The prevalence of gallstones increases with age (Table 50–1). Gallstones are more prevalent in fe-

males than males in all adult age groups, with ratios exceeding 3:1 in women in their reproductive years and falling to under 2:1 in persons over 70. The gender difference is at least partly due to endogenous estrogens, which inhibit the enzymatic conversion of cholesterol to bile acids, thereby increasing the cholesterol saturation of bile. Pregnancy increases the risk of gallstones, and it is common for women to present with symptomatic gallstones for the first time during pregnancy or shortly thereafter (see Chapter 47). Impaired gallbladder emptying, promoted by progesterone, combines with the influence of estrogens to increase the lithogenesis of bile in pregnancy. Pharmacologically administered estrogens also increase the risk of gallstone formation. Patients with extensive ileitis or a history of ileal resection, in whom the enterohepatic circulation is impaired, have a high risk of cholesterol gallstones because of excess loss of bile acids.

Obese persons have an increased risk of cholesterol gallstones associated with excess biliary cholesterol secretion. Certain ethnic groups are also particularly susceptible, most strikingly the Pima Indians of the western United States, in whom the prevalence is over 75%. The prevalence is also relatively high in other Native Americans. Caucasians in the United States and Europe have a higher prevalence than Asians and Africans, in whom pigment stones have historically been more common. More recently, however, cholesterol stones are increasing in prevalence in Asian and African populations, particularly in Japan, where dietary and life-style patterns have become more westernized.

Clinical Findings

Most people with gallstones (approximately 80%) are asymptomatic. The clinical features in symptomatic patients include episodic pain of variable severity and frequency, acute cholecystitis, and complications related to passage of gallstones into the bile duct, including pain, jaundice, cholangitis, and pancreatitis.

A. Symptoms and Signs:

1. Cystic duct obstruction–Most episodes of gallstone-induced pain occur when a stone transiently obstructs the cystic duct. Pain arising from gallstones is usually felt in the right upper quadrant or epigastrium. With right upper quadrant pain particularly, the pain may radiate around to the right side of the back or the right shoulder. Alternatively, pain perceived by the patient as arising in the midline within the epigastrium may radiate to the right side secondarily. Occasionally, pain may be felt in the substernal area, where it may be mistaken for myocardial ischemia. Pain primarily in the left upper quadrant of the abdomen may sometimes be seen.

Gallstone pain is steady rather than wavelike, cramping, or colicky, and therefore the classic description "biliary colic" is somewhat of a misnomer.

Table 50–1. Risk factors for gallstones.

Increasing age
Female gender
Pregnancy
Estrogens
Obesity
Ethnicity (eg, native Americans)
Cirrhosis
Hemolytic anemia (eg, sickle-cell disease, hereditary spherocytosis)
Total parenteral nutrition

Many patients develop pain between 15 minutes and 2 hours after eating, with fatty foods being the most notorious (but far from universal) offender. Indeed, fatty food intolerance is actually no more common in patients with gallstones than in those with other disorders such as nonulcer dyspepsia. Nevertheless, clinicians regularly see patients with gallstones and classic biliary colic whose episodes are brought on by fatty foods and diminished in frequency by avoiding fatty foods, and whose pain is ultimately alleviated by cholecystectomy. Some patients have pain unrelated to eating.

The duration of an episode of biliary colic pain may range from a few minutes to 1–4 hours or even longer. There may be concomitant nausea with or without vomiting. Nocturnal pain awakening the patient is a common presentation.

Gastrointestinal symptoms in the absence of pain conforming to one of the variants described above should not be attributed to gallstones without considering other diagnoses. For example, belching, heartburn, and bloating might indicate reflux or peptic disease. The discovery of gallstones on imaging studies concomitant with these symptoms does not, therefore, mean that cholecystectomy is indicated.

The physical examination in patients with episodic biliary pain is typically normal between episodes. Right upper quadrant tenderness usually is present only in patients with very frequent episodes and usually indicates significant chronic inflammation of the gallbladder.

2. Acute cholecystitis—In acute cholecystitis, unlike biliary colic, there is sustained obstruction of the cystic duct, producing gallbladder distention and a self-perpetuating inflammatory process involving prostaglandins and other inflammatory mediators. Bacterial infection is probably a secondary event occurring later in the course in some patients. Corresponding to its pathogenesis, the pain of acute cholecystitis is distinguished from that of "biliary colic" by its intensity and persistence for more than several hours. Nausea and vomiting are frequent, and there is localization of the pain in the right upper quadrant. The presence of fever in a patient with protracted biliary pain signifies that the process has transcended "biliary colic" and that cholecystitis or another complication, such as cholangitis or pancreatitis, has supervened.

Physical examination in patients with acute cholecystitis reveals right upper quadrant tenderness often extending into the epigastrium. The classic **Murphy's sign** refers to the presence of marked tenderness and inhibition of inspiration on deep palpation under the right subcostal margin.

Mild to moderate leukocytosis is common in acute cholecystitis. Serum liver tests may be mildly abnormal, but substantial elevations should raise the possibility of bile duct obstruction concomitant with, or instead of, acute cholecystitis. Serum amylase levels usually are normal; again, more than minimal elevations raise the possibility of pancreatitis.

3. Bile duct obstruction—Pain arising from obstruction of the bile duct by a gallstone is similar to the pain of cystic duct obstruction. Patients who have had their gallbladders removed and present for the first time with symptomatic common bile duct stones frequently say the pain reminds them of what they felt before surgery. If obstruction of the bile duct by a stone is of sufficient duration and severity, jaundice may develop. Painless jaundice is less common with stones than with tumors that obstruct the bile duct, but it may occur.

If obstruction of the bile duct is accompanied by infection resulting in cholangitis, fever will be present. The temperature often is higher than in patients with cholecystitis, sometimes exceeding 40 °C. In addition, rigors are far more common with cholangitis than with cholecystitis or pancreatitis. Septic patients with cholangitis are commonly hypotensive. The manifestations of pancreatitis are discussed in detail elsewhere (see Chapter 31).

Physical examination in patients with bile duct obstruction by stones is characterized by less abdominal tenderness than in patients with gallbladder inflammation. Fever or jaundice may be pronounced. Murphy's sign is not present.

Most patients with biliary obstruction from stones have elevated liver enzymes, even if the symptoms are transient. The degree of enzyme elevation far exceeds the levels seen in patients with cystic duct obstruction. In acute bile duct obstruction, alanine aminotransferase (ALT) and aspartate aminotransferase (AST) rise quickly, and may reach or exceed levels 10 times the upper limit of normal. Even if obstruction persists, these enzymes fall rapidly toward normal, while the alkaline phosphatase level progressively rises. Hyperbilirubinemia may not occur if obstruction is transient.

B. Diagnostic Studies:

1. Ultrasonography—Ultrasonography is the critical diagnostic procedure in patients with suspected cholelithiasis; its sensitivity in detecting gallstones is greater than 96%. The characteristic finding is an echogenic focus that casts a shadow (Figure 50–1). The mobility of an echogenic focus may help to distinguish gallstones from other filling defects such as polyps. Ultrasonography also demonstrates gallbladder wall thickness, conformation, and size, which all reflect the presence and degree of acute or chronic inflammation (Figure 50–2). Pericholecystic fluid is a highly specific sign of acute rather than chronic cholecystitis. Ultrasonography can also accurately identify common bile duct dilatation, as well as hepatic or pancreatic parenchymal lesions. Common bile duct stones may be identified by ultrasonography, though the sensitivity is no greater than 50% (Figure 50–3).

2. Oral cholecystography—Ultrasonography

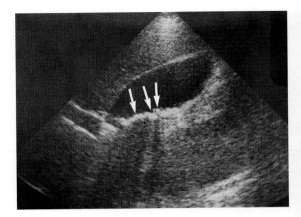

A

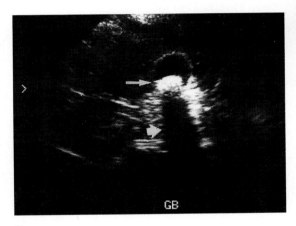

B

Figure 50–1. Sonogram demonstrating multiple small echogenic foci *(arrows)* with shadowing diagnostic of gallstones *(A)*, and single large stone *(thin arrow)* with shadowing *(thick arrow)* in another patient *(B)*.

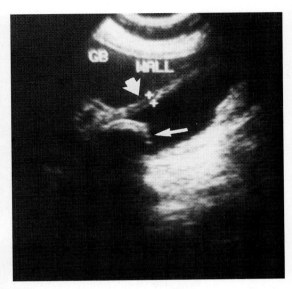

Figure 50–2. Ultrasound demonstrating gallstone in the neck of the gallbladder *(thin arrow)* with thickened gallbladder wall *(thick arrow)*, consistent with acute cholecystitis.

has almost completely replaced oral cholecystography as the initial diagnostic procedure of choice for investigating patients with suspected gallstones, although oral cholecystography may still be valuable in specific situations. It may occasionally detect stones when sonographic studies have been negative, and thus may be appropriate when the clinical suspicion for gallbladder disease is high but sonographic studies have not revealed disease. More commonly, oral cholecystography is useful in assessing patients for nonsurgical therapy of gallstones, because it provides information about gallbladder function, the size and number of gallstones, and gallbladder composition. For example, calcified stones are generally not amenable to dissolution therapy, while small stones that float are likely to be rich in cholesterol and more likely to dissolve.

3. Computed tomography–CT is infrequently used for primary screening for gallstones. It is less sensitive and more expensive than other screening approaches and requires exposure to radiation. CT may, however, reveal gallstones and visualize the biliary system in patients being evaluated for acute abdominal disease or suspected biliary obstruction.

4. ERCP–Endoscopic retrograde cholangiopancreatography (ERCP) reportedly can diagnose gallstones within the gallbladder when noninvasive imaging studies have been negative, but it should rarely if ever be used for this purpose alone if bile duct stones are unlikely.

5. Hepatobiliary scintigraphy–Hepatobiliary scintigraphy is not useful in detecting gallstones, but it is an important procedure in patients with suspected acute cholecystitis. Scintigraphy relies on uptake by the gallbladder of an intravenously administered ^{99m}Tc-labeled iminodiacetic acid (IDA) derivative. The isotope is excreted by the liver into the bile ducts, where it is visualized by gamma counting. Several IDA compounds have been used, including DISIDA, which has the advantage of hepatic uptake even in the presence of hyperbilirubinemia.

Acute cholecystitis is almost always accompanied by cystic duct obstruction. Therefore, a normal DISIDA scan, in which the isotope is seen in the gallbladder within 30–45 minutes, rules out the diagnosis of acute cholecystitis (Figure 50–4). Conversely, failure of the isotope to scan within 4 hours is highly specific for acute cholecystitis (Figure 50–5). The isotope can be seen in intermediate degrees in the gallbladder of patients with chronic

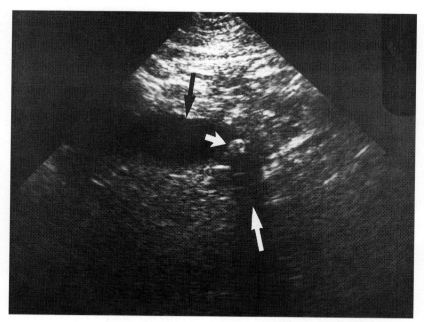

A

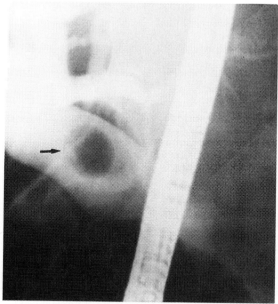

B

Figure 50–3. Ultrasound demonstrating a dilated bile duct with stone *(short arrow)* and shadowing *(long arrow) (A).* ERCP revealed the same findings *(arrow) (B).*

cholecystitis who have partial cystic duct obstruction, a contracted gallbladder, or stasis due to prolonged fasting.

Some clinicians additionally rely upon DISIDA scanning to evaluate patients with suspected bile duct obstruction, but the author's experience does not support the use of this procedure routinely.

Differential Diagnosis

The differential diagnosis of gallstone-related pain includes peptic ulcer disease, gastroesophageal reflux, esophageal dysmotility, nonulcer dyspepsia, irritable bowel syndrome, renal colic, and cardiac disease (Tables 50–2 and 50–3).

The pain of peptic ulcer disease is usually more

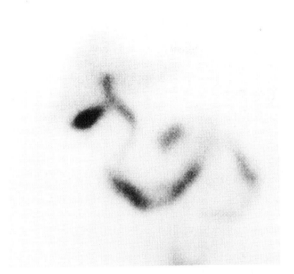

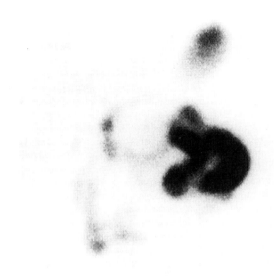

Figure 50–4. DISIDA scan showing normal gallbladder uptake within 30 minutes, ruling out acute cholecystitis.

A

frequent, even occurring daily, and may be relieved by eating, a characteristic almost never shared by gallstone-related pain. Conversely, ulcer pain rarely conforms to the episodic pattern of distinct attacks caused by gallstones. Occasionally, patients with gallbladder disease have a steady ache in the right upper quadrant, but this presentation is less common.

Reflux symptoms are readily distinguished from biliary pain by their burning quality, substernal location, and occasional positional dependence (with symptoms worsening when the patient is supine). Regurgitation is common, and symptoms are usually relieved with antacids or acid-suppressive therapy.

The term **nonulcer dyspepsia** encompasses a variety of symptoms and underlying causes, not all well defined (see Chapter 22). Gastroduodenal dysmotility and gastritis or duodenitis may each contribute. When nonulcer dyspepsia includes epigastric pain, the distinction from gallstone-related pain can be difficult. Nonetheless, biliary pain is distinguished by its sporadic nature, greater intensity, and pattern of radiation to the right upper quadrant or right shoulder. Nocturnal awakenings are uncharacteristic of nonulcer dyspepsia or irritable bowel syndrome, and alterations or irregularities in bowel habits are features of irritable bowel syndrome but not biliary pain. Renal colic may produce pain that predominates in the anterior abdomen rather than the more characteristic location in the back or flank. When renal colic is suspected, urinalysis and imaging studies of the kidneys are indicated. Since biliary pain may appear in the substernal area, it may potentially be confused with angina, although biliary pain is not related to exertion. Any suspicion that chest pain may be car-

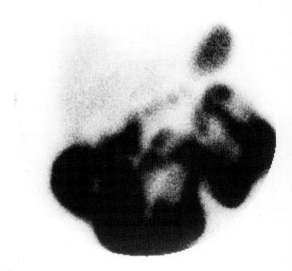

B

Figure 50–5. DISIDA scan with nonvisualization of gallbladder after 2 hours **(A)** and 4 hours **(B),** consistent with acute cholecystitis.

diac in origin, even when gallstones have been documented, warrants rigorous cardiac evaluation.

A dilemma in evaluating patients with suspected biliary pain and documented gallstones is the absence of a test that conclusively establishes gallstones as the source of the pain. Any uncertainly regarding the likelihood of relief from surgery should be shared with the patient. More extensive evaluation may be

Table 50–2. Differential diagnosis of biliary colic.

Peptic ulcer disease
Esophageal spasm
Gastroesophageal reflux
Nonulcer dyspepsia
Irritable bowel syndrome
Renal colic
Coronary artery disease

necessary in patients with less specific symptoms. Therefore, barium studies, endoscopic studies, imaging of the kidneys, cardiac evaluation, and other tests all have a potential role but not an invariable one. In typical patients with documented gallstones, it may be appropriate to proceed directly to cholecystectomy without further testing.

The differential diagnosis of acute cholecystitis includes an acute event related to peptic ulcer disease, such as penetration or perforation, acute pancreatitis, acute hepatitis, Fitz-Hugh-Curtis syndrome, appendicitis, diverticulitis, or acute intestinal diseases. The physical findings in patients with perforated ulcers are usually more diffuse, and the presence of free air on plain films of the abdomen confirms a perforated viscus. Although less often heralded by peritoneal signs, the pain and physical findings in acute pancreatitis are also less focal than in acute cholecystitis. A pattern of pain "boring through" to the back and partially relieved by sitting up is typical of pancreatitis. Fever and leukocytosis may be similar in both diseases, but the serum amylase level is usually far higher in acute pancreatitis than in cholecystitis. In severe pancreatitis, signs of systemic toxicity are more pronounced. A small percentage of patients with gallstone pancreatitis have concomitant acute cholecystitis. In this circumstance, the sonographic appearance of the gallbladder is critical, as a thickened wall or related findings may indicate cholecystitis (see following discussion).

Distinction of hepatitis from cholecystitis should not be difficult. On those occasions when severe pain is present in hepatitis, the pain has a serosal character, since it arises from Glisson's capsule rather than the liver parenchyma itself. A careful physical examination can generally distinguish the tender, enlarged liver from the right subcostal tenderness of cholecystitis, even when the gallbladder is palpably enlarged. Serum chemistry measurements feature much more striking liver enzyme abnormalities in acute hepatitis

Table 50–3. Differential diagnosis of acute cholecystitis.

Acute appendicitis
Acute pancreatitis
Acute bile duct obstruction (with or without cholangitis)
Perforated or penetrating ulcer
Intestinal obstruction
Nephrolithiasis
Acute myocardial infarction

(eg, ALT and AST). Acute hepatitis A, unlike the other forms of acute hepatitis, can cause acute cholecystitis by infecting the gallbladder epithelium. **Fitz-Hugh-Curtis syndrome** should be distinguishable from acute cholecystitis by the presence of adnexal tenderness on pelvic examination and positive findings on cervical gram-stained smears and culture for *Gonococcus* or *Chlamydia*.

Although the pain of appendicitis characteristically evolves in the right lower quadrant, its tendency to begin with pain in the periumbilical area, and the diversity of locations in which the appendix may lie, may occasionally lead erroneously to a diagnosis of acute cholecystitis. Imaging studies, including sonography or CT scanning, or both, should make the distinction.

Occasionally, pulmonary disease involving the right lower lobe may mimic gallbladder disease, and the pain of cholecystitis may have a pleuritic component when there is peritoneal irritation. The differential diagnosis in such cases depends on the presence of other pulmonary signs and symptoms and the findings on chest x-ray.

Treatment & Prognosis

A. Considerations in Planning Treatment: Because most persons with gallstones are asymptomatic, a clear understanding of the natural history of this disorder is essential in formulating management.

1. Asymptomatic gallstones–Prospective cohort studies in the last 15 years have uniformly shown that only a minority of patients with asymptomatic gallstones develop symptoms or biliary complications over many years. In one study of 123 persons with asymptomatic gallstones followed for 11–24 years, biliary pain developed in 2% during each of the first 5 years, followed by a decreasing incidence thereafter. Complications were seen in only three persons and were preceded by pain in all cases. There are occasional patients who present with a complication, especially gallstone pancreatitis, in the absence of prior symptoms, but even in this setting, death is rare.

Based on these data, asymptomatic gallstones should be left alone in otherwise healthy people. Diabetics with gallstones have traditionally been considered high-risk patients, and prophylactic cholecystectomy has been recommended. It appears, however, that the complications of surgery in such patients are related more closely to the systemic complications of the diabetes itself.

Prophylactic cholecystectomy has also been advocated in patients with sickle cell disease, since they are at increased risk of pigment stones. This recommendation is based on the difficulty in distinguishing pain crises from cholecystitis, the likelihood that true cholecystitis will precipitate a pain crisis, and the increased risk of emergent surgery in this population.

One caveat to the expectant management of

asymptomatic gallstones is concern about gallbladder carcinoma (see Chapter 52). Indeed, when carcinoma of the gallbladder develops, it is almost always in persons with gallstones, but most persons with gallstones do not develop carcinoma. In asymptomatic persons, the risk of cancer is not considered sufficient to justify surgical treatment. The main exceptions are patients with calcified or "porcelain" gallbladder and Native Americans with gallstones, since both groups have a higher incidence of gallbladder carcinoma. Prophylactic cholecystectomy should therefore be considered in such persons, even when they are asymptomatic. Gallbladder cancer is more common in persons with symptomatic gallstones. Cohort studies of symptomatic persons revealed a rate of cancer of 0.00078 per year.

2. Symptomatic gallstones–In contrast to those with asymptomatic gallstones, patients with symptomatic stones have a higher risk of future problems, so that cholecystectomy is generally warranted. Up to two-thirds of patients with biliary pain will have recurrent episodes within 1–2 years. Moreover, about 3% will develop biliary complications annually. Decision analysis has indicated that elective cholecystectomy in symptomatic patients produces a small but real increase in life expectancy of 3–4 months.

B. Surgical Treatment: Until the past decade, cholecystectomy by laparotomy was the only treatment for gallstones, with a mortality rate of less than 1%. The need for prolonged hospitalization with this technique and the lengthy period of convalescence have fueled interest in less invasive alternatives.

1. Laparoscopic cholecystectomy–Laparoscopic cholecystectomy, introduced in 1987, has rapidly become the standard method of cholecystectomy in patients with symptomatic gallstones. Despite the absence of controlled trials, its advantages are obvious. Patients are usually discharged within 1–2 days postoperatively, there is decreased scar tissue, and the return to normal activities is rapid. The number of cholecystectomies in the United States has increased recently, and this has been attributed in part to less hesitation on the part of physicians to recommend surgery for "high-risk," reluctant, or mildly symptomatic patients.

Approximately 10% of laparoscopic cholecystectomies must be converted to open procedures in the operating room because of excessive inflammation, adhesions, or complications such as bile duct injuries requiring repair. Laparoscopy was previously contraindicated in patients with acute cholecystitis but is now performed safely in the hands of experienced surgeons.

Although the incidence of wound infections and cardiopulmonary complications appears to be reduced by laparoscopic cholecystectomy, the incidence of bile duct injuries has increased, reportedly to 0.1–0.5%. The risk of bile duct injury is greatest with less experienced surgeons.

Surgical bile duct injuries are either recognized at the time of surgery or become apparent days to months later. The most common short-term postoperative problem is leakage of bile from the cystic duct remnant; this is not a true duct "injury," however. Patients complain of pain and may have low-grade fever or leukocytosis. The diagnosis may be apparent from a fluid collection on ultrasound or CT scanning, and can be confirmed by DISIDA scanning. Large fluid collections may require percutaneous drainage. The preferred treatment is stent placement, with or without sphincterotomy (preferences among endoscopists vary), to diminish the outflow resistance intrinsic to the intact ampulla and divert bile from the leak. This approach usually permits the leak to heal spontaneously.

Late complications of cholecystectomy are more difficult to manage because they usually result from bile duct stricturing. Patients may develop jaundice or cholangitis and are at high risk for secondary biliary cirrhosis if untreated. Endoscopic treatment with balloon dilation and stent placement may be effective, but surgery is often required, especially for proximal lesions involving the hepatic duct bifurcation.

2. Laparotomy (open cholecystectomy)–Currently, cholecystectomy by laparotomy is reserved in most centers for patients in whom laparoscopy is not feasible technically. In addition, patients with common bile duct stones that are not removable by endoscopic means have open cholecystectomy and bile duct exploration, unless they are in a center with surgical expertise in laparoscopic removal of stones from the bile duct. Finally, if there is suspicion of gallbladder cancer, many surgeons advocate open cholecystectomy.

C. Nonsurgical Treatment:

1. Ursodeoxycholic acid–Ursodeoxycholic acid is a bile acid currently approved for gallstone dissolution in appropriate patients. The drug reduces cholesterol saturation by inhibiting HMG CoA reductase, a critical enzyme in cholesterol biosynthesis. Ursodeoxycholic acid also forms highly soluble multilamellar vesicles and prolongs the nucleation time of bile. Its only significant adverse effect is diarrhea, which is unusual. The overall efficacy of this agent in dissolving stones (at a dosage of 10–13 mg/kg/d) is about 50%, with dissolution complete within 6–12 months. The ideal candidate for dissolution therapy has small floating (ie, cholesterol-rich) noncalcified stones in a gallbladder demonstrated to be functional on oral cholecystography. Nonfloating stones are not an absolute contraindication to treatment. Stones over 1.5 cm in size will rarely dissolve. Pigment stones are not responsive to ursodeoxycholic acid.

Despite the initial enthusiasm for ursodeoxycholic acid, the expense, need for serial imaging studies, and high recurrence rates (at least 50%) after completion of therapy have all diminished the interest in this treatment. For these reasons, dissolution therapy with bile acids is limited to patients who are at unusually high risk or who simply refuse surgery.

2. Contact dissolution therapy–Solvents that dissolve cholesterol stones can be instilled directly into the gallbladder via a percutaneously or endoscopically placed catheter. The prototype agent, methyl-tert-butyl ether, dissolves cholesterol gallstones within 1–3 days. Adverse effects include complications of catheter placement, hemorrhagic duodenitis, and sedation related to systemic absorption of the agent. As with oral bile acid dissolution therapy, gallstones may recur. This treatment currently remains experimental.

3. Extracorporeal shock wave lithotripsy (ESWL)–ESWL for gallbladder stone fragmentation was developed because of its initial success in renal stone dissolution. Results in gallstone fragmentation have been less impressive, however. In ESWL, high-amplitude shock waves generated by external electrohydraulic or piezoelectric devices are focused on gallbladder stones by ultrasonographic guidance. The goal of ESWL is the production of tiny fragments, which are then amenable to oral bile acid dissolution therapy. The selection criteria are similar to those for primary bile acid dissolution therapy; preferred patients are those with a small number of stones, ideally a solitary stone. The lower rate of efficacy in patients with multiple stones excludes many patients with gallstones from this therapy. Moreover, gallstones commonly recur even after successful treatment, though less often than with dissolution therapy alone. Adverse effects of ESWL include postprocedure biliary colic, pancreatitis (rarely), and transient injury to the right lung or kidney.

Despite the clear benefit of ESWL in some patients, the expense of the lithotripsy units, limited spectrum of eligible patients, potential for recurrence, and need for subsequent medical therapy have limited enthusiasm for this option.

D. Treatment of Complications:

1. Acute cholecystitis–Patients admitted with suspected acute cholecystitis should initially be made NPO and intravenously hydrated. Administration of broad-spectrum antibiotics early in the course is recommended, because secondary infection often supervenes in what is initially a noninfectious process. If the diagnosis of acute cholecystitis is made within 24–48 hours of onset of symptoms, early surgery leads to reduced morbidity and mortality rates. If the diagnosis has been delayed, surgery may be technically more difficult. Therefore, some surgeons prefer to postpone surgery for several weeks, in the hope that the acute inflammation will subside with medical therapy. Surgery without delay is sometimes necessary in patients who fail to respond to medical therapy. In severely ill or elderly patients with high surgical risk, percutaneously placed cholecystostomy catheters may temporize the situation.

Although complications of cholecystitis almost always require surgery, definitive cholecystectomy may not be feasible in all cases at the time of the initial operation. Such complications can include free or localized perforation, with pericholecystic abscess; fistulization to bowel, most commonly the duodenum or hepatic flexure of colon; gallbladder empyema; emphysematous cholecystitis with gas-producing organisms; or **Mirizzi's syndrome,** in which a stone impacted in the gallbladder neck or cystic duct obstructs the adjacent bile duct. Mirizzi's syndrome frequently is diagnosed by ERCP because of the prominence of biliary obstruction in the patient's presenting illness. Endoscopic stent placement may provide temporary benefit if cholangitis or jaundice is dominating the clinical picture, but cholecystectomy is ultimately required.

Gallstone passage from the gallbladder into the bowel via a fistula may cause intestinal obstruction if the stone is sufficiently large ("gallstone ileus"). Obstruction usually occurs in the ileum, but duodenal obstruction has also been encountered. The clinical presentation is similar to that of obstruction from other causes, although the presence of gallstones and air in the biliary tree may provide clues. At surgery, the obstructing stone must be removed by enterotomy; cholecystectomy can be performed simultaneously if deemed feasible by the surgeon.

2. Common bile duct stones–There are several modes of presentation in patients with common bile duct stones. Most common is the patient presenting with biliary pain accompanied by abnormal liver tests, with or without jaundice. Jaundice from common bile duct stones may be painless, although the possibility of malignant bile duct obstruction must also be considered.

Most patients with symptoms suggestive of bile duct stones have stones in the gallbladder. Thus, treatment plans must consider adjunctive cholecystectomy. Recommendations for cholecystectomy in patients with primarily common bile duct complications have evolved rapidly since the advent of laparoscopic cholecystectomy. There is a low threshold of hesitation to remove the gallbladder given the minimal discomfort and rapid recovery in patients who have undergone this procedure. Therefore, endoscopic stone removal is now often complemented by laparoscopic surgery. The combination of the two techniques is the preferred approach for patients with common duct and gallbladder stones, although no randomized trials have compared this approach with common duct exploration and open cholecystectomy.

Because some patients may have a self-limited episode due to passage of a stone, it may be difficult to determine when further evaluation is essential. Factors favoring persistent choledocholithiasis include imaging of duct stones or dilatation on sonography, or persistent abnormalities in liver tests after presentation, or both. The author has found that patients with transient pain, rapidly resolving liver enzyme abnormalities, and negative sonographic studies of the gallbladder usually have normal cholangiograms; therefore, ERCP is not usually performed in such patients.

The treatment of choice in patients with bile duct stones who have had prior cholecystectomy is endoscopic sphincterotomy and stone extraction. The success rate exceeds 90% at experienced centers. Complications can be anticipated in 5–10%, however, with mortality rates of 0.5–1%. The major complications include iatrogenic pancreatitis, bleeding, perforation, and infection. Infection is a major concern when the bile duct is not drained adequately, either by complete clearing of stones or placement of a biliary stent. Pancreatitis usually resolves with conservative therapy, but in exceptional circumstances, a protracted course with pseudocyst or abscess formation may occur. Perforation is retroperitoneal and usually responds to antibiotics, preferably with nasobiliary drainage if the complication is recognized during ERCP. Surgery may be required, however, and should be considered early if there is any evidence of sepsis or fluid collections.

3. Biliary pancreatitis–This subject is covered in more detail elsewhere (see Chapter 31). The key decision in managing gallstone pancreatitis is whether to intervene early or treat conservatively. Most cases of gallstone pancreatitis resolve spontaneously and can be managed expectantly. Once the acute episode has subsided, it is generally preferable to perform cholecystectomy prior to discharge to prevent recurrent attacks.

Studies have not clearly shown an advantage to early surgery in patients with severe acute gallstone pancreatitis, but early ERCP may be warranted. A study of patients with severe pancreatitis demonstrated that urgent ERCP and sphincterotomy reduced the duration of hospitalization and overall complication rate, and showed a trend toward reduced mortality rates. Another study from Asia documented that early ERCP reduced the incidence of cholangitis in biliary pancreatitis, although the nature of stone disease (ie, more primary bile duct stones and bacterial contamination) may differ from that of Western patients. ERCP in patients with severe pancreatitis does not exacerbate the disease.

4. Cholangitis–ERCP has assumed an important role in the management of acute cholangitis because it provides a prompt, nonsurgical method of bile duct drainage, with or without stone extraction. For septic, acutely ill patients, this offers a distinct advantage over surgery. In particularly unstable patients with cholangitis, placement of a nasobiliary tube may be the most expeditious way to rapidly drain the bile duct without prolonging the procedure.

Some patients with cholangitis are not overtly toxic at presentation, and their acute illnesses resolve with antibiotics. During this time, vigilant observation is required, with endoscopic intervention if the patient fails to defervesce promptly. The likelihood of persistent common bile duct stones in these patients is high even after clinical improvement has occurred, indicating that ERCP is still warranted to clear the ducts.

5. Acalculous cholecystitis–Cholecystitis in the absence of gallstones is seen most often in critically ill patients in intensive care units. Its pathogenesis involves ischemia, with distention of the wall of the gallbladder and bile stasis. Immunocompromised patients, especially those with human immunodeficiency virus (HIV) infection, are also at risk for cytomegalovirus-related acalculous cholecystitis (see Chapter 39).

The presentation of acalculous cholecystitis may be similar to that of gallstone-associated cholecystitis, or it may be more subtle, with fever or leukocytosis but no focal abdominal symptoms or signs. Acalculous cholecystitis is associated with a high mortality rate, in part because patients often have severe underlying multisystem disease. Thus, a high index of suspicion is essential in making a diagnosis early enough to prevent death.

Hepatobiliary scintigraphy with HIDA scanning frequently is abnormal in patients with acalculous cholecystitis. The utility of this test is reduced in severely ill patients, however, because of prolonged fasting. In contrast, sonographic studies and CT scanning may reveal thickening of the gallbladder wall and the presence of pericholecystic fluid even in the absence of stones and should be considered early.

The optimal treatment for acalculous cholecystitis is cholecystectomy, but underlying critical illness may preclude laparotomy. Surgical or percutaneous cholecystostomy is an established alternative, the latter requiring sonographic guidance. Most recently, transpapillary endoscopic drainage of the gallbladder has been reported; this technique may be most appropriate in patients with ascites and coagulopathies. The choice of treatment will depend on local expertise within the institution.

6. Sphincter of Oddi dysfunction–Also called biliary dyskinesia and papillary stenosis, this disorder is recognized most frequently in postcholecystectomy patients with recurrent biliary pain. Its incidence has been much debated, as have diagnostic criteria and appropriate therapy. Sphincter of Oddi dysfunction encompasses both actual stenosis due to fibrosis of the sphincter and spasm of the smooth muscle within the sphincter.

Criteria used by clinicians to diagnose this dysfunction include abnormal liver enzymes not attributable to parenchymal liver disease, dilatation of the bile duct beyond 12 mm in a postcholecystectomy patient, and delayed drainage of contrast material from the biliary tree more than 45 minutes after ERCP (Table 50–4). Sphincter of Oddi manometry

Table 50–4. Proposed criteria for sphincter of Oddi dysfunction.

Biliary pain
Dilated common bile duct over 12 mm (postcholecystectomy)
Delayed drainage of contrast beyond 45 minutes (postcholecystectomy)
Abnormal liver enzymes beyond twice normal
Delayed drainage from bile duct to duodenum on DISIDA scan
Abnormal sphincter of Oddi manometry:
    Basal sphincter of Oddi pressure beyond 40 mm
    Tachyoddia (over 8 sphincter contractions per minute)
    Paradoxical response to cholecystokinin
    Excessive number of retrograde contractions

has become the "gold standard" in diagnosing this disorder, although the technique remains confined to relatively few centers and poses a risk of postprocedure pancreatitis higher than that following routine diagnostic ERCP. In an attempt to reduce the invasiveness of diagnostic testing for this entity, some clinicians use DISIDA scanning to assess the rapidity of flow from the bile duct into the intestine. The level of confidence in this modality varies widely, however, and at best, it furnishes supplementary rather than definitive data on which to base management decisions.

Sphincter of Oddi manometry can help to predict which patients will respond to endoscopic sphincterotomy, usually considered the treatment of choice for this condition. An accurate diagnosis is essential, because the risk of sphincterotomy for sphincter of Oddi dysfunction is greater than when performed for bile duct stones. Investigators in specialized centers have shown that patients who meet the laboratory and radiologic criteria for sphincter of Oddi dysfunction almost always have abnormal sphincter pressures, so that manometry prior to sphincterotomy may not always be necessary. More commonly, however, patients with postcholecystectomy biliary pain have only one or two of these criteria, and the results of manometry cannot be predicted. Manometry findings in patients with an uncertain diagnosis of sphincter of Oddi dysfunction correlate most clearly with the results of sphincterotomy. The approach to patients with biliary pain alone but no other criteria for sphincter of Oddi dysfunction is less well defined. Even in patients with laboratory or imaging abnormalities, many endoscopists prefer to rely on clinical judgment rather than manometry in deciding whether to perform sphincterotomy.

REFERENCES

Abei M et al: Identification of human biliary acid glycoprotein as a cholesterol crystallization promoter. Gastroenterology 1994;106:231.

Everhart JE: Contributions of obesity and weight loss to gallstone disease. Ann Intern Med 1993;119:1029.

Gracie WA, Ransohoff DF: The natural history of silent gallstones: The innocent gallstone is not a myth. N Engl J Med 1982;798.

Johnston DE, Kaplan MM: Pathogenesis and treatment of gallstones. N Engl J Med 1993;328:412.

Leuschner U et al: Gallstone dissolution with methyl-tert-butyl ether in 120 patients: Efficacy and safety. Dig Dis Sci 1991;36:193.

Podda M et al: Efficacy and safety of a combination of chenodeoxycholic acid and ursodeoxycholic acid for gallstone dissolution: A comparison with ursodeoxycholic acid alone. Gastroenterology 1989;96:222.

Sackmann M et al: Gallstone recurrence after shock-wave therapy. Gastroenterology 1994;106:225.

Sackmann M et al: The Munich gallbladder lithotripsy study: Results of the first 5 years with 711 patients. Ann Intern Med 1991;114:290.

Southern Surgeons Club: A prospective analysis of 1518 laparoscopic cholecystectomies. N Engl J Med 1991;324:1073.

Strasberg S, Clavien P-A: Cholecystolithiasis: Lithotherapy for the 1990s. Hepatology 1992;16:820.

Primary Disease of the Bile Ducts

51

Keith D. Lindor, MD

PRIMARY BILIARY CIRRHOSIS

Primary biliary cirrhosis is a chronic cholestatic liver disease characterized by inflammatory destruction of interlobular and septal bile ducts. The disease affects middle-aged women in nine out of 10 cases, and is typically marked by the presence of antimitochondrial antibodies. It is usually slowly progressive, with eventual development of cirrhosis and portal hypertension and its complications.

Primary biliary cirrhosis is uncommon, with an estimated incidence of 10–12 cases per year per million persons, and a prevalence of 100–150 cases per million. Many of these patients are identified because of increased serum alkaline phosphatase levels found during routine health evaluations or during evaluation of unrelated complaints. Most patients at this stage are asymptomatic; some may manifest symptoms specific for primary biliary cirrhosis (see following discussion) or symptoms from diseases known to be associated with primary biliary cirrhosis, such as Hashimoto's thyroiditis or keratoconjunctivitis sicca.

Primary biliary cirrhosis is being recognized with increasing frequency. Promising medical therapy is emerging, but liver transplantation still plays an important role in the management of end-stage disease.

Pathophysiology

Although the cause of primary biliary cirrhosis is not established, immunologic mechanisms may play a primary role. As immunologic destruction of bile ducts progresses, chronic cholestasis ensues. Many of the complications of primary biliary cirrhosis are related to chronic cholestasis and the resultant hepatic dysfunction. Treatment has been used to alter immunologic function and improve the chronic cholestasis.

A. Immunologic Mechanisms: Immunologic mechanisms are most strongly suggested by the presence of T cells, sometimes activated, in the inflammatory infiltrates surrounding the damaged bile ducts. A widespread defect in immune function is suggested by the association of primary biliary cirrhosis with other autoimmune diseases characterized by lymphocytic destruction of glandular epithelial tissues, including thyroid, salivary, and lacrimal glands.

Several immunologic abnormalities have been demonstrated, but it is not known whether these are etiologic or a secondary phenomenon. Precipitating agents such as toxins or viruses have been unsuccessfully sought. Genetic factors do not appear to play a major role in the development of this disease. Abnormalities of cellular immunity include defective suppressor cell function, increased autoreactivity to autoantigens, and aberrant expression of autoantigens on biliary epithelium. As noted previously, however, it is uncertain whether these are primary or secondary phenomena. Similarly, the presence of antimitochondrial antibodies has been recognized as a characteristic and diagnostic feature of this disease. In recent years, characterization of the antigens recognized by this antibody have been greatly advanced, but their role in the pathogenesis of primary biliary cirrhosis is uncertain.

B. Cholestasis: Progressive immunologically mediated destruction of bile ducts leads to impaired intrahepatic bile flow and chronic cholestasis. Animal models indicate that it is likely that cholestasis causes accumulation of hydrophobic and potentially toxic bile acids within the liver, creating a self-perpetuating liver injury. Although copper was once considered to be pathogenically important, it is now recognized that copper accumulation is a passive consequence of cholestasis and is without pathogenic significance.

Clinical Findings

A. Symptoms and Signs: The most common symptom in patients with primary biliary cirrhosis is fatigue (Table 51–1), but this is nonspecific. Of the specific symptoms, pruritus is the most important; it can occur at any stage of the disease, and its intensity does not correlate with the severity of the underlying liver disease. Symptoms of more advanced disease, such as jaundice, variceal bleeding, ascites, or encephalopathy, are rare at presentation but can occur late in the course of the disease. As noted above, an

Table 51–1. Symptoms and signs of primary biliary cirrhosis.

Symptoms and Signs	Incidence (%)
Fatigue	60–70
Pruritus	50–60
Asymptomatic	30–40
Associated with advanced disease	
Jaundice	16
Variceal bleeding	2
Ascites	3

increasing number of patients (in some series, up to 40%) are now being recognized without symptoms. A number of diseases that share a presumed autoimmune basis have been associated with primary biliary cirrhosis (see Table 51–2). There also appears to be an associated increased risk of breast cancer in women with primary biliary cirrhosis.

B. Diagnostic Studies: The diagnosis of primary biliary cirrhosis should be considered particularly in any middle-aged woman with chronic cholestasis. The most characteristic biochemical abnormality is an increase in the serum alkaline phosphatase level to at least three or four times normal or higher. Occasional patients may have nearly normal alkaline phosphatase levels but positive antimitochondrial antibody and liver biopsies consistent with the diagnosis of primary biliary cirrhosis. Antimitochondrial antibodies are usually present in high titers; 90–95% of patients will have an antimitochondrial antibody titer greater than 1:40. Every patient should undergo ultrasound study or CT scanning to exclude biliary obstruction, although the presence of an antimitochondrial antibody is unusual (< 2%) in biliary obstruction from other causes. Liver biopsy is important for confirming the diagnosis histologically as well as providing information regarding histologic staging. Ordinarily, cholangiography is not necessary, unless atypical features are present, such as the absence of an antimitochondrial antibody, occurrence in a male, or the suggestion of biliary obstruction on imaging studies.

1. Laboratory findings–Elevated alkaline

Table 51–2. Diseases associated with primary biliary cirrhosis.

Disease	Incidence (%)
Keratoconjunctivitis sicca	50
Thyroid disease	15
Arthritis	10
Less commonly associated diseases	
Raynaud's phenomenon	9
Scleroderma	2
Renal stones	3
Breast cancer	2

phosphatase is the most commonly found abnormality in patients with primary biliary cirrhosis; usually, this is elevated to four to five times normal or higher. The transaminases are typically only mildly elevated, and most patients have serum bilirubin levels ranging from normal to less than 2 mg/dL at presentation. Serum IgM levels are elevated in approximately 95% of patients. Hypercholesterolemia is common and found in nearly 80% of patients. Serum albumin levels and prothrombin times are usually normal until late in the course of the disease. Antimitochondrial antibodies are present in approximately 95% of patients. The M2 component of this antibody, which recognizes the pyruvate dehydrogenase complex, is the most specific for primary biliary cirrhosis.

Some patients may have features of primary biliary cirrhosis but lack antimitochondrial antibodies. Although previously classified as "antimitochondrial antibody–negative primary biliary cirrhosis," such patients are now considered to have "autoimmune cholangitis," a distinct syndrome (see Chapter 37). Ninety-five percent of antimitochondrial antibody–negative patients will have either antinuclear antibody or anti–smooth muscle antibodies. These patients with autoimmune cholangitis follow a course that is identical to that of primary biliary cirrhosis.

2. Histologic findings–Histologic changes have been divided into four stages, as shown in Figure 51–1.

- The portal stage (stage 1) is characterized by inflammation of the portal tracts surrounding the bile ducts.
- Stage 2 is characterized by more bile duct destruction, proliferation of bile ductules, and piecemeal necrosis, with inflammation spilling from the portal areas into the hepatic parenchyma.
- Stage 3 is characterized by fibrosis extending from the portal tracts.
- The so-called septal stage (stage 4) is defined as the presence of regenerative nodules surrounded by fibrosis.

Histologic progression occurs over many years. At present, most patients have advanced histologic changes at the time of diagnosis, although they may follow a benign asymptomatic course for many years after the diagnosis is established.

3. Imaging studies–The most important imaging studies are those to exclude biliary obstruction. Ordinarily, ultrasound studies and CT scans are adequate for this purpose in a middle-aged woman with chronic cholestasis and a positive antimitochondrial antibody test. In a patient who is antimitochondrial antibody–negative or male, the author routinely recommends endoscopic retrograde cholangiopancreatography to exclude other diagnoses. In the great majority of patients, however, routine cholangiography is not indicated.

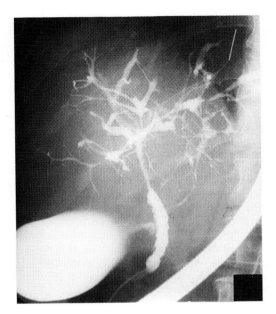

Figure 51–1. The typical cholangiographic features of primary sclerosing cholangitis as seen here include diffuse multifocal stricturing of the intra- and extrahepatic bile ducts.

Differential Diagnosis

The differential diagnosis of patients with chronic cholestasis includes extrahepatic biliary obstruction due to biliary stones, strictures, or tumors; ultrasonography or CT scanning will help exclude these possibilities. Several other conditions may not be excluded by these imaging studies, however, including primary sclerosing cholangitis (see Table 51–7), drug-induced cholestasis, overlap with autoimmune hepatitis, hepatitis C, and, occasionally, sarcoidosis or idiopathic adulthood ductopenia (Table 51–3).

Primary sclerosing cholangitis (see following discussion) should be considered, especially in patients with inflammatory bowel disease. In primary sclerosing cholangitis, cholangiography is the critical diagnostic study. Liver biopsy can suggest primary sclerosing cholangitis but may not adequately distinguish between primary biliary cirrhosis and primary scle-

rosing cholangitis, because both conditions may be associated with periductular inflammation, bile duct injury, and cholestasis.

The use of drugs such as phenothiazines, estrogens, androgens, and those associated with granulomatous involvement of the liver should be considered. Some patients with autoimmune hepatitis may be confused with patients with primary biliary cirrhosis, particularly because up to 25% of these patients may also have antimitochondrial antibodies. In contrast to primary biliary cirrhosis, however, patients with autoimmune hepatitis have antimitochondrial antibody titers of 1:40 or less. Liver biopsy will also help distinguish the condition because patients with autoimmune hepatitis rarely have bile duct destruction.

Hepatitis C must also be considered in the differential diagnosis of patients with primary biliary cirrhosis because the infection is sometimes associated with granulomatous inflammation around bile ducts. Increasingly, cases of hepatitis C associated with a cholestatic profile are being described.

Sarcoidosis may present with cholestasis and hepatic granulomas; however, its histologic features are otherwise different from those of primary biliary cirrhosis. Florid duct lesions are not a part of sarcoidosis. Antimitochondrial antibody tests are negative, and characteristic chest x-ray abnormalities are present in the great majority of patients with sarcoidosis.

Idiopathic adulthood ductopenia is a recently described entity. It typically occurs in men who have normal cholangiography and do not have autoantibodies or a history of colitis. The cholestasis is usually more rapidly progressive than in primary biliary cirrhosis and often results in referral for liver transplantation. As the name implies, the cause of the condition is unknown.

Complications

Complications of primary biliary cirrhosis include those of chronic liver disease, such as portal hypertension with variceal bleeding, ascites, and hepatic encephalopathy, as well as consequences of cholestasis, including osteopenia, fat-soluble vitamin deficiency, and hypercholesterolemia (Table 51–4).

A. Osteopenia: The osteopenia found in patients with primary biliary cirrhosis in North America is nearly always osteoporosis. Osteomalacia has been

Table 51–3. Differential diagnosis of primary biliary cirrhosis.

Extrahepatic biliary obstruction due to stones, strictures, tumors
Primary sclerosing cholangitis
Drug-induced cholestasis
Overlap with autoimmune hepatitis
Sarcoidosis
Idiopathic adulthood ductopenia
Autoimmune cholangitis

Table 51–4. Complications of cholestatic liver disease.

Associated with chronic liver disease
  Portal hypertension
  Variceal bleeding
  Ascites
  Hepatic encephalopathy
Specific for cholestasis
  Osteopenia
  Fat-soluble vitamin deficiency
  Hypercholesterolemia

described primarily from the United Kingdom and has been related to decreased exposure to sunlight. Nevertheless, osteomalacia should be considered in these patients because of the increased risk of vitamin D deficiency in the setting of malabsorption of fat-soluble vitamins (see following discussion). Approximately 35% of patients with primary biliary cirrhosis have bone mineral densities of the lumbar spine below the fracture threshold. The exact incidence of spontaneous compression fractures, however, is not known. No specific measures have yet been identified for management of these patients with osteoporosis of cholestasis. Vitamin D deficiency should be identified and corrected (see following discussion). General measures to treat postmenopausal osteoporosis are recommended, including supplemental calcium and adequate exercise. The utility of estrogens in these patients is less well defined; our experience has shown that estrogens are safe, well tolerated, and lead to stabilization or actual improvement in the bone density. Because of concerns about worsening cholestasis, however, estrogens should be used with caution and at low dosages (ie, transdermal estrogen, 0.05 mg twice weekly), with liver tests carefully monitored after initiating therapy. Supplemental vitamin D in the absence of deficiency does not appear to have a role. Agents such as calcitonin, fluoride, and bisphosphonates have not been adequately evaluated in patients with cholestatic osteopenia.

B. Fat-soluble Vitamin Deficiency: Fat-soluble vitamin deficiency, especially of vitamin A, is common. Although no clinical trials have optimized the approach to vitamin A deficiency, the author's policy has been to measure serum levels in patients with advanced disease and to replace deficiencies as needed with 50,000–150,000 units per week when levels are below normal. Others have followed a less aggressive approach, instead replacing vitamin A only after the onset of changes in dark adaptation. If vitamin A therapy is used, levels should be monitored to ensure adequacy without overreplacement, because of concerns regarding vitamin A hepatic toxicity, with therapy continued as needed to maintain normal serum levels.

Vitamin D deficiency occurs especially in patients with advanced disease. Approximately 12% of the author's patients have had vitamin D deficiency. Vitamin D can be replaced with a dosage of 50,000–150,000 units per week of vitamin D_2 (ergocalciferol). These patients usually do not have difficulty in hydroxylation of 25-hydroxycholecalciferol, and, therefore, do not require the more expensive 1,25-dihydroxycholecalciferol or 25-hydroxyergocalciferol replacement.

Vitamin K deficiency can be inferred from a prolonged prothrombin time. If an elevated prothrombin time responds to vitamin K replacement, chronic therapy with water-soluble vitamin K, 5 mg/d, is indicated.

Vitamin E deficiency is rare. When symptomatic, it causes usually irreversible neurologic abnormalities characterized by areflexia, loss of proprioception, and ataxia. Patients with symptomatic vitamin E deficiency may not respond to replacement therapy, and it has been the author's policy to measure levels, particularly in patients with advanced disease, and institute replacement therapy with 100 mg orally twice daily in those who are deficient.

Treatment

Treatment for primary biliary cirrhosis has been based on measures to reverse abnormalities observed clinically and histologically.

A. Drug Treatment: Drugs that have been tested are those designed to modify cholestasis, suppress the immune response, and alter fibrogenesis.

1. Ursodeoxycholic acid–The most important advance in recent years has been the use of ursodeoxycholic acid. The drug may be effective by displacing hepatotoxic endogenous bile acids. Ursodeoxycholic acid may also have immunomodulatory effects that modify the underlying immunologic abnormalities of primary biliary cirrhosis. Controlled trials have now reported that ursodeoxycholic acid leads to clear-cut biochemical improvement. In some series, symptomatic and histologic improvement has been reported, and a controlled trial cites improvement in survival rates and a decreased need for liver transplantation. Although not yet approved for use for primary biliary cirrhosis, ursodeoxycholic acid holds promise for slowing the progression of this disease, with several prospective long-term follow-up studies in progress.

Several other agents described below have undergone clinical testing with limited success.

2. Corticosteroids–Corticosteroids led to some improvement in symptoms, biochemical measurements, and histologic findings in patients with primary biliary cirrhosis in the only small randomized trial that has been reported. Improvement in the liver disease was offset by worsening of the osteopenia from the corticosteroids. Although, with further follow-up, this osteopenia was less of a problem, the small study size and the large number of dropouts prevent any conclusions to be drawn regarding efficacy. Thus, corticosteroids should be considered experimental and potentially hazardous therapy.

3. Other drugs–Azathioprine has been studied in controlled trials the largest of which showed no benefit with respect to clinical symptoms, biochemical measurements, histologic findings, or survival rates. At present, this treatment is seldom used for patients with primary biliary cirrhosis. Cyclosporine has been tested because of its immunomodulatory activity, but trials to date have shown little benefit and a high risk of drug-induced renal dysfunction. Methotrexate was initially reported in a small series to be effective in slowing primary biliary cirrhosis progression, but recent trials show little benefit. Penicillamine has been tested but found to be of no value. Colchicine has been studied in three large trials and appears to be of limited, if any, benefit in patients with primary biliary cirrhosis.

B. Liver Transplantation: Liver transplantation clearly benefits patients with end-stage primary biliary cirrhosis and is also considered on rare occasions for patients with intractable pruritus or fatigue (see Chapter 54). The osteoporosis associated with primary biliary cirrhosis may be worsened initially following liver transplantation. Thus, patients with severe osteoporosis should probably be referred early to a liver transplantation program.

Prognosis

There has been an increased appreciation of the natural history of primary biliary cirrhosis in recent years. The disease is slowly progressive, with initial asymptomatic presentation followed by the gradual development of symptoms in most patients. Earlier studies suggested that asymptomatic patients with primary biliary cirrhosis had a normal life expectancy; however, continued follow-up studies suggest that such interpretations were based on a lead time bias, so that, ultimately, almost all patients develop progressive, symptomatic disease. The author believes that both asymptomatic and symptomatic patients should be considered for treatment.

In general, the course of primary biliary cirrhosis may exceed 10–15 years, but the prognosis varies among patients. Survival models have been developed that allow for better prediction of the course of the disease and that are particularly useful for timing of liver transplantation. The best-validated model relies on simple clinical features such as age of the patient, serum bilirubin and albumin levels, prothrombin time, and the presence or absence of edema or ascites.

Liver transplantation can now be performed with a 1-year survival rate of 85–90% in most centers and a 5-year survival rate in the 60–70% range. Patients with primary biliary cirrhosis should be considered for liver transplantation when the serum bilirubin level approaches or exceeds 8–10 mg/dL, when hepatic synthetic function deteriorates, or, as noted above, for relief of symptoms such as disabling fatigue or pruritus. Other indications include uncontrolled ascites, hepatic encephalopathy, and variceal bleeding not controlled by endoscopic or pharmacologic means. Recurrence of primary biliary cirrhosis after transplantation has been described in approximately 10% of patients, but the disease in this setting follows a relatively benign course thus far.

PRIMARY SCLEROSING CHOLANGITIS

Primary sclerosing cholangitis is a chronic cholestatic liver disease which, like primary biliary cirrhosis, often progresses to cirrhosis, with complications of portal hypertension. The characteristic pathologic feature of this disease is inflammation, with obliterative fibrosis of intra- and extrahepatic bile ducts. Primary sclerosing cholangitis frequently occurs in association with chronic ulcerative colitis and, less commonly, with Crohn's colitis. The prevalence of primary sclerosing cholangitis is approximately 10–40 persons per million, making it much less common than primary biliary cirrhosis.

The cause of primary sclerosing cholangitis is unknown, and adequate therapy has not yet been defined. Like primary biliary cirrhosis, a variety of complications of cholestasis can occur in patients with primary sclerosing cholangitis. A major problem unique to primary sclerosing cholangitis is the occurrence of cholangiocarcinoma in approximately 10% of patients.

The presentation of primary sclerosing cholangitis can vary greatly, from asymptomatic disease to advanced liver disease. Nearly 70% of patients with primary sclerosing cholangitis have chronic colitis, which usually precedes the development of primary sclerosing cholangitis but may occur years after the onset of liver disease. Moreover, the liver disease can occur even after proctocolectomy. It is estimated that 5% of patients with ulcerative colitis will develop primary sclerosing cholangitis.

Pathogenesis

The cause of primary sclerosing cholangitis is unknown. A variety of mechanisms have been investigated, including toxins, viral agents, and immunologic abnormalities. Environmental toxins have not been found. An attractive hypothesis based on animal studies is that toxins absorbed from an inflamed colon, including bacterial peptides such as N-formylated chemotactic peptides and endotoxins, lead to the release of inflammatory cytokines, which cause bile duct injury.

Several viral infections have been considered as precipitating agents in primary sclerosing cholangitis. Typical hepatitis viruses such as hepatitis A, B, and C do not appear to play a role; *Reovirus* type 3 has also been excluded. Although hepatic artery damage due to chemotherapeutic agents such as floxuridine has been associated with biliary features of sclerosing cholangitis, no such arteriopathy has been identified in the primary disease.

Immunologic mechanisms may be important. Haplotypes HLA-B2 and HLA-DR3 are often present in both primary sclerosing cholangitis and other autoimmune diseases. Autoantibodies and defects in cellular immune function have been described in primary sclerosing cholangitis, but, as in primary biliary cirrhosis, a pathogenic role for such immunologic abnormalities has not been established.

Clinical Findings

A. Symptoms and Signs: Sixty to seventy

percent of patients with primary sclerosing cholangitis are male, with a mean age at diagnosis of 43 years. Symptoms include progressive fatigue, pruritus, and jaundice. One (or more) of these symptoms is present in 75% of patients, whereas 25% may be asymptomatic, with abnormal liver tests noted incidentally (Table 51–5). Other symptoms such as fever, abdominal pain, and cholangitis are less common. Cholangitis is more common after surgical or endoscopic biliary tract manipulation.

B. Diagnostic Studies: Primary sclerosing cholangitis should be considered in patients with chronic cholestasis, particularly in the setting of inflammatory bowel disease. Cholangiography is the most important diagnostic study. Endoscopic retrograde cholangiopancreatography is the preferred method to visualize the biliary system (see following section, "Imaging Studies,"). Transhepatic cholangiography is technically difficult because the intrahepatic bile ducts are often sclerotic. Liver biopsy suggesting primary sclerosing cholangitis is often obtained prior to cholangiography; biopsy obtained even after the diagnosis is established can provide prognostic information. Although autoantibodies are found in primary sclerosing cholangitis, their role in diagnosis is less certain than in primary biliary cirrhosis. Antimitochondrial antibodies are seldom found, and antinuclear antibodies can be found on occasion. Pericytoplasmic antineutrophil cytoplasmic antibodies (p-ANCA) have been described in patients with inflammatory bowel disease as well as primary sclerosing cholangitis, suggesting that these autoantibodies may prove useful diagnostically in the future.

1. Laboratory findings–An elevated serum alkaline phosphatase level is the most important laboratory finding and is seen in nearly all patients at some point in the disease. The alkaline phosphatase levels may fluctuate considerably and, at times, may be normal. Transaminases are almost always elevated to less than three to five times normal. Serum bilirubin levels may rise as the disease progresses. Antinuclear antibody and p-ANCA are being identified more commonly. The antimitochondrial antibody is uncommon. Unlike primary biliary cirrhosis, primary sclerosing cholangitis is not commonly associated with autoimmune diseases.

2. Histologic findings–Surgical biopsies from the extrahepatic bile duct are not specific for primary sclerosing cholangitis, as stricturing conditions may give an identical histologic appearance. Liver biopsy findings may strongly support the diagnosis of primary sclerosing cholangitis by demonstrating the absence of intralobular bile ducts in some portal tracts (ductopenia), with duct proliferation in other tracts. Fibrous cholangitis with duct obliteration is nearly diagnostic for primary sclerosing cholangitis but is an uncommon finding. In some patients, the histologic findings of primary sclerosing cholangitis cannot be distinguished from those of primary biliary cirrhosis; as was noted previously, cholangiographic abnormalities on endoscopic retrograde cholangiopancreatography would establish the diagnosis of primary sclerosing cholangitis in this setting.

Recently, the entity of **small duct primary sclerosing cholangitis** has been described. This condition, which occurs in the setting of chronic colitis, is characterized by an identical histologic appearance to primary sclerosing cholangitis but with cholangiographically normal ducts. Small duct primary sclerosing cholangitis may represent the initial phase of primary sclerosing cholangitis.

A liver biopsy is useful in establishing the diagnosis of primary sclerosing cholangitis and is also indispensable in staging. As in primary biliary cirrhosis, the abnormalities in primary sclerosing cholangitis are divided into four stages:

1. The portal stage, which involves inflammation in the portal triad
2. The periportal stage, in which there is inflammation spilling into the periportal area
3. The septal stage, characterized by septal formation
4. The cirrhotic stage, characterized by the development of regenerative nodules

3. Imaging studies–Cholangiography is the most important diagnostic study. Endoscopic retrograde cholangiopancreatography, as noted above, is the procedure of choice. Typical findings include multifocal stricturing and irregularity usually involving both the intra- and extrahepatic biliary system. These strictures are usually diffuse, short, and annular, with intervening segments of normal to dilated bile ducts giving a beaded appearance. Marked dilation, a polypoid mass, or progressive stricture formation suggest a complicating bile duct carcinoma (see following section, "Complications").

Differential Diagnosis

The differential diagnosis includes primary biliary cirrhosis, drug-induced cholestasis, idiopathic adult-

Table 51–5. Symptoms and signs at presentation of primary sclerosing cholangitis.

Symptoms	Incidence (%)
Fatigue	75
Pruritus	60
Fever	20
Cholangitis	10
Asymptomatic	25
Signs	
Hepatomegaly	50
Splenomegaly	30
Hyperpigmentation	25
Xanthomas	5

hood ductopenia, cholestatic alcoholic hepatitis, or chronic viral hepatitis.

Abnormalities of the bile ducts that may give a similar cholangiographic appearance include the following:

- the cholangiopathy associated with AIDS, which is due to *Cryptosporidium, Microsporidia,* or cytomegalovirus (see Chapter 39);
- the cholangiopathy arising after manipulation of the hepatic artery, such as following infusions of the chemotherapeutic agent floxuridine;
- extrahepatic bile duct obstruction caused by stones, surgical strictures, choledochal cysts, or the presence of cholangiocarcinoma or other malignant tumors involving the bile ducts such as lymphoma or metastatic adenocarcinomas (Table 51–6).

A comparison of the features of primary biliary cirrhosis and primary sclerosing cholangitis is shown in Table 51–7.

Complications

Complications of primary sclerosing cholangitis include those resulting from advancing liver failure, such as variceal bleeding, ascites, and encephalopathy, and sequelae of cholestasis, such as osteopenia and fat-soluble vitamin deficiency (see preceding section, "Complications of Primary Biliary Cirrhosis"). Complications relatively unique to primary sclerosing cholangitis include cholangitis, dominant strictures, biliary stone disease, cholangiocarcinoma, and peristomal varices.

A. Cholangitis: Cholangitis can occur spontaneously but is much more likely following surgical or radiologic manipulation of the biliary tree. Cholangiography should be considered in a patient with an otherwise stable course who develops cholangitis. Clinical features of cholangitis may range from mild fevers, chills, and pain, to life-threatening sepsis with

Table 51–6. Differential diagnosis of primary sclerosing cholangitis.

Primary biliary cirrhosis
Drug-induced cholestasis
Idiopathic adulthood ductopenia
Cholestatic alcoholic hepatitis or chronic viral hepatitis
Abnormalities of bile ducts
  AIDS
    Cryptosporidium
    Microsporidium
    Cytomegalovirus
  Damage to hepatic artery (floxuridine infusions)
  Extrahepatic bile duct obstruction from stones
  Surgical strictures
  Choledochal cysts
  Cholangiocarcinoma
  Lymphoma
  Metastatic adenocarcinoma

Table 51–7. Comparison of the features of primary biliary cirrhosis and primary sclerosing cholangitis.

	Primary Biliary Cirrhosis	Primary Sclerosing Cholangitis
Mean age	53 years	41 years
Sex (M:F)	1:9	2:1
Inflammatory bowel disease	< 1%	70%
Sicca	50%	2%
Biochemical findings	Cholestatic	Cholestatic
Antimitochondrial antibodies	90–95%	< 5%
Cholangiography	Normal (or changes of cirrhosis)	Characteristic multifocal strictures
Liver histologic findings	Paucity of bile ducts, granulomatous cholangitis	Paucity of bile ducts, fibrous obliterative cholangitis

shock. Empiric antibiotic therapy is indicated if cholangitis is suspected. The aggressiveness of the therapy should be matched to the severity of the disease. Some episodes of cholangitis will respond to oral antibiotics that are effective for the most commonly found organisms, such as enterobacteriaceae, enterococcus, and clostridia species; others require intravenous drugs such as the aminoglycosides. Oral agents, including ampicillin (500 mg 4 times daily), trimethoprim-sulfamethoxasole (one double-strength tablet twice daily), ciprofloxacin (500 mg twice daily), and metronidazole (250 mg 3 times daily) have been used. For patients with a more severe clinical presentation, ampicillin or mezlocillin in conjunction with an aminoglycoside is usually used. Cefotaxime or other third-generation cephalosporins can also be used, but these do not cover enterococcus, and metronidazole should probably be added for increased anaerobic coverage if these drugs are chosen.

B. Biliary Tree Strictures: Dominant strictures of the biliary tree in primary sclerosing cholangitis can lead to a rapid but reversible deterioration in liver function. Cholangiography is indicated in this setting, with possible balloon dilatation. Cytologic brushings should be obtained to exclude the presence of complicating cholangiocarcinoma as a cause of the stricture. Dominant strictures may also require stenting for 3–6 months after dilatation to maintain patency of the bile duct.

C. Biliary Stone Disease: Biliary stone disease is also a potential explanation for worsening liver tests, the onset of pruritus, or cholangitis. Endoscopic cholangiography is usually diagnostic and can be combined with sphincterotomy and stone removal.

Biliary stone disease is a common complication in patients with primary sclerosing cholangitis, occurring in approximately one-fourth of these patients, but the stones are usually confined to the gallbladder. patients with recurrent cholangitis may also develop intraductal pigment stones due to recurrent infection.

D. Cholangiocarcinoma: As noted above, cholangiocarcinoma may develop in up to 10–15% of patients with primary sclerosing cholangitis, usually in patients with advanced disease. Differentiation of cholangiocarcinoma from preexisting primary sclerosing cholangitis is difficult, and detection early enough to allow surgical cure is unusual. Liver transplantation is seldom successful for patients with cholangiocarcinoma.

E. Peristomal Varices: Another complication in patients with primary sclerosing cholangitis and portal hypertension is the development of peristomal varices around an ileostomy site in patients with colitis who have had a colectomy. These varices may bleed severely, and local measures are usually unable to control the bleeding. Portacaval shunts have been used but make subsequent liver transplantation more difficult. The role of angiographic portal decompression by transjugular intrahepatic portasystemic shunting (TIPS) is uncertain.

Treatment

A. Surgical Treatment: Aggressive surgical approaches have been attempted to relieve strictures in primary sclerosing cholangitis; however, considerably less enthusiasm now is shared for this approach. Because of the widespread intrahepatic disease, it is unlikely that surgical correction of isolated abnormalities of the extrahepatic biliary system will be sufficient in most cases. Aggressive endoscopic dilatation and stenting is advocated by some but has not been evaluated in controlled studies.

B. Drug Treatment: Ursodeoxycholic acid is under intensive investigation, and preliminary information suggests some benefit to patients with primary sclerosing cholangitis. Biochemical improvement has been reported in several series, and isolated reports have suggested improvement in symptoms, histologic findings, and cholangiographic findings. A regimen of 10–15 mg/kg/d in three or four divided doses has been used in most studies. The results of ongoing, randomized trials should help clarify the role of this agent.

Aggressive control of concurrent inflammatory bowel disease by measures such as colectomy or use of antibiotics has not been successful, as the severity of the biliary and bowel disease does not correlate in most patients. Copper depletion therapy with penicillamine is ineffective. Immunosuppressive therapy with corticosteroids, whether administered topically or systematically, is not beneficial for primary sclerosing cholangitis and may worsen the associated osteopenia. Similarly, methotrexate has no proved effect.

C. Liver Transplantation: Liver transplantation has been reserved for patients with end-stage primary sclerosing cholangitis and is successful in most of these patients (see Chapter 54). Previous colectomy or biliary surgery may make transplantation technically more difficult. In theory, the choledochojejunostomy used in transplantation increases the risks of biliary complications. However, the 5-year survival rate of patients transplanted for primary sclerosing cholangitis is similar to that of patients with primary biliary cirrhosis. Retransplantation is more common in patients with primary sclerosing cholangitis than primary biliary cirrhosis, however. Concern has been raised, as yet unproved, about recurrence of the primary sclerosing cholangitis and accelerated risks of developing colon cancer in patients with underlying inflammatory bowel disease. Monitoring for colon cancer is appropriate but should not influence the decision to perform transplantation in patients with primary sclerosing cholangitis.

Prognosis

The prognosis of primary sclerosing cholangitis varies considerably. The average survival is approximately 10 years, with progression of liver disease over this interval. In a study from the author's institution, one-third of patients followed for 6 years developed liver failure. Progression of disease may be asymptomatic or symptomatic. Models for predicting survival rates and aiding in the timing of transplantation have been developed based on age of the patient, bilirubin levels, histologic staging, and the presence or absence of splenomegaly.

OTHER DISEASES OF THE BILE DUCTS

Other diseases of the bile ducts include extrahepatic biliary obstruction and papillary stenosis. Incomplete mechanical obstruction of the bile duct may be difficult to differentiate from primary biliary cirrhosis and primary sclerosing cholangitis. Frequently, however, dilated bile ducts will be present on abdominal imaging and provide an important diagnostic clue to mechanical obstruction. This diagnosis should not be overlooked, because liver disease is reversible before secondary biliary cirrhosis arises. Secondary biliary cirrhosis can occur within 6 months of the onset of mechanical obstruction, but more typically develops over several years. Cholangiography is usually diagnostic. Liver biopsy may suggest features of mechanical obstruction such as bile infarcts, edema in the portal area, bile duct proliferation, and neutrophilic infiltrates. Mechanical obstruction should be considered when a biopsy shows edema and neutrophilic infiltrates. In contrast, in primary sclerosing cholangitis there is primarily fibrosis rather than edema, and the inflammatory cells are frequently mononuclear rather than neutrophilic.

Papillary stenosis or sphincter of Oddi dysfunction may occasionally be confused with primary problems of the bile duct in a patient complaining of upper abdominal pain who has abnormal liver tests. The existence of this process is controversial, and optimum management has not yet been established. A sphincterotomy has been most often used, but this has not been well studied in controlled trials.

REFERENCES

Crippin JS, Lindor KD: Primary sclerosing cholangitis: Etiology and immunology. Eur J Gastroenterol Hepatol 1992;4:261.

Gershwin ME, Mackay IR: Primary biliary cirrhosis: Paradigm or paradox for autoimmunity. Gastroenterology 1991;100:822.

Kaplan MM: Medical treatment of primary biliary cirrhosis. Semin Liver Dis 1989;9:138.

LaRusso NF, Ludwig J, Wiesner RH: Primary sclerosing cholangitis. Semin Liver Dis 1991;11:1.

Lindor KD: Management of osteopenia of liver disease with special emphasis on primary biliary cirrhosis. Semin Liver Dis 1993;13:367.

Lindor KD et al: Advances in primary sclerosing cholangitis. Am J Med 1990;89:73.

Lindor KD et al: Ursodeoxycholic acid in the treatment of primary biliary cirrhosis. Gastroenterology 1994;106:1284.

Poupon RE et al: The UDCA-PBC Study Group: A multicenter, controlled trial of ursodiol for the treatment of primary biliary cirrhosis. N Engl J Med 1991;324:1548.

Poupon RE et al: The UDCA-PBC Study Group: Ursodiol for the long-term treatment of primary biliary cirrhosis. N Engl J Med 1994;330:1342.

Sherlock S: Pathogenesis of sclerosing cholangitis: The role of nonimmune factors. Semin Liver Dis 1991;11:5.

Triger DR: Update on primary biliary cirrhosis. Dig Dis Sci 1990;8:61.

Wiesner RH et al: Clinical and statistical analysis of new and evolving therapies for primary biliary cirrhosis. Hepatology 1988;8:668.

52

Tumors of the Ampulla & Bile Ducts

Paul M. Basuk, MD

Ampullary and biliary tract neoplasms are uncommon tumors with similar clinical presentations. Extrahepatic biliary obstruction results in jaundice, pruritus, fevers, and weight loss. Most patients develop symptoms when the tumor is in an advanced, frequently incurable stage. This chapter concentrates on gallbladder cancer, cholangiocarcinoma, and ampullary neoplasms (Table 52–1). The diagnostic evaluation for all three tumors is similar (Figure 52–1). Advances in medical technology have resulted in better staging and characterization of these tumors. Despite these advances, the dismal prognosis has remained largely unchanged over the past four decades.

GALLBLADDER CANCER

Gallbladder cancer, the most common of the biliary tract malignant tumors, accounts for approximately 4% of all carcinomas. One to two percent of patients who undergo biliary tract surgery have gallbladder cancer. It is the fifth most common digestive system tumor and is found in 0.40–0.55% of autopsies.

Pathogenesis
The cause of gallbladder cancer is unknown. There are, however, several important risk factors associated with its development. It is more common in women, and in Japanese-Americans, Mexican-Americans, and Native Americans in the southwestern United States. As many as 22% of patients with a calcified gallbladder (**"porcelain" gallbladder**) on x-ray have gallbladder cancer. Carcinomas and adenomas coexist in a small percentage of patients, although the relationship between the two tumors is uncertain. Diminutive adenomas of the gallbladder do not appear to be a precursor to cancer.

A. Anomalies of Pancreaticobiliary Ducts: Some investigators have suggested that anomalous pancreaticobiliary ductal anatomy results in pancreatic fluid reflux, which may induce mucosal metaplasia, a premalignant condition, in the gallbladder. The

anomalous confluence of the pancreatic duct and bile duct may occur in as many as 17% of patients with gallbladder cancer, compared with 3% without cancer.

B. Gallstones: Numerous studies support a relationship between gallstones and gallbladder cancer. Sixty to ninety percent of patients with gallbladder cancer have gallstones. Both are more common in women and in identical ethnic groups. Native Americans living in the southwestern United States, Mexican-Americans, and northeastern Europeans have a higher incidence of gallstones and gallbladder cancer than blacks and Indians living in Bombay, who have a low incidence of both. A decline in the incidence of gallbladder cancer has been correlated with increased numbers of cholecystectomies. In the United States, as cholecystectomy rates increased, the mortality rate from gallbladder cancer fell by over 30% in the 1970s. Despite this association, a causal relationship between cholelithiasis and gallbladder cancer has not been established. Gallstones may result in chronic inflammation and epithelial dysplasia, leading to carcinoma. The chronically inflamed gallbladder epithelium may also be susceptible to the effects of environmental carcinogens. Chronically inflamed tissue may elaborate cytokines, which perpetuate irreversible epithelial injury. Bacterial infection associated with cholecystitis may result in the production of toxic bile acids and local carcinogens.

Pathologic Findings
The vast majority of gallbladder cancers are adenocarcinomas, most of which are scirrhous or papillary. Less common forms include adenoacanthoma, anaplastic tumors, and squamous cell carcinoma. Gallbladder cancer may be discovered incidentally at the time of gallbladder surgery. Many of these tumors are intramucosal or submucosal, with a favorable prognosis. Most gallbladder adenocarcinomas, however, are infiltrating and desmoplastic. The stages of gallbladder cancer illustrate its biologically aggressive behavior (Table 52–2).

Gallbladder cancer is characterized by advanced

Table 52–1. General characteristics of ampullary and biliary tract tumors.

	Gallbladder Cancer	Cholangiocarcinoma	Ampullary Carcinoma
Incidence in autopsy series	0.4–0.55%	0.01–0.46%	0.06–0.21%
Age of onset	7th decade	7th decade	7th–8th decade
Gender (female:male)	3:1	1:1	1:1.5
Risk factors	Native Americans in southwestern US, Japanese-Americans, Mexican-Americans; calcified gallbladder gallstones (?)	Ulcerative colitis, primary sclerosing cholangitis, hepatolithiasis, chole-dochal cysts, *Clonorchis sinensis* infection	Famillial adenomatous poly-posis
% survival at 1 year	< 5%	< 5%	40%

local disease, with extension to the biliary tree and involvement of adjacent vasculature. The cancer spreads via lymphatics to the duodenal, choledochal, and pancreatic nodes and by venous drainage to the liver. Liver invasion occurs in up to 70% of patients and regional lymph node invasion in nearly 50%. Less than 10% have cancer confined to the gallbladder. Two-thirds of patients develop noncontiguous liver metastases. Widespread intraperitoneal metastases are uncommon.

Clinical Findings

A. Symptoms and Signs: The signs and symptoms of gallbladder cancer develop insidiously and are nonspecific. Abdominal pain occurs in at least 75% of patients, followed by jaundice in 40–50% and weight loss in 40%. Patients may present with symptoms of acute cholecystitis unrelated to the malignant tumor; these cancers are usually detected at surgery and at an earlier stage. Patients who present with biliary obstruction have more advanced

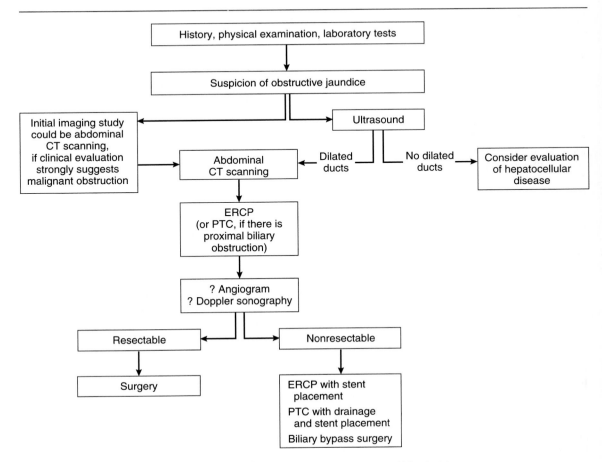

Figure 52–1. Algorithm for evaluation of ampullary and bile duct tumors.

Table 52–2. Stages of gallbladder carcinoma.

Stage I	Intramucosal or submucosal involvement
Stage II	Extending to muscularis
Stage III	Transmural to serosal involvement
Stave IV	Cystic node metastasis
Stage V	Liver or other organ involvement

disease, with nodal and vascular involvement and extension of tumor into the liver. Advanced disease may be associated with an abdominal mass, jaundice, and hepatomegaly.

B. Laboratory Findings: Laboratory blood test abnormalities are nonspecific for gallbladder cancer. Alkaline phosphatase and bilirubin levels are almost always elevated due to bile duct obstruction. Benign causes of biliary obstruction rarely result in bilirubin levels over 10 mg/dL. Occasional patients with anorexia or extensive involvement of the liver by tumor will demonstrate low serum albumin levels. Elevations of aminotransferase levels are more modest than elevations of alkaline phosphatase or bilirubin levels. Elevations of the peripheral white blood cell count may suggest cholangitis. Bleeding from the tumor results in anemia and fecal occult blood. Rarely, massive hemobilia causes significant gastrointestinal blood loss and anemia.

C. Imaging Studies: The history, physical examination, and interpretation of blood test abnormalities often suggest obstructive jaundice. Noninvasive imaging studies define the specific nature of the obstruction. Ultrasonography and CT scanning are appropriate initial imaging studies.

1. Ultrasound—Ultrasound is an excellent tool for visualizing gallstones, gallbladder polyps, or masses and bile duct obstruction. Dilatation of the bile ducts occurs proximal to the obstructing lesion. Ultrasonic patterns of gallbladder cancer include a complex, intraluminal gallbladder; marked gallbladder wall thickening; and a polypoid or fungating tumor. The addition of Doppler imaging to ultrasound may identify vascular involvement of the portal venous system and obviate the need for angiography.

2. CT scanning—When ultrasound demonstrates a gallbladder mass or ductal obstruction, CT scanning of the abdomen provides for a detailed picture of the liver, pancreas, and biliary tree. It can also stage the tumor by demonstrating vascular involvement and metastatic disease (Figure 52–2A). CT findings of gallbladder cancer include diffuse gallbladder wall thickening, intraluminal mass, direct liver invasion, lymphadenopathy, dilated bile ducts, and noncontiguous liver involvement. If CT scanning or ultrasound studies demonstrate a mass, directed biopsy or fine-needle aspiration may confirm the diagnosis of gallbladder cancer. In some cases, an an-

giogram complements the findings of abdominal CT scanning by demonstrating the degree of vascular involvement by tumor.

3. PTC and ERCP—Following ultrasound or CT scanning, or both, a diagnosis of malignant biliary obstruction will typically be made or strongly suspected. Direct imaging of the biliary tree provides specific information about the extent of biliary obstruction. Imaging techniques include percutaneous transhepatic cholangiography (PTC) and endoscopic retrograde cholangiopancreatography (ERCP). These studies reveal the extent of intraductal involvement by tumor. Interventional radiologists perform PTC. A narrow-caliber needle is passed under fluoroscopic guidance intercostally into the liver and one of the dilated biliary radicles. Following injection of contrast medium, a cholangiogram is obtained. PTC is particularly useful in demonstrating proximal ductal obstruction (Figure 52–2B). ERCP is an endoscopic procedure performed with fluoroscopy (see also Chapter 16). A side-viewing duodenoscope is passed into the second portion of the duodenum, and a catheter is guided through the ampullary orifice into the distal bile duct. Injection of contrast medium through the catheter results in a cholangiogram. The advantages of ERCP include visualization of the ampulla to detect ampullary cancer and injection of contrast medium into the pancreatic duct to detect pancreatic cancer. ERCP is a suitable study for all forms of biliary obstruction, especially distal obstructing lesions. Ductal stones are removed at the time of ERCP. Both ERCP and PTC allow for brush cytologic studies of mass lesions. Bile duct obstruction from advanced gallbladder cancer can also be palliated by either approach, using polyethylene or expandable metal stents.

Treatment

Treatment of gallbladder cancer is dictated by the stage of the tumor, which may not be clearly known until surgery. Simple cholecystectomy is adequate therapy for intramucosal gallbladder cancer. Preoperative CT scanning, ERCP, or PTC and angiography may accurately stage gallbladder cancers. Treatment of stage I and II disease is simple cholecystectomy, although some authors advocate radical cholecystectomy for stage II tumors. Treatment of stage III and IV disease may include radical cholecystectomy, consisting of cholecystectomy, resection of the gallbladder fossa, and regional node dissection. Radical cholecystectomy does not clearly improve survival rates in advanced stages of gallbladder carcinoma, however. Patients with stage V disease are candidates for palliative therapy, which includes decompression of an obstructed biliary tree with percutaneous drainage or stents or endoscopic placement of internal biliary stents. There are reports of tumor shrinkage with aggressive chemotherapy or radiation treatment, but without clear-cut clinical benefit.

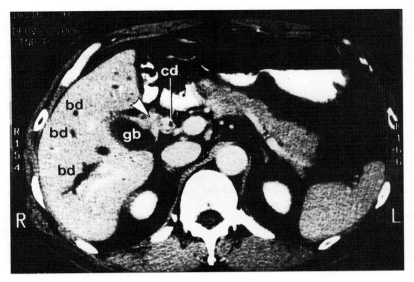

A

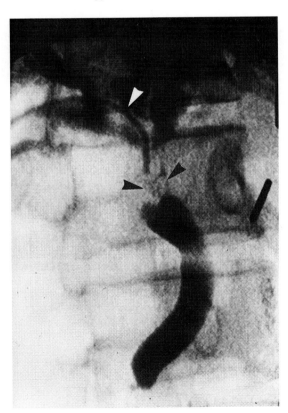

B

Figure 52–2. **A:** CT scan demonstrating dilated intra-hepatic bile ducts **(bd)** and gallbladder cancer **(arrow)** extending into the common bile duct **(cd)**. **B:** Cholan-giogram of the same patient with a bile duct stricture **(dark arrows)** (the transhepatic catheter is identified by the white arrow). On the basis of the cholangiogram alone, it would be impossible to differentiate this lesion from cholangiocarcinoma.

Prognosis

The prognosis of gallbladder cancer depends on its stage (Table 52–3). Overall mean survival rates are less than 6 months, and 5-year survival rates are less than 5%.

CHOLANGIOCARCINOMA

In autopsy series of patients with jaundice, 10% have cholangiocarcinoma as the underlying cause. Most develop jaundice with advanced stages of the tumor, when it is unresectable. Cures of cholangiocarcinoma are uncommon.

Pathogenesis

Cholangiocarcinoma is thought to arise from a pluripotent stem cell or periductal biliary glands; the precipitating event is unknown, but several risk factors are associated.

A. Primary Sclerosing Cholangitis: In Western societies, the disease entity most strongly associated with cholangiocarcinoma is primary sclerosing cholangitis (7–9% of patients develop cholangiocarcinoma). In one autopsy series, 42% of patients with primary sclerosing cholangitis had concomitant cholangiocarcinoma. Despite the exhaustive evaluation of primary sclerosing cholangitis patients during the course of the disease and prior to liver transplantation, as many as 9% are found to have cholangiocarcinoma when undergoing transplantation. Tumor develops following years of disease in patients with primary sclerosing cholangitis.

B. Chronic Ulcerative Colitis: Patients with chronic ulcerative colitis are also at risk of developing cholangiocarcinoma. This association does not apply to Crohn's disease. The relative risk of bile duct carcinoma in chronic ulcerative colitis patients is 31 times that of the general population, probably owing to associated primary sclerosing cholangitis. The mean age of patients with chronic ulcerative colitis and cholangiocarcinoma is 30 years younger than that of patients with chronic ulcerative colitis. The diagnosis of chronic ulcerative colitis precedes the development of cholangiocarcinoma by 19 years. Total colectomy does not reduce the risk of subsequent tumor development.

C. Clonorchis sinensis Infection: Cyprinid fish ingestion may result in transmission of the parasite *Clonorchis sinensis,* which has been associated with cholangiocarcinoma. The parasites enter the bile duct from the duodenum and reside in the intrahepatic ducts, where they mature. In one study, 26% of Asian immigrants to New York City had *Clonorchis* infection. The fluke worm lives for 20–30 years. Suckers on the parasite result in chronic ductal injury and predispose to bacterial infection of damaged epithelium. Saccular or cystic dilatation of the intrahepatic ducts produces a berrylike appearance on cholangiogram. Case reports and a large autopsy series from Thailand demonstrated liver fluke worm infections in 78% of patients with cholangiocarcinoma. Cholangiocarcinoma associated with *Clonorchis* infection is often hilar and intrahepatic where the worm resides.

D. Choledochal Cyst: Carcinomas arising in extrahepatic congenital biliary choledochal cysts occur with an overall frequency as high as 3% (see Chapter 53). The risk of cholangiocarcinoma is greater in those with choledochal cyst that becomes symptomatic later in life. Seventy percent of patients developing cyst-related cholangiocarcinoma are female, with a mean age of 34 years. For this reason, the surgical approach to choledochal cysts usually includes attempts at curative excision and not bypass alone.

E. Gallstones: Thirty percent of patients with cholangiocarcinoma have gallstones. According to epidemiologic data, the risk of cholangiocarcinoma declines following cholecystectomy. It is unclear whether the association of cholangiocarcinoma and gallstones is causal or not. Further study into the role of toxic bile salts, cytokines, and chronic inflammation associated with gallstones may elucidate factors contributing to the development of cholangiocarcinoma.

F. Other Risk Factors: Less commonly seen entities associated with cholangiocarcinoma include a history of Thorotrast injection. Thorotrast was a radiocontrast agent used over 50 years ago, with an unusually long biologic half-life and a propensity to remain within the reticuloendothelial system. Hepatolithiasis and α_1-antitrypsin deficiency may be additional risk factors for cholangiocarcinoma.

Pathologic Findings

Cholangiocarcinomas can be broadly classified into several types: cholangiocellular carcinoma are peripheral tumors that originate along intrahepatic ductal radicles; (bifurcation, hilar, or "Klatskin" tumors [named after Gerald Klatskin, who described 13 patients with these tumors in 1965]) occur at the confluence of the right and left hepatic ducts; and tumors that occur in the middle and distal thirds of the common bile duct.

Over 90% of bile duct tumors are adenocarcinomas. A smaller percentage are squamous cell carci-

Table 52–3. Survival times for gallbladder cancer.

	Survival times (%)[1]	
	1 year	5 years
Stage I	100	96
Stage II	87	56
Stage III	53	15
Stage IV	58	16
Stage V	10	6

[1]Data reproduced, with permission, from Nagorney DM, McPherson GAD: Semin Oncol 1988;15(2):106.

nomas, undifferentiated carcinomas, leiomyosarcomas, granular cell tumors, cystadenocarcinomas, or carcinoid tumors. Benign papillomatous disease of the biliary tract presents as a single papilloma, usually in the distal bile duct, or as multiple papillary tumors throughout the biliary tree.

Adenocarcinomas of the bile duct fall into one of three recognizable forms: the intrahepatic cholangiolocellular or peripheral carcinoma; the scirrhous or sclerosing carcinoma; and the papillary carcinoma. The scirrhous cholangiocarcinoma is a common type and often develops at the bifurcation of the right and left hepatic ducts. It presents as an annular, constricting tumor with a dense fibroblastic reaction. Less than 10% of these tumors are resectable. Papillary cholangiocarcinoma more commonly occurs in the common bile duct, presents at an earlier stage, and has the most favorable prognosis of the three different types of carcinoma. Peripheral cholangiocarcinoma mimics hepatocellular carcinoma, although it arises from bile duct epithelium or peribiliary glands.

The location of the cholangiocarcinoma strongly influences its clinical presentation and prognosis. Approximately 50% of tumors are at the bifurcation of the major hepatic ducts, 20–25% along the mid portion of the common bile duct, and 10–20% in the distal common bile duct. Tumors situated diffusely throughout the biliary tree constitute 5–10% of cholangiocarcinomas. Klatskin tumors are classified into three types, based on the involvement of the bifurcation and extension into the hepatic ducts (Figure 52–3). A hilar carcinoma situated in the proximal common hepatic duct, not obstructing the bifurcation nor extending into either of the major hepatic ducts, is a type I tumor; these may be resectable. A type II hilar carcinoma obstructs the bifurcation but does not extend into the right or left hepatic duct. Type III hilar cholangiocarcinoma extends at least to a secondary right or left ductal radicle. Type II and III hilar tumors are often complex and unresectable.

Metastatic disease from cholangiocarcinoma occurs in 75% of patients. Cholangiocarcinoma spreads to regional lymph nodes in 50% of patients, the liver in 20%, the portal vein in 10–15%, and the lung in 10–15%. Notably, vascular involvement with cholangiocarcinoma is less common than with gallbladder cancer.

Clinical Findings

Obstructive jaundice is the hallmark feature of cholangiocarcinoma. The clinical evaluation and radiographic studies often suggest a malignant tumor; however, it may not be possible to differentiate either biliary obstruction resulting from gallbladder cancer or pancreatic cancer from cholangiocarcinoma. In most patients, these tumors are unresectable, and the distinction is purely an academic one because treatment is palliative and not based on the type of tumor. Sometimes, only surgical exploration determines the

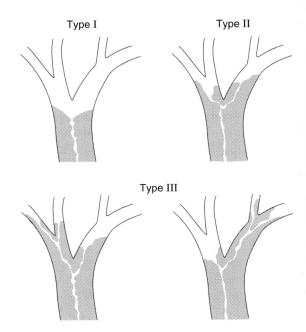

Figure 52–3. Three types of bile duct bifurcation tumors (see text for description).

extent and resectability of a tumor. In some patients, the tumor is resectable or the obstruction is not malignant. A thorough evaluation of obstructive jaundice should identify patients with benign disease who can be treated nonsurgically.

A. Symptoms and Signs: The most common clinical feature of cholangiocarcinoma is jaundice, which occurs in 90% of patients. Other common symptoms include weight loss in 40–50%, abdominal pain in 40–50%, pruritus in 30–40%, and fevers or cholangitis in 10–20%. Patients usually develop symptoms in the seventh or eighth decade, although those with primary sclerosing cholangitis develop cholangiocarcinoma in their thirties or forties. Men and women develop cancer in relatively equal numbers. Besides jaundice, other findings include hepatomegaly in 50–60% of patients, fecal occult blood in 50–60%, and stigmas of portal hypertension in less than 5%.

Distal bile duct carcinomas may result in a markedly distended gallbladder (so-called "Courvoisier gallbladder") or cholecystitis. Bifurcation tumors often present with jaundice, anorexia, weight loss, and hepatomegaly. Tumors obstructing a single hepatic duct or a peripheral type of cholangiolocellular carcinoma may not lead to jaundice.

B. Laboratory Findings: Laboratory blood tests demonstrate elevations of bilirubin and alkaline phosphatase levels in at least 90% of patients. Modest elevations of aminotransferase levels develop in 20–30% and hypoalbuminemia in 30–40%. Patients with tumors obstructing a single hepatic duct or with a peripheral type of cholangiolocellular carcinoma often have elevated alkaline phosphatase levels, with normal or nearly normal bilirubin levels.

Patients with primary sclerosing cholangitis pose a dilemma because of the difficulty in diagnosing an associated cholangiocarcinoma. Progressive clinical deterioration along with worsening jaundice characterize the development of cholangiocarcinoma in these patients. Routine laboratory tests fail to predict or identify the patient with primary sclerosing cholangitis and ductal carcinoma. Measurements of CA 19-9, a tumor-associated antigen, when elevated beyond 100 U/mL, may be a marker of ductal cancer in patients with primary sclerosing cholangitis. CA 19-9 does not predict the development of cholangio-carcinoma. Elevated CA 19-9 levels associated with cholangiocarcinoma indicate advanced disease. The combination of carcinoembryonic antigen and CA 19-9 enhances the predictive value of either individually for cholangiocarcinoma. In a recent study, an index score of [CA 19-9 + (CEA × 40)] over 400 had a positive predictive value for cholangiocarcinoma of 100%.

C. Imaging Studies: The clinical suspicion of obstructive jaundice necessitates imaging studies.

1. CT scanning and ultrasound–If malignant obstruction is strongly suspected, abdominal CT scanning provides valuable information about a malignant tumor that ultrasound frequently does not detect. If there is doubt about the cause of jaundice, ultrasound is a helpful initial imaging study. Ultrasound demonstrates bile duct dilatation and the level of obstruction in over 90% of patients (Figure 52–4A). It less commonly identifies the cause of the obstruction. CT scanning complements ultrasound studies because it more accurately identifies the cause and provides important information about resectability (Figure 52–4B). Because at least 70% of cholangiocarcinomas are unresectable at presentation, CT findings of unresectability may prevent attempts at surgical resection. CT evidence of tumor unresectability includes adenopathy, perivascular fat plane invasion, encasement or occlusion of a major vascular structure, invasion of adjacent organs, ascites, or peritoneal metastases. With 80% certainty, any of these CT findings predict unresectability.

2. Angiography–Angiography may complement CT scanning by demonstrating vascular involvement by tumor. The addition of Doppler sonography to ultrasound may provide information comparable to that obtained with angiography.

3. PTC and ERCP–Following noninvasive imaging studies, cholangiography defines the extent of tumor involvement. For bifurcation tumors, PTC successfully images the proximal biliary tree. For distal bile duct tumors, ERCP should adequately determine the extent of intraductal tumor (Figure 52–4C). Brush cytologic studies of cholangiocarcinoma, performed either percutaneously or endoscopically, often confirm the clinical suspicion of cancer. Cholangiographic evidence of involvement of both hepatic ducts is a sign of unresectability. The combination of unilateral vascular involvement and extensive contralateral spread of tumor is evidence of unresectability.

Treatment

A. Resection: Most cholangiocarcinomas are

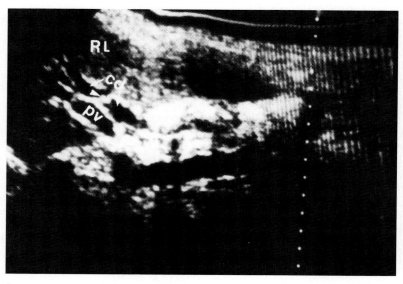

A

Figure 52–4. **A:** Ultrasound of cholangiocarcinoma **(arrow).** The common bile duct is dilated proximal to the tumor. RL, right lobe of liver; cd, common bile duct; pv, portal vein.

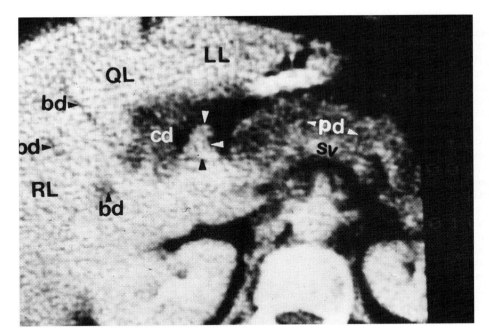

B

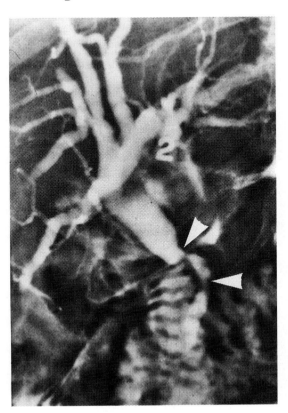

C

Figure 52–4. *B:* CT scan of the same patient, with arrows pointing to a tumor within the common bile duct. RL, right lobe of liver; QL, caudate lobe of liver; LL, left lobe of liver; bd, dilated intrahepatic bile ducts; cd, common bile duct; pd, pancreatic duct; sv, splenic vein. *C:* Cholangiogram of the same lesion *(arrows)* in the mid portion of the common bile duct.

unresectable at the time of diagnosis. Resectability is determined by noninvasive imaging studies, cholangiography, angiography, and, in some patients, surgery. The type of resection depends on the location of the tumor. Surgical resection of distal common bile duct tumors involves pancreaticoduodenectomy. Resection of tumors of the middle third of the bile duct is followed by Roux-en-Y hepaticojejunostomy or choledochojejunostomy. Bifurcation tumors require complicated resections, with a surgical mortality rate of 5–10%. Surgery involves hilar ductal resection, limited hepatic resection, and Roux-en-Y anastomosis of a limb of jejunum to the right and left hepatic duct. Limited hepatic resection is associated with increased rates of complications and death for radical surgery of bifurcation tumors and does not clearly improve survival rates. Mean survival rates following radical surgery are 20–30 months, with or without liver resection.

B. Palliative Therapy: Most patients with cholangiocarcinoma are candidates for palliative, rather than curative, therapy. Surgical palliation involves ductal bypass to a Roux-en-Y limb of jejunum. Nonsurgical palliation includes percutaneous tube drainage and stenting and endoscopic placement of biliary stents. Until recently, endoscopic stenting of malignant bile duct strictures utilized 10 French to 12 French polyethylene stents. Prospective studies comparing endoscopic polyethylene stenting with surgical palliation of malignant biliary obstruction (including patients with pancreatic cancer) failed to demonstrate any difference in long-term survival rates between the two study groups. Rates of short-term complications were greater in the surgery group because of operative complications, while rates of long-term complications were greater in the endoscopic treatment group due to recurrent stent occlusion.

1. Stenting procedures–Technologic advances in stent manufacturing have resulted in the development of expandable metal stents. These stents are permanent, are placed percutaneously or endoscopically, and expand to the size of a 30 French stent following insertion. In preliminary comparisons of 10 French polyethylene stents with 30 French expandable metal stents for malignant biliary obstruction, survival rates were similar in the two study groups. There is a greater frequency of stent occlusion and cholangitis with polyethylene stents. Tumor ingrowth through the mesh of the metal stent can result in stent occlusion, which can be managed by insertion of another metal or polyethylene stent into the original stent (Table 52–4).

2. Chemotherapy and irradiation–There are reports of improvement following chemotherapy or radiation therapy. Single-agent regimens using mitomycin or fluorouracil and combination regimens using doxorubicin hydrochloride, carmustine, and tegafur; or doxorubicin hydrochloride, fluorouracil, and mitomycin have demonstrated shrinkage in tumor

Table 52–4. Randomized clinical trials of metal and polyethylene endoprostheses for malignant biliary obstruction.

	Metal Stent	Plastic Stent	p Value
30-day mortality rates			
Amsterdam (1992)	14%	5%	< 0.05
Germany (1993)	—	—	—
USA Wallstent Group (1993)	5%	5%	NS
Stent occlusion			
Amsterdam (1992)	33%	54%	—
Germany (1993)	22%	43%	NS
USA Wallstent Group (1993)	13%	13%	NS
Time to occlusion USA Wallstent Group (1993)	111 days	62 days	—

[1]Davids PHP et al: Randomised trial of self-expanding metal stents versus polyethylene stents for distal malignant biliary obstruction. Lancet 1992;340:1488.
[2]Knyrin K et al: A prospective, randomized, controlled trial of metal stents for malignant obstruction of the common bile duct. Endoscopy 1993;25:207.
[3]Carr-Locke DL et al: Multicenter, randomized trial of Wallstent biliary endoprosthesis versus plastic stents. Gastrointest Endosc 1993;39:310a.

size without improvement in survival rates. Favorable responses to intraductal irradiation with ^{192}Ir wire have been reported. Chemotherapy and radiation therapy are largely palliative, and their specific role in the management of cholangiocarcinoma awaits large, prospective clinical trials.

C. Orthotopic Liver Transplantation: Results of orthotopic liver transplantation for patients with cholangiocarcinoma are poor. Five-year survival rates are less than 20%, and tumor recurs in most patients. At the current time, transplantation is not a viable treatment option for cholangiocarcinoma.

Prognosis

The prognosis of cholangiocarcinoma depends on its location, histologic characteristics, and stage. Five- year survival rates for proximal tumors are zero to 40%; for middle-third common bile duct tumors, zero to 12%; and for distal-third common bile duct tumors, 20–40%. Papillary tumors have the most favorable prognosis, with a 5-year survival rate of 31%. Scirrhous tumors, more commonly found in bifurcation tumors, have a 5-year survival rate of no more than 20%.

The overall mean survival time for patients with cholangiocarcinoma is 5–22 months. Long-term survival times are dismal; less than 1% of patients live for 10 years.

AMPULLARY CARCINOMA

Tumors at the choledochoduodenal junction are either pancreatic, ampullary, distal bile duct, or duodenal. Distinguishing between these tumors is difficult and occasionally not accomplished until surgery. Ampullary carcinoma comprises 6–12% of all tumors at the choledochoduodenal junction; it often presents clinically at an earlier stage and has the most favorable prognosis of all these tumors.

Pathogenesis

Ampullary neoplasms arise from ampullary epithelium. Initially, the epithelium may undergo neoplastic differentiation and become adenomatous. At least 30% of patients with ampullary carcinoma have areas of adenomatous epithelium within the lesion. Up to 91% of invasive ampullary carcinomas contain adenomas, adenomatous tissue, or intramural adenomas. Eighty-one percent of patients demonstrate epithelial dysplasia in the vicinity of resected ampullary cancers. Ampullary carcinoma may develop from a preexisting adenoma in a large percentage of cases.

Patients with **familial adenomatous polyposis** develop multiple adenomas in the colon and small intestine. The most common cause of death in patients with this disorder who are treated with colectomy is not colorectal cancer but rather duodenal and ampullary carcinoma. Ninety to 100% of patients with familial adenomatous polyposis have ampullary and periampullary adenomas. The risk of developing ampullary adenocarcinoma in patients with familial adenomatous polyposis is 100–200 times greater than that in the general population. Because many ampullary adenomas do not progress to carcinoma, it is not necessary to perform prophylactic surgery on the adenoma. Given the risks of ampullary carcinoma, patients with familial adenomatous polyposis should undertake a program of surveillance endoscopy at regular intervals. Interestingly, when ERCP is used as an additional screening method for pancreaticobiliary adenomas in patients with familial adenomatous polyposis, biliary polyps are detected in as many as 40% of patients.

Pathologic Findings

Ampullary carcinomas are either papillary or ulcerating adenocarcinomas. Tumors smaller than 2 cm and papillary tumors have the most favorable prognosis. Lymph node metastases are present in 20–50% of resected cancers and occur more frequently with ulcerating tumors. The pancreaticoduodenal nodes are most commonly involved. Tumor spread to the duodenum and local venous structures occurs in 30% of patients. Distant metastases are unusual. The staging of ampullary carcinoma is shown in Table 52–5.

Clinical Findings

The history, physical examination, and laboratory tests suggest malignant biliary obstruction. Most causes of malignant obstruction result in a similar clinical appearance. Imaging studies elucidate the specific type of obstruction. Even after imaging stud-

Table 52–5. Stages of ampullary carcinoma (based on TNM classification).

Stage I	Limited to ampulla
Stage II	Extension into duodenal wall, or ≤ 2 cm into pancreas
Stage III	Regional node involvement
Stage IV	> 2 cm invasion into pancreas, or involvement of other organs, or distant metastases

(Reproduced, with permission, from: Hermanek P, Sobel LH [editors]. TNM classification of malignant tumors, 4/e. Springer, 1992.)

ies, it may not be possible to differentiate one choledochoduodenal junction tumor from another. That distinction may not be necessary if the patient has extensive disease and is not suitable for surgery. Sometimes, the distinction is made at surgery, but it is not a critical finding, since the operative approach for choledochoduodenal junction tumors is similar.

A. Symptoms and Signs: Ampullary carcinoma most commonly occurs in the seventh decade of life. The male to female ratio is 1.5:1. The most common clinical manifestation is jaundice due to biliary obstruction. Unlike in cholangiocarcinoma, jaundice may fluctuate early in the course of illness and thus suggest a nonneoplastic cause such as ductal calculi. The intermittent jaundice may be secondary to recurrent sloughing of the central portion of the tumor.

Pruritus, anorexia, intermittent cholangitis, and a palpable gallbladder (Courvoisier gallbladder) may develop. Unfortunately, these symptoms develop in many patients with malignant biliary obstruction and are not specific for ampullary cancer. Anemia and fecal occult blood are more common with ulcerating ampullary tumors. Hepatomegaly is a nonspecific finding in about 50% of patients.

B. Laboratory Findings: As with other causes of biliary obstruction, the principal laboratory findings include marked hyperbilirubinemia and increased alkaline phosphatase levels. Modest elevations of aminotransferase measurements may occur.

C. Imaging Studies: (See also Chapter 15). It is not sufficient to diagnose obstructive jaundice on the basis of clinical judgment alone. Imaging studies confirm the diagnosis of obstruction, identify its cause, and help stage malignant tumors.

1. Ultrasound–Ultrasound is usually the initial imaging study because it provides useful information about the bile ducts, avoids radiation (for some patients this may be a concern), and is inexpensive. Ultrasound reveals extrahepatic bile duct dilatation, usually to the distal bile duct and often the ampulla. It may delineate the ampullary mass between the distal bile duct and the duodenum when luminal fluid or gas is present.

2. CT scanning–Abdominal CT scanning is often ordered after ultrasound studies, since it usually provides more specific information about the ob-

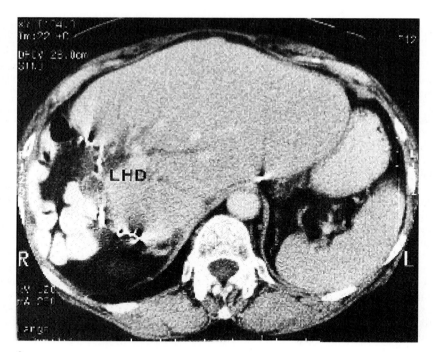

A

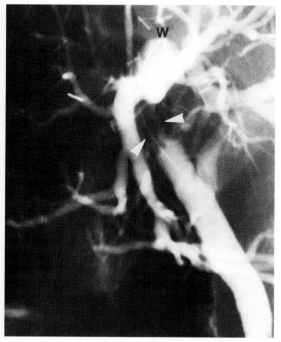

B

Figure 52–5. A 74-year-old patient developed obstructive jaundice 1 year following a right hepatic lobectomy for metastatic colon cancer. **A:** This CT scan demonstrated significant left hepatic ductal **(Lhd)** dilatation, without a discrete hilar mass. **B:** The cholangiogram revealed a stricture in the proximal common hepatic duct **(arrows).** A wire **(W)** was positioned at ERCP across the stricture to facilitate stent placement. Brush cytologic studies of the lesion at ERCP were positive for adenocarcinoma.

struction. If the clinical suspicion strongly favors malignant jaundice (eg, in the elderly patient with painless jaundice, anorexia, and pruritus), CT scanning should replace ultrasound as the initial imaging study. CT scanning provides better imaging of the pancreas than ultrasound and may visualize large ampullary tumors.

3. ERCP and PTC–If the level of biliary obstruction is at the distal choledochus, ERCP should be the next study. ERCP permits inspection and biopsy of the ampulla, visualization of the biliary tree, and contrast study of the pancreatic duct. If the pancreatic duct is normal, pancreatic cancer is unlikely. If the tumor is incurable, palliation of jaundice is possible at the time of ERCP. PTC is an alternative to ERCP in those centers without a biliary endoscopist or when the tumor is so bulky as to prevent cannulation of the bile duct at ERCP. In the setting of biliary obstruction, PTC successfully images the biliary tree in almost all patients. PTC does not permit inspection of the ampulla or contrast study of the pancreatic duct.

4. Endoscopic ultrasound–Endoscopic ultrasound using a transduodenal approach may be helpful in the preoperative assessment of patients with ampullary carcinoma. As a complement to the above studies, it may help in the staging of ampullary tumors by detecting nodal spread, extension through the duodenum, and invasion of local organs and the portal venous circulation.

Treatment

Ampullary carcinoma is more curable at presentation than either gallbladder carcinoma or cholangiocarcinoma. Preoperative imaging studies are most helpful in determining unresectability; however, surgical exploration is the definitive means of establishing resectability. Curative resection of ampullary carcinoma is done by pancreaticoduodenectomy. The operative mortality rate is 5–10%. An alternative procedure is ampullectomy, which in some authors' experience has similar long-term survival rates but less operative risk than pancreaticoduodenectomy. Treatment of ampullary carcinoma is based on the stage of the tumor.

Curative resection is the treatment of choice for stage I and II tumors. Treatment of patients with stage III or IV tumors should be tailored to institutional expertise. Surgical palliation includes choledochoenteric bypass. Nonsurgical palliation involves ERCP or PTC. Endoscopic palliation consists of sphincterotomy, with placement of bile duct stents in most patients. Percutaneous biliary drainage and placement of transpapillary stents are alternatives to endoscopic palliation.

Prognosis

Ampullary carcinoma is resectable in as many as 85% of patients due to its indolent growth and early symptoms. The overall 5-year survival rate is 40%, but this is based on a range of 6–62%. Certain factors portend a more favorable prognosis, including stage I or II tumors, papillary type of histologic findings, and absence of nodal involvement. The mean survival time following pancreaticoduodenectomy is as high as 55 months, although this is halved with nodal involvement. Endoscopic palliation is usually reserved for unresectable tumors and is associated with a mean survival time of 9–12 months. Surgical bypass operations, also reserved for unresectable tumors, result in a mean survival time of 6 months when metastases are present and up to 42 months when they are not.

MISCELLANEOUS TUMORS OF THE AMPULLA & BILE DUCTS

Metastatic Tumors

A number of tumors metastasize to the bile duct and periductal lymph nodes. Advanced colon cancer, breast cancer, gastric cancer, and melanoma are examples of such tumors (Figure 52–5). Non-Hodgkin's lymphoma may also involve the biliary tree. These tumors can mimic bile duct tumors clinically, biochemically, and radiographically. Brush cytologic studies of the ductal lesions, if positive, may not readily characterize the type of tumor. Usually, the history and physical examination provide clues to the presence of a nonpancreaticobiliary tumor. Special staining of cytologic aspirates may facilitate a diagnosis of breast cancer.

Tumors in AIDS Patients

In patients with AIDS, Kaposi's sarcoma and non-Hodgkin's lymphoma may involve the ampulla (see also Chapter 39). Kaposi's sarcoma rarely occurs in the absence of cutaneous involvement. Lymphoma limited to the ampulla or duodenum is unusual.

REFERENCES

Diehl AK, Beral V: Cholecystectomy and changing mortality from gallbladder cancer. Lancet 1981;2:187.

Jones RS: Carcinoma of the gallbladder. Surg Clin North Am 1990;70:1419.

Looser C et al: Staging of hilar cholangiocarcinoma by ultrasound and duplex sonography: A comparison with angiography and operative findings. Br J Radiol 1992;65:871.

Mukai H et al: Evaluation of endoscopic ultrasonography in the preoperative staging of carcinoma of the ampulla of

Vater and common bile duct. Gastrointest Endosc 1992;38:676.

Nichols JC et al: Diagnostic role of serum CA 19-1 for cholangiocarcinoma in patients with primary sclerosing cholangitis. Mayo Clin Proc 1993;68:874.

Nunnerly HB, Karan JB: Intraductal radiation. Radiol Clin North Am 1990;28:1237.

Offerhaus CGA et al: The risk of upper gastrointestinal cancer in familial adenomatous polyposis. Gastroenterology 1992;102:1980.

Ona FV, Dytoc JNT: *Clonorchis*-associated cholangiocarcinoma: A report of two cases with unusual manifestations. Gastroenterology 1991;101:831.

Polydorou AA et al: Palliation of proximal malignant biliary obstruction by endoscopic endoprosthesis insertion. Gut 1991;32:685.

Rabinowitz M et al: Diagnostic value of brush cytology in the diagnosis of bile duct carcinoma: A study in 65 patients with bile duct strictures. Gut 1992;33:1675.

Ramage JK et al: Serum tumor markers for the diagnosis of cholangiocarcinoma in primary sclerosing cholangitis. Gastroenterology 1995;108:865.

Rosen CB, Nagorney DM: Cholangiocarcinoma complicating primary sclerosing cholangitis. Semin Liv Dis 1991;11:26.

Yamaguchi K, Enjoji M: Carcinoma of the ampulla of Vater. Cancer 1987;59:506.

Yeo CJ, Pitt HA, Cameron JL: Cholangiocarcinoma. Surg Clin North Am 1990;70:1429.

Cystic Diseases of the Bile Duct & Liver

53

Rowen K. Zetterman, MD

There is significant clinical overlapping among the fibrocystic diseases of the liver, which include congenital hepatic fibrosis, biliary microhamartomas (Meyenburg's complexes), polycystic liver disease, Caroli's disease, and choledochal cysts. These diseases occur in varying combinations, with congenital hepatic fibrosis the most frequently recurring disorder. Cysts appear to arise from biliary components and may or may not communicate with or be an integral part of the biliary tree. There is an increased risk of carcinoma in patients with fibrocystic diseases, including those with choledochal cysts, Caroli's disease, congenital hepatic fibrosis, and microhamartomas.

Microhamartomas are typically asymptomatic and often found when liver biopsy is obtained for other reasons. On gross examination of the biopsy specimen, they may appear as small white deposits, and on histologic examination, they may be seen as enlarged fibrotic portal areas with increased numbers of bile ducts and nerve fibers (Figure 53–1).

Congenital hepatic fibrosis is characterized by broad bands of fibrosis creating enlarged portal areas, which can result in portal hypertension. When portal hypertension is present, congenital hepatic fibrosis should be considered, although portal hypertension may also occur for other reasons in cystic disease (see Chapter 48).

SOLITARY CYSTS

Essentials of Diagnosis

- Typically unilocular and single in number.
- More common in women.

General Considerations

Solitary liver cysts are common, occurring in more than 2.5% of the adult population. They are more often found in the right lobe than the left, are four times more frequent in women than men, and are usually identified in persons 20–50 years of age. While most are small, cysts as large as 17 L have

been described. If aspirated, cystic fluid is usually clear but may be bile stained.

Pathophysiology

Solitary cysts of the liver are thought to be congenital and arise from aberrant bile duct remnants. Most are true cysts lined by biliary-type epithelium, although "pseudocysts" lined by fibrous tissue also occur.

Clinical Findings

A. Symptoms and Signs: Isolated liver cysts are usually asymptomatic, although vague right upper quadrant discomfort may develop from the mass effect if cysts are large. Compression of adjacent viscera or bile ducts can cause nausea and vomiting or jaundice. If cysts are pedunculated, torsion can result in severe pain, hemorrhage, or rupture. A palpable mass may be rarely noted on physical examination. Large cysts may be mistaken for ascites.

B. Laboratory Findings: There are no abnormalities in biochemical liver tests in the absence of major bile duct compression.

C. Imaging Studies: Cysts are typically round or ovoid, well circumscribed, and more common in the right lobe. The location and size of the cyst will affect radiographic findings, producing elevation of the right diaphragm, displacement of adjacent organs, or compression of major bile ducts. The cyst wall may calcify and be confused with an echinococcal cyst. The absence of daughter cysts in association with a simple liver cyst should assist in the differentiation.

Ultrasound is the best and most cost-effective test. Liver and spleen scans will identify only a cold filling defect, whether the cyst is benign or infectious. Ultrasound will reveal the simple cyst as a well-defined, thin-walled, noncomplex cyst lacking internal echoes. Ultrasound can also exclude cysts in the kidney or pancreas.

CT scanning offers little additional information and need not be completed when ultrasound has identified a simple liver cyst. CT scanning will also

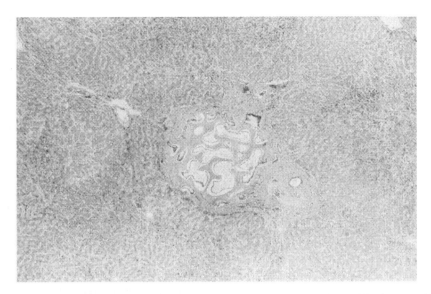

Figure 53–1. Microhamartoma with increased portal area size, multiple enlarged bile ducts, and fibrosis.

define a smooth-walled filling defect that lacks internal structures and has an attenuation similar to that of water. If MRI is used, solitary cysts may be confused with hemangiomas, as both are hyperdense on a T_2-weighted image and hypodense with T_1 weighting. If gadolinium is used, there is no increase in signal intensity in a simple cyst.

Differential Diagnosis

Other diseases may produce solitary cysts with an appearance similar to that of the solitary liver cyst. These include infectious cysts (both bacterial and echinococcal), cystic tumors such as biliary cystadenoma, endometriosis involving the liver, old intrahepatic hematomas, and pseudocysts that arise from the pancreas and erode into the liver. Certain features may assist in differentiation (eg, bacterial and echinococcal cysts are thick walled with coexisting internal echoes, and cystic tumors are often multiloculated). Old hematomas from either endometriosis or trauma may be difficult to differentiate radiographically, although a history of endometriosis or trauma is helpful.

Complications

Complications of solitary cysts are rare. Cystic rupture into the biliary tree or peritoneal cavity, intracystic hemorrhage, infection, and enlargement causing bile duct obstruction, visceral compression, or pain may develop.

Treatment

Treatment of a solitary cyst is usually not required. If symptomatic, smaller cysts of less than 8 cm in diameter may be aspirated and injected with a scle-

rosant such as absolute ethanol. Large cysts may require operation, although some may be excised. The cyst wall, however, may contain large blood vessels, with risk of hemorrhage. Biliary fistulas may also follow resection. Simply unroofing the cyst to permit continuing drainage of contents into the peritoneal cavity may be preferable. Infected cysts should be drained externally with a percutaneously placed catheter.

Prognosis

As solitary cysts are usually asymptomatic, the prognosis is excellent. Aspirated cysts may recur. Recurrence is unusual following resection.

CHOLEDOCHAL CYST

Essentials of Diagnosis

- Single or multiple dilatations of the extrahepatic biliary tree.
- Occurs as concentric bile duct dilatation or a diverticulum.

General Considerations

Choledochal cysts may be identified at any age. Two percent present in infancy, 60% before age 10 years, and 75% by age 20 years. Females are four times more likely to be affected, except in the case of choledochoceles, for which the incidence is similar in males and females. Choledochal cysts may be more prevalent in Asia.

*See also Chapter 48.

There are multiple types of choledochal cysts:

Type I: Fusiform or saccular dilatation of the common bile duct with distal duct narrowing (85%).
Type II: Diverticulum of the common bile duct (1–2%).
Type III: Choledochocele (dilatation of the intraduodenal segment of the common bile duct) (1–5%).
Type IV: Generalized involvement of both the extrahepatic and intrahepatic ducts (> 10%).

Choledochal cysts may be associated with other anomalies of the biliary tree, including common duct or gallbladder duplication and accessory hepatic ducts. There may also be coexisting hypoplastic or polycystic kidneys.

Pathophysiology

An anomalous junction of the pancreatic duct and common bile duct proximal to the sphincter of Oddi is frequently observed in patients with choledochal cysts, creating a common channel of up to 2 cm in length. This permits reflux of pancreatic secretions into the common bile duct and may weaken the duct wall, resulting in enlargement of the duct. Choledochal cysts also appear to be part of the spectrum of fibrocystic disorders, as congenital hepatic fibrosis is frequently associated. Biliary atresia occurs in 2% of cases and raises the possibility of distal obstruction and bile duct weakness as a cause.

Clinical Findings

A. Symptoms and Signs: The classic triad of pain, abdominal mass, and jaundice develops in approximately one-third of patients. Overall, two-thirds will present with jaundice, 60% with a mass, and 55% with pain. The presentation in infants is similar to that of biliary atresia. A palpable mass may extend from the liver to the umbilicus. Cholangitis, typically with enteric organisms, may result in fever and chills. At diagnosis, portal hypertension may be evident due to coexisting biliary cirrhosis or congenital hepatic fibrosis. Recurrent abdominal pain from pancreatitis is described.

B. Laboratory Findings: Cholestasis with elevation of alkaline phosphatase and gamma glutamyltransferase and hyperamylasemia due to pancreatitis and conjugated hyperbilirubinemia are observed. Histologic findings in the liver may be normal or demonstrate cholestasis or biliary cirrhosis. Biliary atresia or congenital hepatic fibrosis may be present.

C. Imaging Studies: Ultrasonography or CT scanning is the preferred diagnostic study and will identify a dilated segment of the common bile duct with an abrupt change between the dilated portion and the normal duct. Biliary scans may show accumulation of isotopes in a dilated common bile duct or

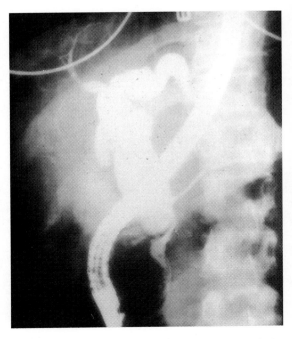

Figure 53–2. Retrograde cholangiography of a choledochal cyst. CBD = common bile duct; PD = pancreatic duct.

a choledochocele. Cholangiography may be used (Figure 53–2). Debris or stones may accumulate within the cyst and result in pancreatitis or cholangitis.

Differential Diagnosis

Other causes of common bile duct obstruction must be excluded. With ultrasound or CT scanning, a pseudocyst of the pancreatic head that causes jaundice from biliary obstruction may be confused with a choledochal cyst.

Complications

Choledochal cysts may develop spontaneous or traumatic rupture, rupture during pregnancy, obstructive jaundice, sludge and stone formation within the cyst, liver abscess, and biliary cirrhosis. Choledochoceles cause obstructive jaundice in one-fourth and pancreatitis in approximately one-third of cases. Portal hypertension may result from secondary biliary cirrhosis, congenital hepatic fibrosis, or compression of the portal vein.

Denudation and ulceration of the cystic mucosa occurs and is associated with development of bile duct neoplasms (usually adenocarcinomas). Up to 15% of patients over age 20 years with choledochal cysts will develop carcinomas, especially those with type I and IV cysts. The presence of an apparently solid mass on ultrasound or CT scanning should alert the clinician to a possible adenocarcinoma in a patient with a known choledochal cyst.

Treatment

Treatment is operative in all but type III cysts (choledochoceles), where the risk of carcinoma is low and adequate drainage may be achieved by sphincterotomy. Internal drainage that does not remove all of the cyst is associated with a continuing risk of carcinoma. When portal hypertension precludes resection, however, internal drainage may be the best treatment option. If resection is attempted, as much duct as possible should be resected, with the remaining biliary epithelium excluded from pancreatic secretions. Complete excision of the cyst with a Roux-en-Y hepaticojejunostomy is preferred.

Prognosis

The prognosis is excellent for those with complete cyst excision.

POLYCYSTIC LIVER DISEASE

Essentials of Diagnosis

- Multiple, uncomplicated nonbiliary liver cysts of varying size.
- Disease may be localized to one area such as the left lobe.

General Considerations

Polycystic liver disease is more prevalent in women and commonly identified with increasing age, typically in the fourth or fifth decade of life. Liver cysts may also be identified during evaluation of worsening renal function due to polycystic kidney disease. Infantile polycystic liver disease results in small cysts at the periphery of portal areas and portal fibrosis. Associated congenital hepatic fibrosis and portal hypertension may also occur.

Pathophysiology

Polycystic liver diseases are inherited disorders. Adult disease is inherited as an autosomal dominant disorder, and infantile disease as an autosomal recessive disorder resulting in embryologic maldevelopment and failed involution of interlobular bile ducts, with cysts in other organs such as the kidney, pancreas, lung, and spleen in 50% of patients. Cerebrovascular aneurysms also occur. Cysts are lined with biliary-type epithelium and filled with fluid similar to the bile-salt independent fraction of bile.

Clinical Findings

A. Symptoms and Signs: Patients are frequently asymptomatic, although large or multiple cysts may result in continuous pain due to stretching, mass effect, or compression of other structures. Nausea from stomach compression and jaundice from bile duct obstruction may develop. Palpation may suggest normal liver size or massive enlargement. The texture may be nodular and firm due to large cysts (adult polycystic disease) or enlarged, smooth, and firm (infantile polycystic disease).

B. Laboratory Findings: Liver tests are usually normal in the absence of bile duct obstruction. Histologic examination of the liver reveals a preserved architecture with cysts. Microhamartomas may be present.

C. Imaging Studies: Multiple uncomplicated liver cysts of varying size (< 10 cm in diameter) are identified by ultrasound or CT scanning. Cysts may also be seen in other organs (eg, in kidneys in 50% of

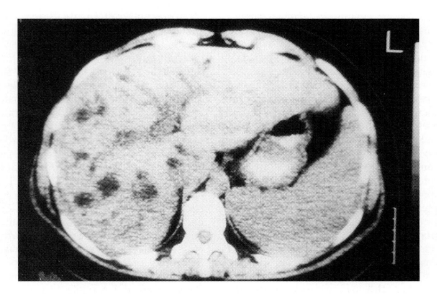

Figure 53–3. CT scan of Caroli's disease, with multiple cystic structures within the liver.

patients). Radionuclide scans, MRI, and arteriography are of little assistance in diagnosis.

Differential Diagnosis

The large nodular liver may be confused with metastatic disease or cirrhosis. Multiple cystic structures are also seen in Caroli's disease and rarely with biliary cystadenomas. If only a few cysts are present, simple cysts may be suggested.

Complications

Cystic rupture, intracystic hemorrhage, and infection (especially with *Klebsiella* or *Enterobacter* species) may develop. Cysts rarely obstruct bile ducts, cause pain, or result in portal hypertension.

Treatment

If the cystic disease is asymptomatic, no therapy is required, but symptomatic disease may require surgical intervention. If there are only a few cysts near the liver surface, symptoms may be controlled by aspiration, ethanol injection, unroofing of the cysts, or surgical cystojejunostomy. Localized collections of cysts can be resected, while severe diffuse symptomatic disease has been treated with orthotopic liver transplantation.

Prognosis

The prognosis is excellent when cysts can be easily controlled by operation or aspiration. The prognosis also depends in part on the severity of cystic disease in other organs such as the kidney, where renal failure may be a larger risk.

CAROLI'S DISEASE

Essentials of Diagnosis

- Documentation of saccular intrahepatic biliary cysts of varying size separated by normal or dilated bile ducts.
- Disease may be diffuse or localized.

General Considerations

Patients with Caroli's disease often have coexisting congenital hepatic fibrosis or sometimes a choledochal cyst or Laurence-Moon-Biedl syndrome. Symptoms usually begin in adulthood, although Caroli's disease should be considered in any child with bacterial cholangitis. One patient with kidney cysts and Caroli's disease of the liver has been described.

Pathophysiology

Caroli's disease is a congenital malformation of the bile ducts. It is unclear if the disease is inherited, although two sisters have been described with the disease. Caroli's disease is associated with other fibrocystic diseases, including choledochal cysts and congenital hepatic fibrosis.

Clinical Findings

A. Symptoms and Signs: Presentation is usually with fever and recurrent sepsis, which sometimes coexists with pain or jaundice. For those with biliary stones, obstruction of the common bile duct may cause jaundice. If congenital hepatic fibrosis coexists, hepatic enlargement or complications of portal hypertension, including variceal hemorrhage, ascites, and edema, may lead to the diagnosis. Right upper quadrant tenderness occurs.

B. Laboratory Findings: Biochemical liver tests are typically normal, although there may be mild elevation of alkaline phosphatase or gamma glutamyltransferase. With sepsis, leukocytosis is also present. Histologic examination of the liver may identify coexisting congenital hepatic fibrosis.

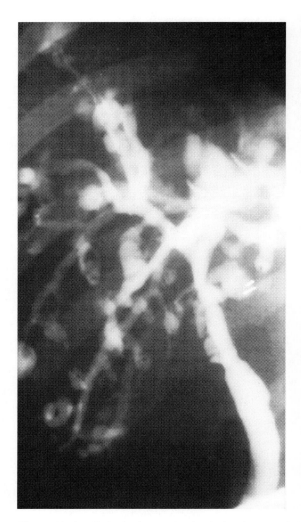

Figure 53–4. Endoscopic retrograde cholangiogram of Caroli's disease, with multiple cystic areas communicating with the bile ducts.

C. Imaging Studies: Hepatobiliary scans may define initially cold areas that become isotope dense with time. Ultrasound and CT scanning will identify low-density saccular structures within the liver, which may be diffuse or localized (Figure 53–3). When localized, the left lobe is more typically involved. Radiographic "dots" within cysts correspond to portal vein branches, which protrude into the cyst lumen. Intracystic stones also occur. Endoscopic retrograde cholangiography identifies the integral nature of the cystic structures within the biliary tree (Figure 53–4). This procedure may lead to infection of the cysts by organisms introduced during contrast injection.

Differential Diagnosis

Polycystic liver disease, dilated ducts due to biliary obstruction, and ectatic ducts associated with primary sclerosing cholangitis may present with similar findings on ultrasound or CT scanning.

Complications

Recurrent bacterial cholangitis with formation of intrahepatic or subdiaphragmatic abscess and septicemia may develop. With recurrent infection, secondary amyloidosis may occur. Intracystic calculi of calcium bilirubinate may serve as a nidus for persisting infection. Pancreatitis and biliary tract carcinoma are associated findings in some patients.

Treatment

Sepsis should be controlled with antibiotics as needed. The ability to intervene surgically is limited, unless there is localized disease and the involved lobe can be resected. Orthotopic liver transplantation following control of sepsis has been successful in management of recurrent cholangitis.

Prognosis

For those with recurrent sepsis, the prognosis is poor, as many die of complications. Stones that form within cysts may migrate to the common bile duct and cause obstruction, cholangitis, or pancreatitis.

REFERENCES

Desmet VJ: What is congenital hepatic fibrosis? Histopathology 1992;20:465.

Dotey JE, Tompkins RK: Management of cystic disease of the liver. Surg Clin North Am 1989;69:285.

Forbes A, Murray-Lyon IM: Cystic disease of the liver and biliary tract. Gut 1991(Suppl):S116.

Harris KM et al: Clinical and radiographic features of simple and hydatid cysts of the liver. Br J Surg 1986;73:835.

Lee SS et al: Choledochal cyst: A report of nine cases and a review of the literature. Arch Surg 1969;99:19.

Mercadier M et al: Caroli's disease. World J Surg 1984;8:22.

O'Neill JA Jr: Choledochal cyst. Curr Probl Surg 1992;29:365.

Sarris GE, Tsang D: Choledochocele: Case report, literature review, and proposed classification. Surgery 1989;105:408.

Vauthey J-N, Maddern GJ, Blumert LH: Adult polycystic disease of the liver. Br J Surg 1991;78:524.

Liver Transplantation

54

Jonathan L. Riegler, MD, & John R. Lake, MD

Orthotopic liver transplantation is now an accepted therapy for hepatic failure resulting from acute or chronic liver disease. It also has a role in the treatment of several inborn errors of metabolism that do not ultimately affect the liver itself. Initially described by Starzl and colleagues in 1963, the procedure did not gain widespread acceptance until improved methods of immunosuppression and refinements in surgical technique led to enhanced patient and graft survival rates. In 1993, there were nearly 6000 liver transplantations performed worldwide about half of which were in the United States. Current 1-year survival rates in this country are 75–90%.

The success of transplantation in treating end-stage liver disease has led to a dramatic increase in the number of patients referred for evaluation and then placed on waiting lists for the procedure (Figure 54–1). Because the pool of potential donors appears to be relatively constant, the shortage of donor organs has become acute, and more patients are dying while awaiting transplantation (Figure 54–2).

The clinical profile of patients transplanted will probably continue to change over the next several years. Until better therapies are developed for managing patients with hepatitis B and hepatobiliary malignant tumors, such patients will continue to be less attractive candidates. Patients with alcoholic liver disease, postnecrotic cirrhosis, and acute liver failure who already have acceptable long-term survival rates will probably undergo transplantation with increasing frequency. As more and more patients are referred for transplantation and then return to the community, it will become increasingly important for physicians in all fields, including primary care, to understand the basic principles involved in patient selection, transplantation surgery, and postoperative complications and management.

INDICATIONS & CONTRAINDICATIONS FOR LIVER TRANSPLANTATION

Indications

A. Treatment of Certain Diseases: Diseases for which liver transplantation might be a therapeutic option are shown in Table 54–1.

1. Hepatocellular diseases—Postnecrotic cirrhosis is the most common cause of end-stage liver disease necessitating orthotopic liver transplantation. In patients with hepatitis B virus-induced cirrhosis, a high incidence of recurrent infection and aggressive posttransplantation liver disease, along with disappointing postoperative survival rates, have led to a reduction in the number of transplanted patients. In contrast, patients with hepatitis C virus-induced cirrhosis have acceptable survival rates, in spite of a high rate of recurrent infection; this reflects a lower incidence of recurrent disease and a more benign course than for recurrent hepatitis B virus (HBV) infection. Alcoholic liver disease is the most common cause of cirrhosis in the Western world and an increasingly frequent reason for transplantation referral. Autoimmune chronic hepatitis with resulting cirrhosis is a relatively uncommon indication for transplantation.

Up to 30% of patients undergoing orthotopic liver transplantation have no discernible cause of cirrhosis and are thus described as having cryptogenic cirrhosis. This group probably includes those with clinically inapparent hepatitis B and C virus infections, autoimmune hepatitis, drug-induced disease, alcoholic liver disease, and various other causes. A yet-to-be-identified viral agent or toxin may also be responsible (see Chapter 37).

Other less common causes of hepatocellular disease that may be effectively treated by transplantation include acute liver failure and Budd-Chiari syndrome, and neonatal hepatitis in the pediatric population (see Chapters 35, 45, and 48).

2. Cholestatic liver diseases—Primary biliary cirrhosis, primary and secondary sclerosing cholangitis, and extrahepatic biliary atresia may all lead to hepatic failure and necessitate orthotopic liver transplantation. Although primary biliary cirrhosis and primary sclerosing cholangitis may recur, this does not seem to be a significant short-term clinical problem following transplantation.

3. Inborn errors of metabolism—Liver transplantation may correct an inborn error of metabolism, even when its effect does not primarily involve the liver, since the liver allograft retains its native metabolic potential. In adults, this is a relatively un-

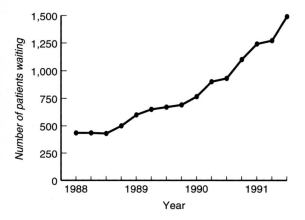

Figure 54–1. Number of patients on the UNOS liver transplantation waiting list, 1988–1991.

Table 54–1. Hepatic disorders successfully treated by liver transplantation.

Hepatocellular disease
Postnecrotic cirrhosis
Alcoholic cirrhosis
Budd-Chiari syndrome
Fulminant liver failure
α_1-antitrypsin deficiency
Autoimmune hepatitis
Wilson's disease
Trauma
Hemochromatosis
Neonatal hepatitis[1]
Congenital hepatic fibrosis[1]
Cholestatic liver disease
Biliary cirrhosis (primary and secondary)
Primary sclerosing cholangitis
Biliary atresia[1]
Inborn errors of metabolism[1]

[1]More common in pediatric patients.

common indication for liver transplantation, but in children, up to one-third of such procedures are performed for this reason. Examples of metabolic diseases necessitating transplantation are shown in Table 54–2.

In the case of α_1-antitrypsin deficiency, the serum phenotype of the recipient will become that of the donor. Patients with concomitant pulmonary disease may achieve stabilization of the lung disease following transplantation. Copper metabolism becomes normal in patients with Wilson's disease, and liver transplantation may reverse neurologic deficits. In contrast, diseases such as genetic hemochromatosis, in which the liver is damaged by enhanced iron uptake by the intestine, are not "cured" by transplantation. The liver disease is corrected, but ongoing enhanced iron uptake may eventually damage the allograft.

B. Improvement of Quality of Life: Symptoms resulting from hepatic dysfunction that markedly impair the quality of life but do not pose an immediate threat to survival are increasingly being considered as indications for liver transplantation (Table 54–3). Some of these symptoms are more common in early cholestatic liver disease, and others in hepatocellular disease or advanced cholestatic liver disease. Determining whether fatigue is a result of hepatic insufficiency may be difficult, and this symptom is seldom the sole indication for transplantation.

C. Prevention of Death in Severe Disease: Patients with certain disorders who have a reduced chance of survival (approximately 50%) within the next year may be candidates for transplantation (Table 54–4). The natural history of many hepatic diseases is poorly defined, and prediction of survival time may be difficult. Few would argue that hepatorenal syndrome (HRS), spontaneous bacterial peritonitis, and marked coagulopathy portend a poor prognosis and suggest the need for liver replacement. Disease severity indications may be influenced by regional waiting times and may vary from one transplantation center to the next.

Contraindications

A. Absolute Contraindications: Commonly

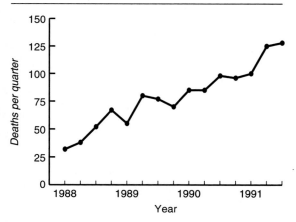

Figure 54–2. Number of patients on the UNOS liver transplantation waiting list who died before transplantation, 1988–1991.

Table 54–2. Inborn errors of metabolism treated by liver transplantation.

α_1-antitrypsin deficiency
Wilson's disease
Tyrosinemia
Type I and IV glycogen storage disease
Niemann–Pick disease
Crigler-Najjar syndrome
Type I hyperoxaluria
Urea cycle enzyme deficiency
C protein deficiency
Hemophilia A, B

Table 54–3. Quality-of-life indications
for liver transplantation.

Cholestatic liver disease
    Intractable pruritus
    Metabolic bone disease with fracture
    Recurrent episodes of biliary sepsis
    Xanthomatous neuropathy
Hepatocellular liver disease
    Intractable ascites
    Hepatic encephalopathy
    Variceal hemorrhage
    Fatigue

Table 54–5. Absolute contraindications
to liver transplantation.

HIV seropositivity
Extrahepatic cancer
Advanced cardiac or pulmonary disease
Chronic hepatitis B with viremia
Medical noncompliance
Active substance abuse
Anatomic abormalities precluding transplantation surgery

accepted absolute contraindications are listed in Table 54–5. The presence of these conditions sufficiently reduces the potential success of transplantation so that long-term benefits are unlikely. In cases of concomitant renal, heart, or pulmonary disease, consideration may be given to multiple-organ transplantation. Contraindications to orthotopic liver transplantation vary widely among different programs and may depend on the experience of the transplantation team (hepatologists, transplantation surgeons, and nursing staff). Contraindications may change not only within centers as experience increases, but also among the transplantation community at large, as surgical techniques and management of these disorders evolve.

B. Relative Contraindications: Relative contraindications (Table 54–6) may also reduce the success of orthotopic liver transplantation or increase its cost, but not to the same extent as absolute contraindications. The presence of extrahepatic infection does not preclude transplantation, but therapy should be initiated prior to the procedure. In patients with spontaneous bacterial peritonitis, a 48-hour course of antibiotics is probably sufficient, whereas other infections should be treated more aggressively for longer periods. Transplantation may be performed successfully in some patients with partially treated infections if antibiotics are continued postoperatively.

The use of thrombectomy and jump grafts has allowed successful transplantation in many patients with portal vein thrombosis, although operative blood loss and overall financial costs may be greater than with conventional therapy. Surgical (ie, portacaval) shunts do not preclude successful transplanta-

tion; however, angiography should be performed preoperatively to help plan vascular anastomoses.

Controversial Indications

A. Alcoholic Liver Disease: Initially, centers were reluctant to perform orthotopic liver transplantation in patients with alcoholic liver disease for several reasons:

- concern that the patient would return to drinking;
- concern that the presence of alcohol-mediated damage to other organs would lead to unacceptable complications; and
- concern about societal disapproval of treating a disease that was perceived to be self-inflicted.

Data from several centers have suggested that recurrent alcoholic liver disease following transplantation is uncommon and death from recurrent drinking rare. Success rates are similar to those of transplantation performed for other causes of liver disease, although some studies suggest that transplantation for alcoholic liver disease may be more costly. Patients with a history of alcohol abuse appear no more likely to be noncompliant with medical therapy than a control group of patients without prior alcohol use.

B. Hepatitis B Virus Infection: The initial enthusiasm for performing orthotopic liver transplantation in patients with chronic HBV infection has been tempered by the high rate of severe, recurrent infection of the allograft. Recurrent infection, defined as the appearance following transplantation of detectable hepatitis B surface antigen (HBsAg) in serum, occurs in 80–90% of patients who are HBsAg positive preoperatively. Reinfection of the allograft

Table 54–4. Disease severity indications
for liver transplantation.

Cholestatic liver disease
    Serum bilirubin > 10 mg/dL
Hepatocellular disease
    Hepatorenal syndrome
    Spontaneous bacterial peritonitis
    Serum albumin concentration < 2.5 mg/dL
    Prothrombin time > 5 seconds prolonged
    Serum bilirubin concentration > 5 mg/dL

Table 54–6. Relative contraindications
to liver transplantation.

Advanced malnutrition
Renal insufficiency
Extrahepatic or hepatobiliary infection
Portal vein thrombosis
Surgical portacaval shunt
Mild impairment of cardiac function
Chronic, unremitting encephalopathy

results primarily from the reservoir of extrahepatic HBV in other solid organs and peripheral mononuclear blood cells. Histologic findings of hepatitis are seen in most patients but may be atypical, including a recently described "fibrosing cytolytic" pattern, characterized by rapid progression to liver failure or cirrhosis, or both. The lesion may develop as early as a few weeks following surgery, and liver failure may occur within several months. The fibrosing cytolytic variant is marked by overexpression of HBV proteins in hepatocytes, with cellular swelling and cholestasis but only minimal inflammation. These observations have suggested that HBV may be directly cytopathic in the posttransplantation setting. Fortunately, most patients who remain HBsAg negative following transplantation have a normal liver on histologic studies and a benign clinical course.

Patients at risk of developing recurrent HBV infection include those with chronic hepatitis and, in particular, those with detectable HBV DNA or hepatitis B "e" antigen (HBeAg) in the serum before transplantation. Patients at lower risk of reinfection include those with fulminant HBV infection and those who are coinfected with hepatitis D, which appears to suppress HBV replication.

Use of recombinant α-interferon prior to transplantation does not clearly reduce the risk of recurrent HBV infection. Several studies have shown that hepatitis B immune globulin given during and following transplantation may substantially reduce the risk of recurrence, with improved survival rates. This approach is more effective in those at lower risk for recurrent infection; however, administration of hepatitis B immune globulin, which is quite costly, may be required for life. The optimal dosage and treatment interval have not been established, nor has the utility of measuring HBsAg titers to monitor therapy. Orthotopic liver transplantation for patients with chronic HBV should ideally be performed in centers with ongoing in clinical trials or by groups experienced in treating posttransplantation hepatitis B.

There is presently no therapy for posttransplantation HBV infection. Based on preliminary studies, it does not appear that interferon is effective. Other antiviral agents such as vidarabine or ganciclovir transiently reduce viral replication but do not eliminate detectable HBsAg from the serum.

C. Hepatitis C Virus Infection: Chronic hepatitis C virus infection (HCV) with cirrhosis is a common indication for orthotopic liver transplantation. As with chronic HBV, recurrent HCV is nearly universal following transplantation. Because antibody tests are not reliable in diagnosing this infection following transplantation, recurrent infection is usually determined by detection of HCV RNA in serum. Reinfection of the allograft may occur either from extrahepatic sites of HCV replication or from circulating virus perioperatively. Recurrent infection less commonly leads to clinical hepatitis than does hep-

atitis B, and, in most cases, the natural history is much more benign than with recurrent hepatitis B. Short-term graft loss secondary to recurrent infection is uncommon. As with hepatitis B virus, recurrent hepatitis C usually does not respond to α-interferon, although circulating virus levels may be transiently reduced.

D. Carcinoma of the Liver and Biliary System:

1. Hepatocellular carcinoma–In principle, orthotopic liver transplantation is an attractive treatment for hepatocellular carcinoma, since tumors are often not amenable to partial hepatectomy, either because the uninvolved liver is cirrhotic or the tumor is too extensive. Unfortunately, hepatocellular carcinoma usually recurs following transplantation, and long-term survival has been uncommon. Early attempts to treat hepatocellular carcinoma with transplantation resulted in 3-year survival rates of only 20–30%, although most patients had extensive tumor bulk pretransplant. Smaller tumors have lower rates of recurrence. In fact, tumors discovered incidentally at the time of transplantation have a good prognosis and rarely recur. Thus, when transplantation is performed for the underlying liver disease rather than as primary therapy for hepatocellular carcinoma, the prognosis is considerably better. Patients with hepatitis B virus–associated hepatocellular carcinoma do especially poorly following transplantation, whereas those with the slower-growing fibrolamellar variant seem to have lower rates of recurrence and a slightly better prognosis.

Posttransplantation recurrence of hepatocellular carcinoma may be reduced through the use of adjuvant chemotherapy given prior to and possibly following transplantation. One recent study reported a 54% tumor-free survival rate at 3 years with this combined approach. Other innovative therapies such as chemoembolization may prove useful in conjunction with transplantation. Although recommendations are evolving, some patients with hepatocellular carcinoma benefit from liver transplantation; however, the procedure should currently be performed only in the setting of clinical trials.

2. Cholangiocarcinoma–Three-year survival rates for patients with cholangiocarcinoma who have undergone transplantation are less than 20%. Unlike hepatocellular carcinoma, cholangiocarcinoma discovered incidentally recurs in most cases, with poor survival rates. Thus, cholangiocarcinoma should not be treated by orthotopic liver transplantation.

3. Epithelioid hemangioendothelioma–This low-grade, uncommon hepatic neoplasm is sometimes curable by orthotopic liver transplantation.

E. Fulminant Hepatic Failure (Acute Liver Failure): Because medical therapy for fulminant hepatic failure is associated with a 40–80% mortality rate, transplantation is a potentially attractive treatment (see Chapter 35). In carefully selected patients, survival rates following transplantation are comparable to those for other indications. Recognition of several indications that predict a poor prognosis has recently optimized patient selection (Table 54–7). These indicators differ significantly, depending on whether liver failure results from acetaminophen toxicity or other causes. Intracranial pressure monitoring, which allows for earlier diagnosis and treatment of elevated pressure, is also a useful adjunct in the preoperative management of potential transplantation candidates. Increased pressure resulting in cerebral perfusion pressures of less than 40 mm Hg for at least an hour results in irreversible neurologic damage; in this situation, transplantation should be withheld.

PRETRANSPLANTATION MEDICAL EVALUATION

The preoperative medical evaluation of potential candidates for liver transplantation includes the following steps:

Evaluation of Cause of Liver Disease

One approach to determining the cause of liver disease in potential transplantation candidates is outlined in Table 54–8, and should include several tests.

A. Serologic Testing: Serologic testing should include tests for hepatitis A, B, C, and D virus, antinuclear antibody, antimitochondrial antibody, and anti–smooth muscle antibody. Antibody testing should be performed for Epstein-Barr virus, cytomegalovirus, HIV, and syphilis.

B. Other Tests: α_1-antitrypsin levels, cerulo-

Table 54–7. Indications for liver transplantation in fulminant (acute) hepatic failure.[1,2]

Patients with acetaminophen-induced FHF
pH < 7.3 (irrespective of stage of encephalopathy)
or
PT > 100 seconds (INR > 6.5) and serum creatinine > 3.4 mg/dL in patients wih stage 3 or 4 encephalopathy
Other causes of FHF
PT > 100 seconds (INR > 6.5) (irrespective of stage of encephalopathy)
or
Any three of the following:
Age < 10 or > 40 years
Any cause other than acetaminophen-induced disease or hepatitis A or B
Duration of jaundice prior to onset of encephalopathy > 7 days
PT > 50 seconds (INR > 3.5)
Serum bilirubin > 17.5 mg/dL

[1]Adapted, with permission, from O'Grady JG et al: Early indicators of prognosis in fulminant hepatic failure. Gastroenterology 1989;97:439.
[2]PT, prothrombin time; INR, international normalized ratio.

Table 54–8. Preoperative evaluation of liver transplantation candidates: evaluation of cause of disease.

Serologic testing
Hepatitis A, B, C, and D
Antinuclear, antimitochondrial, anti–smooth muscle antibodies
Other testing
α_1-antitrypsin phenotype
Ceruloplasmin
Iron studies
When indicated
Liver biopsy
Endoscopic retrograde cholangiopancreatography

---

plasmin levels, and serum iron studies should be obtained. Skin testing for tuberculosis (PPD) with appropriate controls is necessary. Patients without immunity to hepatitis B virus infection should be vaccinated. A liver biopsy may be helpful in determining the cause of hepatic disease but may be nonspecific if cirrhosis is advanced. Endoscopic retrograde cholangiopancreatography (ERCP) is indicated if there is a suspicion of sclerosing cholangitis or cholangiocarcinoma.

Evaluation of Severity of Liver Disease

The severity of hepatic dysfunction is determined by a clinical evaluation for the presence and severity of encephalopathy, ascites, and evidence of muscle wasting. Other helpful studies are shown in Table 54–9. Prothrombin time and measurements of serum albumin, alanine aminotransferase (ALT) and aspartate aminotransferase (AST), alkaline phosphatase, and bilirubin may be helpful in assessing hepatic reserve.

There is no ideal "liver function" test that reliably identifies patients in need of transplantation. Scoring systems such as the Child-Pugh score have been developed, but, except in patients with cholestatic disease, these systems have fallen short of consistent, accurate prediction of prognosis (Table 54–10).

Table 54–9. Preoperative evaluation of liver transplantation candidates: assessment of disease severity.

Laboratory evaluation
Complete blood count
Electrolytes, blood urea nitrogen, creatinine
Serum aminotransferase activities
Alkaline phosphatase activity, total serum bilirubin concentrations
Total protein, albumin serum concentrations
Prothrombin time, partial thromboplastin time
Other testing
Abdominal ultrasound with Doppler studies of hepatic vessels
Endoscopic evaluation where indicated
Liver biopsy where indicated

Table 54–10. Child-Pugh classification.[1]

Variable	1 Point	2 Points	3 Points
Bilirubin (mg/dL)	< 2	2–3	> 3
Albumin (g/dL)	> 3.5	2.8–3.5	< 2.8
Prothrombin time (seconds prolonged)	1–3	4–6	> 6
Ascites	None	Slight	Moderate
Encephalopathy	None	Stages 1–2	Stages 3–4

[1]Class A: 1–6 total points; B: 7–9 points; C: 10–15 points.

Evaluation of Hepatic Reserve & General Health

Determining whether the patient is an appropriate candidate for liver transplantation requires evaluation of both liver reserve and general health. The protocol includes the following evaluations:

A. Hepatic Evaluation: Esophagogastroduodenoscopy may reveal varices or peptic ulcer disease. In the patient with asymptomatic varices, prophylactic sclerotherapy or ligation is not indicated. Patients with primary sclerosing cholangitis should undergo ERCP in most cases for biliary cytologic examination to exclude cholangiocarcinoma as a cause of sudden clinical deterioration. Doppler ultrasonography can exclude mass lesions and ensure patency of the portal vein and other vessels. Any suspected vascular abnormalities should be further evaluated with angiography. Patients with elevated serum α-fetoprotein concentrations (ie, > 100 µg/mL) require CT or MRI scanning to exclude hepatocellular carcinoma.

B. Cardiopulmonary Evaluation: A chest radiograph is necessary, with thorough evaluation of any abnormalities. Pulmonary function testing is indicated, especially in patients with a history of lung disease or tobacco use. Patients with hypoxemia or increased alveolar-arterial oxygen gradients suggesting hepatopulmonary syndrome should have the diagnosis confirmed by contrast echocardiography or injection of radiolabeled albumin microaggregates to document intrapulmonary shunting. Echocardiography is helpful in evaluating general cardiac function. Patients with abnormal echocardiographic examinations or significant risk factors for coronary artery disease should undergo additional testing to exclude coronary artery insufficiency.

C. Psychosocial Evaluation: The potential candidate's social situation should be evaluated to ensure that adequate support mechanisms exist for posttransplantation care and rehabilitation. The patient must be judged likely to comply with medical therapy, postoperative instructions, and evaluations. In patients with a history of substance abuse, the likelihood of recidivism should be estimated, with arrangements made for further rehabilitation prior to transplantation if necessary.

Special Considerations

A. Renal Failure: In patients with pretransplantation renal dysfunction, the cause should be determined using urine electrolyte measurements, glomerular filtration rates, ultrasonography, and renal biopsy where indicated. Patients with HRS usually regain some renal function following transplantation. Patients with chronic renal disease may require combined liver and kidney transplantation.

B. Pulmonary Disorders: Patients with pulmonary infiltrates should be carefully investigated prior to orthotopic liver transplantation. Those with infectious disease should be treated with appropriate antibiotics. Patients with adult respiratory distress syndrome usually have poor survival rates following transplantation. It now appears that the hepatopulmonary syndrome may be reversible with transplantation, but these patients may require oxygen supplementation for some period postoperatively.

Preoperative Management of Complications of Hepatic Failure

A. Variceal Hemorrhage: Esophageal variceal hemorrhage may be managed acutely by variceal sclerotherapy or variceal ligation. In patients who continue to hemorrhage despite these therapies, transjugular intrahepatic portasystemic shunt (TIPS) placement is usually effective in controlling bleeding, and provides an effective "bridge" to transplantation. Optimal therapy for gastric variceal hemorrhage is not defined, but anecdotal experience supports the use of TIPS. Surgical portacaval shunts are also an option in the candidate refractory to other measures, but surgical complications and transfusion requirements during the transplantation procedure are increased compared with healthier patients.

B. Ascites: In patients who do not respond adequately to diuretic therapy, large-volume paracenteses may be necessary to control ascites. Peritoneovenous shunts are another option but can be associated with complications, including shunt occlusion and disseminated intravascular coagulation. TIPS may improve the control of ascites, but further study is needed. Patients with low-protein ascites (< 1 g/dL) benefit from prophylaxis against spontaneous bacterial peritonitis with norfloxacin, 400 mg/d. Patients with a prior history of spontaneous bacterial peritonitis should also receive prophylaxis while awaiting transplantation.

C. Renal Failure: In patients who develop renal insufficiency, it is important to discontinue agents that adversely affect renal function in cirrhosis, particularly nonsteroidal anti-inflammatory drugs (NSAIDs). The development of HRS portends a poor prognosis. Prostaglandins, peritoneovenous shunts, and TIPS have had limited success in treating this complication. Urgent transplantation should be considered while it still may be effective in reversing this condition.

TIMING OF LIVER TRANSPLANTATION

Patients with one or more indications for orthotopic liver transplantation should be referred for evaluation. Appropriate candidates must be placed on the waiting list as soon as possible. Allocation of available donor organs is currently based on a priority system developed by the Unified Network of Organ Sharing (UNOS), in which the sickest patients are given the highest priority. Recent studies suggest, however, that transplantation in these patients is more costly and less successful. Optimal timing of transplantation may allow more efficient use of available donor organs.

Ideally, the timing should be based on detailed information about the natural history of the underlying disease process, with the goal of avoiding transplantation too early (ie, when extended survival time is possible without it) or too late in the course of the illness (ie, when posttransplantation survival time is impaired or the course prolonged). Unfortunately, such information on the natural history is not available for most forms of hepatocellular disease.

Table 54–11 illustrates variables for predicting survival rates in patients with primary biliary cirrhosis or primary sclerosing cholangitis based on the various clinical factors. A formula is used to calculate a risk score, which predicts survival times and thus allows decisions about the timing of transplantation to be made with more precision. Higher-risk scores correlate both with increased costs and reduced survival rates following transplantation. The

Table 54–11. Independent clinical variables predictive of survival in primary biliary cirrhosis and primary sclerosing cholangitis.[1]

Primary Biliary Cirrhosis	Primary Sclerosing Cholangitis
Age	Age
Bilirubin	Bilirubin
Albumin	Histologic stage
Prothrombin time	Hemoglobin
Edema	Inflammatory bowel disease

[1]Reproduced, with permission, from Weisner RH et al: Selection and timing of liver transplantation in primary biliary cirrhosis and primary sclerosing cholangitis. Hepatology 1992; 16:1291.

implication is that patients should be considered for the procedure before the risk becomes unacceptably high. Similar models might be developed for examining other chronic liver diseases.

SURGICAL CONSIDERATIONS

Donor Operation

A. Donor Suitability: Livers from older patients are more prone to preservation injury and primary graft nonfunction. Most studies suggest, however, that when carefully selected, these organs are as effective as livers from younger donors.

The donor should be hemodynamically stable prior to organ donation. Long-term, high-dosage vasopressor support may lead to ischemic liver damage and increase the risk of posttransplantation graft dysfunction. Serologic testing for HIV and hepatitis B and C viruses should be performed. Elevated liver tests do not necessarily preclude donation of the organ, but histologic evidence of significant steatosis or viral hepatitis should exclude it.

The use of organs from donors testing positive for HCV is controversial. There is a clear risk of transmission to the recipient, but the likelihood of significant hepatitis and subsequent graft loss is small. In an elective situation, these organs should probably not be used. In severely ill patients, however, use of these organs may be preferable to a prolonged wait for a more desirable one. In some cases, the decision to use the organ will depend on the extent of histologic damage.

B. Organ Retrieval and Preservation: The donor liver is inspected at time of harvest, with biopsy performed to evaluate the parenchyma. Cold preservation solution is flushed through the arterial supply and portal vein prior to removal. The liver, together with its vascular and biliary structures, is then removed en bloc. Immediately prior to transplanting the organ into the recipient, all extraneous tissues are removed and vascular structures prepared for anastomosis.

The preservation solution most commonly used is the University of Wisconsin solution, which allows storage times of up to 24 hours. The risk of preservation injury, primary graft nonfunction, and biliary complications increases with time, however, so the cold-ischemia time should be minimized.

Recipient Operation

The underlying goal is to replace the diseased liver with a donor graft matched as closely as possible for size and blood group. The liver is devascularized, the biliary tree ligated, and the portal vein dissected. The inferior vena cava is clamped. The resulting reduction in cardiac output may not be well tolerated. Underlying portal hypertension makes the surgery more difficult; to circumvent this problem, many programs

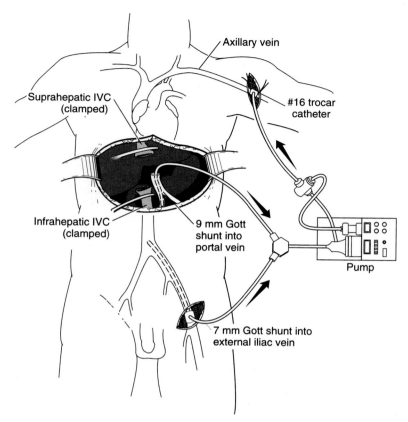

Axillary vein

Suprahepatic IVC
(clamped)

#16 trocar
catheter

Infrahepatic IVC
(clamped)

9 mm Gott
shunt into
portal vein

Pump

7 mm Gott shunt into
external iliac vein

Figure 54–3. Venovenous bypass. Bypass may be initiated at any time during the procedure and is usually most helpful in situations where very high portal pressures create bleeding problems. (Reproduced, with permission, from Miller CM et al: Operative techniques and strategies in liver transplantation. In: *Guide to Liver Transplantation.* Fabry TL, Klion FM (editors). Igaku-Shoin, 1992.)

use a venovenous bypass (Figure 54–3), which decompresses the venous system below the diaphragm, shunting the blood to the superior vena cava via the axillary vein. This procedure allows for more stable hemodynamic status and blood volume and less bowel edema. Venovenous bypass may reduce intraoperative bleeding, according to some, but not all, studies.

Following removal of the diseased liver, the donor liver is placed into the abdominal cavity and the anastomoses are performed in the following order:

1. Suprahepatic vena cava
2. Intrahepatic vena cava
3. Portal vein
4. Hepatic artery
5. Bile duct.

Adequate hepatic arterial flow is usually assessed intraoperatively by Doppler ultrasound or flowmeters. A portal vein thrombosis can be managed by thrombectomy or iliac vein grafts. The biliary anastomosis is most commonly a choledochocholedochos-

tomy, with choledochojejunostomy being used more commonly in patients with known disease of the biliary tree (Figure 54–4). Most centers use a T tube to stent the anastomosis; this reduces leakage from the fresh anastomosis, prevents stricture as the anastomosis heals, and allows assessment of bile production and duct patency during the immediate postoperative course. The T tube is usually clamped 3–4 days following transplantation and removed 2–5 months later. The transplantation operation usually lasts 4–8 hours.

Newer Surgical Techniques

The large number of patients awaiting orthotopic liver transplantation has prompted innovative approaches to expand the donor pool. Using livers from older donors is one option (see preceding discussion). More promising is the use of reduced-size liver grafts.

A. Split-liver Transplantation: In this operation, a single donor liver is used to provide grafts to two patients with end-stage liver disease. The smaller recipient receives the left lobe or left lateral segment of the donor organ. Thus far, biliary complications

A

B

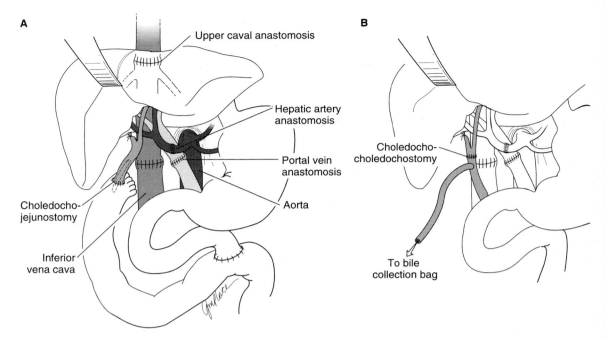

Figure 54–4. Types of biliary anastomoses performed. **A:** Choledochojejunostomy, most commonly performed in patients with prior biliary tract abnormalities. **B:** Choledochocholedochostomy with T tube drainage. (Reproduced, with permission, from Miller CM et al: Operative techniques and strategies in liver transplantation. In: *Guide to Liver Transplantation.* Fabry TL, Klion FM (editors). Igaku-Shoin, 1992.)

have been a major postoperative factor, and survival rates have been less than those of conventional orthotopic liver transplantation.

B. Auxiliary Liver Transplantation: A portion of the diseased liver is removed, usually the left lobe lateral segment, and the reduced-size graft is implanted alongside the remaining native organ. This operation can correct metabolic defects in pediatric patients with otherwise normally functioning livers. Another indication is fulminant liver disease in adults, where the graft provides metabolic support until the native liver has recovered function.

C. Live Donor Transplantation: This technique is used primarily in pediatric patients but may ultimately be appropriate in carefully selected adults. A portion of the left lobe from the donor is resected and placed into the recipient following removal of the diseased liver. The resected lobe must be of adequate size to support the smaller patient. Experienced programs report donor survival rates of 100%, and recipient survival rates of 80–90% after 1 year. Hepatic artery thrombosis was once the major postoperative complication, but in a recent series reported by Emond, the incidence was about 10%, similar to that seen in adults. The incidence of rejection and graft loss is similar to that in patients undergoing cadaveric liver transplantation.

POSTOPERATIVE COMPLICATIONS & MANAGEMENT

Complications following orthotopic liver transplantation may be divided into those occurring early (within the first 10 days) and later, although there is significant overlap in the timing. A basic approach to evaluating liver dysfunction following transplantation is outlined in Figure 54–5.

Early Complications

A. Primary Graft Nonfunction: Primary graft nonfunction occurs in 2–23% of transplants and often results in death if retransplantation is not performed immediately. The wide range of reported incidence likely reflects differences in definition. Technical problems are the cause in less than 10% of adults but are more common in children. Primary nonfunction is usually the result of ischemic damage of the allograft sustained during harvest and transport, but the exact mechanisms are not well characterized. Less common causes are hepatic artery thrombosis, portal vein thrombosis, and hyperacute rejection. Risk factors for primary nonfunction have been recently identified by Ploeg et al (Table 54–12). Primary nonfunction should be suspected if coagulopathy does not resolve following transplantation, if encephalopathy

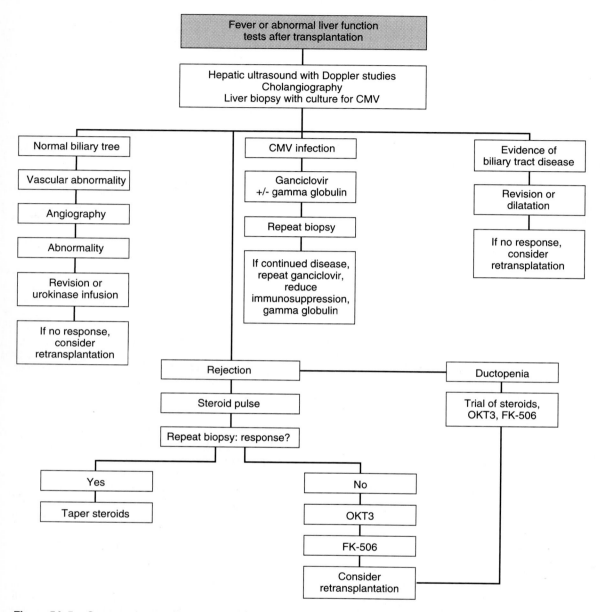

Figure 54–5. Suggested algorithm for evaluation of abnormal liver function tests or fevers following liver transplantation. See text for details.

occurs or does not clear, if serum transaminase activities remain persistently elevated, or if lactic acidosis develops. Reduced bile production in the first 24–48 hours following transplantation may also suggest poor graft function. Primary nonfunction may be seen immediately postoperatively or may develop within 2–3 days. Prostaglandin E_1 may be of some benefit, but further studies are needed.

B. Initial Poor Function: This term has been used by some investigators to describe a marginally functioning graft that recovers adequate function only after days to weeks. Sometimes these organs fail, and retransplantation is required. The risk factors for initial poor function are similar to those for primary nonfunction.

C. Preservation Injury: This refers to hepatocyte injury that results from cold preservation or reperfusion of the allograft. Some degree of preservation injury is common following orthotopic liver transplantation, but severe injury may result in initial

Table 54–12. Risk factors for the development of primary graft nonfunction following liver transplantation.

Reduced-size livers
Donor liver steatosis
Older donor age
Retransplantation
Renal insufficiency
Prolonged cold ischemia time

poor function or primary nonfunction. Typical laboratory abnormalities include a marked increase in serum transaminase activities during the first 24–48 hours following surgery, with a subsequent slow decrease. Later, elevated serum alkaline phosphatase and bilirubin levels also develop. These changes occur in the absence of other recognized causes of graft failure. The diagnosis may be made by liver biopsy, but vascular thrombosis can cause a similar histologic appearance and must be excluded by Doppler studies.

D. Hyperacute Rejection: Preformed antidonor antibodies may cause arterial endothelial damage resulting in hepatic necrosis and liver failure within days of transplantation. This type of rejection is seen more commonly following kidney transplantation and can be distinguished histologically from other causes of early graft loss by the presence of portal inflammatory infiltrates, which are not typically seen in primary nonfunction or preservation injury. Fortunately, hyperacute rejection is uncommon following orthotopic liver transplantation.

Later Complications

A. Allograft Rejection: This is the most common problem seen in the posttransplantation setting. Because of overlap in the timing of different types of rejection following transplantation, terms such as acute and chronic rejection are being replaced by more descriptive ones such as cellular and ductopenic rejection. Characteristics of cellular and ductopenic rejection are summarized in Table 54–13.

1. Mechanisms of rejection–Both cellular and ductopenic rejection appear to be T cell-mediated. Host CD4-positive T cells recognize donor class II major histocompatibility antigens on biliary epithelial and vascular endothelial cells. Activated CD4-positive cells produce cytokines such as interleukins 1 and 6, tumor necrosis factor-α, and interferon-γ, which stimulate maturation and proliferation of CD8-positive cytotoxic T cells. These effector cells damage the biliary epithelium and vasculature. Elaboration of adhesion molecules also plays a role in the final pathologic response. Because of the relative paucity of major histocompatibility antigens on the hepatocytes, these cells are often left undamaged during rejection. Despite the apparent importance of the major histocompatibility antigens in this process, there has been no consistent benefit demonstrated of HLA matching of donor with recipient.

2. Cellular rejection–Cellular rejection is usually seen in the first 3 weeks (average 10 days) following orthotopic liver transplantation, but may occur at any time. Acute cellular rejection is seen in about two-thirds of patients; risk factors include dual immunosuppressive therapy (versus triple therapy using cyclosporine, azathioprine, and prednisone), young age, and complete HLA-DR donor-recipient mismatching.

Episodes of rejection may be asymptomatic or associated with fevers, malaise, abdominal pain, or, occasionally, manifestations of elevated portal pressure such as ascites. Protocol liver biopsies may be useful in diagnosing rejection in the early postoperative period, since biochemical changes are relatively nonspecific during this time. Histologically, cellular rejection is characterized by a mixed infiltrate containing neutrophils, eosinophils, and lymphocytes in the portal tracts. Destructive nonsuppurative cholangitis or centrilobular necrosis also may be seen. Inflammatory changes around the endothelial cells of the portal or hepatic vein branches (endothelialitis) is less commonly seen but relatively specific for the diagnosis of rejection. Therapy is additional immunosuppression with steroids or OKT3 (see following discussion).

3. Ductopenic rejection–This type of rejection occurs in 5–10% of patients undergoing orthotopic liver transplantation and is usually diagnosed between 6 weeks and 6 months postoperatively. Risk factors include recurrent bouts of acute rejection, primary sclerosing cholangitis as the indication for transplantation, dual immunosuppression, and, possibly, a positive cytotoxic lymphocyte cross-match. The process tends to be progressive and responds poorly to additional immunosuppression. Retransplantation may be required, but ductopenic rejection tends to recur in subsequent allografts. Histologically, this type of rejection is characterized by little inflammation, with the loss of interlobular and septal bile ducts in at least 50% of examined portal tracts. A

Table 54–13. Hepatic allograft rejection: terminology and characteristics.

	Acute Cellular Rejection	Chronic Ductopenic Rejection
Histology	Mixed, but predominantly mononuclear portal-based infiltrate, with bile duct damage with or without endotheliitis	Duct loss, arteriopathy
Timing	Earlier, but may occur any time	Later, but may occur any time
Reversibility	Usually reversible	Rarely reversible

so-called foam cell arteriopathy also suggests ductopenic rejection but is seen in only a minority of cases.

4. Prevention of rejection–Prophylaxis against rejection involves starting immunosuppression immediately after transplantation of the donor organ (primary or induction immunosuppression). Use of a triple-drug regimen that includes prednisone, cyclosporine, and azathioprine reduces the risk of subsequent rejection episodes and is currently standard practice at most centers. OKT3 is a mouse-derived antihuman antibody directed at the CD3 determinant on human T cells. Its administration (sequential therapy) may delay the onset of cellular rejection, but the overall incidence of rejection appears to be unaffected. Polyclonal antilymphocyte preparations have similar effects. Some studies suggest OKT3 administration may be associated with an increased risk of subsequent bacterial, fungal, and cytomegalovirus infections as well as posttransplantation lymphoproliferative disorders. In addition, the development of anti–murine antibodies can prevent its subsequent use for the treatment of rejection. Many physicians reserve OKT3 for use in the early postoperative period in patients with renal insufficiency who may not tolerate cyclosporine because of potential nephrotoxicity.

5. Treatment of rejection episodes–Because of the risks involved with additional immunosuppressive therapy, liver biopsy should be performed to confirm rejection. A biopsy is also commonly performed following the completion of treatment to document an adequate response. Cellular rejection often responds to additional immunosuppression with corticosteroids, usually in two or three daily boluses, followed by tapering of the prednisone dosage. Episodes of cellular rejection that are refractory to steroid pulse therapy (about 15% of patients) usually respond to a 7- to 14-day course of OKT3. It is often useful to follow the number of circulating CD3-positive cells to ensure adequate T cell depletion during OKT3 treatment.

FK-506 (tacrolimus), a macrolide antibiotic, inhibits the proliferation of cytotoxic T lymphocytes and the elaboration of cytokines by a mechanism of action similar to that of cyclosporine. Side effects are also similar to those of cyclosporine. FK-506 is as effective as cyclosporine when used as primary therapy. It is especially useful as "rescue" therapy when conventional therapy has failed to control rejection, and can be effective when rejection has not responded to steroids and OKT3 therapy.

Medications used to treat rejection are associated with many potential adverse reactions. Common side effects of cyclosporine are listed in Table 54–14. Cyclosporine-induced hypertension is usually managed with calcium channel blockers, since angiotensin-converting enzyme inhibitors may exacerbate cyclosporine-induced hyperkalemia or fluid retention.

Table 54–14. Adverse effects of cyclosporine therapy.

Nephrotoxity
Hypertension
Hypertrichosis
Gastrointestinal symptoms: anorexia, nausea, vomiting, gingival hyperplasia
Neurotoxicity: headache, tremors, seizures, cortical blindness, quadriplegia, coma
Opportunistic infections
Cancer: B cell lymphoma

Some patients may also require long-term magnesium supplementation. Drug interactions are important to consider because many commonly used medications alter blood levels through their effect on the metabolism of cyclosporine by the cytochrome P450 system, leading to either rejection or toxicity. Common drug interactions are shown in Table 54–15.

The side effect profile of FK-506 is similar to that of cyclosporine, but hypertension may be less common. Drug interactions with FK-506 are also related to interference with cytochrome P450–mediated metabolism.

Use of OKT3 usually causes fever, diarrhea, and headache and additionally may cause rigors, hypotension, pulmonary edema, aseptic meningitis, or seizures.

B. Infectious Complications: Infections are the most common cause of death following orthotopic liver transplantation. Most patients develop a bacterial infection, 30–50% develop a clinically recognized viral infection, and fungal infections may also occur. In particular, *Aspergillus* infections can be quite difficult to manage. Virtually any pathogen can cause infection following transplantation; this underscores the need to thoroughly investigate fevers in these patients.

1. Cytomegalovirus infection–Infection with cytomegalovirus is the most frequent viral infection following transplantation, with an overall incidence of 25–85%. This infection may be fatal and may also increase the risk of superinfection with other organisms and chronic rejection. Patients at highest risk include seronegative patients who receive an organ

Table 54–15. Common cyclosporine drug interactions.

Drugs that may decrease cyclosporine concentrations
  Carbamazepine
  Phenobarbital
  Phenytoin
  Rifampin
Drugs that may increase cyclosporine concentrations
  Bromocriptine
  Diltiazem
  Erythromycin
  Fluconazole
  Itraconazole
  Ketoconazole
  Metoclopramide
  Verapamil

from a cytomegalovirus-positive donor, those who receive antilymphocyte therapy for rejection, and those undergoing retransplantation.

Because of the potential for illness and death associated with cytomegalovirus infection, there have been attempts to use prophylactic antiviral therapy. Ganciclovir, administered early in the postoperative course and followed by high-dosage acyclovir when the patient is taking oral medications, may reduce the incidence and severity of cytomegalovirus disease. The administration of intravenous immunoglobulin directed at cytomegalovirus may also be helpful in high-risk patients such as cytomegalovirus-negative recipients of cytomegalovirus-positive donor organs, but this therapy is expensive and the overall impact on patient and graft survival rates is unclear. Nevertheless, many programs use some form of prophylaxis against cytomegalovirus infection during the first 6 months following transplantation.

Cytomegalovirus infection occurs an average of 30–50 days following transplantation and may be diagnosed by detecting anticytomegalovirus IgM antibody; seroconversion from negative to positive indicates infection. Recovery of virus in urine or blood cultures also represents infection, but cytomegalovirus "disease" is a term used to describe end-organ damage, such as cytomegalovirus pneumonitis, hepatitis, esophagitis, or colitis. Patients may present with fever, malaise, shortness of breath, problems in swallowing, diarrhea, or abdominal pain. Laboratory abnormalities may include elevated liver tests and leukopenia. Diagnosis is made by biopsy of the involved organ.

Treatment of cytomegalovirus requires intravenous ganciclovir, which eradicates disease in approximately 85% of patients. The usual dose is 5 mg/kg intravenously every 12 hours, with adjustment for renal dysfunction. Resistance to this agent has been reported. In patients not responding to ganciclovir, another antiviral agent, foscarnet, may be used. An attempt should be made to reduce immunosuppression in conjunction with antiviral therapy if possible.

2. Posttransplantation viral hepatitis–Hepatitis B virus infection can either recur following orthotopic liver transplantation or can result from inapparent infection of blood products or the donor liver. Several groups have reported transmission from donors who have serologic evidence of past infection only. The infection is difficult to manage, and treatment with currently available antiviral medications such as interferon is usually unsuccessful (see preceding discussion). The same appears to be true for HCV infection, but this infection is less likely to lead to graft loss. Other viruses that may cause hepatitis following transplantation include Epstein-Barr virus, herpes simplex virus, and adenovirus. Diagnosis of these infections is usually made on the basis of histologic appearance and increases in antibody titers from pretransplantation levels. Herpes simplex virus

hepatitis and Epstein-Barr virus hepatitis may respond to treatment with acyclovir, but treatment for adenovirus is largely supportive.

3. Bacterial infections–These usually occur within 2 months following orthotopic liver transplantation and are most often due to gram-positive aerobic bacteria. The risk of bacterial infection increases with the length of the operation and the need for retransplantation. The source of infection is often related to use of a catheter or to pneumonia; abdominal abscess and peritonitis are less common. Early use of empiric broad-spectrum antibiotics, such as a third-generation cephalosporin, is usually indicated in patients with fever, pending the results of further studies and cultures. Following discharge, transplanted patients most commonly develop infections with community-acquired bacteria (eg, pneumococcus).

A few published studies suggest that selective bowel decontamination using a drug combination against gram-negative and fungal organisms may reduce the incidence of these infections. Regimens used include oral quinolones alone or gentamycin, nystatin, and polymyxins in combination. The impact of this approach on graft and patient survival rates is unclear.

4. Fungal infections–Patients receiving immunosuppression or prolonged antibiotic therapy are susceptible to fungal infections. The incidence declines with time following discharge from the hospital. Superficial infections involving the skin or mouth may be treated with topical antifungals such as mycostatin or chlortrimazole. Candidal urinary tract infections are responsive to oral fluconazole or amphotericin B bladder irrigation. Invasive infections, however, must be treated with systemic amphotericin B, often for prolonged periods. The role of newer antifungal agents, such as itraconazole, is under investigation.

Aspergillus infection may involve the lung, skin, or central nervous system. In contrast to persons with intact immune systems, immunosuppressed patients develop a diffuse, patchy infiltrate on chest radiography, rather than a fungus ball. Hematogenous spread is possible, and central nervous system infection is difficult to treat and usually fatal. Prolonged courses of amphotericin are usually required, and combination therapy with flucytosine may be helpful.

Infections with *Cryptococcus, Mucor,* or *Rhizopus* may also be seen, but are less common. Treatment involves the combination of systemic amphotericin, surgical debridement of infected tissue where possible, and reduced immunosuppression.

6. Other infections–*Pneumocystis carinii* infections usually occur 2–3 months following transplantation and are eliminated by prophylactic trimethoprim-sulfamethoxazole, inhaled pentamidine, or dapsone. *Mycobacterium tuberculosis* infection may develop or reactivate following transplantation and often presents atypically.

C. Biliary Complications: Once a major cause

of illness following orthotopic liver transplantation, biliary problems are becoming less frequent because of improved surgical techniques and liver preservation. They are currently seen in 10–25% of patients.

1. Anastomotic leak–These usually occur either early in the postoperative course or much later following removal of the T tube. Corticosteroids may mask symptoms and signs, but patients often present with right upper quadrant pain, fever, or other signs of peritonitis. The diagnosis is typically suggested by the presence of a biloma on ultrasonography or CT scanning. Any new fluid collection seen in the porta hepatis, even if the imaging studies was performed for other reasons, should prompt an investigation for a biliary leak. A cholangiogram should be obtained to rule out biliary obstruction or identify the site of leakage. A Doppler study is indicated to rule out hepatic artery thrombosis, which may lead to biliary ischemia and anastomotic leaks.

Management of an anastomotic leak includes antibiotics and opening the T tube if it is still in place. For leakage at the exit site of the T tube, successful therapy can include insertion of a biliary stent to allow bile diversion, or placement of a nasobiliary drain. Endoscopic sphincterotomy also can be effective. Associated fluid collections require percutaneous drainage if technically feasible.

2. Anastomotic stricture–Strictures at the site of anastomosis occur in 4–10% of patients following orthotopic liver transplantation. Patients may present with right upper quadrant pain or fevers following removal of the T tube, or, more commonly, with asymptomatic increased measurements in liver tests. Ultrasonography may demonstrate dilated intrahepatic ducts. Liver biopsy, which is commonly abnormal, reveals a portal infiltrate composed of periductular neutrophils, suggesting cholangitis and proliferation of intralobular bile ductules. Percutaneous cholangiography or ERCP is usually diagnostic. Hepatic artery thrombosis can also explain these abnormalities. These strictures may be treated with balloon dilatation or stent placement, but surgical revision to a choledochojejunostomy is often required.

3. Nonanastomotic biliary strictures–These strictures occur predominantly at the bifurcation of the right and left hepatic ducts and in intrahepatic bile ducts. In one series, nonanastomotic strictures were seen following 19% of liver transplantations. Important associations include hepatic artery thrombosis, transplantation across ABO blood barriers, ductopenic vascular rejection, extended cold preservation times (> 10–14 hours) and pretransplantation primary sclerosing cholangitis. They typically occur 1–4 months after transplantation; those occurring earlier usually have a worse prognosis. Patients with these types of strictures have lower 1-year graft survival rates and a higher rate of retransplantation, but their overall survival rate appears to be similar to that of other patients. The Mayo Clinic has described successful nonoperative management of these ischemic-type biliary strictures using percutaneously placed stents and serial dilatations, but approximately one-fourth of these patients eventually required retransplantation.

D. Pulmonary Complications: Pulmonary effusions are extremely common following orthotopic liver transplantation but are usually not clinically significant. They typically occur on the right side and usually resolve within 1–2 weeks after surgery. Rarely, pleurodesis may be required for persistent symptomatic effusions. Atelectasis is common and also is usually right-sided.

Pulmonary infiltrates occur in 12–50% of patients, with about half of these being infectious. Early pulmonary infections more commonly result from bacteria, with gram-negative organisms predominating. Opportunistic infections tend to occur later in the postoperative course; causes include *Pneumocystis carinii, Cryptococcus, Aspergillus,* and *Candida.* Cytomegalovirus is the most common viral pathogen. Bronchoscopy with bronchoalveolar lavage and, rarely, open-lung biopsy may be required to make a diagnosis. Noncardiogenic pulmonary edema has been reported with the use of OKT3. *Pneumocystis* and cytomegalovirus pneumonitis can be prevented using trimethoprim-sulfamethoxazole and ganciclovir prophylaxis, respectively.

In one retrospective study, preoperative pulmonary testing did not accurately predict postoperative pulmonary infections or pulmonary-related deaths. It is important to realize that the hypoxemia associated with the hepatopulmonary syndrome may take weeks to months to resolve after successful liver transplantation.

E. Neurologic Complications: Neurologic complications occur in up to one-third of patients undergoing orthotopic liver transplantation and are more common following retransplantation. Alterations in mental status may be related to electrolyte abnormalities, metabolic encephalopathy suggesting graft dysfunction, situational psychoses, or medications. In patients receiving immunosuppression prior to transplantation, the possibility of central nervous system infection must be considered in the early postoperative period. Cyclosporine may cause tremor, confusion, cortical blindness, and seizures; this is more common in patients with reduced serum cholesterol and magnesium levels. Similar adverse effects have been reported with FK-506. Less common causes of neurologic dysfunction include cerebral infarction, central pontine myelinolysis, and nonspecific psychoses. Management includes treatment of the underlying condition where possible; drug withdrawal or dose reduction, particularly in the case of corticosteroid-induced neurologic complications; and use of antiepileptics and antipsychotics when necessary. Treatment for seizures is needed for only a limited period (ie, 3 months).

F. Renal Complications: Pretransplantation

renal dysfunction is a risk factor for the development of posttransplantation renal complications. Acute renal failure requiring hemodialysis occurs in 10–20% of patients. Most commonly, intraoperative hypotension or drug toxicity (eg, cyclosporine) results in renal ischemia and acute tubular necrosis. Management includes withdrawal of the offending drug or dose reduction and, occasionally, dialysis. Survival rates in patients requiring dialysis are reduced, particularly in the presence of concomitant multisystem organ failure or if hemodialysis is required for prolonged periods. Despite the prevailing notion that renal function in patients with HRS is normal after successful transplantation, many patients with pretransplantation functional renal failure are at increased risk for developing posttransplantation renal failure and commonly develop long-standing renal insufficiency.

G. Other Complications:

1. Bone disease–Bone loss is maximal during the first 3–6 months following orthotopic liver transplantation due to the effects of high-dosage corticosteroid therapy, bed rest, and, possibly, increased cytokine levels. In the absence of significant pretransplantation bone disease, this loss is generally not clinically significant. Osteonecrosis can also occur, particularly of the hip. In patients with preexisting osteopenia, posttransplantation calcium and vitamin D supplementation may be used but is of uncertain benefit. The role of pre- or posttransplantation biphosphate administration in preventing bone resorption is being investigated.

2. Graft-versus-host disease–Although common following bone marrow transplantation (see Chapter 49), graft-versus-host disease occurs only rarely following orthotopic liver transplantation. The clinical syndrome typically is skin rash, diarrhea, neutropenia, and fever occurring 1–2 months following transplantation. The pathophysiology involves the migration of donor lymphocytes from the transplanted organ into the recipient, with a subsequent immune response against the host. Diagnosis of graft-versus-host disease requires biopsy of the involved organ, usually the skin or colon, and, if possible, HLA typing of peripheral mononuclear blood cells. Therapy usually includes increased immunosuppression with corticosteroids and antilymphocyte preparations, but few patients respond.

3. Posttransplantation lymphoproliferative disorder–This disorder occurs in 2–3% of liver transplantation recipients, as early as 1 month or as late as 11 years following operation. The clinical presentation is variable, from an infectious mononucleosis-like illness with fevers and lymphadenopathy, to weight loss and symptoms suggestive of bowel obstruction or perforation. Extrahepatic manifestations are common. The development of posttransplantation lymphoproliferative disorder is thought to reflect the unrestricted proliferation of B cells stimulated by Epstein-Barr virus infection. Both polyclonal and mon-

oclonal B cell proliferation have been described. The major risk factors are exposure to greater amounts of immunosuppression and lack of previous Epstein-Barr virus exposure. Posttransplantation lymphoproliferative disorder may respond to reduced immunosuppression and initiation of anti-Epstein Barr virus therapy (eg, acyclovir) in some patients.

4. Ascites–Ascites may be a persistent problem for several weeks or months following transplantation, but resolves in the absence of complications. Worsening ascites usually indicates allograft rejection, hepatic venous outflow obstruction, or portal vein thrombosis.

5. Gastrointestinal complications–Gastrointestinal complications include gastrointestinal bleeding following a Roux-en-Y choledochojejunostomy biliary reconstruction, intestinal obstruction secondary to adhesions or posttransplantation lymphoma, hemorrhage related to varices that may persist for days to weeks following transplantation, or peptic ulceration. Liver biopsy has a number of associated complications, but these appear to be no more common in posttransplantation patients than in other patients. Pancreatitis may occur secondary to operative trauma or medications.

Retransplantation

Approximately 10–20% of transplantations performed in the United States are retransplantations. The indications are listed in Table 54–16, with primary nonfunction the most common. Patients undergoing retransplantation have reduced survival rates compared with those of patients undergoing a first transplantation. Some recurrent disorders, such as hepatitis B and C infection and ductopenic rejection, have such a high risk of recurrence following retransplantation that the appropriateness of retransplantation is under debate. There is theoretically no limit on the number of transplantations that may be performed in an individual patient, but, in reality, limits are imposed by concerns over worsening prognosis after retransplantation and the diversion of donor organs away from other deserving recipients.

Disease Recurrence

A. Viral Hepatitis: As was noted previously, patients undergoing orthotopic liver transplantation for chronic hepatitis B or C infection frequently de-

Table 54–16. Indications for retransplantation.

Primary graft nonfunction
Chronic rejection
Nonresponsive acute rejection
Hepatic artery thrombosis
Portal vein thrombosis
Recurrent viral hepatitis
Biliary strictures

velop recurrent infection of the allograft. Herpes simplex virus infection is an uncommon indication for transplantation, and significant recurrent disease is uncommon. Hepatitis D virus infection may recur, even in the absence of detectable HBsAg, but is usually associated with only minor hepatitis on histologic studies and appears to be self-limited.

B. Hepatobiliary Cancer: Recurrence of carcinoma, even the fibrolamellar variant, is the rule following orthotopic liver transplantation. Transplantation for these patients should be provided only in the setting of well-designed research protocols.

C. Alcoholic Liver Disease: Although the recidivism rate following orthotopic liver transplantation appears to be 10–20%, recurrent alcoholic liver disease is relatively uncommon. Patients who return to alcohol abuse are also less likely to comply with medical therapy, and this may lead to graft loss.

D. Other Recurrent Diseases: Recurrence of Budd-Chiari syndrome has been reported but may be prevented by use of anticoagulants following transplantation. Controversy exists as to whether primary biliary cirrhosis recurs. Although titers of antimitochondrial antibodies may become negative immediately following transplantation, they reappear in nearly 100% of patients. Defining histologic evidence of recurrent disease is difficult because there is overlap with the histologic changes associated with rejection. Nevertheless, characteristic histologic findings such as the florid duct lesion have been reported. Given the natural history of primary biliary cirrhosis, it may be years before clear-cut evidence of recurrent disease is seen. Similarly, recurrent primary sclerosing cholangitis is difficult to prove, since similar cholangiographic abnormalities may be caused by a number of events (eg, ischemia). Patients undergoing orthotopic liver transplantation for primary sclerosing cholangitis do have a higher incidence of biliary complications than those without the disorder. As with primary biliary cirrhosis, recurrent disease may become more evident with longer follow-up. It appears unlikely that recurrent primary biliary cirrhosis or primary sclerosing cholangitis will be a major problem in the early years following transplantation. Recurrent autoimmune hepatitis following transplantation is rare.

Diseases Transmitted by Donor Organs

Diseases transmitted by donor organs include hepatitis B and C, HIV infection, factor XI deficiency, idiopathic thrombocytopenic purpura, Gilbert syndrome, and various malignant tumors. Donor organs are carefully screened for such diseases, but given the imperfect sensitivities of current assays, a small risk of transmission will likely persist. The use of HCV-positive donor livers is controversial, but they may be used in severely ill recipients whose survival is otherwise in jeopardy (see Surgical Considerations above). Donors with readily treatable infectious diseases such as syphilis are acceptable if antibiotics are administered following transplantation.

Multiple-Organ Transplantation

Liver transplantation may be performed in conjunction with renal transplantation in the presence of advanced renal dysfunction without adding significantly to rates of complications or death. The liver may also be transplanted in combination with the pancreas, heart, and lung. Visceral organ cluster transplantation involving the liver, pancreas, and entire gastrointestinal tract or a portion of intestine has also been performed.

Development of Cellular Chimerism

Migration of donor lymphocytes into recipients frequently results in the formation of a chimeric state, with donor cells demonstrable in a number of different organs as well as in the blood. The emergence of this chimerism may be important for the development of immune tolerance to the allograft. Indeed, it has been suggested that patients who develop sufficient chimerism may no longer require immunosuppression.

COSTS & OUTCOME OF LIVER TRANSPLANTATION

Costs of Liver Transplantation

The total expense of performing a liver transplantation includes the costs of pretransplantation evaluation, hospital charges, costs associated with acquisition of the donor organ, and professional fees. The costs of medications and treatment of complications can be substantial but are difficult to analyze and therefore not usually included in published cost estimates. The cost of hospitalization for transplantation itself appears to be declining, possibly as a result of better candidate selection and improved postoperative management.

In a recent review of expenses, Evans and coworkers determined that the average cost of a liver transplantation in the United States is $145,795 of which $104,049 was hospital charges and the remainder professional fees and donor acquisition costs. Private insurance pays for orthotopic liver transplantation in about 70% of cases, and government programs pay for most other cases. No reliable information is available on the long-term costs of caring for patients following transplantation.

Patient Outcomes

The rate of complications and death in patients surviving more than 1 year after liver transplantation is relatively low. Late deaths, occurring after more than 5 years, are most commonly related to disease recurrence, chronic rejection, or a malignant tumor.

In a study from the Mayo Clinic, 91% of patients surviving 1 year following transplantation reported subjective feelings of well-being and satisfaction with life. Of patients followed for 2 years, over 90% reported no health problems or only minor difficulties. More than 85% of patients working prior to transplantation were able to return to work and said they could perform their jobs well. Hence, despite debate regarding the costs of this procedure, it is clear that liver transplantation rehabilitates patients with advanced liver disease and contributes to an improved quality of life.

REFERENCES

Pimstone NR et al: Liver transplantation. In: *Hepatology: A Textbook of Liver Disease,* 2/e. Zakim D, Boyer TD (editors). Saunders, 1990.

UNOS Scientific Registry: Liver allocation data examined. UNOS Update 1991;7(issue 10):11.

INDICATIONS & CONTRAINDICATIONS FOR LIVER TRANSPLANTATION

Abu-Elmagd KM et al: Cholangiocarcinoma and sclerosing cholangitis: Clinical characteristics and effect on survival after liver transplantation. Transplant Proc 1993;25:1124.

Ascher NL et al: Liver transplantation for fulminant hepatic failure. Arch Surg 1993;128:677.

Benner KG et al: Fibrosing cytolytic liver failure secondary to recurrent hepatitis B after liver transplantation. Gastroenterology 1992;103:1307.

Chazouilleres O et al: Quantitation of hepatitis C virus RNA in liver transplant recipients. Gastroenterology 1994;106:994.

Cohen C, Benjamin M: Alcoholics and liver transplantation. JAMA 1991;265:1299.

David E et al: Recurrence of hepatitis D (delta) in liver transplant patients: Histopathologic aspects. Gastroenterology 1993;104:1122.

Delcore R et al: Risk of occult carcinomas in patients undergoing orthotopic liver transplantation for end-stage liver disease secondary to primary sclerosing cholangitis. Transplant Proc 1993;25:1883.

Ferrell LD et al: Hepatitis C viral infection in liver transplant recipients. Hepatology 1992;16:865.

Gordon RD, Van Thiel DH, Starzl TE: Liver Transplantation. In: *Diseases of the Liver,* 7/e. Schiff L, Schiff ER (editors). Lippincott, 1993.

Gores GJ: Liver transplantation for malignant disease. Gastroenterol Clin North Am 1993;22:285.

Gores GJ, Steers JL: Progress in orthotopic liver transplantation for hepatocellular carcinoma. (Editorial.) Gastroenterology 1993;104:317.

Gugenheim J et al: Long-term immunoprophylaxis of B virus recurrence after liver transplantation in HBs antigen–positive patients. Transplant Proc 1993;25:1349.

Konig V et al: Hepatitis C virus reinfection in allografts after orthotopic liver transplantation. Hepatology 1992;16:1137.

Kumar S et al: Orthotopic liver transplantation for alcoholic liver disease. Hepatology 1990;11:159.

Lake JR: Changing indications for liver transplantation. Gastroenterol Clin North Am 1993;22:213.

Lake JR, Wright TW: Liver transplantation for patients with hepatitis B: What have we learned from our results? Hepatology 1991;13:796.

Lake JR et al: Hepatitis B and C in liver transplantation. Transplant Proc 1993;25:2006.

Lidofsky SD: Liver transplantation for fulminant hepatic failure. Gastroenterol Clin North Am 1993;22:257.

Lidofsky SD et al: Intracranial pressure monitoring and liver transplantation for fulminant hepatic failure. Hepatology 1992;16:1.

Lucey MR: Liver transplantation for the alcoholic patient. Gastroenterol Clin North Am 1993;22:243.

Martin P, Munoz SJ, Friedman LS: Liver transplantation for viral hepatitis: Current status. Am J Gastroenterol 1992;87:409.

Moss AH, Siegler M: Should alcoholics compete equally for liver transplantation? JAMA 1991;265:1295.

O'Grady JG et al: Early indicators of prognosis in fulminant hepatic failure. Gastroenterology 1989;97:439.

O'Grady JG et al: Hepatitis B virus reinfection after orthotopic liver transplantation. J Hepatol 1992;14:104.

Osario RW et al: Orthotopic liver transplantation for end-stage alcoholic liver disease. Transplant Proc 1993;25:1133.

Pageaux GP et al: Results and cost of orthotopic liver transplantation for alcoholic cirrhosis. Transplant Proc 1993;25:1135.

Rakela J: Hepatitis C viral infection in liver transplant patients: How bad is it really? (Editorial.) Gastroenterology 1992;103:38.

Samuel D, Bismuth H: Liver transplantation for hepatitis B. Gastroenterol Clin North Am 1993;22:271.

Samuel D et al: Liver transplantation in European patients with the hepatitis B surface antigen. N Engl J Med 1993;329:1842.

Shah G et al: Incidence, prevalence, and clinical course of hepatitis C following liver transplantation. Gastroenterology 1992;103:323.

Starzl TE, Demetris AJ, Van Thiel D: Liver transplantation. (Part 1 of 2 parts). N Engl J Med 1989;321:1014.

Starzl TE et al: Orthotopic liver transplantation for alcoholic cirrhosis. JAMA 1988;260:2542.

Stone MJ et al: Neoadjuvant chemotherapy and liver transplantation for hepatocellular carcinoma: A pilot study in 20 patients. Gastroenterology 1993;104:196.

Tan CK et al: Orthotopic liver transplantation for preoperative early-stage hepatocellular carcinoma. Mayo Clin Proc 1994;69:509.

Wright H, Gavaler JS, Van Thiel DH: Preliminary experience with alpha 2b interferon therapy of viral hepatitis in liver allograft recipients. Transplantation 1992;53:121.

Wright TL: Liver transplantation for chronic hepatitis C viral infection. Gastroenterol Clin North Am 1993;22:231.

Wright TL et al: Recurrent and acquired hepatitis C viral infection in liver transplant recipients. Gastroenterology 1992;103:317.

PRETRANSPLANTATION MEDICAL EVALUATION

Conn HO: Transjugular intrahepatic portalsystemic shunts: The state of the art. Hepatology 1993;17:148.

Fabry TL, Klion FM (editors): *Guide to Liver Transplantation.* Igaku-Shoin, 1992.

Gines P et al: Paracentesis with intravenous infusion of albumin as compared with peritovenous shunting in cirrhosis with refractory ascites. N Engl J Med 1991;325:829.

Hoefs JC: Spontaneous bacterial peritonitis: Prevention and therapy. (Editorial.) Hepatology 1990;12:776.

Ring EJ et al: Using transjugular intrahepatic portasystemic shunts to control variceal bleeding before liver transplantation. Ann Intern Med 1992;116:304.

Rossle M et al: The transjugular intrahepatic portasystemic stent-shunt procedure for variceal bleeding. N Engl J Med 1994;330:165.

Runyon B: Care of patients with ascites. N Engl J Med 1994;330:337.

Scott V et al: Reversibility of the hepatopulmonary syndrome by orthotopic liver transplantation. Transplant Proc 1993;25:1787.

TIMING OF LIVER TRANSPLANTATION

Starzl TE, Demetris AJ, Van Thiel D: Liver transplantation. (Part 1 of 2 parts). N Engl J Med 1989;321:1014.

Wiesner RH et al: Selection and timing of liver transplantation in primary biliary cirrhosis and primary sclerosing cholangitis. Hepatology 1992;16:1290.

SURGICAL CONSIDERATIONS

Adam R et al: Liver transplantation from elderly donors. Transplant Proc 1993;25:1556.

Belzer FO et al: Update on preservation of liver grafts. Transplant Proc 1993;25:2010.

Broelsh CE et al: Application of reduced-size liver transplants as split grafts, auxiliary orthotopic grafts, and living related segmental transplants. Ann Surg 1990;212:368.

Emond JC: Clinical application of living-related liver transplantation. Gastroenterol Clin North Am 1993;22:301.

Gottesdiener KM: Transplanted infections: Donor-to-host transmission with the allograft. Ann Intern Med 1989;110:1001.

Kalayoglu M et al: Surgical refinements in liver transplantation. Transplant Proc 1993;25(Suppl 3):48.

Langnas AN et al: The results of reduced-size liver transplantation, including split livers, in patients with end-stage liver disease. Transplantation 1992;53:387.

Masatoshi M et al: Donor hepatectomy for living related partial liver transplantation. Surgery 1993;113:395.

Miller CM et al: Operative techniques and strategies in liver transplantation. In: *Guide to Liver Transplantation.* Fabry TL, Klion FM (editors). Igaku-Shoin, 1992.

Moreno-Gonzalez E et al: Utilization of split liver grafts in orthotopic liver transplantation. Hepatogastroenterology 1993;40:17.

Pereira BJG et al: Transmission of hepatitis C virus by organ transplantation. N Engl J Med 1991;325:454.

Ringe B et al: An update of partial liver transplantation. Transplant Proc 1993;25:2198.

Zaballos JM et al: Venovenous bypass versus no bypass in orthotopic liver transplantation: Metabolic values during reperfusion. Transplant Proc 1993;25:1865.

POSTOPERATIVE COMPLICATIONS & MANAGEMENT

Adams DH, Neuberger JM: Treatment of acute rejection. Semin Liver Dis 1992;12:80.

Ascher NL: Immunosuppression and rejection in liver transplantation. Transplant Proc 1993;25:1744.

Chazouilleres O et al: Preservation-induced liver injury: Clinical aspects, mechanisms, and therapeutic approaches. J Hepatol 1993;18:123.

Clavien PA et al: Preservation and reperfusion injuries in liver allografts. Transplantation 1992;53:957.

de Groen P: Cyclosporin: A review and its specific use in liver transplantation. Mayo Clin Proc 1989;64:680.

Donaldson P et al: Influence of human leukocyte antigen matching on liver allograft survival and rejection: "The dualistic effect." Hepatology 1993;17:1008.

Greig PD et al: Treatment of primary liver graft nonfunction with prostaglandin E_1. Transplantation 1989;48:447.

Krams SM, Ascher NL, Martinez OM: New immunologic insights into mechanisms of allograft rejection. Gastroenterol Clin North Am 1993;22:381.

Lake JR, Roberts JP, Ascher NL: Maintenance immunosuppression after liver transplantation. Semin Liver Dis 1992;12:73.

Mor E et al: Acute cellular rejection following liver transplantation: Clinical pathologic features and effect on outcome. Semin Liver Dis 1992;12:28.

Peters DH et al: Tacrolimus: A review of its pharmacology, and therapeutic potential in hepatic and renal transplantation. Drugs 1993;46:746.

Ploeg RJ et al: Risk factors for primary dysfunction after liver transplantation: A multivariate analysis. Transplantation 1993;55:807.

Schwartz ME et al: Immunosuppression and rejection. In: Guide to Liver Transplantation. Fabry TL, Klion FM (editors). Igaku-Shoin, 1992.

Vierling JM: Immunologic mechanisms of hepatic allograft rejection. Semin Liver Dis 1992;12:16.

Wiesner R et al: Hepatic allograft rejection: New developments in terminology, diagnosis, prevention, and treatment. Mayo Clin Proc 1993;68:69.

INFECTIOUS COMPLICATIONS

Chazouilleres O et al: Quantitation of hepatitis C virus RNA in liver transplant recipients. Gastroenterology 1994;106:994.

Cuevas-Mons V et al: Bacterial infections in liver transplant patients under selective decontamination with norfloxacin. Transplant Proc 1989;21:3558.

Dummer JS: Cytomegalovirus infection after liver transplantation: Clinical manifestations and strategies for prevention. Rev Infect Dis 1990;12(Suppl 7):S767.

Dunn DL et al: A prospective randomized study of acyclovir versus ganciclovir plus human immune globulin prophylaxis of cytomegalovirus infection after solid organ transplantation. Transplantation 1994;57:876.

Gorensek MJ et al: Selective bowel decontamination with quinolones and nystatin reduces gram-negative and fungal infections in orthotopic liver transplant recipients. Cleve Clin J Med 1993;60:139.

Kizilisik TA, Preiksaitis JK, Kneteman NM: Cytomegalovirus disease in liver transplant recipients: Impact of acyclovir prophylaxis. Transplant Proc 1993;25:2282.

Mollison L et al: High-dose oral acyclovir reduces the incidence of cytomegalovirus infection in liver transplant recipients. J Infect Dis 1993;168:721.

O' Grady JG et al: Hepatitis B virus reinfection after orthotopic liver transplantation: Serological and clinical implications. J Hepatol 1992;14:104.

Paya CV et al: Incidence, distribution, and outcome of episodes of infection in 100 orthotopic liver transplantations. Mayo Clin Proc 1989;64:555.

Saliba F et al: Randomized controlled trial of acyclovir for the prevention of cytomegalovirus infection and disease in liver transplant recipients. Transplant Proc 1993;25:1444.

Snydman DR et al: Cytomegalovirus immune globulin prophylaxis in liver transplantation: A randomized, double-blind, placebo-controlled trial. Ann Intern Med 1993;119:984.

Stratta RJ et al: A randomized prospective trial of acyclovir and immune globulin prophylaxis in liver transplant recipients receiving OKT3 therapy. Arch Surg 1992;127:55.

Wright HI, Gavaler JS, Van Thiel DH: Preliminary experience with alpha-2b-interferon therapy of viral hepatitis in liver allograft recipients. Transplantation 1992;53:121.

Wright TL et al: Recurrent and acquired hepatitis C viral infection in liver transplant recipients. Gastroenterology 1992;103:317.

BILIARY COMPLICATIONS

Colonna JO et al: Biliary strictures complicating liver transplantation: Incidence, pathogenesis, management, and outcome. Ann Surg 1992;216:344.

Donovan J: Nonsurgical management of biliary tract disease after liver transplantation. Gastroenterol Clin North Am 1993;22:317.

Li S et al: Diffuse biliary tract injury after orthotopic liver transplantation. Am J Surg 1992;164:536.

Sanchez-Urdazpal L et al: Diagnostic features and clinical outcome of ischemic-type biliary complications after liver transplantation. Hepatology 1993;17:605.

Sanchez-Urdazpal L et al: Increased bile duct complications in liver transplantation across the ABO barrier. Ann Surg 1993;218:152.

Sanchez-Urdazpal L et al: Ischemic-type biliary complications after orthotopic liver transplantation. Hepatology 1992;16:49.

Wolfsen HC et al: Role of endoscopic retrograde cholangiopancreatography after orthotopic liver transplantation. Am J Gastroenterol 1992;87:955.

OTHER COMPLICATIONS

Adams DH et al: Neurological complications following liver transplantation. Lancet 1987;ii:949.

Afessa B et al: Pulmonary complications of orthotopic liver transplantation. Mayo Clin Proc 1993;68:427.

de Groen PC et al: Central nervous system toxicity after liver transplantation: The role of cyclosporine and cholesterol. N Engl J Med 1987;317:861.

Gordon RD, Van Thiel DH, Starzl TE: Liver transplantation. In: *Diseases of the Liver.* Schiff L, Schiff ER (editors). Lippincott, 1993.

Hay JE: Bone disease in liver transplant patients. Gastroenterol Clin North Am 1993;22:337.

Ishitani M et al: Outcome of patients requiring hemodialysis after liver transplantation. Transplant Proc 1993;25:1762.

Krowka MJ, Cortese DA: Pulmonary aspects of liver disease and liver transplantation. Clin Chest Med 1989;10:593.

Lopez OL et al: Neurological complications after liver retransplantation. Hepatology 1992;16:162.

McCauley J et al: Dialysis in liver failure and liver transplantation. Transplant Proc 1993;25:1740.

Penn I: Cancers complicating organ transplantation. N Engl J Med 1990;323:1767.

Randhawa PS et al: Expression of Epstein-Barr virus–encoded small RNA (by the EBER-1 gene) in liver specimens from transplant recipients with posttransplantation lymphoproliferative disease. N Engl J Med 1992;327:1710.

Renard TH, Andrews WS, Foster ME: Relationship between OKT3 administration, EBV seroconversion, and the lymphoproliferative syndrome in pediatric liver transplant recipients. Transplant Proc 1991;23:1473.

Roberts JP et al: Graft versus host disease after liver transplantation. Hepatology 1991;14:274.

Wiesner RH et al: Long-term management of liver transplant recipients. Semin Gastrointest Dis 1993;4:151.

DISEASE RECURRENCE & RETRANSPLANTATION

Anthuber M et al: Liver retransplantation: Indications, frequency, and results. Transplant Proc 1992;24:1965.

Crippen J et al: Retransplantation in hepatitis B: A multicenter experience. Transplantation 1994;57:823.

Ezio D et al: Recurrence of hepatitis D (delta) in liver transplants: Histopathologic aspects. Gastroenterology 1993;104:1122.

Gores GJ: Liver transplantation for malignant disease. Gastroenterol Clin North Am 1993;22:285.

Halff G et al: Liver transplantation for Budd-Chiari syndrome. Ann Surg 1990;211:43.

Lucey MR: Liver transplantation for the alcoholic patient. Gastroenterol Clin North Am 1993;22:243.

Perrillo R, Mason AL: Hepatitis B and liver transplantation: Problems and promises. (Editorial.) N Engl J Med 1993;329:1885.

Shah GA et al: Incidence, prevalence, and clinical course of hepatitis C following liver transplantation. Gastroenterology 1992;103:323.

Starzl TE, Demetris AJ, Van Thiel D: Liver transplantation. (Part 2 of 2 parts.) N Engl J Med 1989;321: 1014.

Wright TL et al: Recurrent and acquired hepatitis C viral infection in liver transplant patients. Gastroenterology 1992;103:317.

DISEASES TRANSMITTED BY DONOR ORGANS & CELLULAR CHIMERISM

Aeder et al: Incidence and clinical impact of hepatitis C virus–positive donors in cadaveric transplantation. Transplant Proc 1993;25:1469.

Collins RH et al: Brief report: Donor-derived long-term mutilineage hematopoiesis in a liver transplant recipient. N Engl J Med 1993;328:762.

Gottesdiener KM: Transplanted infections: Donor-to-host transmission with the allograft. Ann Intern Med 1989;110:1001.

Pereira BJG et al: Prevalence of hepatitis C virus RNA in organ donors positive for hepatitis C antibody and in recipients of their donor organs. N Engl J Med 1992;327:910.

Pereira BJG et al: Transmission of hepatitis C virus by organ transplantation. N Engl J Med 1991;325:454.

Starzl TE et al: Cell migration and chimerism after whole-organ transplantation: The basis of graft acceptance. Hepatology 1993;17:1127.

Starzl TE et al: Chimerism after liver transplantation for type IV glycogen storage disease and type I Gaucher's disease. N Engl J Med 1993;328:745.

Starzl TE et al: Systemic chimerism in human female recipients of male livers. Lancet 1992;340:876.

Steinman RM, Inaba K, Austyn JM: Donor-derived chimerism in recipients of organ transplants. (Editorial.) Hepatology 1993;17:1153.

COSTS & OUTCOME OF LIVER TRANSPLANTATION

Eid A et al: Beyond 1 year after liver transplantation. Mayo Clin Proc 1989;64:446.

Evans RW, Manninen DL, Dong FB: An economic analysis of liver transplantation: Costs, insurance coverage, and reimbursement. Gastroenterol Clin North Am 1993;22:451.

Krom RAF: Organ donation: Are we moving in the right direction? (Editorial.) Mayo Clin Proc 1989;64:705.

Starzl TE, Demetris AJ, Van Thiel D: Liver transplantation. (Part 2 of 2 parts.) N Engl J Med 1989;321:101

Index

NOTE: A *t* following a page number indicates tabular material and an *f* following a page number indicates a figure. Drugs are listed under their generic names. When a drug trade name is listed, the reader is referred to the generic name.

(more on reverse)

Clinical Cardiology, 6/e
Cheitlin, Sokolow, & McIlroy
1993, ISBN 0-8385-1093-0, A1093-2
Fluid & Electrolytes
Physiology & Pathophysiology
Cogan
1991, ISBN 0-8385-2546-6, A2546-8
Basic & Clinical Biostatistics, 2/e
Dawson-Saunders & Trapp
1994, ISBN 0-8385-0542-2, A0542-9
Basic Gynecology and Obstetrics
Gant & Cunningham
1993, ISBN 0-8385-9633-9, A9633-7
Review of General Psychiatry, 4/e
Goldman
1995, ISBN 0-8385-8421-7, A8421-8
**Principles of Clinical
Electrocardiography, 13/e**
Goldschlager & Goldman
1990, ISBN 0-8385-7951-5, A7951-5
Basic & Clinical Endocrinology, 4/e
Greenspan & Baxter
1994, ISBN 0-8385-0560-0, A0560-1
Occupational Medicine
LaDou
1990, ISBN 0-8385-7207-3, A7207-2
Primary Care of Women
Lemcke, Pattison, Marshall, & Cowley
1995, ISBN 0-8385-9813-7, A9813-5
Clinical Anesthesiology, 2/e
Morgan & Mikhail
1996, ISBN 0-8385-1381-6, A1381-1
Dermatology
Orkin, Maibach, & Dahl
1991, ISBN 0-8385-1288-7, A1288-8
Rudolph's Fundamentals of Pediatrics
Rudolph & Kamei
1994, ISBN 0-8385-8233-8, A8233-7
Genetics in Clinical Medicine and Primary Care
Seashore
1995, ISBN 0-8385-3128-8, A3128-4
Smith's General Urology, 14/e
Tanagho & McAninch
1995, ISBN 0-8385-8612-0, A8612-2
Clinical Oncology
Weiss
1993, ISBN 0-8385-1325-5, A1325-8
General Ophthalmology, 14/e
Vaughan, Asbury, & Riordan-Eva
1995, ISBN 0-8385-3127-X, A3127-6

CURRENT Clinical References

**CURRENT Critical Care Diagnosis &
Treatment,**
Bongard & Sue
1994, ISBN 0-8385-1443-X, A1443-9
**CURRENT Diagnosis & Treatment in
Cardiology**
Crawford
1995, ISBN 0-8385-1444-8, A1444-7

**CURRENT Diagnosis & Treatment in
Vascular Surgery**
Dean, Yao, & Brewster
1995, ISBN 0-8385-1351-4, A1351-4
CURRENT Obstetric & Gynecologic Diagnosis & Treatment, 8/e
DeCherney & Pernoll
1994, ISBN 0-8385-1447-2, A1447-0
**CURRENT Diagnosis & Treatment in
Gastroenterology**
Grendell, McQuaid, & Friedman
1996, ISBN 0-8385-1448-0, A1448-8
**CURRENT Pediatric Diagnosis &
Treatment, 12/e**
Hay, Groothuis, Hayward, & Levin
1995, ISBN 0-8385-1446-4, A1446-2
**CURRENT Emergency Diagnosis &
Treatment, 4/e**
Saunders & Ho
1993, ISBN 0-8385-1347-6, A1347-2
**CURRENT Diagnosis & Treatment in
Orthopedics**
Skinner
1995, ISBN 0-8385-1009-4, A1009-8
**CURRENT Medical Diagnosis &
Treatment 1996**
Tierney, McPhee, & Papadakis
1996, ISBN 0-8385-1465-0, A1465-2
CURRENT Surgical Diagnosis & Treatment, 10/e
Way
1994, ISBN 0-8385-1439-1, A1439-7

LANGE Clinical Manuals

Dermatology
Diagnosis and Therapy
Bondi, Jegasothy, & Lazarus
1991, ISBN 0-8385-1274-7, A1274-8
Practical Oncology
Cameron
1994, ISBN 0-8385-1326-3, A1326-6
Office & Bedside Procedures
Chesnutt, Dewar, Locksley, & Tureen
1993, ISBN 0-8385-1095-7, A1095-7
Psychiatry
Diagnosis & Therapy 2/e
Flaherty, Davis, & Janicak
1993, ISBN 0-8385-1267-4, A1267-2
Neonatology
*Management, Procedures, On-Call
Problems, Diseases and Drugs, 3/e*
Gomella
1994, ISBN 0-8385-1331-X, A1331-6
Practical Gynecology
Jacobs & Gast
1994, ISBN 0-8385-1336-0, A1336-5
Drug Therapy, 2/e
Katzung
1991, ISBN 0-8385-1312-3, A1312-6

Ambulatory Medicine
The Primary Care of Families
Mengel & Schwiebert
1993, ISBN 0-8385-1294-1, A1294-6
Poisoning & Drug Overdose, 2/e
Olson
1994, ISBN 0-8385-1108-2, A1108-8
Internal Medicine
Diagnosis and Therapy, 3/e
Stein
1993, ISBN 0-8385-1112-0, A1112-0
Surgery
Diagnosis & Therapy
Stillman
1989, ISBN 0-8385-1283-6, A1283-9
Medical Perioperative Management
Wolfsthal
1989, ISBN 0-8385-1298-4, A1298-7

LANGE Handbooks

**Handbook of Gynecology &
Obstetrics**
Brown & Crombleholme
1993, ISBN 0-8385-3608-5, A3608-5
HIV/AIDS Primary Care Handbook
Carmichael, Carmichael, & Fischl
1995, ISBN 0-8385-3557-7, A3557-4
Pocket Guide to Diagnostic Tests
Detmer, McPhee, Nicoll, & Chou
1992, ISBN 0-8385-8020-3, A8020-8
Handbook of Poisoning
*Prevention, Diagnosis & Treatment,
12/e*
Dreisbach & Robertson
1987, ISBN 0-8385-3643-3, A3643-2
**Handbook of Clinical Endocrinology,
2/e**
Fitzgerald
1992, ISBN 0-8385-3615-8, A3615-0
Clinician's Pocket Reference, 7/e
Gomella
1993, ISBN 0-8385-1222-4, A1222-7
Surgery on Call, 2/e
Gomella & Lefor
1996, ISBN 0-8385-8746-1, A8746-8
Internal Medicine On Call
Haist & Robbins
1991, ISBN 0-8385-4052-X, A4052-5
Obstetrics & Gynecology On Call
Horowitz & Gomella
1993, ISBN 0-8385-7174-3, A7174-4
**Pocket Guide to Commonly
Prescribed Drugs**
Levine
1993, ISBN 0-8385-8023-8, A8023-2
Handbook of Pediatrics, 17/e
Merenstein, Kaplan, & Rosenberg
1994, ISBN 0-8385-3657-3, A3657-2

 Appleton & Lange • P.O. Box 120041 • Stamford, CT • 06912-0041 • 1-800-423-1359